Springhouse Review for

NCLEX-RN®

6th edition

Springhouse Review for NCLEX-RN®

6th edition

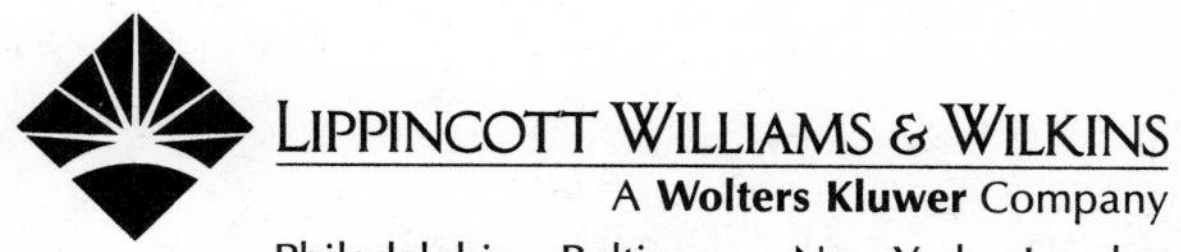

Philadelphia • Baltimore • New York • London
Buenos Aires • Hong Kong • Sydney • Tokyo

STAFF

Executive Publisher
Judith A. Schilling McCann, RN, MSN

Senior Acquisitions Editor
Elizabeth Nieginski

Editorial Director
David Moreau

Clinical Director
Joan M. Robinson, RN, MSN

Senior Art Director
Arlene Putterman

Editorial Project Manager
Tracy S. Diehl

Clinical Project Manager
Collette Bishop Hendler, RN, BS, CCRN

Editors
Laura Bruck, Diane Labus, Brenna H. Mayer

Clinical Editor
Joanne Bartelmo, RN, MSN

Copy Editors
Thomas DeZego, Josephine Donofrio, Danielle Michaely, Dorothy P. Terry

Digital Composition Services
Diane Paluba (manager), Donna S. Morris (project manager), Joyce Rossi Biletz

Manufacturing
Patricia K. Dorshaw (director), Beth J. Welsh

Editorial Assistants
Megan L. Aldinger, Karen J. Kirk, Linda K. Ruhf

Indexer
Barbara Hodgson

The clinical treatments described and recommended in this publication are based on research and consultation with nursing, medical, and legal authorities. To the best of our knowledge, these procedures reflect currently accepted practice. Nevertheless, they can't be considered absolute and universal recommendations. For individual applications, all recommendations must be considered in light of the patient's clinical condition and, before administration of new or infrequently used drugs, in light of the latest package-insert information. The authors and publisher disclaim any responsibility for any adverse effects resulting from the suggested procedures, from any undetected errors, or from the reader's misunderstanding of the text.

 Printed in the United States of America. For information, write Lippincott Williams & Wilkins, 323 Norristown Road, Suite 200, Ambler, PA 19002-2756.

SHNCLEXRN6011205 — D
07 06 05 10 9 8 7 6 5 4 3 2 1

Library of Congress Cataloging-in-Publication Data

Springhouse review for NCLEX-RN. — 6th ed.
p. ; cm.
Includes bibliographical references and index.
1. Nursing — Examinations, questions, etc. 2. National Council Licensure Examination for Registered Nurses — Study guides. I. Lippincott Williams & Wilkins. II. Title: Review for NCLEX-RN.
[DNLM: 1. Nursing — Examination Questions. WY 18.2 S7697 2006]
RT55.S65 2006
610.73076 — dc22
ISBN 1-58255-829-9 (alk. paper) 2005026310

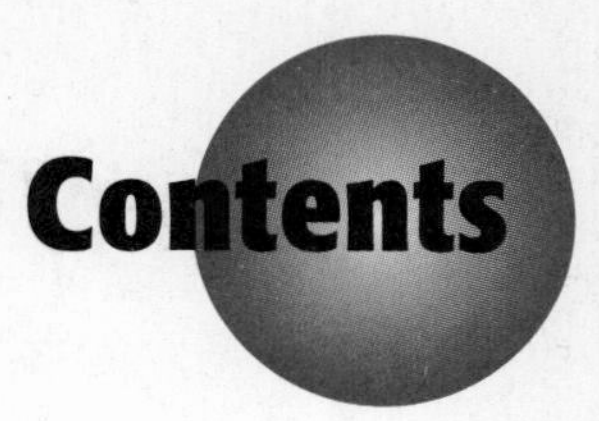
Contents

PART IV APPENDICES

Advisory board

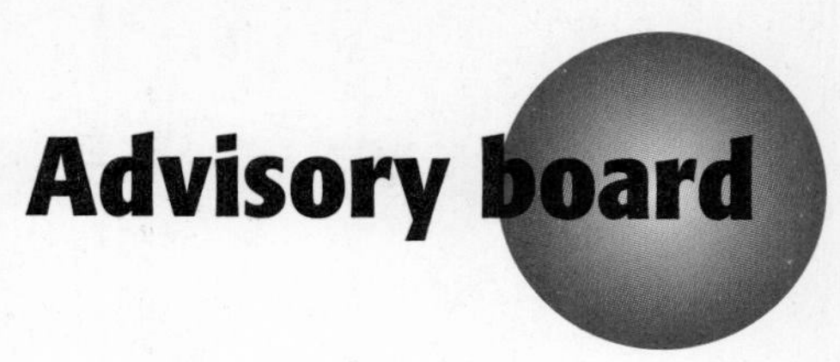

Ivy Alexander, PhD, CANP
Assistant Professor
Yale University
New Haven, Conn.

Susan E. Appling, RN, MS, CRNP
Assistant Professor
Johns Hopkins University School of Nursing
Baltimore

Paul M. Arnstein, PhD, APRN-BC, FNP-C
Assistant Professor
Boston College

Bobbie Berkowitz, PhD, CNAA, FAAN
Chair & Professor
Psychosocial & Community Health
University of Washington
Seattle

Michael A. Carter BSN, MNSC, DNSC, FAAN, APRN-BC
University Distinguished Professor
University of Tennessee
Memphis

Karla Jones, RN, MSN
Nursing Faculty
Treasure Valley Community College
Ontario, Ore.

Manon Lemonde, RN, PhD
Associate Professor
University of Ontario (Oshawa) Institute of Technology

Sheila Sparks Ralph, DNSC, RN, FAAN
Director & Professor
Division of Nursing & Respiratory Care
Shenandoah University
Winchester, Va.

Kristine Anne Scordo, PhD, RN, CS, ACNP
Director, Acute Care Nurse Practitioner Program
Wright State University
Dayton, Ohio

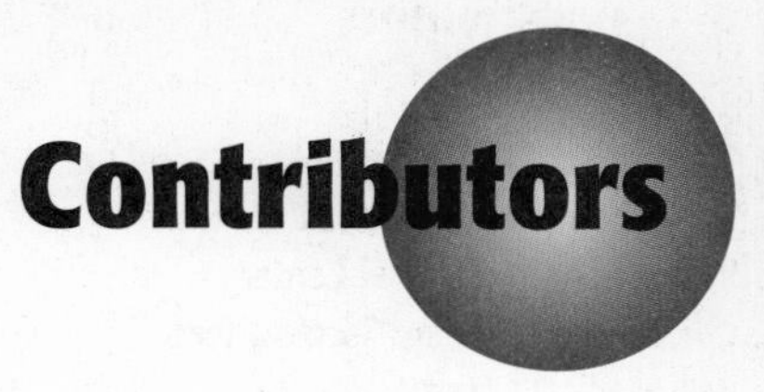

Contributors

Judith Alexander, RN, DNS
Associate Professor
Armstrong Atlantic State University
Savannah, Ga.

Rita Bates, RN, MSN
Assistant Professor
University of Arkansas
Fort Smith

Peggy Bozarth, RN, MSN
Professor
Hopkinsville (Ky.) Community College

Michelle Byrne, RN, PhD, CNOR
Associate Professor of Nursing
North Georgia College & State University
Dahlonega

Esther M. Conner, RN, MSN
Assistant Professor
Southwest Missouri State University
West Plains

Marsha L. Conroy, RN, MSN, APN
Nursing Educator
Cuyahoga Community College
Cleveland

Celeste Cook, RN, MSN
Community & Family Health
Nursing Professor
University of Arkansas
Ft. Smith

Kim Cooper, RN, MSN
Nursing Department Program Chair
Ivy Tech State College
Terre Haute, Ind.

Linda Carman Copel, RN, PhD, CPG, CS, DAPA
Associate Professor, College of Nursing
Villanova (Pa.) University

Lillian Craig, RN, MSN, CS, FNP
Instructor of Nursing
Oklahoma Panhandle State University
Goodwell

James S. Davis, IV, RN, BSN
Clinical Leader, Intensive Care
Abington (Pa.) Memorial Hospital

Carrin L. Dvorak, RN, MSN
Assistant Professor of Nursing
Cuyahoga Community College
Cleveland

Ken W. Edmisson, RN, RNC, ND, EdD, FNP
Associate Professor
Middle Tennessee State University
Murfreesboro

Jennifer L. Embree, RN, MSN, CCRN, CNABC, CCNS
Chief Clinical Officer
Dunn Memorial Hospital
Bedford, Ind.
Faculty
Indiana University of Pennsylvania School of Nursing
Indianapolis

Laura R. Favand, RN, MS
Chief, Education and Training
Army Trauma Training Center
Miami

Athena A. Foreman, RN, MSN
Nursing Coordinator – Senior Level
Stanly Community College
Albemarle, N.C.

Janice D. Hausauer, RN, MS, FNP
Adjunct Assistant Professor
Montana State University
Bozeman

Timothy Hudson, RN, MS, MEd, CCRN, CHE, CNA
Nurse Manager, Intensive Care Unit
Womack Army Medical Center
Chief Nurse, Forward Surgical Team
44th Medical Command
Fort Bragg, N.C.

Julia Anne Isen, RN, MS, FNP-C
Family Nurse Practitioner
University of California, San Francisco

Karla Jones, RN, MS
Nursing Faculty
Treasure Valley Community College
Ontario, Ore.

David C. Keller, RN, MS, APRN
Assistant Professor
Utah Valley State College
Orem

Sharon Lee, RN, MS, BSN, FNP, CCRN
Family Nurse Practitioner
Bryan LGH Medical Center
Lincoln, Neb.

Elizabeth Molle, RN, MS
Nurse Educator
Middlesex Hospital
Middletown, Conn.

Jill Morsbach, RNC, CBE, MSN
Adjunct Instructor
Pikes Peak Community College
Colorado Springs, Colo.

Donna Nielsen, RN, CCRN, MSN
RN Educator
Pasadena (Ca.) City College

Tracy S. Patil, RN, MSN
Nursing Faculty
Lincoln Memorial University
Harrogate, Tenn.

Elizabeth Petit De Mange, RN, PhD
Assistant Professor
Drexel University College of Nursing and Health Professions
Philadelphia

Melody F. Pope, RN, C/LNHA, MSEd, MSN
Assistant Professor
Community College of Denver, Lowry Campus

Sherry L. Rogman, RN
Staff and Charge Nurse
BryanLGH Medical Center
Lincoln, Neb.

Doris J. Rosenow, RN, PhD, CCRN, CNS-M-S
Associate Professor
Texas A&M International University
Laredo

Betty Sims, RN, MSN
Nurse Consultant
Board of Nurse Examiners
Austin, Tex.
Adjunct Faculty
St. Philips College
San Antonio, Tex.

Belinda L. Spencer, RN, MSN, CCRN, ACNP-BC
Chief Nurse, Army Trauma Training Center
Ryder Trauma Center
Miami

Beryl Stetson, RNC, MSN
Assistant Professor, Nursing
Raritan Valley Community College
Somerville, N.J.

Colleen R. Walsh, RN, MSN, ONC, CS, ACNP-BC
Faculty, Graduate Nursing
University of Southern Indiana School of Nursing
Evansville

E. Monica Ward-Murray, RN, SRN, RMN, BSN, EdD, EdM
Assistant Professor
Medical University of South Carolina College of Nursing
Charleston

Mary E. Weyer, RN, EdD, APN, CS
Associate Professor, Deicke Center for Nursing Education
Elmhurst (Ill.) College

Sharon Wing, RN, MSN
Assistant Professor
Cleveland State University

How to use this book

This brand new sixth edition of *Springhouse Review for NCLEX-RN®* has been completely revised and updated to help you organize your review, check your understanding of the examination process and, finally, help you achieve success on the NCLEX-RN®.

To begin, you'll find two pretests — each includes 75 questions and answers, that are formatted to reflect the latest test plan of the NCLEX-RN, including alternate-format questions, such as multiple-response, multiple-choice; fill-in-the-blank; drag-and-drop; chart-exhibit; and hot-spot questions.

This way, you'll get a feel for which areas you need to concentrate on *before* beginning your review for the examination. Chapters 1 and 2 cover specific information to help you understand the test plan of the NCLEX-RN and how it's organized. Test-taking hints are presented as well as ideas to help you prepare for the examination and to organize your own review. You'll find that setting aside a routine block of time to review, developing a plan to organize the review, and following through consistently to meet the review schedule goals will lead you toward the good study habits you'll need to pass the NCLEX-RN.

After the introduction to the NCLEX-RN, chapter 3, an overview of the fundamentals of nursing, introduces key topics and test points on nursing concepts and skills. New to this edition are chapter 4: Leadership and management, and chapter 5: Ethical and legal issues. Chapters 6 through 12 outline the relevant nursing topics (including perioperative, mental health, oncologic, pediatric, maternal-neonatal, and adult nursing) that are tested on the examination.

Overall, the book contains new review content in all major clinical areas and key facts about the NCLEX-RN examination. The disorders for each chapter are presented in an easy-to-use format that includes the nursing process. For example, Parkinson's disease includes a description, and the *possible causes* are presented with *assessment findings* and *diagnostic evaluation.* This is followed by *nursing diagnoses; treatment; drug therapy options;* and *planning and goals.* Most important, the *implementation* is broken down in a bulleted list with *rationales* that are clearly identified in italics for each intervention. An *evaluation* summary follows.

You can finish your study sessions by testing yourself with the 4 comprehensive (75 questions each) and challenging question-and-answer posttests. They're set in the same format as the pretests — a format identical to that of the NCLEX-RN.

Not only does *Springhouse Review for NCLEX-RN®* have a brand new design but it also offers features you won't find in any other NCLEX-RN review book. Our study icons help you organize your review sessions and facilitate retention of information. Some of the features that were specifically designed to promote your learning in preparation for the NCLEX-RN include:

Fast fact — Key information is set off in boxes throughout the text to help you rehearse and remember important review material.

Spot check — As you progress in your review, questions are sprinkled throughout the text to verify that you understand the material.

Quick study — Limericks, mnemonics, and other creative strategies are used in a boxed format to present easy ways to help you remember information.

Clinical situation — A variety of clinical situations that focus on the nurse's role promote your understanding of nursing practice. Questions are posed for you to reflect on, and nursing principles are applied to promote your understanding. You'll incorporate the valuable information you've learned in this book with the information you've learned in the classroom to solve some of these questions. Questions for further thought are included at the end of each clinical situation to promote expanded learning.

Lastly, the bonus CD-ROM gives you an additional 1,500 questions — not found in this book — that are written in the format you can expect on the NCLEX-RN examination. You can practice and become comfortable with the same format that you'll see on the actual examination — including alternate-format questions. You can select questions to answer by subject, or you can answer questions in random order. After answering each question, you'll immediately receive feedback about your answers. Practicing in this format will help you increase your knowledge and understanding of key information as well as enhance your familiarity with the testing format.

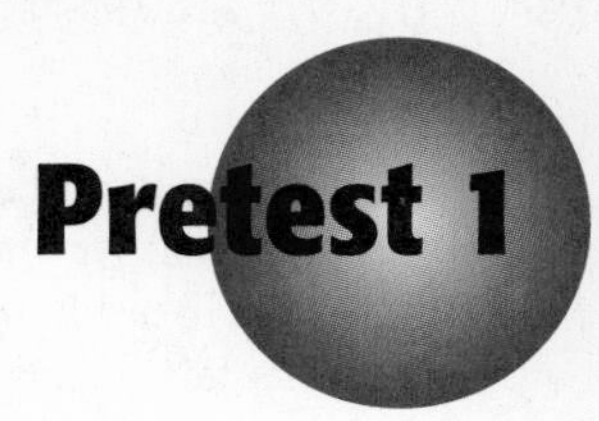

Pretest 1

Instructions

The two pretests have been designed to determine your current knowledge base before you begin your study program for the NCLEX-RN. By analyzing the results, you can identify the areas in which you may wish to do more comprehensive study.

Each pretest contains 75 questions, written in the format used in the computerized examination. In the traditional multiple-choice questions, there are four possible answers for each question. Read each question and all possible answers carefully; then select the best answer. For alternate-format questions, you may be asked to identify multiple correct responses; fill-in-the-blank with the correct numerical answer; choose an answer based on a chart or exhibit; place answers in sequential, ascending order; or identify an area in an illustration or graphic.

Take no more than 75 minutes to complete each pretest. If you have difficulty understanding a question or aren't sure of the answer, place a small mark next to the question number—but still select an answer, even if you have to guess. The mark will help you recall that you had trouble with that question. However, be aware that on the computerized examination, you will *not* be able to go back to a question or go on to the next question without selecting an answer choice.

In the pretests, possible answers are labeled 1, 2, 3, and 4 to help identify the correct answer and the rationale. These numbers don't appear in the actual computerized NCLEX-RN.

The pretest questions appear as:

1. Atonic
2. Dystonic
3. Hypotonic
4. Hypertonic

The NCLEX-RN questions appear as:

Atonic
Dystonic
Hypotonic
Hypertonic

Now, select a quiet room where you'll be undisturbed, set a timer for 75 minutes, and begin the first pretest. After you've completed the first pretest or the 75-minute time limit expires, check your responses against the correct answers provided. Repeat these same steps for the second pretest.

Questions

1. A 60-year-old male client with a history of angina has been taking nitroglycerin. He states, "Everything is fine, except that I get chest pain while having sex with my wife." Which response by a nurse would be best?

☐ **1.** "Have you thought of seeing a sex therapist for counseling?"
☐ **2.** "You'll have to limit your sexual activity."
☐ **3.** "You should expect that intercourse at your age may pose some problems."
☐ **4.** "You may be helped by taking a nitroglycerin tablet just before intercourse."

2. A client has been placed on a low-cholesterol diet. A nurse should advise the client to reduce intake of which food?

☐ **1.** Cottage cheese
☐ **2.** Eggs
☐ **3.** Veal
☐ **4.** Chicken

3. A client is admitted to a psychiatric facility for treatment of agoraphobia. For the past 3 months, she has been afraid to leave her home, and she and her husband have agreed that hospitalization is necessary. When the staff nurse introduces herself, the client starts to cry and says, "I'm so afraid to be here. I'm not crazy. I just want to go home." Which response by the nurse would be most appropriate?

☐ **1.** "Try not to be so upset now. Let's get busy helping you."
☐ **2.** "You seem upset. I'll sit here with you."
☐ **3.** "You can't go home until we've helped you with your fears."
☐ **4.** "Is there some way I can help you?"

4. A nursing assistant asks the nurse why a client's physician doesn't just force an agoraphobic client to get out of the house to help her get over her fears. Which understanding of the treatment of phobias should the nurse's response include?

☐ **1.** People must gain a sense of control over the feared object—they can't be forced when they aren't ready.
☐ **2.** People use their fears to consciously avoid taking responsibility for their lives.
☐ **3.** The treatment approach is intentionally slow to help lull the client into a sense of fearlessness.
☐ **4.** Forcing people into fearful situations can cause acute psychosis.

5. A nurse finds an agoraphobic client standing in front of a sign-up sheet for a field trip to a shopping mall. The client says, "If I had any guts, I'd sign up for this trip. What do you think I should do?" Which comment by the nurse would help the client make an appropriate decision?

☐ **1.** "You have plenty of guts! Why not sign up now?"
☐ **2.** "I'm not here to tell you what to do, but if I were you, I'd go."
☐ **3.** "It sure is a great trip. I think you'd enjoy it."
☐ **4.** "Let's discuss what you're thinking about this trip."

6. A 15-year-old female client with bulimia nervosa tells the nurse she doesn't like the other teenagers on the ward. A nurse senses the client's disdain toward her peers. Which nursing action would best help the teenager with peer relationships?

☐ **1.** Point out to the client how she affects others.
☐ **2.** Ask the client why she doesn't like her peers.
☐ **3.** Carefully select same-age peers to include in an activity with the client.
☐ **4.** Have the client choose an activity that would include herself, the nurse, and some peers as participants.

7. When approaching an alcoholic client who is having visual hallucinations, a nurse should do what first?

☐ **1.** Seek the client's permission to discuss the hallucinations.
☐ **2.** Explain the reason for the hallucinations.
☐ **3.** Avoid discussion of the hallucinations and present reality.
☐ **4.** Administer an antipsychotic medication.

8. What's the best way to deal with a toddler who is having a temper tantrum?

☐ **1.** Reason with the child.
☐ **2.** Threaten the child.
☐ **3.** Spank the child.
☐ **4.** Ignore the child's outburst.

9. A client visits the prenatal clinic for the first time after missing two menstrual periods. She suspects she may be pregnant and tells a nurse that the 1st day of her last menstrual period was June 30, 2005. According to Nägele's rule, which of these dates is the client's expected date of delivery?

☐ **1.** March 14, 2006
☐ **2.** March 30, 2006
☐ **3.** April 6, 2006
☐ **4.** April 13, 2006

10. A client has a positive pregnancy test. Which hormone is related to this finding?

☐ **1.** Luteinizing hormone
☐ **2.** Follicle-stimulating hormone
☐ **3.** Human chorionic somatomammotropin
☐ **4.** Human chorionic gonadotropin

11. In addition to the hormonal changes indicated by a positive pregnancy test, which physiological change would have occurred by the time a client had missed two menstrual periods?

☐ **1.** Diastasis recti
☐ **2.** Decreased glomerular filtration rate
☐ **3.** Bluish discoloration of the vaginal vault
☐ **4.** Blood volume increased by 50%

12. A pregnant client who received dietary instructions during her first visit to the prenatal clinic returns for a follow-up. The nurse asks her what she had for lunch that day. Which response would indicate that the client followed the dietary instructions?

☐ **1.** Cheeseburger, salad, fruit, and milk
☐ **2.** Bouillon, crackers, fruit, and milk
☐ **3.** Ham sandwich, pickles, pie, and iced tea
☐ **4.** Cottage cheese, tomatoes, crackers, and coffee with cream

13. A client has questions about exercise during pregnancy. Which approach would be the most appropriate for a nurse to take?

☐ **1.** Recommend that the client follow an exercise routine.
☐ **2.** Assure the client that her pregnancy is normal and she need not adjust her usual activities.
☐ **3.** Give the client a pamphlet explaining recommended exercises.
☐ **4.** Explore the amount and type of exercise the client is doing.

14. A physician has ordered ferrous sulfate 100 mg three times per day for a pregnant client. Which instruction should the client be given for optimal absorption?

☐ **1.** "Take the medication just before meals and with plenty of fluid."
☐ **2.** "Take the medication with milk at mealtimes."
☐ **3.** "Take the medication with an antacid after meals."
☐ **4.** "Take the medication with orange juice between meals."

15. At 28 weeks' gestation, a pregnant client's laboratory values include blood: hemoglobin, 11 g/dl; hematocrit, 36%; urine: glucose, trace; acetone, negative; albumin, negative. These results probably indicate which disorder?

☐ **1.** Iron deficiency anemia
☐ **2.** Preeclampsia
☐ **3.** Diabetes mellitus
☐ **4.** Pseudoanemia of pregnancy

16. A male client is receiving an antihypertensive agent. Which of these potential adverse reactions would be most important for the nurse to discuss with him?

☐ **1.** Impotence
☐ **2.** Nausea and vomiting
☐ **3.** Nasal stuffiness
☐ **4.** Postural hypotension

17. Infants achieve structural control of the head before the trunk and extremities. Which of these universal principles of development does this reflect?

☐ **1.** Development proceeds in a cephalocaudal direction.
☐ **2.** Development proceeds in a proximal-distal fashion.
☐ **3.** The sequence of development is from simple to complex.
☐ **4.** The sequence of development is from general to specific.

18. A male client has been on glucocorticoid therapy for the past year. He calls a nurse to report that he has been vomiting for the past 2 days and hasn't taken his "hormone" pills. The nurse should plan the client's care based on which potential effect of glucocorticoids?

☐ **1.** The client may develop adrenal insufficiency.
☐ **2.** The client is at risk for developing pituitary syndrome.
☐ **3.** The client's own adrenal glands will start to produce more glucocorticoids immediately.
☐ **4.** The client's pituitary gland will increase production of corticotropin immediately.

19. A divorced computer programmer is admitted after taking 15 secobarbital sodium (Seconal) capsules. Three days later, the client is transferred from the intensive care unit to the psychiatric unit. Quiet and withdrawn, the client refuses to get out of bed for breakfast. Which response by a nurse would be most appropriate?

☐ **1.** "It's a beautiful day today. Time to get up."
☐ **2.** "It's time to get up. I'll help you get ready for breakfast."
☐ **3.** "It's time to get up for breakfast. Let's get ready."
☐ **4.** "It's the policy on this unit to be up and dressed for breakfast."

20. A nurse has been working with a depressed male client for 1 week. This morning, the client comes to the dining room with his hair uncombed and shirt unbuttoned. Which of these actions should the nurse take first?

- ☐ **1.** Approach the client and offer to help him finish getting dressed.
- ☐ **2.** Ignore the client's appearance and help him find his place at the table.
- ☐ **3.** Sit with the client and help him eat the food.
- ☐ **4.** Walk with the client until he notices that his shirt is unbuttoned.

21. A client who has recovered from second- and third-degree burns is being discharged. Which comment demonstrates the client has understood the discharge teaching?

- ☐ **1.** "I need to wear the pressure stockings to decrease scarring on my legs."
- ☐ **2.** "I only need to do physical therapy once per week."
- ☐ **3.** "I can take off the pressure garments for 4 hours per day."
- ☐ **4.** "I don't need to worry about contractures because if I was going to get them, I would have gotten them by now."

22. A depressed client participates in unit activities and meets regularly with a nurse. One morning, the client asks the nurse to get the comb from the bedside table. Next to the comb, the nurse finds 10 Xanax tablets. After confiscating the capsules, what should the nurse do next?

- ☐ **1.** Report the finding to the other team members.
- ☐ **2.** Tell the client about finding the capsules and ask if the client was planning to commit suicide.
- ☐ **3.** Sit with the client for the rest of the day and increase suicide precautions.
- ☐ **4.** Give the client the comb; then suggest that the client and nurse go for a walk.

23. Which measure should a nurse take when providing care to a client in Buck's traction?

- ☐ **1.** Maintain the head of the bed at a 45-degree angle.
- ☐ **2.** Ensure that the client's right heel touches the bed.
- ☐ **3.** Remove the weights when bathing the client's lower extremities.
- ☐ **4.** Allow the weights to hang freely at the foot of the bed.

24. A client admitted with pulmonary edema is improving. The physician's current orders include digoxin (Lanoxin) 0.25 mg daily, furosemide (Lasix) 40 mg daily, and nasal oxygen at 2 L/minute. To evaluate the effectiveness of digoxin, a nurse should observe for:

- ☐ **1.** increased urine output.
- ☐ **2.** increased pulse rate.
- ☐ **3.** decreased respiratory rate.
- ☐ **4.** lowered blood pressure.

25. A client with pulmonary edema is receiving furosemide (Lasix). When planning the client's care, a nurse would include which action?

- ☐ **1.** Monitor magnesium levels.
- ☐ **2.** Report a heart rate less than 60 beats/minute.
- ☐ **3.** Record amount and characteristics of urine output.
- ☐ **4.** Assess for neurologic intention tremor.

26. A client with pulmonary edema is receiving continuous oxygen therapy and daily doses of furosemide (Lasix) and digoxin. When the client complains of no appetite and asks to have the food tray removed, a nurse's best action should be based on knowledge that:

- ☐ **1.** many clients dislike hospital food.
- ☐ **2.** anorexia is common in clients receiving oxygen.
- ☐ **3.** furosemide causes decreased appetite in many clients.
- ☐ **4.** anorexia may be an early sign of digoxin toxicity.

27. A boy, age 7, recently was diagnosed with juvenile-onset diabetes mellitus. He takes NPH and regular insulin. His mother asks a nurse if he can go on an afternoon hike during an upcoming weekend camp-out. Which response by the nurse would be the best?

- ☐ **1.** "He should have a snack, such as a cheese sandwich and a glass of milk, 1 hour before the hike and should carry a fast-acting source of glucose."
- ☐ **2.** "He shouldn't go on the hike. The possible effects of extraordinary activities are just too unpredictable."
- ☐ **3.** "He should increase his morning dosage of NPH insulin by approximately one-third to cover his increased metabolic rate during the hike."
- ☐ **4.** "Do you feel it's really appropriate for him to participate in a weekend camp-out when he has physical limitations?"

28. A client with hypertension is receiving chlorothiazide (Diuril) to reduce blood pressure. The nurse should instruct the client to consume which food regularly?

☐ **1.** Apples
☐ **2.** Liver
☐ **3.** Low-fat milk
☐ **4.** Dried fruits

29. A client visits the company nurse for treatment of a minor cut on her right arm. The nurse is aware that the client had a right mastectomy 5 years ago. Further action by the nurse should be based on which understanding?

☐ **1.** Previous removal of lymph nodes places the client at increased risk for complications such as infection.
☐ **2.** After 5 years, the client is no longer at risk for complications.
☐ **3.** Only underlying psychological problems could cause someone to be concerned with a minor cut.
☐ **4.** On-the-job stress is probably the real cause of the client's visit.

30. Laboratory results for a client who's receiving chemotherapy include: hematocrit, 34%; hemoglobin, 11 g/dl; platelet count, 48,000/µl; and white blood cell count, 4,000/µl. All of the following goals are indicated in the care plan. Which goal should take priority?

☐ **1.** To prevent infection
☐ **2.** To prevent bleeding
☐ **3.** To prevent anemia
☐ **4.** To prevent alopecia

31. A client is told that a tuberculin skin test is positive. Which statement would indicate that the client understands the test results?

☐ **1.** "I've had previous exposure to tuberculosis."
☐ **2.** "I have immunity and can't develop the disease."
☐ **3.** "I currently have active tuberculosis."
☐ **4.** "I have a reactivation of a healed primary lesion."

32. A client, age 14, has been sexually abused by her father for the past 2 years. Now she's 8 weeks pregnant and asks a nurse what she should do about the pregnancy. Which reply would be best?

☐ **1.** "Because you're so young, you stand a good chance of having a miscarriage."
☐ **2.** "That's a decision only you and your mother can make."
☐ **3.** "I think it would be all right for you to have an abortion. Is that what you'd like to do?"
☐ **4.** "Making a sound decision isn't always easy. What are your thoughts about the pregnancy?"

33. A 15-month-old boy is admitted to the pediatric unit with a diagnosis of bilateral serous otitis media and bacterial meningitis. In which room on the pediatric unit should a nurse plan to put the client?

☐ **1.** An isolation room off the main hallway
☐ **2.** A private room two doors away from the nurses' station
☐ **3.** A semiprivate room with a 15-month-old child who has meningitis
☐ **4.** A four-bed room with two toddlers who have croup

34. To best meet the developmental needs of a 15-month-old hospitalized boy, a nurse should take which measure?

☐ **1.** Ask his mother to stay with him overnight.
☐ **2.** Turn on the television to his favorite cartoons.
☐ **3.** Arrange for other staff to visit him at regular intervals throughout the day.
☐ **4.** Tape a bright red punching balloon onto the side of his crib.

35. Which statement by the mother of a 15-month-old boy with bacterial meningitis would indicate that she understands the nurse's discharge teaching?

☐ **1.** "I wish I had brought my child to the doctor sooner. The next time, I'll be more careful."
☐ **2.** "We'll need to see the doctor every week or so until we're sure everything is all right."
☐ **3.** "Next time he pulls on his ears or won't lie down, I'll take him to the doctor right away."
☐ **4.** "I'm glad we'll be going home soon and that all of this business with infections and meningitis is behind us."

36. A client who has been diagnosed with conductive deafness is scheduled for a stapedectomy and has been taught about the condition. Which statement by the client would indicate a need for further instruction?

☐ **1.** "Bone conduction of sound is still effective."
☐ **2.** "My acoustic nerve is injured."
☐ **3.** "Otosclerosis is a cause of my condition."
☐ **4.** "Air conduction of sound is impaired."

37. Two days after a left-eye cataract extraction, a client complains of nausea, vomiting, and seeing halos around lights. Which complication should a nurse suspect?

☐ **1.** Detached retina
☐ **2.** Increased intraocular pressure
☐ **3.** Dislocated lens
☐ **4.** Corneal abrasion

38. After an above-the-knee amputation, a client returns to the unit from the recovery room. A nurse helps transfer the client from the stretcher to the bed. Before leaving the bedside, the nurse should make sure the client and the stump are in which positions?

- ☐ **1.** The client should be lying in a prone position, and the stump shouldn't be elevated.
- ☐ **2.** The stump should be abducted with a pillow between the client's legs.
- ☐ **3.** The client should be in a side-lying position, with the stump externally rotated.
- ☐ **4.** The client should be lying on his back, with the stump elevated slightly on a pillow.

39. A nurse accompanies a client who is having an intravenous pyelogram (IVP). Which reaction, if it were to occur, should the nurse report to the physician immediately?

- ☐ **1.** Angioedema
- ☐ **2.** A feeling of warmth
- ☐ **3.** Flushing of the face
- ☐ **4.** Salty taste

40. A client has been treated for cirrhosis of the liver for 3 years. Now he's hospitalized for treatment of recently diagnosed esophageal varices. Which instruction should a nurse give the client?

- ☐ **1.** Eat foods quickly so they don't get cold and cause distress.
- ☐ **2.** Avoid straining at stool to keep venous pressure low.
- ☐ **3.** Decrease fluid intake to avoid ascites.
- ☐ **4.** Avoid exercise because it may cause bleeding of the varices.

41. A client is in acute renal failure. A nurse must assess the client carefully for which complication?

- ☐ **1.** Tetany
- ☐ **2.** Hypernatremia
- ☐ **3.** Vascular collapse
- ☐ **4.** Cardiac arrhythmias

42. Several hours after a leg amputation, a client complains of cramping pain in the toes of the amputated foot. When discussing this pain with the client, which approach would be best for a nurse to take?

- ☐ **1.** Explain to the client that he can't feel pain in an amputated limb.
- ☐ **2.** Tell the client that the phantom pain will lessen in 2 to 3 days.
- ☐ **3.** Review the reasons for phantom pain with the client.
- ☐ **4.** Mention that phantom pain is a common occurrence.

43. A client sees a physician, complaining he has no energy and fears he has a terrible disease. He reports he has had trouble sleeping and completing his normal daily work for the past 3 months. The physical examination is normal. The client denies any recent losses. He seeks psychiatric care and is admitted to a psychiatric facility. After meeting with a nurse for 3 weeks, the client starts the one-on-one session again by saying, "I'm such a failure. I can't earn a living. I'm never successful." Which response by the nurse would be most therapeutic?

- ☐ **1.** "We all feel discouraged at times."
- ☐ **2.** "I'd like to discuss your plans for today."
- ☐ **3.** "You aren't a failure. Look at what a successful salesman you've been."
- ☐ **4.** "It's hard to feel like you're a failure. Let's talk about your plans for the future."

44. A depressed client is sitting in the activities room, staring at the wall. Which nursing intervention would be the most appropriate?

- ☐ **1.** Give the client free access to the activities materials, and ask what he wants to do.
- ☐ **2.** Give the client time to select an activity, and sit with him until he gets busy.
- ☐ **3.** Give the client equipment for making a collage, and show him how to do it.
- ☐ **4.** Give the client a 500-piece jigsaw puzzle, and tell him to do the best he can.

45. A client on the psychiatric unit slams down the phone after talking with his wife. He says, "She's the reason why I'm here." Which response by a nurse would be most appropriate?

- ☐ **1.** Tell him he has a lovely wife.
- ☐ **2.** Tell him we all get angry with our loved ones at times.
- ☐ **3.** Ask the client if he'd like to talk about it and show interest in his further comments.
- ☐ **4.** Suggest that they take a walk to work off some of his anger.

46. A client with type I diabetes mellitus is admitted to the hospital for reevaluation. Approximately 3 hours after the client receives 20 units of regular insulin, a nurse assists with morning care. Which assessment findings would lead the nurse to suspect the client is having an insulin reaction?

☐ **1.** Air hunger and acetone breath
☐ **2.** Vomiting and flushed skin
☐ **3.** Nausea and headache
☐ **4.** Confusion and diaphoresis

47. During a hypoglycemic (insulin) reaction, a client is alert but can't swallow. Which would be the best nursing action to take?

☐ **1.** Give orange juice.
☐ **2.** Administer 50% glucose I.V.
☐ **3.** Administer epinephrine subcutaneously.
☐ **4.** Administer glucagon I.M.

48. A client is admitted to the nursing unit in acute abdominal pain. A physician diagnoses peritonitis. Which finding on an abdominal assessment occurs with peritonitis?

☐ **1.** High-pitched bowel sounds
☐ **2.** Pain radiation from the flank
☐ **3.** Diffuse abdominal pain
☐ **4.** Diarrhea

49. A client with peritonitis has a Salem sump that's connected to low suction. Which strategy should a nurse include in the care plan?

☐ **1.** Turn the client from side to side every 4 hours.
☐ **2.** Irrigate the nasogastric (NG) tube through the blue opening.
☐ **3.** Measure NG drainage every 24 hours.
☐ **4.** Increase the suction control to high if no drainage appears.

50. A neonate, 1 hour old, is admitted to the neonate nursery from the delivery room. The mother had polyhydramnios, and the health care team suspects the neonate has a tracheoesophageal fistula. The nurse should assess the neonate for which symptom?

☐ **1.** Meconium stool
☐ **2.** Bile-stained vomitus
☐ **3.** Coughing, cyanosis, and choking
☐ **4.** Excessive vomiting

51. A neonate undergoes surgery that consists of repair of a tracheoesophageal fistula and a gastrostomy. Between the 3rd and 14th postoperative days, the neonate receives feedings through the gastrostomy tube. Which action should a nurse perform as part of the gastrostomy feeding?

☐ **1.** Inject 1 to 5 ml of air through the tube and listen over the stomach with a stethoscope.
☐ **2.** Feed through the gastrostomy tube with the neonate positioned on his left side.
☐ **3.** After the feeding, leave the gastrostomy tube unplugged and elevated above the level of the stomach.
☐ **4.** Immediately after the feeding, turn the neonate onto his right side and plug the gastrostomy tube.

52. When assessing a client with chronic obstructive pulmonary disease (COPD), a nurse would expect which laboratory finding?

☐ **1.** Elevated red blood cell (RBC) count
☐ **2.** Decreased platelet count
☐ **3.** Increased Pao_2 and decreased $Paco_2$ levels
☐ **4.** Elevated serum cholesterol

53. A pediatric client is about to have skin traction applied. The client's mother says, "I thought everyone who needed traction had to have skeletal traction." When discussing traction with her, the nurse can mention that skin traction has which advantage over skeletal traction?

☐ **1.** It's easier to apply.
☐ **2.** It causes no complications.
☐ **3.** It prevents rotation of the extremity.
☐ **4.** It can be maintained for longer periods.

54. A client with rheumatoid arthritis is receiving ibuprofen (Motrin). Which statement would indicate that the client has a correct understanding of ibuprofen?

☐ **1.** "I should take the medicine between meals."
☐ **2.** "The medicine will increase my appetite."
☐ **3.** "The medicine may cause diarrhea."
☐ **4.** "I should stop the medicine if my joints start to swell."

55. A child, age 2, is brought to the emergency department (ED) by his parents, who state that he refuses to move his right arm. X-rays reveal a dislocated right shoulder and a simple fracture of the right humerus. During the child's stay in the ED, a nurse observes all of the following behaviors by the child. Which behavior most strongly suggests the child has been abused and should be carefully documented by the nurse?

☐ **1.** The child tries to sit up on the stretcher.
☐ **2.** The child tries to move away from the nurse.
☐ **3.** The child doesn't answer the nurse's questions.
☐ **4.** The child doesn't cry when he's being moved.

56. A hospitalized child, age 2½, hasn't tried to feed himself. The primary nurse notes a poor nutritional intake. To increase the child's food intake, the nurse should attempt which action?

☐ **1.** Giving the child pudding
☐ **2.** Talking to the physician about enteral feedings
☐ **3.** Providing nutritious snacks between meals
☐ **4.** Keeping a 6-oz (175-ml) bottle of milk in the crib between feedings

57. During a health care team meeting to discuss a pediatric client suspected of having been abused, a nursing assistant says, "We shouldn't let that child's parents visit her at all. After all, they put her here in the first place!" A nurse's response to the assistant should be based on which understanding about abusive parents?

☐ **1.** They shouldn't visit their child in the hospital.
☐ **2.** They shouldn't visit until the child is ready for discharge.
☐ **3.** They should visit on a limited schedule set up by the health care team and should be supervised during all visits.
☐ **4.** They should be encouraged to visit frequently and should be welcomed by the staff.

58. During a visit to the pediatric outpatient clinic, a mother says her 3-year-old son hasn't yet received any "shots." A nurse's response should be based on which understanding?

☐ **1.** The child will need double the number of immunizations now because he's no longer an infant.
☐ **2.** Immunizations can safely be delayed until the child enters nursery school.
☐ **3.** At his age, immunizations are contraindicated.
☐ **4.** Up to age 6, the same immunizations are given.

59. In a client with a spinal cord injury, which clinical finding would indicate spinal shock?

☐ **1.** Loss of sweating
☐ **2.** Urinary incontinence
☐ **3.** Normal blood pressure
☐ **4.** Muscle spasticity

60. A client with a spinal cord injury has autonomic dysreflexia. Which action should a nurse take first?

☐ **1.** Call the physician.
☐ **2.** Place the client in reverse Trendelenburg's positon.
☐ **3.** Administer a sedative on a standing order.
☐ **4.** Check the client for a fecal impaction.

61. A 10-year-old child who has scoliosis is being discharged after the placement of a Harrington rod. A nurse anticipates the child may require which community resource at discharge?

☐ **1.** Family support group
☐ **2.** Outpatient psychiatric care
☐ **3.** Physical therapy and rehabilitation
☐ **4.** Social service

62. The use of isolation in the hospital is intended to:

☐ **1.** discourage a client with an infection from ambulating.
☐ **2.** keep an infection from becoming endemic.
☐ **3.** maintain a sterile environment.
☐ **4.** prevent the further spread of an infection to others.

63. When a client is being treated for a renal calculus, a nurse anticipates:

☐ **1.** checking specific gravity.
☐ **2.** collecting a 24-hour urine sample.
☐ **3.** measuring urine output.
☐ **4.** straining the urine.

64. Upon a client's admission to the hospital, a nurse provides the client with a document written by the American Hospital Association (AHA) that defines patients rights. This document is called:

☐ **1.** an informed consent.
☐ **2.** a legal competence.
☐ **3.** the Patient's Bill of Rights.
☐ **4.** the right to know.

65. A client who is 10 weeks pregnant is seen in a clinic for a prenatal visit. She tells a nurse that she has had nausea and vomiting every morning for the last week. The nurse should instruct the client to:

☐ **1.** restrict fluid intake during the afternoon.
☐ **2.** drink a glass of juice before bedtime.
☐ **3.** eat a high-protein snack after arising.
☐ **4.** eat dry crackers before arising.

66. A client diagnosed with gestational diabetes is admitted for induction of labor at 38 weeks' gestation. Which intervention would a nurse expect to perform on admission?

☐ **1.** Test the client's urine for protein with a dipstick.
☐ **2.** Measure the client's fundal height with a tape measure.
☐ **3.** Administer the client's oral hypoglycemic.
☐ **4.** Assess the client's glucose level with a fingerstick.

67. Each morning in the unit, the head nurse assigns clients and additional tasks to the nurses to be completed that day. During the shift, a crisis develops and one of the staff nurses doesn't complete the additional tasks. The next day, the staff nurse is reprimanded. When the staff nurse tries to explain, the head nurse replies that the tasks should have been completed anyway. Which of these leadership styles is the head nurse exhibiting?

☐ **1.** Democratic
☐ **2.** Permissive
☐ **3.** Laissez-faire
☐ **4.** Authoritarian

68. A 10-month-old infant with recurrent otitis media is brought to the clinic for evaluation. To help determine the cause of the infant's condition, a nurse should ask the parents:

☐ **1.** "Does water ever get into the baby's ears during shampooing?"
☐ **2.** "Do you give the baby a bottle to take to bed?"
☐ **3.** "Have you noticed a lot of wax in the baby's ears?"
☐ **4.** "Can the baby combine two words when speaking?"

69. When developing a postoperative care plan for an infant scheduled for cleft lip repair, a nurse should assign highest priority to which intervention?

☐ **1.** Comforting the infant as quickly as possible
☐ **2.** Maintaining the infant in a prone position
☐ **3.** Restraining the infant's arms at all times, using elbow restraints
☐ **4.** Avoiding disturbing crusts that form on the suture line

70. A man has been diagnosed with benign prostatic hyperplasia. A transurethral prostatic resection (TURP) under spinal anesthesia is planned under spinal anesthesia. A nurse informs the client that postoperative discomfort will probably manifest as:

☐ **1.** back pain.
☐ **2.** pain radiating from bladder area to shoulders.
☐ **3.** bladder spasms.
☐ **4.** leg cramps resulting from the position the client is in during surgery.

71. A nurse is preparing an 86-year-old client diagnosed with iron deficiency anemia and diabetes mellitus for discharge. The nurse suggests that the client increase her intake of which iron-rich foods?

☐ **1.** Fortified wheat products and red meat
☐ **2.** Fish and white rice
☐ **3.** Dairy products and sardines
☐ **4.** Eggs and cheese

72. A client with chest pain receives nitroglycerin en route to the hospital. Based on an electrocardiogram obtained on admission, a physician suspects a myocardial infarction (MI) and prescribes I.V. morphine to relieve continuing pain. A primary goal of nursing care for this client is to recognize life-threatening complications of an MI. The major cause of death after an MI is:

☐ **1.** cardiogenic shock.
☐ **2.** cardiac arrhythmias.
☐ **3.** heart failure.
☐ **4.** pulmonary embolism.

73. A client is returning to a clinic to have the results of a Western blot test explained. The results are positive; therefore a nurse should include which statement when discussing results with the client?

☐ **1.** "You have AIDS."
☐ **2.** "You're immune to the HIV."
☐ **3.** "You can't transmit the virus to others."
☐ **4.** "Antibodies to HIV are present in your blood."

74. A client is prescribed 2 tsp Bactrim (trimethoprim and sulfamethoxazole) by mouth twice per day. How many milliliters of the drug should the nurse administer?

____

75. The physical examination of a client reveals exophthalmos, a classic sign of Graves' disease. Which other assessment findings are associated with Grave's disease? Select all that apply.

☐ **1.** Dry, waxy swelling and abnormal mucin deposits in the skin
☐ **2.** Heat intolerance and diarrhea
☐ **3.** A wide, staggering gait
☐ **4.** More than 10 beats/minute difference between the apical and radial pulse rates
☐ **5.** Nervousness and weight loss

Answers and rationales

In the pretest answers, the question number appears in boldface type, followed by the number of the correct answer. Rationales for correct answers and incorrect options follow. To help you evaluate your knowledge base and application of nursing behaviors, each rationale is classified as:

- nursing process step
- client needs category
- client needs subcategory
- cognitive level.

1. CORRECT ANSWER: 4
A client with angina is commonly taught to take a nitroglycerin tablet before intercourse to prevent anginal pain caused by an increased cardiac workload. Nitroglycerin dilates the coronary arteries, increasing circulation to the myocardium.
Nursing process step: Implementation
Client needs category: Physiological integrity
Client needs subcategory: Reduction of risk potential
Cognitive level: Application

2. CORRECT ANSWER: 2
The nurse should advise the client to limit intake of eggs, which are high in cholesterol. The other foods would be recommended on this client's diet.
Nursing process step: Implementation
Client needs category: Physiological integrity
Client needs subcategory: Reduction of risk potential
Cognitive level: Application

3. CORRECT ANSWER: 2
The most appropriate response would be to acknowledge the client's feelings and offer support. Options 1 and 3 slight the client's feelings. Option 4 is unrealistic; a client experiencing high anxiety would have trouble giving a specific response.
Nursing process step: Implementation
Client needs category: Psychosocial integrity
Client needs subcategory: None
Cognitive level: Application

4. CORRECT ANSWER: 1
A client can best deal with a phobia by gaining a sense of control over the feared object. People don't consciously use phobias. Instilling a sense of fearlessness is an unrealistic expectation. People experience high anxiety or panic, not acute psychosis, when forced into fearful situations.
Nursing process step: Implementation
Client needs category: Psychosocial integrity
Client needs subcategory: None
Cognitive level: Comprehension

5. CORRECT ANSWER: 4
Encouraging the client to discuss feelings would help the nurse elicit more information. Giving advice would be inappropriate. The nurse doesn't know that the client would enjoy the trip.
Nursing process step: Implementation
Client needs category: Psychosocial integrity
Client needs subcategory: None
Cognitive level: Application

6. CORRECT ANSWER: 4
Allowing the client to select the activity would give her some control over the situation. Because clients with eating disorders struggle with issues of control, they can benefit when given the chance to have input in their treatment program. Option 1 would put the client on the defensive. The client may not know why she doesn't like her peers (option 2). Option 3 would take control away from the client.
Nursing process step: Implementation
Client needs category: Psychosocial integrity
Client needs subcategory: None
Cognitive level: Analysis

7. CORRECT ANSWER: 1
Respect is a major component of a trusting relationship. Without a trusting relationship, interactions can't be therapeutic. Providing reassurance and explaining the reason for the hallucination may not be received if the client

doesn't trust the nurse. Denying the hallucinations may increase the client's anxiety. Administering antipsychotic drugs isn't the initial approach.
Nursing process step: Planning
Client needs category: Psychosocial integrity
Client needs subcategory: None
Cognitive level: Analysis

8. CORRECT ANSWER: 4
Ignoring the child's outburst (while reducing external stimulation and removing objects that could cause injury) is the most appropriate management technique. During a tantrum, an upset toddler is incapable of dealing with reason or threats (options 1 and 2). The tantrum results from loss of control; spanking the child (option 3) would increase insecurity, which already is present.
Nursing process step: Implementation
Client needs category: Health promotion and maintenance
Client needs subcategory: None
Cognitive level: Knowledge

9. CORRECT ANSWER: 3
Using Nägele's rule (the most common method for estimating the date of delivery), the nurse would take the 1st day of the last normal menstrual period (June 30), subtract 3 months (March 30), and add 7 days (April 6).
Nursing process step: Assessment
Client needs category: Health promotion and maintenance
Client needs subcategory: None
Cognitive level: Application

10. CORRECT ANSWER: 4
Human chorionic gonadotropin is produced by the trophoblastic tissue of the placenta and secreted into the urine and serum of a pregnant woman shortly after the onset of pregnancy. Luteinizing hormone (option 1) and follicle-stimulating hormone (option 2) are anterior pituitary hormones necessary for developing and releasing the mature ovum and for synthesizing estrogen and progesterone. Human chorionic somatomammotropin (option 3) is a placental hormone that acts similarly to the pituitary growth hormone. It produces a diabetogenic effect in pregnant women and isn't diagnostic of pregnancy.
Nursing process step: Assessment
Client needs category: Health promotion and maintenance
Client needs subcategory: None
Cognitive level: Knowledge

11. CORRECT ANSWER: 3
Chadwick's sign, a bluish discoloration of the vaginal vault, occurs from increased vascularity and would be evident by the time a client had missed two menstrual periods. Diastasis recti (option 1) occurs in late pregnancy. The glomerular filtration rate (option 2) increases by approximately 50% during the second trimester. Blood volume (option 4) peaks at 30% to 50% above normal during the second trimester.
Nursing process step: Assessment
Client needs category: Health promotion and maintenance
Client needs subcategory: None
Cognitive level: Knowledge

12. CORRECT ANSWER: 1
A nutritionally sound lunch includes two servings of a grain and one serving each of protein, fruit, vegetable, and milk or a milk product. The cheeseburger, salad, fruit, and milk contain sufficient protein, minerals, and vitamins to meet the pregnant client's nutritional needs. The other options are nutritionally inadequate. In addition, options 2 and 3 are high in sodium, which can cause fluid retention.
Nursing process step: Evaluation
Client needs category: Physiological integrity
Client needs subcategory: Basic care and comfort
Cognitive level: Application

13. CORRECT ANSWER: 4
Because moderate exercise is encouraged during pregnancy, the best approach is to assess the amount and type of exercise in which the client currently engages. The other options don't provide for assessment of the client's individual needs, nor do they explore possible client concerns.
Nursing process step: Planning
Client needs category: Health promotion and maintenance
Client needs subcategory: None
Cognitive level: Application

14. CORRECT ANSWER: 4
The client should be told to take ferrous sulfate between meals with orange juice. Food and antacids inhibit absorption of iron.
Nursing process step: Implementation
Client needs category: Physiological integrity
Client needs subcategory: Pharmacological and parenteral therapies
Cognitive level: Knowledge

15. Correct answer: 4
Hemoglobin level and hematocrit may decline slightly from hemodilution, resulting in the pseudoanemia of pregnancy. This is most noticeable during the second and third trimesters. In true anemia (option 1), caused by inadequate iron intake, hemoglobin level and hematocrit are lower than the values given. The client's laboratory values don't indicate preeclampsia (option 2). During pregnancy, the renal threshold decreases, allowing glucose to spill into the urine. Lactosuria also may occur as the breasts prepare for lactation. Thus, a small amount of glucose in a pregnant woman's urine isn't unusual and doesn't indicate diabetes (option 3), although it should be reported.
Nursing process step: Assessment
Client needs category: Health promotion and maintenance
Client needs subcategory: None
Cognitive level: Analysis

16. Correct answer: 4
Potential adverse reactions of antihypertensive agents include postural hypotension, impotence, nausea, vomiting, and nasal stuffiness. Of these, postural hypotension is the most hazardous because the client could fall and suffer a serious injury.
Nursing process step: Implementation
Client needs category: Physiological integrity
Client needs subcategory: Pharmacological and parenteral therapies
Cognitive level: Analysis

17. Correct answer: 1
Control of the head before the trunk and extremities is best described as cephalocaudal, or development from head to tail.
Nursing process step: Assessment
Client needs category: Health promotion and maintenance
Client needs subcategory: None
Cognitive level: Comprehension

18. Correct answer: 1
Glucocorticoid therapy will have caused the client's adrenal glands to have atrophied. If the client suddenly stops this therapy, acute adrenal insufficiency (Addison's crisis) may occur.
Nursing process step: Planning
Client needs category: Physiological integrity
Client needs subcategory: Pharmacological and parenteral therapies
Cognitive level: Application

19. Correct answer: 2
This response gives the client direction and support. Option 1 is incorrect because of the client's depression — the client doesn't care if it's a beautiful day. Saying "let's" (option 3) implies fusing between client and nurse. Option 4 offers no support.
Nursing process step: Implementation
Client needs category: Psychosocial integrity
Client needs subcategory: None
Cognitive level: Application

20. Correct answer: 1
A depressed client may find it difficult to do even the simplest things, such as combing his hair, and may need direction and support in performing these tasks. Options 2 and 3 ignore the fact that the client's personal grooming hasn't been performed. Option 4 is incorrect because the client may not notice that his shirt is unbuttoned; this offers no help with personal grooming needs.
Nursing process step: Implementation
Client needs category: Psychosocial integrity
Client needs subcategory: None
Cognitive level: Application

21. Correct answer: 1
Pressure stockings reduce the redness of the scar, soften the tissue, and decrease the vascularity of the involved tissue, thus improving its appearance. Physical therapy at home or at the hospital or clinic is needed until recovery is complete. The pressure garments are kept on as ordered by the physician. Contractures may occur until recovery is complete, up to 1 year postinjury.
Nursing process step: Evaluation
Client needs category: Safe, effective care environment
Client needs subcategory: Management of care
Cognitive level: Application

22. Correct answer: 2
By telling the client about the found pills and then asking about the client's intentions, the nurse provides for the client's safety needs and directly addresses the issue of suicide with the client. The other options only remove a source of danger; they don't directly address the issue of suicide.
Nursing process step: Implementation
Client needs category: Safe, effective care environment
Client needs subcategory: Safety and infection control
Cognitive level: Analysis

23. CORRECT ANSWER: 4
Weights on a traction apparatus should hang freely and unobstructed. Option 1 is incorrect because the head of the bed should be elevated no more than 30 degrees. Option 2 is incorrect because the affected heel should be raised off the bed. Option 3 is incorrect because the weights shouldn't be removed from traction.
Nursing process step: Planning
Client needs category: Physiological integrity
Client needs subcategory: Basic care and comfort
Cognitive level: Application

24. CORRECT ANSWER: 1
Increased urine output indicates greater cardiac output. The pulse rate decreases as digoxin slows the rate of conduction through the heart. Digoxin wouldn't significantly alter respirations or blood pressure.
Nursing process step: Evaluation
Client needs category: Physiological integrity
Client needs subcategory: Pharmacological and parenteral therapies
Cognitive level: Analysis

25. CORRECT ANSWER: 3
Because furosemide is a diuretic, the nurse should record the amount and characteristics of urine output. Furosemide doesn't affect magnesium levels or heart rate. Intention tremor is irrelevant to the client's condition.
Nursing process step: Planning
Client needs category: Physiological integrity
Client needs subcategory: Physiological adaptation
Cognitive level: Analysis

26. CORRECT ANSWER: 4
Anorexia and gastric irritation are early, and sometimes overlooked, signs of digoxin toxicity. A client who dislikes hospital food (option 1) would say so. Oxygen administration and Lasix therapy (options 2 and 3) don't cause anorexia.
Nursing process step: Analysis
Client needs category: Physiological integrity
Client needs subcategory: Pharmacological and parenteral therapies
Cognitive level: Application

27. CORRECT ANSWER: 1
A snack with intermediate-acting sugars (such as lactose in milk) ensures adequate blood glucose levels during the expected peak action of NPH insulin taken in the morning. Increasing the morning NPH insulin dosage (option 3) increases the risk for a hypoglycemic reaction. Options 2 and 4 discourage the mother from promoting a normal life for her diabetic child.
Nursing process step: Implementation
Client needs category: Physiological integrity
Client needs subcategory: Reduction of risk potential
Cognitive level: Analysis

28. CORRECT ANSWER: 4
A client who is receiving Diuril should be instructed to increase potassium intake because thiazide diuretics cause potassium and sodium excretion during diuresis. Dried fruits are the only high-potassium item among the options listed.
Nursing process step: Implementation
Client needs category: Physiological integrity
Client needs subcategory: Pharmacological and parenteral therapies
Cognitive level: Application

29. CORRECT ANSWER: 1
Removal of axillary lymph nodes places the postmastectomy client at increased risk for infection for the rest of her life. All mastectomy clients are taught to prevent injury, to avoid blood pressure checks and venipunctures on the arm on the side of surgery, and to seek prompt treatment if a problem results.
Nursing process step: Implementation
Client needs category: Physiological integrity
Client needs subcategory: Reduction of risk potential
Cognitive level: Comprehension

30. CORRECT ANSWER: 2
The primary goal should be to prevent bleeding. A platelet count below 50,000/µl indicates a severe platelet deficiency. The client is at great risk for bleeding and probably requires a platelet transfusion. The other laboratory values are only slightly below normal and don't place the client at great risk.
Nursing process step: Planning
Client needs category: Physiological integrity
Client needs subcategory: Reduction of risk potential
Cognitive level: Analysis

31. CORRECT ANSWER: 1
A positive reaction indicates a person has been exposed to tuberculosis in the past. Although this person may be at

increased risk for developing active tuberculosis, a positive skin test doesn't indicate active tuberculosis.
Nursing process step: Evaluation
Client needs category: Physiological integrity
Client needs subcategory: Physiological adaptation
Cognitive level: Application

32. CORRECT ANSWER: 4
Asking the client to discuss how she feels about her pregnancy enables the nurse to elicit more information and provides an opportunity to explore all possible alternatives before any decision is made. Options 1 and 2 evade the issue. Option 3 puts the nurse in charge; the client may feel coerced into making a decision to please the nurse.
Nursing process step: Implementation
Client needs category: Psychosocial integrity
Client needs subcategory: None
Cognitive level: Application

33. CORRECT ANSWER: 2
The best room for this client is a private room two doors away from the nurses' station. During the initial acute phase, he should be as close as possible to the nurses' station for maximum observation.
Nursing process step: Planning
Client needs category: Safe, effective care environment
Client needs subcategory: Safety and infection control
Cognitive level: Application

34. CORRECT ANSWER: 1
The child's developmental needs would best be met by having his mother stay with him overnight. At 15 months, he's at maximum risk for experiencing separation anxiety.
Nursing process step: Implementation
Client needs category: Health promotion and maintenance
Client needs subcategory: None
Cognitive level: Comprehension

35. CORRECT ANSWER: 3
His mother shows full understanding of discharge teaching when she repeats the specific signs to watch for. Pulling on the ears, refusing to lie down, and shaking the head back and forth are common signs of otitis in toddlers. If they occur, the child should be checked promptly by a physician. Option 1 expresses guilt. Option 2 only indicates understanding of the need for follow-up care. Option 4 doesn't indicate a realistic understanding of the condition.
Nursing process step: Evaluation
Client needs category: Health promotion and maintenance
Client needs subcategory: None
Cognitive level: Application

36. CORRECT ANSWER: 2
In conductive deafness, the acoustic nerve isn't damaged. Although air conduction of sound waves is impaired, bone conduction isn't. Otosclerosis can cause conductive deafness.
Nursing process step: Evaluation
Client needs category: Physiological integrity
Client needs subcategory: Physiological adaptation
Cognitive level: Comprehension

37. CORRECT ANSWER: 2
Nausea, vomiting, seeing halos around lights, and pain are signs and symptoms of increased intraocular pressure. The client's signs and symptoms don't suggest the other options.
Nursing process step: Assessment
Client needs category: Physiological integrity
Client needs subcategory: Physiological adaptation
Cognitive level: Comprehension

38. CORRECT ANSWER: 4
Stump elevation increases venous return and decreases edema. Abduction and external rotation should be avoided.
Nursing process step: Evaluation
Client needs category: Physiological integrity
Client needs subcategory: Physiological adaptation
Cognitive level: Application

39. CORRECT ANSWER: 1
Angioedema is a severe allergic reaction to iodine in the dye used during an IVP; it can cause edema of the larynx and difficulty in breathing. The other options are unlikely to arise as reactions to the dye.
Nursing process step: Implementation
Client needs category: Physiological integrity
Client needs subcategory: Reduction of risk potential
Cognitive level: Analysis

40. CORRECT ANSWER: 2
Straining during a bowel movement raises venous pressure and could cause rupture of the varices. Eating quickly (option 1) could irritate the varices; the client should eat slowly and chew foods well. Option 3 is incorrect because the client doesn't have ascites. Option 4 is incorrect be-

cause exercise isn't contraindicated unless the varices are bleeding.
Nursing process step: Implementation
Client needs category: Physiological integrity
Client needs subcategory: Reduction of risk potential
Cognitive level: Application

41. CORRECT ANSWER: 4
An elevated serum potassium level (hyperkalemia) is common in acute renal failure and puts the client at risk for cardiac arrhythmias. Option 1 results from a below-normal serum calcium level (hypocalcemia); although hypocalcemia may occur in acute renal failure, it doesn't cause signs or symptoms because the acidosis that occurs with renal failure keeps more calcium in an ionized form. Option 2 isn't a complication of acute renal failure because damaged renal tubules can't conserve sodium; therefore, sodium excretion increases, causing a normal or below-normal serum sodium level. Option 3 suggests shock, which hasn't been identified as a complication of acute renal failure.
Nursing process step: Assessment
Client needs category: Physiological integrity
Client needs subcategory: Reduction of risk potential
Cognitive level: Comprehension

42. CORRECT ANSWER: 3
To learn to cope with the phantom pain, the client first needs to understand the reasons for the pain. Telling the patient that he can't feel pain in an amputated limb is inaccurate. Phantom pain may last longer than 2 to 3 days. Telling the client that phantom pain is a common occurrence will not help him cope with the pain.
Nursing process step: Implementation
Client needs category: Physiological integrity
Client needs subcategory: Physiological adaptation
Cognitive level: Analysis

43. CORRECT ANSWER: 2
The most therapeutic response would be to focus the client's thoughts on the present. Option 1 diminishes the client's feelings by giving the impression that everyone feels this way. Option 3 refutes the client's feelings and calls attention to something the client currently doesn't believe. Option 4 doesn't address the client's present needs.
Nursing process step: Implementation
Client needs category: Psychosocial integrity
Client needs subcategory: None
Cognitive level: Application

44. CORRECT ANSWER: 3
Making a collage is easy and doesn't require great concentration. Options 1 and 2 call for the client to make a decision, and option 4 demands that he concentrate carefully, both of which would be difficult in his depressed state.
Nursing process step: Implementation
Client needs category: Psychosocial integrity
Client needs subcategory: None
Cognitive level: Comprehension

45. CORRECT ANSWER: 3
Using therapeutic communication encourages the client to discuss his feelings further. Options 1 and 2 minimize or ignore his feelings. Option 4 implies that he needs to work off his anger without talking about it.
Nursing process step: Implementation
Client needs category: Psychosocial integrity
Client needs subcategory: None
Cognitive level: Application

46. CORRECT ANSWER: 4
Confusion occurs when the brain is deprived of needed glucose, and diaphoresis results from the developing shocklike state. Air hunger, acetone breath, nausea, vomiting, and flushed skin are signs and symptoms of ketoacidosis.
Nursing process step: Assessment
Client needs category: Physiological integrity
Client needs subcategory: Physiological adaptation
Cognitive level: Comprehension

47. CORRECT ANSWER: 2
The nurse should administer an I.V. bolus of 50% glucose to a hospitalized client who's having a hypoglycemic reaction and can't swallow. Epinephrine, an adrenergic agent, would stimulate the pancreas to increase insulin in the blood, further decreasing the blood glucose level. Glucagon, a substance produced by the pancreas to increase the blood glucose level, could be administered I.M. but is usually in an outpatient setting, if the client can't swallow but remains conscious.
Nursing process step: Implementation
Client needs category: Physiological integrity
Client needs subcategory: Pharmacological and parenteral therapies
Cognitive level: Analysis

48. CORRECT ANSWER: 3
Diffuse abdominal pain occurs in peritonitis. Bowel sounds are absent in peritonitis. Pain radiating from the

flank may indicate pyelonephritis or kidney stones. Constipation, not diarrhea, also may occur in peritonitis.
Nursing process step: Assessment
Client needs category: Physiological integrity
Client needs subcategory: Physiological adaptation
Cognitive level: Comprehension

49. CORRECT ANSWER: 1
Turning the client will aid suctioning. For the NG tube to be effective, the blue opening should remain open and clear of solution or secretions. Drainage is measured every 8 hours. Increasing the suction control to high may cause gastric mucosal damage.
Nursing process step: Planning
Client needs category: Physiological integrity
Client needs subcategory: Basic care and comfort
Cognitive level: Application

50. CORRECT ANSWER: 3
Coughing, choking, cyanosis, and drooling are classic signs of tracheoesophageal fistula. Passing of meconium stool is normal in the neonate. Tracheoesophageal fistula doesn't cause bile-stained vomitus. In the most common type of tracheoesophageal fistula, the distal esophagus is attached to the trachea and can't receive food or fluid; therefore, vomiting shouldn't occur.
Nursing process step: Assessment
Client needs category: Physiological integrity
Client needs subcategory: Physiological adaptation
Cognitive level: Comprehension

51. CORRECT ANSWER: 3
After the gastrostomy tube feeding, the nurse should elevate the tube and leave it unplugged to allow reflux of stomach contents through the tube instead of through the newly repaired esophagus. Before feeding, placement of the gastrostomy tube should be checked by aspirating stomach contents with a syringe and measuring pH, not injecting air through the tube and listening over the stomach with a stethoscope. The gastrostomy tube is kept in place in the stomach with an inflated bulb at the end of the catheter. The neonate should be placed on his right side, with the head of the bed slightly elevated, to provide for gravity drainage. The gastrostomy tube shouldn't be plugged after feeding because gastric reflux may occur over the fresh operative site or be aspirated.
Nursing process step: Implementation
Client needs category: Physiological integrity
Client needs subcategory: Reduction of risk potential
Cognitive level: Application

52. CORRECT ANSWER: 1
The RBC count increases to help carry hemoglobin to offset chronic hypoxia, which is common in clients with COPD. Platelet count and serum cholesterol levels aren't affected by COPD. Pao_2 levels are usually decreased and $Paco_2$ levels are increased.
Nursing process step: Assessment
Client needs category: Physiological integrity
Client needs subcategory: Physiological adaptation
Cognitive level: Comprehension

53. CORRECT ANSWER: 1
Of all traction types, skin traction is the easiest to apply because no pins are inserted into bones. Specially prepared nurses can apply skin traction but not skeletal traction. Both types of traction can cause complications and prevent rotation of the extremity. Skeletal traction is usually maintained for longer periods.
Nursing process step: Implementation
Client needs category: Physiological integrity
Client needs subcategory: Reduction of risk potential
Cognitive level: Comprehension

54. CORRECT ANSWER: 3
Common GI adverse reactions of ibuprofen include anorexia, nausea, and diarrhea. Ibuprofen should be taken with milk or meals to reduce adverse GI reactions. Ibuprofen will not increase appetite, it may decrease it. Ibuprofen relieves inflammation and swelling; it doesn't cause it.
Nursing process step: Evaluation
Client needs category: Physiological integrity
Client needs subcategory: Pharmacological and parenteral therapies
Cognitive level: Comprehension

55. CORRECT ANSWER: 4
The behavior that most strongly suggests child abuse is that the child doesn't cry when being moved. A victim of child abuse typically doesn't complain of pain, even with obvious injuries, for fear of further displeasing the abuser.
Nursing process step: Assessment
Client needs category: Psychosocial integrity
Client needs subcategory: None
Cognitive level: Comprehension

56. CORRECT ANSWER: 3
Nutritious snacks should be provided. Instead of soft foods, such as puddings or soups, finger foods should be provided to promote independence. Enteral feeding would be inappropriate at this time. At age 2, the child is capable of drinking from a cup and should be encouraged to do so. Toddlers left with bottles in their cribs may develop nursing bottle syndrome.
Nursing process step: Planning
Client needs category: Health promotion and maintenance
Client needs subcategory: None
Cognitive level: Comprehension

57. CORRECT ANSWER: 4
The nurse working with abusive families needs to understand that abusive parents should be encouraged to visit their child and should be welcomed to the unit by the staff. Many abusive parents love their children but lack effective parenting skills. During the child's hospitalization, the staff has the opportunity to model appropriate parenting behaviors for the parents.
Nursing process step: Planning
Client needs category: Health promotion and maintenance
Client needs subcategory: None
Cognitive level: Analysis

58. CORRECT ANSWER: 4
According to the recommended schedule of immunizations from the American Academy of Pediatrics, the same immunizations are given up to age 6.
Nursing process step: Planning
Client needs category: Health promotion and maintenance
Client needs subcategory: None
Cognitive level: Knowledge

59. CORRECT ANSWER: 1
Loss of sweating occurs below the level of the cord lesion. Spinal shock also causes urine retention, a marked reduction in blood pressure, and motor paralysis.
Nursing process step: Assessment
Client needs category: Physiological integrity
Client needs subcategory: Physiological adaptation
Cognitive level: Comprehension

60. CORRECT ANSWER: 4
Autonomic dysreflexia can be caused by a full bowel or bladder or by a urinary infection. Removing the cause of the dysreflexia will relieve symptoms.
Nursing process step: Implementation
Client needs category: Physiological integrity
Client needs subcategory: Physiological adaptation
Cognitive level: Analysis

61. CORRECT ANSWER: 3
The child will require physical therapy and rehabilitation to ensure continued recovery and mobility. Although the other options may be needed, option 3 is the best answer.
Nursing process step: Planning
Client needs category: Safe, effective care environment
Client needs subcategory: Management of care
Cognitive level: Comprehension

62. CORRECT ANSWER: 4
Isolation protocols are used in the hospital setting to contain an organism to one area and reduce the spread of infection to others. Clients may ambulate while on isolation protocols, but they are required to follow the precautions specified by the specific type of isolation in effect. Isolation protocols may not prevent an infection from becoming endemic, nor will they maintain a sterile environment.
Nursing process step: Implementation
Client needs category: Safe, effective care environment
Client needs subcategory: Safety and infection control
Cognitive level: Application

63. CORRECT ANSWER: 4
To determine whether the stone has been passed, the urine must be strained and the stone must be collected to confirm that it has been passed. Checking specific gravity, collecting a 24-hour urine sample, or measuring urine output won't confirm that the stone has been passed.
Nursing process step: Planning
Client needs category: Safe, effective care environment
Client needs subcategory: Management of care
Cognitive level: Knowledge

64. CORRECT ANSWER: 3
The Patient's Bill of Rights is a document developed by the AHA. Informed consent, legal competence, and right to know are all addressed in the Patient's Bill of Rights.
Nursing process step: Implementation
Client needs category: Safe, effective care environment
Client needs subcategory: Management of care
Cognitive level: Knowledge

65. CORRECT ANSWER: 4
When nausea occurs most frequently in the morning, the nurse should suggest that the client eat dry crackers or toast before arising. Nausea and vomiting typically cease by the fourth missed menstrual period or earlier. Restricting fluid intake, drinking a glass of juice, or eating a high-protein snack won't decrease the episodes of nausea and vomiting.
Nursing process step: Planning
Client needs category: Physiological integrity
Client needs subcategory: Basic care and comfort
Cognitive level: Analysis

66. CORRECT ANSWER: 4
Care for the client with gestational diabetes would include an assessment of her blood glucose level. The urine is tested for protein in the client with preeclampsia. Because the client is at 38 weeks' gestation, measuring her fundal height isn't necessary. The fetus of the client with gestational diabetes tends to be larger than the average fetus. Oral hypoglycemics are contraindicated during pregnancy because they may cause adverse effects to the fetus; clients with gestational diabetes are maintained on insulin during the pregnancy.
Nursing process step: Implementation
Client needs category: Safe, effective care environment
Client needs subcategory: Safety and infection control
Cognitive level: Application

67. CORRECT ANSWER: 4
The authoritarian leader retains all authority and responsibility and is concerned primarily with completing tasks and accomplishing goals. The democratic leader is people-centered, allows greater individual participation in decision making, and maintains open communication. The permissive and the laissez-faire leaders deny responsibility and abdicate authority to the group.
Nursing process step: Assessment
Client needs category: Safe, effective care environment
Client needs subcategory: Management of care
Cognitive level: Knowledge

68. CORRECT ANSWER: 2
In an infant, the eustachian tube is relatively short, wide, and horizontal, promoting drainage of secretions from the nasopharynx into the middle ear. If the infant takes a bottle to bed and drinks while lying down, fluids may pool in the pharyngeal cavity, increasing the risk of otitis media. Cerumen in the external ear canal doesn't promote the development of otitis media. However, during shampooing, water may become trapped in the external ear canal by large amounts of cerumen, possibly causing otitis externa. Persistent fluid in the middle ear may impair language development and hearing; however, a 10-month-old infant isn't expected to combine two words when speaking.
Nursing process step: Assessment
Client needs category: Health promotion and maintenance
Client needs subcategory: None
Cognitive level: Analysis

69. CORRECT ANSWER: 1
After surgery to repair a cleft lip, the primary goal of nursing care is to maintain integrity of the operative site. Crying causes tension on the suture line, so comforting the infant as quickly as possible is the highest nursing priority. Parents may help by cuddling and comforting the infant. The prone position is contraindicated after surgery because rubbing on the sheet may disturb the suture line. Elbow restraints may cause agitation; if used to prevent the infant from disturbing the suture line, they must be removed, one at a time, every 2 to 4 hours so that the infant can exercise and the nurse can assess for skin irritation. Crusts forming on the suture line contribute to scarring and must be cleaned carefully.
Nursing process step: Planning
Client needs category: Physiological integrity
Client needs subcategory: Reduction of risk potential
Cognitive level: Application

70. CORRECT ANSWER: 3
Bladder spasms are the usual type of postoperative discomfort of a transurethral prostatic resection because of instrumentation and the presence of a large-sized indwelling urinary catheter. Other types of pain aren't usually experienced after this type of surgery.
Nursing process step: Implementation
Client needs category: Physiological integrity
Client needs subcategory: Basic care and comfort
Cognitive level: Knowledge

71. CORRECT ANSWER: 1
Eating green leafy vegetables, fortified and whole grains, and organ and red meats and using cast iron cookware will increase dietary intake of iron. Fish and white rice are suggested for a low-residue diet. Dairy products and sardines add calcium to the diet. Eggs and cheese are dietary sources of vitamin B_{12}.

Nursing process step: Implementation
Client needs category: Physiological integrity
Client needs subcategory: Basic care and comfort
Cognitive level: Knowledge

72. CORRECT ANSWER: 2
Cardiac arrhythmias cause roughly 40% to 50% of deaths after MI. Heart failure accounts for 33% and cardiogenic shock for 9% of post-MI deaths. Pulmonary embolism, another potential complication of an MI, is less common.
Nursing process step: Planning
Client needs category: Physiological integrity
Client needs subcategory: Physiological adaptation
Cognitive level: Knowledge

73. CORRECT ANSWER: 4
The client has been infected with the human immunodeficiency virus (HIV) and as a compensatory mechanism, the body has produced antibodies. The client may not have AIDS, the client isn't immune to HIV, and the client can transmit the virus to others.
Nursing process step: Implementation
Client needs category: Health promotion and maintenance
Client needs subcategory: None
Cognitive level: Application

74. CORRECT ANSWER: 10
A teaspoon is equivalent to 5 ml; therefore, 2 tsp is equivalent to 10 ml. The nurse should adminiser 10 ml of the drug.
Nursing process step: Planning
Client needs category: Physiological integrity
Client needs subcategory: Pharmacological and parenteral therapies
Cognitive level: Application

75. CORRECT ANSWER: 2, 5
Exophthalmos is characterized by protruding eyes and a fixed stare is a characteristic finding in Grave's disease. Other findings include: weight loss despite increased appetite, nervousness, heat intolerance, diarrhea, palpitations, and tremors. Dry, waxy swelling and abnormal mucin deposits in the skin typify myxedema, a condition resulting from advanced hypothyroidism. A wide, staggering gait and a differential between the apical and radial pulse rates aren't specific signs of thyroid dysfunction.
Nursing process step: Assessment
Client needs category: Physiological integrity
Client needs subcategory: Reduction of risk potential
Cognitive level: Application

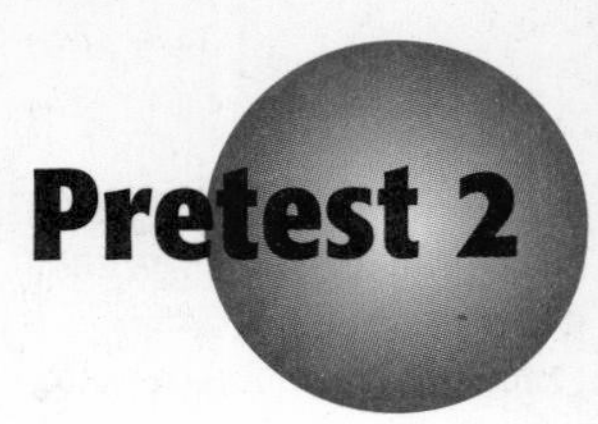

Pretest 2

Questions

1. On the first postoperative day of a traditional cholecystectomy, a client complains of pain 1 hour after receiving meperidine (Demerol) 75 mg I.M. A nurse notes that the client's position hasn't been changed for 2 hours. Which statement would be most appropriate for the nurse to make while turning the client?

☐ **1.** "I can't imagine why the pain medicine didn't work. I'll call the physician as soon as I leave here."
☐ **2.** "Let's turn you onto your other side. Maybe that will help."
☐ **3.** "This change in position will make you more comfortable and help the medication relieve your pain."
☐ **4.** "The physician should be here in 30 minutes. I'll have him check on you then."

2. A postpartum client observes a nurse in the nursery perform a neonatal examination on her daughter. Later, the nurse sees the client, who is bottle-feeding, hold the neonate closely and talk to her quietly as she feeds her. Which action would be the nurse's best response to the client's behavior?

☐ **1.** Show her how to burp the neonate.
☐ **2.** Provide her with positive support.
☐ **3.** Ask if she's starting to have feelings for the neonate.
☐ **4.** Show her how to stimulate the neonate's sucking reflex.

3. A paranoid client refuses to eat with the other clients. A nurse finds him circling a table and staring intently at one client. Which action by the nurse would be most appropriate?

☐ **1.** Call the client by name and suggest he accompany the nurse to another area of the unit.
☐ **2.** Alert other staff members and ask the client to go with the nurse to another area of the unit.
☐ **3.** Sit down at the table and invite the client to sit at the table with the nurse.
☐ **4.** Quickly leave the room to get more help.

4. A client is scheduled for excretory urography. In preparation for this test, a nurse should assess the client for an allergy to:

☐ **1.** milk and cheese.
☐ **2.** seafood and iodine.
☐ **3.** wheat glutens and eggs.
☐ **4.** molds and antibiotics.

5. An infant, age 7 months, is admitted to the hospital with diarrhea and hyponatremic dehydration. His mother tells a nurse she can't afford to buy infant formula and has been feeding him only water by bottle for the past 2 days. When monitoring the infant's hydration status, the nurse should assess and document all of the following at regular intervals. Which one is most important?

☐ **1.** Body weight
☐ **2.** Intake and output
☐ **3.** Urine specific gravity
☐ **4.** Anterior fontanel status

6. An elderly client with Alzheimer's disease has been living with his adult son's family for the past 6 months. He wanders at night and needs help with activities of daily living (ADLs). Which statement by his son suggests that the family is successfully adjusting to this living arrangement?

- ☐ **1.** "It's difficult dealing with Dad. It's a thankless job."
- ☐ **2.** "We had no idea this would be so difficult. It's our cross to bear."
- ☐ **3.** "Dad really seems to be making progress. We're hoping he'll be able to move back into his house soon."
- ☐ **4.** "Dad has presented many challenges. We have alarms on all the outside doors now. Respite care gives us a break."

7. A client is admitted to the emergency department after being sexually assaulted. She's accompanied by a policewoman. The nurse realizes that several important tasks should be done in sexual assault cases. Which nursing intervention should receive first priority?

- ☐ **1.** Assisting with medical treatment
- ☐ **2.** Collecting and preparing evidence for the police
- ☐ **3.** Attempting to reduce the client's anxiety from panic to a moderate level
- ☐ **4.** Providing anticipatory guidance to the client about normal responses to sexual assault

8. A client who is 30 weeks pregnant has a corrected atrial septal defect and minor functional limitations. Which pregnancy-related physiological change places her at greatest risk for more severe cardiac problems?

- ☐ **1.** Decreased heart rate
- ☐ **2.** Increased plasma volume
- ☐ **3.** Decreased cardiac output
- ☐ **4.** Increased blood pressure

9. Which strategy can help make a nurse a more effective teacher?

- ☐ **1.** Including the client in discussions
- ☐ **2.** Using technical terms
- ☐ **3.** Providing detailed explanations
- ☐ **4.** Using loosely structured teaching sessions

10. After a third arrest for abusing a neighbor's cat, a client is admitted to the psychiatric unit for treatment of antisocial personality disorder. Which action is most appropriate for a nurse assigned to the client?

- ☐ **1.** Examining personal feelings toward the client
- ☐ **2.** Encouraging the client to use problem-solving techniques
- ☐ **3.** Insisting the client obey all unit rules and attend all unit activities
- ☐ **4.** Administering antianxiety medication as prescribed

11. A healthy 6-month-old infant is brought to the well-baby clinic for a check-up. When assessing the infant's anterior fontanel the nurse expects it to be:

- ☐ **1.** open.
- ☐ **2.** sunken.
- ☐ **3.** closed.
- ☐ **4.** bulging.

12. A client admitted to the emergency department states that she fell down a flight of stairs. On initial physical assessment, a nurse finds cuts and bruises on her face, neck, and forearms. X-rays reveal a spiral fracture of the right arm. The client seems severely anxious and upset. After her physical needs are met, what's the most important intervention for the nurse to take?

- ☐ **1.** Gather more information about her emotional state from family members.
- ☐ **2.** Take steps to reduce her level of anxiety.
- ☐ **3.** Initiate health care teaching about at-home care of her injuries and cast.
- ☐ **4.** Have the client explain again how she got hurt.

13. A client is in the 1st trimester of pregnancy. During her visit to the physician's office today, a nurse is to instruct her concerning nutritional needs during pregnancy. Which objective is most important to accomplish during this initial interview?

- ☐ **1.** Planning a 1-week menu with the client
- ☐ **2.** Obtaining a diet history from the client
- ☐ **3.** Providing a list of nutrient requirements
- ☐ **4.** Emphasizing the importance of a balanced diet

14. A client who is breast-feeding her neonate is to be discharged from the postpartum unit. The client has been found to have no immunity to rubella and has orders to receive rubella vaccine on the day of discharge. What's the most important instruction for a nurse to include in the discharge plan?

- ☐ **1.** Practice contraception and avoid conception for at least 3 months.
- ☐ **2.** Discontinue breast-feeding to prevent the infant from becoming infected with the rubella virus.
- ☐ **3.** Avoid contact with women who are pregnant or who suspect they may be pregnant for at least 2 months.
- ☐ **4.** Have the infant screened for active rubella virus every 2 weeks for at least 2 months.

15. A child with acute asthma is to receive aminophylline. Immediately before and during administration of this drug, which nursing assessment is most important?
- ☐ **1.** Pupil size
- ☐ **2.** Temperature
- ☐ **3.** Apical pulse
- ☐ **4.** Bilateral breath sounds

16. Which position would be best for a client showing signs of shock?
- ☐ **1.** Semi-Fowler's
- ☐ **2.** High Fowler's
- ☐ **3.** Trendelenburg's
- ☐ **4.** Modified Trendelenburg's

17. Which instruction should a nurse give a client who is going to have a chest tube removed?
- ☐ **1.** "Hyperventilate just before the tube is removed."
- ☐ **2.** "Inhale as the tube is being pulled out."
- ☐ **3.** "Take a deep breath and hold it."
- ☐ **4.** "Avoid the Valsalva maneuver."

18. What's the best position for a child, age 5, who is 2 hours postoperative of a tonsillectomy?
- ☐ **1.** On his back, with his head turned to the side
- ☐ **2.** On either side, with his neck extended
- ☐ **3.** In semi-Fowler position, with his neck hyperextended
- ☐ **4.** On his abdomen, in low Fowler position

19. A client with heart palpitations and dizziness is referred by his family physician for outpatient mental health counseling. As counseling progresses, the nurse senses that the client has ambivalent feelings about his recent promotion to a high-level management position. How can the nurse best promote the client's ability to examine these feelings?
- ☐ **1.** Tell him it's normal for a person to experience upheaval when changing positions.
- ☐ **2.** Ask him why he's upset about such an important promotion.
- ☐ **3.** Have him describe in detail his old position and his new position.
- ☐ **4.** Share with him the experiences others have had when they changed positions.

20. To aid respirations, a nurse should place a preterm neonate in which position?
- ☐ **1.** Prone
- ☐ **2.** Supine
- ☐ **3.** Head slightly elevated
- ☐ **4.** Head slightly lowered

21. A client has a Sengstaken-Blakemore tube in place to treat esophageal varices. Which action is most appropriate to include in the client's care plan?
- ☐ **1.** Offer the client sips of water to swallow every 2 hours.
- ☐ **2.** Deflate the gastric balloon to prevent an upset stomach.
- ☐ **3.** Check pressure in the balloons by deflating and reinflating them every 4 hours.
- ☐ **4.** Observe for restlessness and increased respirations.

22. A client's labor doesn't progress. After ruling out cephalopelvic disproportion, the physician orders I.V. administration of 1,000 ml normal saline solution with 10 units of Pitocin to run at 2 milliunits/minute. Two milliunits/minute is equivalent to how many ml/minute?
- ☐ **1.** 0.002
- ☐ **2.** 0.02
- ☐ **3.** 0.2
- ☐ **4.** 2

23. Which foods would be best for a postoperative tonsillectomy client?
- ☐ **1.** Toast, jelly, and ice cream
- ☐ **2.** Clear soup, apple juice, and gelatin
- ☐ **3.** Creamed tuna fish, root beer, and cake
- ☐ **4.** Hot tea, wiener and roll, and sherbet

24. A client is admitted to the hospital with acute urinary retention caused by benign prostatic hyperplasia. A Foley catheter is inserted. After 750 ml of urine are drained, the catheter is clamped because rapid bladder decompression can cause which condition?
- ☐ **1.** Dysuria
- ☐ **2.** Hematuria
- ☐ **3.** Oliguria
- ☐ **4.** Albuminuria

25. Which activity would best meet the diversional needs of a client who is markedly impaired with Alzheimer's disease?

- ☐ **1.** Playing a simple card game
- ☐ **2.** Working with play dough
- ☐ **3.** Singing familiar songs
- ☐ **4.** Putting a puzzle together

26. Within 48 hours after being admitted to the hospital for acute gastritis, a client seems agitated and states that he can feel bugs crawling on his body. A nurse should suspect that the client most likely is:

- ☐ **1.** having an acute episode of schizophrenia.
- ☐ **2.** in the beginning stages of alcohol withdrawal delirium.
- ☐ **3.** reacting to ingestion of an hallucinogenic substance.
- ☐ **4.** entering a preconvulsive state.

27. A client has been receiving oxytocin (Pitocin) to aid her labor progress. A nurse notes that a contraction has remained strong for more than 90 seconds. Which action should the nurse take first?

- ☐ **1.** Stop the Pitocin.
- ☐ **2.** Notify the physician.
- ☐ **3.** Monitor fetal heart tones.
- ☐ **4.** Turn the client onto her left side.

28. A 2-year-old child, diagnosed with cystic fibrosis as an infant, is admitted to the hospital with pneumonia. He's placed in a high-humidity tent with oxygen and receives aerosol treatments followed by percussion and postural drainage four times daily. Which nursing diagnosis takes priority in planning this child's care?

- ☐ **1.** Imbalanced nutrition: Less than body requirements
- ☐ **2.** Impaired urinary elimination
- ☐ **3.** Risk for injury
- ☐ **4.** Ineffective airway clearance

29. A client who had cataract surgery in the morning is to be discharged that afternoon. Which statement would indicate that the client understands instructions about wearing the eye shield?

- ☐ **1.** "I don't need to wear the eye shield after I'm discharged."
- ☐ **2.** "I'll wear the eye shield day and night for 3 weeks."
- ☐ **3.** "I'll wear the eye shield at night for 1 month."
- ☐ **4.** "I can stop wearing the eye shield after 2 weeks."

30. When caring for a client with glaucoma who's scheduled for eye surgery, it's imperative that the nurse:

- ☐ **1.** not administer acetazolamide (Diamox) before the surgery.
- ☐ **2.** stay alert for any mydriatic medications ordered for the client.
- ☐ **3.** give preoperatively ordered meperidine and atropine on time.
- ☐ **4.** instill cycloplegic eye drops every 15 minutes for 1 hour.

31. A new mother is interested in seeing what her neonate's eyes look like. Which is the most effective way for a nurse to stimulate the neonate to open his eyes?

- ☐ **1.** Gently separate the neonate's eyelids with the fingers.
- ☐ **2.** Stimulate the Moro reflex.
- ☐ **3.** Hold the neonate in an upright position.
- ☐ **4.** Shine a penlight toward the neonate's face.

32. When caring for a client who has just undergone a transsphenoidal hypophysectomy, a nurse must stay most alert for:

- ☐ **1.** respiratory depression.
- ☐ **2.** gastric distention.
- ☐ **3.** cardiac arrhythmias.
- ☐ **4.** excessive urine output.

33. After a car accident, a client exhibits signs of a head injury and is admitted to the hospital for observation. A nurse sees the client take several Percodan tablets he brought from home. Which action by the nurse indicates understanding of the potential adverse reactions to Percodan for this client?

- ☐ **1.** Notifying the client's physician
- ☐ **2.** Raising the side rails of the client's bed
- ☐ **3.** Turning off the client's television and room lights
- ☐ **4.** Monitoring the client's blood pressure every 2 hours

34. A preterm neonate is diagnosed with respiratory distress syndrome. Which pathophysiological problem is most clearly associated with respiratory distress syndrome?

- ☐ **1.** Hypocalcemia
- ☐ **2.** Hypoglycemia
- ☐ **3.** Inadequate synthesis of lecithin
- ☐ **4.** Inadequate storage of glycogen and fat

35. An Rh-negative client delivers her second child at 40 weeks' gestation. She had a rising antibody titer during pregnancy and her Coombs' test result was positive. Her neonate son, of average weight for gestational age, is admitted to the neonate nursery for initial care. Sixteen hours after his birth, the nurse receives the following laboratory report: serum bilirubin, 10 mg/100 ml; Coombs' test of cord blood is positive. Based on the these laboratory values for the neonate, which action should the nurse take first?

☐ **1.** Assess him for signs of hypoglycemia.
☐ **2.** Increase his fluid intake.
☐ **3.** Place him under the bilirubin lights.
☐ **4.** Notify his physician.

36. Which activity would be most appropriate for a client who's in a manic state?

☐ **1.** Tearing rags to make a rug
☐ **2.** Playing a table game
☐ **3.** Doing vigorous aerobic dancing
☐ **4.** Reading light, entertaining stories

37. A client is scheduled for a routine gynecologic examination by her private physician. Which action would be appropriate for a nurse who's assisting with the pelvic examination?

☐ **1.** Staying with the client throughout the examination
☐ **2.** Instructing the client in shallow breathing to aid relaxation
☐ **3.** Reminding the client that, should she feel embarrassed, many women have the same experience
☐ **4.** Leaving the room after draping the client to ensure her privacy

38. A client is receiving external beam radiation on an outpatient basis. A nurse instructs him in the care of his skin within the port marks. Which response by the client would indicate that he understands the instructions?

☐ **1.** "I'll wash the area every day with soap and water."
☐ **2.** "I can use a little talcum powder to help soothe my skin."
☐ **3.** "I can use A & D ointment if my skin becomes dry."
☐ **4.** "I'll be sure to wash between the marks."

39. When caring for a pregnant client with a lactose intolerance, a nurse should pay special attention to the client's need for:

☐ **1.** iron.
☐ **2.** calcium.
☐ **3.** folic acid.
☐ **4.** carbohydrates.

40. In a neonate, which sign indicates developing hydrocephalus?

☐ **1.** A pulsating anterior fontanel
☐ **2.** Closure of the suture lines in the skull
☐ **3.** Orthopneic positioning
☐ **4.** "Setting sun" sign

41. A client is to be discharged after a total hip replacement. Which statement indicates that the client understands the discharge instructions?

☐ **1.** "I have to do special exercises several times per day."
☐ **2.** "I should take frequent rides in the car to increase my activity."
☐ **3.** "I should wear loose clothes so my hip movements aren't restricted."
☐ **4.** "I should walk at least 2 miles per day."

42. A pregnant client is being coached by her husband during early labor. She complains of discomfort during contractions. To help his wife cope with the discomfort, which technique should the husband suggest?

☐ **1.** Normal breathing
☐ **2.** Slow chest breathing
☐ **3.** Accelerated breathing
☐ **4.** Pant-blow breathing

43. A client with second-degree burns covering 40% of her body has a nursing diagnosis of *Imbalanced nutrition: Less than body requirements related to large burn area and pain.* She enjoys all of the following foods. Which foods would be the best choices to help her regain nutritional balance?

☐ **1.** Steak and french fries
☐ **2.** Peanut butter and raisins
☐ **3.** Orange juice and carrots
☐ **4.** Corn and milk

44. A client who has been struck by a car is being observed in the hospital for signs of injury. Present orders read:

- Vital signs q1h
- NPO for 24 hours
- Nasal O_2 at 2 L/minute p.r.n.
- Foley catheter to straight drainage, if needed
- 5% dextrose in 0.45% saline solution at 100 ml/hour
- Call physician for any signs of shock or increased intracranial pressure.

A nurse determines that the client is showing early signs of shock. Which action should the nurse take first?

☐ **1.** Call the physician.
☐ **2.** Start nasal oxygen.
☐ **3.** Increase the intravenous rate.
☐ **4.** Insert the Foley catheter.

45. A pediatric client is to be discharged after recovering from an acute asthmatic attack. A nurse plans to teach the child and his family all of the following methods involved in managing the asthmatic client. Which one should the nurse emphasize?

☐ **1.** Activity limitations
☐ **2.** Dietary restrictions
☐ **3.** Postural drainage
☐ **4.** Breathing exercises

46. A primigravida client is admitted to the maternity unit at 4 a.m. Five hours later, a summary report of her progress reads:

Time	Dilated	Effaced	Station	Membranes
4 a.m.	3 cm	60%	-1	Intact
6 a.m.	5 to 6 cm	80%	0	Ruptured
8 a.m.	6 cm	80%	0	Ruptured
9 a.m.	6 cm	80%	0	Ruptured

At the same times as listed above, her contractions were:

Time	Severity	Interval	Duration
4 a.m.	Moderate	q 4 to 5 minutes	30 seconds
6 a.m.	Moderate	q 4 minutes	45 seconds
8 a.m.	Moderate	q 5 to 8 minutes	35 seconds
9 a.m.	Mild	q 10 minutes	20 seconds

This assessment data indicate dystocia. Which term best describes the type of contraction pattern?

☐ **1.** Atonic
☐ **2.** Dystonic
☐ **3.** Hypotonic
☐ **4.** Hypertonic

47. A client with increased intracranial pressure is receiving mannitol. To evaluate the effectiveness of this drug, a nurse should assess the client for which sign?

☐ **1.** Decreased pulse rate
☐ **2.** Increased temperature
☐ **3.** Increased urine output
☐ **4.** Increased pupillary reaction

48. A depressed and withdrawn client approaches a nurse, who is busy working with a social worker in the conference room. Which would be the best response by the nurse?

☐ **1.** Tell the client that the nurse will see him in 10 minutes.
☐ **2.** Tell the client he'll have to wait until the nurse and social worker are finished.
☐ **3.** Ask the client if what he wants is urgent.
☐ **4.** Ask the client how the nurse can help him.

49. When administering oxytocin (Pitocin), a nurse should observe for which potential adverse reaction?

☐ **1.** Decreased pulse rate
☐ **2.** Elevated blood pressure
☐ **3.** Generalized rash
☐ **4.** Increased urine output

50. Which sign would alert a nurse to possible hemorrhage in a client immediately after a tonsillectomy?

☐ **1.** Mouth breathing
☐ **2.** Stertorous respirations
☐ **3.** Frequent swallowing
☐ **4.** Dark brown emesis

51. The primary cause of abdominal ascites in a client with cirrhosis of the liver is:

☐ **1.** an increased vasopressin level.
☐ **2.** an increased serum sodium level.
☐ **3.** a decreased serum aldosterone level.
☐ **4.** a decreased serum albumin level.

52. A client delivers a child spontaneously after oxytocin (Pitocin) induction. One minute after the birth, a nurse makes these observations of the neonate:
- pulse above 100 beats/minute
- respiratory effort good
- active motion
- body pink, extremities blue.

Which Apgar score should the neonate receive?

☐ **1.** 4
☐ **2.** 6
☐ **3.** 8
☐ **4.** 10

53. A child, age 4, is admitted to the hospital with acute myelogenous leukemia. He has many bruises and petechiae over his legs and arms. Which nursing measure would best prevent additional bruising?

☐ **1.** Brushing his teeth only once per day
☐ **2.** Trimming his nails short
☐ **3.** Handling him with the palms of the hands
☐ **4.** Placing him in a caged crib with padded rails

54. During admission to the pediatric unit, a 2-year-old child clings to his blanket from home. This behavior is an example of:

☐ **1.** ritualism.
☐ **2.** negativism.
☐ **3.** dawdling.
☐ **4.** regression.

55. A client is 1 day postoperative of a transurethral resection. The client also has chronic glaucoma. Postoperative orders read:
- Maintain continuous bladder irrigation at 100 ml/hour.
- Administer belladonna and opium suppositories q4h p.r.n.
- Administer pilocarpine eye drops 1% q6h in each eye.

The client develops painful bladder spasms. Which action would be most appropriate for a nurse to take?

☐ **1.** Call the physician and question the orders.
☐ **2.** Administer the belladonna and opium suppositories.
☐ **3.** Suggest that the client try to void around the catheter.
☐ **4.** Decrease the flow rate of the continuous bladder irrigation.

56. A farmer with Alzheimer's disease is admitted to the gerontology unit. His wife asks a nurse what she should do when her husband doesn't recognize her. What would be the nurse's best response?

☐ **1.** Read books to him dealing with farm activities.
☐ **2.** Tell him who she is and then walk with him on the unit.
☐ **3.** Bring family pictures with her when she visits.
☐ **4.** Show him her wedding ring and remind him she's his wife.

57. When caring for a client with bulimia, the best way for a nurse to determine if the client has stopped purging after meals is to:

☐ **1.** observe what she does after every meal.
☐ **2.** monitor her electrolyte laboratory values.
☐ **3.** weigh her before and 2 hours after each meal.
☐ **4.** not allow her to leave the unit right after meals.

58. A client who's receiving a phenothiazine medication has become restless and fidgety and has paced the hallway continuously for the past hour. This behavior suggests that the client may be experiencing:

☐ **1.** dystonia.
☐ **2.** akathisia.
☐ **3.** parkinsonian effects.
☐ **4.** tardive dyskinesia.

59. A girl, age 12, has scoliosis with a curve greater than 40 degrees. She's admitted for treatment with halo-pelvic traction, to be followed by surgical insertion of a Harrington rod. Given her age and condition, which activity would be most appropriate for her to select during her hospitalization?

☐ **1.** Playing Monopoly with a child her age
☐ **2.** Doing crossword puzzles
☐ **3.** Reading a novel such as *Little Women*
☐ **4.** Playing a card game such as Old Maid

60. A neonate has just been admitted to the nursery. Nursing assessment reveals all of the following findings. Which finding should the nurse consider a deviation from normal?

☐ **1.** Visible jaundice
☐ **2.** Cyanosis of the hands and feet
☐ **3.** Mongolian spots on the buttocks
☐ **4.** Respiratory rate of 42 breaths/minute

61. One month after undergoing a subtotal gastrectomy, a client complains of dizziness, sweating, and tachycardia occurring within 30 minutes after eating. These signs and symptoms most likely result from:

☐ **1.** pernicious anemia.
☐ **2.** pyloric stenosis.
☐ **3.** dumping syndrome.
☐ **4.** a recurring ulcer.

62. During a screening of first graders for the presence of sickle cell disease, a 6-year-old girl is found to be positive. Which of these assessments would support that diagnosis?

☐ **1.** She has a beefy-red tongue.
☐ **2.** She has joint nodules.
☐ **3.** She has scleral icterus.
☐ **4.** She has edema of the legs.

63. A 14-year-old boy who has a history of asthma is being seen in a physician's office. Which of these observations would indicate that his condition is worsening?

☐ **1.** He's sitting upright with his shoulders in a hunched position.
☐ **2.** He's having paroxysmal, productive coughing spells.
☐ **3.** He's breathing slowly and deeply.
☐ **4.** He's using his intercostal and diaphragmatic muscles to breathe.

64. A staff nurse on a busy surgical unit suspects that another nurse on the unit is abusing drugs. She documents her observations as follows: "When the unit was extremely busy during the evening shift of June 21, 2005, Ms. Brown couldn't be located on three separate occasions for 20 minutes. When she returned, her pupils were constricted and she was euphoric." The nurse's documentation of the colleague's behavior is best described as:

☐ **1.** conclusive.
☐ **2.** interpretive.
☐ **3.** objective.
☐ **4.** digressive.

65. An elderly client has been taking digoxin (Lanoxin) at home for heart failure. The client is admitted to the hospital because of cardiac arrhythmias. His digoxin blood level is 5 mg/ml. A diagnosis of digoxin toxicity is made. The nurse determines that the client has been taking the prescribed dose of digoxin as well as furosemide (Lasix). A nurse also learns that all of the following facts pertain to the client. Which one most likely caused the digoxin toxicity?

☐ **1.** He has periodic episodes of constipation.
☐ **2.** He's been taking potassium supplements.
☐ **3.** He's been overeating for the past week.
☐ **4.** Laboratory studies show renal insufficiency.

66. A client who is 28 weeks pregnant tells the nurse, "I had to have my rings cut off because my hands were so puffy." Based on this data, the nurse should seek additional information concerning the:

☐ **1.** height of the fundus.
☐ **2.** fetal heart rate.
☐ **3.** presence of protein in the urine.
☐ **4.** blood level of human placental lactogen.

67. A nurse is interviewing a client who is in the 2nd trimester of her pregnancy. Which of these questions would provide information about the client's mastery of the primary developmental task during the 2nd trimester?

☐ **1.** "Does your baby seem to be a separate person now?"
☐ **2.** "Does your pregnancy seem real to you now?"
☐ **3.** "Have you started to prepare yourself for labor and delivery?"
☐ **4.** "Have you given your baby a name yet?"

68. A 14-year-old girl with structural scoliosis is fitted with a Milwaukee brace. Because of the brace, which of these potential nursing diagnoses should be given priority in her care plan?

☐ **1.** Ineffective breathing pattern
☐ **2.** Activity intolerance
☐ **3.** Impaired skin integrity
☐ **4.** Acute pain

69. A postpartum client is planning to breast-feed. To keep the nipples in good condition for breast-feeding and to prevent infection, a nurse should include which of these measures in the client's care plan?

☐ **1.** Wash the nipples with soap and water before each feeding.
☐ **2.** Expose the nipples to air and sunlight for short periods of time.
☐ **3.** Use a plastic bra liner to handle leakage.
☐ **4.** Clean the nipples with a mild antiseptic solution.

70. A nurse is orienting a new staff nurse about the care of a client who is to have temporary internal radiation therapy for cancer of the cervix. The nurse should give the staff nurse which of these instructions about the client's care after the implantation of the radiation?

☐ **1.** "Make sure that an aluminum-lined container with long forceps is in the room at all times in case the radiation source becomes dislodged."
☐ **2.** "Collect all of the client's soiled linen in her room until it's determined that they don't contain radiation."
☐ **3.** "To minimize exposure to the radiation, pregnant staff members should plan to accomplish their direct care activities for the client in 15 minutes."
☐ **4.** "Because the client's body wastes are considered irradiated, they should be discarded down the toilet with three flushes."

71. A client who has increased intracranial pressure (ICP) from a head injury is to receive mannitol (Osmitrol) intravenously. The mannitol is prescribed for which of these purposes?

☐ **1.** To restore electrolytes
☐ **2.** To stimulate kidney function
☐ **3.** To increase circulating blood volume
☐ **4.** To reduce cerebral edema

72. A common adverse effect of diphtheria, tetanus, and a cellular pertussis (DTaP) vaccine given to an infant would most likely be manifested by which of these symptoms?

☐ **1.** Vomiting
☐ **2.** Hematuria
☐ **3.** Sudden elevated temperature
☐ **4.** Swelling at the injection site

73. A nurse's aide, who appears intoxicated, reports for duty on the pediatric unit. Which of these actions would be appropriate for a nurse to take initially?

☐ **1.** Send the aide home to sleep it off.
☐ **2.** Advise the aide to seek help from Alcoholics Anonymous.
☐ **3.** Assign the aide to nonclient care tasks.
☐ **4.** Discuss the aide's condition with a supervisor.

74. Which action is effective in obtaining a postoperative client's cooperation with the treatment plan? Select all that apply.

☐ **1.** Providing adequate pain control
☐ **2.** Having thorough preoperative teaching
☐ **3.** Giving the client a sense of control
☐ **4.** Reducing unfamiliar external stimuli
☐ **5.** Making sure informed consent form is signed

75. A 12-year-old child begins choking. Place the following steps in ascending, sequential order of how the nurse should intervene. Use all the options.

Unordered response

1. Make a fist with one hand, and place the thumb of her fist above the client's navel.
2. Assess for airway obstruction.
3. Stand behind the client and wrap her arms around the client's waist.
4. Grasp the fist with her other hand.
5. Perform quick, upward and inward thrusts with her fists.

Ordered response

Answers and rationales

In the pretest answers, the question number appears in boldface type, followed by the number of the correct answer. Rationales for correct answers and, where appropriate, for incorrect options follow. To help you evaluate your knowledge base and application of nursing behaviors, each rationale is classified as follows:

- nursing process step
- client needs category
- client needs subcategory
- cognitive level.

1. CORRECT ANSWER: 3
Option 3 promotes the client's belief in the effectiveness of the intervention, which may help potentiate its effect. Option 1 is inappropriate because the nurse should attempt nursing measures before notifying the physician. Option 2 doesn't suggest strongly enough that the position change will bring relief. Option 4 suggests that the nurse should wait for the physician to arrive instead of trying to relieve discomfort through nursing measures and positive suggestion.
Nursing process step: Implementation
Client needs category: Physiological integrity
Client needs subcategory: Basic care and comfort
Cognitive level: Application

2. CORRECT ANSWER: 2
Positive reinforcement of attachment behaviors promotes such behaviors. Options 1 and 4 are inappropriate because there's no indication that the client needs help with burping or stimulating the sucking reflex. Option 3 isn't appropriate at this time because the client's behavior suggests she has positive feelings; it may confuse or threaten the client.
Nursing process step: Implementation
Client needs category: Psychosocial integrity
Client needs subcategory: None
Cognitive level: Analysis

3. CORRECT ANSWER: 2
The nurse should provide safety and take measures to defuse the potentially violent reaction between the clients. If a client shows a potential for violence, the nurse should obtain help rather than try to manage the situation alone (option 1). Option 3 would increase the risk of violence by bringing the two clients closer together. Option 4 is inappropriate because the nurse shouldn't leave unattended a room with a potentially violent client.
Nursing process step: Implementation
Client needs category: Psychosocial integrity
Client needs subcategory: None
Cognitive level: Analysis

4. CORRECT ANSWER: 2
The nurse should check the client's history for an allergy to seafood and iodine because the dye used for excretory urography contains iodine. The other options aren't iodine sources.
Nursing process step: Assessment
Client needs category: Safe, effective care environment
Client needs subcategory: Safety and infection control
Cognitive level: Application

5. CORRECT ANSWER: 1
Body weight provides a baseline for fluid and electrolyte replacement; the percentage of weight gained or lost is the best indicator of hydration status. Although the other options are important to monitor when assessing hydration status, weight changes are more accurate.
Nursing process step: Assessment
Client needs category: Physiological integrity
Client needs subcategory: Reduction of risk potential
Cognitive level: Application

6. CORRECT ANSWER: 4
This statement in option 4 demonstrates a realistic understanding of the client's disorder and effective family coping with the challenges it presents. Options 1 and 2 indicate that the family is having difficulty adjusting. Option 3 suggests that the family is in denial or has an unrealistic view of the prognosis for a client with Alzheimer's disease.
Nursing process step: Evaluation
Client needs category: Psychosocial integrity
Client needs subcategory: None
Cognitive level: Comprehension

7. CORRECT ANSWER: 3
Reducing anxiety will help the client participate in medical, forensic, and legal follow-up activities. Option 1 should be done as soon as the client's anxiety decreases below the panic level. Option 2 doesn't take high priority. Option 4 is of little use until the client's anxiety level decreases.
Nursing process step: Implementation
Client needs category: Psychosocial integrity
Client needs subcategory: None
Cognitive level: Analysis

8. CORRECT ANSWER: 2
Pregnancy increases plasma volume and expands the uterine vascular bed, possibly increasing the heart rate and boosting cardiac output. These changes may cause cardiac stress, especially during the 2nd trimester. Blood pressure during early pregnancy may decrease by 5 to 10 mm Hg, reaching its lowest point during the second half of the 2nd trimester. During the 3rd trimester, it gradually returns to first-trimester levels.
Nursing process step: Assessment
Client needs category: Health promotion and maintenance
Client needs subcategory: None
Cognitive level: Comprehension

9. CORRECT ANSWER: 1
An effective teacher always involves the student in discussions. Using technical terms and providing detailed explanations usually confuse the student and act as barriers to learning. Using loosely structured teaching sessions permits distraction and deviations from the teaching goals.
Nursing process step: Implementation
Client needs category: Safe, effective care environment
Client needs subcategory: Management of care
Cognitive level: Application

10. CORRECT ANSWER: 1
When caring for a client with a personality disorder, the nurse must examine personal feeling toward the client. If negative feelings exist, the client will sense this and may "act out" the feelings. Also, conveying negative feelings could jeopardize the therapeutic relationship. Clients with antisocial personality disorders aren't motivated to problem-solve because they lack remorse and have no regard for the truth. Although the nurse must set limits on manipulative behavior, insisting the client obey all unit rules and attend all unit activities would make the client feel increasingly threatened. Drug therapy is rarely effective in treating personality disorders, except in cases of extreme distress such as severe anxiety (which this client doesn't have).
Nursing process step: Implementation
Client needs category: Safe, effective care environment
Client needs subcategory: Management of care
Cognitive level: Application

11. CORRECT ANSWER: 1
The anterior fontanel is open in a healthy 6-month-old infant. Normally it closes between the ages of 9 and 18 months. It should feel flat and firm. A sunken fontanel indicates dehydration. Although coughing or crying may cause temporary bulging, persistent bulging and tenseness of fontanel signals increased intracranial pressure.
Nursing process step: Assessment
Client needs category: Physiological integrity
Client needs subcategory: Basic care and comfort
Cognitive level: Knowledge

12. CORRECT ANSWER: 2
Once the client's anxiety level is reduced, she'll be able to cooperate with treatment and express her needs. Option 1 is inappropriate because no further information is needed for initial evaluation of the client's emotional state. The client is too anxious to accept teaching (option 3) or to give additional information (option 4).
Nursing process step: Implementation
Client needs category: Psychosocial integrity
Client needs subcategory: None
Cognitive level: Analysis

13. CORRECT ANSWER: 2
For teaching to be effective, the nurse must assess the client's usual dietary habits. The other options are also important but should be done *after* obtaining the diet history.
Nursing process step: Assessment
Client needs category: Physiological integrity
Client needs subcategory: Basic care and comfort
Cognitive level: Analysis

14. CORRECT ANSWER: 1
The client shouldn't become pregnant soon after being immunized because the rubella virus is teratogenic. Rubella from the vaccine isn't communicable, so the client need not discontinue breast-feeding (option 2), need not avoid contact with pregnant women (option 3), and need not worry about transmitting the virus to her infant because of receiving the vaccine (option 4).
Nursing process step: Evaluation
Client needs category: Physiological integrity
Client needs subcategory: Reduction of risk potential
Cognitive level: Application

15. CORRECT ANSWER: 3
The nurse should assess the child's apical pulse because overdose or rapid administration of aminophylline can cause cardiac arrhythmias. Aminophylline doesn't affect pupil size (option 1) or temperature (option 2). Although the child's breath sounds (option 4) should improve after aminophylline administration, this isn't the most important assessment.

Nursing process step: Assessment
Client needs category: Physiological integrity
Client needs subcategory: Physiological adaptation
Cognitive level: Comprehension

16. CORRECT ANSWER: 4
The modified Trendelenburg position allows full respiratory excursion by slightly elevating the head and increases venous return by elevating the feet. Full respiratory excursion is crucial to assume maximum ventilation capacity; the client is going into shock and needs all the air he can get. Options 1 and 2 promote respiratory excursion but don't improve venous return. Option 3 promotes venous return but doesn't aid respiratory excursion.
Nursing process step: Implementation
Client needs category: Physiological integrity
Client needs subcategory: Physiological adaptation
Cognitive level: Application

17. CORRECT ANSWER: 3
To prevent atmospheric air from rushing into the thoracic cavity, the nurse should instruct the client to take a deep breath and then hold it. Options 1 and 2 would allow air to enter the thoracic cavity. The Valsalva maneuver is helpful when a chest tube is removed; the nurse shouldn't tell the client to avoid it (option 4).
Nursing process step: Implementation
Client needs category: Physiological integrity
Client needs subcategory: Reduction of risk potential
Cognitive level: Application

18. CORRECT ANSWER: 2
A side-lying position with the neck extended allows secretions to drain and maintains a patent airway. The other options increase the risk of aspiration of blood, secretions, and vomitus.
Nursing process step: Implementation
Client needs category: Physiological integrity
Client needs subcategory: Reduction of risk potential
Cognitive level: Application

19. CORRECT ANSWER: 3
Having the client describe the old and new positions allows him to explore his experience objectively. Options 1 and 4 minimize his experience and don't focus on his distress. Option 2 is judgmental and implies that the client should be grateful for the promotion.
Nursing process step: Planning
Client needs category: Psychosocial integrity
Client needs subcategory: None
Cognitive level: Analysis

20. CORRECT ANSWER: 3
Slightly elevating the neonate's head keeps the weight of the abdominal contents off the diaphragm and aids breathing. Option 1 would place the neonate's full weight on the chest and abdomen, compromising respiratory excursion. Option 2 wouldn't aid respirations, unless the neonate's head is elevated and the neck extended. Option 4 would place the weight of the abdominal contents on the diaphragm, impeding respirations.
Nursing process step: Implementation
Client needs category: Safe, effective care environment
Client needs subcategory: Safety and infection control
Cognitive level: Application

21. CORRECT ANSWER: 4
Restlessness and increased respirations may indicate hemorrhage. Introducing water into the stomach (option 1) may cause metabolic alkalosis from loss of chloride or hydrogen ions. The balloon holds the tube in place and shouldn't be deflated (option 2) until just before tube removal. The esophageal balloon controls esophageal bleeding and therefore should be kept inflated at all times; the nurse shouldn't deflate and reinflate it periodically (option 3).
Nursing process step: Planning
Client needs category: Safe, effective care environment
Client needs subcategory: Safety and infection control
Cognitive level: Analysis

22. CORRECT ANSWER: 3
Use the following equation:

$$10{,}000 \text{ milliunits} : 1{,}000 \text{ ml} = 2 \text{ milliunits} : X \text{ ml}$$

$$\frac{10{,}000}{1{,}000} = \frac{2}{X}$$

$$10{,}000X = 2{,}000$$

$$X = \frac{2{,}000}{10{,}000}$$

$$X = 0.2 \text{ ml}$$

Each unit of Pitocin contains 1,000 milliunits. Therefore, 1,000 ml of I.V. fluid contains 10,000 milliunits (10 units) of Pitocin.
Nursing process step: Implementation
Client needs category: Physiological integrity
Client needs subcategory: Pharmacological and parenteral therapies
Cognitive level: Application

23. CORRECT ANSWER: 2
These foods aren't irritating to the tonsil bed. The other options include solid or hard foods, which would irritate the tonsil bed.
Nursing process step: Evaluation
Client needs category: Health promotion and maintenance
Client needs subcategory: None
Cognitive level: Application

24. CORRECT ANSWER: 2
Rapid emptying of a distended bladder can cause shock and hemorrhage into the bladder as blood rushes to fill previously compressed blood vessels. The other options don't occur with rapid bladder decompression.
Nursing process step: Implementation
Client needs category: Physiological integrity
Client needs subcategory: Basic care and comfort
Cognitive level: Comprehension

25. CORRECT ANSWER: 3
Typically, the client with Alzheimer's disease responds favorably to music, especially selections that recall pleasant times and memories. The other options would give the client something to put in the mouth, which could cause choking.
Nursing process step: Implementation
Client needs category: Psychosocial integrity
Client needs subcategory: None
Cognitive level: Application

26. CORRECT ANSWER: 2
The client's symptoms are consistent with early alcohol withdrawal delirium, which occurs 2 to 5 days after alcohol withdrawal. Gastritis is a result of increased alcohol intake; when hospitalized, the alcohol level goes to zero and the client goes into withdrawal. His symptoms aren't typical of schizophrenia (option 1). A reaction to an hallucinogenic substance (option 3) would occur within minutes of ingestion. Although seizures (option 4) may occur if delirium tremens isn't treated promptly, they aren't likely to arise during early stages.
Nursing process step: Assessment
Client needs category: Psychosocial integrity
Client needs subcategory: None
Cognitive level: Analysis

27. CORRECT ANSWER: 1
A contraction that remains strong for more than 90 seconds with no sign of letting up signals approaching tetany and could cause rupture of the uterus. Pitocin stimulates contractions and, therefore, should be stopped. The nurse also should take the actions described in the other options, but only *after* stopping the Pitocin.
Nursing process step: Implementation
Client needs category: Physiological integrity
Client needs subcategory: Pharmacological and parenteral therapies
Cognitive level: Analysis

28. CORRECT ANSWER: 4
Adequate respiratory function is essential to maintain life; a nursing diagnosis related to respiratory dysfunction takes priority over all other nursing diagnoses.
Nursing process step: Analysis
Client needs category: Physiological integrity
Client needs subcategory: Reduction of risk potential
Cognitive level: Comprehension

29. CORRECT ANSWER: 3
The client should wear the eye shield at night for 1 month after surgery to guard against rubbing or hitting the eye while sleeping.
Nursing process step: Evaluation
Client needs category: Health promotion and maintenance
Client needs subcategory: None
Cognitive level: Comprehension

30. CORRECT ANSWER: 2
Mydriatic agents cause pupil dilation and therefore may affect the size of the pupil desired by the surgeon during surgery. Option 1 is incorrect because acetazolamide and other carbonic anhydrase inhibitors are given preoperatively to restrict the action of the enzyme necessary to produce aqueous humor. Option 3 is incorrect because atropine is a mydriatic agent and wouldn't be ordered preoperatively for a client with glaucoma. Option 4 is incorrect because cycloplegic eye drops also are mydriatic agents and therefore are contraindicated for this client.
Nursing process step: Implementation
Client needs category: Physiological integrity
Client needs subcategory: Reduction of risk potential
Cognitive level: Application

31. CORRECT ANSWER: 3
When held upright, an neonate will open his eyes reflexively. Stimulation, such as by separating the eyelids (option 1), induces the blink reflex, which causes the eyes to close. Option 2 also causes the eyes to close. Option 4 is incorrect because infants are sensitive to light and will frown and close their eyes if a bright light is flashed at them.

Nursing process step: Implementation
Client needs category: Health promotion and maintenance
Client needs subcategory: None
Cognitive level: Application

32. CORRECT ANSWER: 4
Pituitary gland removal may lead to signs of diabetes insipidus by decreasing production of antidiuretic hormone (ADH). With insufficient ADH production, the client may lose up to 15 L/day of urine and may be at risk for severe dehydration. Although the nurse also must assess for respiratory depression, gastric distention, and cardiac arrhythmias, these changes are less significant than excessive urine output in a client recovering from a transsphenoidal hypophysectomy.
Nursing process step: Assessment
Client needs category: Physiological integrity
Client needs subcategory: Reduction of risk potential
Cognitive level: Analysis

33. CORRECT ANSWER: 1
For a client with a head injury, use of any central nervous system (CNS) depressant is potentially dangerous and must be reported to the physician. Option 2 doesn't address this danger. Option 3 is unnecessary. Option 4 may be important but doesn't address the risks of CNS depressant use in this client.
Nursing process step: Implementation
Client needs category: Physiological integrity
Client needs subcategory: Reduction of risk potential
Cognitive level: Application

34. CORRECT ANSWER: 3
Lecithin is a surfactant that's necessary for alveolar stability, lung expansion, and adequate respiration. The other options ultimately may lead to metabolic imbalances but aren't directly related to neonate respiratory distress syndrome.
Nursing process step: Assessment
Client needs category: Physiological integrity
Client needs subcategory: Physiological adaptation
Cognitive level: Knowledge

35. CORRECT ANSWER: 4
In a neonate younger than 24 hours old, the laboratory values reported indicate clinical hemolytic disease. The nurse should notify the physician, who will determine further management. Options 1 and 2 are appropriate but don't take precedence over notifying the physician. Option 3 may be indicated but requires a physician's order.
Nursing process step: Implementation
Client needs category: Physiological integrity
Client needs subcategory: Reduction of risk potential
Cognitive level: Analysis

36. CORRECT ANSWER: 1
During a manic state, the client has severe anxiety; the broad muscle activity involved in tearing rags will help drain off excess energy. Option 2 requires concentration and problem solving: abilities a manic client lacks. Option 3 is highly stimulating and could exhaust the client. Option 4 requires too much concentration for this client.
Nursing process step: Implementation
Client needs category: Psychosocial integrity
Client needs subcategory: None
Cognitive level: Application

37. CORRECT ANSWER: 1
Staying with the client during the examination offers the most support. Option 2 is inappropriate because deep, not shallow, breathing usually aids relaxation. Option 3 is too general and doesn't acknowledge the client's individuality. Option 4 is inappropriate because the nurse should always remain in the room during a pelvic examination.
Nursing process step: Implementation
Client needs category: Safe, effective care environment
Client needs subcategory: Safety and infection control
Cognitive level: Application

38. CORRECT ANSWER: 3
Although skin care instructions may vary among facilities, most permit the use of A & D ointment but not talcum powder and baby oil to ease drying and desquamation. Port marks must be retained because they guide the radiation therapist. Within the port marks, skin is red, tender, and dry and shouldn't be washed; soap may erase marks and contribute to dry skin.
Nursing process step: Evaluation
Client needs category: Safe, effective care environment
Client needs subcategory: Safety and infection control
Cognitive level: Analysis

39. CORRECT ANSWER: 2
A client with a lactose intolerance may have a calcium deficiency, from difficulty digesting milk and dairy products. The other options aren't diminished in clients with lactose intolerance.
Nursing process step: Planning
Client needs category: Health promotion and maintenance
Client needs subcategory: None
Cognitive level: Application

40. Correct answer: 4
"Setting sun" sign (downward deviation of the eyes, so that the sclera is visible above each iris) is a classic sign of hydrocephalus. A pulsating anterior fontanel (option 1) is normal. Swelling cranial contents causes suture lines to widen, not close (option 2). Orthopneic positioning (option 3) isn't related to hydrocephalus.
Nursing process step: Assessment
Client needs category: Physiological integrity
Client needs subcategory: Physiological adaptation
Cognitive level: Comprehension

41. Correct answer: 1
After a total hip replacement, the client must do specially designed exercises to help regain muscle strength. Riding in a car should be discouraged because it may cause injury or dislocation of the prosthesis. The client need not wear loose clothes because most ordinary clothes don't restrict movement. Walking 2 miles per day is excessive; at first, the client should walk for short distances, then gradually increase the distance.
Nursing process step: Evaluation
Client needs category: Health promotion and maintenance
Client needs subcategory: None
Cognitive level: Analysis

42. Correct answer: 2
Slow, rhythmic chest breathing is the most relaxing and requires the least concentration of the learned breathing techniques. Option 1 wouldn't provide relief. Options 3 and 4 should be reserved for later stages of labor.
Nursing process step: Implementation
Client needs category: Health promotion and maintenance
Client needs subcategory: None
Cognitive level: Application

43. Correct answer: 2
Peanut butter provides protein and fat, while raisins provide iron. Option 1 provides adequate nutrients but too much fat. Options 3 and 4 don't provide adequate protein or iron.
Nursing process step: Planning
Client needs category: Physiological integrity
Client needs subcategory: Basic care and comfort
Cognitive level: Comprehension

44. Correct answer: 2
Shock causes tissue hypoxia. The first action should be to start nasal oxygen to promote tissue oxygenation. Option 1 is appropriate after oxygen therapy is initiated. Before implementing option 3, the nurse would need further data. Option 4 is important, but doesn't take precedence over starting oxygen.
Nursing process step: Implementation
Client needs category: Physiological integrity
Client needs subcategory: Reduction of risk potential
Cognitive level: Analysis

45. Correct answer: 4
Breathing exercises help establish normal breathing patterns, strengthen the respiratory muscles, and remove mucus from the lungs. The physician may not order options 1 or 2. Option 3 is used to manage an acute attack; it's not a preventive measure.
Nursing process step: Planning
Client needs category: Physiological integrity
Client needs subcategory: Reduction of risk potential
Cognitive level: Application

46. Correct answer: 3
Hypotonic contractions are irregular and poor in quality; they commonly occur during the active phase of stage one of labor. An atonic pattern is characterized by lack of tone. In a dystonic pattern, contractions are painful, ineffective, and asymmetrical. In a hypertonic pattern, contractions are strong, painful, and uncoordinated and occur in the latent phase of labor in primigravidas.
Nursing process step: Assessment
Client needs category: Physiological integrity
Client needs subcategory: Physiological adaptation
Cognitive level: Analysis

47. Correct answer: 3
An osmotic diuretic, mannitol increases urine output. The other options aren't adverse effects of mannitol.
Nursing process step: Evaluation
Client needs category: Physiological integrity
Client needs subcategory: Pharmacological and parenteral therapies
Cognitive level: Comprehension

48. Correct answer: 4
The client is attempting to interact with the nurse, who shouldn't squander this opportunity for therapeutic intervention. The other options aren't therapeutic responses because a depressed client can't problem solve and is capable of following only simple directions.

Nursing process step: Implementation
Client needs category: Psychosocial integrity
Client needs subcategory: None
Cognitive level: Analysis

49. CORRECT ANSWER: 2
Pitocin causes vasoconstriction, resulting in hypertension. Option 1 is incorrect because Pitocin is associated with an increased pulse rate (tachycardia). The drug doesn't cause a rash (option 3). Option 4 is incorrect because the drug's antidiuretic effect may decrease urine output.
Nursing process step: Assessment
Client needs category: Physiological integrity
Client needs subcategory: Pharmacological and parenteral therapies
Cognitive level: Application

50. CORRECT ANSWER: 3
Blood trickling down the throat stimulates the swallowing reflex; therefore, frequent swallowing indicates bleeding. Option 1 is common after a tonsillectomy. Option 2 is also a common posttonsillectomy finding and results from moderate edema of the nasopharynx. Option 4 indicates old blood swallowed during surgery.
Nursing process step: Assessment
Client needs category: Physiological integrity
Client needs subcategory: Reduction of risk potential
Cognitive level: Application

51. CORRECT ANSWER: 4
With a decrease in serum albumin, hydrostatic pressure of the blood pushes fluid and electrolytes into the extracellular space, thus causing ascites. An increased vasopressin level contributes to fluid retention but doesn't cause ascites. An increased serum sodium level leads to fluid retention but isn't the primary cause of ascites. In cirrhosis, the serum aldosterone level increases, not decreases.
Nursing process step: Assessment
Client needs category: Physiological integrity
Client needs subcategory: Physiological adaptation
Cognitive level: Comprehension

52. CORRECT ANSWER: 3
The neonate receives a score of 2 for a pulse above 100 beats/minute, 2 for good respiratory effort, 2 for active motion, 1 for pink body and blue extremities, and 1 for a grimace. Added together, these scores result in an Apgar score of 8. Options 1 and 2 are too low; option 4 is too high.
Nursing process step: Assessment
Client needs category: Health promotion and maintenance
Client needs subcategory: None
Cognitive level: Analysis

53. CORRECT ANSWER: 3
Handling the child with the palms of the hands will prevent further bruising (which results from a decreased platelet count). The client's teeth should be brushed more than once per day to prevent gum infection. Trimming his nails short may cause bleeding. A 4-year-old child probably would object to being placed in a crib.
Nursing process step: Implementation
Client needs category: Physiological integrity
Client needs subcategory: Reduction of risk potential
Cognitive level: Analysis

54. CORRECT ANSWER: 1
During the toddler stage, the child begins to develop autonomy and needs rituals and specific objects to gain a sense of consistency and order. Option 2 is typical toddler behavior — saying no to everything and doing nothing — neither of which has anything to do with clinging to his blanket. Option 3 is also characteristic toddler behavior and has nothing to do with clinging to his blanket. Clinging to a blanket is age-appropriate; so it isn't a sign of regression.
Nursing process step: Assessment
Client needs category: Psychosocial integrity
Client needs subcategory: None
Cognitive level: Comprehension

55. CORRECT ANSWER: 1
Although belladonna decreases bladder spasms when given with opium (option 2), it's contraindicated in the presence of glaucoma because its anticholinergic effect would increase intraocular pressure. Therefore, the nurse should question the physician's orders. If the indwelling urinary catheter is functioning properly, urine will drain through it from the bladder; therefore, voiding around the catheter (option 3) shouldn't be possible. Option 4 wouldn't relieve the spasms.
Nursing process step: Implementation
Client needs category: Physiological integrity
Client needs subcategory: Reduction of risk potential
Cognitive level: Analysis

56. CORRECT ANSWER: 2
This action orients the client directly and meets his need for diversional activity. Before the client's wife can inter-

act with him further, such as by reading books to him (option 1) or showing him family pictures (option 3), the client needs to be oriented to her. Showing him her wedding ring (option 4) would provide only an indirect reference to her identity; this client needs direct orientation.
Nursing process step: Implementation
Client needs category: Psychosocial integrity
Client needs subcategory: None
Cognitive level: Application

57. CORRECT ANSWER: 2
Laboratory values are valid and reliable indicators of the client's electrolyte status and would be altered by purging. No client can be watched every minute after every meal (option 1). Weighing her (option 3) wouldn't determine accurately if she's still purging. Restricting her movement (option 4) wouldn't be therapeutic; she could always find a way to get rid of food while on the unit.
Nursing process step: Assessment
Client needs category: Safe, effective care environment
Client needs subcategory: Management of care
Cognitive level: Analysis

58. CORRECT ANSWER: 2
The client's behavior suggests akathisia — an adverse reaction of phenothiazines. Dystonia would manifest as excessive salivation, difficulty speaking, and involuntary movements of the face, neck, arms, and legs. Parkinsonian effects include a shuffling gait, hand tremors, drooling, rigidity, and loose arm movements. Tardive dyskinesia is characterized by odd facial and tongue movements, difficulty swallowing, and a stiff neck.
Nursing process step: Assessment
Client needs category: Physiological integrity
Client needs subcategory: Pharmacological and parenteral therapies
Cognitive level: Comprehension

59. CORRECT ANSWER: 1
Children in this age range have a strong interest in competitive games such as Monopoly, which provide the socializing so important to children in this age group. Solitary activities, such as doing crossword puzzles and reading, are less desirable than those that encourage socialization. Playing Old Maid is appropriate for much younger children.
Nursing process step: Planning
Client needs category: Psychosocial integrity
Client needs subcategory: None
Cognitive level: Application

60. CORRECT ANSWER: 1
Jaundice during the first 24 hours after birth is always considered pathological. The other options are considered normal in the neonate.
Nursing process step: Analysis
Client needs category: Physiological integrity
Client needs subcategory: Physiological adaptation
Cognitive level: Application

61. CORRECT ANSWER: 3
Dumping syndrome is the rapid emptying of gastric contents into the small intestine, causing a decrease in circulating blood volume and a blood glucose elevation. The resulting insulin oversecretion leads to hypoglycemia, which may manifest as dizziness, sweating, and tachycardia. Pernicious anemia wouldn't cause the client's signs and symptoms. Pyloric stenosis would cause projectile vomiting. A recurring ulcer would result in pain.
Nursing process step: Assessment
Client needs category: Physiological integrity
Client needs subcategory: Physiological adaptation
Cognitive level: Comprehension

62. CORRECT ANSWER: 3
Frequently, the first signs of sickle cell disease are lack of appetite, irritability, and an increased susceptibility to infection. The child might be small for her age and might gain weight slowly. The mucous membranes are pale, and scleral icterus is evident. Option 1 is a sign of scarlet fever. Option 2 is seen in rheumatic fever. Option 4 is a sign of cardiac or renal disease or water overload, not sickle cell anemia.
Nursing process step: Assessment
Client needs category: Health promotion and maintenance
Client needs subcategory: None
Cognitive level: Comprehension

63. CORRECT ANSWER: 1
During an acute attack of asthma, older children tend to sit upright with their shoulders in a hunched-over position, with hands on the bed or chair and arms braced to facilitate the use of accessory muscles of respiration. Option 2 is incorrect because an asthmatic episode begins with a hacking, paroxysmal, nonproductive cough caused by bronchial edema. Option 3 is incorrect because the child with a severe attack is short of breath and tries to breathe more deeply. The expiratory phase becomes prolonged and is accompanied by wheezing. Option 4 is incorrect because intercostal and diaphragmatic muscles are normally used for breathing.

Nursing process step: Assessment
Client needs category: Physiological integrity
Client needs subcategory: Physiological adaptation
Cognitive level: Analysis

64. CORRECT ANSWER: 3
The documentation objectively describes the nurse's observations of her colleague. It doesn't draw conclusions (option 1), interpret the colleague's behavior (option 2), or digress from the topic of concern (option 3).
Nursing process step: Assessment
Client needs category: Safe, effective care environment
Client needs subcategory: Management of care
Cognitive level: Analysis

65. CORRECT ANSWER 4
About 80% to 90% of digoxin is excreted by the kidneys. If the kidneys aren't functioning properly, large amounts of the drug aren't eliminated, which can cause digoxin toxicity. Option 1 is incorrect because diarrhea (not constipation) may be an adverse effect of the drug. Option 2 is incorrect because potassium supplements are frequently prescribed with furosemide to prevent digoxin toxicity. Option 3 is incorrect because excessive food intake for 1 week wouldn't cause digoxin toxicity.
Nursing process step: Assessment
Client needs category: Physiological integrity
Client needs subcategory: Pharmacological and parenteral therapies
Cognitive level: Analysis

66. CORRECT ANSWER: 3
The client is reporting symptoms that suggest gestational hypertension. Therefore, her urine should be checked for the presence of protein. Fundal height, fetal heart rate, and presence of human placental lactogen in maternal blood have lower priorities in assessing this client.
Nursing process step: Analysis
Client needs category: Health promotion and maintenance
Client needs subcategory: None
Cognitive level: Application

67. CORRECT ANSWER: 1
The main developmental task of the 2nd trimester is to recognize the fetus as a separate being. Accepting the pregnancy (option 2) is the major task of the 1st trimester, and preparing for childbirth (option 3) is the main task of the 3rd trimester. Selecting a name for the baby (option 4) is begun during pregnancy, but a definite decision is made after birth.
Nursing process step: Assessment
Client needs category: Health promotion and maintenance
Client needs subcategory: None
Cognitive level: Comprehension

68. CORRECT ANSWER: 3
Impaired skin integrity related to the corrective device is the nursing diagnosis that should be given priority. The goal is to prevent skin irritation and breakdown. Other nursing diagnoses related to the brace in this condition include *Risk for injury* and *Disturbed body image*. Options 1, 2, and 4 are incorrect.
Nursing process step: Planning
Client needs category: Safe, effective care environment
Client needs subcategory: Safety and infection control
Cognitive level: Application

69. CORRECT ANSWER: 2
Exposing the nipples to air and sunlight will help toughen them. Soap (option 1) and antiseptics (option 4) should not be used on the nipples because they remove protective oils that keep nipples supple. Plastic bra liners (option 3) aren't recommended because they retain moisture against the nipples.
Nursing process step: Planning
Client needs category: Health promotion and maintenance
Client needs subcategory: None
Cognitive level: Comprehension

70. CORRECT ANSWER: 2
Soiled linens should be kept in the client's room until radiation monitoring determines that they don't contain a source of radiation that has become dislodged from the site of placement. Options 1, 3, and 4 are incorrect. The container should be lined with lead (not aluminum). Persons younger than age 18 and those who are pregnant or lactating shouldn't visit or care for a client who has internal radiation. Body excreta aren't irradiated, so no special precautions (besides universal precautions) are required for their disposal.
Nursing process step: Implementation
Client needs category: Safe, effective care environment
Client needs subcategory: Safety and infection control
Cognitive level: Application

71. CORRECT ANSWER: 4
Mannitol, an osmotic diuretic, is prescribed to reduce increased ICP, which will then reduce cerebral edema. Options 1, 2, and 3 are incorrect. Many diuretics put the client at risk for electrolyte imbalance. Although mannitol is sometimes used to prevent or treat the oliguric phase of acute renal failure, no evidence in the question indicates that the client has that problem. A diuretic will tend to reduce blood volume rather than increase it.
Nursing process step: Planning
Client needs category: Physiological integrity
Client needs subcategory: Pharmacological and parenteral therapies
Cognitive level: Comprehension

72. CORRECT ANSWER: 4
With inactivated antigens, such as DTP, adverse reactions are most likely to occur within a few hours or days of administration and are usually limited to local tenderness, erythema, and swelling at the injection site; low grade fever; and behavior changes. Options 1, 2, and 3 are incorrect.
Nursing process step: Evaluation
Client needs category: Physiological integrity
Client needs subcategory: Pharmacological and parenteral therapies
Cognitive level: Comprehension

73. CORRECT ANSWER: 4
Chemically impaired staff members place clients at risk for harm and the employing agency at risk for liability for negligent actions. Therefore, the nurse's supervisor should be informed about the situation and should help verify perceptions and clarify procedures. Sending the aide home isn't the best action initially. The supervisor should first be consulted. More information should be obtained before referring the aide to Alcoholics Anonymous. Assigning the aide to nonclient care tasks, such as sterilizing equipment, could harm clients or the aide and also would foster denial of the problem.
Nursing process step: Implementation
Client needs category: Safe, effective care environment
Client needs subcategory: Management of care
Cognitive level: Analysis

74. CORRECT ANSWER: 2
Providing adequate pain control (option 1) is important. Knowing what to expect is an effective way to allay fear and reduce anxiety. A client who is well informed can anticipate what's likely to take place postoperatively and cooperate in the care. Giving the client a sense of control (option 3) isn't realistic while the client is in the postanesthesia recovery unit or intensive care unit. Reducing unfamiliar external stimuli (option 4) isn't always possible and would have little effect on promoting a client's cooperation. Making sure that the client's informed consent form is signed is important in ensuring that the client understands the procedure but it doesn't help ensure postoperative client cooperation.
Nursing process step: Implementation
Client needs category: Psychosocial integrity
Client needs subcategory: None
Cognitive level: Analysis

75. CORRECT ANSWER:

2. Assess for airway obstruction.
3. Stand behind the client and wrap her arms around the client's waist.
1. Make a fist with one hand, and place the thumb of her fist above the client's navel.
4. Grasp the fist with her other hand.
5. Perform quick, upward and inward thrusts with her fists.

Nursing process step: Implementation
Client needs category: Physiological integrity
Client needs subcategory: Physiological adaptation
Cognitive level: Application

Analyzing the pretest

Total the number of incorrect responses on the pretest. A score of 1 to 10 indicates that you have an excellent knowledge base; 11 to 15, good; 16 to 20, fair. If your incorrect responses total 21 or more, you'll need intensive study; review this book carefully and see how well you do on the posttests.

Part I

Taking the NCLEX-RN

Understanding the NCLEX-RN

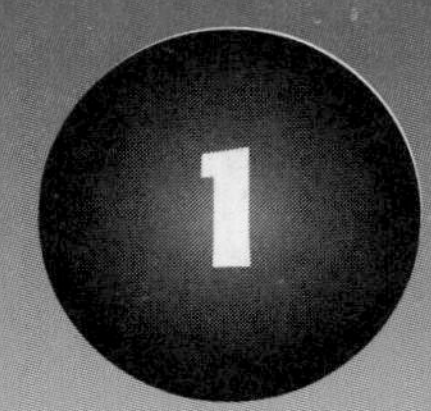

INTRODUCTION

Anyone who wants to practice as a registered nurse (RN) in the United States must be licensed by the nursing licensure authority in the state or territory in which she intends to practice. In January 2005, Hong Kong, London, and Seoul, South Korea, also began administering the NCLEX®. To obtain this license, you must pass the National Council Licensure Examination for Registered Nurses (NCLEX-RN®). The NCLEX-RN is designed for one purpose: to determine whether it's appropriate for you to receive a license to practice as a nurse. By passing the NCLEX-RN, you demonstrate that you possess the minimum level of knowledge necessary to practice nursing safely and effectively.

Your success on the NCLEX-RN depends on three key elements:

- ◆ your nursing knowledge base
- ◆ your study program for the test
- ◆ your confidence level.

You also must understand the test administration method — the computerized adaptive testing (CAT) method.

Understandably, you may feel anxious about taking the examination on a computer, especially if you haven't had much practice with one. This chapter provides helpful information about applying for your license, registering for the NCLEX-RN, following the test plan, and using the computerized format.

To become more acquainted with taking a computerized examination and to obtain additional experience with NCLEX-RN questions, be sure to practice with the 1,200 review questions on the CD-ROM included with this book. You can select review or practice test modes or focus on a specific subject, nursing process step, or client needs category and subcategory. The questions are presented in a format similar to the actual examination and aren't included in this review book.

APPLICATION FOR LICENSURE AND REGISTRATION

Obtaining an RN license is actually a three-step process. You must:

- ◆ apply for licensure in the state or territory in which you want to be licensed
- ◆ meet the Board of Nursing's eligibility requirements to take the NCLEX
- ◆ complete the registration form in the NCLEX-RN Candidate Bulletin.

The following key steps can help make the road to taking the NCLEX-RN smoother:

- ◆ Make sure you're in good standing with your school financially. That way, you won't have any trouble getting the school to release your transcript. After graduation, your school will send your transcript to the Board of Nursing.
- ◆ Contact your Board of Nursing for an application for licensure. Your school may also provide you with an application. Make sure you're aware of the licensure requirements of the state where you plan to practice. Ask your school's nursing department or check with the appropriate Board of Nursing.
- ◆ Fill out an application for a limited permit if you plan to start working before you take the NCLEX-RN.
- ◆ Read the application instructions carefully. Be aware that individual states require different materials at the time of application. These may include:
  - 2″ × 2″ photograph
  - completed fingerprint card
  - additional form if you're requesting verification of receipt of your application
  - proof that you have completed a course or have been trained in the identification and reporting of child abuse, infection control, and barrier precautions
  - your notarized signature.
- ◆ Submit your application or a certificate of nursing education, if required, to your nursing school for completion of appropriate sections.

◆ Register with the appropriate educational testing service by going to the NCLEX Candidate Web site (*www.pearsonvue.com/nclex*) and select the REGISTRATION option. Answer the questions as directed and be prepared to pay for your registration with an acceptable credit card (VISA, MasterCard, or American Express). Use the registration form within the NCLEX-RN Candidate Bulletin to register by mail. Be sure to include a certified check, cashier's check, or money order for the fee. Call NCLEX Candidate Services if you need more information or if you want to register by phone. Be aware that registering by phone using your credit card is quicker but it costs more.
◆ If registering by mail, consider sending your application by certified mail so you have confirmation of its delivery and receipt.
◆ Await receipt of your Authorization to Test (ATT) form before making your appointment to take the test. You'll receive it from the educational testing group after they've been notified by your state board of nursing that you're eligible. If you have an e-mail address, it will be used to deliver your confirmation of registration, your ATT, and the confirmation of your examination appointment. Paper copies of these documents will also be sent through the U.S. mail.
◆ Schedule your examination appointment through the NCLEX Candidate Web site (*www.pearsonvue.com/nclex*) or by calling the Candidate Services center of your choice within the United States or its territories. Schedule your test keeping in mind that the testing session may last a maximum of 6 hours.

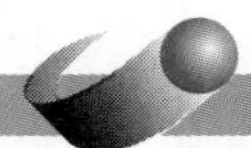

FAST FACT

Additional security measures are now being taken at the test centers, including a digital fingerprint, signature, and photograph taken at the test center, which will accompany your examination result. Your fingerprint, signature, and photograph may also be used to confirm your identity for licensure by the Board of Nursing. You'll also be observed directly during the test as well as by video and audio recordings of your examination session.

◆ Keep the ATT form for the day of testing. It's required at the testing center on the day of the test. You'll also need a form of current identification with your signature and recent photograph of yourself, such as a valid driver's license or passport.

COMPUTERIZED ADAPTIVE TESTING

Since 1994, the NCLEX-RN has been a computerized test in which a candidate must answer enough questions of various levels of difficulty to demonstrate minimum competence as an entry-level RN. The CAT differs from the standard paper-and-pencil test in other ways as well. The most obvious difference is that, instead of sitting at a table with a test book and a pencil, you'll sit in front of a computer terminal, interacting with it as you take the examination.

The CAT chooses test items based on your response to the previous question; the computer will "adapt" to your answers, correct or incorrect, by selecting harder or easier items for the next question. For example, at the start of the examination, a question of low-level difficulty may appear on the screen. If you answer this question correctly, the computer will then ask a more difficult question; if you answer incorrectly, the computer will ask an easier question. (See *Sample NCLEX questions*, pages 4 and 5.)

The database contains thousands of questions, each categorized according to the NCLEX-RN test plan and assigned a level of difficulty using a complex statistical formula. Every time you answer a question, the computer will search the database for the next appropriate question based on the difficulty level of the previous question and the accuracy of your response. This process continues until the computer can determine your competence in all areas of the test plan. Because each test is individualized, the number of questions can range from 75 to 265.

MECHANICS OF TAKING THE CAT

The CAT begins with brief instructions and an opportunity to answer a few practice questions. Keep in mind:
◆ Computer experience isn't necessary. You'll be using only the button on the mouse to answer questions. This allows you to focus on the questions and not the keyboard.
◆ Two small boxes are located at the bottom of the screen of each question. They include a CALCULATOR button and a NEXT button. A tutorial will precede the examination to review how to use these buttons.
◆ One question at a time will appear on the screen. After you've confirmed your answer, the question will disappear; you can't return to the question.
◆ Answer every question. You can't skip questions, and you aren't penalized for wrong answers.
◆ The test will end when the computer has determined your competence level.

Sample NCLEX questions

Sometimes, getting used to the format is as important as knowing the material. Try your hand at these sample questions and you'll have a leg up when you take the real test!

Sample four-option, multiple-choice question

A client's arterial blood gas (ABG) results are as follows: pH, 7.16; $Paco_2$, 80 mm Hg; Pao_2, 46 mm Hg; HCO_3^-, 24 mEq/L; Sao_2, 81%. This ABG result represents which condition?

1. Metabolic acidosis
2. Metabolic alkalosis
3. Respiratory acidosis
4. Respiratory alkalosis

Correct answer: 3

Sample multiple-response, multiple-choice question

The nurse is caring for a 45-year-old married woman who has undergone hemicolectomy for colon cancer. The woman has two children. Which concepts about families should the nurse keep in mind when providing care for this client? Select all that apply:

1. Illness in one family member can affect all members.
2. Family roles don't change because of illness.
3. A family member may have more than one role at a time in the family.
4. Children typically aren't affected by adult illness.
5. The effects of an illness on a family depend on the stage of the family's life cycle.
6. Changes in sleeping and eating patterns may be signs of stress in a family.

Correct answer: 1, 3, 5, 6

Sample hot-spot question

An elderly client has a history of aortic stenosis. Identify the area where the nurse should place the stethoscope to best hear the murmur.

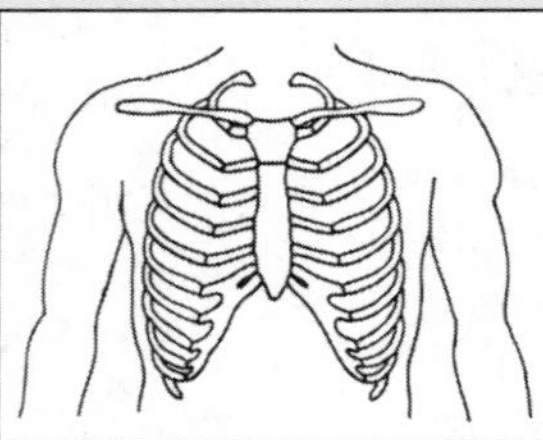

Correct answer:

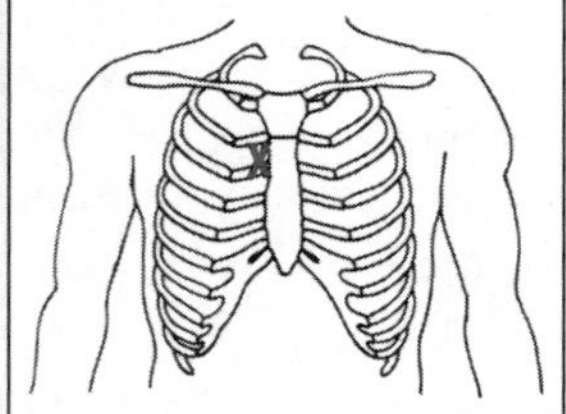

Sample NCLEX questions *(continued)*

Sample fill-in-the-blank calculation question

An infant who weighs 8 kg is to receive ampicillin (Omnipen) 25 mg/kg I.V. every 6 hours. How many milligrams should the nurse administer per dose?

____

Correct answer: 200

Drag-and-drop question

When teaching an antepartal client about the passage of the fetus through the birth canal during labor, the nurse describes the cardinal mechanisms of labor. Place these events in ascending sequential order. Use all the options.

Unordered options

1.	Flexion	
2.	External rotation	
3.	Descent	
4.	Expulsion	
5.	Internal rotation	
6.	Extension	

Ordered options

3.	Descent
1.	Flexion
5.	Internal rotation
6.	Extension
2.	External rotation
4.	Expulsion

◆ Your State Board of Nursing will notify you of your results approximately 2 weeks to 1 month after testing. No test results are given over the phone.

NCLEX-STYLE QUESTIONS

Most of the questions on the NCLEX are traditional four-option, multiple-choice items with only one correct answer. However, in April 2004, the National Council of State Boards of Nursing (NCSBN) added alternate-format items to the examination. Certain strategies can help you understand and answer any type of NCLEX question.

Alternate formats

There are four types of alternate-format questions currently on the NCLEX-RN:

- multiple-response, multiple-choice
- "hot-spot"
- fill-in-the-blank
- "drag and drop."

Unlike a traditional multiple-choice question, each multiple-response, multiple-choice question has more than one correct answer for every question, and it may contain more than four possible answers. You'll recognize this type of question because it will ask you to select all answers that apply — not just the best answer (as may be requested in the more traditional multiple-choice questions).

The so-called "hot-spot" question asks you to identify an area on an illustration or graphic. For these questions, the computerized examination will ask you to place your cursor and click over the correct area on an illustration or graph. Try to be as precise as possible when marking the location. As with the fill-in-the-blank questions, the identification questions on the computerized examination may require extremely precise answers to be considered correct.

Fill-in-the-blank questions require you to provide the answer yourself, rather than selecting it from a list of options. This type of question will require you to perform a calculation and type your answer (a number, without any

Client needs categories on NCLEX

The NCLEX-RN assigns each question a certain category based on client needs. This chart lists client needs categories and subcategories and the approximate percentages of each type of question on the NCLEX-RN. The NCLEX recently deleted the subcategories for Health promotion and maintenance and Psychological integrity.

CATEGORY	SUBCATEGORIES	PERCENTAGE OF NCLEX-RN QUESTIONS
Safe, effective care environment	Management of care	13% to 19%
	Safety and infection control	8% to 14%
Health promotion and maintenance	None	6% to 12%
Psychosocial integrity	None	6% to 12%
Physiological integrity	Basic care and comfort	6% to 12%
	Pharmacological and parenteral therapies	13% to 19%
	Reduction of risk potential	13% to 19%
	Physiological adaptation	11% to 17%

words, commas, or spaces) in the blank space after the question.

The "drag and drop" type of question requires you to place the answer options in the correct order using the mouse to drag and drop them.

The NCSBN hasn't yet established a percentage of alternate-format items to be administered to each candidate. In fact, your examination may contain only a few of them. So relax; the standard, four-option, multiple-choice format questions constitute the bulk of the test.

NCLEX-RN TEST PLAN

All questions on the CAT NCLEX-RN adhere to a test plan, or blueprint. The NCLEX-RN draws questions from four categories of client needs that were developed by the NCSBN, the organization that sponsors and manages the NCLEX-RN. Client needs categories ensure that a wide variety of topics appear on every NCLEX-RN examination.

The NCSBN developed the client needs categories after conducting a work-study analysis of new RNs. All aspects of nursing care observed in the study were broken down into categories. (See *Client needs categories on NCLEX.*)

Categories were broken down further into subcategories. The four main client needs categories for the NCLEX-RN are:

- safe, effective care environment
- health promotion and maintenance
- psychosocial integrity
- physiological integrity.

Client needs categories and subcategories

The categories and subcategories are used to develop the NCLEX-RN test plan, which are the content guidelines for the distribution of test questions. The people who write the questions and put the NCLEX-RN examination together use the test plan and client needs categories to make sure that a full spectrum of nursing activities are covered in the NCLEX-RN. Client needs categories appear in most NCLEX-RN review and question-and-answer review books, including this one. The truth is, however, that as a test-taker you don't have to concern yourself with client needs categories. You'll see those categories for each question and answer in this book and on the CD-ROM, but they aren't identified on the actual NCLEX-RN.

An integrated examination

In nursing school, you may have had courses organized by the medical model. Courses were separated into such subjects as medical-surgical, pediatric, and psychiatric nursing. By contrast, the NCLEX-RN is integrated, meaning that different subjects are mixed together. As you answer the NCLEX-RN questions, you may encounter questions about clients (the NCLEX-RN term for patients) in any stage of life, from neonatal to geriatric. These clients may be of any background and may be completely healthy or extremely ill and have a variety of disorders.

The following processes are integrated into all Client needs categories of the NCLEX-RN Test Plan:

- caring
- communication and documentation
- teaching and learning.

Planning for success

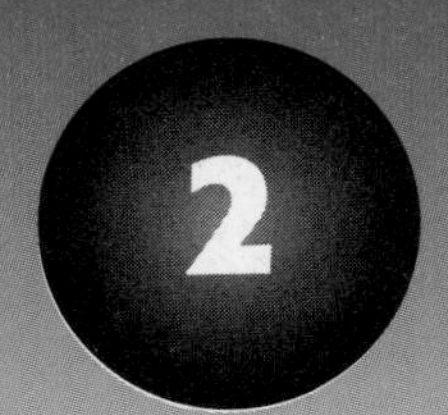

PREPARING FOR THE EXAMINATION

To prepare for the examination, you must study thoroughly, plan carefully, and master test-taking strategies. These tips can help ensure your success on the NCLEX-RN.

Create a good study plan

◆ You may know more about some topics than others. Identify topics you feel less secure about. Become well versed in all topics the examination is likely to cover. When you're done studying, you should feel well prepared in every topic area.

◆ Study when you're alert. Study the difficult topics when you're most alert and energized. Study for topics that only require some refreshing during times when you're less alert. (See *Finding the right study space.*)

◆ Set up a basic schedule for studying. Using a calendar or organizer, determine how much time remains before you'll take the NCLEX-RN and set up a schedule. Set realistic goals. However, make sure you set aside time for normal activities.

> **Finding the right study space**
>
> Having the right study space can be conducive to effective learning. Find a quiet, inviting study space that:
>
> ◆ is located in a convenient place, away from normal traffic patterns
>
> ◆ uses comfortable, soft lighting with which you can see clearly without eye strain
>
> ◆ has a temperature between 65° and 70° F
>
> ◆ contains flowers or green plants, familiar photographs or paintings, and easy access to soft instrumental background music
>
> ◆ doesn't have a television
>
> ◆ contains a solid chair that encourages good posture (avoid studying in bed – you'll be more likely to fall asleep and not accomplish your goals).

◆ Become familiar with all parts of a test question.

◆ Take a review course or organize a study group with others planning to take the examination.

◆ Ask a nursing instructor or colleague for help or clarification if you encounter material that's unfamiliar or difficult to understand.

Keep focused

When you're faced with reviewing the amount of information covered by the NCLEX-RN, it's easy to become distracted and lose your concentration. When you lose concentration, you make less effective use of valuable study time. To help stay focused, keep these tips in mind:

◆ Alternate the order of the subjects you study during the day to add variety. Try alternating between topics you find most interesting and those you find least interesting.

◆ Approach studying with enthusiasm, sincerity, and determination.

◆ After you have decided to study, begin immediately. Don't let anything interfere with your thought processes after you've begun.

◆ Concentrate on accomplishing one task at a time.

◆ Don't watch television or converse with friends while studying.

◆ Work continuously without interruption for a while, but don't study for such a long time that the whole experience becomes grueling or boring.

◆ Allow time for periodic breaks to give yourself a change of pace. Use these breaks to ease your transition into studying a new topic.

◆ When studying in the evening, wind down from your studies slowly. Don't move directly from studying to sleeping.

Take care of yourself

Don't neglect your physical and mental well-being in favor of studying longer hours. Maintaining your physical and mental health is critical for success in taking the NCLEX-RN. (See *Keeping yourself healthy.*)

Be prepared the day of testing

- Get a good night's sleep before the test.
- Eat a nutritious breakfast.
- Know your testing site location and arrive at least 20 minutes early.
- Wear comfortable clothing.
- Make hotel arrangements in advance if you must travel and stay overnight.
- Take your admission ticket and identification with you. You *must* present your Authorization to Test form, along with a valid form of identification with your signature and a recent photograph.
- Try to relax as much as you can but know that mild anxiety is normal.
- Be aware that a proctor will help you begin and will monitor security during the test.
- Know that the maximum time for the examination is 6 hours.
- Remember that the number of questions can range from 75 to 265. Of these questions, 15 are pretest questions that aren't scored.

ANSWERING NCLEX-RN QUESTIONS

NCLEX-RN questions are commonly long. As a result, it's easy to become overloaded with information. To focus on each question and avoid becoming overwhelmed, apply proven approaches to answer NCLEX-RN questions that include:

- determining what the question asks
- identifying relevant facts about the client described
- rephrasing the question
- choosing the best option.

Determine what the question asks

Read the question twice. If the answer isn't apparent, break it down into easier, less intimidating terms to help you focus more accurately on the correct answer.

For example, a question might be, "A 74-year-old client with a history of heart failure is admitted to the coronary care unit with pulmonary edema. He's intubated and placed on a mechanical ventilator. Which parameters should the nurse monitor closely to assess the client's response to a bolus dose of furosemide (Lasix) I.V.?" The options for this question — numbered 1 to 4 — include:

1. daily weight
2. 24-hour intake and output
3. serum sodium levels
4. hourly urine output.

> **Keeping yourself healthy**
>
> You can increase your likelihood of passing the NCLEX-RN by establishing these simple health rules:
>
> - Get plenty of rest – You can't think deeply or concentrate for long periods when you're tired.
> - Eat nutritious meals – Maintaining your energy level is impossible when you're undernourished.
> - Exercise regularly – Regular exercise helps you work harder and think more clearly. As a result, you'll study more efficiently, increasing the likelihood of success on the all-important NCLEX-RN.

Read the question again, ignoring all details except what's being asked. Focus on the last line of the question. It asks you to select the appropriate assessment for monitoring a client who received a bolus of furosemide I.V.

Identify the relevant facts

Sort out the relevant client information. Start by asking whether any of the information provided about the client isn't relevant.

For instance, do you need to know that the client has been admitted to the coronary care unit? Probably not; his reaction to I.V. furosemide won't be affected by his location in the hospital. Determine what you do know about the client. In the example, you know that:

- he just received an I.V. bolus of furosemide, a crucial fact
- he has pulmonary edema, the most fundamental aspect of the client's underlying condition
- he's intubated and placed on a mechanical ventilator, suggesting his pulmonary edema is serious
- he's 74 years old and has a history of heart failure, a fact that may or may not be relevant.

Rephrase the question

After you've determined relevant information about the client and the question being asked, consider rephrasing the question to make it clearer. Here's how you might rephrase it: "My client has pulmonary edema. He requires intubation and mechanical ventilation. He's 74 years old and has a history of heart failure. He received an I.V. bolus of furosemide. What assessment parameter should I monitor?"

The nursing process

The nursing process is a scientific method of applying nursing principles to client care. Understanding the different steps in the nursing process can help you determine which answer takes priority. Here's a list of common activities in nursing practice for each step of the nursing process.

Assessment: Gathering subjective and objective information about a client

- Collect information by reading hospital records and observing verbal and nonverbal interactions among the client, family, friends, hospital staff, and other reliable sources.
- Examine common data sources for information.
- Recognize symptoms and findings.
- Assess the client's ability to perform activities of daily living (ADLs).
- Assess the client's environment.
- Assess the client's knowledge of his health problem.
- Assess the nurse's reaction to the client.
- Confirm all observations and perceptions by gathering additional data.
- Monitor the client personally rather than relying solely on machines.
- Communicate gathered information to other team members.

Nursing diagnosis: Identifying real or potential health care needs and problems based on assessment findings

- Organize, interpret, and validate assessment data.
- Gather additional data when necessary.
- Identify and communicate nursing diagnoses to the health care team.
- Determine the client's needs and the staff's ability to meet them.

Planning: Establishing goals to meet client needs

- Include the client, family, friends, and other health team members in setting goals.
- Mutually establish goal priorities.
- Prepare a teaching plan appropriate for the client's ability.
- Anticipate the client's needs.
- Involve the client, family, friends, and other health care team members in developing care strategies.
- Document all information needed to manage the client's needs.
- Plan for the client's comfort and the maintenance of optimal functioning.
- Select the best nursing measures to deliver effective care.
- Identify community resources to assist the client and his family.
- Coordinate the client's care with other providers.
- Delegate care responsibilities to other providers.
- Formulate outcomes of nursing interventions.

Implementation: Carrying out actions that accomplish established goals

- Organize and manage the client's care.
- Perform or aid the client in performing ADLs.
- Provide comfort to the client.
- Help the client maintain optimal functioning.
- Teach the client and his family about the client's condition, treatment, and care, and provide other instruction as appropriate.
- Apply proper technique in giving client care.
- Initiate lifesaving measures in life-threatening emergencies.
- Provide care that enables the client to achieve self-care and optimal independence.
- Supervise and validate the activities of other health care team members.
- Document all appropriate information.

Evaluation: Measuring the success of goal achievement

- Compare actual outcomes with expected outcomes.
- Evaluate client compliance with the prescribed therapy.
- Record the client's response to care.
- Change the care plan, and reorder priorities as needed.

Choose the best option

After you develop a strategy by applying the above steps, choose the best option for the question being asked.

You know that the client received an I.V. bolus of furosemide, a diuretic. You know that monitoring fluid intake and output is a key nursing intervention for a client taking a diuretic, a fact that eliminates options 1 and 3 (daily weight and serum sodium levels), narrowing the answer down to option 2 or 4 (24-hour intake and output or hourly output).

You also know that the drug was administered by I.V. bolus, suggesting rapid effect. In fact, furosemide administered by I.V. bolus takes effect almost immediately. Monitoring the client's 24-hour intake and output would be appropriate for assessing the effects of repeated doses of furosemide. Hourly urine output, however, is *most* appropriate in this situation because it monitors the immediate effect of this rapid-acting drug.

USING KEY STRATEGIES

Regardless of the types of questions, there are four key strategies that will help you determine the correct answer for each question. Consider the nursing process, apply Maslow's hierarchy, consider patient safety, and consider verbal and nonverbal therapeutic communication.

Consider the nursing process

The nursing process steps include assessment, nursing diagnosis, planning, implementation, and evaluation:

- Remember that assessment comes before nursing diagnosis, which comes before planning, which comes before implementation, which comes before evaluation.
- If your question asks you to assess, you can immediately eliminate options that aren't assessment options.
- Clearly understand what the question is asking. Are you assessing? Implementing? Remember you must assess before you can diagnose. (See *The nursing process.*)

Apply Maslow's hierarchy

Following Maslow's hierachy of needs will help establish priorities:

- Physiologic needs are the most basic and the first need to be met.
- Safety and security, the second level of needs to be met, are followed by loving and belonging, then self-esteem, and finally self-actualization.
- Always satisfy the lowest-level need first.
- Always ask yourself, "Does this choice make sense for this client?" Eliminate choices, even those that might normally take priority, if they don't make sense for a particular client's situation. (See *Maslow's hierarchy of needs,* page 12.)

Consider patient safety

- Use patient safety criteria for situations involving laboratory values, drug administration, or nursing care procedures.

Consider verbal and nonverbal therapeutic communication

- Listen to the client.
- Try to understand the client's needs.
- Promote clarification and insight about the client's condition.

MORE TEST-TAKING HINTS

- Read case studies carefully. They contain information you'll need to answer the question correctly.
- Pay special attention to such words as *best, most, first,* and *not* when reading the question (stem). These words, which may be italicized, capitalized, or otherwise highlighted, usually provide clues to the correct response. For example, consider the question, "What should the nurse do *first?*" All of the listed options may be appropriate nursing actions for the given circumstances, but only *one* action can take top priority.
- Try to predict the correct answer as you read the stem. If your predicted answer is among the four options, it's probably the correct response.
- Read each question and all options carefully before making your selection or selections. Remember, some questions request that you select "all" appropriate answers.
- If two options seem equally correct, reread them; they must differ in some way. Also reread the stem. You may notice something you missed before that will aid your selection. If you're still unsure, make an educated guess. The computer won't let you skip a question.
- If the question asks for delegation, make sure that what you delegate to others is within their job descriptions. In general, don't delegate activities that involve assessment, evaluation, or nursing judgment.
- Choices that involve notifying the physician are usually incorrect. Remember, the NCLEX-RN wants to see you, the nurse, at work.
- Memorize common laboratory values so you can make an informed decision.
- Remain calm if a question focuses on an unfamiliar topic. Try to recall clients who have had problems similar to those in the question. Determine the nursing principles involved in your client's care and how they may apply to the test question. This may help you eliminate some options and may increase your chances of choosing the right answer.
- Take the necessary time for each question without spending excessive time on any one item. You'll have up to 6 hours to take the test. Pace yourself accordingly.
- Pay no attention to other candidates or the time they take to complete their tests. Because each test is individualized, some tests contain more questions than others.
- Take advantage of breaks during the test to give your mind and body a needed rest. The first optional break is given after 2 hours of testing and lasts 10 minutes. Candidates may take a second optional break ater 3½ hours of

Maslow's hierarchy of needs

Maslow's hierarchy of needs is a vital tool for establishing priorities on the NCLEX-RN. This list provides a description of what constitutes each stage. The stages are arranged from the most basic to the most complex.

NEED	DESCRIPTION
Physiologic needs	◆ Oxygen ◆ Food ◆ Elimination ◆ Temperature control ◆ Sex ◆ Movement ◆ Rest and comfort
Safety and security	◆ Safety from physiologic and psychological threat ◆ Protection ◆ Continuity ◆ Stability ◆ Lack of danger
Love and belonging	◆ Affiliation ◆ Affection ◆ Intimacy ◆ Support ◆ Reassurance
Self-esteem	◆ Sense of self-worth ◆ Self-respect ◆ Independence ◆ Dignity ◆ Privacy ◆ Self-reliance
Self-actualization	◆ Recognition and realization of one's potential growth, health, and autonomy

testing. All breaks count against testing time. Do some stretching exercises during breaks to help you relax.

Developing and following an organized study plan will provide the best assurance that you're fully prepared to succeed on the NCLEX-RN. Approach the test with confidence. Good luck, and congratulations on choosing nursing as a career!

Introduction to nursing fundamentals

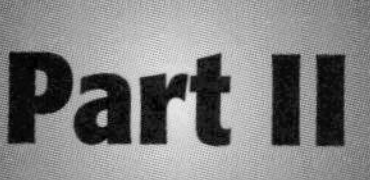

Part II

Nursing concepts and skills

3

FUNDAMENTALS: AN OVERVIEW

Nursing concepts and nursing skills are important in preparing for the NCLEX-RN. Use this chapter as the basis for your review of the patient care problems that will be covered in the remainder of this book. The basic nursing concepts and skills contained in this chapter are essential for your understanding and application of the information contained in the subsequent chapters.

Taking the NCLEX-RN is a daunting challenge, so some degree of apprehension is normal. By organizing your efforts into a well-planned review, you can channel your energy to decrease your anxiety and improve your preparation for passing this critical examination. Remember that every registered nurse (RN) has gone through this experience and survived — and you can, too!

NURSING CONCEPTS

Understanding critical nursing concepts is essential to effective nursing practice. These concepts include:

- nursing process
- nursing practice
- therapeutic communication
- growth and development
- family as the primary unit of health care
- rehabilitation
- grieving
- gerontologic nursing
- case management
- home health care
- infection control
- cultural and spiritual dimensions of care.

THE NURSING PROCESS

The nursing process — a scientific, systematic method of problem solving — forms the organizing framework for effective nursing practice. Using the nursing process in an ongoing, interactive way with the client assures a scientific approach to, and continuous monitoring of, the nursing care received. (See *Steps of the nursing process.*)

Five steps make up the nursing process:

- *Assessment* involves collecting data, establishing a comprehensive database, and recording subjective and objective data, including diagnostic test results.
- *Diagnosis* involves analyzing the data collected, identifying specific client needs, and establishing nursing diagnoses according to a prescribed format and nomenclature.
- *Planning and goal setting* involves planning for how to solve client problems according to priority and identify goals or client outcomes to measure the effectiveness of nursing actions. (Goal setting is a mutual activity performed by the nurse and the client.)
- *Implementation* involves nursing actions based on the plans that have been established to achieve the desired client outcomes and includes everything a nurse does to meet client needs, such as health promotion, administering treatments and medications, providing support and comfort to the client and family, documenting all client care, and compensating for the client's inability to perform certain activities as necessary. It also implies that the nurse understands the rationale for all nursing actions.
- *Evaluation* focuses on the effectiveness of care the client receives and includes a review of the extent to which the nursing process has met its goals. For goals achieved, no further action is necessary. For goals not achieved, the nurse retraces the nursing process steps to reassess the goals.

Steps of the nursing process

The nurse should proceed through the five steps of the nursing process, moving from assessment to evaluation. Depending on the evaluation findings, the nurse may update or change any of the previous steps.

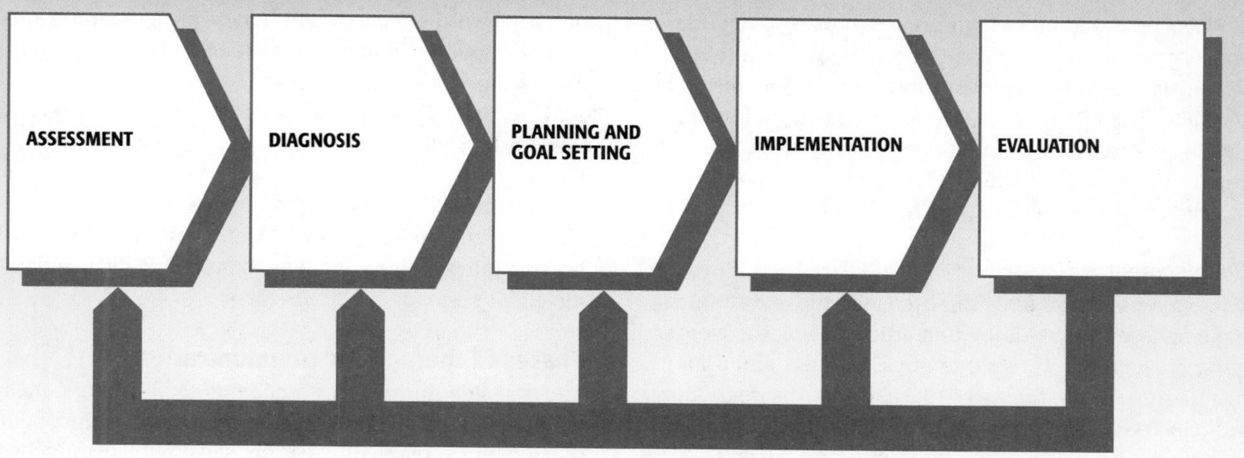

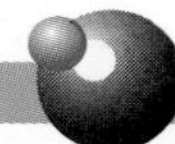

SPOT CHECK

Why is it important to follow the steps of the nursing process? What might happen if you were to perform an action, even one that appeared critical, without the preliminary steps of assessment, identification, and planning? Even in critical situations and emergencies that require rapid action, it's always essential to accurately assess what's happening with the client first – before taking action. Assessing the client's needs allows for identifying an appropriate nursing diagnosis and planning necessary, relevant interventions – keeping the focus on the most important factors, especially when time is so critical. Intervene only after taking these initial steps and you'll avoid worsening an already serious situation.

Nursing diagnosis: A critical part of the nursing process

The nursing diagnoses derived from the physical assessment and history data collected during the assessment step of the nursing process provide the basis for all subsequent nursing care.

Definition

A nursing diagnosis includes a clinical judgment about an individual, family, or community that has been reached through a deliberate, systematic process of data collection and analysis. The diagnosis provides the basis for prescribed, definitive therapy (for which the nurse is accountable) and concisely states the cause of the client's condition if the cause is known.

Components

A nursing diagnosis has these components:

- word or phrase about the degree or amount of change noted, indicated by such words as *deficient, disturbed, imbalanced, impaired, ineffective, interrupted,* or *dysfunctional*
- immediacy of the problem, commonly indicated by *acute* or *risk*
- tissue or system involved, such as skin, bowel, cerebral, or GI system
- type of problem, such as injury, nausea, or rape
- activity affected, such as mobility, coping, interaction, or home maintenance
- cause or etiology, indicated by *related to.*

A well-constructed nursing diagnosis, therefore, sets the direction for the client's care plans and goals and clearly relates:

- *priority.* The words *acute* and *risk* help the nurse and the client to prioritize goals. For example, *acute pain related to a stab wound to the chest* indicates the need to set an immediate goal that *the client will express a feeling of comfort and relief from pain.*

◆ *relation.* The initial nursing diagnosis should refer to the tissue or system most in need of corrective care. Thus, a client with a myocardial infarction warrants an initial nursing diagnosis related to the cardiac and circulatory systems.
◆ *client needs.* Another high-priority nursing diagnosis concerns the client's deficient knowledge related to the diagnosis, treatment regimen (including its benefits and risks), and self-care needs. Teaching related to these factors is an initial and ongoing nursing activity: as the client's treatment regimen proceeds, the condition changes, and the client regains independence.

Development

The efforts of many individuals created the current nursing diagnoses. Some of the first articles using the words *nursing diagnosis* were written by Chambers and Komorita and appeared in the early 1960s in the *American Journal of Nursing.* Others associated with nursing diagnoses include Ackley, Carpenito, Kim, McFarland, Sparks, Taylor, and Gordon, each of whom has published books on nursing diagnoses.

NANDA

The leading force in reviewing and developing new nursing diagnoses is North American Nursing Diagnosis Association (NANDA), whose membership includes nursing experts from the various nursing disciplines. Refer to the appendix piece, *NANDA Nursing Diagnoses,* which contains the most current list of nursing diagnoses approved by NANDA.

NANDA members meet yearly to review and refine established nursing diagnoses and develop new ones. NANDA bases its diagnoses on human response patterns of exchanging, communicating, relating, valuing, choosing, moving, perceiving, knowing, and feeling. Other nursing diagnoses are derived from functional health patterns, such as activity and exercise, elimination, nutrition and metabolism, sleep and rest, cognition, perception, and coping and stress tolerance.

The categories of nursing diagnoses consider the physical, social, emotional, cognitive, spiritual, cultural, and environmental sources of disequilibrium experienced by each client. A nursing diagnosis focuses on the client's health care needs, whereas a medical diagnosis focuses on the client's disease.

The nursing process offers a way of thinking related to nursing care. The nursing diagnosis forms a vital and integral part of that process to make each client's care specific and individualized.

THERAPEUTIC COMMUNICATION

Therapeutic communication has a purpose and is goal-directed. Nonverbal and verbal therapeutic communication enhances the client's self-esteem, self-worth, and ability to function. Verbal communication includes speech patterns, word selection, and honest presentation. Nonverbal communication includes touch, eye contact, facial expression, appearance, and gait.

The goals of therapeutic communication are directed toward the client's needs. The nurse should clarify the client's thoughts, feelings, and actions as well as explore new coping skills or behavior patterns. By utilizing the phases of therapeutic communication and focusing on nursing interventions and actions, the nurse can achieve the client's goal of self-discovery.

Phases of therapeutic communication

The first step in caring for a client is establishing a therapeutic relationship. Like other relationships, a therapeutic relationship is marked by caring, sensitivity, genuineness, and empathy. However, it also must be goal-oriented, purposeful, time-limited, and focused on the client's needs and growth. A therapeutic relationship evolves naturally into three distinct phases:
◆ *Orientation and initiation* establishes the initial introduction of client and nurse. Guidelines of this relationship are formed, roles are clarified, and the setting, frequency, and duration of the relationship are defined. (See *Characteristics of therapeutic and social relationships.*)
◆ *Working and continuation* involves dynamic interaction between the nurse and the client. The nurse assists the client to reach certain goals.
◆ *Termination and separation* involves the evaluation of the goals as met or unmet. The client is able to express his emotional state at this stage.

Focus of therapeutic communication

To be effective, therapeutic communication should be tailored to focus on the needs of the individual, group, and family.

Individual

Focusing on the individual needs of the client when communicating is particularly helpful. It encourages the client to concentrate on his feelings, thoughts, and actions and helps him develop valuable insight into his life. Therapeutic communication is especially effective when dealing with a client who is highly anxious or disorganized.

Characteristics of therapeutic and social relationships

In an effective nurse-client relationship, the nurse uses therapeutic communication to shed light on and promote healthy changes in the client's behavior. This chart contrasts important differences between a therapeutic relationship and a purely social one.

THERAPEUTIC RELATIONSHIP	SOCIAL RELATIONSHIP
◆ Focuses on the client, with the nurse giving and the client receiving	◆ Focuses on mutual sharing, with each participant giving and receiving
◆ Promotes client healing	◆ Promotes mutual pleasure
◆ Is time-limited	◆ Has no time constraints
◆ Involves a contract between nurse and client	◆ Doesn't involve a contract
◆ Requires the nurse to have a sound understanding of human behavior and to examine the nurse's and the client's behaviors from a theoretical perspective	◆ Doesn't require the participants to examine their behavior or possess a specialized knowledge base

Group

Communication should also emphasize the needs of the group, including coworkers and other staff. Communicating effectively as a group promotes efficiency and ensures continuity of care. For example, a nurse who has an emergency with one of her assigned clients must be able to relate the situation clearly and effectively to the staff, enabling another nurse to render assistance or to fill in where needed.

Staff meetings that enable group members to exchange information freely about client care and nursing practices also illustrate the way in which communication strategies help promote quality client care.

Family

The client's family must also be considered when providing therapeutic communication. Nurses have long recognized the effect that a client's physical and psychological needs have on the entire family (including significant others). Effective communication allows for identification of dysfunctional family situations, providing opportunities for individual family members to alter and improve communication patterns, define desired relationships, and clarify roles.

Therapeutic communication techniques

Much of communication involves spoken words which, when chosen thoughtfully and with the client's best interest in mind, can promote healing. (See *The communication continuum.*) However, many other aspects of communication (including nonverbal approaches) are often equally effective and crucial to the therapeutic nurse-client relationship.

Regardless of the specific communication technique used, nurses need to focus attention on the client and his needs. This includes:

The communication continuum

Words can help the nurse create a healing atmosphere. However, when poorly chosen, they can jeopardize nurse-client rapport and even harm the client's emotional well-being. Think of verbal communication as a continuum from destructive to constructive. Destructive communication can damage a client's self-esteem; constructive communication builds and preserves it.

DESTRUCTIVE COMMUNICATION	CONSTRUCTIVE COMMUNICATION
◆ Erodes self-esteem	◆ Promotes self-esteem
◆ Conveys disrespect	◆ Aids self-discovery
	◆ Conveys respect

Techniques that facilitate communication

These techniques can help facilitate communication between the nurse and the client. Each technique is listed along with its description and an example.

TECHNIQUE	DESCRIPTION	EXAMPLE
Silence	Refraining from speech to give the client (and nurse) time to sort out thoughts and feelings	*Client:* "I hate you and everyone else." The nurse remains silent, with her body in an open position, and observes the client.
Self-disclosure	Sharing personal information at an opportune moment to convey understanding	*Client:* "My husband's death was like losing a major part of my life." *Nurse:* "I had a similar feeling when my husband died."
Suggestion	Posing alternatives for client consideration	*Client:* "I won't see a shrink!" *Nurse:* "Have you ever thought about…?" *Client:* "I don't like that, either." *Nurse:* "What would happen if you…?"
Confrontation	Acknowledging discrepancies in the client's verbal and nonverbal behaviors; calling attention to evasions, distortions, smoke screens, and game playing	*Client:* "I don't have a problem with alcohol." *Nurse:* "You say that alcohol hasn't created any problems for you, yet you have had two DUIs and your wife nags you about your drinking."
Concreteness	Clarifying the meaning of the client's communication; being clear, direct, and to the point	*Client:* "They said…" *Nurse:* "Who said that?"
Genuineness	Giving honest feedback when the client is ready; acting in a congruent manner with the client	*Client:* "You look bored." *Nurse:* "I'm not bored, but I do feel very tired." *Client:* "Do you think I'm weird?" *Nurse:* "Sometimes."
Immediacy	Acknowledging what's occurring between the nurse and the client as it happens	*Client:* "I think I have the right to know as much about you as you know about me." *Nurse:* "It sounds as if you may not be too sure that I'll be able to understand what you're experiencing."
Empathy	Experiencing another's feelings temporarily	*Client:* "This whole thing is a mistake. I shouldn't even be here." *Nurse:* "It sounds as if it's difficult for you to be here."
Respect	Conveying openness, a nonjudgmental attitude, and a desire to hear what the client has to say	*Client:* "What difference does it make? You just think I'm wrong, anyway." *Nurse:* "Try me. I'd like to hear about what's been happening."
Reflection	Paraphrasing what the client has said	*Client:* "The cop was out to get me. He had no reason to pull me over. It was a real setup." *Nurse:* "You believe that it was unfair for the police to pull you over."
Broad opening	Using a general statement or question to encourage the client to set the direction for the session	The client enters the room, takes a seat, and looks expectantly at the nurse. *Nurse:* "How has it gone since we last met?" or "How are you today?"
Restating	Repeating what the client has said to indicate that the nurse is listening and interested; possibly encouraging the client to elaborate	*Client:* "I don't belong here." *Nurse:* "You don't belong here?" *Client:* "Of course not. I'm not like the others here. I'm educated and have a good job."
Focusing	Assisting the client to explore a specific topic	*Client:* "I don't know where to begin." *Nurse:* "What's your biggest problem now?" *Client:* "I can't decide about…" *Nurse:* "Let's talk about that. Perhaps more discussion will help you decide."

◆ noting the client's behavioral patterns
◆ responding in a way that enhances the client's self-esteem and functioning
◆ using active listening skills, such as maintaining open body posture; appearing alert, relaxed, and attentive; and gesturing appropriately (See *Techniques that facilitate communication.*)
◆ ensuring that communication is culturally sensitive, including demonstrating an awareness of appropriate eye contact, posture, and personal space
◆ avoiding role conflicts.

Of course, not all communication is therapeutic. Nurses must be especially aware of situations that can impede therapeutic communication and take measures to prevent it. (See *Nontherapeutic communication.*)

Nontherapeutic communication

Characteristics of nontherapeutic communication include:
◆ focusing on the caregiver
◆ giving advice, rather than seeking information
◆ changing the subject, rather than pursuing clarification or elaboration
◆ confronting the subject in an untimely or hostile manner
◆ failing to hear or acknowledge the client
◆ blaming the client, which suggests that the client is wrong
◆ using trite expressions or clichés or ignoring the problem
◆ talking more than listening
◆ focusing on why instead of what we can do now.

GROWTH AND DEVELOPMENT

Understanding the client's physical, cognitive, psychosocial, and nutritional status in relation to "normal" levels of growth and development is critical to nursing care. Various renowned psychiatrists, including Erikson and Piaget, developed theories that define personality and cognitive development. Their theories, along with other widely accepted integrated views addressing the physical, social, and nutritional aspects of health, help nurses to assess the client's maturity and overall level of functioning.

Erikson's theory of personality development

Erik Erikson postulated a theory of personality development that begins with Freudian theory but emphasizes the healthy aspects of personality development rather than the pathologic ones, building from predictable, age-related stages. Erikson describes key conflicts or core problems from which, after successful completion or mastery of one problem, the individual moves on to the next problem. Each conflict has a favorable and unfavorable component. No core problem is ever solved in its entirety. With each new situation, the core problem demands another resolution. (See *Psychosocial development,* pages 22 and 23.)

Piaget's theory of cognitive development

Jean Piaget developed the best known and most comprehensive theory regarding children's thinking, or *cognition.* The development of cognition represents a continuous and orderly process. Piaget postulated four major stages, each derived from and based on accomplishments of the previous stage.

The following information reviews psychosocial and cognitive development together with physical-motor and social-play development throughout the life span. Ages listed are approximate.

Sensorimotor: Birth to age 2

◆ The sensorimotor stage is one of simple learning.
◆ The child progresses from reflex activity to repetitive behavior, and then to imitative behavior.
◆ The child displays a high level of curiosity.
◆ The child begins to develop a sense of self as different and separate from the environment.
◆ The child learns that objects have permanence and existence even if they aren't visible.

Examples of this development are the emerging social smile and differentiated cry of the infant, progressing to the self-exploration of hands, then feet. The infant imitates patty-cake and then peek-a-boo, finally realizing that the hidden object is still there.

Preoperational: Ages 2 to 7

◆ The young child can't empathize.
◆ The child interprets objects and events solely in relationship to himself.
◆ The child can't make deductions or generalizations. Learning and thinking embrace only what the child sees, hears, feels, or experiences.
◆ The child begins elaborate concepts and "correct" experiences with increasing language skills, imaginative play, questioning, and interacting.
◆ Near the end of this stage, reasoning becomes intuitive and the child begins to work with problems of weight, length, size, and time.

Psychosocial development

This chart outlines key points for psychosocial development through the life span. It lists each developmental stage along with the psychosocial skills appropriate for that stage and possible nursing interventions.

DEVELOPMENTAL STAGE	PSYCHOSOCIAL SKILLS	NURSING INTERVENTIONS
Birth to age 1 Sense of trust versus mistrust	◆ Learns basic needs will be met ◆ Develops self-trust and trust in others ◆ Learns mistrust when care is inconsistent or basic needs are unmet	◆ Educate the parents on infant care techniques.
Ages 1 to 3 Sense of autonomy versus shame and doubt	◆ Focuses on autonomy (independence) and body control (trust) ◆ Gains physical and motor ability to be independent and can manipulate environment and others ◆ Holds on to or lets go such as with sphincter control ◆ Demonstrates uncertainty with gaining mastery and control as displayed by rituals, negativism, and temper tantrums	◆ Assess through family history the child's usual routine, physical security objects, and sensorimotor independence. ◆ Facilitate maximum consistency in the above areas. ◆ Assist caregivers in offering choices and in not chastising or shaming the child in response to negative behaviors. ◆ Accept and explain regressive behaviors in response to illness and stress.
Ages 3 to 6 Sense of initiative versus guilt	◆ Displays vivid imagination, magical thinking, sense of right and wrong ◆ Becomes increasingly aware of body parts ◆ Displays anxiety that gives rise to night terrors, fears of bodily mutilation, physical aggression, and acting out behaviors	◆ Provide a concrete explanation and demonstration of treatments and procedures. ◆ Provide the opportunity for acting out participatory play. ◆ Avoid threatening terminology, such as "cutting off," when referring to surgical procedures. ◆ Encourage outward expression of fear, anxiety, anger, and pain. ◆ Avoid labeling behavior as good or bad.
Ages 6 to 12 Sense of industry versus inferiority	◆ Becomes success-oriented worker and producer ◆ Aspires to be the best at everything, doesn't like to fail ◆ Gradually learns social skills of cooperation, compromise, negotiation, completion, and achievement ◆ Learns to play and live by rules ◆ Feels inadequate and inferior	◆ Promote activities that the child can complete independently. ◆ Foster the child's self-esteem by praising his achievements and appropriate behavior.
Ages 12 to 19 Sense of identity versus role diffusion	◆ Seeks to gain personal identity ◆ May demonstrate negativism, ritualism, and emotional lability, reflecting emotional turmoil evolving from body changes and the question, "Who am I?" ◆ Allows peers to influence decision making ◆ May experience role diffusion caused by unresolved answers to complex questions about adolescence	◆ Involve the adolescent in decision making as much as possible. ◆ Mutually set goals. ◆ Encourage active participation in implementing the care plan. ◆ Provide the supplies needed to enhance body image when possible. ◆ Impose as few limits as possible. ◆ Be aware of the effect of any threat to body image. ◆ Use therapeutic communication skills.

Psychosocial development *(continued)*

DEVELOPMENTAL STAGE	PSYCHOSOCIAL SKILLS	NURSING INTERVENTIONS
Ages 20 to 40 Sense of intimacy versus isolation	◆ Shares and forms commitments with other persons without fearing identity loss ◆ Focuses on individual needs, excluding all other interests, when intimacy isn't achieved	◆ Assess stresses and changes experienced. ◆ Provide teaching and resources to help the client maintain health. ◆ Be aware that, with hospitalization, the client may face loss of employment benefits, disrupted lifestyle, and decreased self-esteem. ◆ Be nonjudgmental about the client's needs and lifestyle. Don't impose personal attitudes.
Ages 40 to 65 Sense of generativity versus stagnation	◆ Helps the next generation become adults ◆ Assumes work, family, and community responsibilities ◆ If no responsibilities developed, client becomes egocentric, caring only about himself ◆ May not develop further if the above occurs	◆ Consider the stresses and responsibilities that are affecting the client. ◆ Assess a client in relation to these stresses. ◆ Provide resources and emotional support to the client, his family, and his friends.
Ages 65 and older Sense of integrity versus despair	◆ Reviews life events ◆ Displays satisfaction if content with his life ◆ Displays hopelessness and desperation if not content with his life	◆ Recognize physical and social changes and the limitations they may cause. ◆ Promote independence and use of skills the client retains. ◆ Stimulate functioning senses. ◆ Treat a client as an adult even if the client behaves as an adolescent or a child. ◆ Provide emotional support when needed for life events such as the deaths of friends and family.

Concrete operations: Ages 7 to 11

◆ Increasingly logical and coherent thoughts are present.
◆ The child can sort, classify, order, and organize facts about the world.
◆ The child collects and saves everything from stamps to crickets and toads.
◆ Although containers may differ, the child realizes that weight, volume, and number may be the same.
◆ Problem solving proceeds in a concrete manner.
◆ The child can handle several aspects of a situation at one time.
◆ Abstractions remain incomprehensible.
◆ The child can now recognize other points of view, as evidenced by a stronger desire for companionship and teamwork.

Formal operations: Ages 12 to 15

◆ The formal operations period is characterized by flexibility.
◆ The adolescent learns to deal with abstractions and abstract symbols.
◆ Arriving at answers, the adolescent may confuse the ideal world with the real world but can nevertheless solve problems, develop hypotheses, test them, and reach conclusions.
◆ The adolescent, working through moral, ethical, religious, and social issues, begins to achieve an adult identity.

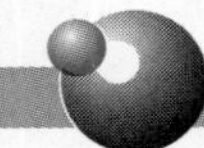

SPOT CHECK

According to Piaget, at which stage would an individual accomplish the following processes?

A. Learn that objects have permanence even when invisible
B. Learn to deal with abstractions
C. Interpret the world solely in relationship to himself
D. Learn to classify, sort, and organize

Answers:

A. Sensorimotor
B. Formal operations
C. Preoperational
D. Concrete operations

Physical-motor and social-play development

Normal physical and motor development is usually categorized by age level (although each person's development is ongoing and unique), and progress in one level may overlap another. Such overlap also occurs with social or play behaviors, which correspond with physical-motor developmental levels.

At some point during early middle-age, maximum physical strength and physiological functioning peak and the health continuum begins to slowly decline. No longer growing and developing, the body begins degenerating and displaying the normal characteristics of aging.

Birth to age 3 months

Physical-motor development

- At age 1 month, the infant's eyes follow bright, moving objects.
- At age 2 months, the crossed-eye reflex disappears.
- At age 3 months, a stimulus evokes a social smile response. The infant can rest on his forearms, keeps his head in midline, and discovers his hands and stares at them. The stepping reflex disappears and Landau reflex appears. Now able to lift his head and chest, the infant holds a rattle and stares at it and can follow moving objects with his eyes.

Social-play development

- The infant responds when a caregiver shakes a rattle or dangles a bright, moving object (such as a mobile).
- The infant also responds favorably to the caregiver's smiles, caresses, and speech. When the infant is awake, the caregiver should rock, pat, and play with the infant and change his position regularly.
- The infant usually reacts positively to a busy box and enjoys the freedom to kick.
- The infant expresses demands by crying, enjoys sucking, and reacts affectionately to all who approach.
- By age 3 months, the infant coos, babbles, gurgles, and laughs aloud; responds to his name; shows pleasure; and makes sounds and faces in reaction to the social play of others.

Ages 4 to 6 months

Physical-motor development

- The infant holds his head up for longer periods, displays improved eye coordination, and turns from his back to his side.
- At age 5 months, the infant can sit with support.
- At age 6 months, the infant can turn over completely.
- By age 6 months, birth weight doubles and the infant begins to turn his head toward familiar sounds.

Social-play development

- The 4-month-old infant recognizes his parents, demands attention by fussing, grasps objects with both hands, and shows excitement with his whole body.
- By age 5 months, the infant plays with his toes and smiles at a mirror image.
- At age 6 months, the infant holds out his arms to be picked up and shows definite likes and dislikes.

Age 6 months

Physical-motor development

- The 6-month-old infant can raise his chest and upper abdomen, keeping his weight on his hands.
- The infant can sit in a high chair with a straight back.
- The infant can turn from his back to his abdomen.
- The infant can hold a bottle or eat a cracker independently.
- The infant can grasp his feet and pull them to his mouth.
- Teething may begin.

Social-play development

- The infant may exhibit loud laughter.
- The infant demonstrates the ability to distinguish familiar and strange faces.
- The infant exhibits the desire to be picked up and held.
- The infant enjoys rattles and stuffed toys.
- The infant displays frequent mood swings.
- The infant begins imitating others (for instance, by coughing or sticking out his tongue).

Age 7 months

Physical-motor development

◆ The infant can sit and lean forward on his hands and can transfer objects from one hand to the other.

◆ The infant's upper central incisors typically erupt during this period.

Social-play development

◆ The infant begins to display a fear of strangers.

◆ The infant displays oral aggressiveness (biting), and he'll reject disliked foods by keeping his mouth closed.

Age 8 months

Physical-motor development

◆ The infant shows increased bowel and bladder regularity.

◆ The infant sits steadily.

◆ The infant releases objects at will.

◆ The infant exhibits a beginning pincer grasp.

Social-play development

◆ The infant shows his dislikes, such as for getting dressed or having a diaper changed.

Age 9 months

Physical-motor development

◆ The infant can typically pull to a standing position, and upper lateral incisors may erupt.

Social-play development

◆ The infant begins to exhibit a fear of being left alone.

Age 10 months

Physical-motor development

◆ Although crawling most of the time, the infant can step with one foot if supported by a person or an object.

◆ The infant has a neat pincer grasp but a crude release.

◆ New social-play behavior patterns emerge and others continue.

Social-play development

◆ Fear of strangers increases, and scolding elicits a strong reaction.

◆ The infant continues to imitate others (as when waving "bye-bye").

◆ The infant looks at and follows pictures in a book.

Age 11 months

Physical-motor development

◆ The child is creeping, with the abdomen off the floor.

◆ The child can stroll while holding on to a person or an object.

◆ The child can put objects into a container and remove them.

Social-play development

◆ The child also begins to drop objects deliberately — either to marvel at their sound or to gain the attention of others.

◆ During this period, the child begins to learn self-feeding and will help with dressing. Playing games, such as peek-a-boo, and shaking the head "no" are common.

Age 12 months

Physical-motor development

◆ The child's weight will have tripled from birth.

◆ The 1-year-old child can sit alone and can roll over.

◆ The child usually has eight teeth by the end of the first year.

◆ If not already evident, the child develops a fear of strangers and clings to the mother.

◆ The child can understand simple commands.

◆ The child can help with dressing and points to indicate desired objects.

Social-play development

◆ The child discriminates in giving affection and shows fear, anxiety, and sympathy.

◆ Having learned to repeat behaviors that elicit laughter, the child continues to imitate, wave "bye-bye," and shake his head "no."

Ages 10 to 14 months

Physical-motor development

◆ Creeping and crawling for locomotion, the child can pull up to a standing position independently and can stand for extended periods with support.

◆ By the end of this stage, the child is walking with a broad, stiff-legged gait.

Social-play development

◆ The child makes attempts at self-feeding with a spoon, poking and probing with the index finger, and develops a fondness for finger foods.

Ages 13 to 15 months

Physical-motor development

◆ The child likes to empty containers, fill boxes, and drop objects intentionally.

◆ The child can put a spoon to his mouth and drink from a cup.
◆ The child can hand objects to people.
◆ The child demonstrates the ability to creep upstairs; however, he can't come down. Attempts to back downstairs begin at 15 to 16 months.
◆ The child can build two-block towers and put a round peg in a round hole.

Social-play development
◆ The child wants to be with adults but also enjoys playing alone, exploring kitchen cupboards and imitating housekeeping duties.
◆ The child doesn't differentiate sex roles.
◆ The child displays a fondness for kissing pictures and mirrored reflections and asks for things by pointing and grunting.
◆ The child can remove his own shoes and perform self-feeding.
◆ The child wants and enjoys an audience and is capable of affection and sympathy, especially in the form of sympathetic crying.

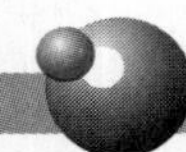
SPOT CHECK

At what age would a child begin to play with blocks?
13 to 15 months

Ages 16 to 24 months
Physical-motor development
◆ The child explores his entire physical world and is all over the house.
◆ The child falls less frequently.
◆ The child walks backward with a wide-based gait; walks forward and runs with a stiff, wide-based gait.
◆ The child stoops to pick up toys.
◆ The child can throw a ball and unzip zippers; loves to push, pull, tug, bang, carry, and hug toys; and can manage a spoon without rotation.
◆ By 15 to 18 months, the anterior fontanel closes.

Social-play development
◆ The child continues to play alone.
◆ The child is profoundly ritualistic and exerts control with temper tantrums.
◆ At 18 months, sphincter control begins. (The child controls adults through toileting.) The child likes to clean up messes, flush the toilet, run water, and put things in their place.
◆ The child uses push-pull, noisy toys; points to body parts on request; shows sustained interest; and imitates others.
◆ The child finds security in thumb-sucking or in a favorite blanket or toy; and becomes easily frustrated and angry.
◆ Personal identity begins, with differentiation between "you" and "me."

Age 2
Physical-motor development
◆ The child can put on his shoes and pants, wash and dry his hands, begin to use scissors and string large beads, and undress himself.
◆ The 2-year-old child tries to dance; pinches, kicks, hits, and bites; goes up and down steps one at a time; and can turn pages.

Social-play development
◆ Still ritualistic, the child engages in solitary and some parallel play; imitates older children; uses three-word phrases; is shy with strangers (negativism peaks at 24 months); develops fears of bedwetting, animals, and being deserted; may become a fussy eater; and displays slower growth.

Age 3
Physical-motor development
◆ The child can ascend steps with alternating feet, ride a tricycle, copy a circle, build a nine- to ten-cube tower, and perform self-feeding completely.
◆ The child's pulse rate is about 95 beats/minute; respiratory rate, about 24 breaths/minute; and blood pressure, 100/67 (±25) mm Hg.

Social-play development
◆ The child has developed a vocabulary of about 900 words, displays telegraphic speech, and constantly asks questions.
◆ The child knows his own sex and identifies with it, engages in parallel and associative play.
◆ The child can better tolerate brief separation from his parents or his primary caregiver.

Age 4
Physical-motor development
◆ The child hops on one foot, skips, catches a ball, throws overhand, uses scissors, and can lace (but not tie) his shoes.

Social-play development

◆ Questioning reaches a peak during this time, and exaggerated stories and mild profanity are typical.
◆ The child can't conceive that, although an object's shape may change, its mass remains the same; judges by one dimension (centering).
◆ The child has developing sense of right and wrong; identifies strongly with parent of opposite sex; and still experiences many fears.

Age 5

Physical-motor development

◆ The eruption of the child's permanent teeth may begin. The child jumps rope and can tie shoelaces.

Social-play development

◆ The child can identify coins and name at least four colors; knows the days of the week.
◆ The child engages in cooperative play, attempts to resolve fears and anxieties through play, and tries to be brave.
◆ The child is independent in self-care activities, such as bathing and dressing.

Age 6

Physical-motor development

◆ With increased activity, the child's appetite increases; plain food, snacking, and eating on the run are favored by the 6-year-old child.
◆ The child begins to dislike bathing.
◆ Possessing more poise and greater control of motor abilities, the child is in constant motion, practicing coordination of large and fine motor groups.

Social-play development

◆ Temper tantrums reappear at age 6.
◆ The child becomes more self-centered, boastful, and bossy.
◆ The child enjoys dramatic play to enact feelings and commonly is "fresh," rude, and ready to fight.
◆ The child develops fear concerning the supernatural, unusual noises, the mother's death, and any self-injury, and persistent night terrors are common.

Ages 7 to 9

Physical-motor development

◆ The child begins to lose baby teeth at age 6 to 7, with first molars coming in at around age 7.
◆ Physical-motor changes at ages 7, 8, and 9 are subtle, but the child develops better coordination of physical and motor skills and practices to achieve perfection.
◆ Less brisk and wiggly than at age 6, the child's movements are more fluid and graceful.

Social-play development

◆ During this time, the child is more likely to shout than act out.
◆ The child resists bathing less and shows little interest in clothes.
◆ The child prefers to play with the same sex; competes but doesn't like to lose; and withdraws from situations rather than resists.
◆ More contemplative than before, the child can be moved by sad stories and is becoming a real family member with chores and responsibilities.
◆ The gang stage begins; close relationships with peers begin to take shape.
◆ The child begins to collaborate and compromise; the major fear is failure.

Ages 10 to 12

Physical-motor development

◆ Rapid changes in height, weight, body contour, and physiology typically coincide with an increased appetite and awkwardness in motor ability.
◆ With rapid growth, the child begins to envision adulthood.
◆ Onset of secondary sex characteristics occurs in some boys.
◆ Girls can no longer compete with boys in physical strength.
◆ The child requires an adequate explanation of body changes, and one who lags behind in physical development needs special understanding as he compares body changes with those of classmates and friends.

Social-play development

◆ During this stage, girls usually seem wiser and more poised than boys.
◆ For both sexes, companionship becomes more important than play as a social behavior. Club membership and teamwork play increasingly significant roles, although the sexes tend to remain separated.
◆ The child likes to run errands, enjoys crafts and music, and seeks others' ideas and opinions.

Ages 13 to 16

Physical-motor development

◆ The early teenager may be awkward and uncoordinated, with poor posture, and may tire easily because heart and lung growth doesn't keep pace with that of the rest of the body.
◆ Although the adolescent has a large appetite, a preference for fast foods and fad diets can lead to poor nutrition and lethargy.
◆ Physiologic problems that concern the teenager include acne, increased perspiration, and a propensity to blush easily.
◆ The teenager develops a full growth of pubic and axillary hair.

Social-play development

◆ The adolescent likes parties, dances, movies, daydreaming, telephone conversations, books, and hobbies.
◆ The peer group becomes extremely important.
◆ While beginning to become emancipated from the parents, the adolescent develops crushes on or attachments to neighbors or teachers.
◆ The adolescent typically shows increased interest in the opposite sex, and strong friendships develop with one or two friends.
◆ Concerns embrace morality, ethics, religion, and social customs.
◆ The adolescent requires help in adjusting to and accepting body changes.

Ages 17 to 19

Physical-motor development

◆ A young man has a beginning beard, his structural growth is near completion, and his physique is that of a mature male, including genital size and pubic hair.
◆ A young woman may grow 2″ to 4″ taller after menarche; breasts and pubic hair have reached adult development, and she's capable of reproduction about 1 year after menses begin.
◆ Both the young man and the young woman have more energy as the growth spurt slows.

Social development

◆ The young adult is more mature and begins to enjoy an interdependent relationship with the parents while finding increasingly less satisfaction from the peer group.
◆ Learning to balance pleasure and responsibility, the young adult engages in romantic love affairs and may still daydream about adult life but also begins to establish career goals and plans how to achieve them.

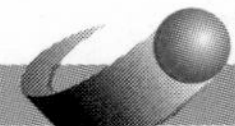

FAST FACT

As an adolescent passes into the 17- to 19-year-old age-group, parents may need assistance facing the loss of their dependent child.

Ages 20 to 30

Physical-motor development

◆ Physical strength and physiologic reserve are at a maximum, and the person's health needs usually aren't significant.

Social development

◆ Body image and sexuality are extremely important during this time.
◆ Selection of a marriage partner — and perhaps the decision to have children — commonly occurs.
◆ Marriage and parenthood necessarily entail periods of adjustment fraught with increased stresses, such as changing one's lifestyle to accommodate children and socializing the children into the family.
◆ Optional lifestyles (celibacy, childless marriage, single parenthood, homosexuality, communal living) may also develop; each has inherent stresses and periods of adjustment, compromise, and change.

Ages 30 to 40

Physical-motor changes

◆ As physical strength, physiologic reserve, and systemic functioning begin to diminish, proper nutrition becomes more important.
◆ The person requires fewer fats and calories in the diet and may require more vitamins and iron.
◆ Exercise is essential to regulate appetite, release tension, enhance rest and sleep, increase muscle tone, and improve well-being.

Social development

◆ Choice of vocation and career successes and failures largely determine the person's social status and roles.
◆ Unemployment or unsatisfying employment may lower self-esteem.
◆ Hectic schedules and limited income during this phase may contribute to an unhealthful diet.
◆ To attain career goals, the person may work or worry excessively at the expense of needed sleep and relaxation.

Ages 40 to 65

Physical-motor changes

◆ Physical strength, physiologic reserve, and systemic functioning continue to diminish, mandating a low-calorie, high-vitamin diet with limited saturated fat.
◆ Exercise is still important but should be less strenuous.
◆ During this stage, the person may have concerns about stiff joints, wrinkles, gray hair, baldness, dentures, poor hearing or vision, menopause, osteoporosis, nervousness, or depression.
◆ Angina and coronary occlusion, cancer, hypertension, peptic ulcer, and (if the person smokes) respiratory disease are common.
◆ Stresses during this phase may lead to substance abuse or insomnia.
◆ Sexual problems may also develop; mutilating surgery, chronic disease, or menopause can dramatically lower the person's self-esteem, particularly if the sexual partner doesn't provide emotional support.

Social development

◆ Assuming more significant and varied roles at this stage than at any other stage in the life span, the adult is now responsible not only for the self, spouse, and children but for parents, coworkers, and community members.
◆ As children grow up and begin their own families, the adult in this stage may need to rethink goals and consider lifestyle changes. The empty-nest syndrome may occur, causing depression.
◆ A woman sometimes sees this period as an opportunity to continue education and enter or resume a career; a man may need to prepare for a second vocation.

Age 65 and over

Physical-motor changes

◆ Physical strength, physiologic reserve, and systemic functioning continue to decline.
◆ Hearing and vision loss may be more pronounced, and cataracts may require surgery. Other common geriatric problems include immobility, constipation, indigestion, arteriosclerosis, stroke, peripheral vascular disease, hypertension, coronary occlusions, and cancer.
◆ A man may have benign prostatic hypertrophy or experience the climacteric.
◆ A woman may have osteoporosis, resulting in bone fractures.
◆ The elderly person may have multiple chronic illnesses, with accompanying exacerbations and remissions.
◆ Prolonged bed rest proves highly detrimental during this stage — lack of exercise can impair digestion, circulation, muscle and joint function, and mental alertness.
◆ Decreased sensitivity of taste buds and olfactory receptors typically causes the elderly adult to overseason foods (high blood pressure is a major concern).
◆ Exercise, although important, must be tailored to individual needs.

Social development

◆ Having worked hard to achieve career goals, the elderly adult wants to enjoy the carefree leisure of retirement.
◆ Pursuing hobbies, spending time with family and friends, and participating in community events can provide enjoyment and satisfaction.
◆ The new lifestyle usually means living on a fixed income; thus, the person with an inadequate income worries about the present and the future and may live with other persons on fixed incomes simply to make ends meet.
◆ Declining health and the loss of family and friends can result in grieving, loneliness, and depression during this stage, and some persons withdraw from society (disengagement).
◆ Because reconciliation is important to many elderly adults, misunderstandings may be forgotten and relationships improved.

Nutrition and energy needs

Nutrition is the process by which foods are selected and ingested and their nutrients are absorbed and used by the human body. Foods contain the nutrients and energy that the body requires for growth, activity, and health promotion and maintenance. The essential nutrients are:
◆ carbohydrates
◆ lipids
◆ protein
◆ vitamins and minerals
◆ water.

Carbohydrates

Carbohydrates occur mainly as sugars, starches, and fiber; all carbohydrates must be modified to simple sugars before the body can absorb and use them. The body requires at least 100 grams of carbohydrates daily because the central nervous system needs a constant supply of glucose. Ideally, 50% to 60% of total calories should be carbohydrates.

Sugars and starches

Sugars and starches provide the body with its primary source of energy. Glucose, also called blood sugar, is the form in which carbohydrates circulate in the bloodstream, providing energy to individual cells. Although glucose is an energy source for the brain, consuming foods with added sugars may be harmful. New dietary guidelines suggest avoiding foods that contain added sugars.

Lipids

Chemically similar to carbohydrates and commonly known as *fats,* lipids provide the most concentrated source of energy for the body. Linoleic acid, the essential fatty acid, must be obtained from dietary sources and is necessary for normal growth of infants. In addition to serving as an energy source, dietary fats carry fat-soluble vitamins, cushion vital body organs, insulate the body, and add a feeling of fullness and satisfaction at the completion of a meal.

Fat requirements

Ideally, fats should be limited to 22% to 29% of total calories. In choosing dietary fats, consider the benefits of fish (such as mackerel or tuna) that contain omega-3 fatty acids and oils (such as peanut, canola, or olive oil) that contain monounsaturated fatty acids. Both groups of fatty acids help reduce the risk of coronary heart disease.

Protein

Protein is the building block of all body cells. It's broken down by the body into its individual components, amino acids.

Amino acids

Essential amino acids can't be made by the body and must be obtained from food. Nonessential amino acids can be synthesized within the body. The principal function of protein is to provide the amino acids needed for growth and the formation of enzymes, hormones, antibodies, muscles, hemoglobin, and other body tissues.

Protein requirements

The adult requirement for protein is 0.8 g/kg of ideal body weight. Protein is 16% nitrogen. In a healthy adult (except one who's pregnant or lactating), nitrogen intake equals nitrogen output. With disease, tissue wasting occurs, and nitrogen losses exceed nitrogen intake; this negative nitrogen balance ceases when tissue repair begins. Insufficient protein intake can compromise the immune system, impairing the body's response to stress and infection.

Vitamins and minerals

Vitamins are needed daily in small quantities to sustain growth and health; they're classified as water-soluble or fat-soluble. (See *Reviewing selected vitamins.*)

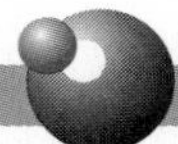

SPOT CHECK

Match the vitamin deficiency with the appropriate vitamin or nutrient.

Vitamin	**Clinical deficiency**
1. Vitamin A (retinol)	A. Hemorrhage
2. Vitamin B_1 (thiamine)	B. Scurvy
3. Vitamin B_2 (riboflavin)	C. None identified
4. Vitamin B_6 (pyridoxine)	D. Leg cramps
5. Vitamin C	E. Rickets
6. Vitamin D (cholecalciferol)	F. Mouth lesions
7. Vitamin E (tocopherol)	G. Night blindness
8. Vitamin K (menadione)	H. Pellagra
9. Niacin	I. Pernicious anemia
10. Folic acid	J. Slow growth
11. Vitamin B_{12} (cyanocobalamin)	K. Skin lesions

Answers: 1-G, 2-D, 3-F, 4-K, 5-B, 6-E, 7-C, 8-A, 9-H, 10-J, 11-I

Minerals are inorganic elements that help with many vital body functions and give the body its structural strength and rigidity. (See *Reviewing selected minerals,* page 33.)

Water

Water, essential to sustain life, transports nutrients throughout the body and may contribute minerals when consumed. Water has no calories, fat, caffeine, or cholesterol; therefore, it's the best fluid to consume under normal circumstances.

To maintain fluid balance, a person's daily fluid intake should equal fluid output. On average, an adult loses about 1,450 to 2,800 ml of water daily from sensible and insensible losses. Roughly speaking, an adult needs 1 to 1.5 ml of water per calorie consumed. So someone who consumes 2,000 calories daily needs a total fluid intake of 2,000 to 3,000 ml. Of this, at least 60% should be consumed as water, with the remainder obtained from foods and metabolism.

Food selection guidelines

Individual food preferences are influenced not only by the taste and odor of specific foods but also by the availability of foods, family economic status, cultural and religious preferences and restrictions, and the food purchaser's

Reviewing selected vitamins

This chart lists common vitamins along with their major functions, primary sources, clinical deficiencies, and adverse effects when taken at toxic doses.

VITAMIN	MAJOR FUNCTIONS	PRIMARY SOURCES	CLINICAL DEFICIENCIES	TOXICITIES
Water-soluble vitamins				
Vitamin C	Collagen formation, wound healing, resistance to stress and infection, blood vessel elasticity	Citrus fruit, strawberries, broccoli, cabbage, green peppers	Easy bruising, bleeding gums, delayed wound healing, scurvy	GI upset, diarrhea, renal calculi
Thiamine (B_1)	Carbohydrate metabolism, nerve transmission	Pork, peanuts, whole grains	Poor appetite, leg cramps, depression	None
Riboflavin (B_2)	Carbohydrate, protein, and fat metabolism; normal appetite	Milk, meat, wheat germ	Mouth lesions, scaly skin, glossitis	None
Niacin	Carbohydrate, protein, and fat metabolism; healthy skin	Meat, peanuts, whole grains	Pellagra, dermatitis, diarrhea, depression	Flushing, tingling, vision disturbances
Pyridoxine (B_6)	Amino acid synthesis, fatty acid metabolism	Meat, whole grains, nuts	Skin lesions, depression, seizures	None
Folic acid	Nucleic acid synthesis, amino acid breakdown, red blood cell (RBC) formation	Green, leafy vegetables; asparagus; broccoli	Slow growth, megaloblastic anemia	None
Cyanocobalamin (B_{12})	Formation of nucleic acids, bone marrow, and RBCs	Meat, eggs, fish	Pernicious anemia, nervousness, weakness	None
Fat-soluble vitamins				
A (retinol)	Normal vision and growth, healthy epithelium, aid to reproduction	Dark green and yellow fruits and vegetables, margarine and butter, whole milk and cheeses	Night blindness; thickened, cracked skin; poor growth; reduced resistance to infection	Skin rashes, hair loss, vomiting, abnormal bone growth, increased intracranial pressure
D (cholecalciferol)	Absorption and utilization of calcium and phosphorus, bone matrix formation	Sunlight, fortified milk	Rickets (in children), osteomalacia (in adults)	Elevated serum calcium, kidney damage, growth retardation, vomiting, diarrhea

(continued)

Reviewing selected vitamins *(continued)*

VITAMIN	MAJOR FUNCTIONS	PRIMARY SOURCES	CLINICAL DEFICIENCIES	TOXICITIES
Fat-soluble vitamins *(continued)*				
E (tocopherol)	Antioxidant (protects cell membrane)	Vegetable oils, margarine, nuts, whole grains	None	Headache, nausea, fatigue, dizziness, blurred vision
K (menadione)	Blood clotting (prothrombin formation)	Intestinal bacteria (synthesize adequate vitamin K)	Hemorrhage	Excessive breakdown of RBCs (synthetic form)

knowledge of nutrition. Several guidelines have been developed to help individuals plan and evaluate food intake.

Dietary guidelines for Americans

Dietary Guidelines for Americans were revised in 2005 by the Department of Health and Human Services and the U.S. Department of Agriculture (USDA). These guidelines emphasize health improvement by adhering to diets that provide all of the nutrients needed for growth and health. The key recommendations include:

- consuming a variety of nutrient-dense foods and beverages within the basic food groups
- choosing foods that limit the intake of saturated and trans fats, cholesterol, added sugars, salt, and alcohol
- balancing recommended intakes with energy needs by adopting an eating plan, such as the USDA Food Guide or the DASH eating plan. (Meeting nutrient recommendations must go hand-in-hand with keeping calorie intake under control.)

Specific populations

The new guidelines also offer key recommendations for specific populations:

- People over age 50 should consume vitamin B_{12} in fortified foods or supplements.
- Women of childbearing age who may become pregnant should eat foods high in iron along with a food that increases the absorption of iron such as those rich in vitamin C.
- Women of childbearing age who may become pregnant and those in the first trimester of pregnancy should consume adequate amounts of synthetic folic acid daily in addition to varied foods that contain folate.
- Older adults, people with dark skin, and people exposed to insufficient ultraviolet band radiation (such as that found in sunlight), should consume extra vitamin D from fortified foods or supplements.

Energy needs and balance

Energy is required for basal metabolism — ongoing internal processes, such as respiration, heartbeat, and glandular activity.

Basal metabolic rate

The basal metabolic rate (BMR) is the rate at which the body burns calories at rest. It's influenced by sex, age, body composition, and physiologic status.

Energy value of foods

The energy value of foods is measured in kilocalories, commonly known as *calories.* Calories come from carbohydrates, fats, and protein (the only nutrients that supply calories):

- Carbohydrates and protein each provide 4 calories per gram; fats provide 9 calories per gram.
- Carbohydrates and fats are the preferred energy sources, leaving protein for its important role in tissue maintenance.
- In addition to basal metabolism, calories are necessary for physical activity and for the 10% increase in BMR that occurs after eating.

When the number of calories consumed matches the number used for energy, an individual achieves energy balance. Calories in excess of energy needs are stored as fat in the body's adipose tissue. If insufficient calories are consumed, weight loss occurs.

Reviewing selected minerals

This chart lists common minerals along with their major functions, primary sources, and clinical deficiencies.

MINERAL	MAJOR FUNCTIONS	PRIMARY SOURCES	CLINICAL DEFICIENCIES
Calcium	Bone and tooth formation, blood clotting, muscle contraction, transmission of nerve impulses, normal heart rhythm	Milk, cheese, yogurt, broccoli, collards, kale, greens, canned salmon with bones	Osteoporosis, slow blood clotting, tetany, poor tooth formation
Phosphorus	Bone and tooth formation, carbohydrate and fat metabolism, pH buffer systems	Cheese, meat, milk and milk products, carbonated beverages	Osteoporosis, slow blood clotting, tetany, poor tooth formation
Magnesium	Carbohydrate, fat, and protein metabolism; adenosine triphosphate formation; nerve transmission; muscle contraction	Grains, green vegetables, milk, meat	Fluid and electrolyte imbalance, skin breakdown
Sodium	Fluid balance, nerve transmission, muscle contraction	Table salt, processed and preserved foods, milk and dairy products, protein foods	Headache, nausea, muscle spasm, mental confusion, fluid and electrolyte imbalance, cardiac disturbances, hypertension, edema
Potassium	Fluid balance, muscle activity	Widespread in all food groups, especially fruits and vegetables	Fluid and electrolyte imbalance, muscle weakness, tachycardia, cardiac arrhythmia, renal failure, severe dehydration
Trace elements			
Iron	Hemoglobin formation (as component of myoglobin)	Meats, whole grains, dried fruit, legumes	Iron deficiency anemia
Iodine	Regulation of basal metabolic rate (as component of thyroxin)	Iodized salt, saltwater fish	Goiter
Zinc	Protein synthesis, normal growth and sexual maturation, wound healing, normal senses of taste and smell, enzyme formation	Meats, legumes, nuts	Slow wound healing, altered senses of taste and smell, poor growth, delayed sexual development
Fluoride	Strengthening of tooth enamel	Fluoridated drinking water, fluoride supplementation	50% to 70% increase in tooth decay

Undernutrition and overnutrition

Resulting from a sustained deficit in nutrient intake, undernutrition depletes stored protein and compromises the immune system. Overnutrition leaves an individual vulnerable to the toxic effects of nutrient overdoses as well as to excess weight gain with associated health risks.

Nutrition requirements through the life cycle

Nutrition requirements vary among individuals, depending primarily on the person's age, state of health, and activity level.

Infant

An infant's nutritional needs are greater than those of any other age-group; for example:

◆ Protein and fluid needs are two to three times greater than those of an adult.

◆ Breast milk or formula alone is satisfactory for the first 5 to 6 months of life, at which time solid foods should be incorporated into the daily diet.

Childhood and adolescence

Childhood and adolescence are characterized by growth spurts that demand a gradual increase in intake of all nutrients. Snacking, commonly thought to be a problem, can contribute significantly to nutritional quality, particularly in adolescent years.

Adults

Nutritional needs of most adults under age 65 remain largely unchanged, with two exceptions:

◆ Caloric and iron requirements generally decrease.

◆ Pregnancy and lactation warrant special attention:

– Sound nutritional practices during pregnancy usually lead to a higher birth weight.

– Daily nutritional needs during pregnancy include increases in calories (+300) and iron (+15 mg); protein intake increases to 60 g/day and calcium to 1,200 mg/day.

– The need for folic acid doubles during pregnancy and usually requires a vitamin supplement.

– A weight gain of 24 to 30 lb (11 to 14 kg) is recommended, although a gradual gain over the last two trimesters is more important than the total amount gained.

– Lactation requires an additional 2 quarts (2 L) of fluid daily to prevent dehydration and to produce an adequate milk supply.

Adults older than age 65

For those over age 65, adequate protein to maintain the immune system and muscle strength becomes increasingly important:

◆ Vitamin D requirements increase for an older adult.

◆ Energy needs may be lower because of gradual decreases in basal metabolism.

◆ Fluid needs are especially critical in this age-group; because of a lost sense of thirst, many older adults fail to recognize the thirst mechanism and are prone to dehydration.

FAMILY: THE PRIMARY UNIT OF HEALTH CARE

The family is the basic social unit — the primary unit of health care. Although not all families include the traditional functional unit of husband, wife, and children (American nuclear family), they generally share the same common characteristics:

◆ usually loving, affectionate relationships

◆ long-term associations

◆ consideration of members as unique individuals.

Function of families

Families also have common functions, including:

◆ care and rearing of children

◆ transmission of cultural values, traits, and rituals from one generation to another

◆ socialization

◆ provision of food, shelter, clothing, safety, and comfort

◆ communication and decision making.

Types of families

There are several types of families, including:

◆ beginning nuclear (husband and wife)

◆ single parent

◆ nuclear (husband, wife, and minor children)

◆ extended (three or more generations forming a kinship network)

◆ blended (parents with unrelated children of previous relationships brought together)

◆ expanded (various age or kinship groups or unrelated family members)

◆ communal (formed for specific ideologic or societal purposes; may comprise nuclear, extended, or expanded family units).

Developmental tasks and stages

Evelyn Duvall's theory of family development focuses on the tasks of the family unit and the characteristics and needs of the family at different stages in the life cycle. These stages are marked by the growth of members (expanding family) or loss of individual members (contracting family) and by their needs and ability to function as a unit.

Developmental tasks

Families function as a basic unit as well as a system within a larger society. Developmental tasks of a family include:

- physical maintenance of the family unit
- allocation of resources
- division of labor
- socialization of family members
- reproduction or recruitment and release of family members
- maintenance of order
- placement of members into the larger society
- maintenance of motivation and morale.

Expanding family stages

An expanding family is one in the stages between marriage and parenthood and the time when children leave home. The family typically grows and develops increasingly complex relationships during the following stages:

- childless couple establishing first home
- expectant family or childbearing family (from first pregnancy through the first 30 months of the child's life)
- family with preschool children
- family with school-age children
- family with teenagers.

Contracting family stages

During these stages, the family unit typically decreases, becoming less complex but with different needs:

- family with young adults
- middle-age parent family
- aging family.

Family assessment data

Nurses must gather sufficient information about the client and other family members in order to meet the client's needs. This includes asking about:

- family constellation (names, relationships, ages, sexes)
- education levels
- occupations
- communication patterns
- finances
- residences
- transportation needs
- family goals and functioning
- typical daily activities
- religious preferences
- avocation and recreational interests
- health resources
- strengths and coping mechanisms
- weaknesses and problems
- goals.

REHABILITATION

Rehabilitation is the restoration of a person to an optimal level of functioning in the physical, mental, spiritual, and social aspects of life. The short-term goals of rehabilitation include regaining mobility, retaining remaining abilities and, when possible, preventing further incapacity or disability. The long-term goals of rehabilitation include returning to a normal capacity. Factors affecting rehabilitation include:

- severity or extent of injury (loss of some or all nerve pathways, muscles, bones, or circulation to a portion of the body)
- treatment and facilities (immediacy, adequacy, and continuity of medical, surgical, nutritional, and pharmacologic treatments)
- client's age, education, and psychological response to injury (all of which influence the client's ability to understand and participate in rehabilitative efforts)
- health care personnel (those skilled in various disciplines to develop and administer a rehabilitation program)
- financial resources (to pay for the facilities, treatments, and personnel services required for rehabilitation)
- legislation (to protect the rights of clients requiring rehabilitation).

Initiating therapy

Regaining and retaining the client's mobility involves initiating various therapies, including exercise, heat or cold treatment, and use of ambulatory and respiratory aids as well as genitourinary (GU) and speech therapy. Additionally, the client may require occupational, physical, and nutritional therapy that helps to restore his ability to perform such tasks as activities of daily living (ADLs).

Activities of daily living

ADLs include the abilities to:

- breathe

- dress, feed, bathe, move and transfer oneself
- eliminate
- communicate.

Exercise

Exercise works muscles and joints, allowing the client to regain mobility. It typically requires time and repetition to help the client regain or increase muscle tone, strength, and precision. The client may need the help of various therapists, family members, nurses, or other health care personnel to exercise, depending on his needs and the level of expertise required to perform the regimen.

Forms of exercise include:

- active exercise (performed by the client)
- active-assisted exercise (performed by the client with therapist assistance)
- resistive-active exercise (performed by the client with resistance provided by weights or devices)
- passive exercise (performed without the client's active participation)
- selective or special exercise (individualized to meet a client's needs to exercise a particular group of muscles for particular activities — for example, breathing exercises).

Heat or cold therapy

Heat or cold therapy must be intermittent to allow for tissue recovery. (Clients with impaired circulation have decreased tolerance for heat or cold therapy.) This therapy may also:

- be moist or dry
- involve short-term or long-term application for vasoconstriction or vasodilation.

Ambulatory aids

The client may need an ambulatory aid during rehabilitation. Such aids include:

- walkers, which are lightweight, foldable, height-adjustable devices that assist with weight bearing or mobility (The client must be cautioned about the safe degree of weight bearing and must be taught to turn, sit, or stand to prevent falls and injury.)
- crutches, which can be wood or aluminum; axillary-supported or forearm-supported; with two-, three-, or four-point gaits (The client must learn to walk, sit, rise, and go up and down stairs with one or both crutches.)
- canes, which can be wood or metallic supports with one-, three-, or four-point bottoms (If using only one cane, the client should hold it in the hand *opposite* the affected leg.)
- wheelchairs, which can be metal or wood and metal, with detachable arm or leg rests, straps, and other supports and may be battery-operated or manually pushed (The client must learn to transfer correctly from the chair to a bed, car, and home.)
- braces, which can be cloth, foam, or metallic supports for one or more joints (may be worn continuously or intermittently)
- utensils, which are aids used by disabled clients (such as handles that may be lengthened, enlarged, swiveled, hinged, or otherwise adapted for individual need).

Respiratory aids

Respiratory aids include:

- postural drainage to increase excretion of respiratory secretions
- incentive spirometry to improve respiratory ventilation
- machine-assisted breathing apparatus to increase respiratory depth and prevent atelectasis.

Genitourinary rehabilitation

GU rehabilitation may include:

- continuous bladder catheterization
- self-catheterization and bladder training
- bowel-training programs
- penile prosthesis to help maintain an erection
- sexual counseling to help the client cope with necessary adjustments.

Speech rehabilitation

Speech rehabilitation may include:

- speech therapy to relearn the language or alternate speech methods
- mechanical speech-amplifying aids.

Occupational therapy

The client may require occupational therapy for:

- home management, such as preparation, assistance, and learning
- craft preparation and education for muscle use
- occupational retraining of muscles, joints, and the entire body.

Physical therapy

Physical therapy may be needed to provide:

- specialized retraining for muscle use or muscle substitution to regain or maintain muscle strength
- assistance in any of the previous rehabilitation techniques.

Nutritional therapy

Nutritional therapy may include:

- ◆ individualized dietary teaching for a client with a modified diet (high- or low-calorie, high-vitamin, high- or low-protein, acid ash, or low-sodium regimens or modifications, as needed)
- ◆ modifications for home cooking and other food preparation and eating.

Responses to rehabilitation

Factors that influence the client's response to rehabilitation include:

- ◆ age and personality
- ◆ severity or extent of injuries
- ◆ potential for partial or full recovery
- ◆ client's stress response pattern
- ◆ initial and continued medical, nursing, and rehabilitative care.

Common response pattern

Clients commonly respond to rehabilitation in a similar pattern, which can be broken down into five phases.

First phase

The first phase of response to rehabilitation is disbelief. Characteristics of this phase include:

- ◆ primary behaviors — anger, hostility, withdrawal, apathy, denial
- ◆ other symptoms — irritability, sleeplessness, tension, numbness, fears, and vague pains.

Nursing interventions

- ◆ Allow the client to express feelings.
- ◆ Accept dependency behaviors and provide care as needed.
- ◆ Encourage participation by the client and his family if appropriate.
- ◆ Refer the client for vocational rehabilitation if appropriate.

Second phase

The second phase of response to rehabilitation involves awareness, transition, impact, and perception of the event. Characteristics of this phase include:

- ◆ gradual realization of the extent of injury or disability
- ◆ possible behaviors — depression, anxiety, anger, silence, sadness, and grief. (Grief, sadness, and crying may or may not directly correlate with the injury or disability but they represent the client's personal responses to developing awareness.)

Nursing interventions

- ◆ Keep the lines of communication open.
- ◆ Accept the client's outward expressions of grief, sadness, anger, and guilt.
- ◆ Encourage and teach self-care as the client becomes able.
- ◆ Seek a psychiatric consultation if the client prolongs reactions.
- ◆ Refer the client for vocational rehabilitation, if appropriate.

Third phase

The third phase of response to rehabilitation involves the use of coping mechanisms, including resistance, reorganization, disequilibrium, and retreat. Characteristics include:

- ◆ gradual realization of the disability's permanence, wavering between acceptance and rejection
- ◆ possible behaviors — self-pity (even while actively participating in care), bargaining (for relief from pain, physical therapy, and so forth), and extreme dependence on others for detailed care.

Nursing interventions

- ◆ Continue to accept the client's expressions and behaviors.
- ◆ Encourage active participation in physical therapy, occupational therapy, hydrotherapy, and so forth, as the client's condition dictates.
- ◆ Teach the client and his family techniques for providing self-care.

Fourth phase

The fourth phase of response to rehabilitation is resolution, convalescence, and acknowledgment. Characteristics include certainty of the disability's permanence, as seen by a vacillation between rejection and acquiescence (with the client gradually leaning more toward tolerance and acceptance if reactions are "normal" or "healthy").

Nursing interventions

- ◆ Accept the client's vacillations while preparing and teaching self-care.
- ◆ Allow sufficient time and opportunities for the client and his family to become confident and proficient in care procedures.
- ◆ Follow up on vocational rehabilitation referrals.

Fifth phase

The fifth phase of response to rehabilitation is recognition of a positive change, restored equilibrium, recovery, or exhaustion (in which no further improvement is possible) and the regaining of as much health as possible. Common characteristics include:

- active participation of the client in self-care and preparation for discharge
- preparation of the family for the client's return home or transfer to a rehabilitation unit.

Nursing interventions

- Make sure that the client and his family can perform self-care.
- Complete continuity-of-care referrals as needed.

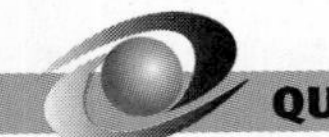

QUICK STUDY

How can you best remember the psychological factors that influence client responses to rehabilitation efforts?

Remember ***ASPRI.***

Age and personality
Severity or extent of injury
Potential for partial or full recovery
Response to stress
Initial and continuing care

GRIEVING

Grieving is a normal human response to loss that may be real or perceived. It may also be anticipatory, such as grief when a child is terminally ill. It's a psychological process that allows one to cope with a loss and accept it as a reality. Grieving may last from 2 months to 1 year or longer.

Stages of grief

Elisabeth Kübler-Ross, a psychiatrist who was an expert on death and dying, identified five phases of grief:

- denial and isolation
- anger
- bargaining
- depression
- acceptance.

Theorist George Engel further identified three stages a person goes through in the acute grieving state:

- shock and disbelief, characterized by rejection or denial
- developing awareness, characterized by weeping and lashing out at loved ones and others
- restitution or resolution, characterized by integration of negative and positive aspects of the lost person or object so that the individual can confront the loss comfortably.

Losses that cause grief

Many types of losses cause grief, including:

- client's impending death
- loss of health, such as in cancer or another debilitating disease
- loss of a body organ or part
- loss or impending loss of a loved one (family member, friend, or pet)
- major events precipitating a loss, such as job loss, divorce, loss of financial security, or one's home. (See *Comparing grief and clinical depression.*)

Nursing interventions

- Be available to the client.
- Use therapeutic communication, especially active listening.

Comparing grief and clinical depression

A client who appears to be suffering from clinical depression may actually be experiencing a phase of grieving. This chart shows the major distinctions between the two conditions.

CHARACTERISTICS OF GRIEF	CHARACTERISTICS OF CLINICAL DEPRESSION
Healthy response	Unhealthy response
Self-resolution	No self-resolution of depressive state
Little if any guilt	Overwhelming guilt
Intact self-esteem	Loss of self-esteem
Sadness	Hopelessness, despair, and helplessness
Intact ability to meet life's demands	Impaired ability to meet life's demands
No biochemical imbalance	Possible biochemical imbalance
Temporary loss of interest in pleasurable activities (anhedonia)	Pervasive anhedonia

- Encourage the client to express feelings and concerns.
- Assist the client in identifying coping mechanisms, such as support from significant others as well as cultural, religious, and spiritual support.
- Help the client to remember comfortably negative and positive aspects of the lost person or object.

Factors that affect grieving

Some factors that may affect the grieving process include:
- developmental stage
- cultural and spiritual beliefs
- loss of a child
- gender
- cause of the loss
- unresolved issues with the deceased.

PRINCIPLES OF GERONTOLOGIC NURSING

Since the early 1970s, the number of Americans over age 65 has been increasing dramatically; the U.S. government projects that there will be 70 million Americans over age 65 by 2030. As the population ages, more demands are put on the health care delivery system by elderly clients, forcing greater focus on their special needs.

The normal aging process leads to a steady deterioration in physical strength and the development of chronic illnesses that threaten an older person's quality of life and independence. Gerontologic nursing concerns itself with the care of elderly clients and the development of processes that meet older adults' special needs.

Nursing practice focuses on helping elderly clients maintain optimum autonomy despite physiologic, pathologic, and psychosocial changes that occur during aging.

Theories of the aging process

There are many different developmental and social theories regarding the aging process.

Developmental theories

In 1963, Erikson postulated that the major developmental task of elderly clients was to choose either ego integrity or despair. *Ego integrity* is the act of accepting one's lifestyle and the choices made during life. *Despair* refers to being dissatisfied with one's life and wishing for another chance to make different choices about how to live it.

In 1972, theorist Robert Havighurst formulated his developmental task theory in which he identified tasks that need to be completed during one's life. If these tasks are completed, the person is content. If they remain unfulfilled, the person becomes dejected and believes he's a failure.

Social theories

Two social theories — the activity theory and the continuity theory — attempt to explain the aging process. According to the activity theory, satisfaction with becoming older means living a middle-age lifestyle. According to the continuity theory, adjusting successfully to the aging process requires continuing the patterns of living that have been established over one's lifetime — for example, old habits and ethical values provide continuity as one moves from one age phase to another.

Changes associated with the aging process

With aging, the client undergoes many physiologic and psychosocial changes. Nurses should be aware of the various changes because they directly affect nursing care.

Physiologic changes

Physiologic changes due to aging affect every body system:
- *integumentary* — wrinkled, dry, thin, pale skin, tendency toward sunburn, and easy bruising
- *cardiovascular* — decreased cardiac output and stroke volume, slow pulse rate, increased blood pressure, and weakened peripheral pulses, especially in the legs
- *respiratory* — increased respiratory rate, decreased lung expansion, and diminished effective coughing
- *musculoskeletal* — diminished muscle mass and strength, trunk shortening, decreased joint mobility, and bone demineralization
- *neurologic* — slowed reflexes, reduced ability to respond to multiple stimuli, and reduced cerebral circulation
- *gastrointestinal* — dry mouth, swallowing difficulties, decreased production of digestive enzymes, decreased peristalsis, increased flatulence, and increased constipation
- *genitourinary* — decreased kidney efficiency, voiding difficulties, urine retention, nocturia, and incontinence
- *reproductive* — dyspareunia in women, vaginal itching and irritation, decreased estrogen, decreased size of penis and testes, delayed erection, and decreased sperm count
- *sensory* — diminished hearing, taste, smell, and vision; reduced ability to adapt to darkness; and increased sensitivity to glare.

Psychosocial changes

Psychosocial changes due to aging include:
- stress about retirement and reduced income

- development of feelings of unworthiness because of perceived loss of productivity
- potential for social isolation, including *attitudinal isolation* (societal rejection because of age bias), *presentational isolation* (social withdrawal because of changes in body image, mental or physical functional loss, or self-consciousness), and *behavioral isolation* (social withdrawal because of unacceptable social behavior, such as confusion, incontinence, or erratic behavior)
- reduced memory retention
- changes to the environment, including moving from a house or an apartment to a retirement community and reorganization of one's living environment to prevent falls
- fear of dying (elderly people aren't always prepared to die; some desire to live until all of their life goals are achieved)
- stress from loss of a significant other.

Gerontologic nursing process

The gerontologic nursing process follows the same steps as for other areas of nursing and includes assessment, nursing diagnoses, planning and goals, implementation, and evaluation.

Assessment

- Assess the client's developmental level to identify how he feels about aging.
- Assess the client's functional level so appropriate goals and outcomes can be developed.
- Assess the client's living environment to evaluate if adjustments are needed.
- Determine if the client has health complaints that may need immediate attention to ensure optimal health.
- Note financial and support resources available to assist the client in maintaining an optimal level of independent function.
- Evaluate the client's coping skills so a realistic care plan can be developed.

Nursing diagnoses

Nursing diagnoses are developed from data obtained during the initial interview and physical assessment. Commonly expressed concerns by the older adult that may warrant a nursing diagnosis include:

- sexual functioning difficulties
- changes in physical appearance and function
- concerns about social interaction
- problems with grieving over loss of spouse
- specific physical complaints.

Planning and goals

When planning care, priority should be given to the client's perception of the problem's importance. Goals should be prioritized according to the nature of the problem; they should:

- always be realistic
- allow the client to achieve an optimal level of independent function.

Implementation

Appropriate interventions used to implement the care plan may include the following:

- Promote socialization *to help the client build secondary social relationships.*
- Use therapeutic communication *to build a trusting nurse-client relationship.*
- Use reality orientation *to maintain or restore the client's sense of awareness.*
- Promote positive body image *to build the client's self-confidence and to foster the willingness of others to interact with the client.*
- Inform the client and his family of the availability of health care services *to ensure that health problems are adequately treated.*
- Teach family members about respite care (short-term care given to a dependent client *so that the permanent caregivers may have a break from the stress of continual-care responsibility).*
- Teach the client and his family how to make their home safe and comfortable *to minimize the risk of injury from falls and maximize the client's comfort at home.*
- Promote ambulation and range-of-motion exercises *to maintain muscle strength, stimulate circulation, and reduce the risk of pressure ulcers.*
- Promote urinary and bowel continence *to foster self-esteem and minimize the risk of institutionalization.*

Evaluation

Evaluation should focus on measuring the client's response to interventions against the goals set in the care plan. When outcomes don't match established goals, a revised care plan should be developed.

Desired outcomes in a gerontologic nursing care plan may include:

- The client maintains proper body alignment when sitting and walking.
- The client actively engages in a planned activity program with others.
- The client seeks out and maintains social contacts.
- The client maintains urinary and bowel continence.

◆ The client is oriented to time, place, and person.
◆ The client is free from bodily injury.
◆ The client knows how to seek health care and does so when needed.

PRINCIPLES OF CASE MANAGEMENT

The concept of managed care dominated health care delivery in the 1990s and is expected to continue well into the 21st century. Within the U.S. health care delivery system, there are health maintenance organizations, preferred provider organizations, and managed care.

Managed care has its roots in the public health nursing model, which provided for one nurse to assume responsibility for meeting (managing) the health care needs of a number of clients and families. Professional nurses, by virtue of the breadth of their education and experience, are ideal case managers.

Case management model

Case management is a systematic approach to delivering total client care within specified time frames and economic resources. Case management includes the client's entire illness episode, crosses all care settings in which care is received, and involves collaboration of all health care personnel who care for the client.

Case managers focus on coordinating care for a client group with complex care requirements. The clients usually have similar diagnoses and needs, and they require common therapies.

Goals of case management

The goals of case management remain the same regardless of the care setting. Case management attempts to direct client care to ensure:
◆ quality of care
◆ appropriateness of care
◆ timeliness of services rendered
◆ cost-effectiveness of care given.

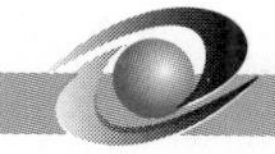

QUICK STUDY

What are the chief goals of case management?
To provide quality care
To provide appropriate care
To provide timely care
To provide cost-effective care

Clinical pathways in case management

Clinical pathways are interdisciplinary plans of care that must be carried out for a group of clients (caseload). These tools enable nurses to monitor caseloads to make sure that clients reach desired outcomes regardless of the health care setting.

Clinical pathways are placed in one of two groups:
◆ medical-drug orders, diagnostic procedures, prescriptions for therapies
◆ nursing comfort interventions, client-teaching activities, self-care activities.

Roles of case managers

Case managers assume various roles and responsibilities, including:
◆ being accountable for the appropriate delivery of health care services in a timely and cost-effective manner
◆ ensuring that desired client outcomes are achieved, using critical pathways
◆ facilitating referrals to the multidisciplinary care team
◆ supervising discharge planning
◆ providing the client with appropriate resources to meet the care plan and troubleshooting for the client if problems occur
◆ evaluating the quality, timeliness, and cost-effectiveness of client care, using quality assurance programs.

Characteristics of case managers

According to current guidelines established by the American Nurses Association, nurse case managers should:
◆ hold a baccalaureate degree in nursing and a master's degree and certification as a clinical nurse specialist in the client's disease area
◆ have 3 years of clinical nursing experience.

Case managers must possess expert knowledge to set client goals and outcomes, must clearly understand and be willing to work within the financial constraints of current health care systems, and must be skilled at developing strategies for quality improvement. They must also have highly developed skills of communication, negotiation, and collaboration with other health care providers. Finally, case managers must know which resources are available in health care facilities and the client's community.

PRINCIPLES OF HOME HEALTH CARE

Home health care is the delivery of multidisciplinary health services to clients and their families wherever they live. The focus of such service is to restore the optimal level of client and family independence.

The introduction of managed care to the U.S. health care delivery system has accelerated the need for providing more health care in the home. Reasons for this increased need include the following:

◆ Chronic health problems that used to receive periodic care in a hospital now are cared for exclusively at home.

◆ Early discharge of clients who have had surgery or an acute illness has raised the acuity level of clients in home care.

◆ Elderly clients with chronic illnesses are being treated at home with greater frequency, thereby raising the level of skills required by the caregivers.

Home health care services

Several types of home health care services are available to clients, including:

◆ *professional services* — skilled nursing care, teaching health care, interdisciplinary collaboration among professional health care providers (which ensures cooperation, continuity of care, and compliance with government eligibility requirements), and identification and communication of community resources (which help the client and his family achieve care plan outcomes)

◆ *ancillary services* — home health aides, housekeepers, and companions

◆ *equipment services* — beds and ambulatory aids, portable dialysis units, and ventilators and infusion pumps.

Factors that influence home health care

Numerous factors can influence the effectiveness of home health care, including:

◆ thorough family education about the health problem

◆ educated professionals trained in the relevant skills to deal with the health problem

◆ effective social support services

◆ appropriate living environment

◆ reliable transportation and local emergency health facility

◆ competent case managers.

Role of nurses in home care

Nurses, the traditional providers of community-based care, are being called on by the federal government, through Medicare regulations, home health agencies, and insurance providers, to direct the delivery of skilled and unskilled home health care. Providing effective home health care requires enhanced clinical skills and an understanding of home care rules and regulations.

Clinical responsibilities

The clinical responsibilities of a home health nurse to the client include maintaining wound care, complying with drug therapy, maintaining nutrition, making sure elimination needs are met, assisting with mobility, and controlling the spread of infection. Specific responsibilities are outlined in this section.

Wound care

◆ Debriding and irrigating wounds

◆ Assessing wound healing

◆ Teaching wound care

Drug therapy compliance

◆ Teaching drug actions, adverse effects, and administration schedules

◆ Monitoring drug therapy effectiveness

◆ Monitoring client compliance

Nutrition

◆ Assessing the client's nutritional status

◆ Administering tube and parenteral feedings

◆ Teaching proper nutrition habits

◆ Monitoring diet compliance

Elimination

◆ Providing enterostomal care

◆ Teaching the client and his family use of irrigation catheters and proper skin care

◆ Monitoring the client for infection

Mobility

◆ Demonstrating use of assistive devices

◆ Performing range-of-motion exercises

Infection control

◆ Teaching the family infection-control precautions

◆ Monitoring the home environment to identify areas that promote infection

Psychosocial responsibilities

The psychosocial responsibilities of the home health nurse include being aware of the client's psychosocial needs, understanding the legal and ethical issues, and maintaining personal safety, as outlined in this section.

Psychosocial needs

◆ Being aware of socioeconomic factors and cultural and family dynamics in the client's home

◆ Recognizing that the home health nurse is a guest in the client's home
◆ Remaining nonjudgmental about the client's beliefs
◆ Accepting the client's ability to learn and willingness to follow directions

Legal and ethical responsibilities
◆ Complying with the laws and regulations regarding home care
◆ Working within an approved care plan
◆ Making sure that physician collaboration on the treatment plan has been obtained
◆ Making sure that the client's or his family's written permission to enter the home has been obtained
◆ Maintaining confidentiality about the client's condition and treatment when asked by family, friends, or neighbors
◆ Providing documentation of care to ensure continued and optimal reimbursement for the client
◆ Understanding when and how to withdraw services when reimbursement authorization expires

Personal safety precautions
◆ Knowing the neighborhood and the safest route in and out
◆ Carrying agency, police, and emergency facility telephone numbers
◆ Informing the agency of a daily visit schedule, with telephone numbers of each client
◆ Reporting in to the agency by phone after each visit
◆ Refrain from driving an expensive automobile, wearing expensive jewelry, or showing a lot of money
◆ Avoiding entering the home if anyone is intoxicated, hostile, or demonstrating obnoxious behavior
◆ Never entering a home until invited, and leaving if feeling unsafe

PRINCIPLES OF INFECTION CONTROL

As primary caregivers, nurses play a major role in preventing the onset and spread of infection. For an infection to occur, a series of events must be completed:
◆ A causative organism must be present.
◆ A reservoir host for the organism must exist.
◆ A transmission route from the reservoir host to a susceptible host must be present.
◆ A means of entry into the new host must exist.
◆ The new host must be susceptible to the organism.

Preventing and controlling the spread of infection requires eliminating or blocking one or more of these events. (See *CDC isolation precautions,* page 44.)

Well-established and proven interventions can prevent and control infection. Nurses must always follow the measures outlined in infection-control programs and should teach clients and their families appropriate methods to avoid spreading infection.

Preventing transmission

To prevent transmission of infection, follow these steps:
◆ Wash hands thoroughly before and after each client contact, after handling body fluids and wastes, and after handling contaminated equipment.
◆ Use protective barriers, including:
– gloves when handling body substances and substances soiled with body fluids (such as open wounds, dressings, or contaminated equipment)
– mask or respirator when caring for clients with airborne infections
– gown, goggles, and hair and shoe covers during potential exposure to sprayed body fluid.
◆ Use isolation techniques, including:
– isolating a client suspected of or with a communicable disease or one who could endanger the immediate environment with body fluids
– placing body substances in a leakproof or puncture-proof container, and bagging soiled linen.

Maintaining natural defenses

The nurse is responsible for maintaining the client's natural defense against infection. This includes the following steps:
◆ Ensure intact, healthy skin by:
– promoting regular bathing to remove organisms
– suggesting the use of lubricants to keep skin hydrated and prevent cracking
– encouraging the client to practice regular oral hygiene, including tartar and plaque control, to reduce oral pathogens.
◆ Maintain adequate nutrition and fluid intake by:
– suggesting a high fluid intake to promote frequent urination, which helps flush the client's system of microorganisms
– encouraging the client to follow a well-balanced diet, which promotes homeostasis and general resistance to infection.

Teaching infection-control measures

Teaching the client and his family ways to prevent or limit the spread of infection is critical, especially for those at high risk for communicable diseases. Teaching should include these steps:

CDC isolation precautions

To help hospitals maintain up-to-date isolation practices, the Centers for Disease Control and Prevention (CDC) and the Hospital Infection Control Practices Advisory Committee revised the CDC's *Guideline for Isolation Precautions in Hospitals.* These guidelines are summarized below.

Standard precautions

The revised guidelines contain two tiers of precautions. The first – called *standard precautions* – are those designated for the care of all hospital clients, regardless of their diagnosis or presumed infection. Standard precautions are the primary strategy for preventing nosocomial infection and take the place of *universal precautions.* These precautions apply to:

- ◆ blood
- ◆ all body fluids, secretions, and excretions except sweat, regardless of whether they contain visible blood
- ◆ skin that isn't intact
- ◆ mucous membranes.

Transmission-based precautions

The second tier of precautions are known as *transmission-based precautions.* These precautions are instituted for clients who are known to be or suspected of being infected with a highly transmissible infection – one that needs precautions beyond those set forth in the standard precautions. There are three types of transmission-based precautions: airborne, droplet, and contact.

Airborne precautions

Airborne precautions are designed to reduce the risk of airborne transmission of infectious agents. Microorganisms carried through the air can be dispersed widely by air currents, making them available for inhalation or deposit on a susceptible host in the same room or a longer distance away from the infected client. Airborne precautions include special air handling and ventilation procedures to prevent the spread of infection. They require the use of respiratory protection, such as a mask – in addition to standard precautions – when entering an infected client's room.

Droplet precautions

Droplet precautions are designed to reduce the risk of transmitting infectious agents through large-particle (exceeding 5 micrometers) droplets. Such transmission involves the contact of infectious agents with the conjunctivae or the nasal or oral mucous membranes of a susceptible person. Large-particle droplets don't remain in the air and generally travel short distances of 3′ or less. They require the use of a mask – in addition to standard precautions – to protect the mucous membranes.

Contact precautions

Contact precautions are designed to reduce the risk of transmitting infectious agents by direct or indirect contact. Direct-contact transmission can occur through client care activities that require physical contact. Indirect-contact transmission involves a susceptible host coming in contact with a contaminated object, usually inanimate, in the client's environment. Contact precautions require the use of gloves, a mask, and a gown – in addition to standard precautions – to avoid contact with the infectious agent. Stringent hand washing is also necessary after removal of the protective items.

- ◆ Assess the client's and family's knowledge level about infection.
- ◆ Teach control measures to use in the home to prevent transmission, such as:
  - frequent hand washing
  - using separate dishes and utensils
  - maintaining a clean environment
  - keeping vaccinations current.

Additionally, it's important to update staff members as needed by teaching them:

- ◆ how to maintain immunizations
- ◆ about the infection process
- ◆ how to use standard precautions in client care.

Infection-control programs

Each facility or institution is responsible for setting up its own infection-control program that adheres to recommended guidelines. An infection-control department composed of specially educated professionals typically develops a formal program, and all health care workers, including nurses, have a duty to know what the guidelines are.

The infection-control department is responsible for:

- ◆ ensuring staff education
- ◆ establishing infection-control procedures
- ◆ conducting research on infection-control measures
- ◆ providing a liaison to community and other health agencies.

Questions for cultural and spiritual assessment

A client's cultural and religious background can provide a powerful positive influence for healing when supported by caregivers. Taking the time to assess a client's cultural and spiritual background allows the nurse to render sensitive, effective care.

Critical questions to ask include:

- What language is spoken by the client and his family? Is an interpreter needed?
- Is there a religious preference identified by the client and his family?
- What cultural and religious supports are available to the client and his family? Have appropriate clergy been notified as requested by the client?
- How do cultural and religious views influence dietary habits? What implications does this have for treatment?
- What restrictions regarding treatment may the client and his family have, based on religious beliefs?
- What religious observances (prayers, blessings, ceremonies) might the client and his family desire? Who would assist with these observances?
- What does the client do to maintain health? What religious or cultural beliefs affect health care behaviors?
- How does the client conceptualize illness? What religious or cultural beliefs may influence receptivity to medical or surgical treatment?
- What special cultural or religious medals, icons, texts, clothing or other emblems of belief are important to the client? If not available, how can they be obtained?
- What alternate health care practices may be utilized? Are herbal or other natural remedies routinely taken? Are other nontraditional healers participating in care?

CULTURAL AND SPIRITUAL DIMENSIONS OF CARE

A critical part of the nursing process involves the assessment of cultural and spiritual needs, followed by appropriate planning and implementation. Too often these vital components of client care are neglected in the urgency to address critical physical needs.

Important components to address in identifying cultural and spiritual needs of clients include:

- *identifying the dominant cultural and religious background of the client and his family.* Culture, including religion, helps to determine a person's role and status in the family and community. It influences the availability of social and material supports, how illness and health are viewed, and how individuals who are sick are expected to behave.
- *performing a cultural and spiritual assessment.* This assessment may be brief or may require considerable evaluation depending on the circumstances of the patient care situation. (See *Questions for cultural and spiritual assessment.*
- *involving the client and his family in planning to meet cultural and spiritual needs.* Identify institutional barriers, which may need to be addressed. Identify alternate means of meeting cultural or spiritual needs when in conflict with institutional barriers. For example, when caring for a Jehovah's Witness client, be aware that blood transfusions are unacceptable, as they're considered against God's will. What alternative treatments are available and acceptable? What legal ramifications need to be considered?
- *intervening as the advocate for the client and his family.* Make sure that cultural and religious views are taken into account as physical care is rendered. For example, when caring for a Latter-day Saint (Mormon) client, allow for the retention of special undergarments whenever possible.
- *evaluating the effectiveness of the plan to include cultural and spiritual dimensions of care.* Does the client feel supported and validated? Are there areas of concern or conflict? Can these be mitigated or can the difficulties be discussed sufficiently with the client and family so that they feel their concerns are understood?

NURSING SKILLS

Various basic nursing skills are needed to provide quality care for most clients in any setting. These skills are important in the care of clients with various health needs and for promoting health and wellness for clients of all ages. These essential skills include:

- physical assessment
- blood transfusion
- cardiac rhythm interpretation
- cardiopulmonary resuscitation
- anticipatory guidance
- discharge planning.

PHYSICAL ASSESSMENT

Physical assessment constitutes an important part of the assessment phase of the nursing process. Physical assessment:

◆ must be accurate and thorough to produce appropriate nursing diagnoses

◆ requires effective communication techniques and interviewing skills

◆ should be holistic and include a comprehensive health history that explores biopsychosocial factors relevant to the client's health status

◆ consists of four physical examination techniques in which the nurse uses the senses to gather information about the client:

– INSPECTION, which uses sight and smell to collect data (for example, observing the client's gait or detecting a fruity breath odor)

– PALPATION, which uses touch (fingers and hands) to collect data (for example, taking a radial pulse)

– AUSCULTATION, which uses hearing (primarily with the aid of a stethoscope) to detect sounds produced by certain body organs (for example, taking an apical pulse)

– PERCUSSION, which uses the striking of one object against another to generate a vibration that produces an audible sound wave (for example, percussing the lung fields) and is the technique least likely to be used by the novice nurse.

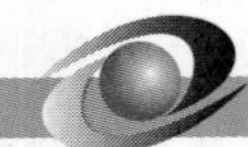

QUICK STUDY

When trying to remember the correct order of nursing assessment steps, think ***IPAP.***

Inspection
Palpation
Auscultation
Percussion

Health history

The health history can provide valuable information regarding present and past health conditions (including the primary reason the client is seeking care) as well as other factors that may affect the client's health, such as family and social histories. It's usually taken during the initial examination.

A thorough health history covers the following areas:

Present health history

◆ Allergies
◆ Diet
◆ Exercise
◆ Alcohol intake
◆ Tobacco use
◆ Sleep pattern
◆ Medications, including prescription and nonprescription
◆ Appliances (for example, dentures, prostheses, glasses)

Past health history

◆ Childhood illnesses
◆ Immunizations
◆ Surgeries
◆ Injuries
◆ Hospitalizations
◆ Obstetric and menstrual history
◆ Adult illnesses
◆ Psychiatric illnesses

Family history

◆ Diabetes mellitus
◆ Heart disease
◆ Cancer

Social history

◆ Lifestyle
◆ Relationships with family and friends
◆ Occupation
◆ Leisure-time activities
◆ Residence (for example, urban or rural, one-story house or high-rise apartment, rent or own)

Perceptions of health

As part of the health history, record the client's perception of his own health and assess how his family and friends perceive his health.

Physical examination

After obtaining the client's health history, the nurse conducts a physical examination that includes noting apparent state of health, signs of distress, motor activity, weight, facial expression, grooming, mood, and state of awareness. To perform the physical examination, assess the client's vital signs, body systems, and motor function, as outlined here:

Vital signs

◆ Blood pressure (in both arms in lying, sitting, and standing positions)

◆ Pulses (including carotid, abdominal aortic, femoral, tibial, and pedal — taken bilaterally when possible)

Body systems

◆ Skin (inspection of color, moisture, temperature, turgor, presence of lesions compared bilaterally)
◆ Nails (compared bilaterally on hands and feet)
◆ Hair (dry or oily texture)
◆ Eyes (inspection of visual acuity of central and peripheral vision), noting use of glasses, contact lenses, prosthesis, and the presence of eye discharge, inflammation, swelling, or redness
◆ Ears (hearing acuity, presence of cerumen, condition of the tympanic membrane)
◆ Nose (palpation of the nose and sinuses; note the presence of discharge)
◆ Mouth and pharynx (inspection of the lips, mucosa of the mouth, gums, teeth, and tongue; ability to swallow and taste; and movement of the uvula)
◆ Neck (palpation of the lymph nodes [preauricular, posterior auricular, occipital, tonsillar, submaxillary, submental, superficial cervical, posterior cervical, deep cervical, and supraclavicular], thyroid gland, and trachea)
◆ Back (inspection and palpation of the spine and muscles, observing for curvatures)
◆ Thorax and lungs (inspection, percussion, and auscultation of thorax and lungs, palpating for respiratory excursion and noting the presence and type of cough)
◆ Breasts and axillae (palpation of breasts and nodes in axillae, observing for symmetry, discharge, and pain)
◆ Heart (auscultation of the heart, observing for palpitations, thrills, and heaves; taking the heart rate at the point of maximal impulse)
◆ Abdomen (auscultation for bowel sounds, palpation of the liver and kidneys, noting symmetry)
◆ Genitalia (penis and scrotum in men; external genitalia and vagina in women) and groin (checking for hernia)

Motor function

◆ Range of motion for all joints
◆ Ability to contract all muscles (check muscle tone and strength)
◆ Coordination of movements
◆ Gait
◆ Ability to speak and write
◆ Reflexes
◆ Sensation (pain and vibration in the hands, feet, arms, and legs, while touching lightly on the abdomen, arms, and legs)
◆ Level of consciousness (LOC) (orientation) and mental status (mood, cognitive functions)
◆ Presence of seizures, tremors, or tics
◆ Secondary sex characteristics (hair distribution, voice)
◆ Activity level (noting pain, dyspnea, fatigue, or weakness)
◆ Voiding and bowel patterns
◆ Fluid, electrolyte, and acid-base balance
◆ Pain, infection, bleeding, and lesions (noting presence and location)

BLOOD TRANSFUSION

A blood transfusion is the I.V. infusion of blood or blood products into the bloodstream. The transfusion can be autologous (the client's blood) or homologous (donor blood).

QUICK STUDY

When trying to remember the difference between autologous and homologous, just remember that:
Auto means self. Blood comes from self.
Homo means man. Blood comes from any man (person).

One or more blood transfusions may be performed to replenish the client's blood volume or erythrocytes (red blood cells) or to provide platelets or other coagulation factors. The procedure carries risks that can be minimized by carefully assessing the donor's health status, following safe blood administration practices, and knowing how to recognize and manage transfusion reactions.

Donor history and screening

A donor history must be obtained, and proper screening, including blood typing and crossmatching, must be performed before a blood transfusion can take place. Donor blood is unacceptable for use if the donor's history includes:
◆ viral hepatitis or contact with a hepatitis client within the previous 6 months
◆ blood transfusion within the previous 6 months
◆ previous or current I.V. drug use
◆ exposure to human immunodeficiency virus
◆ recent allergies or hives.

Donor blood shouldn't be used if screening tests yield positive results for:
◆ hepatitis
◆ acquired immunodeficiency syndrome
◆ syphilis
◆ cytomegalovirus.

Blood typing and cross matching

Blood tests are necessary before transfusions to determine the client's blood type and the suitability of blood to be transfused.

ABO typing

ABO blood typing is a test that identifies the client's blood group (A, B, O, or AB) to check compatibility of donor and recipient blood before transfusion:

- Type A blood is that of a person whose erythrocytes contain isoagglutinin (antigen) A and antibody anti-B (about 40% of the population).
- Type B blood is that of a person whose erythrocytes contain isoagglutinin (antigen) B and antibody anti-A (about 10% of the population).
- Type O blood is that of a person whose erythrocytes contain neither isoagglutinin A nor B but do contain antibodies anti-A and anti-B (about 40% to 45% of the population, known as *universal donors*).
- Type AB blood is that of a person whose erythrocytes contain isoagglutins A and B but no antibodies (about 5% to 10% of the population, known as *universal recipients*).

Rh typing

Rh typing is a test that determines the presence or absence of the Rho(D) antigen on the surface of red blood cells. An Rh-positive result indicates isoagglutins D, C, and E in erythrocytes.

Crossmatching

Crossmatching is a test in which the donor's erythrocytes are exposed to the recipient's serum and the donor's serum is exposed to the recipient's erythrocytes. The test is performed to evaluate for agglutination.

Hazards and complications of blood transfusion

The recipient of a blood transfusion is at risk for contracting a bloodborne disease, such as serum hepatitis, syphilis, malaria, or acquired immunodeficiency disease. Transmission of incompatible or contaminated blood produces agglutination and hemolysis of the donor's erythrocytes by isoagglutination in the recipient's plasma.

Too-rapid administration can produce circulatory overload. Massive transfusions (5 L in less than 12 hours) can cause acidosis, hypothermia, citrate overload, hyperkalemia, and dilutional coagulation defects.

Complications of blood transfusion cause about 3,000 deaths annually in the United States, primarily through serum hepatitis or a hemolytic transfusion reaction. Transfusion reactions usually develop during, immediately after, or within 96 hours of the transfusion.

Delayed complications, which may develop 10 to 120 days after the last transfusion, typically result from disease transmission or sensitization to previous transfusions.

Procedures for safe administration

Always follow standard precautions and facility protocol when administering blood or blood products.

- Wear gloves when handling any blood or blood products.
- Properly collect and label blood and blood products.
- Provide detailed information labels for typing and crossmatching samples.
- Obtain appropriate authorization to remove blood from the blood bank.
- Ensure proper client identification by having two nurses compare the recipient's identification using two client identifiers (client's full name, birth date, telephone number, or medical record number), both identifiers may be contained on the client's identification band, with matching information on the blood label. Some facilities use barcoding as a means of client identification.
- Prepare all necessary equipment in advance:
  - Y-type administration set
  - large-gauge needle (20G or larger)
  - blood filter.

Symptoms of transfusion reaction

Common symptoms of a transfusion reaction include:

- fever (possibly as high as 103° F [39.4° C])
- chills
- itching
- flushing
- urticaria
- nausea
- vomiting
- headache
- dyspnea
- stridor
- wheezing.

In severe cases, hemolytic reactions can develop. Signs and symptoms include:

- chest, flank, or back pain
- apprehension or a feeling of impending doom
- severe hypotension
- spontaneous diffuse bleeding
- anuria.

Managing transfusion reactions

If a client shows signs and symptoms of a transfusion reaction, the following steps should be taken:

◆ Stop the transfusion immediately. Infuse normal saline solution at a keep-vein-open rate, being careful not to infuse any of the blood that remains in the blood administration tubing into the client.
◆ Notify the physician.
◆ Obtain a urine sample from the client and send it to the laboratory for analysis; continue to measure and assess urine output hourly.
◆ Draw a fresh sample of the client's blood, and send it to the blood bank or laboratory for analysis.
◆ Return unused blood to the blood bank for incompatibility and contamination testing.
◆ Reduce the client's temperature by giving a sponge bath, administering acetaminophen, or lowering the room temperature, if necessary. Measure the client's temperature every 30 minutes until it's normal.
◆ To treat an allergic reaction, administer antihistamines (and possibly epinephrine or steroids), as ordered.
◆ To treat a hemolytic reaction, infuse an osmotic diuretic (possibly with sodium bicarbonate and hydrocortisone) and administer vasopressors as ordered.

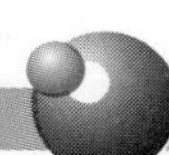

SPOT CHECK

What's the first intervention you should perform if you suspect your client is having a transfusion reaction?

Answer: Your first priority is to stop the transfusion immediately. You should also infuse normal saline solution at a keep-vein-open rate.

CARDIAC RHYTHM INTERPRETATION

Nurses who work outside specialty care areas are now routinely assigned to monitor clients for cardiac arrhythmias, whether during an emergency or while on a regular nursing unit. With this duty comes the responsibility of knowing and understanding basic cardiac anatomy and physiology as well as the fundamental components of the electrocardiogram (ECG). Indeed, the health care team's ability to initiate prompt treatment may depend on the nurse's ability to recognize potentially life-threatening ECG changes.

The following text reviews the heart's normal conduction system, basic components of the ECG, methods to calculate heart rate, ECG lead placement, and characteristics of and treatment measures for five life-threatening arrhythmias.

Cardiac conduction system

Electrical impulses travel through the heart along a pathway called the conduction system. The cardiac conduction system consists of the sinoatrial (SA) and atrioventricular (AV) nodes along with the bundle of His and right and left bundle branches.

Sinoatrial node

The SA node has these characteristics:

◆ On the ECG, its electrical activity is represented by the P wave.
◆ It contains specialized conduction cells.
◆ Electrical impulses originate here.
◆ It's located in right atrium near the junction of the superior vena cava.
◆ It discharges at a rate of 60 to 100 beats/minute.
◆ Its impulses spread through atrial tissue via specialized interatrial and internodal pathways, causing atrial depolarization (P wave).
◆ Atria contract with depolarization.
◆ Blood flows to the ventricles. (See *The heart's conduction system,* page 50.)

Atrioventricular node

The AV node has these characteristics:

◆ On the ECG, the electrical activity is represented by the straight line following the P wave.
◆ Impulses arrive at the AV node.
◆ There's a brief delay (0.07 to 0.10 second) for the atria to contract completely and blood to flow into the ventricles.
◆ If the SA node fails, the AV node can serve as a backup pacemaker with a rate of 40 to 60 beats/minute.

Bundle of His and bundle branches

The bundle of His and bundle branches have these characteristics:

◆ On the ECG, the electrical activity of this area is represented by the QRS wave.
◆ Impulses leave the AV node and travel down the bundle of His and the left and right bundle branches, terminating in the Purkinje system.
◆ Conduction through the His-Purkinje system produces ventricular depolarization with ventricular contraction immediately following.
◆ Blood propels through the pulmonary artery to the lung and through the aorta to the body.
◆ If the SA node or AV junction fails, the His-Purkinje system can initiate impulses usually at a rate of 20 to 40 beats/minute.

The heart's conduction system

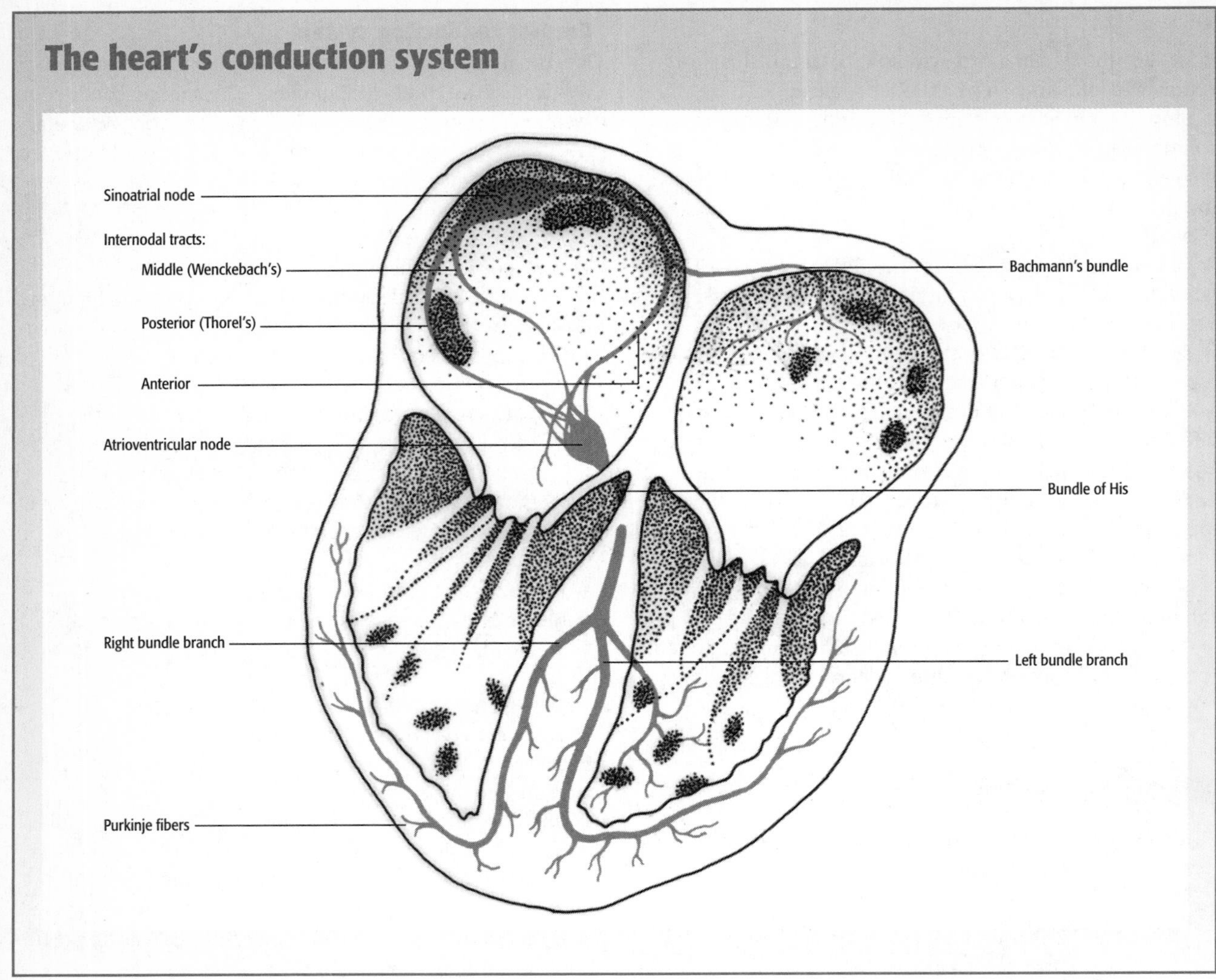

Normal ECG complex

A normal ECG complex has these characteristics:

- *P wave* — atrial depolarization (the electrical impulse spreading throughout the atrial musculature)
- *PR interval* — atrial depolarization plus brief delay of the electrical impulse at the AV node, measured from the beginning of the P wave to the beginning of the QRS complex, with normal duration 0.12 to 0.20 second
- *QRS complex* — ventricular depolarization, measured from the beginning of the Q wave to the end of the S wave, normally lasting 0.06 to 0.10 second with Q wave as first negative deflection, R wave as first positive deflection, and S wave as first negative deflection after the R wave
- *T wave* — ventricular repolarization. (The point on or near the peak of the T wave, the vulnerable period, may produce dangerous rhythm disturbances, such as tachycardia and ventricular fibrillation.) (See *Components of an ECG waveform.*)

Calculating heart rates

An ECG records the heart's electrical activity on graph paper at a constant rate. The graph paper contains small and large boxes that represent time: 0.04 second for each small box and 0.20 second for each large box. Thus, 1,500 small boxes or 300 large boxes represent 1 minute. Also, at the top of the paper, vertical lines appear at 3-second intervals.

Components of an ECG waveform

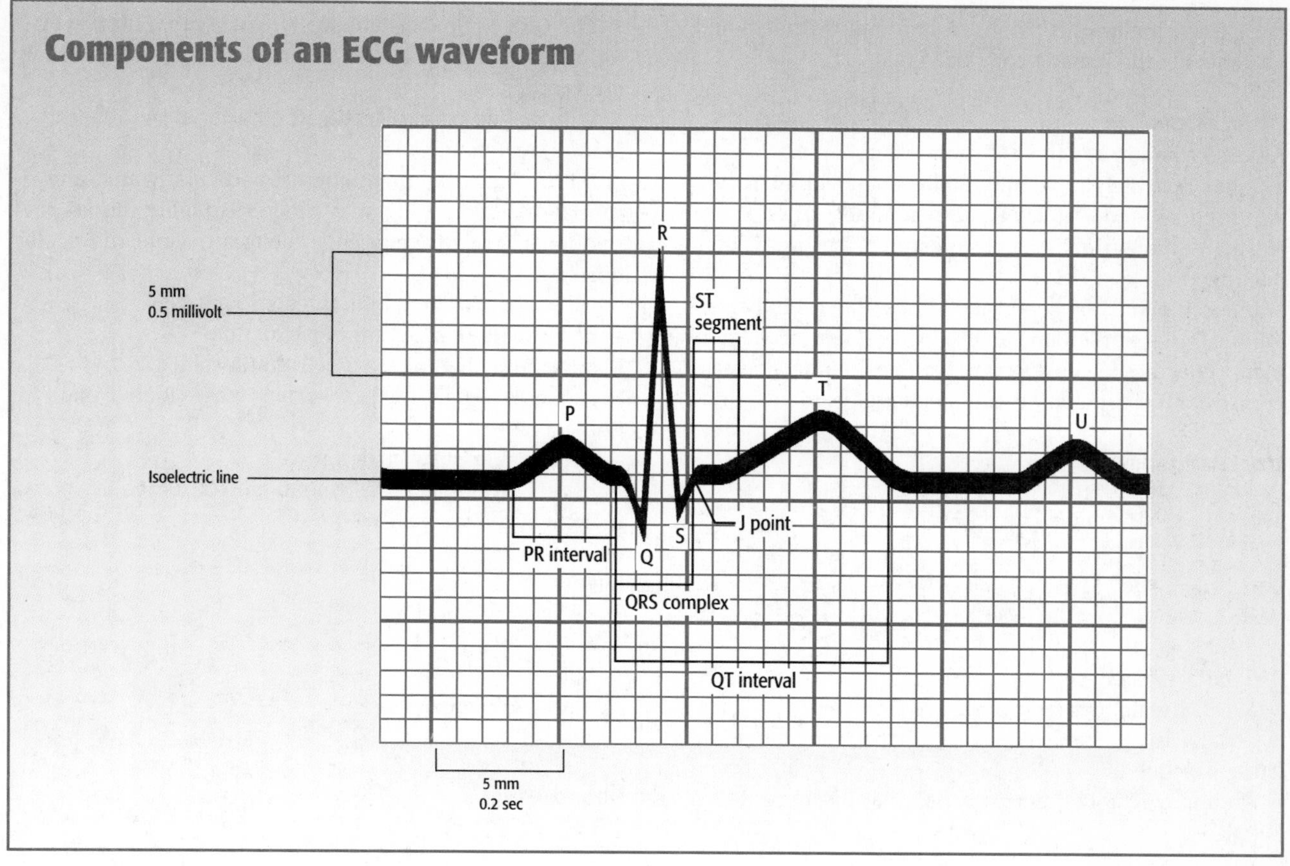

Various methods are used to calculate the heart rate. For example:

◆ To measure the atrial rate (P-P interval), calculate the time between two regular consecutive P waves.

◆ To measure the ventricular rate (R-R interval), calculate the time between two regular consecutive R waves.

The actual calculation can usually be accomplished by one of two methods that involve counting the boxes that appear on the ECG strip.

◆ Count the number of large boxes between the two complexes (P-P or R-R) and divide by 300. (For example, if there are three large boxes between the two P waves, then the atrial rate is 100 beats/minute.) This method is faster but not as accurate as counting small boxes.

◆ Count the number of small boxes between the two complexes (P-P or R-R) and divide by 1,500. (For example, if there are 15 small boxes between two R waves, then the ventricular rate is 100 beats/minute.) This method is more accurate but takes longer.

Note that if the client's rhythm is irregular, neither of these methods is accurate. For irregular rates, count the QRS complexes in a 6-second strip and multiply by 10. (For example, if the rate is 8 QRS complexes in a 6-second strip, then the heart rate is 80 beats/minute.)

ECG lead placement

Standard placement of ECG leads is to position the leads on the right arm, left arm, right leg (used to ground the system), and left leg. An alternative placement of ECG leads is to position arm leads on the side of chest under the clavicles and leg leads on the upper abdomen under the ribs — which provides better access to the client in an emergency, permits monitoring of a three-limb lead (I, II, III), and reduces interference from client movement.

Lead II is commonly used to monitor cardiac rhythm because it provides the best visualization of a P wave.

Arrhythmia interpretation

Some potentially lethal cardiac arrhythmias include atrial fibrillation, premature ventricular contraction, ventricular tachycardia, ventricular fibrillation, and complete heart block (third-degree AV block). Being able to recognize these arrhythmias quickly ensures prompt treatment and prevents life-threatening complications.

Atrial fibrillation

Atrial fibrillation has these characteristics:
- It has extremely rapid and totally chaotic atrial activity.
- It occurs without effective atrial contraction.
- The AV node usually blocks most impulses from conducting to the ventricles.
- If accompanied by a ventricular rate above 150 beats/minute, atrial fibrillation can produce deleterious hemodynamic effects, such as decreased stroke volume, decreased effective atrial contraction, and decreased cardiac output.

ATRIAL FIBRILLATION

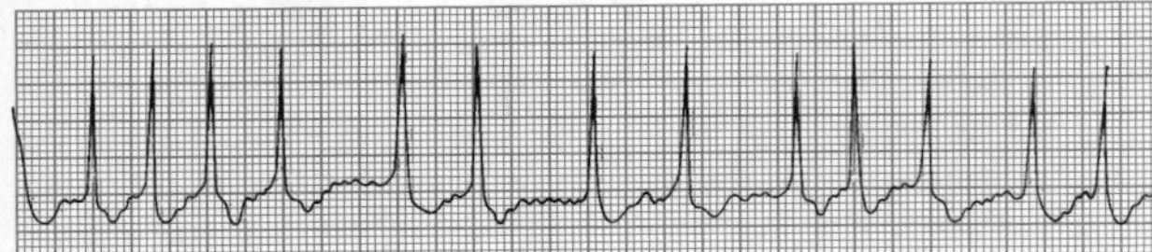

ECG characteristics

- No clearly defined or measurable P waves
- Atrial activity characterized by a wavy, irregular, undulating baseline
- An unpredictably irregular ventricular response (R-R interval)

Nursing interventions

- Notify the physician.
- Assess the client for signs of decreased cardiac output, including falling blood pressure, decreased urine output, and altered LOC.
- Prepare emergency equipment, including a defibrillator, oxygen, and drugs (crash cart).

Emergency medical treatments

- Assist with cardioversion, if necessary (initially, 50 to 100 joules, which may be increased for subsequent attempts).
- Administer drugs, such as verapamil (Isoptin), digoxin (Lanoxin), diltiazem (Cardizem), and amiodarone (Cordarone), if ordered.
- Assist in treating the underlying cause.

Premature ventricular contraction

Premature ventricular contraction (PVC) has these characteristics:
- It causes early discharge from an irritable focus in the ventricles.
- The QRS complex is unusually wide with a bizarre distorted configuration due to electrical activity conducted in the ventricles.
- If there's no heart disease, an occasional PVC doesn't require treatment.
- If it occurs with other patterns, particularly after a myocardial infarction, PVCs may progress to more serious arrhythmias, such as ventricular tachycardia and ventricular fibrillation.
- PVCs are considered life-threatening if they:
  - occur more than six times per minute
  - have more than one source (multifocal PVCs)
  - occur on or near the preceding T wave (R-on-T phenomenon)
  - appear at least twice in a row
  - have a bigeminal or trigeminal pattern (when every second or third beat is a PVC).

PAIRED PVCs

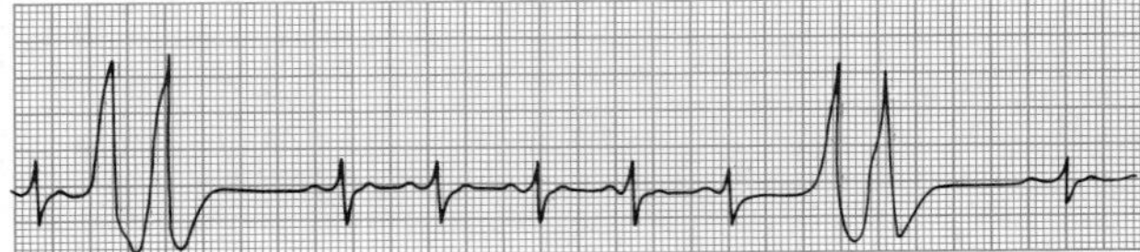

MULTIFORM PVCs

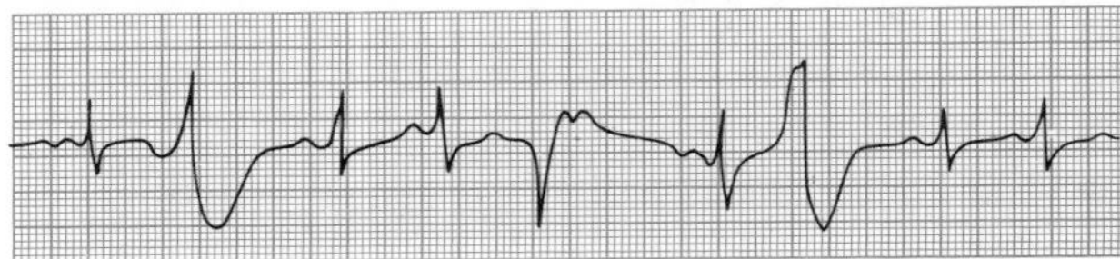

BIGEMINY

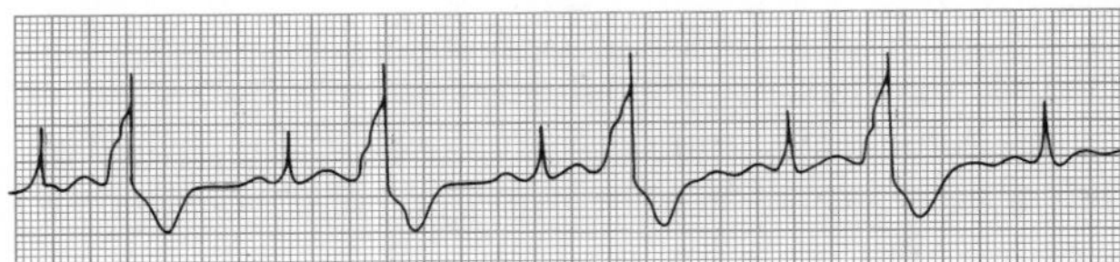

R-ON-T PHENOMENON

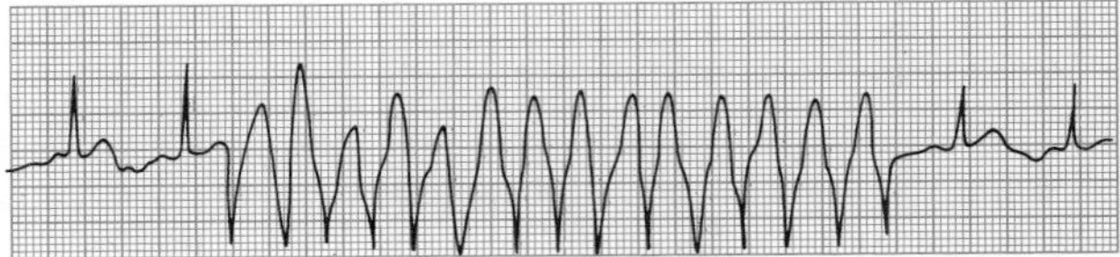

ECG characteristics

- Not preceded by a P wave
- Wide, distorted QRS complex (greater than 0.12 second)

◆ Large T wave in the opposite direction of the QRS complex

Nursing interventions
◆ Notify the physician.
◆ Assess the client for signs of decreased cardiac output, including falling blood pressure, decreased urine output, and altered LOC.
◆ Prepare emergency equipment, including a defibrillator, oxygen, and drugs.

Emergency medical treatments
◆ Administer drugs, such as lidocaine (Xylocaine), procainamide (Pronestyl), and amiodarone (Cordarone), if ordered.
◆ Assist in treating the underlying cause.

Ventricular tachycardia
Ventricular tachycardia has these characteristics:
◆ It develops when an irritable ventricle focus, firing 150 to 250 beats/minute, takes control of the heart's normal pacing pattern.
◆ Ventricle beating is unrelated to atrial mechanism.
◆ It's also used to describe when three or more PVCs occur consecutively.
◆ It produces significant hemodynamic effects.
◆ It commonly accompanies heart disease.
◆ It commonly precedes ventricular fibrillation.

VENTRICULAR TACHYCARDIA

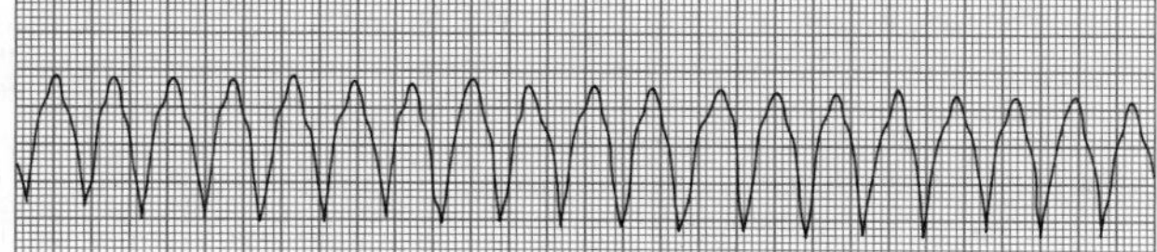

ECG characteristics
◆ Rapid ventricular rate, either regular or slightly irregular
◆ No relationship to atrial activity
◆ Wide, distorted QRS complex (greater than 0.12 second)
◆ Possibly intermittent P waves unrelated to ventricular activity

Nursing interventions
◆ Assess the client's LOC; if the client is unconscious, begin cardiopulmonary resuscitation.
◆ Notify the physician.
◆ Assess the client for signs of decreased cardiac output, including falling blood pressure, decreased urine output, and altered LOC.
◆ Prepare emergency equipment, including a defibrillator, oxygen, and drugs.

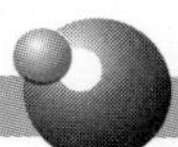

SPOT CHECK

What's the first intervention if your client has ventricular tachycardia?
Answer: Assess the client's LOC. If the client is unconscious, begin cardiopulmonary resuscitation.

Emergency medical treatments
◆ Treatment of ventricular tachycardia depends on the degree to which the client is tolerating the rhythm. Unless the client is hemodynamically unstable, drug therapy is preferred over cardioversion.
◆ If the rhythm resolves, the team starts a maintenance infusion of the drug that aided resolution.
◆ Phenytoin may be administered I.V. to resolve ventricular tachycardia induced by digoxin toxicity.
◆ If the client is awake and alert, administer drugs, such as sotalol (Betapace), lidocaine, procainamide, and amiodarone, if ordered.
◆ If the client is unconscious or hypotensive or shows signs of angina or heart failure, assist with cardioversion or defibrillation if necessary (initially, 50 joules, which may be increased up to 360 joules). Then administer amiodarone or lidocaine, if ordered.
◆ Assist in treating the underlying cause.

Ventricular fibrillation
Ventricular fibrillation has these characteristics:
◆ Ventricular fibrillation is considered an emergency.
◆ When multiple irritable foci in the ventricles fire rapidly, the heart can't respond with effective contraction and cardiac output ceases.
◆ Death will occur in 3 to 5 minutes without intervention.

VENTRICULAR FIBRILLATION

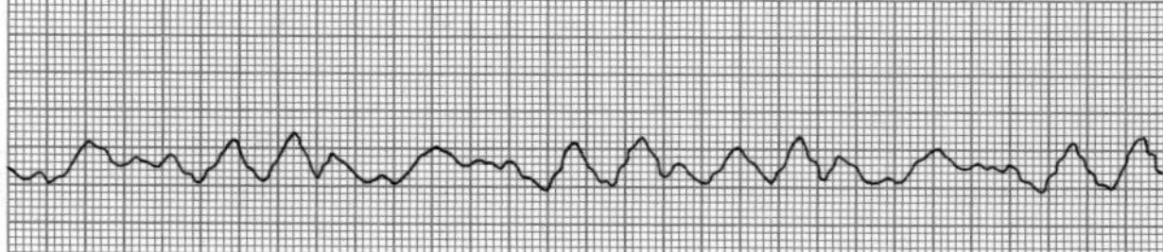

ECG characteristics
◆ Totally disorganized, chaotic pattern
◆ No discernible waves or complexes

Nursing interventions
◆ Call a code.
◆ Begin cardiopulmonary resuscitation and continue until help arrives.
◆ Prepare emergency equipment, including defibrillator, oxygen, and drugs.

Emergency medical treatments
◆ Assist with defibrillation if necessary (initially, 200 joules, which may be increased up to 360 joules).
◆ Administer drugs, such as epinephrine, vasopressin, lidocaine, procainamide, or amiodarone, if ordered.
◆ Draw a sample of the client's blood for arterial blood gas analysis, and administer sodium bicarbonate according to the client's pH level.
◆ Help identify and treat the underlying cause.

Complete heart block

Complete heart block, also called third-degree AV block, has these characteristics:
◆ It prevents the conduction of all atrial impulses to the ventricles.
◆ It's usually caused by an underlying disease or drug toxicity.
◆ An escape mechanism from the junctional tissue or ventricles takes over and paces the ventricles.
◆ The atria and ventricles are controlled by two independent pacemakers, firing at two independent rates with no relationship to each other.

COMPLETE HEART BLOCK

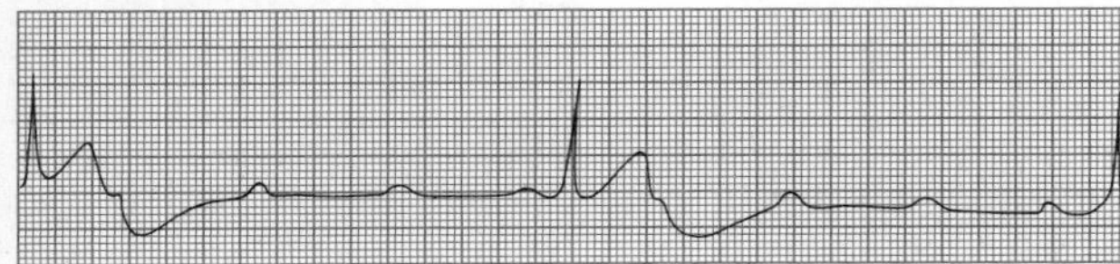

ECG characteristics
◆ Regular atrial rate (P-P interval), usually 60 to 100 beats/minute
◆ Regular ventricular rate, usually 40 to 60 beats/minute (junctional escape rhythm) or 20 to 40 beats/minute (ventricular escape rhythm)
◆ No relationship of P waves to QRS complexes

Nursing interventions
◆ Notify the physician.
◆ Assess the client for signs of decreased cardiac output, including falling blood pressure, decreased urine output, and altered LOC.
◆ Prepare emergency equipment, including oxygen and drugs.

Emergency medical treatments
◆ Insert a temporary or permanent transvenous pacemaker.
◆ Administer atropine, dopamine, or epinephrine, as ordered, if the client is showing signs of decreased cardiac output. These drugs speed up the effective heart rate and improve cardiac output until cardiac pacing is accomplished.

CARDIOPULMONARY RESUSCITATION

Cardiopulmonary resuscitation (CPR) is an emergency procedure that consists of artificial respiration and external cardiac massage, instituted after cardiopulmonary arrest. CPR provides tissue oxygenation until normal cardiac function is restored. The basic principles of life support center on the ABCs of CPR:
◆ **A**irway
◆ **B**reathing
◆ **C**irculation.

Performing CPR

Follow these steps when performing CPR:
◆ Determine the client's responsiveness by calling, "Are you OK?"
◆ If the client doesn't respond, call for help (911).
◆ Place the client in the supine position (flat on his back) on a hard surface, supporting the head and neck.
◆ Open the airway by using the head tilt–chin lift maneuver.
◆ Look, listen, and feel for signs of breathing.
◆ If the client isn't breathing, pinch the client's nose and, with your mouth, establish a tight seal over the client's mouth.
◆ Ventilate twice using a microshield; then pause to see whether the client's chest rises.
◆ If the client's breaths are blocked, reposition the head and try again. If still blocked, perform the Heimlich (abdominal thrust) maneuver.
◆ Palpate for the carotid pulse on the near side. (Keep the client's head tilted with your hand on the forehead.)

◆ If the client has no pulse, begin cycles of ventilations with sternal compressions:
- Check landmarks before placing the heel of your hand on the client's sternum.
- Perform vertical compressions without bouncing.
- Try to establish a rate of 100 beats/minute by counting 4 cycles of 15 compressions to 2 ventilations.
- Make compressions and relaxations of equal duration.
- Assess each ventilation for proper chest expansion.

◆ Periodically assess the client for return of pulse and spontaneous breathing; don't interrupt resuscitation efforts for longer than 5 seconds.

◆ Continue CPR until another rescuer relieves you, the client responds, you become too exhausted to continue, or you receive instructions to terminate CPR.

ANTICIPATORY GUIDANCE

Anticipatory guidance refers to the initiation of interventions before an event occurs to prevent potential problems. If an event can be anticipated, guidance (teaching) increases the likelihood that the event will have a favorable outcome (for example, preparing parents for their child's impending developmental tasks or discussing the ramifications of upcoming surgery with a client). Anticipatory guidance is inherent in all levels of prevention related to health care. (See *Levels of illness prevention.*)

Client-teaching responsibilities

The nurse's primary client-teaching responsibilities with hospitalized patients include:

◆ orienting the client to the hospital environment

◆ explaining all nursing procedures that will be performed as part of the client's care

◆ explaining all diagnostic tests, treatments, and medical procedures that the client will undergo, including a discussion of what the client can expect before, during, and after the test, treatment, or procedure

◆ providing written and oral explanations and instructions

◆ determining the client's understanding and perception of health care management

◆ providing feedback as needed to clarify any concerns or correct any misconceptions the client may have.

DISCHARGE PLANNING

Preparing the client for eventual discharge involves individualized planning that reflects the client's special health needs and identifies available and appropriate facilities and services. The overall purpose of discharge planning is to ensure continuity of client care.

Through effective discharge planning, the nurse can accomplish numerous goals:

◆ helping the client find efficient, timely, and economical solutions to anticipated health problems

Levels of illness prevention

This chart lists levels of illness prevention along with their purpose and examples of anticipatory guidance that you can use to prevent illness.

LEVEL	PURPOSE	EXAMPLES OF ANTICIPATORY GUIDANCE
Primary	To prevent trauma or disease	◆ Child education ◆ Infant immunization ◆ Health screening programs ◆ Accident prevention programs ◆ Parent education classes
Secondary	To delay or stop the progress of an established disease or injury	◆ Diabetic teaching ◆ Discharge planning ◆ Return demonstration by the client
Tertiary	To maintain an incurably ill client at maximal activity level	◆ Referral to self-help groups ◆ Preparation of family for grieving patterns

- ensuring uninterrupted therapy, which may start in one institution (such as a hospital) but continue in other settings (such as a clinic, the client's home, the physician's office, or a nursing home)
- ensuring quality care by coordinating interventions provided by multidisciplinary team members
- assisting the client's family or significant others with necessary home care preparations, including teaching aids (such as for treatments and medications), referrals, and follow-up appointments.

The discharge planning process

Discharge planning should begin on admission, when the client enters the health care system. For discharge planning to be effective, the nurse uses a five-step problem-solving approach:

- Assess discharge planning needs based on the client's problems.
- Design a goal-directed plan.
- Test the plan.
- Evaluate test results.
- Redesign the plan as indicated.

The client and family must assist in the planning process and must receive information about available resources and services. A coordinated team approach ensures reliable information and uninterrupted care, initiates interagency communication (through referrals or written agreements), and establishes contact between the client and the resources and services best suited to the client's needs. Integrated discharge planning can resolve complex health problems and produce optimal client recovery.

Clients with special needs

Although every client requires some type of discharge planning, some clients have critical needs that warrant more complex planning. Examples of such special needs clients include:

- children with chronic health problems (asthma, hemophilia, neurologic conditions, scoliosis, seizures)
- children with social problems (such as parental rejection or battered child syndrome)
- neonates at risk for complications (prematurity, weighing more than 10 lb [4.5 kg], Apgar score of 7 or lower, major congenital deformities or disabling birth injuries)
- infants and children with severe weight loss (10%) or failure-to-thrive syndrome
- women with a complicated pregnancy, labor, delivery, or postpartum period
- pregnant or recently delivered adolescents
- anyone lacking a support system, especially elderly clients
- medical-surgical clients with acute problems that require follow-up (drainage tubes, extensive casts, injections, medications requiring special considerations such as insulin, open or infected wounds, ostomies, special diet instructions or exercises)
- clients who have had radical surgery with lifestyle changes (bilateral amputation, bilateral nephrectomy, cardiovascular surgery, radical neck surgery)
- clients with chronic illnesses or multiple diagnoses (cancer, diabetes mellitus, heart disease)
- emotionally disturbed clients
- impoverished clients.

Special needs services

For clients with special needs, the nurse, case manager, or social worker should arrange community or home health services as part of the discharge plan, as indicated. Examples of special needs services include:

- extended care facility, nursing home, skilled care, or home care
- medical supervision and follow-up
- physical, occupational, speech, and other therapies or rehabilitation
- periodic laboratory testing
- inhalation therapy
- homemaker services
- transportation (ambulance or other special vehicles, as required)
- special equipment and supplies.

Client transfers

Part of discharge planning includes arranging for the safe transfer of the client from:

- one hospital unit to another (for example, from acute care to progressive care)
- the hospital (or facility) to the client's home
- the hospital (or facility) to another private or community institution.

Additionally, the nurse must provide for the transfer of client records and other essential information from one care level to another.

Leadership and management

Leadership and management are two very different but related roles within nursing. Leaders are those individuals who have the ability or power to influence others to achieve goals. Managers direct or empower leaders to achieve organizational or corporate goals.

ROLES OF LEADERS AND MANAGERS

Although their functions are inherently different, leaders and managers must coexist and function as a seamless force to attain shared goals.

The primary functions of leaders include:

◆ communicating effectively to members of a group in various situations
◆ motivating group members to achieve goals
◆ modifying individual and group behavior to achieve goals
◆ providing tools, resources, and education to individuals in order to accomplish assigned tasks that contribute to overall goals
◆ integrating the group's ideas into a format that can be easily implemented by those assigned, or who volunteer, to accomplish the goals.

The primary functions of managers include:

◆ planning and mapping out how a goal will be achieved
◆ organizing a structure of leadership to carry out the plan
◆ staffing and scheduling workers so that the plan can be accomplished
◆ controlling and monitoring performance according to the established plan while adhering to its time frame, standards, and goals. (See *Leader and manager characteristics.*)

Leader and manager characteristics

This chart compares important characteristics of leaders and managers.

LEADERS	MANAGERS
Communicate	Plan
Motivate	Organize
Initiate	Staff
Facilitate	Direct
Integrate	Control

ROLE THEORY IN NURSING

Role theory, a theoretical framework for describing, analyzing, and comprehending social interaction, includes five basic concepts:

◆ A *role* is the set of behavior patterns that ideally flow from a person in a particular position (such as a job) in a particular social system (such as the workplace). For example, the role of a staff nurse involves such behaviors as caring for clients, ensuring client safety, and serving as a client advocate.
◆ *Role expectations* are the behavior patterns that an individual and those around them would expect from a person in that particular position, in that particular social system. Nurses' role expectations evolve from various sources, including:
- standards of professional nursing practice
- ethical and legal standards
- work environment
- nursing care delivery systems
- client base
- other health care disciplines and ancillary staff
- other nurses, leaders, and managers
- an individual's own beliefs, status, personality, needs, and values.

Role conflict in leadership

The types of role conflict that arise in leadership are varied. Here are a few instances in which a role conflict can occur:
- A person's behavior may differ from how others uniformly perceive that the person should behave in a given role.
- Others may disagree about how a person should behave in a given role.
- One person may perform multiple roles that compete for the person's time and energy.
- A person may have mixed feelings about a chosen role.
- A person may be uncertain about which role to choose.

- *Role enactment* or *role performance* refers to the individual's (in this case, the nurse's) actual behavior.
- *Role conflict* emerges when an individual (nurse) must conform to mutually exclusive, contradictory, or inconsistent expectations. (See *Role conflict in leadership.*)
- Resolution of role conflict (*conflict resolution*) may benefit or harm the social system (workplace) and those individuals working within it. In nursing, a role conflict may lead to better client care or improved morale among staff, or it can have the opposite effect, depending on the circumstances.

For instance, complaints about having insufficient staff to care for complex critically ill clients may compel administrators to add staff to decrease the workload, benefiting both staff and clients. Conversely, management's failure to address such complaints may lead to anger and frustration among staff members, causing job dissatisfaction, diminished performance, substandard client care, and even resignations.

Conflict resolution

Nursing leaders and managers can apply the principles of role theory to resolve conflicts when they arise. When individual nurses or groups of staff become dissatisfied, angry, or stressed, a leader or manager can assess their roles by asking several pertinent questions:
- What are the sources of conflict?
- Has conflict developed because roles weren't clearly defined?
- Do the individuals within the group have different expectations for the role?

Depending on the answers to these assessment questions, the leader may use one or more combined strategies to resolve conflict, such as:
- having the individuals in the group describe their role expectations
- clarifying for the group what their expectations should be
- helping the group set priorities
- identifying measures to diffuse anger and alleviate stress.

LEADERSHIP AND MANAGEMENT STYLES

Three basic leadership styles dominate leadership and management:
- *Autocratic* — The leader is the keeper of centralized power and limits subordinate input, is capable of unilateral decision making, and has a high priority for task accomplishment rather than who performs the task. This leadership style is commonly effective in crisis situations.
- DEMOCRATIC — This type of leader involves subordinates in the decision-making process, is masterful at delegation, and values feedback as a tool for change. This leadership style is typically preferred in most work settings because people usually perform more effectively when they have an equal voice in decision making.
- LAISSEZ-FAIRE — The leader who uses this style typically gives the group complete freedom to make decisions about how tasks are to be completed. This style is usually successful in highly motivated or creative work environments.

Power

Managers and leaders must use power appropriately to accomplish tasks and goals. Nursing is recognized as a profession that isn't subordinate to other disciplines and, as such, has an obligation to exercise its power. The modulation of an appropriate amount of power is an important part of being a professional nurse.

Forms of power

Power exists in many different forms:
- *Expert power* results from the individual's ability to influence actions and decisions based on expert knowledge. Nurses increase expert power by developing professionally and remaining current in their area of practice.

◆ *Position power* results from an individual's position or job title. It's important to have appropriate titles or designations in order to define the scope of a nurse's ability or increasing responsibility.
◆ *Economic power* is rooted in the ability to generate or otherwise alter resources and revenue. A change in nursing practice can influence cost savings. Collective bargaining can influence compensation and working conditions.
◆ *Political power* is the ability to gain public exposure or rally support for an important cause. Political power is a manifestation of nursing groups and organizations that lobby for reform.
◆ *Referent power,* or *charismatic power,* resides in the individual and is a combination of one's personal, professional, and other dimensions. A nurse who's ethical and uses her position in the workplace and community to influence political or economic power possesses referent power.

The power of nursing

When caring for clients, nurses use several other forms of power that are associated with the art of nursing:
◆ TRANSFORMATIONAL POWER is the ability to assist clients in changing their self-image or self-care strategies.
◆ INTEGRATIVE POWER is the ability to return clients to their baseline functionality, while providing methods and adaptations necessary because of illness or injury.
◆ ADVOCACY POWER is the ability to protect the client. Nurses possess intuitive insight into their clients' needs and wishes, as well as an ability to be proactive in clinical situations, removing obstacles to care or correcting misperceptions about providing care.
◆ *Healing power* is the ability to encourage, provide for, and support physical and emotional healing.
◆ *Participative power* is power derived from caring for others. Nurses use a holistic approach to care, using all of their clinical skill, experience, insight, and healing power to promote a positive client outcome.

COMMUNICATION IN NURSING

Effective communication is necessary at all nursing levels — from upper management to staff nurses. It can dramatically influence the organization's effectiveness and perception within the community, as well as the individual nurse's role and job performance — which ultimately affects client care. For example:
◆ Effective change-of-shift communication between nurses can improve continuity of care and promote individualized care planning.
◆ Accurate and thorough documentation creates a permanent record of care and actively communicates information to other health care disciplines involved with the client's care.
◆ Communication between a client and a nurse may bring to light issues that are vital to the client's well-being.

THE COMMUNICATION PROCESS

Communication follows six basic steps:
1. *Formulation* — The sender formulates a message, which should be clear and complete.
2. *Encoding* — The sender encodes the message with verbal and nonverbal information (in which emotion or tone is encoded in the message).
3. *Transmission* — The sender transmits the message (memo, speech, e-mail, phone, etc.).
4. *Decoding* — The receiver interprets meaning from the sent message.
5. *Action* — The receiver takes action based on his interpretation of the message.
6. *Feedback* — The sender and receiver of the message provide feedback, continually exchanging and clarifying information.

COMMUNICATION METHODS

To achieve organizational goals, management must communicate effectively and clearly to the nursing staff. This is accomplished through two basic methods:
◆ *interpersonal communication,* in which a message is transmitted from one person to another, or to a very small group, with the intent that the message will be received and understood
◆ *organizational communication,* the system of choice used by an organization to communicate with its members, in which messages may be transmitted formally and informally.

With *formal communication,* information flows through established channels whereby messages are received and sent to people inside and outside the organization. Examples of formal communication include newsletters, departmental meetings, and written minutes or memos.

With *informal communication,* messages are sent and received through social interaction that's typically outside the formal channels of communication (for example, information that's heard through the "grapevine").

Interpretation and clarification

Communication is capable of travel in any direction and by any vehicle. What's important is interpreting communication correctly and evaluating the source. Messages (formal and informal) should always be clarified at the formal level. Formal clarification prevents corruption of goals and may limit role conflict.

Feedback as a management tool

Feedback to staff members about job performance serves as a control measure for managers. Feedback about performance should be:

- helpful to staff
- objective rather than judgmental
- specific rather than general
- timely.

DELEGATION

Delegation is another skill of a competent nurse leader. By appropriately delegating, a nurse can:

- make better use of time
- focus on higher-order priorities
- foster teamwork
- develop staff skills
- compensate for staffing shortages
- distribute time and skill evenly across the client load
- use all available staff to their fullest potential.

Delegation enables a leader to entrust authority to someone else. Thus, the designee can act independently and assume responsibility with the leader for the assigned tasks. However, if something goes awry while the designee performs the task, the leader is responsible for problem-solving the situation. Whether the leader is held accountable for the problem depends on the appropriateness of the delegated task.

AUTHORITY TO DELEGATE

The authority to delegate is based on law and regulation. It's essential to adhere to the state's standard for delegation as found in the nurse practice act. When making the decision to delegate, ask:

- Is delegation permitted in this institution?
- How is delegation defined in the culture in which you practice?
- Do you have the authority to delegate?
- Are the roles of ancillary staff defined?
- How is the scope of practice of ancillary staff defined?
- What tasks should be delegated and what tasks shouldn't be delegated?
- Does the nurse practice act indicate the consequences of inappropriate delegation?

Appropriate delegation should take place at the following practice levels:

- Managers delegate to leaders, and leaders to managers.
- Registered nurses (RNs) can delegate to other RNs, licensed practical nurses (LPNs), or unlicensed assistive personnel (UAPs).
- LPNs delegate to other LPNs and UAPs.
- UAPs delegate to UAPs.

Overall, the delegated skill or task must match the designee's level of training and remain within the realm of that practitioner's lawful scope of practice.

DELEGATING AT THE RN LEVEL

The following guidelines can be used for successful delegation in the clinical setting:

- Tasks that are to be delegated must fall within your own scope of practice as an RN.
- Delegated tasks can't exceed the scope of practice of the staff member to whom the task is delegated.
- The delegated task can be assigned only to those competent to perform the task.
- Delegated tasks must be consistent with legal requirements, the nurse practice act, professional standards of practice, and the policies and procedures of the facility.
- The decision to delegate must consider the client's needs, including maintaining safety, availability of resources, and the particular circumstances under which the delegated care is to be performed.

PRINCIPLES OF DELEGATION

All nurse leaders must master these basic principles to guide and empower subordinates effectively:

- Provide clear, specific instructions about the delegated task to the staff member; include objectives, a time frame for completion, and expectations.
- Periodically check on progress, and provide support as needed.
- Discuss anticipated problems and possible solutions.
- Be available for consultation and continued guidance.

◆ Allow the staff member some latitude on how to complete the task.
◆ Instill confidence and provide feedback.
◆ Expect errors, especially with new tasks; provide constructive suggestions for improvement when a task isn't completed as expected.
◆ Provide praise for a job well done.

STAFF DEVELOPMENT

Nurse leaders and managers should take an active role in the professional development of their staff. Staff members should be motivated to learn and be held accountable for acquiring new knowledge, skills, and abilities.

Effective teaching is most likely to occur when the teacher follows these learning principles:
◆ Learner satisfaction increases learning potential.
◆ Active participation enhances learning.
◆ Learning increases motivation.
◆ Relevant learning experiences augment clinical expertise.
◆ Provision of educational opportunities assigns value to staff.
◆ The learner's experience and knowledge can enhance future learning.
◆ Mutual goal setting produces meaningful learning.
◆ Critical thinking will proliferate.
◆ Quality of care will increase.
◆ Mild anxiety may benefit the learner.
◆ Clinical skills can be validated and measured.

AGENTS OF CHANGE

An essential function of managers and leaders is to act as agents of change. An agent of change is someone who can innovate and bring change successfully. In order to bring change to the working environment, the manager or leader must be willing to take risks and, more important, must plan changes that are appropriate for the group.

An agent of change uses one or both of the following behaviors to initiate change:
◆ *Directive behavior* — One-way communication is employed to explain what subordinates should do and how it is to be done.
◆ *Supportive behavior* — Two-way communication is employed to provide emotional support to subordinates, thus, facilitating task accomplishment.

PHASES OF CHANGE

There are three primary phases of change. All nurse leaders, managers, and subordinates experience these phases to some degree when change has begun.

Phase 1: Unfreezing

The leader challenges and limits customary or traditional behavior and introduces new behaviors and alternatives. Evaluation of past failures helps ensure success.

Phase 2: Changing

Subordinates exhibit behavior in one of three ways:
◆ They identify with and emulate the alternative behavior provided by the environment of change.
◆ They internalize new behaviors when success depends on it.
◆ They reject change and suffer the effects of role conflict.

Phase 3: Refreezing

Subordinates integrate new behaviors and concepts into their work styles. This takes place only if phases one and two are successful. Maintaining the new behavior requires reinforcement from the leader or manager.

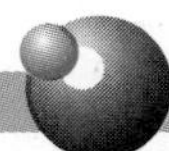

SPOT CHECK

What are the three phases of change?

1. Unfreezing
2. Changing
3. Refreezing

ENSURING QUALITY CARE

Two accepted methods for ensuring quality services and care are quality control and total quality management.

Quality control refers to monitoring the safety and efficacy of client care that has already been rendered. It occurs when operations, standards, and procedures are periodically reviewed. Other characteristics include:
◆ provides a traditional approach to quality management
◆ focuses on clinical errors or mistakes

- has limited potential because it addresses quality of care at its end-point rather than preventively or as it occurs.

Total quality management offers a comprehensive way of monitoring client care as issues arise or preventively, before they happen. It operates on the following principles:

- identifying risk of error in the care continuum and employing benchmarking
- emphasizing error prevention
- empowering health team members from all levels to improve the quality of care
- continual process focused on client care improvement.

PERFORMANCE IMPROVEMENT

In nursing, performance improvement refers to the systems a facility uses to monitor the outcomes of its services by comparing them with established standards. The data gathered by performance improvement activities helps to guide quality control and total quality management.

The level of nursing care provided and its effects on clients are assessed by examining the nursing process and client outcomes. The nursing process is the scientifically organized sequence of activities undertaken by nurses in caring for clients. Client outcomes are the end result of nursing care. The focus of performance improvement is to assess and measure the effectiveness of the nursing process upon client outcome.

Methods of assessment include:

- open and closed chart review
- peer review
- client questionnaire
- staff observations
- auditing tools
- rating scales
- national benchmarking.

Quality of care and services in nursing are universally defined by standards set forth by:

- state nursing boards
- nurse practice acts
- rules and regulations that legally define nursing
- The Standards of Practice promulgated by the American Nurses' Association or specialty agencies such as the American Association of Critical Nurses
- The Standards for Nursing Services of the Joint Commission on Accreditation of Health Care Organizations
- state and federal agencies.

Performance improvement procedures that are routinely enacted by progressive managers and leaders include:

- identifying standards, goals, and methods of completing performance improvement activities
- measuring actual performance
- comparing results of performance with standards, goals, and practices
- taking action to correct poor outcome
- identifying good outcomes and making sure that they're reproducible.

RISK MANAGEMENT

Risk management provides a formal method for predicting problems and providing resources to ensure safe care delivery. It includes a system of responding to clinical errors and changing organizational policies and procedures to prevent the repetition of other similar occurrences.

Numerous risk factors can be found in various nursing settings that can prompt or initiate the involvement of risk management:

- facility or organizational procedures that don't comply with standards or state nurse practice acts
- client injuries that result from nursing errors
- delays in client treatment
- insufficient documentation of nursing care
- insufficient documentation of a significant event
- poor communication among departments that causes harm or the potential for harm
- staffing concerns
- equipment failure.

THE ROLE OF STAFF

The staff nurse plays a valuable role in quality assurance and risk management. Focus groups of staff can be used to:

- define performance goals guided at improving care delivery and reducing risk to clients
- identify problems and formulate solutions
- develop methods for attaining standards
- assert change in order to correct deficiency.

CLINICAL PRACTICE STRUCTURE

The structure of the work environment significantly influences the role of nurse managers and leaders. An efficient structure enables the staff to achieve the tasks and goals at hand in the most time-efficient, cost-effective manner.

Common care delivery systems include:

◆ *Functional nursing* — Nurses are assigned to specific tasks, such as medication administration, multidisciplinary rounds, and direct client care. Accountability rests primarily with the nurse manager.
◆ *Team nursing* — Nurses share responsibility for a group of clients. The team can include RNs, LPNs, UAPs, and other ancillary staff. Accountability rests with the team leaders and the nurse manager. This style is common in many emergency department settings.
◆ *Primary nursing* — Each nurse has her own caseload and is responsible for every aspect of her clients' care. The staff nurse and nurse manager share accountability for the care of this group of patients. This patient care delivery style is common in critical care settings.

NURSING GROUP MANAGEMENT

Nursing groups exist for a variety of reasons, including problem solving, goal development, and new project initiation and management. A group depends on the leadership skills of its leader for success. To be successful, the group leader must take on primary roles, which include:
◆ getting to know, then accept group members
◆ securing agreements from the group members about the purpose of the group
◆ establishing structures, rules, and procedures for accomplishing the group's goals.

To be an effective member of a group, members must:
◆ relate well to others inside and outside the group
◆ provide clear directions and information
◆ make sound decisions
◆ use effective problem-solving techniques.

Groups are most successful when their goals are clearly defined and measurable, each member is committed to the goals, and the members of the group have the resources to achieve their goals.

DISASTER MANAGEMENT

The terrorist attack against the United States on September 11, 2001, forever changed the way disaster management is perceived. The constant threat of attack requires health care leaders to develop and maintain plans to counter disaster and manage its consequences. In addition to the threat of a terrorist attack, health care personnel must be ready to respond to natural disasters, biological disasters, accidental hazardous material releases, and mass casualty incidences. (See *When disaster strikes.*)

When disaster strikes

Regardless of the type of disaster, the health care team must be prepared to mobilize all available personnel and resources. This includes triaging already hospitalized clients to make room for those who are more seriously ill or injured.

The key to successful disaster management is planning. Facilities must perform disaster exercises regularly to ensure that the team is prepared whenever disaster strikes. Such planning includes preparations for the following types of disasters:

Natural disasters
◆ Fire
◆ Flood
◆ Earthquake
◆ Mudslide
◆ Hurricane
◆ Tornado
◆ Blizzard
◆ Tsunami

Civil catastrophes
◆ Explosion
◆ Building collapse
◆ Infrastructure failure
◆ Civil uprising
◆ Epidemic outbreak

Toxic exposure
◆ Biologic agent release or attack
◆ Radiologic agent release or attack
◆ Chemical agent release or attack

PLANNED RESPONSE

Each facility must devise a plan that includes the four phases of disaster management:
◆ planning for the disaster
◆ mitigation of the disaster
◆ response to the disaster
◆ recovery from the disaster.

Health care teams can't respond to a disaster unless they're properly prepared. Managers and leaders must work together to develop a plan. After the plan is developed, each staff member must be adequately trained. To ensure the highest level of preparedness, facilities must conduct disaster drills to make sure that their plan can be implemented in an efficient manner. Moreover, staff members must also be trained to properly use equipment and maintain it so that it's readily available should disaster strike. After the leadership and management team devises a hospital-wide plan, they must work with the community to make sure they're prepared and informed in the event of a disaster. They must also coordinate their plan with other local, state, and federal agencies.

To be effective, the disaster plan must include:

- measures to control and direct all of the appropriate resources
- ways to establish and maintain communication within the facility and outside with neighboring responders and agencies
- interventions to protect as many lives as possible
- methods to protect property
- resources for the community
- road map for recovery of the facility and staff after the disaster.

IMPLEMENTING A DISASTER PLAN

Nurse leaders must be available to implement the disaster response plan. They must provide direction for mobilizing staff and equipment while ensuring that the needs of hospitalized clients are met. They must also plan with neighboring facilities to transfer clients to other facilities to make resources available for those involved in the disaster.

Leaders also play a key role in the recovery phase that follows the activation of the disaster plan. Tasks include:

- calculating damages
- prioritizing the replenishment of supplies
- preparing for future disasters
- assessing staffing needs
- devising plans to relieve frontline personnel
- preparing for staff debriefing
- preparing for leadership debriefing
- evaluating the effectiveness of the disaster plan and response
- identifying measures to improve the disaster plan.

Ethical and legal issues

5

ETHICAL PRINCIPLES AND NURSING PRACTICE

The basic premise of addressing ethical issues is to promote good and avoid harm. Although nurses strive to do the right thing, good intentions alone aren't enough. Nurses must use a systematic approach to solving ethical dilemmas. Ethical dilemmas occur when there's a conflict between two ethical principles. These ethical principles include:

- autonomy, a person's right to self-determination (the right to make decisions about one's own health care)
- nonmalificence, the obligation to do no harm
- beneficence, the promotion of good and prevention of harm
- justice, the provision of equal treatment and resources for everyone.

There's usually no right or wrong decision when it comes to ethical decision making. It's important for the nurse to understand the client's wishes and to advocate for him. Sometimes that means putting personal beliefs aside to best represent the client. Nurses have a responsibility to support a client's decisions. The American Nurses Association Code of Ethics and the Code for Nurses developed by the International Council of Nurses provide guidelines for conduct by professional nurses. These documents aren't legally binding; however, many State Boards of Nursing consider these principles standards of behavior.

The Joint Commission on Accreditation of Healthcare Organizations (JCAHO) mandates that hospitals must provide ethics consultation. Such consultation can be accomplished by a multidisciplinary committee (made up of nurses, physicians, hospital legal council, community members, and clergy) or an ethics consultant. Committees and consultants may be voluntary or may be a service done for a fee.

With the advent of new technology and research advances, ethical decision making has become a part of everyday care. These ethical decisions are commonly difficult ones because they spark emotions from families, clients, and their designated caregivers. Such emotions may be fueled by each individual's past experiences, religious and cultural backgrounds, and developmental stage.

TECHNOLOGY

In addition to advances in client care technology, there has been an explosion in health care information technology, or *informatics*. Computerized charting systems and physician order entry have been developed to decrease the number of medical errors. These computerized charting systems pose new ethical issues for nurses.

For example, hospital personnel potentially have access to all inpatient records from any computer terminal. It's important that all hospital computer systems be password protected. Users shouldn't share passwords. Users should only have access to information pertinent to their positions; other information should be designated as "read only" or blocked. Terminals should be set to log off automatically when not accessed for 3 to 5 minutes. Screens should be turned away from public viewing. Systems should have a tracking information log that shows who has accessed information. Nurses shouldn't access information for clients other than those assigned to their care.

RESEARCH

Agencies that participate in research should have access to an Institutional Review Board (IRB). The IRB is usually made up of volunteers who include members of the community. The purpose of the IRB is to protect human subjects from harm when participating in research projects. All research involving humans and animals should be approved by the IRB.

PATIENT SELF-DETERMINATION ACT

The Patient Self-Determination Act of 1990 mandates that all clients must be asked whether they have an advance directive. An ADVANCE DIRECTIVE, which may include a *living will,* is legally binding and should become part of the medical record. This document gives instructions for which treatments should or shouldn't be provided if the client becomes incapacitated.

A DURABLE POWER OF ATTORNEY is a legal document that identifies the client's proxy, or surrogate decision maker, in case the client becomes incapacitated. This document should also become part of the medical record. If no such document exists, state law mandates who may give consent if the client becomes incapacitated. If a surrogate decision maker can't be determined, the court may appoint a suitable surrogate.

The Patient Self-Determination Act also mandates that clients must be informed of their right to refuse treatment at any time regardless of whether they have given informed consent.

END-OF-LIFE CARE

Clients with terminal diseases or in the end stages of a chronic illness commonly have concerns about the dying process. They fear pain, abandonment, and powerlessness most when making end-of-life decisions. It's important for the nurse to reassure the client that pain will be addressed, care will continue, and no treatment will begin or end without the client's consent or that of the designated decision maker. The nurse is commonly the health care provider most aware of clients' wishes and family dynamics because of the time spent with clients and their loved ones at the bedside.

Hospice care

HOSPICE focuses on providing comfort and care to the client with a terminal illness. Hospice uses a multidisciplinary team approach to care that encompasses medical care, pain management, and emotional and spiritual support based on the client's needs and wishes. Hospice care providers support the client and family. The goal of hospice and palliative care is to ensure a person's right to die pain free and with dignity.

Hospice care is covered by Medicare and most insurance companies and usually takes place in the client's home or in a hospice facility. Medicare requires clients to have a terminal prognosis of 6 months or less, although length of care can be reevaluated. Unfortunately, most clients are referred for hospice care in the last few weeks of life and aren't able to take advantage of the full benefits of hospice care.

Palliative care

PALLIATIVE care also improves a client's quality of life in the final stages of a terminal disease. It focuses on making the client as comfortable as possible, not on curing the underlying disease. The client may transition into hospice care when the timing is appropriate.

When planning palliative care, all treatments are considered; however, the choice of treatments is based on the client's desires. Treatment plans are constantly reevaluated and revised as needed and approved by the client.

DO-NOT-RESUSCITATE ORDERS

A do-not-resuscitate (DNR) order indicates that the client doesn't want any treatment if his respirations cease and his heart stops beating. This order must be signed by a physician. Some hospitals have different levels of treatment for cardiac arrest. It's the nurse's responsibility to know what treatments the client wishes when the DNR order is in effect. Providing treatment for a client who wants nothing done is considered battery, and the nurse is liable for treatment without the client's consent.

ORGAN DONATION

The Uniform Anatomical Gift Act was adopted by all 50 states and the District of Columbia, ensuring uniform laws regarding organ and tissue donation and compliance with donors' wishes. Many states have a "required request," mandating that all clients or family members be given the opportunity for organ donation. Anyone older than age 18 can execute an anatomical gift. Consent is usually indicated on a driver's license or in an advance directive. A minor may also make a gift with a parent's or legal guardian's consent. It's the nurse's responsibility to notify the local organ procurement organization about potential donors.

LEGAL PRINCIPLES AND NURSING PRACTICE

Law is a set of rules and principles derived from several sources and enforceable by legal processes. Laws provide a means of settling disputes, compensating for injuries caused by another, and disciplining and isolating individuals for wrongdoing as defined by society. Essential to any society's progress and survival, laws form an important basis for nursing practice.

Each state has a nurse practice act and board of nursing rules and regulations that are designed to protect the public by broadly defining the legal scope of nursing practice. The state legislature enacts the nurse practice act and any amendments. The board of nursing, in accordance with the nurse practice act, publishes its rules and regulations. These rules and regulations, which are generally more specific than what's found in the nurse practice act, establish procedure and carry the same weight as the nurse practice act.

Every nurse is expected to care for clients within these defined practice limits — the most important one affecting nursing care; if she gives care beyond these limits, she becomes vulnerable to charges of violating the law and losing her licensure. These laws, rules, and regulations also serve to exclude untrained or unlicensed people from practicing nursing.

JUDICIAL OPINIONS

A judicial opinion is the court's official position on a legal dispute, written by the judge who presides over the court case. Usually, judicial opinions emanate from appeals or higher courts in the state or federal court system as a result of disputes brought before lower courts by the litigants (those who bring the lawsuit or are otherwise involved in it). These opinions, published in what's usually called the legal reporter system, are also referred to as *case law* or *case decisions.*

Judicial opinions form *precedent,* a body of law that commonly serves as the basis for future decisions. Judicial opinions also address nursing practice in such areas as employment, licensure, malpractice and negligence, and crimes.

LEGISLATION

Legislation is the set of rules created by the legislative branch of government at the federal, state, or local (city or county) level. The legislative branch of government, which meets periodically, is elected by the people. Also called *statutes* or *statutory law,* legislation is published and made available to the public; some states publish legislation in a book called a *code* or an *annotated code.*

Legislation results from the legislative process, which involves the study of issues, drafting of a bill, discussion, compromise, redrafting, and voting for or against the bill's passage. A bill — the proposed law — usually becomes law when more votes are for passage than against, and after the governor (in state legislation) or the president (in federal legislation) signs the bill. (In some circumstances, legislation can become law without the governor's or the president's approval.) Nursing practice is shaped by many pieces of legislation, particularly the state nurse practice act and state and federal public health laws.

REGULATIONS

Regulations are the rules created by the executive branch of government. The executive branch is headed by the governor of a state or the president of the United States. The legislative branch enacts laws granting the executive branch the authority to write regulations.

Regulations are created through the regulatory process, which involves the study of issues, publication of the proposed rule, a period of public input (through written opinions or testimony at hearings), possible redrafting, and publication of the final regulation. Federal regulations are found in the Code of Federal Regulations, and state regulations are usually found in the state's Code of Regulations.

The government agency created by the state nurse practice act, usually called the *State Board of Nursing,* has the power to write specific rules that govern and control nursing practice within its jurisdiction.

TYPES OF LAW

The three types of law are civil, administrative, and criminal law.

Civil law

CIVIL LAW refers to a wide range of legal issues that are unrelated to criminal acts. Usually, civil law involves disputes between two or more individuals or entities. Civil disputes related to safe nursing practice may involve an employment contract, a tort, or a violation of a client's rights. (See "Administrative disputes and nursing practice," page 73.)

Administrative law

ADMINISTRATIVE LAW deals with enforcement of government agencies' rules and regulations. Licensure and the state's power to discipline nurses involve the administrative law and process. A state can make rules that govern nursing based on its "police power," the power to act to protect public health, safety, and welfare. For example, a state can prohibit a nurse from practicing nursing if the nurse is found guilty of unprofessional conduct.

Criminal law

Crimes involve public wrongs (wrongs against society). CRIMINAL LAW refers to a set of laws that define wrongs against society. The criminal justice and law enforcement systems exist to investigate, prosecute and, if the accused is found guilty, punish the offender.

CIVIL DISPUTES AND NURSING PRACTICE

The law of the nurse's workplace is derived from federal and state statutes and judicial opinions, employer personnel handbooks, civil service rules, employer practice, collective bargaining agreements, and employment contracts.

A CONTRACT is a written or oral agreement between two or more individuals that includes several elements regarding formation, interpretation, and enforcement. A contract can be individual or collective (such as a union contract). It can specify the period within which the conditions of the agreement must be met. A contract may also include the elements *offer, acceptance,* and *consideration* (usually monetary compensation). In nursing practice, civil disputes can arise that may involve torts and client rights.

Torts

A TORT is a private wrong or a breach of a legal duty to the rights and interests of others. An injured litigant (usually called a *plaintiff*) can receive remedy for a tort, commonly in the form of damages, if the litigant presents adequate evidence to prove that an injury occurred. Courts recognize three types of torts: unintentional, intentional, and quasi-intentional.

Unintentional tort

An UNINTENTIONAL TORT is an act that fails to meet a duty owed to another person (the plaintiff) and leads to the person's injury. In nursing, the two most common types of unintentional torts are negligence and malpractice. Both types also involve some form of liability.

Negligence

NEGLIGENCE is an unintentional tort that involves four elements:

- *DUTY* — refers to the nurse's legal obligation to provide nursing care to a client. The nurse has the duty to meet a reasonable and prudent standard of care under the circumstances. The nurse must also deliver care as any other reasonable and prudent nurse would under similar circumstances. Standards of care are found in policy and procedure manuals, nursing education materials, and publications of professional associations and accreditation groups.
- *BREACH OF DUTY* — refers to the failure to provide the expected reasonable standard of care under the circumstances; it can take two forms. The nurse may fail to provide care (breach by omission of the duty) or the nurse may provide care in an unreasonable manner (breach by commission of the duty).
- *PROXIMATE CAUSE* — refers to the causal connection between the breach of duty and the resulting injury. Proximate cause doesn't necessarily involve a direct cause-and-effect relationship, but the plaintiff must produce evidence that the nurse's action or inaction led to the plaintiff's injury. State laws vary in the language used to define proximate cause:
  - If the definition uses the term "but for," the plaintiff must prove that the injury wouldn't have occurred "but for" the nurse's breach of duty.
  - If the definition uses the term "substantial factor," the plaintiff must prove that the nurse's breach of duty was a "substantial factor" in the injury.
  - If the definition uses the term "foreseeability," the plaintiff must prove that the nurse's breach of duty "foreseeably" led to the plaintiff's injury — that is, that the nurse should have known what would happen.
- *DAMAGES* — refers to physical and psychological injuries and monetary compensation awarded to the plaintiff for incurring the injuries. The plaintiff must prove that an injury occurred and present evidence showing its monetary value. The plaintiff can request:
  - *COMPENSATORY DAMAGES,* which are awarded to reimburse the plaintiff for the expenses, rehabilitation, and pain and suffering related to the injury
  - *NOMINAL DAMAGES,* which are awarded to indicate a defendant's wrongdoing when little if any injury occurred
  - *PUNITIVE DAMAGES,* which are awarded to the plaintiff in special circumstances, usually to punish the defendant for an especially egregious or outrageous act.

Malpractice

MALPRACTICE is a specific form of negligence committed by a member of a profession (such as nursing). It differs from negligence only in that the standard or duty owed is a professional one, based on special knowledge and skills. The plaintiff in a malpractice action must prove all the elements of negligence, usually with an expert witness to testify about the professional duty owed and whether it was breached. However, not all states automatically apply a professional standard to nurses; some states still apply a nonprofessional one, and other states apply a professional standard only when the nurse's act required special knowledge and skill.

Intentional tort

An INTENTIONAL TORT is a willful act that injures another person or the person's property. These acts include:

- ASSAULT — the threat of imminent harmful or offensive bodily contact (for example, threatening comments made by a nurse to a client)
- BATTERY — bodily contact with another person without the person's permission or consent (such as forcing a client to submit to injections)
- FALSE IMPRISONMENT — unlawful restraint of a person against his will (for instance, refusing to let a client return home from a clinical setting)
- INTENTIONAL INFLICTION OF EMOTIONAL DISTRESS — extreme, outrageous, or intolerable conduct toward another, causing emotional harm (for example, making false statements about a client to a third person, which damages the client's reputation)
- INVASION OF PRIVACY — the release of private information to an unauthorized third party without the client's consent (such as allowing an unauthorized staff member to read a client's medical record).

Quasi-intentional tort

A quasi-intentional tort is an act that interferes with a person's intangible interests, such as privacy and reputation. A nurse may be charged with invasion of privacy and breach of confidentiality for revealing personal information about a client to an unauthorized person. A nurse may also be charged with defamation for injuring the plaintiff's reputation in the community as the result of a false statement, either spoken (slander) or written (libel). False statements about another person's professional competence can lead to a defamation lawsuit. However, truth is a viable defense against a defamation charge.

Liability

Negligence and malpractice lawsuits also involve legal principles about who bears LIABILITY (responsibility) for resultant injuries. Two types of liability are:

- personal liability, or responsibility for one's acts
- vicarious liability, or responsibility for another person's acts, which can take one of two forms:
  - *RESPONDEAT SUPERIOR LIABILITY* addresses an employer's responsibility for injuries caused by an employee's negligent acts, if those acts were performed within the scope of employment and when an employment relationship existed. For example, if a hospital-employed nurse fails to detect a hematoma under the blood pressure cuff of a heavily heparinized client in the intensive care unit, both the hospital and the nurse are liable.
  - *CORPORATE LIABILITY* refers to an employer's responsibility for injury caused by an employee who acted according to the employer's decisions. For example, because a hospital determines its budget, staff, and client population, the hospital — not the nurse — is liable for injury that results from understaffing.

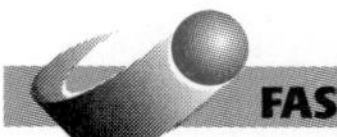

FAST FACT

If a client sustains injuries because a staff nurse administers the wrong drug or fails to monitor the client properly, the nurse can be found liable for those acts.

DOCUMENTATION

The client's medical record is the only document that details the nurse's interaction with the client during care. Medical records are legal documents and can be the best defense against allegations of negligence or malpractice — if documentation is done properly. Remember, your charting is a reflection of your care. If your charting is incomplete, people will assume the same of your care. Chart so the person reading the record has a visual picture of the client's condition and the care you've provided.

Tips for complete documentation

Here are some tips to ensure that your documentation is complete:

- Record observations rather than interpretations; use accurate measurements to describe lesions or wounds.
- Avoid generalizations; use approved assessment scales when available.
- Note client problems in an orderly, sequential manner.
- Record all consultations and physician visits.
- Document responses from physicians, nursing supervisors, and others.
- Use approved medical terminology, date and time entries, and don't skip lines.
- Use only the standardized list of abbreviations, acronyms, and symbols that are used throughout your facility. Avoid using any abbreviations deemed "dangerous" by JCAHO.

◆ Sign every entry with your first initial, last name, and title.
◆ If you make a mistake, draw a single line through the error and write *error in charting* above or beside the error with your initials, the date, and the time.
◆ Avoid telephone orders except in emergency situations; always repeat the order back to the prescriber, and have another nurse verify the order.
◆ Use approved formats for verbal and telephone orders.

PATIENT RIGHTS

A Patient's Bill of Rights, written by the American Hospital Association, contains a sample list of patient (client) rights. Although not law, this code lists many rights of clients legally recognized through sources of law previously mentioned. (See *A Patient's Bill of Rights.*) Client rights include:
◆ informed consent
◆ freedom from unreasonable restraint
◆ right to refuse treatment
◆ right to privacy and confidentiality.

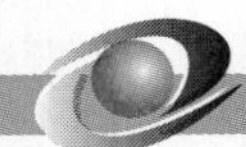

QUICK STUDY

Want an easy way to remember client rights as listed in a Patient's Bill of Rights? Remember this sentence: ***I**ngrid **F**ries **R**ed **P**eppers.*

Informed consent
Freedom from unreasonable restraint
Right to refuse treatment
Privacy and confidentiality right

Informed consent

INFORMED CONSENT refers to the client's involvement in and agreement with treatment decisions based on careful consideration of all information pertinent to his condition. For informed consent to be recognized by the court, several conditions must be met:
◆ The consent must be voluntary.
◆ The information given to the client must include the nature of the proposed treatment, its foreseeable risks and benefits, alternatives to the proposed treatment, and the consequences of choosing to do nothing.
◆ The consent must be given by a person who's legally competent to do so.

The physician has the legal obligation to obtain a client's informed consent to medical treatment. Nurses are commonly assigned the task of obtaining a signed consent form and witnessing the client's signature. Doing so legally obligates the nurse, if called later, to testify about anything relating to what she saw, heard, or knew about the consent. A nurse who's concerned about the validity of an informed consent has a legal obligation to tell the physician and the nursing supervisor about the concerns and to document that she has done so.

Competency considerations

Before informed consent is obtained, the client's legal competence must be determined. Be aware that legal competence differs from medical or mental competence. It's a presumption established by the state legislatures (usually a chronological age, such as 18 years); thus, everyone older than age 18 is presumed legally competent, and everyone younger than age 18 is presumed legally incompetent.

For those younger than age 18 (known as *minors*), legislatures have established exceptions to the rule of presumed incompetency; unless one of these exceptions applies, informed consent for treatment of a minor must be obtained from the minor's parent or legal guardian.

Consent from a parent or guardian usually isn't required if the minor is married, has a child, lives independently, or seeks certain types of health care services (such as for pregnancy, substance abuse, or a mental health problem).

After reaching the legal age of competence, one can lose the legal capacity to consent only through a formal judicial process. In this proceeding, a court determines, usually on the basis of medical and psychiatric testimony, whether the person is incompetent. If the court finds the person incompetent, the court appoints a guardian (who becomes the person authorized to give informed consent).

In some situations, the court not only must rule on incompetency but also must determine whether the individual needs involuntary commitment to an institution for treatment. Before the court orders involuntary commitment, it must receive clear and convincing evidence that the individual poses a danger to self or others with no other less restrictive treatment available. The rules to make these determinations from state to state.

When consent isn't required

Under certain circumstances, informed consent may not be required, such as:
◆ life-threatening emergencies, in which client consent is implied.
◆ a WAIVER, in which a client tells the physician that he doesn't want to know the appropriate information

A Patient's Bill of Rights

Introduction

Effective health care requires collaboration between patients and physicians and other health care professionals. Open and honest communication, respect for personal and professional values, and sensitivity to differences are integral to optimal patient care. As the setting for the provision of health services, hospitals must provide a foundation for understanding and respecting the rights and responsibilities of patients, their families, physicians, and other caregivers. Hospitals must ensure a health care ethic that respects the role of patients in decision making about treatment choices and other aspects of their care. Hospitals must be sensitive to cultural, racial, linguistic, religious, age, gender, and other differences as well as the needs of persons with disabilities.

The American Hospital Association presents A Patient's Bill of Rights with the expectation that it will contribute to more effective patient care and be supported by the hospital on behalf of the institution, its medical staff, employees, and patients. The American Hospital Association encourages health care institutions to tailor this bill of rights to their patient community by translating or simplifying the language of this bill of rights as may be necessary to ensure that patients and their families understand their rights and responsibilities.

Bill of rights*

1. The patient has the right to considerate and respectful care.

2. The patient has the right to and is encouraged to obtain from physicians and other direct caregivers relevant, current, and understandable information concerning diagnosis, treatment, and prognosis.

Except in emergencies when the patient lacks decision-making capacity and the need for treatment is urgent, the patient is entitled to the opportunity to discuss and request information related to the specific procedures and/or treatments, the risks involved, the possible length of recuperation, and the medically reasonable alternatives and their accompanying risks and benefits.

Patients have the right to know the identity of physicians, nurses, and others involved in their care as well as when those involved are students, residents, or other trainees. The patient also has the right to know the immediate and long-term financial implications of treatment choices, insofar as they're known.

3. The patient has the right to make decisions about the plan of care prior to and during the course of treatment and to refuse a recommended treatment or plan of care to the extent permitted by law and hospital policy and to be informed of the medical consequences of this action. In case of such refusal, the patient is entitled to other appropriate care and services that the hospital provides or transfer to another hospital. The hospital should notify patients of any policy that might affect patient choice within the institution.

4. The patient has the right to have an advance directive (such as a living will, health care proxy, or durable power of attorney for health care) concerning treatment or designating a surrogate decision maker with the expectation that the hospital will honor the intent of that directive to the extent permitted by law and hospital policy.

Health care institutions must advise patients of their rights under state law and hospital policy to make informed medical choices, ask if the patient has an advance directive, and include that information in patient records. The patient has the right to timely information about hospital policy that may limit its ability to implement fully a legally valid advance directive.

5. The patient has the right to every consideration of privacy. Case discussion, consultation, examination, and treatment should be conducted so as to protect each patient's privacy.

6. The patient has the right to expect that all communications and records pertaining to his/her care will be treated as confidential by the hospital, except in cases such as suspected abuse and public health hazards when reporting is permitted or required by law. The patient has the right to expect that the hospital will emphasize the confidentiality of this information when it releases it to any other parties entitled to review information in these records.

7. The patient has the right to review the records pertaining to his/her medical care and to have the information explained or interpreted as necessary, except when restricted by law.

8. The patient has the right to expect that, within its capacity and policies, a hospital will make reasonable response to the request of a patient for appropriate and medically indicated care and services. The hospital must provide evaluation, service, and/or referral as indicated by the urgency of the case. When medically appropriate and legally permissible, or when a patient has so requested, a patient may be transferred to another facility. The institution to which the patient is to be transferred must first have accepted the patient for transfer. The patient must also have the benefit of complete information and explanation concerning the need for, risks, benefits, and alternatives to such a transfer.

9. The patient has the right to ask and be informed of the existence of business relationships among the hospital, educational institutions, other health care providers, or payers that may influence the patient's treatment and care.

(continued)

A Patient's Bill of Rights *(continued)*

10. The patient has the right to consent to or decline to participate in proposed research studies or human experimentation affecting care and treatment or requiring direct patient involvement, and to have those studies fully explained prior to consent. A patient who declines to participate in research or experimentation is entitled to the most effective care that the hospital can otherwise provide.

11. The patient has the right to expect reasonable continuity of care when appropriate and to be informed by physicians and other caregivers of available and realistic patient care options when hospital care is no longer appropriate.

12. The patient has the right to be informed of hospital policies and practices that relate to patient care, treatment, and responsibilities. The patient has the right to be informed of available resources for resolving disputes, grievances, and conflicts, such as ethics committees, patient representatives, or other mechanisms available in the institution. The patient has the right to be informed of the hospital's charges for services and available payment methods.

The collaborative nature of health care requires that patients, or their families/surrogates, participate in their care. The effectiveness of care and patient satisfaction with the course of treatment depend, in part, on the patient fulfilling certain responsibilities. Patients are responsible for providing information about past illnesses, hospitalizations, medications, and other matters related to health status. To participate effectively in decision making, patients must be encouraged to take responsibility for requesting additional information or clarification about their health status or treatment when they do not fully understand information and instructions. Patients are also responsible for ensuring that the health care institution has a copy of their written advance directive if they have one. Patients are responsible for informing their physicians and other caregivers if they anticipate problems in following prescribed treatment.

Patients should also be aware of the hospital's obligation to be reasonably efficient and equitable in providing care to other patients and the community. The hospital's rules and regulations are designed to help the hospital meet this obligation. Patients and their families are responsible for making reasonable accommodations to the needs of the hospital, other patients, medical staff, and hospital employees. Patients are responsible for providing necessary information for insurance claims and for working with the hospital to make payment arrangements, when necessary.

A person's health depends on much more than health care services. Patients are responsible for recognizing the impact of their lifestyle on their personal health.

Conclusion

Hospitals have many functions to perform, including the enhancement of health status, health promotion, and the prevention and treatment of injury and disease; the immediate and ongoing care and rehabilitation of patients; the education of health professionals, patients, and the community; and research. All these activities must be conducted with an overriding concern for the values and dignity of patients.

*These rights can be exercised on the patient's behalf by a designated surrogate or proxy decision maker if the patient lacks decision-making capacity, is legally incompetent, or is a minor.

- a situation in which the physician's professional judgment may dictate that fully informing a client would be a substantial detriment to the client and cause harm (known as the *physician's therapeutic privilege*).

Freedom from unreasonable restraint

Freedom from unreasonable restraint recognizes the client's autonomy and freedom of movement. The client must receive care in a safe, prudent manner. Health care providers can legally restrain a client under certain conditions previously defined by law and by the health care facility's policies and procedures.

- The restraints must be necessary to meet the client's therapeutic needs or to ensure the safety of the client or others.
- The least restrictive type of restraint must be used first.
- Use of restraints must be accompanied by the physician's orders except in an emergency.

◆ Health care providers must closely monitor the client, release the restraints periodically, and remove them when the client's condition no longer warrants their use.
◆ Accurate and thorough documentation must reveal all pertinent details of the care given to the client, including how and why restraints were applied and removed.

Right to refuse treatment

The right to refuse treatment enables every competent adult to refuse treatment — even life-sustaining treatment. Also known as the *right to withhold consent,* this right and all the requirements of informed consent apply to a client's decision to refuse treatment.

Similar to other client rights, the right to refuse treatment isn't absolute and must be considered by the court in relation to the interests of society. Thus, the client's right to refuse treatment may be outweighed by the court's responsibility to preserve human life, protect innocent third parties, prevent suicide, or maintain the ethical integrity of the medical profession.

Many states have enacted legislation that permits a client to make health care decisions in advance, including the use of a LIVING WILL (document in which the client instructs family and health care professionals about specific medical measures that should or shouldn't be provided if he becomes incapacitated) or a *durable power of attorney* (legal document in which the client identifies a proxy, or surrogate, decision maker in the event he becomes incapacitated). Both types of documents should be included in the client's medical record.

State laws vary on the issue of SUBSTITUTED CONSENT; if the client lacks the capacity to make informed decisions, health care professionals usually turn to the client's family members and close friends, and the court may formally appoint these surrogate decision makers.

Right to privacy and confidentiality

The Health Insurance Portability and Accountability Act of 1996 (HIPAA) is federal legislation enacted to protect client privacy and assure access to health care. The right to privacy and confidentiality recognizes a client's autonomy and right to be left alone. Because the client and the health care provider have a relationship based on trust, the client may reveal private information that will enhance treatment. In return, the health care provider must keep the information confidential.

The client has the right to access personal health records and obtain a copy of the records. Health care providers have the responsibility to maintain health records in a secure, controlled manner. Information can be revealed only with the client's permission or when required by law. For example, physicians must report acquired immunodeficiency syndrome and other communicable diseases to the federal and state governments, but they must still keep such reports confidential.

ADMINISTRATIVE DISPUTES AND NURSING PRACTICE

State governments regulate nursing practice through an executive branch office, a state board of nursing. The state nurse practice act creates the state board. Each state typically regulates several areas of nursing practice, including:
◆ nursing profession's licensure examination — by determining the rules and requirements for admission or entry into nursing practice
◆ in most states, the nurse practice act that defines the legal scope of nursing practice — by addressing such issues as discipline, fines, censure, or other appropriate steps against anyone who practices nursing without meeting the state requirements
◆ professional conduct of licensed nurses — by defining unprofessional conduct (A nurse who's charged with unprofessional conduct has the right to due process, including notice of the specific charges, an opportunity to present evidence to counter the charge, and representation by an attorney hired by the nurse.)
◆ initiation of investigations, bringing charges of misconduct, and levying of disciplinary measures (investigations include chemical impairment, including drug or alcohol abuse, which is the most common reason for disciplinary action against a nurse)
◆ nursing education — by establishing the requirements of and approving the educational programs for nurse preparation.

CRIMINAL DISPUTES AND NURSING PRACTICE

In nursing practice, criminal disputes can arise that result in the conviction of nurses for such crimes as murder, fraud, client abuse, and illegal use of controlled substances. Most states recognize two types of crimes: felonies and misdemeanors. Some states use the generic term *offenses,* categorizing felonies as crimes and misdemeanors as violations. The primary difference between these types of crimes lies in the crime's degree of severity and, thus, in the length and type of sentence or penalty imposed on the convicted criminal.

Felonies entail more serious offenses and warrant lengthy prison sentences. Misdemeanors, which are less serious, usually result in a short prison sentence, a fine, or both. Keep in mind that, although the defendant in a criminal case may have committed a crime, he has constitutionally provided rights, such as the right to legal counsel.

Criminal codes or statutes define the elements of each crime; the prosecutor must prove the existence of these elements beyond a reasonable doubt. For an act to be considered criminal, the prosecutor must prove the defendant's culpability — that is, the defendant committed the act intentionally, knowingly, recklessly, or in a criminally negligent manner. However, mental impairment precludes the possibility of culpability; thus, the law doesn't support convicting a person who was affected by mental disease or a mental defect when committing the act. A person who's found not guilty by reason of insanity is committed to a treatment facility and is released after recovery. Definitions of mental impairment differ among jurisdictions.

Criminal intent

Nurses occasionally face criminal charges. When they do, the prosecutor needs to prove criminal intent. Showing such intent involves:

- proving that the nurse knew (or should have known) that what she did or failed to do would harm the client, and that she failed to take necessary action to prevent the harm (for example, a registered nurse might ignore the observations made by a licensed practical nurse about a client's worsening condition, then fail to appropriately assess the client to determine necessary intervention and follow-up; if the registered nurse's inaction leads to a severe worsening of the client's condition, she could face criminal charges)
- proving that the nurse intentionally harmed a client (for example, a nurse might commit a violent act that caused either physical or mental harm to a client, such as wrongfully restraining him in a way that caused injury).

Maintaining homeostasis

INTRODUCTION

HOMEOSTASIS — a state of constancy or equilibrium within the body — is essential for the preservation of life. The body maintains homeostasis through a system of internal control mechanisms that regulate vital functions, including blood pressure, temperature, pH, heart rate, respiratory rate, glandular secretion, and fluid and electrolyte balance.

CONTRIBUTING FACTORS

Various factors may adversely affect homeostasis. These include:

- acute illness
- chronic illness
- trauma
- pressures of everyday life.

The degree to which these stressors alter the body's normal balance depends on the individual's adaptability and ability to cope. Typically, the body responds to stress by activating various regulatory mechanisms (primarily within the vascular system, brain, kidneys, liver, and endocrine system) that produce physiologic changes to bring the body back to normal functional levels.

Understanding physiologic responses to stress is crucial to providing appropriate nursing care. This chapter focuses on major physiologic stressors that can disrupt homeostasis as well as the internal mechanisms by which the body responds to maintain normalcy.

INFLAMMATION

INFLAMMATION is defined as the body's response to cellular injury. It's an immediate, defensive, beneficial response.

Cardinal signs

- Redness from dilation of arterioles, which increases blood flow to the injured area
- Heat from increased blood supply to and increased metabolism in the injured area
- Pain from the release of chemicals, pH changes, and pressure on nerve endings caused by swelling and trauma
- Edema from accumulation of fluids in the interstitial tissues of the injured area
- Loss of function from culminaton of inflammatory changes
- Migration and extravasation of leukocytes into the injured area
- Phagocytosis (engulfing and destruction of irritants, primarily by polymorphonuclear neutrophils, monocytes, and lymphocytes)
- Walling off by leukocytes to keep the inflammation localized (By cleaning up cellular debris, leukocytes also help resolve inflammation.)
- Exudate formation, produced by the accumulation of interstitial fluids (Exudates dilute noxious chemicals in the inflamed area and bring antibodies to the tissue's defense.)

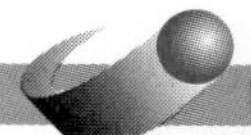

FAST FACT

Types of exudate include:
– clear (serous)
– purulent (pus-containing)
– bloody (sanguineous).

- Cellular size changes (metaplasia)
  – Increased cell size or number (hypertrophy or hyperplasia)
  – Decreased cell size (atrophy)
- Migration of the inflammation (metastasis) into contiguous tissues (signaled by red streaks radiating along blood vessels)

Systemic signs

- Fever (from the release of pyrogens in the body)
- LEUKOCYTOSIS (increased production of white blood cells [WBCs])

◆ Malaise, anorexia, and disability (varies with individuals)
◆ Increased sedimentation rate (from changes in blood proteins and effects on red blood cells [RBCs])

Factors affecting inflammation

◆ Blood supply (Inadequate blood supply may prolong inflammation and impair healing.)
◆ Increased number of leukocytes (Leukocytes localize inflammation and produce phagocytosis.)
◆ Nutritional status of the client (Cellular regeneration requires adequate nutrients.)
◆ Foreign material in the inflamed area (Such material prevents healing and leads to infection.)
◆ Age (Children and young adults generally exhibit faster healing and recovery than older adults.)

Complications

◆ CONTRACTURE (shortening or tightening of tissues, causing deformity)
◆ STRICTURE (scar tissue that encircles a tubular structure, such as the esophagus, producing a narrowing)
◆ ADHESION (band of granulation [or scar] tissue that binds tissues and organs, causing loss of function or other complications)
◆ HERNIA (outward bulging of scars)
◆ KELOID (excessive growth of scar tissue)
◆ GRANULOMA (accumulation of scar tissue within scar tissue)

Resolution of inflammation

◆ Resolution (complete remission of signs and symptoms)
◆ Repair (replacement of lost cells with new cells)
◆ Scar formation (organization of connective tissue cells to form scar tissue)

Implementation

◆ Monitor vital signs for indications of developing inflammation and report any findings to the physician, including:
- fever
- spiking temperatures
- increased pulse rate
- early signs of soreness, redness, edema, and rash
- changes in respiratory rate or breath sounds
- pain on respiration
- changes in level of consciousness, especially in the older adult (occasionally first sign noted before fever).

◆ Assess wound sites and report any findings to the physician, including:
- color changes
- edema
- increased redness or tenderness
- increased drainage. (Purulent drainage signals infection.)

◆ Assess other drainage and report any findings to the physician, including:
- yellow sputum
- cloudy urine
- diarrhea.

◆ Be alert for client complaints and report any findings to the physician, including:
- malaise
- fatigue
- anorexia
- increasing pain
- dysuria, burning, or frequent urination.

◆ Be alert for blood chemistry (signs of inflammation or infection), including:
- high WBC count
- high sedimentation rate.

◆ Document all assessment findings and data on the client's chart, including nursing interventions, and notification of the physician.

SHOCK DISORDERS

Shock is a clinical syndrome characterized by excessive reduction of circulating blood volume, resulting in inadequate cell perfusion to tissues and vital organs. Cell death can occur because cells don't receive adequate nutrition and oxygen. Reduced organ perfusion eventually leads to organ dysfunction and failure.

SHOCK CLASSIFICATIONS

Shock can be classified into four major categories based on the precipitating factors: distributive shock, which includes anaphylactic shock, neurogenic shock, and septic shock; cardiogenic shock; hypovolemic shock; and obstructive shock.

Assessment findings

Some general physical changes that may be found on assessment include:
◆ altered level of consciousness
◆ changes in skin temperature (cool and clammy, or hot and flushed)
◆ decreased or absent bowel sounds
◆ decreased renal output

> **Shared goals**
>
> Shock classifications share some of the same planning goals, such as:
> - The client will have adequate cellular perfusion.
> - The client will retain renal function.
> - The client will suffer no complications.
> - The client's and family's anxiety will decrease.
>
> Corresponding evaluative statements include:
> - The client's normal blood pressure has been restored.
> - The client's fluid and electrolyte levels fall within reference limits.
> - The client doesn't experience complications, such as pulmonary edema or metabolic acidosis.
> - The client's and family's anxieties have decreased satisfactorily.

- elevated respiratory rate
- hypotension
- metabolic acidosis
- nausea or vomiting
- restlessness, anxiety, apprehension
- thirst. (See *Shared goals.*)

Distributive shock

- Caused by decreased vascular volume or tone
- Possible neural-induced factors include:
  - pain
  - anesthesia
  - stress
  - spinal cord injury
  - head trauma.
- Possible chemical-induced factors:
  - anaphylaxis
  - sepsis
  - capillary leak
  - burns
  - extensive trauma.

Cardiogenic shock

- Caused by direct pump failure
- Possible factors include:
  - myocardial infarction (MI)
  - cardiac arrest
  - ventricular arrhythmias
  - cardiomyopathies.

Hypovolemic shock

- Caused by a decrease in total body fluid
- Possible factors include:
  - hemorrhage
  - trauma
  - surgery
  - GI ulcer
  - dehydration
  - vomiting
  - diarrhea
  - nasogastric (NG) suctioning
  - diabetes insipidus
  - hyperglycemia.

Obstructive shock

- Caused by indirect pump failure, including conditions that may cause an obstruction of blood flow
- Possible factors include:
  - cardiac tamponade
  - pulmonary embolus
  - pulmonary hypertension
  - tension pneumothorax.

ANAPHYLACTIC SHOCK

Anaphylatic shock or ANAPHYLAXIS is a dramatic and widespread acute atopic reaction. It's a type of distributive shock that's marked by the sudden onset of rapidly progressive urticaria and respiratory distress. A severe anaphylactic reaction may cause vascular collapse, leading to systemic shock and, sometimes, death.

Possible causes

Possible causes of anaphylaxis include systemic exposure to or ingestion of sensitizing drugs or other substances, such as:

- allergen extracts
- diagnostic chemicals (sulfobromophthalein, sodium dehydrocholate, and radiographic contrast media)
- enzymes (such as L-asparaginase)
- foods (legumes, nuts, berries, seafood, meat proteins, and egg albumin) and sulfite-containing food additives
- hormones
- insect venom (honeybees, wasps, hornets, yellow jackets, fire ants, mosquitoes, and certain spiders)
- local anesthetics
- penicillin and other antibiotics
- polysaccharides
- ruptured hydatid cyst (rarely)
- salicylates

- serums (usually horse serum)
- sulfonamides
- vaccines.

Assessment findings

The severity of the reaction is inversely related to the interval between exposure to an allergen and the onset of symptoms (the longer the interval, the less severe the reaction).

- Cardiovascular symptoms (hypotension, shock, cardiac arrhythmias); may precipitate circulatory collapse if untreated
- GI and genitourinary symptoms (severe stomach cramps, nausea, diarrhea, urinary urgency and incontinence)
- Persistent or delayed reaction (may occur up to 24 hours after exposure to allergen)
- Respiratory symptoms (nasal mucosal edema; profuse watery rhinorrhea; itching; nasal congestion; sudden sneezing attacks; edema of upper respiratory tract that causes hoarseness and stridor; and dyspnea, an early sign of acute respiratory failure)
- Sudden physical distress within seconds or minutes after exposure to an allergen (may include feeling of impending doom or fright, weakness, sweating, sneezing, shortness of breath, hives, nasal pruritus, urticaria, and angioedema, followed rapidly by symptoms in one or more target organs)

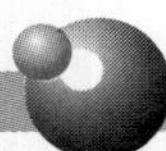

SPOT CHECK

Name two signs of physical distress a client may exhibit almost immediately after being exposed to an allergen.

The client may exhibit one or more of the following signs:

- feeling of impending doom or fright
- weakness
- sweating
- sneezing
- shortness of breath
- nasal pruritus
- urticaria
- angioedema.

Diagnostic evaluation

- Anaphylaxis can be diagnosed by the rapid onset of severe respiratory or cardiovascular symptoms after ingestion or injection of a drug, vaccine, diagnostic agent, food, or food additive, or after an insect sting.
- If symptoms occur without a known allergic stimulus, other possible causes of shock (such as acute MI, status asthmaticus, or heart failure) must be ruled out.

Nursing diagnoses

- Ineffective breathing pattern
- Risk for suffocation
- Decreased cardiac output
- Anxiety

Treatment

- Cardiopulmonary resuscitation (CPR) in case of cardiac arrest
- Endotracheal tube insertion or a tracheotomy and oxygen therapy in case of laryngeal edema
- Other therapy as indicated by clinical response

Drug therapy options

Immediate

- Epinephrine: immediate injection of 1:1,000 aqueous solution, 0.1 to 0.5 ml by the subcutaneous (subQ) or I.M. routes repeated every 10 to 15 minutes as necessary; I.V. route if the client loses consciousness

After initial emergency

- Vasopressors: norepinephrine (Levophed), phenylephrine (Neo-Synephrine), and dopamine (Intropin) if hypotensive
- Corticosteroid: methylprednisolone (Solu-Medrol) I.V.
- Diphenhydramine (Benadryl) I.V.

Planning and goals

- The client will exhibit patent airway and adequate breathing patterns.
- The client will regain and maintain adequate blood pressure.
- The client will state that anxiety is decreased.

Implementation

- In the early stages of anaphylaxis when the client hasn't lost consciousness and is still normotensive, give epinephrine I.M. or subQ and massage the injection site *to help it move into the circulation faster.* In severe reactions when the client has lost consciousness and is hypotensive, give epinephrine I.V. *to prevent crisis.*
- Maintain airway patency. Observe for early signs of laryngeal edema (stridor, hoarseness, and dyspnea), and prepare for endotracheal tube insertion or tracheotomy and oxygen therapy *to prevent cerebral anoxia.*
- In case of cardiac arrest, begin CPR and advanced cardiac life support *to prevent irreversible organ damage.*
- If client is hypotensive, prepare to administer volume expanders (plasma, plasma expanders, saline solution, and albumin) as ordered *to maintain circulatory volume.* Stabilize blood pressure with the I.V. vasopressors norepi-

nephrine, phenylephrine, and dopamine *to prevent altered tissue perfusion.* Monitor blood pressure, central venous pressure (if a central venous catheter is in place), and urine output *to monitor response to treatment.*

◆ After the initial emergency, administer other medications such as corticosteroids and diphenhydramine I.V. for long-term management *to prevent recurrence of symptoms.*

◆ Make sure a client who must receive a drug to which he's allergic undergoes careful desensitization with gradually increasing doses of the antigen or advance administration of steroids *to prevent a severe reaction.*

◆ Be aware that a person with a known history of allergies should receive a drug with a high anaphylactic potential only after cautious pretesting for sensitivity. Closely monitor the client during testing, and make sure that resuscitative equipment and epinephrine are ready *to prevent a severe reaction that may lead to cardiopulmonary arrest.*

◆ Make sure that any client who needs a drug with high anaphylactic potential (particularly parenteral drugs) receives each dose under close medical observation *to prevent a severe reaction.*

◆ Closely monitor a client undergoing diagnostic tests that use radiographic contrast dyes, such as cardiac catheterization, excretory urography, and angiography, *to detect early signs of anaphylaxis.*

◆ Review key teaching topics with the client *to ensure adequate knowledge about the condition and treatment,* including:

– risks of delayed symptoms and the need to report any recurrence of shortness of breath, chest tightness, sweating, angioedema, or other symptoms

– preventing anaphylaxis (avoiding exposure to known allergens, including all forms of the offending food or drug; avoiding open fields and wooded areas during the insect season in case of a reaction to an insect bite or sting; carrying an anaphylaxis kit containing epinephrine, an antihistamine, and a tourniquet)

– wearing medical identification jewelry identifying the client's allergies.

Evaluation

◆ The client maintains adequate oxygenation.

◆ The client has vital signs within normal limits.

◆ The client is free of anxiety.

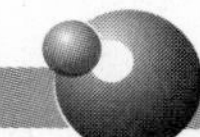

SPOT CHECK

Name three specific substances that can cause an anaphylactic reaction.

Examples of these substances are:

- penicillin and other antibiotics
- salicylates
- polysaccharides
- radiographic contrast media
- seafood
- nuts.

For additional examples, see "Possible causes," page 77.

NEUROGENIC SHOCK

NEUROGENIC SHOCK is sometimes referred to as *spinal shock.* It's a form of distributive shock. In distributive shock, vasodilation causes a state of hypovolemia. A loss of sympathetic vasoconstrictor tone in the vascular smooth muscle and reduced autonomic function lead to widespread arterial and venous vasodilation. Venous return is reduced as blood pools in the venous system, leading to a drop in cardiac output and hypotension.

Possible causes

◆ Nervous system damage, including damage to the medulla oblongata

◆ Spinal anesthesia

◆ Spinal cord injury

Assessment findings

◆ Bradycardia

◆ Warm, dry skin

◆ Hypotension

Diagnostic evaluation

◆ Hemodynamic monitoring may indicate a decrease in systemic vascular resistance, right atrial pressure, pulmonary artery pressure, and PAWP.

◆ Spinal X-rays reveal fracture.

◆ Computed tomography and magnetic resonance imaging show the fracture location and the site of compression, and reveal spinal cord edema and possible spinal cord tumor.

Nursing diagnoses

◆ Ineffective breathing pattern

◆ Ineffective airway clearance

◆ Ineffective tissue perfusion (peripheral)

- Impaired physical mobility
- Risk for autonomic dysreflexia

Treatment

- Trauma resuscitation as indicated
- Oxygen therapy and endotracheal intubation as needed
- Spinal immobilization

Drug therapy options

- Atropine if bradycardia is present
- High-dose corticosteroid: methylprednisolone (Solu-Medrol) administered I.V. within 8 hours of a spinal cord injury; loading dose of 30 mg/kg; then, after 45 minutes, continuous infusion of 5.4 mg/kg for 23 hours
- Vasopressors: dopamine (Intropin), phenylephrine (Neo-Synephrine), norepinephrine (Levophed)

Planning and goals

- The client will maintain a patent airway.
- The client will demonstrate adequate circulation.
- The client will not develop neurogenic complications.

Implementation

- Maintain a patent airway. Monitor oxygen level with pulse oximetry *to prevent hypoxemia.* Maintain cervical immobilization *to prevent injury.*
- Administer oxygen, as ordered, *to increase the amount of oxygen in the blood.* Prepare for intubation, as needed.
- Monitor ABG results and pH levels *to detect acidosis and inadequate oxygenation. Shock decreases the partial pressure of oxygen (PaO_2) and pH.*
- Apply a cardiac monitor *for continuous monitoring. Fluid and electrolyte imbalances can cause arrhythmias.*
- Maintain the client in the supine position or, if possible, use a modified Trendelenburg's position, with the lower end of the bed elevated about 45 degrees and the client's head slightly elevated *to promote increased respiratory exchange and increased venous return.*
- Encourage deep breathing and coughing *to help prevent respiratory complications. Clients have a poor cough due to insufficient intrathoracic pressure.*
- Apply antithrombolytic stockings. Pneumatic compression devices may also be used *to prevent deep vein thrombosis.*
- Assess the client's neurologic status and observe for autonomic hyperreflexia (autonomic dysreflexia), which usually begins in 3 to 6 weeks as neurogenic shock resolves. *Prompt recognition of complications prevents treatment delay.*

Evaluation

- The client maintains adequate oxygenation and hemodynamic status.
- Complications are minimized.

SEPTIC SHOCK

SEPTIC SHOCK is usually the result of a bacterial infection. It causes inadequate blood perfusion and circulatory collapse.

Septic shock occurs most commonly among hospitalized clients, especially men over age 40 and women ages 25 to 45. It's second only to cardiogenic shock as the leading cause of shock death. About 25% of clients in whom gram-negative bacteremia develops go into shock. Unless vigorous treatment begins promptly, preferably before symptoms fully develop, septic shock rapidly progresses to death (commonly within a few hours) in up to 80% of these clients.

Possible causes

- Infection with gram-positive bacteria: *Streptococcus pneumoniae, S. pyogenes*, and *Actinomyces*
- Infection with gram-negative bacteria (in two-thirds of clients): *Escherichia coli, Klebsiella, Enterobacter, Proteus, Pseudomonas*, and *Bacteroides*

Assessment findings

Indications of septic shock vary according to the stage of the shock, the organism causing it, and the age of the client.

Early stage

- Chills
- Sudden fever (over 101° F [38.3° C])
- Oliguria
- Nausea
- Vomiting
- Diarrhea
- Prostration

Late stage

- Altered level of consciousness
- Anuria
- Apprehension
- Hyperventilation
- Hypotension
- Hypothermia
- Irritability
- Restlessness

- ◆ Tachycardia
- ◆ Tachypnea
- ◆ Thirst from decreased cerebral tissue perfusion

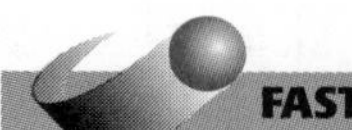

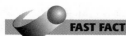

FAST FACT

Infants and elderly people may have only these signs of septic shock:

- Altered level of consciousness
- Hyperventilation
- Hypotension.

Diagnostic evaluation

◆ Arterial blood gas (ABG) analysis indicates respiratory alkalosis (low partial pressure of carbon dioxide [$PaCO_2$], low or normal bicarbonate [HCO_3^-] level, and high pH) that may progress to metabolic acidosis.

◆ Blood cultures isolate the organism.

◆ Blood tests show decreased platelet count and leukocytosis (15,000 to 30,000/µl), increased blood urea nitrogen (BUN) and creatinine levels, decreased creatinine clearance, and abnormal prothrombin time (PT), International Normalized Ratio (INR), and partial thromboplastin time (PTT).

◆ Electrocardiography (ECG) shows ST-segment depression, inverted T waves, and arrhythmias resembling MI.

◆ Hemodynamic monitoring reveals increased cardiac output and low systemic vascular resistance.

Nursing diagnoses

◆ Decreased cardiac output

◆ Deficient fluid volume

◆ Ineffective tissue perfusion (renal, cerebral, cardiopulmonary, GI)

Treatment

◆ Removing and replacing I.V., intra-arterial, or urinary drainage catheters that may be the source of infection

◆ Oxygen therapy (may require endotracheal intubation and mechanical ventilation)

◆ Colloid or crystalloid infusion to increase intravascular volume

◆ Blood transfusion if anemia is present

◆ Surgery to drain abscesses, if present

Drug therapy options

◆ Antibiotics: according to sensitivity of causative organism

◆ Vasopressors: dopamine (Intropin), norepinephrine (Levophed), phenylephrine (Neo-Synephrine) if fluid resuscitation fails to increase blood pressure

◆ Diuretics: furosemide (Lasix) after sufficient fluid volume has been replaced to maintain urine output above 20 ml/hour

◆ Drotrecogin alfa (Xigris) in severe sepsis with acute organ dysfunction

◆ Insulin infusion to maintain glycemic control

Planning and goals

◆ The client will regain and maintain adequate blood pressure.

◆ The client will exhibit stable vital signs and adequate urine output.

Implementation

◆ Remove I.V., intra-arterial, or urinary drainage catheters and send them to the laboratory *for culture of the causative organism.* New catheters can be reinserted *to provide access for fluid resuscitation and ensure accurate measurement of urine output.*

◆ Start an I.V. infusion with normal saline solution or lactated Ringer's solution, usually with a large-bore (14G to 18G) catheter, *to allow easier infusion.*

◆ When the client's blood pressure drops below 80 mm Hg, increase oxygen flow rate and call the physician immediately *to prevent a progressive drop in blood pressure accompanied by a thready pulse, which generally signifies inadequate cardiac output from reduced vascular volume.*

◆ Carefully maintain the pulmonary artery catheter *to monitor fluid volume status and cardiac output.*

◆ Check ABG values for adequate oxygenation and gas exchange, watching for any changes, *to prevent hypoxemia.*

◆ Keep accurate intake and output records. Maintain adequate urine output (0.5 to 1 ml/kg/hour) and systolic pressure *to prevent kidney damage and fluid overload.*

◆ Administer broad-spectrum antibiotics, initially I.V., *to achieve effective blood levels quickly,* and monitor drug levels *to prevent toxicity.* When the cause of the infection is identified, more specific antibiotics may be administered.

◆ Watch closely for complications of septic shock: disseminated intravascular coagulation (abnormal bleeding), renal failure (oliguria, increased specific gravity), heart failure (dyspnea, edema, tachycardia, distended neck veins), GI ulcers (hematemesis, melena), and hepatic abnormalities (jaundice, hypoprothrombinemia, and hypoalbuminemia) *to prevent crisis.*

◆ Review key teaching topics with the client and family members *to ensure adequate knowledge about the condition and treatment,* including:
– risks associated with blood transfusion
– disease process and treatment options.

◆ Administer drotrecogin alfa as prescribed. Monitor the client closely for signs of bleeding, *an adverse effect of therapy.*

Evaluation

◆ The client's vital signs are within normal limits.
◆ The client has adequate urine output.

CARDIOGENIC SHOCK

CARDIOGENIC SHOCK occurs when the heart fails to pump adequately, thereby reducing cardiac output and compromising tissue perfusion.

Here's how cardiogenic shock progresses:

◆ Decreased stroke volume results in increased left ventricular volume.
◆ Blood pooling in the left ventricle backs up into the lungs, causing pulmonary edema.
◆ To compensate for falling cardiac output, heart rate and contractility increase.
◆ These compensating mechanisms increase the demand for myocardial oxygen.
◆ An imbalance between oxygen supply and demand results, increasing myocardial ischemia and further compromising the heart's pumping action.

Possible causes

◆ Advanced heart block
◆ Cardiomyopathy
◆ Heart failure
◆ MI
◆ Myocarditis
◆ Papillary muscle rupture

Assessment findings

◆ Anxiety, restlessness, disorientation, and confusion
◆ Cold, clammy skin
◆ Crackles in lungs
◆ Hypotension, narrow pulse pressure
◆ Jugular venous distention
◆ Oliguria (urine output of less than 30 ml/hour)
◆ S_3 and S_4 heart sounds
◆ Tachycardia or other arrhythmias
◆ Tachypnea, hypoxia
◆ Weak, thready pulse

Diagnostic evaluation

◆ ABG levels show respiratory alkalosis initially. As shock progresses, metabolic acidosis develops.
◆ Blood chemistry tests show increased BUN and creatinine levels.
◆ ECG shows possible evidence of acute MI, ischemia, or ventricular aneurysm.
◆ Hemodynamic monitoring reveals decreased stroke volume and decreased cardiac output; it also shows increased pulmonary artery pressure, increased pulmonary artery wedge pressure (PAWP), and increased central venous pressure (CVP).
◆ Echocardiography is used to determine left ventricular function and reveals valvular abnormalities.

Nursing diagnoses

◆ Decreased cardiac output
◆ Ineffective tissue perfusion (cardiopulmonary, renal)

Treatment

◆ Intra-aortic balloon pump

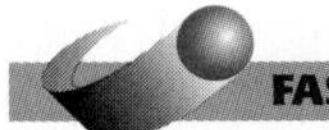

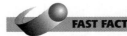

FAST FACT

An intra-aortic balloon pump helps improve coronary artery perfusion and reduce cardiac workload.

◆ Ventricular assist device until transplantation is possible
◆ Activity changes, including maintaining bed rest and implementing passive range-of-motion (ROM) and isometric exercises
◆ Oxygen therapy, including intubation and mechanical ventilation, if necessary
◆ Continuous renal replacement therapy
◆ Dietary changes, including withholding food and oral fluids

Drug therapy options

◆ Adrenergic agent: epinephrine (Adrenalin Chloride)
◆ Cardiac glycoside: digoxin (Lanoxin)
◆ Cardiac inotropes: dopamine (Intropin), dobutamine (Dobutrex), inamrinone (Inocor), milrinone (Primacor)
◆ Diuretics: furosemide (Lasix), bumetanide (Bumex), metolazone (Zaroxolyn)
◆ Vasodilators: nitroprusside (Nitropress), nitroglycerin (Nitro-Bid)

Drugs used in cardiogenic shock

One or more drugs may be used in the treatment of cardiogenic shock. Here are some facts about key drugs that may be used.

Dobutamine (Dobutrex)

◆ Increases cardiac output
◆ Produces selective $beta_1$-receptor activation, which results in increased output with only minimal increases in heart rate
◆ Stimulates $beta_1$ receptors on the vascular beds, which also causes vasodilation, decreasing left ventricular end-diastolic pressure and further improving the pumping efficiency of the heart
◆ One of the most useful drugs in treating cardiogenic shock

Dopamine (Intropin)

◆ Dilates coronary, intracerebral, mesenteric, and renal arteries and increases urine output
◆ Dose-dependent effects
– Low doses activate only dopamine receptors
– Higher doses activate $beta_1$ receptors, stimulating the heart
– Still higher doses activate alpha receptors, causing vasoconstriction
◆ Especially useful when low cardiac output is complicated by hypotension and low renal output

Norepinephrine (Levophed)

◆ Increases blood pressure and cardiac output but usually decreases heart rate because of a reflex increase in vagal tone
◆ Stimulates mostly alpha receptors but will also activate $beta_1$ receptors; has no $beta_2$-receptor activity
◆ Especially useful when dobutamine or dopamine can't maintain blood pressure
◆ Because it increases myocardial work and oxygen consumption, may cause arrhythmias

Phenylephrine (Neo-Synephrine)

◆ Causes vasoconstriction by acting on alpha-adrenergic receptors
◆ Doesn't stimulate the myocardium

Vasodilators: nitroglycerin (Nitro-Bid) or nitroprusside (Nitropress)

◆ Cause peripheral vasodilation, which decreases the force against which the heart has to pump
◆ Net effect is decreased myocardial work and oxygen consumption

◆ Vasopressors: norepinephrine (Levophed), phenylephrine (Neo-Synephrine) (See *Drugs used in cardiogenic shock.*)

Planning and goals

◆ The client will demonstrate blood pressure within normal parameters.
◆ The client will have adequate urine output.

Implementation

◆ Assess cardiovascular status, including hemodynamic variables, vital signs, heart sounds, capillary refill, skin temperature, and peripheral pulses, *to monitor effects of drug therapy and detect cardiac decompensation.*
◆ Assess respiratory status, including breath sounds and ABG analysis, *to identify signs of pulmonary edema, such as tachypnea, crackles, and hypoxemia.*
◆ Monitor fluid balance, including intake and output, *to monitor kidney function and detect fluid overload leading to pulmonary edema.*
◆ Monitor level of consciousness *to detect cerebral hypoxia caused by reduced cardiac output.*
◆ Monitor laboratory studies *to detect evidence of MI, evaluate renal function, and assess the oxygen-carrying capacity of the blood.*
◆ Monitor glucose levels frequently if epinephrine infusion is prescribed *to prevent drug-induced hyperglycemia.*
◆ Withhold food and fluids, as directed, *to reduce the risk of aspiration with a reduced level of consciousness.*
◆ Administer I.V. fluids, oxygen, and medications, as prescribed, *to maximize cardiac, pulmonary, and renal functioning.*
◆ Provide suctioning *to aid in the removal of secretions and reduce the risk of aspiration.*
◆ Encourage the client to express feelings, such as a fear of dying, *to reduce the client's anxiety.*
◆ Review key teaching topics with the client and family members *to ensure adequate knowledge about the condition and treatment,* including:
– recognizing early signs and symptoms of fluid overload
– maintaining activity limitations, including alternating rest periods with activity
– maintaining a low-fat, low-sodium diet.

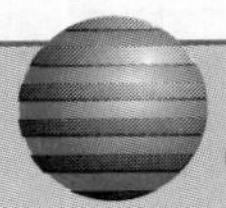

CLINICAL SITUATION

Caring for the client with shock

Evaluate the clinical situation described here. See if you're able to answer the questions as you go.

A male client, age 19, was driving home from a college fraternity party. A drunk driver struck his car. The client sustained major trauma. Upon assessment, the nurse finds the following injuries: a laceration on the scalp, repetitive verbalization, abdominal pain with tenderness on palpation, a lack of neurologic response below the nipple line, and a fractured tibia. The client could have hypovolemic shock, distributive shock, or both.

What should be included in the client assessment?

Assess, monitor, and observe the client for:

- restlessness
- anxiety
- apprehension
- altered level of consciousness
- color changes (pallor, cyanosis, flushing)
- blood pressure (Systolic readings below 80 mm Hg can be caused by decreased circulating blood volume or cardiac output.)
- tachycardia
- elevated respiratory rate
- urine output (Output below 25 ml/hour can be caused by decreased renal perfusion.)
- skin temperature (cool and clammy, or flushed and hot to touch)
- bowel sounds (decreased or absent)
- nausea or vomiting
- thirst.

What are appropriate nursing diagnoses?

- Decreased cardiac output related to left ventricular failure, volume depletion, or vasodilation
- Ineffective tissue perfusion (cardiopulmonary, cerebral, renal, GI, peripheral) related to decreased myocardial contractility, hypovolemia, or fluid shift from vascular spaces
- Deficient fluid volume related to excessive fluid loss
- Ineffective individual coping related to critical situation
- Ineffective family coping: Compromised, related to critically ill family member
- Risk for injury related to sensorimotor deficits or hypotension
- Impaired gas exchange related to altered ventilation-perfusion ratio

What are appropriate goals for this client?

- The client will have adequate cellular perfusion.
- The client will retain renal function.
- The client will suffer no complications.
- The client's and family's anxiety will decrease.

Questions for further thought

- What's the importance of fluid resuscitation if a client has hypovolemia?
- How can you determine if the client is getting adequate oxygenation?
- What evaluation findings would indicate that client goals are met?

Evaluation

- The client has stable vital signs.
- The client has adequate urine output.

HYPOVOLEMIC SHOCK

HYPOVOLEMIC SHOCK is a shock state resulting from decreased intravascular volume due to fluid loss. This volume decrease causes circulatory dysfunction and inadequate tissue perfusion. Without sufficient blood or fluid replacement, hypovolemic shock syndrome may lead to irreversible cerebral and renal damage, cardiac arrest and, ultimately, death.

Hypovolemic shock requires early recognition of signs and symptoms and prompt, aggressive treatment to improve the prognosis. (See *Caring for the client with shock.*)

Possible causes

- Acute blood loss (approximately one-fifth of total volume)
- Acute pancreatitis, ascites, peritonitis
- Burns
- Diabetes insipidus
- Diarrhea or vomiting
- Severe dehydration
- Severe edema
- Surgery
- Trauma

Assessment findings

- Tachycardia
- Cold, clammy skin
- Decreased urine output: less than 30 ml/hour
- Hypotension with narrowing pulse pressure
- Rapid, shallow respirations
- Decreased level of consciousness
- Arrhythmias
- Thirst
- Decreased capillary refill
- Dilated, sluggish reacting pupils

Diagnostic evaluation

- Hemoglobin and hematocrit levels decrease.
- Cardiac enzyme (CK-MB, cTn-1) levels rise.
- BUN and creatinine levels increase.
- Liver enzyme (aspartate aminotransferace [AST], alanine aminotransferase [ALT]) and bilirubin levels increase.
- Coagulation studies show prolonged PT, INR, and PTT.
- Urine specific gravity and urine osmolality increase.
- ABG analysis reveals metabolic acidosis.
- Gastroscopy, aspiration of gastric contents (through an NG tube), and X-rays identify internal bleeding sites.

Nursing diagnoses

- Deficient fluid volume
- Decreased cardiac output
- Ineffective tissue perfusion (cardiopulmonary, cerebral, or renal)

Treatment

- Blood and fluid replacement
- Control of bleeding
- Pneumatic antishock garment is sometimes used

Drug therapy options

- Inotrope: dopamine (Intropin) used only when vigorous fluid resuscitation is no longer effective

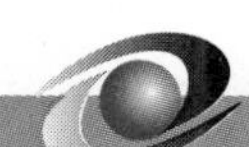

QUICK STUDY

When trying to remember the main treatment focus for hypovolemic shock, think about **Replacement Control:**
- blood and fluid **replacement**
- **control** bleeding.

Planning and goals

- The client will regain and maintain adequate urine output and stable vital signs.
- The client will maintain adequate oxygenation and hemodynamic status.

Implementation

Management of hypovolemic shock necessitates prompt, aggressive supportive measures and careful assessment and monitoring of vital signs. Follow these priorities:

- Check for a patent airway and adequate circulation. If blood pressure and heart rate are absent, start CPR *to prevent irreversible organ damage and death.*
- Record blood pressure, pulse rate, peripheral pulses, respiratory rate, and other vital signs every 15 minutes and monitor the ECG continuously *to monitor the client for changes in condition. A progressive drop in blood pressure accompanied by a thready pulse generally signals inadequate cardiac output from reduced intravascular volume.* Notify the physician immediately.
- Start I.V. lines with normal saline or lactated Ringer's solution using a large-bore catheter (14G), which allows easier administration of later blood transfusions *to correct fluid volume deficit.*
- An indwelling urinary catheter may be inserted *to measure hourly urine output.* If output is less than 30 ml/hour in adults, increase the fluid infusion rate but watch for signs of fluid overload, such as an increase in PAWP. Notify the physician if urine output doesn't improve. An osmotic diuretic, such as mannitol (Osmitrol), may be ordered *to increase renal blood flow and urine output.*
- Check blood pressure, urine output, CVP, and PAWP *to determine how much fluid to give.*
- Draw an arterial blood sample to measure ABG values. Administer oxygen by face mask and adjust the oxygen flow rate to a higher or lower level as ABG measurements indicate *to ensure adequate oxygenation of tissues.*
- Draw venous blood for complete blood cell (CBC) count and electrolyte levels, typing and crossmatching, and coagulation studies *to guide the treatment regimen.*
- During therapy, assess skin color and temperature and note any changes *to identify changes in the client's condition. Cold, clammy skin may be a sign of continuing peripheral vascular constriction, indicating progressive shock.*
- Explain all procedures and their purposes. Throughout these emergency measures, provide emotional support to the client and his family members *to help them cope with the overwhelming situation.*
- Review key teaching topics with the client and family members *to ensure adequate knowledge about the condition and treatment,* including causes of hypovolemia and treatment options.

Evaluation

- Fluid volume is maintained.
- Oxygenation and hemodynamic status is adequate.

PAIN

THEORETICAL OVERVIEW

Pain is universally feared — the strongest human fear after fear of death. It serves as a bodily protective mechanism. (Superficial fibers are rich in pain receptors; viscera aren't.) Pain is a highly complex mechanism that comprises perception and interpretation. Two theories, *specificity* and *gate control,* attempt to explain how pain is perceived and interpreted by the body.

Specificity theory

SPECIFICITY THEORY is the traditional theory of pain perception and interpretation. First, the onset of pain begins with a mechanical, hormonal, or chemical stimulus that interacts with receptor molecules located at the tips of nociceptive primary afferent neurons (commonly called *free nerve endings*). As a result, sodium channels open and extracellular sodium flows in, causing the receptor molecule to depolarize, which creates an action potential. Electrical energy then travels to the spinal cord and on to the brain, signaling pain.

Gate control theory

The GATE CONTROL THEORY is based on the idea that only one major stimulus can be transmitted at a time. First, the onset of pain begins with a stimulus that triggers an open and closed "gate" response within the spinal cord. Next, pain travels through the neural pathways where it's met by conflicting large fibers that close the gate or small fibers that open the gate. This open and closed gate response occurs as a response to impulses from the brain stem.

Reactions to pain perception and interpretation

There are several ways that the body reacts to pain perception and interpretation.

Autonomic

- Stress response
- Increased skeletal muscle activity
- Reflexes (withdrawal from source)
- Reflex muscular rigidity over affected areas; guarding (protective reflex)
- Muscle spasms after a fracture

Voluntary

- Grimacing
- Clenching fists and teeth
- Pacing floor
- Twisting and turning
- Decreasing activity
- Altering body position

Psychological

- Anxiety, fear, and apprehension (Anxiety increases the intensity of pain, which further increases anxiety.)
- Anger and verbalization
- Decreased sense of control

Severe physical or psychological conditions

- Shock
- Panic
- Prolonged pain resulting from fear, depression, insomnia, anorexia, or tension

TYPES OF PAIN

Pain is typically classified as acute or chronic.

Acute pain characteristics

- Caused by tissue damage due to injury or disease
- Varies in intensity from mild to severe
- Lasts briefly (up to 6 months)
- May result from traumatic injury, surgical or diagnostic procedure, or medical disorder

Chronic pain characteristics

- Lasts 6 months or longer and is ongoing
- May be as intense as acute pain
- Examples include arthritis pain, chronic back pain, and pain caused by cancer

ASSESSING PAIN

The most valid pain assessment comes from the client's own reports of pain. A pain assessment includes questions about:

- *location.* Ask the client to tell you where the pain is; there may be more than one area of pain.
- *intensity.* Ask the client to rate the pain using a pain scale. (See *Common pain-rating scales.*)
- *quality.* Ask how the pain feels — sharp, dull, aching, or burning.

Common pain-rating scales

These scales are examples of the rating systems you can use to help a client quantify pain levels.

Visual analog scale

To use the visual analog scale, ask the client to place a line across the scale to indicate the current level of pain. The scale is a 10-cm line with "No pain" at one end and "Pain as bad as it can be" at the other end. The pain rating is determined by using a ruler to measure the distance, in millimeters, from "No pain" to the client's mark.

No pain ____ **Pain as bad as it can be**

Numeric rating scale

To use the numeric rating scale, ask the client to choose a number from 0 (indicating no pain) to 10 (indicating the worst pain imaginable) to indicate the current pain level. The client may circle the number on the scale or verbally state the number that best describes the pain.

No pain | 0 1 2 3 4 5 6 7 8 9 10 | **Pain as bad as it can be**

Faces scale

A pediatric or adult client with language difficulty may not be able to describe the current pain level using the visual analog scale or the numeric rating scale. In that case, use a faces scale like the one below. Ask the client to choose the face on a scale from 1 to 6 that best represents the severity of current pain.

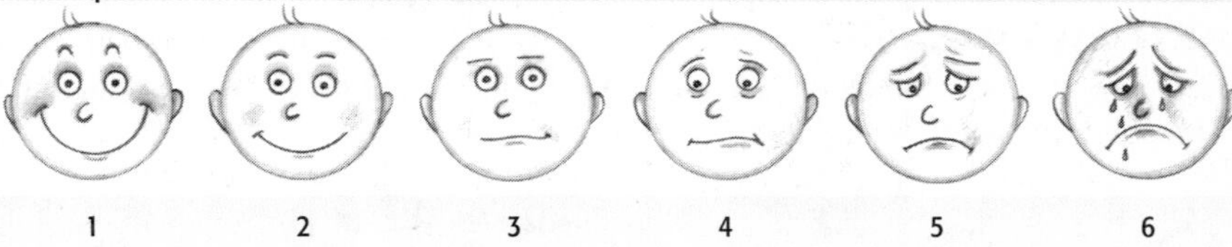

1 2 3 4 5 6

◆ *onset, duration, and frequency.* Ask when the pain started, how long it lasts, and how often it occurs.
◆ *alleviating and aggravating factors.* Ask what makes the pain feel better and what makes it worse.
◆ *associated factors.* Ask whether other problems are associated with the pain, such as nausea and vomiting.
◆ *effects on lifestyle.* Ask whether appetite, sleep, relationships, emotions, or work is affected.

PAIN MANAGEMENT

Unrelieved pain has physiologic and psychological consequences; therefore, managing pain is very important.

Pharmacologic intervention

◆ Nonopioids
◆ Opioids

Nonpharmacologic intervention

◆ Transcutaneous electrical nerve stimulation — electronic stimulation of the large fibers to close the gate to painful stimuli (based on the gate-control theory)
◆ Acupuncture — Chinese method of inserting fine needles at certain sites on the body (How acupuncture works is uncertain.)
◆ Relaxation techniques (Biofeedback, visualization, meditation, and hypnosis can all be useful interventions in pain management.)

ACID-BASE IMBALANCES

Acid base imbalances occur when hydrogen ion concentration is unable to be maintained. The result is a systemic increase (acidosis) or decrease (alkalosis) of hydrogen ion concentration.

KEY CONCEPTS

- Normal pH in the body's blood and extracellular fluids is 7.35 to 7.45.
- The concentration of carbon dioxide (CO_2) is directly related to the concentration of hydrogen (H^+) ions.
- An acid gives up H^+ in solution.
- A base binds H^+ in solution.
- Acid-base balance is regulated by chemical, respiratory, and renal mechanisms.
- Chemical buffers correct acid-base imbalances immediately.
- The lungs regulate the amount of CO_2 retained or exhaled.
- The kidneys control the amount of H^+ and HCO_3^- ions retained or excreted by the body.
- Compensation is the process in which the body uses its three regulatory mechanisms to correct any changes in the pH of body fluids.

KEY POINTS ABOUT ABG VALUES

- pH reflects the number of H^+ ions in the blood. The lungs and the kidneys respond to alterations in the pH levels by retaining or excreting CO_2 and HCO_3^-. (See *Assessing ABG values.*)
- Pao_2 denotes the partial pressure of oxygen in the blood.
- $Paco_2$ denotes the partial pressure of CO_2 in the blood, which is regulated by the lungs.
- HCO_3^- denotes the bicarbonate ion concentration in the blood, which is regulated by the kidneys.

Assessing ABG values

Arterial blood gas (ABG) analysis assesses the client's acid-base balance. The chart below lists typical adult ABG reference values. Normal values may vary slightly among different institutions.

ABG REFERENCE VALUES

pH	7.35 to 7.45
Pao_2	75 to 100 mm Hg
$Paco_2$	35 to 45 mm Hg
HCO_3^-	22 to 26 mEq/L
Sao_2	96% to 100%
Base excess	+1 to −2 mEq/L

- Oxygen saturation denotes the oxygen content of the blood.
- Base excess denotes the difference between the normal serum HCO_3^- level and the client's HCO_3^- level.

RESPIRATORY ACIDOSIS

RESPIRATORY ACIDOSIS is an acid-base disturbance characterized by excess CO_2 in the blood (hypercapnia), indicated by a $Paco_2$ greater than 45 mm Hg. It results from reduced alveolar ventilation. It can be acute (from a sudden failure in ventilation) or chronic (as in long-term pulmonary disease).

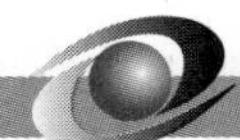

QUICK STUDY

To remember what happens to $Paco_2$ in respiratory acidosis, just look at the "C" and the "I" in the word acidosis. Think of the "C" as standing for $Paco_2$ and the "I" for increase. $Paco_2$ increases in respiratory acidosis.

Possible causes

- Airway obstruction or parenchymal lung disease
- Central nervous system (CNS) trauma
- Chronic metabolic alkalosis
- Drugs, such as opioids, anesthetics, hypnotics, and sedatives
- Neuromuscular disease, such as myasthenia gravis, Guillain-Barré syndrome, and poliomyelitis

Assessment findings

- Restlessness
- Dyspnea and tachypnea with papilledema and depressed reflexes
- Headaches
- Confusion
- Cardiovascular abnormalities, such as tachycardia, hypertension, atrial and ventricular arrhythmias and, in severe acidosis, hypotension with vasodilation
- Coma
- Fine or flapping tremor (asterixis)
- Hypoxemia

Diagnostic evaluation

- ABG measurements confirm respiratory acidosis. $Paco_2$ exceeds the normal level of 45 mm Hg, and pH is usually below the normal range of 7.35 to 7.45. The client's HCO_3^- level is normal in the acute stage and elevated in the chronic stage.

Nursing diagnoses

◆ Anxiety
◆ Impaired gas exchange
◆ Ineffective breathing pattern
◆ Ineffective tissue perfusion (cardiopulmonary)

Treatment

Treatment of respiratory acidosis is designed to correct the underlying source of alveolar hypoventilation. It may include:

◆ endotracheal intubation and mechanical ventilation
◆ dialysis to remove toxic drugs in severe cases or if other treatments fail
◆ removal of foreign body, if appropriate.

Drug therapy options

◆ Antibiotic (if pneumonia is present)
◆ Bronchodilator
◆ Sodium bicarbonate (in severe cases)
◆ Antidotes: naloxone (Narcan) to reverse the effects of opioids, flumazenil (Romazicon) to reverse the effects of benzodiazepines, general anesthesia, or moderate sedation

Planning and goals

◆ The client won't experience preventable complications.
◆ The client's blood pH will remain within normal limits.
◆ As the client's condition improves, the client's and family's anxiety will decrease.

Implementation

◆ Closely monitor the client's blood pH level *to guide the treatment plan.*
◆ Be alert for critical changes in the client's respiratory, CNS, and cardiovascular functions. Also watch closely for variations in ABG values and electrolyte status. Maintain adequate hydration. *These measures help detect life-threatening complications.*
◆ If acidosis requires mechanical ventilation, maintain a patent airway and provide adequate humidification *to ensure adequate oxygenation.* Perform suctioning regularly and vigorous chest physiotherapy if needed. Continuously monitor ventilator settings and respiratory status.
◆ Closely monitor the client with chronic obstructive pulmonary disease and chronic CO_2 retention *to detect signs of acidosis.* Also, administer oxygen at low flow rates and closely monitor all clients who receive opioids and sedatives *to prevent respiratory acidosis.*
◆ Instruct the client who has received a general anesthetic to turn, cough, perform deep-breathing exercises, and use incentive spirometry frequently *to prevent the onset of respiratory acidosis.*
◆ Review key teaching topics with the client and family members *to ensure adequate knowledge about the condition and treatment,* including:
– home oxygen use
– coughing and deep-breathing exercises and incentive spirometry
– medication regimen and possible adverse reactions.

Evaluation

◆ The client doesn't have atelectasis or other respiratory complications.
◆ The client's blood pH ranges between 7.35 and 7.45 and the $Paco_2$ level is between 35 and 45 mm Hg.

RESPIRATORY ALKALOSIS

RESPIRATORY ALKALOSIS is characterized by a deficiency of CO_2 in the blood (hypocapnia), as indicated by a $Paco_2$ below 35 mm Hg (normal level is between 35 and 45 mm Hg). This condition is caused by alveolar hyperventilation. Elimination of CO_2 by the lungs exceeds the production of CO_2 at the cellular level, leading to CO_2 deficiency in the blood. Uncomplicated respiratory alkalosis leads to a decrease in H^+ concentration, which causes elevated blood pH.

Possible causes

Respiratory alkalosis can result from pulmonary or nonpulmonary causes.

Pulmonary causes

◆ Acute asthma
◆ Interstitial lung disease
◆ Pneumonia
◆ Pulmonary vascular disease

Nonpulmonary causes

◆ Anxiety
◆ Aspirin toxicity
◆ CNS disease (inflammation or tumor)
◆ Fever
◆ Hepatic failure
◆ Metabolic acidosis
◆ Pregnancy
◆ Sepsis

Assessment findings

◆ Deep, rapid breathing, possibly exceeding 40 breaths/minute (cardinal sign)
◆ Light-headedness or dizziness (from decreased cerebral blood flow)
◆ Agitation
◆ Circumoral or peripheral paresthesia (prickling sensation around the mouth or extremities)
◆ Muscle weakness
◆ Carpopedal spasms (spasms affecting the wrist and foot)
◆ Twitching (possibly progressing to tetany)
◆ Seizures (severe respiratory alkalosis)
◆ Cardiac arrhythmias that fail to respond to conventional treatment (severe respiratory alkalosis)

Diagnostic evaluation

◆ ABG analysis confirms respiratory alkalosis and rules out respiratory compensation for metabolic acidosis. In the acute stage, $PaCO_2$ is below 35 mm Hg, and pH is elevated in proportion to the fall in $PaCO_2$, but pH drops toward normal in the chronic stage. HCO_3^- level is normal in the acute stage but below normal in the chronic stage.

Nursing diagnoses

◆ Impaired gas exchange
◆ Ineffective breathing pattern
◆ Anxiety

Treatment

Treatment seeks to eradicate the underlying condition. It may include:
◆ removal of ingested toxins
◆ treatment of CNS disease
◆ treatment of fever or sepsis.

Drug therapy options

◆ Antibiotic (specific for type of infectious agent)

In severe respiratory alkalosis

◆ Having the client breathe into a paper bag, which helps relieve acute anxiety and increases CO_2 levels

Planning and goals

◆ The client's blood pH will return to normal.
◆ The client won't have preventable complications.
◆ The client and family will have decreased anxiety.

Implementation

◆ Watch for and report any changes in neurologic, neuromuscular, or cardiovascular functions *to ensure prompt recognition and treatment.*
◆ Remember that twitching and cardiac arrhythmias may be associated with alkalemia and electrolyte imbalances. Monitor ABG and serum electrolyte levels closely, watching for any variations *to detect early changes and prevent complications.*
◆ Review key teaching topics with the client and family members *to ensure adequate knowledge about the condition and treatment,* including:
- relaxation techniques
- breathing into a paper bag during an acute anxiety attack.

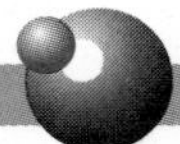

SPOT CHECK

What ABG changes should you expect in acute uncomplicated respiratory alkalosis?
- Decreased $PaCO_2$ (below 35 mm Hg)
- Elevated blood pH (greater than 7.45)
- Normal HCO_3^- (22 to 26 mEq/L)

Evaluation

◆ The client's blood pH ranges between 7.35 and 7.45, and the $PaCO_2$ level is between 35 and 45 mm Hg.
◆ The client has normal breath sounds.
◆ The client and family have decreased anxiety.

METABOLIC ACIDOSIS

METABOLIC ACIDOSIS refers to a state of excess acid accumulation and deficient base HCO_3^-. It's produced by an underlying pathologic disorder. Symptoms result from the body's attempts to correct the acidotic condition through compensatory mechanisms in the lungs, kidneys, and cells.

Metabolic acidosis is more prevalent among children, who are vulnerable to acid-base imbalance because their metabolic rates are faster and their ratios of water to total-body weight are lower than those of adults. Severe or untreated metabolic acidosis can be fatal.

Possible causes

◆ Anaerobic carbohydrate metabolism
◆ Chronic alcoholism
◆ Diabetic ketoacidosis
◆ Diarrhea or intestinal malabsorption
◆ Low-carbohydrate, high-fat diet

- Malnutrition
- Renal insufficiency and failure

Assessment findings

- Headache
- Lethargy
- Drowsiness
- Kussmaul's respirations
- CNS depression
- Stupor

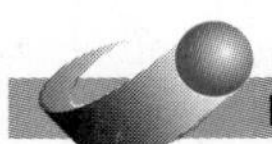

FAST FACT

Kussmaul's respirations are respirations that are fast and deep, without pauses. They characteristically sound labored, with deep breaths that sound like sighs. This breathing pattern develops when the respiratory centers in the medulla detect decreased blood pH, thereby triggering compensatory fast and deep breathing to remove excess CO_2 and restore pH balance.

Diagnostic evaluation

- ABG analysis reveals pH below 7.35 and HCO_3^- level less than 22 mEq/L.

Nursing diagnoses

- Ineffective breathing pattern
- Ineffective tissue perfusion (renal, cerebral, GI)
- Decreased cardiac output

Treatment

- Correcting the underlying cause
- Endotracheal intubation and mechanical ventilation to ensure adequate respiratory compensation (in severe cases)

Drug therapy options

- Insulin: if diabetic ketoacidosis is the cause administer insulin by I.V. infusion until blood glucose levels reach 250 mg/dl, then switch to the subcutaneous route.
- Sodium bicarbonate: I.V. or orally for chronic metabolic acidosis

Planning and goals

- The client's blood pH will return to within normal limits.
- The client won't have preventable complications.

Implementation

- Keep sodium bicarbonate ampules handy *for emergency administration.* Frequently monitor vital signs, laboratory results, and level of consciousness *to identify changes, which can occur rapidly.*
- In diabetic acidosis, watch for secondary changes due to hypovolemia, such as decreasing blood pressure, *to prevent complications of hypoperfusion.*
- Record intake and output accurately *to monitor renal function.*
- Watch for signs of excessive serum potassium — weakness, flaccid paralysis, and arrhythmias — *to detect a life-threatening situation possibly leading to cardiac arrest.* After treatment, check for overcorrection to hypokalemia *to prevent complications of potassium imbalance.*
- Prepare for possible seizures with seizure precautions *to prevent injury.*
- Provide good oral hygiene and lubricate the client's lips *to prevent skin breakdown.*
- Carefully monitor clients receiving I.V. therapy or clients with intestinal tubes in place as well as those suffering from shock, hyperthyroidism, hepatic disease, circulatory failure, or dehydration *to prevent metabolic acidosis.*
- Review key teaching topics with the client and family members *to ensure adequate knowledge about the condition and treatment,* including:
  - testing urine for glucose and acetone
  - encouraging strict adherence to insulin or oral antidiabetic therapy
  - medication therapy and possible adverse reactions.

Evaluation

- The client's fluid and electrolyte levels return to within normal limits.
- The client's blood pH falls between 7.35 and 7.45, and the serum (HCO_3^-) level is between 22 and 26 mEq/L.

METABOLIC ALKALOSIS

METABOLIC ALKALOSIS is a clinical state marked by decreased amounts of acid or increased amounts of base (HCO_3^-). It causes metabolic, respiratory, and renal responses, producing characteristic symptoms — most notably hypoventilation. This condition always occurs secondary to an underlying cause. With early diagnosis and prompt treatment, the prognosis is good; however, untreated metabolic alkalosis may lead to coma and death.

Possible causes

- Loss of acid from vomiting, NG tube drainage, or lavage without adequate electrolyte replacement; fistulas; the use of steroids and certain diuretics (furosemide, thiazides,

and ethacrynic acid); or hyperadrenocorticism (Cushing's syndrome)
◆ Retention of base from excessive intake of bicarbonate of soda or other antacids (usually for treatment of gastritis or peptic ulcer), excessive intake of absorbable alkali (as in milk-alkali syndrome), administration of excessive amounts of I.V. fluids containing bicarbonate or lactate, or respiratory insufficiency

Assessment findings

◆ Hypoventilation
◆ Irritability
◆ Picking at bedclothes (carphology)
◆ Nausea
◆ Vomiting
◆ Diarrhea
◆ Cyanosis
◆ Confusion
◆ Atrial tachycardia
◆ Twitching
◆ Apnea

Diagnostic evaluation

◆ ABG analysis reveals pH greater than 7.45 and HCO_3^- level above 26 mEq/L.

Nursing diagnoses

◆ Decreased cardiac output
◆ Disturbed thought processes
◆ Risk for injury

Treatment

◆ Correcting the underlying cause

Drug therapy options

◆ Acidifying agent: ammonium chloride I.V.
◆ Potassium supplement: Potassium chloride I.V.

Planning and goals

◆ The client's blood pH will return to within normal limits.
◆ The client will learn how to prevent alkalosis.
◆ The client will remain free from injury.

Implementation

◆ When administering ammonium chloride 0.9%, limit the infusion rate to 1¼ hours; *faster administration may cause hemolysis of RBCs.* Avoid overdosage *because it may cause overcorrection to metabolic acidosis.* Don't give ammonium chloride to a client with signs of hepatic or renal disease *to avoid toxicity.*
◆ Monitor vital signs frequently, and record intake and output *to evaluate respiratory, fluid, and electrolyte status.* Respiratory rate usually decreases in an effort to compensate for alkalosis. Hypotension and tachycardia may indicate electrolyte imbalance, especially hypokalemia.
◆ Irrigate NG tubes with isotonic saline solution instead of plain water *to prevent loss of gastric electrolytes.* Monitor I.V. fluid concentrations of HCO_3^- or lactate *to prevent acid-base imbalance.*
◆ Review key teaching topics with the client and family members *to ensure adequate knowledge about the condition and treatment,* including:
– recognizing signs of milk-alkali syndrome (for clients with ulcers), including a distaste for milk, anorexia, weakness, and lethargy
– avoiding overuse of alkaline agents.

Evaluation

◆ The client's blood pH ranges between 7.35 and 7.45 and serum HCO_3^- between 22 and 26 mEq/L.
◆ The client knows how to prevent alkalosis.
◆ The client and family have decreased anxiety.

ELECTROLYTE IMBALANCES

Electrolyte balance is the body's maintenance of normal electrolyte levels. The three electrolytes that have the most frequent imbalances are:
◆ sodium (normal range, 135 to 145 mEq/L)
◆ potassium (normal range, 3.5 to 5.0 mEq/L)
◆ calcium (normal range, 8.2 to 10 mg/dl).

The primary extracellular electrolyte, sodium, is responsible for intracellular and extracellular movement of water, and a close relationship exists between water balance and sodium concentration. The kidneys regulate the amount of sodium excreted.

Potassium, the primary intracellular electrolyte, affects neuromuscular functioning and must be ingested daily. Serum pH directly affects the body's serum potassium concentration.

The most plentiful of the electrolytes, calcium plays a major role in bone and tooth formation, affects blood coagulation, and influences cell membrane permeability (specifically, cardiac and neuromuscular functioning). An electrolyte imbalance — an abnormally high or low level of sodium, potassium, or calcium — can result in dehydration, altered nutrition, and other complications for the client.

SODIUM IMBALANCE

Sodium is the major cation (positively charged ion) in extracellular fluid. Its functions include maintaining tonicity and concentration of extracellular fluid, acid-base balance (reabsorption of sodium ions and excretion of hydrogen ions), nerve conduction and neuromuscular function, glandular secretion, and water balance.

A sodium-potassium pump is constantly at work in every body cell. Potassium is the major cation in intracellular fluid. According to the laws of diffusion, a substance moves from an area of high concentration to an area of lower concentration. Sodium ions, normally most abundant outside the cells, want to diffuse inward. Potassium ions, normally inside the cells, want to diffuse outward. The sodium-potassium pump works to combat this ionic diffusion and maintain normal sodium-potassium balance.

During repolarization, the sodium-potassium pump continually shifts sodium into the cells and potassium out of the cells; during depolarization, it does the reverse.

The body requires only 2 to 4 g of sodium daily. However, most Americans consume 6 to 10 g daily (mostly sodium chloride as table salt), excreting excess sodium through the kidneys and skin.

A low-sodium diet or excessive use of diuretics may induce hyponatremia (decreased serum sodium concentration); dehydration may induce hypernatremia (increased serum sodium concentration).

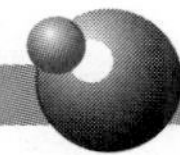

SPOT CHECK

True or False? Sodium is the major cation in intracellular fluid.
Answer: False. Sodium is the major cation in *extra*cellular fluid. Potassium is the major cation in *intra*cellular fluid.

Possible causes

Hyponatremia

- ◆ Diarrhea
- ◆ Excessive perspiration or fever
- ◆ Excessive water intake
- ◆ Low-sodium diet
- ◆ Malnutrition
- ◆ Potent diuretics
- ◆ Starvation
- ◆ Suctioning
- ◆ Trauma, wound drainage, or burns
- ◆ Vomiting

Hypernatremia

- ◆ Decreased water intake
- ◆ Diabetes insipidus
- ◆ Excess adrenocortical hormones, as in Cushing's syndrome
- ◆ Severe vomiting and diarrhea with water loss that exceeds sodium loss

Assessment findings

Hyponatremia

- ◆ Abdominal cramps
- ◆ Anxiety
- ◆ Cold, clammy skin
- ◆ Cyanosis
- ◆ Headaches
- ◆ Hypotension
- ◆ Muscle twitching and weakness
- ◆ Nausea and vomiting
- ◆ Oliguria or anuria
- ◆ Renal dysfunction
- ◆ Seizures
- ◆ Tachycardia

Hypernatremia

- ◆ Agitation and restlessness
- ◆ Circulatory disorders
- ◆ Decreased level of consciousness
- ◆ Dry, sticky mucous membranes
- ◆ Dyspnea
- ◆ Excessive weight gain
- ◆ Fever
- ◆ Flushed skin
- ◆ Hypertension
- ◆ Intense thirst
- ◆ Oliguria
- ◆ Pitting edema
- ◆ Pulmonary edema
- ◆ Rough, dry tongue
- ◆ Seizures
- ◆ Tachycardia

Diagnostic evaluation

- ◆ Serum sodium level less than 135 mEq/L indicates hyponatremia.
- ◆ Serum sodium level greater than 145 mEq/L indicates hypernatremia.

Nursing diagnoses

Hyponatremia

◆ Deficient fluid volume
◆ Risk for injury

Hypernatremia

◆ Excess fluid volume
◆ Disturbed thought processes

Treatment

Hyponatremia

◆ Saline solution: I.V. infusion
◆ Potassium supplement: potassium chloride (K-Lor)

Hypernatremia

◆ Diet: sodium restrictions
◆ Salt-free solution (such as dextrose in water), followed by infusion of half-normal saline solution to prevent hyponatremia

Planning and goals

◆ The client's serum sodium level will return to normal limits. (See *Salty foods.*)

Implementation

For hyponatremia

◆ Watch for extremely low serum sodium and accompanying serum chloride levels. Monitor urine specific gravity and other laboratory results. Record fluid intake and output accurately, and weigh the client daily *to guide the treatment plan.*
◆ During administration of isosmolar or hyperosmolar saline solution, watch closely for signs of hypervolemia (dyspnea, crackles, engorged neck or hand veins) *to prevent respiratory distress.*
◆ Note conditions that may cause excessive sodium loss — diaphoresis, prolonged diarrhea or vomiting, or severe burns — *to prevent hyponatremia.*
◆ Refer the client receiving a maintenance dosage of diuretics to a dietitian for instruction about dietary sodium intake *to increase sodium intake and decrease the risk of hyponatremia.*
◆ Review key teaching topics with the client with hyponatremia and his family members *to ensure adequate knowledge about the condition and treatment,* including:
- the rationale for fluid restriction, if necessary
- increasing dietary intake of sodium
- the medication regimen and possible adverse reactions.

Salty foods

Instruct the client with hypernatremia to avoid these high-sodium foods:
◆ Baking soda and baking powder
◆ Bottled soft drinks, especially those with sodium or sodium saccharin
◆ Canned soups, broth, or vegetables
◆ Condiments, such as salted butter and margarine, ketchup, mustard, and salad dressing
◆ Fast foods
◆ Foods that contain monosodium glutamate
◆ Instant foods such as cereal
◆ Lunch meats and cheeses
◆ Over-the-counter medications such as antacids
◆ Pickles and pickled foods
◆ Potato chips, pretzels, and other snack foods
◆ Prepared foods such as TV dinners.

For hypernatremia

◆ Measure serum sodium levels every 6 hours or at least daily. Monitor vital signs for changes, especially for rising pulse rate. Watch for signs of hypervolemia, especially in the client receiving I.V. fluids, *to guide the treatment regimen.*
◆ Record fluid intake and output accurately, checking for body fluid loss *to prevent dehydration and accompanying hypernatremia.* Weigh the client daily *to monitor fluid volume status.*
◆ Obtain a drug history *to check for drugs that promote sodium retention.*
◆ Review key teaching topics with the client and family members *to ensure adequate knowledge about the condition and treatment,* including the importance of sodium restriction and how to plan a low-sodium diet.

Evaluation

◆ The client has a serum sodium level above 135 mEq/L (hyponatremia) and below 145 mEq/L (hypernatremia).

POTASSIUM IMBALANCE

Potassium is the major cation of intracellular fluid. Because of the high concentration of potassium inside the cells, potassium exerts some control over intracellular osmolarity and volume. Maintaining the difference in the potassium concentration between intracellular fluid and extracellular fluid is critical for enabling excitable tissues to generate action potentials and transmit impulses. Because extracellular fluid potassium levels are extremely low, any alteration in the concentration is poorly tolerated by the body and profoundly affects physiologic activities.

Potassium intake averages about 2 to 20 g/day for most people. Almost all foods contain some amount of potassium, but some foods are higher in potassium than others. The healthy body keeps plasma potassium levels within the narrow range of normal values required for physiologic function.

The sodium-potassium pump within every body cell membrane is the primary controller of extracellular potassium concentration. Some potassium regulation also takes place through renal function. The kidney excretes 80% of potassium from the body. There's no identified hormone that directly controls renal resorption of potassium, so the kidney doesn't conserve potassium directly.

Possible causes

Hypokalemia

- Alkalosis
- Corticosteroids
- Diarrhea
- Digoxin
- Diuretics
- Inappropriate or excessive use of drugs
- No oral intake for an extended period
- Prolonged NG suctioning
- Vomiting

Hyperkalemia

- Acidosis
- Dehydration
- Overeating of potassium-containing foods
- Potassium-sparing diuretics
- Rapid infusion of potassium-containing I.V. solutions
- Renal failure

Assessment findings

Hypokalemia

- Nausea, vomiting
- Leg cramps
- General skeletal muscle weakness
- Orthostatic hypotension
- Constipation
- Abdominal distention
- Anxiety, lethargy, confusion, coma
- Hypoactive or absent bowel sounds
- Decreased breath sounds
- Polyuria
- Low specific gravity

Hyperkalemia

- Irregular, slow heartbeat
- Muscle twitches, cramps, paresthesia (early hyperkalemia)
- Hypotension
- Hyperactive bowel sounds
- Diarrhea
- Ascending flaccid paralysis (progresses distal to proximal with extremities)
- Profound weakness (late hyperkalemia)

Diagnostic evaluation

Hypokalemia

- Serum potassium less than 3.5 mEq/L
- ECG reveals ST depression, inverted T wave, prominent U wave, or heart block, ventricular arrfhythmias, tachycardia, or cardiac arrest

Hyperkalemia

- Serum potassium greater than 5.0 mEq/L
- ECG reveals widened QRS complex, flattened P wave, prolonged PR interval, depressed ST segment or heart block, ventricular arrhythmias, and asystole

Nursing diagnoses

Hypokalemia

- Imbalanced nutrition: Less than body requirements
- Ineffective tissue perfusion (cardiopulmonary)
- Risk for deficient fluid volume
- Impaired physical mobility

Hyperkalemia

- Imbalanced nutrition: More than body requirements
- Ineffective tissue perfusion (cardiopulmonary)
- Diarrhea
- Activity intolerance

Treatment

Hypokalemia

- Potassium supplements (oral or I.V.)
- Potassium-sparing diuretics
- Increased potassium in diet

Hyperkalemia

- Potassium-excreting diuretics (furosemide)
- Sodium polystyrene sulfonate (Kayexalate)
- Insulin I.V. given with I.V. hypertonic dextrose solution (typically 50% dextrose solution)
- Dialysis, if needed
- Bicarbonate

◆ Calcium gluconate I.V. or calcium chloride I.V. to counteract myocardial efects of hyperkalemia

Planning and goals

◆ The client's serum potassium level will return to normal.
◆ The client will be aware of the appropriate foods to include in his daily diet.
◆ The client won't have cardiac complications, such as ventricular tachycardia.
◆ The client will have normal muscle function when potassium levels return to normal.

Implementation

Hypokalemia

◆ Monitor potassium levels frequently *to guide the treatment plan.*
◆ Monitor for arrhythmias *to assess for cardiac involvement.*
◆ Administer potassium supplements as needed. Oral supplements must be diluted in at least 4 oz of fluid *to prevent stomach irritation.* I.V. supplements shouldn't be infused faster than 20 mEq/hour *because rapid infusion can cause life-threatening arrhythmias.*
◆ Review key teaching topics with the client and family members *to ensure adequate knowledge about the condition and treatment,* including:
– importance of having potassium levels drawn at regular intervals when client is taking diuretics
– diet, and foods high in potassium
– awareness of problems with weakness and leg cramps
– importance of follow-up care.

Hyperkalemia

◆ Monitor potassium levels frequently *to guide the treatment plan.*
◆ Monitor for arrhythmias *to assess for cardiac involvement.*
◆ Monitor diet and decrease foods high in potassium *to prevent increase of hyperkalemia.* (See *High-potassium foods.*)
◆ Review key teaching topics with the client and family members *to ensure adequate knowledge about the condition and treatment,* including:
– the need to avoid salt substitutes, which usually contain potassium
– diet and foods to avoid that contain high levels of potassium
– the importance of follow-up evaluation.

High-potassium foods

Instruct the client with hyperkalemia to avoid these high-potassium foods:

◆ Apricots
◆ Bananas
◆ Dark, green leafy vegetables
◆ Dried fruits
◆ Oranges
◆ Peanuts
◆ Strawberries
◆ Tomatoes.

Evaluation

◆ The client's potassium level is within normal limits (between 3.5 and 5 mEq/L).
◆ The client has no cardiovascular complications.
◆ The client knows which foods are high in potassium and what diet to follow.
◆ The client demonstrates normal neuromuscular function.

CALCIUM IMBALANCE

Calcium plays an indispensable role in cell permeability, formation of bones and teeth, blood coagulation, transmission of nerve impulses, and normal muscle contraction.

Nearly all (99%) of the body's calcium is found in the bones. The remaining 1% exists in ionized form in serum; maintaining ionized calcium in the serum is critical to healthy neurologic function.

The parathyroid glands regulate ionized calcium and determine its resorption into bone, absorption from the GI mucosa, and excretion in urine and stool. Severe calcium imbalance requires emergency treatment because a deficiency (hypocalcemia) can lead to tetany and seizures; an excess (hypercalcemia), to cardiac arrhythmias and coma.

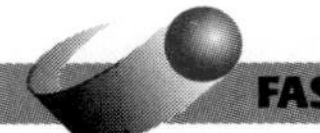

FAST FACT

When calcium levels are too high, the thyroid releases calcitonin. High levels of calcitonin inhibit bone resorption, which causes a decrease in the amount of calcium available from bone, thereby decreasing serum calcium levels. Calcitonin may also be administered as a drug to treat hypercalcemia.

Possible causes

Hypocalcemia

- Hypomagnesemia
- Hypoparathyroidism
- Inadequate intake of calcium and vitamin D
- Malabsorption or loss of calcium from the GI tract
- Overcorrection of acidosis
- Pancreatic insufficiency
- Renal failure
- Severe infections or burns
- Hyperphosphatemia
- Multiple blood transfusions

Hypercalcemia

- Hyperparathyroidism
- Hypervitaminosis D
- Multiple fractures and prolonged immobilization
- Multiple myeloma
- Other causes (milk-alkali syndrome, sarcoidosis, hyperthyroidism, adrenal insufficiency, and thiazide diuretics)
- Tumors
- Hypophosphatemia

Assessment findings

Hypocalcemia

- Perioral paresthesia
- Twitching
- Carpopedal spasm
- Tetany
- Seizures
- Cardiac arrhythmias
- Chvostek's sign
- Trousseau's sign

Hypercalcemia

- Muscle weakness
- Decreased muscle tone
- Anorexia
- Constipation
- Nausea
- Vomiting
- Polydipsia
- Dehydration
- Polyuria
- Cardiac arrhythmias and eventual coma with severe hypercalcemia (serum levels greater than 14 mg/dl)

Diagnostic evaluation

- A serum calcium level less than 8.2 mg/dl confirms hypocalcemia; a level greater than 10.2 mg/dl confirms hypercalcemia. (Because approximately one-half of serum calcium is bound to albumin, changes in serum protein must be considered when interpreting serum calcium levels.)
- ECG reveals a lengthened QT interval, a prolonged ST segment (which places the client at risk for torsades de pointes), and arrhythmias in hypocalcemia; in hypercalcemia, a prolonged PR interval, flattened T waves, a shortened QT interval, and heart block.

Nursing diagnoses

Hypocalcemia

- Imbalanced nutrition: Less than body requirements
- Acute pain
- Decreased cardiac output

Hypercalcemia

- Impaired physical mobility
- Impaired urinary elimination

Treatment

Hypocalcemia

- Diet: adequate intake of calcium, vitamin D, and protein

Drug therapy options

- Ergocalciferol (vitamin D_2), cholecalciferol (vitamin D_3), calcitriol, dihydrotachysterol (synthetic form of vitamin D_2) for severe deficiency
- I.V. calcium gluconate, calcium chloride for immediate correction of acute hypocalcemia (an emergency)
- Vitamin D in multivitamin preparation for mild hypocalcemia
- Vitamin D supplements to facilitate GI absorption of calcium to treat chronic hypocalcemia

Hypercalcemia

- Hydration with normal saline solution to eliminate excess serum calcium through urine excretion
- Diet: Low calcium with increased oral fluid intake

Drug therapy options

- Calcitonin (Calcimar)
- Corticosteroids: prednisone (Deltasone), hydrocortisone (Solu-Cortef) for treating sarcoidosis, hypervitaminosis D, and certain tumors
- Loop diuretics: ethacrynic acid (Edecrin), furosemide (Lasix) to promote calcium excretion (thiazide diuretics are contraindicated in hypercalcemia because they inhibit calcium excretion)

◆ Plicamycin (Mithracin) to lower serum calcium level (especially against hypercalcemia secondary to certain tumors)
◆ Sodium phosphate solution administered by mouth or by retention enema (promotes calcium deposits in bone and inhibits absorption from the GI tract)

Planning and goals

For hypocalcemia

◆ The client will identify food sources rich in calcium and vitamin D.
◆ The client will consume a diet high in calcium and vitamin D.
◆ The client will attain a total serum calcium level within the reference range.
◆ The client will state and carry out appropriate interventions for pain relief.
◆ The client will experience relief from muscle cramps.

For hypercalcemia

◆ The client will have a total serum calcium level within the reference range.
◆ The client will maintain a normal balance between intake and output.
◆ The client will show no evidence of complications related to impaired physical mobility, such as contractures, venous stasis, thrombus formation, or skin breakdown.
◆ The client will adhere to his treatment regimen, which will prevent or minimize further elevations in serum calcium level.

Implementation

Hypocalcemia

◆ Watch for hypocalcemia in clients receiving massive transfusions of citrated blood and in those with chronic diarrhea, severe infections, and insufficient dietary intake of calcium and protein (especially elderly clients). *Identifying clients at risk can ensure early treatment intervention.*
◆ Monitor serum calcium levels every 12 to 24 hours *to identify normal calcium levels;* a calcium level below 8.2 mg/dl requires immediate attention. When giving calcium supplements, frequently check the pH level; *an alkalotic state that exceeds a pH of 7.45 inhibits calcium ionization.* Check for Trousseau's and Chvostek's signs, *which indicate hypocalcemia.*
◆ Administer calcium gluconate slow I.V. in dextrose 5% in water (*never* in saline solution, which encourages renal calcium loss). Don't add calcium gluconate I.V. to solutions containing HCO_3^- to avoid precipitation.

> ## Calcium sources
>
> Instruct the client to eat these calcium-rich foods:
> ◆ Broccoli, turnip greens, and spinach
> ◆ Dairy products, tofu, and low-fat yogurt
> ◆ Dried beans and apricots
> ◆ Salmon and sardines.

◆ When administering calcium solutions, watch for anorexia, nausea, and vomiting, *which are possible signs of overcorrection to hypercalcemia.*
◆ Monitor the client closely for a possible drug interaction if he's receiving cardiac glycosides, such as digoxin, with large doses of oral calcium supplements. *Administration of digoxin concomitantly with calcium supplements may cause synergistic effects of digoxin that precipitate arrhythmias.* Watch for signs of digoxin toxicity (anorexia, nausea, vomiting, yellow vision, and cardiac arrhythmias). Administer oral calcium supplements 1 to 1¼ hours after meals or with milk *to promote absorption.*
◆ Provide a quiet, stress-free environment for the client with tetany *to prevent seizure activity.* Observe seizure precautions for clients with severe hypocalcemia, which may lead to seizures, *to prevent client injury.*
◆ Review key teaching topics with the client and family members *to ensure adequate knowledge about the condition and treatment,* including:
– the importance of calcium for normal bone formation and blood coagulation
– eating foods rich in calcium, vitamin D, and protein, such as fortified milk and cheese, to prevent hypocalcemia (see *Calcium sources*)
– avoiding chronic laxative use and overuse of antacids to prevent hypocalcemia.

Hypercalcemia

◆ Monitor serum calcium levels frequently *to identify abnormal calcium levels.* Watch for cardiac arrhythmias if the serum calcium level exceeds 10.2 mg/dl. Increase fluid intake *to dilute calcium in serum and urine and to prevent renal damage and dehydration.*
◆ Watch for signs of heart failure in clients receiving normal saline solution. *Infusion of large volumes of normal saline solution may cause fluid volume excess, leading to heart failure.*

◆ Administer loop diuretics (not thiazide diuretics) *to promote diuresis and rid the body of excess calcium.* Monitor intake and output, and check the urine for renal calculi and acidity. Provide acid-ash drinks, such as cranberry or prune juice, because calcium salts are more soluble in acid than in alkali.
◆ Check the client's ECG and vital signs frequently *to assess for changes in the client's condition.* In the client receiving cardiac glycosides such as digoxin, watch for signs of toxicity, such as anorexia, nausea, vomiting, and bradycardia (commonly with arrhythmia). Fatal arrhythmias may result when digoxin is administered in hypercalcemia.
◆ Help the client walk as soon as possible *to promote mobility.* Handle the client with chronic hypercalcemia gently *to prevent pathologic fractures.*
◆ If the client is bedridden, reposition him frequently *to monitor for changes in the client's condition,* and encourage ROM exercises *to promote circulation and prevent urinary stasis and calcium loss from bone.*
◆ Review key teaching topics with the client and family members *to ensure adequate knowledge about the condition and treatment,* including:
– the importance of calcium for normal bone formation and blood coagulation
– eating a low-calcium diet and increasing fluid intake to prevent recurrence of hypercalcemia.

Evaluation

◆ The client's calcium level is within reference limits (8.2 to 10.2 mg/dl).
◆ The client can identify foods rich in calcium and vitamin D, and verbalizes the appropriate foods to include in his daily diet.
◆ The client demonstrates an absence of muscle discomfort with the return of calcium to a normal level.
◆ The client demonstrates no complications as a result of impaired physical mobility.

FLUID IMBALANCES

Sodium balance vitally affects fluid balance. Equivalent amounts of sodium and water that are lost or gained won't change serum osmolarity (tonicity), but the client may show signs of deficient fluid volume or excess.

DEFICIENT FLUID VOLUME

Deficient fluid volume (dehydration) results from excessive loss of water and electrolytes from extracellular fluid.

Possible causes

◆ Excessive fluid loss through secretions or excretions
◆ Insufficient intake of water and electrolytes (can occur simultaneously with excessive fluid loss)
◆ Third-space fluid shifting

Assessment findings

◆ Collapsed neck and hand veins
◆ Decreased CVP, pulmonary artery pressure, and cardiac output
◆ Dizziness, syncope, weakness
◆ Dry skin, decreased skin turgor, dry mucous membranes

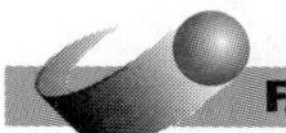

FAST FACT

To assess skin turgor in an adult, pick up a small fold of skin over the sternum or the arm. (In an infant, roll a fold of loosely adherent skin on the abdomen between your thumb and forefinger.) Then release it. Normal skin will immediately return to its previous contour. In decreased skin turgor, the fold of skin will "tent" for up to 30 seconds.

◆ Hypotension
◆ Increased thirst
◆ Nausea, vomiting
◆ Oliguria
◆ Orthostatic blood pressure differences
◆ Tachycardia

Diagnostic evaluation

◆ BUN and creatinine ratio are elevated.
◆ Hematology studies reveal increased hematocrit levels.
◆ Serum sodium is above 145 mEq/L.
◆ Serum osmolality is above 300 mOsm/kg.
◆ Urine specific gravity is above 1.030.

Nursing diagnoses

◆ Deficient fluid volume
◆ Ineffective tissue perfusion (cardiopulmonary, renal, cerebral)

Treatment

Treatment depends on the cause and can vary from shock treatment (See "Shock disorders," page 76.) to replacing fluids by oral supplementation and I.V. therapy. (See "Acid–base imbalances," page 87, and "Electrolyte imbalances," page 92.)

Drug therapy options

- ◆ Albumin
- ◆ Blood transfusion
- ◆ Dextrose 5% in normal saline solution

Planning and goals

◆ The client will achieve and maintain adequate hydration.

◆ The client will achieve and maintain adequate tissue perfusion (adequate urine output, blood pressure, and heart rate).

Implementation

◆ Monitor intake and output *to assess fluid balance.* Normally, the body maintains a balance of about 2,300 ml of intake as fluids and food and 2,300 ml of output as sensible or insensible fluid loss.

◆ Weigh the client daily at the same time, on the same scale, and with the same amount of linens or clothes *to ensure accurate measurements.* Each 2-lb weight loss reflects a 1-L fluid loss.

◆ Measure urine specific gravity as needed *to evaluate the client's fluid status and response to therapy.*

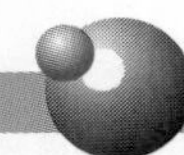

SPOT CHECK

If a client is being treated for deficient fluid volume and the nurse notes that his urine specific gravity has decreased, is this client responding to treatment?

Answer: Yes. Deficient fluid volume causes the urine specific gravity to increase. A decrease indicates a positive response to treatment.

◆ Assess hemodynamic parameters, such as CVP, pulmonary artery pressure, and cardiac output if condition is severe, *to monitor the client's fluid status and response to therapy.*

◆ Review key teaching topics with the client and family members *to ensure adequate knowledge about the condition and treatment,* including:
- diet instruction regarding sodium-containing foods
- signs of deficient fluid volume.

Evaluation

◆ The client has a urine output of at least 30 ml/hour.

EXCESS FLUID VOLUME

Excess fluid volume reflects an increased accumulation of water and electrolytes in extracellular fluid. It usually results from an increase in total sodium concentration, causing more water to be drawn into extracellular fluid to reestablish the proper sodium-water ratio.

Possible causes

◆ Diminished homeostatic mechanisms, such as those occurring in heart failure, cirrhosis, or excessive corticosteroid therapy

◆ I.V. replacement therapy using normal saline or lactated Ringer's solution

◆ Blood or plasma replacement

◆ High intake of dietary sodium

Assessment findings

- ◆ Bounding pulses
- ◆ Crackles on auscultation
- ◆ Dependent edema (such as pedal, sacral, or scrotal edema)
- ◆ Dyspnea
- ◆ Elevated CVP, pulmonary artery pressure
- ◆ Hypertension
- ◆ Neck vein distention

Diagnostic evaluation

- ◆ BUN level is decreased.
- ◆ Hematocrit is decreased due to hemodilation.
- ◆ Serum sodium level is normal or decreased.
- ◆ Serum and urine osmolality are decreased in clients with normal renal function.
- ◆ ABG analysis results reveal hypoxia.
- ◆ Chest X-ray reveals pulmonary congestion.

Nursing diagnoses

◆ Excess fluid volume

Treatment

Drug therapy options

◆ Diuretics act to increase the excretion of water and sodium and other electrolytes through the kidneys. Types of diruetics include:
- loop — bumetanide (Bumex), furosemide (Lasix)
- osmotic — mannitol (Osmitrol)
- potassium-sparing — spironolactone (Aldactone)
- thiazide — chlorothiazide (Diuril), hydrochlorothiazide (HydroDIURIL).

Planning and goals

The client's circulating blood volume will be within reference limits.

Implementation

- Administer diuretics, as ordered, *to decrease fluid volume.*
- Maintain fluid restrictions *to promote fluid balance.*
- Monitor intake and output hourly *to assess for changes in fluid status.*
- Measure urine specific gravity as needed *to evaluate the client's fluid status and response to therapy.*
- Weigh the client daily at the same time and on the same scale with the client wearing the same amount of clothing *to evaluate fluid balance.* Significant weight gain reflects excess fluid volume.
- Assess the client for distended neck and hand veins, *which indicate excess fluid volume.*
- Monitor the client for signs of heart failure or pulmonary edema *to identify changes in physical condition.*
- Assess hemodynamic parameters, such as CVP or pulmonary artery pressure, if excess is severe *to evaluate for changes in fluid status.*
- Review key teaching topics with the client and family members *to ensure adequate knowledge about the condition and treatment,* including:
  - diet instruction regarding sodium-containing foods
  - signs of excess fluid volume, including weight gain, shortness of breath, and swelling of the feet or ankles.

Evaluation

- The client maintains a stable body weight.
- The client displays no overt signs of edema or dehydration.

IMMOBILITY

IMMOBILITY is a temporary or permanent decrease in the client's ability to move all or part of the body easily or comfortably. Immobility can be caused by:

- loss of motor function
- loss of sensory function
- combined loss of motor and sensory function.

The client can also lose proprioception (awareness of one's position, weight, posture, or equilibrium).

LOSS OF MOTOR FUNCTION

Loss of motor function can produce weakness or paralysis of the muscles, as in quadriplegia (paralysis of all extremities), paraplegia (paralysis of the legs), and hemiplegia (paralysis of one side of the body).

LOSS OF SENSORY FUNCTION

Loss of sensory function can result in blindness, hemianopsia (blindness in half of the field of vision in one or both eyes), agnosia (inability to comprehend or recognize an object), deafness, anesthesia (inability to feel pain or touch), and aphasia (inability to speak intended words or to understand words).

Possible causes

- Anoxia (loss of oxygen to cells, resulting in cell death; may accompany hemorrhage or blood loss, excessive swelling, or acid-base imbalances)
- Certain medications (such as anesthetics) and poisons
- Degenerative conditions (such as myasthenia gravis and amyotropic lateral sclerosis) that gradually cause tissues to lose function
- Immobility from surgery or serious illness
- Infectious agents (microorganisms exerting toxic effects on cells — from the organisms themselves or from the toxins they produce)
- Severe anxiety
- Trauma (cutting or transection of nerve pathways or muscle fibers to or from affected tissues)
- Treatment for a medical condition (for example, MI, surgery, or cast application)

Assessment findings

Immobility can affect all of the major body systems:

- Respiratory changes affect the rate, depth, and strength of respiratory effort, predisposing the client to anoxia, atelectasis, and pneumonia.
- Integumentary effects of immobility, which result from pressure and stasis, include atrophy, tissue breakdown, and pressure ulcers.
- Decreased energy expenditure predisposes the client to anorexia, altered intake, and altered nutrient use and metabolism, resulting in diarrhea, hemorrhoids, and malnutrition.
- Decreased fluid intake and urinary stasis predispose the client to urinary tract infections and formation of renal calculi.
- Loss of innervation and sensation predisposes the client to muscle spasticity or flaccidity, with neurologic conse-

quences, such as altered pain perception, autonomic dysreflexia, confusion, and disorientation.

◆ Endocrine metabolic effects of immobility include predisposition to weight loss; acid-base, fluid, and electrolyte imbalances; anemia; osteoporosis; pathologic fractures; prolonged healing; amenorrhea; impotence; and loss of libido.

◆ Psychological effects, such as anxiety, fear, depression, and even death, may occur. The client may not be able to obtain employment. Immobility, especially if chronic, can adversely affect the ability to develop and maintain social relationships.

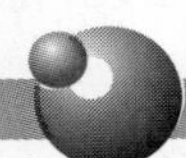

SPOT CHECK

Name three adverse effects of immobility.

Answer: A few examples include atelectasis, pneumonia, muscle atrophy, tissue breakdown, pressure ulcers, urinary tract infections, and muscle spasticity. For a more complete list, see "Assessment findings."

Diagnostic evaluation

◆ The suspected source of the sensory loss guides the evaluation. If a neurologic cause is suspected, electromyography shows nerve disease.

Nursing diagnoses

◆ Impaired physical mobility

◆ Social isolation

Treatment

Treatment focuses on preventive measures and the treatment of specific complications, should they arise.

Planning and goals

◆ The client will maintain function in unaffected tissues.

◆ The client will regain maximal function in affected tissues.

◆ The client will fulfill usual or new roles within the family and society.

Implementation

◆ Instruct the client to use an incentive spirometer and perform regular deep-breathing and coughing exercises *to prevent pulmonary complications.*

◆ Initiate ROM exercises to affected areas *to help maintain muscle tone.* As needed, perform neurologic checks and obtain physical or occupational therapy consultation.

◆ Frequently change the client's position *to maintain joint and body function.* Turn the client from side to side by logrolling if the spinal cord has been damaged.

◆ Perform proper hygiene, including baths and use of lotions, and use support surfaces, protective barriers, and rails *to prevent skin breakdown or tissue trauma.*

◆ Apply antiembolism stockings and a sequential compression device *to prevent thrombus formation.*

◆ Provide appropriate foods and dietary supplements *to ensure adequate nutrition.* Adequate protein intake is necessary *to promote healing and prevent skin breakdown.* The client may need to increase nutrient intake by tube feeding or total parenteral nutrition.

◆ Encourage increased intake of fluids (unless contraindicated), especially fruit juices, and foods that increase dietary bulk (unless contraindicated) *to prevent constipation.*

◆ Keep the head of the client's bed elevated to at least 30 degrees *to prevent aspiration pneumonia.*

◆ Administer a stool softener or laxative, if ordered, *to maintain adequate elimination.* If ordered, administer an enema if the client doesn't have a bowel movement within 3 days.

◆ Monitor the client's weight *to ensure adequate nutrition.*

◆ If appropriate, reduce dietary calcium intake, as ordered, *to prevent renal calculi.*

◆ Regularly observe the client for adverse effects of immobility *so the need for prompt interventions is identified.*

◆ Provide emotional support to the client and family members *to decrease anxiety. The client needs emotional support and reassurance from both the family and health professionals.* Psychiatric consultation may help during prolonged anxiety and depression.

◆ Include family members in the client's care, as feasible, and teach them client care before discharge *to facilitate home support of the client.*

◆ Arrange vocational counseling and education as the client requires and requests *to provide an opportunity for the client to assume his previous role or a new role in the family or society.*

◆ Initiate continuity of care referrals before the client's transfer or discharge home *to promote adequate follow-up care.*

Evaluation

◆ The client demonstrates no adverse effects from immobility.

◆ Interventions have been taken to treat any adverse effects.

◆ The client verbalizes appropriate ways to avoid effects of immobility after discharge.

Perioperative nursing

INTRODUCTION

Perioperative nursing — nursing care provided for a surgical client — encompasses three phases:

- ◆ Preoperative period (before surgery)
- ◆ Intraoperative period (during surgery)
- ◆ Postoperative period (after surgery).

Because clients experience varying degrees of anxiety and deficient knowledge related to surgery, careful planning by the nurse can help ensure a positive outcome.

Standards of perioperative nursing practice based on the nursing process have been developed to provide guidance to those who work in this important nursing specialty. This section, therefore, uses the nursing process to review the three phases of perioperative nursing.

PREOPERATIVE PERIOD

The preoperative period begins when the client decides to have surgery and ends when the client is transferred to the operating room. This period is used to physically and psychologically prepare the client for surgery. The nurse plays a major role in client teaching and in relieving the client's and the family's anxieties.

NURSING RESPONSIBILITIES

Assessment

◆ Assess the client for signs of anxiety, including:
- anger
- elevated pulse and respiratory rates
- increased verbalization
- quiet or withdrawn behavior
- restlessness
- sleeplessness
- sweating.

Virtually every client about to undergo surgery experiences anxiety in some form, from mild to severe.

◆ Assess the client's knowledge about the upcoming surgery and solicit questions about the procedure. Questions are normal, and knowledge will help speed the client's recovery. Depending on the surgical procedure, the client may experience various stages of loss, including depression and anger.

Diagnostic evaluation

◆ Hematology studies analyze a sample of blood for red blood cell count, white blood cell count, hemoglobin level, hematocrit, and platelet count. These studies are used to detect infection, blood disorders, or anemia.

◆ Urinalysis examines a urine specimen to check for bacteria, blood, glucose, and ketone bodies, and to determine specific gravity and urine pH. This test is performed to detect bleeding, infection, kidney disease, or metabolic disorders.

◆ Blood chemistry examines a blood sample to measure levels of potassium, sodium, chloride, calcium, phosphorus, glucose, ketones, blood urea nitrogen, and creatinine. These studies detect fluid and electrolyte imbalances, kidney disease, and diabetes.

◆ Chest radiography may be performed to detect pulmonary or heart disease.

◆ Electrocardiography may be performed to detect heart disease.

◆ Coagulation studies, such as prothrombin time, International Normalized Ratio, partial thromboplastin time, and bleeding time are performed to detect bleeding disorders.

◆ Typing and crossmatching for blood is performed to make sure compatible blood products are available if needed during or immediately after surgery.

Nursing diagnoses

- ◆ Anxiety
- ◆ Deficient knowledge (surgical procedure and recovery)

Planning and goals

- ◆ The client will express concerns freely.

◆ The client will be calm and relaxed.
◆ The client will verbalize an understanding of the perioperative routine.
◆ The client will demonstrate activities and exercises to promote postoperative recovery.

Implementation

◆ Increase time spent privately with the client, and encourage the client to express feelings openly. *A nurse's presence indicates a concern for the client's well-being, which reduces the client's anxiety.*
◆ Encourage the client to participate in decision making *to increase the client's sense of control and help maintain self-esteem.*
◆ Make sure that an informed consent is signed before administering any preoperative sedation. *Sedation prevents the client from making an informed decision.*
◆ Provide the client with necessary information about surgery *to promote trust and ensure that the client's rights are being upheld.*
◆ Provide teaching, as indicated, related to postoperative care, such as coughing, deep-breathing, leg exercises, use of incentive spirometry, use of sequential compression device, and splinting of the anticipated surgical area *to decrease the client's anxiety, which promotes well-being and comfort.* Usually, a client who knows what to expect and how to comply has fewer complications.
◆ Administer sedatives or antianxiety agents, as ordered, the night before surgery *to decrease anxiety and allow the client restful sleep.*
◆ Make sure that blood is available for the client in the blood bank *to prevent treatment delay should the client require blood during surgery.*
◆ When appropriate, inform the client about autologous blood transfusions, which are increasingly used *to eliminate the risk of acquiring bloodborne infections* (although the risk of acquiring infections is low).

Close observation

◆ Observe the client for effects of sedatives or antianxiety agents *to detect potential adverse reactions to medication.*
◆ Administer preoperative medications, such as opioids (morphine) and anticholinergics (atropine, glycopyrrolate), as ordered. *Opioids sometimes are given to decrease anxiety and tension and aid anesthesia induction. Anticholinergic agents decrease secretions, vomiting, laryngospasm, and bronchospasm.*

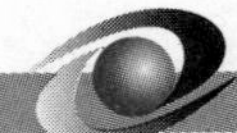

QUICK STUDY

The word **TEACH** is a good way to remember information to include in preoperative teaching:

Turn, cough, and deep-breathe
Exercises to perform after surgery
Administration of medication for pain and nausea
Concerns of the client should be addressed
Healing of the wound

Evaluation

The client approaches surgery with only mild anxiety and freely expresses concerns, and knows about future care.

INTRAOPERATIVE PERIOD

The intraoperative period begins when the client enters the surgical suite and ends with the completion of the surgical procedure.

NURSING RESPONSIBILITIES

◆ Maintaining safety by properly identifying the client and the surgical site according to facility policy
◆ Monitoring physiologic responses to surgery
◆ Keeping the client comfortable

In the operating room, the client is usually sedated and under the care of anesthesia personnel. Depending on the surgical procedure, a regional or general anesthetic is administered. Expect to assist anesthesia personnel or monitor the client when moderate sedation, local, and certain regional anesthesia techniques are used. (See *Types of anesthesia.*) Check whether the client banked his own blood before admission.

Nursing care during the intraoperative period includes:
◆ meeting the client's physical needs
◆ meeting the client's needs for safety and dignity.

Types of anesthesia

Regional anesthesia

Effects on the client

- Produces intact consciousness
- Produces loss of motor and sensory perception to a particular area of the body

Common types

- *Spinal* – injection of a local anesthetic into the subarachnoid space between the second and third or the third and fourth lumbar vertebrae
- *Epidural* – injection of a local anesthetic into the epidural space

Uses

- Surgical procedures involving the legs, lower abdomen, or perineum

Potential complications

- Sympathetic preganglionic block of fibers in the anterior root of the spinal cord, causing vasodilation and reduced venous blood return to the heart
- Spinal headache
- Respiratory depression (if thoracic, intercostal, or accessory muscles are inadvertently anesthetized)
- Over-anesthetization of the spinal cord (resulting in the client's inability to breathe and requiring oxygen and ventilatory support)
- Other complications: hypotension, depressed myocardium, anaphylactic reaction, seizures, ringing in the ears, facial numbness or twitching, nausea and vomiting

Nursing implementations

- Assess the client for hypotension; have a vasopressor, such as ephedrine sulfate (EPhed II) or phenylephrine (Neo-Synephrine), available.
- Record the client's respiratory rate, depth, and oxygen saturation.
- Protect the anesthetized area until full sensation has returned.
- Assess for return of sensation and motor function below the level of anesthesia; ask the client to move the anesthetized part and to report any perception of touch.
- Keep the client flat in bed for about 8 hours after regional anesthesia to prevent spinal fluid leakage into the epidural space, which is thought to cause spinal headache.
- Tell the client not to strain when moving in bed or having a bowel movement; straining increases intracranial pressure, which can exacerbate loss of cerebrospinal fluid.
- If spinal headache occurs, administer an analgesic as ordered, keep the client flat, and report the headache to the physician.
- Provide adequate hydration to help replace spinal fluid and prevent venous stasis. Note that oral intake is commonly avoided during the early postoperative period.
- Have resuscitation equipment available at all times.
- Know the toxic dose of each local anesthetic used during a procedure.

General anesthesia

Effects on the client

- Produces unconsciousness
- Blocks motor and sensory pathways to major nerve and muscle groups

Administration methods

- Inhalation gas
- I.V. injection

Nursing implementations

- Close operating room doors. Check for proper positioning of the safety belt. Have suction equipment available and working. Minimize room noise.
- Stay with the client.
- Avoid stimulating the client. Be available to provide protection or restraint.
- Be available to assist anesthesia personnel with intubation. Confirm with them the appropriate times for positioning and scrubbing the client. To prevent impaired circulation, make sure that the client's feet aren't crossed.
- Be ready to assist in treating cardiac or respiratory arrest. Have emergency drugs and defibrillation equipment available. Document the drug administration.

Moderate sedation

Effects on the client

- Produces an altered level of consciousness in which the client can speak and follow commands
- Produces a brief period of amnesia so the client has no recollection of the procedure

Administration methods

- I.V. injection

Nursing implementations

- Monitor airway, breathing, and circulation.
- Have resuscitation equipment close by.
- Remain with the client.
- Monitor vital signs and pulse oximetry.

SPOT CHECK

Which nursing action is the highest priority for a client under general anesthesia?

A. Ensure that the surgeon is handed the correct instruments.

B. Focus lights to enhance visualization.

C. Monitor urinary output.

D. Meet the client's safety needs.

Answer: D. The highest priority for the nurse is meeting the client's safety needs.

POSTOPERATIVE PERIOD

The postoperative period begins with the completion of the surgical procedure and continues after discharge from the hospital or ambulatory surgical facility. Usually, clients are transferred from the surgical suite to the postanesthesia care unit (PACU) until their condition stabilizes and consciousness returns. Clients in the PACU require intensive care, and nursing actions must maintain basic priorities that are applicable to all clients.

During the postoperative period, the client must be monitored carefully for complications, some of which can be life-threatening.

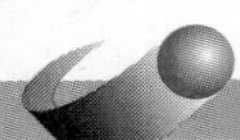

FAST FACT

Potential complications for postoperative clients include:

- altered respiratory function
- altered or decreased mental status
- discomfort and pain
- altered GI function
- decreased urine output
- impaired skin integrity
- impaired peripheral circulation
- hemorrhage
- deficient fluid volume.

This section covers routine postoperative nursing care for all surgical clients. It includes potential postoperative problems and complications, with appropriate nursing diagnoses and interventions listed for each.

NURSING RESPONSIBILITIES

Implementation

◆ Check the client's airway regularly, and position the client *to prevent aspiration.* The side-lying position (unless contraindicated) best prevents aspiration.

◆ Check the client's vital signs, including temperature, every 15 minutes until the client is stable *to identify labile vital signs after surgery.* Monitor for malignant hyperthermia, which can occur in some people as an adverse reaction to certain anesthetic agents.

◆ Check the client's neurologic status *to identify return of neurologic function.* Note orientation to person, place, and time; check reflexes, sensations, and motor functions. *The client can't be discharged from the PACU until neurologic functions have returned to normal.*

◆ Carefully inspect the client's dressing and bedclothes to *detect hemorrhage and ensure prompt treatment.* Inspect underneath the client; *gravity may carry drainage under the client.*

◆ Connect all tubes and catheters *to ensure drainage and proper tube functioning.*

◆ Promote client comfort and relieve pain as needed *to decrease discomfort.* Don't overlook pain unrelated to the surgical procedure. In addition to surgery, the client's discomfort may be caused by body position, a full bladder, flatus, hypoxemia, and tight dressings, casts, or bandages.

◆ Administer opioids with great care, and don't administer them if the client's respiratory rate is less than 12 breaths/minute. *Opioids administered during the postoperative period can decrease the client's respiratory rate and inhibit recovery from anesthetia.*

◆ Ensure the client's safety by keeping the side rails up at all times *to prevent the risk of falling out of bed* until the client is fully recovered from anesthesia.

◆ Apply sequential compression devices if not applied during the immediate preoperative or intraoperative period. (Some institutions apply these devices before surgery *to prevent blood from pooling the lower extremities during surgery, which may cause thrombus formation.*)

ALTERED RESPIRATORY FUNCTION

Ensuring an open airway and efficient respiratory function is imperative. An endotracheal tube, a laryngeal mask airway, or an oral airway may be in place until consciousness returns.

Causes

◆ Airway obstruction

◆ Anesthesia, moderate sedation, and opioids

◆ Atelectasis
◆ Chronic obstructive pulmonary disease
◆ Pain

Assessment

Observe the client for signs of:

◆ dyspnea or hypoxemia, which indicate impaired ventilation
◆ tachycardia, which may indicate hypoxia
◆ decreased breath sounds, which may indicate atelectasis because of alveolar collapse
◆ crackles, rhonchi, and labored snoring respirations, which indicate airway secretions and, possibly, an airway obstruction
◆ pallor, which indicates poor oxygenation and a reduced hemoglobin level
◆ anxiety and restlessness, which are early signs of hypoxia caused by cerebral irritability
◆ temperature greater than 100.4° F (38° C), which may indicate atelectasis. (Higher temperature elevations may indicate malignant hyperthermia.)

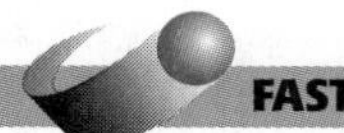

FAST FACT

Atelectasis is the most common cause of increased body temperature during the first 24 hours after surgery.

Diagnostic evaluation

◆ Arterial blood gas (ABG) analysis evaluates a blood sample to check for hypoxemia, hypercapnia, and metabolic or respiratory acidosis or alkalosis.
◆ Pulse oximetry places a sensor on a finger, the bridge of the nose, a toe, or an earlobe to determine hemoglobin saturation and oxygen delivery.

Nursing diagnoses

◆ Impaired gas exchange
◆ Ineffective airway clearance

Planning and goals

◆ The client will be free from postoperative respiratory complications.

Implementation

◆ Review preoperative teaching of coughing and deep-breathing exercises, incentive spirometry, and how and when to change positions *to promote the client's participation in recovery and avoid postoperative complications.*
◆ Tell the client to turn, perform coughing and deep-breathing exercises, and use the incentive spirometer every 1 to 2 hours. Be sure to splint the incision during these exercises by holding a pillow over the dressing and applying slight pressure to the incision site. *Turning, using the incentive spirometer, and coughing and breathing deeply prevent atelectasis and ventilate the distal alveoli. External splinting decreases pain and allows for increased chest expansion.*
◆ Ensure that the client gets out of bed and ambulates as soon as possible and as tolerated *to facilitate full chest expansion.*
◆ Administer analgesics (as ordered), splint the incision site, and reposition the client *to relieve the client's pain.* The client will be unable to perform deep-breathing exercises, cough, use the incentive spirometer, or ambulate if pain is too severe.

Evaluation

◆ The client is free from pulmonary complications.
◆ The client's pulse oximetry readings, ABG levels, and pulmonary function remain within reference limits.

DECREASED CARDIAC OUTPUT

Medication use and fluid loss during surgery can reduce cardiac output, placing the client at risk for shock. Therefore, maintaining adequate cardiac output is essential to prevent shock.

Causes

◆ Fluid volume deficit
◆ Hemorrhage
◆ Vasodilation

Assessment

◆ Monitor the client for decreased blood pressure
◆ Monitor central venous pressure and cardiac output for trends; decreased values indicate decreased perfusion
◆ Monitor the client's urine output and note any decrease, which indicates hypovolemia or poor renal perfusion.
◆ Observe the client for a weak, thready, rapid pulse. As stroke volume decreases, heart rate increases to maintain the same cardiac output.
◆ Monitor the client for decreased heart sounds, which indicate hypovolemia.
◆ Observe the client's skin for pallor or cyanosis, which indicates decreased peripheral circulation.
◆ Observe the client for restlessness, which is an early sign of hypoxia from cerebral irritability.

◆ Monitor the client for profuse perspiration and increased drainage from dressings, which may indicate fluid loss.
◆ Monitor for signs of hemorrhage, such as:
- bleeding
- decreased blood pressure
- increased pulse rate
- pallor or cyanosis.

The risk of hemorrhage is greatest during the first 48 hours after surgery.

Diagnostic evaluation

◆ Electrocardiography to detect heart rate
◆ Cardiac output monitoring through thermodilution catheter to determine functioning of the heart

Nursing diagnoses

◆ Decreased cardiac output
◆ Deficient fluid volume
◆ Ineffective tissue perfusion (cardiopulmonary, cerebral, renal, GI, peripheral)

Planning and goals

◆ The client's blood pressure will stabilize 1 to 2 hours after surgery.
◆ The client's pulse rate will remain at 60 to 100 beats/minute.
◆ The client's urine output will be 30 to 50 ml/hour.

Implementation

◆ Check vital signs every 15 minutes until the client is stable, then every half hour for 2 hours, then every 4 hours for 24 hours *to identify changes in the client's condition. Shock may occur as a result of anesthesia, blood loss, or medication.* As vital signs become more stable, changes occur less frequently.

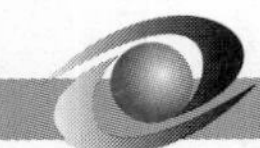

QUICK STUDY

When caring for a postoperative client, remember your **ABC**s:

Airway
Breathing
Circulation

◆ Encourage the client to ambulate as soon as ordered, *to stimulate cardiovascular function and prevent complications of immobility.*
◆ Check the client's dressing and bedclothes, including underneath the client, for evidence of hemorrhage. *Hemorrhage or fluid loss may lead to shock. Gravity may carry drainage under the client.*
◆ Monitor urine output *to assess renal perfusion* (hourly initially, then every 4 hours for 24 hours)

Evaluation

◆ Vital signs are stable and urine output is adequate.
◆ Cardiac output is adequate.
◆ Oxygenation and hemodynamic status is maintained.

ALTERED MENTAL STATUS

Regardless of the type of surgical procedure, the client's mental status will most likely be affected. Protecting the client from injury is important while mental status is altered.

Causes

◆ Anesthesia, moderate sedation, and opioids
◆ Hypoxia
◆ Sedatives
◆ Anxiety

Assessment

◆ Assess the client's level of consciousness. A client who can't be aroused hasn't fully recovered from the anesthesia or may have neurologic damage.
◆ Observe the client for decreased reflexes; gag, cough, swallow, and deep-tendon reflexes can indicate the client's state of alertness.
◆ Observe the client for decreased pupillary response. Normally, pupils are the same size and constrict equally to light.
◆ Observe the client for neuromuscular irritability. After surgery and anesthesia, the client may have an increased response to stimuli.
◆ Observe the client for decreased neuromuscular response to stimuli, which indicates that the client may not have recovered fully from anesthesia; thus, safety precautions should be taken.

Nursing diagnoses

◆ Ineffective tissue perfusion (cerebral)
◆ Disturbed sensory perception (kinesthetic)

Planning and goals

◆ The client will be mentally alert and oriented after surgery.
◆ The client will regain all reflex activity.

Implementation

◆ Assess the client's orientation, neuromuscular reflex response, and ability to follow commands *to help determine whether the client has fully recovered from anesthesia.*
◆ Administer opioids in small doses, as ordered, *to determine the client's response.*

Evaluation

◆ The client is oriented to time, place, and person.
◆ The client's reflexes return.

INEFFECTIVE THERMOREGULATION

Body temperature is usually decreased during the perioperative period. Hypothermia has been associated with an increase in postoperative wound infection, an alteration in metabolism, coagulopathy, cardiac arrhythmias and infarctions, and prolonged recovery time. In rare cases, patients may exhibit signs and symptoms of malignant hyperthermia, which is a familial genetic disorder characterized by hypermetabolism with hyperpyrexia developing in the intraoperative or postoperative period.

Causes

◆ Anesthesia effects
◆ Cold intraoperative environment
◆ Cold irrigation of wounds
◆ I.V. fluids
◆ Elderly or young client
◆ Lack of body fat
◆ Body exposure
◆ Skin disruption or impairment
◆ Circulatory impairment
◆ Stress response

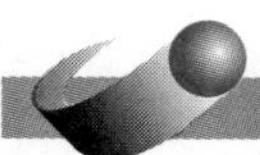

FAST FACT

There are four types of heat loss:

Evaporation – Conversion of a liquid to a vapor, causing the dissipation of heat

Conduction – Heat exchange occurring between two materials that are in direct contact with each other

Radiation – Transfer of heat between two surfaces without direct contact

Convection – Dissipation of heat by air currents

Assessment

Observe the client for:
◆ shivering
◆ hypothermia or hyperthermia
◆ tachypnea
◆ cardiac arrhythmias.

Diagnostic evaluation

◆ Temperature detection through approved facility method (core temperature through thermodilution catheter or in-line ventilator circuit; rectal temperature).

Nursing diagnoses

◆ Ineffective thermoregulation: Hypothermia
◆ Ineffective thermoregulation: Hyperthermia

Planning and goals

◆ The client will maintain a core body temperature of 97.6° to 99° F (35° to 37° C).

Implementation

◆ Control the environmental temperature by decreasing air currents, excess humidity, and contact with cold surfaces *to eliminate heat loss through convection, radiation, and conduction.*
◆ Cover the client's body and head and reduce bodily exposre *to eliminate heat loss.*
◆ Provide an extra heat source, such as convection or warming blankets, mattresses, or pads; heated oxygen; I.V. fluids; or radiant heat lamps *to maintain normal body temperature.*
◆ Keep the client and linens dry *to eliminate chilling from evaporation.*

Evaluation

◆ The client's core body temperature is within normal limits and stable.
◆ The client's skin is warm and dry.

DISCOMFORT AND PAIN

The postoperative client almost always reports some discomfort or pain. Surgical pain usually peaks on the second postoperative day when the client has fully recovered from anesthesia.

Causes

◆ Client's position
◆ Distended bladder
◆ Edema
◆ Flatus
◆ Intraoperative positioning
◆ Surgical incision

- Tissue trauma and inflammatory resonse

Assessment

- Ask the client to rate pain on a scale of 1 to 10, which allows comparison of the client's level of pain from one time to another.
- Reassess the client at regular intervals to monitor effectiveness of therapy.

Diagnostic evaluation

- Electrocardiography to detect heart rate (may increase with pain level)
- Blood pressure monitoring to detect alteration from baseline (may increase with pain or discomfort)

Nursing diagnoses

- Acute pain

Planning and goals

- The client's postoperative pain will be minimal.

Implementation

- Reposition the client as necessary, at least every 2 hours, *to help relieve pain. The client's position may be a source of discomfort. Repositioning the client and explaining its purpose usually helps.*
- If appropriate, relieve tension on the urinary catheter, loosen bedclothes, and reposition the nasogastric (NG) tube. *Relieving these sources of discomfort helps achieve the nurse's primary goal: to minimize the client's postoperative pain.*
- Provide comfort measures and other nonpharmacologic interventions, such as gentle back massage, encouraging participation in diversional activities, teaching relaxation techniques, and reducing external stimuli, *to reduce anxiety and allow the client to relax and rest.*
- Administer opioids or other analgesics, as ordered. Make sure the client understands how to use patient-controlled analgesia, if ordered. *Opioids act on the central nervous system to reduce pain perception. Many clients who use patient-controlled analgesia fear giving themselves too much medication and need reinforcement about the correct use of patient-controlled analgesia.*

Evaluation

- The client's pain is relieved.

ALTERED GI FUNCTION

The usual intake of food and fluids is disrupted for almost all surgical procedures. For some clients, maintaining fluid and electrolyte balance can be a challenge.

Causes

- Anesthesia
- Bacterial overgrowth
- Bowel manipulation
- Infection
- Obstruction
- Paralytic ileus
- Surgery
- Total cessation of bowel function

Assessment

- Observe the client for anorexia. Decreased peristalsis from surgical stress increases the potential for poor nutrition.
- Observe the client for nausea and vomiting. Oral fluids given too soon after surgery may lead to nausea and vomiting because of decreased peristalsis.
- Observe the client for abdominal distention and gas pains, which are common postoperative problems as peristalsis returns.
- Assess the client for absence of bowel sounds, which indicate a lack of peristalsis and may signal paralytic ileus.
- Assess the client for diarrhea and incontinence, which may result from increased peristalsis or bacterial overgrowth.
- Assess the client for dehydration. Dry mucous membranes and "tenting" of skin indicate dehydration.

Diagnostic evaluation

- Electrolytes analyze a blood sample for potassium, sodium, chloride, and magnesium levels.

Nursing diagnoses

- Diarrhea
- Bowel incontinence
- Deficient fluid volume
- Imbalanced nutrition: Less than body requirements

Planning and goals

- The client's GI function will resume a normal pattern.
- The client's fluid and electrolyte balance will be restored.

Implementation

◆ Withhold food and fluids until bowel sounds return (possibly 2 to 3 days after abdominal surgery) *to prevent complications of decreased peristalsis resulting from the effects of anesthesia, opioids, and the stress response, particularly after abdominal surgery.*

◆ Maintain I.V. access and administer fluids and electrolytes, as ordered, *to allow for fluids and electrolytes to be administered* until the client's oral intake is adequate.

◆ Gradually change the client's diet from clear liquids to regular *to provide nutrition consistent with the return of normal bowel functions.*

◆ Ensure that the client drinks 2 to 3 L of fluid daily (unless contraindicated) *to provide adequate hydration for bowel movement.*

◆ Ensure that the client walks as tolerated *to help prevent constipation and other immobility problems.*

◆ Note signs and symptoms of paralytic ileus: absence of bowel sounds, abdominal distention and discomfort, and nausea and vomiting. *Clients with altered GI function are at risk for paralytic ileus.* Measures designed to provide rest for the GI tract include food and fluid restrictions, NG tube drainage, I.V. therapy, and pharmacologic interventions.

Evaluation

◆ The client's bowel sounds return.

◆ The client passes stool or flatus.

◆ The client's electrolyte levels are within reference limits.

DECREASED URINE OUTPUT

The nothing-by-mouth status required for surgery can impact urinary output. Accurately recording all intake and output while the client is at risk for fluid imbalances is critical.

Causes

◆ Anesthesia

◆ Hypovolemia or hypoperfusion

◆ Increased antidiuretic hormone (ADH) levels

◆ Poor position for voiding

◆ Urine retention

◆ Stress

Assessment

◆ Monitor the client's urine output. If the client is well hydrated, allow voluntary control of urine output. Voiding should resume within 6 to 10 hours after surgery or after an indwelling urinary catheter is discontinued. Urine output should be greater than or equal to 30 ml/hour with voiding.

◆ Palpate the bladder above the symphysis pubis to check for distention. A bladder that isn't palpable isn't distended.

Diagnostic evaluation

◆ Blood chemistry studies to determine presence of electrolyte imbalance

◆ ECG to detect arrhythmias (can be tachycardic if hypovolemic)

Nursing diagnoses

◆ Impaired urinary elimination

Planning and goals

◆ The client's voluntary control of urine output will resume within 6 to 10 hours after surgery.

Implementation

◆ Provide eight to twelve 8-oz glasses (2,000 to 3,000 ml) of fluid daily *to ensure adequate hydration, which prevents urinary stasis.* Initially, urine output may be less than 1,500 ml because of body fluid losses and increased ADH levels; however, it should stabilize within 48 hours.

◆ Institute measures to induce voiding if urine retention occurs *to prevent fluid imbalance.* Running water stimulates voiding, as does pouring warm water over the perineum, which relaxes the sphincter.

◆ Insert an indwelling urinary or straight catheter, as ordered, *to enable urine output if urine retention occurs.*

Evaluation

◆ The client's urine output is greater than 30 ml/hour.

◆ The client voids without difficulty.

IMPAIRED SKIN INTEGRITY

The preoperative health status of the client will impact the healing of the surgical incision. Clients who are smokers, are older than age 65, obese, or have impaired immune systems may have more problems with impaired skin integrity.

Causes

◆ Immobility

◆ Surgical incision

Assessment

◆ Note signs of wound healing. The clean surgical wound heals by primary intention and may take more than 1 year to completely heal.
◆ Note signs of infection. Fever and incisional redness and swelling after the third postoperative day indicate infection.
◆ Assess the client for signs of insufficient wound healing, including dehiscence (separation of surgical wound layers, producing pink serous drainage; the client feels a pull at the wound site) and evisceration (such as outright protruding of abdominal contents). A client with poor nutrition, cancer, or wound infection is prone to ineffective wound healing. Dehiscence and evisceration indicate a complete separation of the wound edges, a medical emergency.
◆ Assess all pressure points for evidence of skin breakdown.

Nursing diagnoses

◆ Impaired skin integrity
◆ Risk for infection

Planning and goals

◆ The client's incision will heal without complications.
◆ The client's skin will remain intact without signs of breakdown.

Implementation

◆ Keep the incision clean and dry *to help prevent bacterial infection. Bacteria thrive in a moist environment.*
◆ Encourage ambulation. If the client is unable to ambulae, turn and reposition the client every 2 hours while in bed. *Movement stimulates vascular perfusion, which promotes wound healing.*
◆ Instruct the client to splint the incision when coughing or moving *to avoid putting stress on the incision, which could impair healing or cause wound dehiscence or evisceration.*
◆ If dehiscence or evisceration occurs, notify the physician immediately and cover the wound with sterile saline solution. Stay with the client, and instruct him not to move or cough. Administer antibiotics if ordered. *Evisceration is a medical emergency. Covering the evisceration prevents drying and necrosis of abdominal contents. Antibiotics prevent infection.*

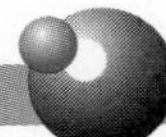

SPOT CHECK

Which statement by a client indicates that additional discharge teaching is needed after surgery?

A. "I'm really looking forward to going outside for short walks."
B. "I can hardly wait to get home and pick up my 18-month-old baby."
C. "I will call my physician if I have a fever or notice drainage from my incision."
D. "I will clean my incision every morning in the shower and pat it dry with a clean towel."

Answer: B. Lifting an 18-month-old child would place stress on the incision.

Evaluation

◆ The client's wound heals without infection.
◆ The client's skin remains dry and intact, without erythema or skin breakdown.

IMPAIRED PERIPHERAL CIRCULATION

Immobility during and after surgery is a predisposing factor to impaired peripheral circulation. A potentially dangerous situation can occur if a clot forms, dislodges, and travels to the lungs.

Causes

◆ Phlebitis
◆ Thrombosis

Assessment

◆ Observe the client for HOMANS' SIGN, which can indicate thrombophlebitis.
◆ Assess the client for pain, warmth, and tenderness in the calf muscles, which indicates thrombophlebitis.

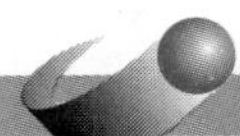

FAST FACT

To test for Homans' sign:

- support the client's thigh with one hand and his foot with the other
- bend the leg slightly at the knee
- firmly and abruptly dorsiflex the ankle.

Diagnostic evaluation

◆ Doppler ultrasound to detect adequacy of peripheral circulation

Nursing diagnoses

◆ Ineffective tissue perfusion (peripheral)
◆ Risk for injury

Planning and goals

◆ The client will have adequate peripheral circulation.

Implementation

◆ Take the following preventive antithrombus measures *to promote peripheral circulation:*
– Provide elastic antiembolism stockings and a sequential compression device *to compress the superficial veins, increase blood flow through the deep veins, and prevent venous pooling.*
– Don't put pressure on the popliteal space, *which causes blood stasis.*
– Don't massage the client's legs, *which may dislodge a clot.*
– Ensure that the client exercises and ambulates soon after surgery *to prevent venous stasis.*
– Administer a prophylactic anticoagulant, such as subcutaneous heparin, *to prevent thrombus formation.*
◆ Treat thrombophlebitis with bed rest, heat, elastic bandages, and anticoagulant drugs. *Bed rest promotes healing and prevents clot dislodgment. Heat and elastic bandages increase circulation to the area. Anticoagulant drugs prevent blood clotting.*

Evaluation

◆ The client shows no signs of circulatory stasis.

DISCHARGE INSTRUCTIONS

Early discharge, which has become common, typically increases client teaching needs. Be sure to provide information about wound care, activity restrictions, dietary management, medication administration, symptoms to report, and follow-up care. Document the care provided during the perioperative period as well as any specific client teaching measures and the client's understanding of discharge instructions.

A client recovering from same-day surgery in an outpatient surgical unit must be in stable condition before discharge. This client must not drive home; make sure a responsible adult takes the client home.

Oncologic nursing

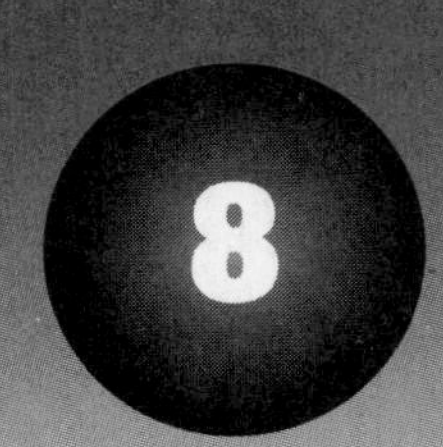

INTRODUCTION

The term CANCER represents a large group of diseases characterized by a malfunction of the cell growth process, which causes the uncontrolled growth of abnormal cells. Cancer is currently second to heart disease as the major cause of death in Americans. Cancer causes morbidity through:

- local extension
- METASTASIS, or spread, from the primary site through the blood or lymphatic circulation to distant, fertile sites in the body, such as the lungs, brain, liver, lymph nodes, or skeleton, where the cancer cells infiltrate and grow into new tumors
- systemic effects of the disease.

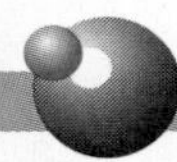

SPOT CHECK

How does cancer spread from a primary site?

Answer: Cancer can spread from the primary site through the blood and lymphatic circulation or through direct, or local, extension.

CANCER SCREENING AND ASSESSMENT

Human carcinogenesis is usually a multistep process involving progressive alteration in cellular deoxyribonucleic acid (DNA) following carcinogenic exposure. Altered genetic makeup initiates the process of malignant expression in a normal cell. The second stage of carcinogenesis, called *promotion,* increases the risk of malignant expression in initiated cells and is related to the dose and duration of carcinogenic exposure.

The relationship between the various carcinogens that initiate malignant transformation is the subject of continuing study. One relationship being studied is the strong positive association between the carcinogens in tobacco smoke and the risk of developing lung cancer. Increased survival rates for many cancers are linked closely to:

- individual awareness of risk factors and preventive measures
- surveillance through self-examination, screening, and early detection.

RISK FACTORS

Here's a list of some of the risk factors for cancer. Be aware that the list isn't all-inclusive.

Chemical carcinogenesis

- Hydrocarbon adducts in tobacco, and tobacco quids (smokeless tobacco, such as chewing tobacco and snuff), and pipe smoking
- Asbestos
- Arsenic, chromium, and nickel compounds
- Vinyl chloride
- Radon gas
- Diethylstilbestrol
- Alkylating agents in cancer chemotherapy protocols
- Estrogen (endogenous and exogenous)

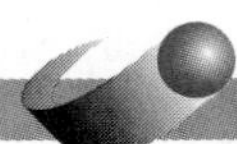

FAST FACT

Lifestyle and personal habits account for the majority of cancer incidence and mortality.

Familial carcinogenesis

Many inherited cancers manifest as autosomal-dominant traits, such as:

- breast cancer
- retinoblastoma
- familial polyposis

◆ dysplastic nevi and congenital melanocytic nevi
◆ xeroderma pigmentosum
◆ Wilms' tumor.

Physical carcinogenesis

◆ Ultraviolet radiation, ionizing radiation, and asbestos
◆ Precancerous lesions, such as oral leukoplakia, dysplastic nevi, senile keratoses, any chronically irritated skin site, cervical dysplasia, and colorectal polyps
◆ Acquired disorders, such as pernicious anemia, ulcerative colitis, cirrhosis, hepatitis, hiatal hernia, and reflux esophagitis
◆ Foods containing high levels of fat (causing colon, breast, or prostate cancer); food additives, such as cyclamates, nitrites, and saccharin; heavy food seasoning; smoked or salted foods (causing esophageal or stomach cancer); foods contaminated with anatoxin (causing gastric cancer)
◆ Obesity (being 40% or more overweight) (causing colon, breast, uterine, or prostate cancer)

Viral carcinogenesis

◆ Hepatitis B virus and hepatocellular carcinoma
◆ Hepatitis C virus and hepatocellular cardinoma
◆ Human T-cell leukemia virus-1 and adult T-cell leukemia or lymphoma
◆ Herpes virus (DNA virus) and Burkitt's lymphoma
◆ Herpes simplex type 2 and human papillomavirus (HPV)

ASSESSMENT FINDINGS

Health history and physical examination includes:
◆ assessing the client's family medical history to identify familial risks
◆ assessing the client's personal habits and lifestyle behaviors to identify risks for cancer development
◆ assessing the client's screening activities, including monthly breast self-examination (BSE), mammography, monthly self-testicular examination, monthly self-skin examination, digital rectal examination (DRE), sigmoidoscopy, and annual pelvic and Papanicolaou (Pap) tests.

Skin

◆ Irregular hyperkeratotic areas (rough areas that scab over, rescab, or fail to heal)
◆ Loss of skin markings
◆ Change in persistent ulcer (any change in color, size, shape, elevation, surface, surrounding skin, sensation, or consistency)
◆ Pruritus (prevalent in Hodgkin's disease)
◆ Variation in pigmentation
◆ Persistent reddish or whitish patch

Head and neck

◆ Difficulty chewing, swallowing, or moving tongue or jaw
◆ Firm, unilateral lymph nodes in neck

Oral cavity

◆ Otalgia
◆ Swelling or ulcer that fails to heal, indurated ulcer, or ipsilateral-referred ulcer

Oropharynx

◆ Dysphasia, local pain, pain on swallowing, or referred otalgia

Hypopharynx

◆ Dysphasia, odynophagia, referred otalgia, or neck mass

Larynx

◆ Persistent hoarseness, pain, referred otalgia, dyspnea, or stridor

Nasopharynx

◆ Bloody nasal discharge, obstructed nostril, conductive deafness, neurologic problems (such as atypical facial pain, diplopia, hoarseness, or Horner's syndrome), or neck mass

Nose and sinuses

◆ Bloody nasal discharge, nasal obstruction, facial pain, facial swelling, or diplopia

Parotic and submandibular glands

◆ Painless local swelling or hemifacial paralysis

Breasts

◆ Axillary lymphadenopathy
◆ Bloody discharge
◆ Unilateral serous nipple discharge
◆ Change in contour of breast
◆ Dimpling of skin in breast
◆ Edema or erythema of breast skin
◆ Fixation of a mass to pectoral fascia or chest wall
◆ Nipple retraction
◆ Painless lump or mass

Lungs

◆ Change in pulmonary habits (such as cough, hoarseness, chest pain, rust-streaked or purulent sputum production, hemoptysis, and dyspnea)
◆ Paresthesia
◆ Pleural effusion
◆ Recurrent pneumonitis
◆ Shoulder and arm pain

GI

Esophagus

◆ Subtle changes in health (such as weight loss, malaise, and anorexia), dysphagia to solid foods followed by dysphagia to liquids, unexplained choking, or gastroesophageal reflux

Stomach

◆ Complaints of indigestion or epigastric distress, loss of appetite, unintentional weight loss or anorexia, dysphagia, abdominal mass, colonic obstruction, ulcer-type pain, or iron-deficiency anemia

Liver

◆ Painful hepatomegaly, liver tenderness with nodular enlargement, splenomegaly, esophageal varices, ascites, jaundice, GI bleeding, fever, or edema

Gallbladder

◆ Acute or chronic cholecystitis, abdominal pain, anorexia, unintentional weight loss, jaundice, nausea, vomiting, or occasional fever

Pancreas

◆ Insidious onset of asthenia (weakness), anorexia, weight loss, gaseousness, or nausea

Colon and rectum

◆ Change in bowel habits (such as constipation or diarrhea), rectal bleeding, tenesmus (feeling of incomplete evacuation), or iron-deficiency anemia

Female genitalia

Vulva

◆ Pruritus vulvae, pain, bleeding, an ulcerated lesion, a mass, or unusual pigmentation

Cervix

◆ Painful intercourse; postcoital, coital, or intermenstrual bleeding; or a watery, foul-smelling discharge

Endometrium

◆ Persistent irregular premenstrual bleeding (especially in obese women) or postmenopausal bleeding (6 months or longer after menopause)

Ovaries

◆ Persistent vague GI complaints, abdominal discomfort, indigestion, early satiety, or mild anorexia as well as ascites, pain, or a pelvic mass, which usually signal advanced disease

Vagina

◆ Abnormal vaginal bleeding (postmenopausal, postcoital, or intermenstrual), changes in urination patterns, or a foul-smelling discharge

Fallopian tubes

◆ Abnormal vaginal bleeding, abdominal pain, or a vaginal discharge

Male genitalia

Penis

◆ Painless ulcer or growth, or persistent discharge (Make sure to retract the foreskin to ensure a thorough assessment.)

Prostate

◆ Bone pain and continuous pain in lower back, pelvis, or upper thighs
◆ Renal insufficiency, hematuria, weak or interrupted urine flow, difficulty in stopping or starting urination, nocturia, or painful, burning urination

Testes

◆ Painless enlargement of one testicle or a testicular lump or nodule (mass that doesn't transilluminate), a feeling of heaviness or dragging in the lower abdomen or scrotum, a change in a preexisting hydrocele, an attack resembling epididymitis (fails to respond to medical treatment within 14 days), fatigue, pallor (from anemia), cough, or hemoptysis

TEACHING THE CLIENT

Provide the client with a copy of the American Cancer Society's seven warning signs of cancer, prevention strategies, and health-screening recommendations.

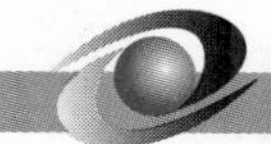

QUICK STUDY

Use the word **CAUTION** to help you remember the American Cancer Society's seven warning signs of cancer when assessing a client:

Change in bowel or bladder habits
A sore that doesn't heal
Unusual bleeding or discharge
Thickening or lump in the breast or elsewhere
Indigestion or difficulty swallowing
Obvious change in a wart or mole
Nagging cough or hoarseness

Health screening recommedations

Low-risk and asymptomatic clients

◆ For clients ages 20 to 40, recommend physical examination with health counseling every 3 years; older than age 40, every year.
◆ Teach and encourage monthly skin self-examination for all adult clients to detect and monitor lesions, especially nevi (mole mapping)
◆ Recommend semiannual dental oral examination.

High-risk or symptomatic clients

◆ Reinforce the need fore more frequent physical or diagnostic examinations, which may be recommended by the health care provider for screening and early detection.

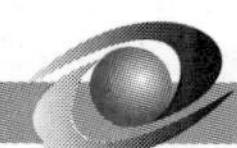

QUICK STUDY

Use **ABCD** to remember the characteristics of malignant melanoma:

Asymmetry
Border irregularity
Color variation
Diameter generally greater than 6 mm

Female clients

◆ Encourage BSE (monthly is optional for clients older than age 20).
◆ Teach the client that BSE should be done 3 to 5 days after her menstrual period ends; for a hysterectomized or postmenopausal woman, teach her to perform BSE on the same day each month (for example, on the first day of the month); encourage the client to report asymmetry, dimpling, abnormal contour, or a painless mass immediately.
◆ Clinical breast examinations should be performed every 3 years between ages 20 and 40, and every year for clients older than age 40.
◆ Initial mammography should be performed between ages 35 and 39 for baseline; and yearly beginning at age 40. Baseline mammogram should be performed at age 25 for genetically predisposed women.
◆ Colposcopic examination should be performed in women with a history of HPV.
◆ Pelvic examination and a Pap test should be performed about 3 years after a client begins vaginal intercourse, but no later than age 21. Screening should be done annually with the regular Pap test or every 2 years with the newer liquid-based Pap test. Beginning at age 30, women who have had three normal Pap tests in a row may be screened every 2 to 3 years.
◆ Endometrial biopsy should be performed at menopause.
◆ DRE should be performed every year in clients older than age 40.
◆ Sigmoidoscopy (preferably flexible) should be performed in clients older than age 50 every 3 to 5 years.

Male clients

◆ Teach the client that DRE should be performed every year for clients older than age 50.
◆ Prostate-specific antigen (PSA) testing and DRE should be performed every year for men at high risk, beginning at age 45.
◆ Sigmoidoscopy (preferably flexible) should be performed for clients older than age 50 every 3 to 5 years.
◆ Young men should be encouraged to perform monthly testicular self-examination from puberty through age 40; teach them how to do the examination and encourage them to report a nontender, enlarged testis or mass immediately.

CHEMOTHERAPY

CHEMOTHERAPY uses cytotoxic drugs to destroy cancer cells. While surgery and radiation therapy are used to treat localized disease, chemotherapy is systemic therapy to prevent cancer cells from multiplying, invading adjacent tissue, or metastasizing to distant sites. Chemotherapy is administered on a schedule that maximizes tumor cell kill while minimizing toxicity by allowing normal cells to recover.

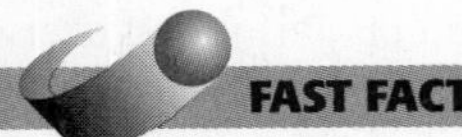

FAST FACT

Vascular access devices are used for administration of chemotherapy and blood products, parenteral nutrition, and obtaining blood specimens. Examples include right atrial catheters, peripherally inserted central venous catheters, and implanted infusion ports or pumps.

TYPES OF CHEMOTHERAPY

- ◆ Adjuvant therapy (treats micrometastases)
- ◆ Neoadjuvant therapy (shrinks a tumor before its surgical removal)
- ◆ Primary therapy (treats a localized tumor when there's an alternative, but less effective treatment)
- ◆ Induction therapy (treats a form of cancer for which there's no alternative treatment)
- ◆ Combination chemotherapy (enhances or synergizes the therapeutic actions of other cytotoxic drugs)
- ◆ Prophylactic therapy (to prevent micrometastasis)

Nursing diagnoses

- ◆ Risk for infection
- ◆ Ineffective tissue perfusion (renal, cerebral, cardiopulmonary, gastrointestinal, peripheral)
- ◆ Social isolation
- ◆ Imbalanced nutrition: Less than body requirements
- ◆ Deficient fluid volume
- ◆ Disturbed body image
- ◆ Impaired skin integrity
- ◆ Decreased cardiac output

Goals and implementation

This section provides key nursing actions for selected goals during chemotherapy treatment.

Goal

- ◆ The client will remain free from local or systemic infection.

Interventions

- ◆ Monitor the client's temperature and report any elevation greater than 100° F (37.8° C) *to detect early risk of infection.*
- ◆ Monitor the client's white blood cell count and granulocyte count at nadir (period of maximal neutropenia); calculate the absolute neutrophil count (ANC) *to assess the relative risk of infection.*

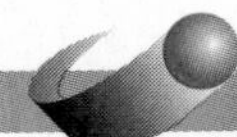

FAST FACT

The pattern of neutropenia varies, depending on the specific antineoplastic agent. An example of one pattern that can occur after chemotherapy treatment is:

- minimal neutropenia 4 to 7 days after treatment
- nadir 8 to 12 days after treatment
- return of normal number of neutrophils 14 to 18 days after treatment.

- ◆ Instruct the client or family member about signs and symptoms of infection, such as temperature greater than 100° F, cough, sore throat, shaking chills, painful or frequent urination, and vaginal discharge *so early treatment can be provided.*
- ◆ Instruct the client or family member about proper handwashing techniques and other measures *to prevent transmission of infection,* such as not cleaning animal litter boxes, using sanitary pads instead of tampons, and preventing trauma to skin and mucous membranes.
- ◆ Avoid invasive procedures if ANC is less than 1,000/mm^3 *to avoid infection.*
- ◆ Administer filgrastim (Nupogen, G-CSF) or sargramostim (Leukine, GM-CSF) as ordered, and monitor the client's response *to promote immune response.*
- ◆ Instruct the client to avoid raw fruits and uncooked vegetables by eating a "cooked diet" only *to avoid infection.*
- ◆ Initiate and administer antibiotic therapy as prescribed *to treat infection.*

Goal

- ◆ The client will remain free from problems associated with thrombocytopenia.

Interventions

- ◆ Monitor platelet count and report abnormal values (normal, 150,000 to 350,000 mm^3) *to detect bleeding tendency.*
- ◆ Test stool, urine, and emesis for occult blood as ordered, and report positive results *to detect bleeding.*
- ◆ Advise the client to avoid trauma to skin and mucous membranes *to avoid bleeding and to promote intact skin.*
- ◆ Instruct the client with throat or mouth sores to avoid rough foods, such as granola or croutons, and to choose soft foods, such as bananas, macaroni and cheese, and pudding *to avoid abraiding mucous membranes.*
- ◆ Teach the client safe personal hygiene, such as using an electric razor, using a soft toothbrush, using sanitary pads

instead of tampons, and avoiding enemas and rectal suppositories *to avoid trauma.*

- Instruct the client to avoid use of drugs containing aspirin *to prevent bleeding.*
- Instruct the client to avoid invasive procedures and I.M. injections *to avoid inducing trauma.*
- Teach the client or family member about signs and symptoms of thrombocytopenia; for example, change in mental status, bleeding nose or gums, increased bruising, petechiae, purpura, hypermenorrhea, bloody or tarry-colored stools, blood in urine, or coffee-ground emesis *to detect early bleeding.*
- Administer platelet transfusion as ordered, and monitor the client's response *to promote normal platelet counts.*
- Administer stool softener *to avoid straining.*
- Apply firm pressure to venipuncture sites for 3 to 5 minutes *to assist blood clotting.*

Goal

- The client will maintain adequate oxygenation of tissue and be able to perform activities of daily living (ADLs).

Interventions

- Monitor hemoglobin level and hematocrit, and report abnormal values *to optimize oxygen-carrying capacity.*
- Instruct the client to conserve energy, finding a balance between rest and exercise *to reduce oxygen needs.*
- Instruct the client or family member to report the following signs and symptoms promptly to the physician: fatigue, dizziness, shortness of breath, palpitations, chest pain, and headache *to avoid complications.*
- Administer epoetin alfa (Erythropoietin, Procrit, EPO) subcutaneously as ordered, and monitor the client's response *to optimize oxygenation of cells.*
- Administer red blood cell transfusion as ordered, and monitor the client's response *to optimize oxygen-carrying capacity of blood.*

Goal

- The client will maintain daily nutritional and fluid requirements and weight within 5% of baseline.

Interventions

- Assess the client's nutritional status, including height and weight, eating habits, skin turgor, and serum albumin and total lymphocyte count *to determine baseline.* (See *Clinical signs of malnutrition.*)
- Administer antiemetic medications as ordered *to avoid vomiting,* and monitor effectiveness.

Clinical signs of malnutrition

The malnourished client may display these signs:

- Beefy and scarlet tongue
- Bleeding and receding gums
- Brittle nails
- Dry, flaky skin
- Dry, red fissures at angles of the lips (cheilosis)
- Poor dentition
- Thin, dull, dry hair.

- Use behavioral techniques, such as relaxation therapy, visual imagery, or distraction, *to help reduce nausea and vomiting.*
- Instruct the client to minimize stimuli (such as sights, sounds, and odors) *to avoid stimulating nausea and vomiting.*
- Instruct the client to use interventions that have relieved nausea during previous illness or stress *to reduce vomiting episodes.*
- Encourage the client to eat several small meals throughout the day *to promote nutrition.*
- Instruct the client to include nutritional supplements (such as Ensure Plus) in his diet, if necessary, *to maintain nutritional status.*
- Instruct the client to consume foods high in protein and calories, unless contraindicated, *to promote healing.*
- Administer medications such as progestational agents or corticosteroids, as ordered, *to stimulate appetite.*
- Encourage fluid intake of 2,000 to 3,000 ml/day, unless contraindicated, *to maintain fluid requirements.*
- Encourage physical exercise and ambulation, as tolerated, *to stimulate appetite.*
- Record weight weekly; report weight loss and trends *to monitor weight.*
- Encourage mouth care before meals *to freshen the oral cavity.*

Goal

- The client will cope effectively with altered body image.

Interventions

- Tell the client that chemotherapy-induced hair loss is temporary and that hair will regrow when the drug is stopped *to provide reassurance.* (Usual hair growth returns in 2 to 6 months.)

◆ Encourage the client to select a wig, cap, scarf, or turban before hair loss occurs (usually 10 to 21 days after initiation of therapy) *to promote positive self-esteem.*
◆ Encourage the client to set small goals that are achievable daily *to promote independence.*
◆ Encourage the client to share feelings and concerns with someone she trusts, such as a family member or clergy member *to reduce stress.*
◆ Encourage the client to participate in enjoyable and diversionary activities, such as hobbies, as tolerated, *to promote positive self-esteem.*
◆ Assess the client for nature and frequency of sexual dysfunction *to determine effect on body image.*
◆ Counsel the female client to avoid pregnancy before and during chemotherapy, and counsel the male client about sperm banking before chemotherapy *to provide information.*
◆ Teach the client or family member that fatigue is a temporary side effect of chemotherapy (and radiation therapy) and may affect libido or cause sexual dysfunction *to maintain hope and positive feelings.* Stress that fatigue will gradually disappear when the treatment is completed.
◆ Evaluate the need for referral for psychological or sexual counseling, when indicated, *to maintain optimum outcomes.*

Goal

◆ The client will maintain intact skin and mucous membranes.

Interventions

◆ Assess skin daily; report onset, location, and description of cutaneous reactions *to avoid complications.*
◆ Instruct the client about hygienic and preventive measures, such as using mild soap and tepid water, avoiding tight-fitting clothing or irritating fabrics, avoiding exposing skin to extreme heat or cold, avoiding scratching any irritated areas, and avoiding chemical irritants such as scented sprays *to promote intact skin.*
◆ Instruct the client to apply topical medication as ordered *for pain or irritation control.*
◆ Instruct the client to avoid exposure to sunlight and other forms of ultraviolet light by using a sunscreen with a sun protection factor of 15 or higher and wearing protective clothing *to maintain skin integrity.*
◆ Instruct the client that hyperpigmentation may occur with certain drugs and will gradually disappear when therapy is discontinued *to reduce stress.*
◆ Assess oral mucosa with and without dental appliances in place, and teach the client how to perform daily self-assessment of the oral cavity *to detect early complications.*
◆ Instruct the client in daily oral hygiene measures, such as gently brushing his teeth after meals and before bedtime and, unless contraindicated, gently flossing daily with unwaxed floss *to prevent dental complications.*
◆ Instruct the client to use preventive oral measures, such as baking soda or saline rinse and mouthwash that contains no alcohol *to soothe oral mucosa.*
◆ Encourage the client to follow a high-protein, high-calorie diet, unless contraindicated, *to promote healing.*
◆ Tell the client to avoid hard, hot, spicy, acidic, or other irritating foods *to avoid dyspepsia or oral ulceration.*
◆ Discourage the client in the use of tobacco and alcohol *to avoid irritating the oral cavity.*
◆ Tell the client to apply a lip balm several times daily *to maintain skin integrity.*
◆ Instruct the client to report pain, tingling, dryness, numbness, or burning of the oral cavity *to detect early complications.*
◆ Instruct the client to report white patches on the tongue, back of the throat, or gums immediately (candidiasis) *so treatment can be provided.*
◆ Tell the client to avoid douching and the use of tampons and deodorant-containing sanitary pads or panty liners *to avoid irritating the skin.*
◆ Instruct the client to increase intake of high-fiber foods and fluids, unless contraindicated, and follow prescribed use of stool softener *to treat constipation.*

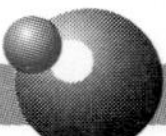

SPOT CHECK

Which factor may precipitate the development of constipation in a client with cancer?

A. Administration of opioids for pain control
B. Daily intake of high-fiber foods
C. Optimal levels of physical activity
D. Depression due to the psychological impact of the diagnosis of cancer

Answer: A. Administration of opioids for pain control may precipitate the development of constipation.

◆ For diarrhea, instruct the client to:
– avoid eating high-roughage, greasy, and spicy foods (a low-residue diet that's high in protein and calories) *to reduce episodes of diarrhea*
– avoid alcoholic beverages and caffeine products *to reduce episodes of diarrhea*

– increase daily fluid intake to 3,000 ml, with fluids such as weak, tepid tea or bouillon *to promote adequate fluid intake*
– follow prescribed medication schedule if the problem persists beyond 1 day *to avoid dehydration*
– clean rectal area after each bowel movement and apply A & D ointment or Desitin *to promote skin healing*
– use nutritional supplements *to increase protein and calorie intake.*

Goal

◆ The client will remain free from potential alterations in cardiac output related to toxicities of antineoplastic agents.

Interventions

◆ Instruct the client or family member about potential cardiac alterations specific to treatment regimen *to detect early signs of complications.*
◆ Instruct the client or family member about early signs and symptoms of cardiac alterations to report to his health care provider *to allow early detection of problems.*
◆ Provide written learning materials *to reinforce teaching.*
◆ Obtain cardiac function studies as ordered, such as electrocardiogram, multiple gated acquisition scan, or echocardiogram *to obtain baseline.*
◆ Assess cardiac function for rate and quality of apical pulse, blood pressure, skin color and turgor, capillary refill, peripheral pulses, mental status, peripheral or periorbital edema, breathing pattern, lung sounds, and jugular vein distention *to assess cardiac status.*
◆ Monitor electrolytes and cardiac enzymes as ordered and report abnormal values *to detect early cardiac problems.*
◆ *To prevent or minimize orthostatic hypotension,* instruct the client to move gradually from a lying to sitting or sitting to standing position.
◆ Administer diuretic or cardiac glycoside as ordered *to promote cardiac output,* and assess results.

Goal

◆ The client will be able to perform daily self-care functions independently or with minimal assistance.

Interventions

◆ Instruct the client or family member about potential neurologic alterations specific to the treatment regimen that may limit independence *to provide early detection.*
◆ Discuss safety measures *to minimize injury should neurologic alterations develop.*
◆ Monitor completion of bathing and hygiene daily, and praise accomplishments *to help the client achieve highest level of functioning.*
◆ Provide assistive devices, such as a long-handled brush for bathing, *to encourage independence.*
◆ Facilitate consultation with home care or hospice as appropriate *to help meet the client's needs.*

RADIATION THERAPY

RADIATION THERAPY is a localized treatment that uses high-energy, ionizing radiation to destroy cancer cells. Radiation therapy sterilizes cancer cells by depositing energy into the cells — a direct "hit" on DNA, causing the strand to break. Tumor cells lose their capacity to repair damage. As damaged cells try to replicate, they die due to the DNA damage. Normal, healthy cells in the area being irradiated are also affected by ionizing radiation but will attempt to repair the DNA damage. The challenge is to eradicate cancer cells while sparing healthy tissue.

Radiation therapy may be used alone or in conjunction with other forms of cancer treatment, such as surgery, chemotherapy, or both. Chemotherapy used in combination with radiation therapy may improve cure rates by enhancing the local effect of radiation (synergism) or reducing radioresistance.

USES FOR RADIATION THERAPY

◆ Eradicates radiocurable disease, such as early-stage breast cancer following lumpectomy
◆ Controls the growth and spread of disease, such as adjuvant therapy for late-stage chest wall recurrence
◆ Acts as prophylactic treatment to prevent microscopic disease, such as whole brain irradiation with lung cancer
◆ Improves quality of life in advanced disease, such as pain from bone metastasis or pressure from spinal cord compression

RADIATION-PROTECTION MEASURES

Radionuclide factors determine the type and amount of radiation-protection measures required. Depending on specific radionuclides, radiation emission consists of alpha, beta, or gamma particles:
◆ ALPHA PARTICLES travel at great speed but have poor penetrating ability; that is, their maximum distance is less

than 5 cm in the air, thus limiting their therapeutic usefulness.

◆ BETA PARTICLES used in therapy, such as phosphorus-32 or yttrium-90, have greater penetration than alpha particles but can be shielded by thick plastic or by the body's surface. If beta particles are instilled or injected into the body, the body usually provides adequate shielding.

◆ GAMMA RAYS are emitted by a radionuclide as an unstable nucleus decays. Gamma rays have a wide range of energies and penetrating abilities. The higher the energy, the thicker the absorbing material required for shielding between the radioactive source and the person receiving the exposure. For example, the thickness of a material required to reduce the radiation exposure of cesium-137 to one-half of its original activity is 6 mm of lead or 10 cm of concrete.

Time and distance

In addition to recommended shielding, continuing to use the principles of time and distance will further reduce radiation exposure. The amount of exposure received is directly proportional to the amount of time spent near the source.

The inverse square law principle applies to the distance from the gamma radionuclide source; by doubling the distance from the source, radiation exposure is decreased by a fraction of 4 (2^2). For example, if health care provider A stands 2′ (61 cm) from the source and health care provider B stands 4′ (122 cm) from the source, then exposure to B is one-quarter that of A. Thus, standing at the head of the bed of a client with a gynecologic implant or talking from the doorway will decrease exposure to the gamma radionuclide source. Consistently wearing a dosimetry monitor is required to measure cumulative exposure.

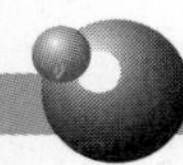

SPOT CHECK

True or false? A personal radiation-monitoring device, such as a film badge or pocket dosimeter, will protect the nurse from radiation exposure.

Answer: False. The device only detects radiation. Using the principles of time, distance, and shielding protects the nurse.

High-energy, gamma-emitting radionuclides, such as radium-226 and cesium-137, require specified distances and shielding, such as radiation isolation and lead shields to reduce the exposure risk. However, low-energy or weak gamma emitters, such as iodine-125, don't require these same radiation-safety protection measures.

ADMINISTRATION OF RADIATION THERAPY

Radiotherapy in the treatment of cancer is delivered using an external beam (teletherapy), in which the treatment machine is placed at some distance from the body or a sealed radioactive source is implanted in or near a tumor (brachytherapy), either temporarily or permanently. Radioactive materials can also be injected or ingested for systemic, radiopharmaceutical therapy (unsealed sources).

Radiolabeled antibodies

RADIOLABELED ANTIBODIES, which are tumor-specific antibodies coupled with radioactive isotopes, can be used to maximize tumor cell kill while sparing healthy tissue. Injected I.V., these antibodies travel in the bloodstream to specific antigens on tumor cells to directly destroy malignant cells. Bone marrow suppression, particularly thrombocytopenia, usually occurs 4 to 6 weeks following antibody administration.

Brachytherapy

In BRACHYTHERAPY, sealed radionuclide sources are placed within or in close proximity to malignant tumors. Intracavitary brachytherapy, such as for lung or gynecological malignancies, is temporary and usually "afterloaded." Interstitial brachytherapy, used for cancers of the prostate and breast, is temporary or permanent ("seeds").

Stereotactic external-beam irradiation

STEREOTACTIC EXTERNAL-BEAM IRRADIATION directs a small, pencil-thin beam of radiation at abnormalities within the head. It's used in the treatment of relatively small intracranial benign tumors, or malignant astrocytomas and brain metastases. A stereotactic frame is fixed to the skull to target the treatment beam. A single fraction is usually delivered to the skull with gamma units using cobalt ("gamma knife"), modified cobalt, or linear accelerator units. Steroid medication is administered to minimize cerebral edema.

PREPARING FOR TREATMENT

Before beginning therapy, localization procedures are performed. These procedures include using a simulator to determine the best approach for delivering treatment and performing radiographic studies, such as computed tomography scans or magnetic resonance imaging, to help define the exact body area to be irradiated. Marks or tattoos placed on the body facilitate proper positioning for treatment, thus promoting consistent delivery. Blocks, made of lead or high-density alloys, may be used to shield normal tissues near the treatment field. The actual treatment takes only about 2 to 5 minutes.

Adverse reactions

◆ The adverse reactions of radiation may be acute and immediate, occurring within the first 6 months after exposure, or late and chronic, occurring more than 1 year after exposure.
◆ Acute adverse reactions reflect cell damage and the accumulation of waste products of tissue destruction, such as anorexia.
◆ Most treatment-related adverse reactions are site-specific and dependent on volume, dose fractionation, total dose, and individual differences.

Site-specific adverse reactions

Brain

◆ Cerebral edema (steroid therapy indicated)
◆ Alopecia
◆ Changes in hair texture and color
◆ Scalp pruritus (dryness or peeling)

Head and neck

◆ Stomatitis (irritation of the mucosa in the mouth and oropharynx)
◆ Xerostomia (dryness of the mouth)
◆ Tooth decay and caries
◆ Taste changes
◆ Osteoradionecrosis (usually occurs in the mandible)
◆ Hypopituitarism (symptoms reflect decreased secretions of cortisol, thyroxine, and sex hormones)

Chest

◆ Esophagitis
◆ Cough
◆ Radiation pneumonitis
◆ Radiation fibrosis

Abdomen

◆ Gastritis
◆ Nausea and vomiting

Pelvis

◆ Diarrhea
◆ Cystitis
◆ Erectile dysfunction
◆ Vaginal stenosis
◆ Ovarian failure
◆ Testicular dysfunction

Nursing diagnoses

◆ Impaired skin integrity
◆ Risk for infection
◆ Activity intolerance
◆ Imbalanced nutrition: Less than body requirements
◆ Impaired swallowing
◆ Ineffective coping
◆ Disturbed body image
◆ Impaired verbal communication

Goals and implementation

Goals and nursing interventions for many adverse effects of radiation therapy are similar to those for chemotherapy. Here are a few additional goals to focus on.

Goal

◆ The client will learn measures to help relieve xerostomia.

Interventions

◆ Teach the client *how to lubricate oral mucous membranes,* such as by drinking water and other nonirritating liquids at frequent intervals throughout the day.
◆ Recommend that the client apply artificial saliva, such as Oral Balance or XeroLube, as often as necessary, *to reduce mouth dryness.*
◆ Recommend lubricating the lips with K-Y Jelly, cocoa butter, or Chapstick, *to maintain intact mucous membranes.*
◆ Advise the client to suck on smooth, flat substances, such as sugarless candy or lozenges *to reduce mouth dryness.* (Sour substances usually stimulate saliva production.)
◆ Recommend humidifying environmental air, such as by using a pan of water near the source of heat, a cold steam vaporizer, or a humidifier installed as part of the central heating system *to reduce dryness.*
◆ *To prevent or minimize the formation of dental caries,* advise the client to:
– clean the oral cavity every 2 hours by brushing his teeth with a soft, nylon-bristle toothbrush and a nonirritating substance such as a baking soda solution
– avoid lemon and glycerin as cleaning agents, which promote dryness and irritation of mucous membranes
– remove and clean dentures, if present

– avoid commercial mouthwashes containing alcohol
– swish and gently gargle with a hydrogen peroxide and saline (1:2), hydrogen peroxide and water (1:4), or baking soda and water (1 tsp in 500 ml) solution.

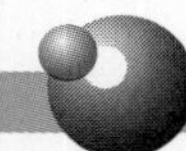

SPOT CHECK

Adverse reactions from radiation to skin are least *likely to include which of the following?*

A. Mild erythema and moist desquamation
B. Fibrosclerotic changes that make skin taut, smooth, and shiny
C. Permanent tanning
D. Complete or patchy alopecia

Answer: D. The adverse reactions from radiation to skin aren't likely to include complete or patchy alopecia.

Goal

◆ The client will maintain skin integrity and take measures to avoid skin breakdown.

Interventions

◆ Assess the client's skin integrity before treatment begins and at frequent intervals throughout irradiation *to detect alteration in baseline.*

◆ Instruct the client *to minimize trauma and protect the skin within the treatment field* by cleaning the skin with lukewarm water as needed, and avoiding the use of soaps, powders, perfumes, cosmetics, and deodorants.

◆ Advise the client to avoid shaving; use an electric razor, if necessary, *to avoid trauma.*

◆ Advise the client to protect his skin from heat, cold, wind, and sun; use sunblock (sun protection factor 15 or greater) when sun exposure is unavoidable *to avoid trauma.*

◆ Instruct the client to wear loose-fitting clothes over the treatment site. Have the client use a gentle detergent, such as Dreft or Ivory Snow, to launder clothes that will come in contact with skin in the treatment field *to avoid skin irritation.*

◆ Advise the client to avoid adhesive tape on irradiated skin *to avoid trauma.*

◆ Assess the client's skin for signs of infection and culture suspicious lesions or drainage *to provide early treatment of infection.*

◆ Instruct the client to use a systemic analgesic *to promote comfort and rest, as necessary.*

Review of clinical nursing

Part III

Mental health nursing

INTRODUCTION

When experiencing the stressors of life, a person tends to respond in a characteristic manner. The person's overall flexibility or rigidity in using this characteristic behavior determines whether the behavior is healthful, unhealthful, or somewhere in between.

A healthy person uses numerous and diverse behaviors to manage daily stressors; a person with compromised mental health doesn't. Instead, the unhealthy person responds to stress by exhibiting a narrow range of behaviors in a manner symptomatic of psychopathology. Using the principles of the nursing process and therapeutic communication, as outlined in chapter 3, this chapter focuses on clients who demonstrate various types of psychopathology or behavioral problems. After reviewing this chapter, you'll be better prepared to apply mental health concepts and principles in any clinical setting.

Therapeutic communication

The nurse who provides care for a client with a mental illness uses therapeutic communication to convey acceptance, preserve the client's self-esteem, and gain a greater understanding of how the client perceives the situation. Therapeutic responses encourage the client to continue talking. Examples include:

- "Tell me about..."
- "What happened after...?"
- "I'm not sure what you're saying."
- "And then...?"

In contrast, evaluative statements ("You must have felt sad" or "I'll bet you miss your children") close off communication and convey lack of understanding. (For a more detailed review of therapeutic communication, see chapter 3, Nursing concepts and skills.)

THE NURSE-CLIENT RELATIONSHIP

Any therapeutic relationship, including the nurse-client relationship, passes through four phases:

- Preinteraction phase
- Introductory phase
- Exploration phase
- Termination phase.

Preinteraction phase

During the preinteraction phase, which may last a few seconds to several weeks, the nurse assesses the client for unresolved problems. The client may not be actively involved at this point.

Introductory phase

During the introductory phase, previously known as the *orientation phase,* the nurse establishes certain parameters for the relationship, such as the time and duration of nurse-client visits, the responsibilities that each must bear, and the types of issues that they'll address.

Exploration phase

During the exploration phase, previously known as the *working phase,* the client actively works on issues germane to managing daily affairs. Although this phase may be emotionally painful, the client must be willing to examine issues with the nurse.

Termination phase

During the termination phase, the client and the nurse summarize their work, and the client plans for the future. If the client and the nurse have become emotionally attached, the termination phase may be painful for both of them. Ideally, termination begins during the first meeting with the nurse, when the parameters of the relationship are negotiated.

Responses to anxiety

EMOTIONAL RESPONSES	COGNITIVE RESPONSES	PHYSICAL RESPONSES
◆ Worry	◆ Rumination	◆ Restlessness
◆ Irritability, hypersensitivity	◆ Forgetfulness	◆ Tremulousness
◆ Apprehension	◆ Poor concentration	◆ Increased pulse and respiratory rates
◆ Vague discomfort	◆ Blocking of thoughts	◆ Elevated blood pressure
◆ Expectation of danger	◆ Inattentiveness	◆ Muscle tightness
◆ Tendency to cry easily	◆ Distractibility	◆ Nausea
◆ Lack of self-confidence	◆ Preoccupations	◆ Dizziness
◆ Strong startle response		◆ Fatigue
		◆ Urinary urgency or frequency, or both
		◆ Constipation or diarrhea

How anxiety affects behavior

Anxiety is unexplained discomfort, apprehension, or uneasiness. The energy generated by anxiety can be used constructively or destructively.

Anxiety can be precipitated in several ways, as:

◆ unmet expectations that are important to one's self-worth.

◆ an actual or perceived threat to one's values, status, prestige, biological integrity, or body image.

◆ psychological or physiologic stress.

◆ an adverse reaction to chemical substances (for example, a bad "trip" after taking D-lysergic acid diethylamide [LSD]).

Anxiety has emotional, cognitive, and physical manifestations that the nurse must consider when planning care. (See *Responses to anxiety.*) Defense mechanisms are used to cope with anxiety. They operate on an unconscious level (except for suppression) and allow the client to deny or distort reality.

Regardless of the underlying psychopathology, the nurse must assess the client's anxiety level because this guides the choice of nursing interventions. (See *Anxiety levels and nursing implications,* page 134.)

◆ A client with mild anxiety can function well and needs no assistance from the nurse.

◆ A client with moderate anxiety will require some assistance because of selective inattention and an inability to provide the self-structure needed to remain focused.

◆ A client with severe anxiety will require much assistance from the nurse because of an inability to solve problems and a preoccupation with internal experience.

◆ A client at the panic level of anxiety is at risk for harming himself or others because of distortions of reality.

Research and technology

As health care professionals strive to understand what causes mental illness, research and technology continue to play significant roles. Despite advances, a simple explanation for mental illness hasn't been revealed; causation appears to be multidimensional, with psychological, biological, social, and cultural factors affecting human behavior.

WORKING WITH GROUPS

Nurses are expected to have group skills so they can work therapeutically with clients in a group setting. Nurses can facilitate educational groups, skills-in-living groups, parenting groups, support groups, and socialization groups.

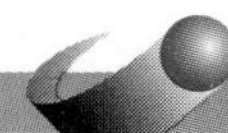

FAST FACT

Having group skills does *not* mean the nurse is permitted to conduct group psychotherapy. Conducting group psychotherapy requires a master's degree and at least 2 years' experience with supervision in psychotherapy.

Working with clients in small groups has many benefits for the nurse and clients. Because the nurse works with several clients simultaneously, the technique is cost-effective. Also, it allows the nurse to observe interaction patterns and permits situation repetition. Being in a group allows clients to:

Anxiety levels and nursing implications

This chart presents manifestations of and nursing implications for the four primary levels of anxiety.

ANXIETY LEVEL	MANIFESTATIONS	NURSING IMPLICATIONS
Mild	◆ Alertness ◆ Maximal ability to solve problems ◆ Enhanced learning	◆ Allow the client to be fully responsible for himself.
Moderate	◆ Selective inattention ◆ Impaired ability to solve problems ◆ Complaints of feeling uptight, on edge, or nervous	◆ Help the client talk through the situation and label feelings. ◆ Use relaxation techniques.
Severe	◆ Narrowed attention span ◆ Inability to grasp meanings ◆ Inability to solve problems ◆ Distorted view ◆ Self-absorption ◆ Inability to connect events or details ◆ Clingy or demanding behavior ◆ Many physiologic signs, including increased blood pressure, dry mouth, restlessness, and muscular tightness	◆ Provide structure and direction. ◆ Don't force the client to make decisions. ◆ Provide one-on-one supervision. ◆ Give as-needed medication for escalating anxiety, as ordered. ◆ Provide a nonstimulating environment. ◆ Use touch carefully. Don't physically touch the client without first obtaining permission or explaining what you're doing; a severely anxious client may misinterpret touch as an attack. ◆ Maintain a calm, soothing tone of voice. ◆ Act as a focal point, taking over the interaction and actively directing the client's attention to you, which usually has a calming effect on the client. ◆ Dress conservatively to maintain a soothing environment; brightly colored clothing can overstimulate severely anxious and manic clients.
Panic	◆ Inability to solve problems ◆ Feeling detached from body or unreal ◆ Many physiologic signs, such as those previously mentioned in severe anxiety and breathing problems ◆ Withdrawal, loss of contact with reality ◆ Inability to communicate ◆ Insomnia ◆ Inability to recognize familiar objects, persons, or environment ◆ Erratic behavior ◆ Terror-stricken behavior	◆ See nursing implications for severe anxiety.

- receive feedback from peers
- learn information about themselves
- practice new interactional and coping skills
- express their feelings
- see that others have had similar experiences.

It also helps them meet unfulfilled needs for belonging and acceptance and gives them a chance to network.

To work with groups, the nurse must understand group dynamics and therapeutic communication. The nurse also must establish group standards or rules — for example, who has access to what group members say (confidentiality), who's responsible for determining content and keeping the group focused (leadership and responsibility), and whether smoking, eating, drinking, interrupting, or swearing will be permitted (norms). What's said in a group is referred to as *group content.* The meeting of individual needs while meeting group goals is called *group process.*

Standard group protocol

- Designated group leaders
- Purpose and goals of group
- Framework to guide group
- Content for discussion
- Methods for keeping group working
- Determining appropriate participants
- Measuring outcomes by specific evaluation methods
- Documents group work and participant progress

Roles of group members

- Opinion giver or seeker
- Information giver or seeker
- Initiator
- Elaborator
- Coordinator
- Evaluator
- Summarizer

Goals of group therapy

- To reduce or modify symptoms
- To mitigate disturbed behavior patterns
- To promote positive behaviors

Phases of a group

According to some practitioners, the goals of group therapy are achieved in four phases:

1. Boundaries and dependence on the group leader are established.
2. Conflict emerges.
3. The group becomes cohesive and new behaviors begin.
4. Support for group members becomes evident as roles change, effective work is done, and goals are accomplished.

GROUP FACILITATION

To facilitate a therapeutically oriented group, the nurse can use various strategies. For example, to start a new session, briefly review the last session, and then ask how things have gone since then. When appropriate, respond to themes. For instance, say, "At least three people have talked about staying balanced. Perhaps it would be useful to examine what staying balanced means to each of us."

Leading a group

The group leader, or *facilitator,* has multiple functions:

- to keep the group focused
- to monitor established group rules or norms
- to facilitate the group process (how members respond to one another and the topic being discussed), when appropriate
- to address problems that occur in the group
- to screen group members, when appropriate
- to evaluate outcomes.

Problems within a group

When a group is cohesive, members have the potential to experience maximal growth because they're committed to themselves as well as to fellow participants. This commitment allows members to risk dealing with sensitive issues within the group. Threats to group cohesion include:

- transient group members
- poorly selected group members
- cliques
- competition
- transference and countertransference
- unacknowledged conflict
- lack of privacy
- irregular meetings.

Interventions for group problems

Threats to cohesion can be diffused through various interventions:

- Screen the participants before the first group meeting to determine their suitability.
- Stress consistent attendance if it's important. (This requirement should be made known during the first group meeting, and members who can't commit to regular attendance should be excluded.)
- Acknowledge the presence of any cliques, and assist clique members and others in analyzing this phenomenon. If competition or unacknowledged conflict exists among group members, acknowledge it, state observations, and seek feedback about what's happening.
- Identify transference, in which unresolved issues of group members are projected onto other members or the group leader, and assist members in responding to the issues.
- Identify countertransference, in which unresolved issues of the nurse interfere with the ability to work objectively with the group. Solving this problem requires imme-

Problem behaviors in a group

Common problems encountered within groups are listed here along with possible causes. It's important for the nurse to remember that these behaviors are intended to protect the person who's engaging in them.

PROBLEM BEHAVIOR	POSSIBLE CAUSES
Conflict	◆ Attempt to focus attention elsewhere ◆ Lack of knowledge about how to resolve issues in a healthy manner ◆ Highly charged issue ◆ Transferences and countertransferences
Group gets sidetracked	◆ Unclear focus ◆ Group members with limited intellectual capacity or inability to consider a wide range of ideas ◆ Lack of group structure ◆ Avoidance of painful issues ◆ Leader doesn't effectively assist group members in analyzing what's happening within the group
Member approaches group leader outside group to discuss group business	◆ Inability to confront issues directly ◆ Attempt to manipulate leader to gain power ◆ Lack of understanding about how groups work ◆ Lack of clarity about group rules ◆ Testing behavior ◆ Fear of reprisal within group ◆ Attempt to seek attention to fill inner void
Member uses strong or offensive language	◆ Attempt to control others ◆ Testing behavior ◆ Self-protection ◆ Poor communication skills
Member exhibits minimal or no active participation	◆ Anxiety ◆ Opinions or views previously squelched ◆ Uncertainty of group rules ◆ Fear that expressed ideas may lead to more work
Member dominates group interaction	◆ Anxiety or discomfort with silence ◆ Feeling overly responsible for outcome ◆ Attempt to feel important ◆ Avoidance of painful issues ◆ Attempt to control outcome through bulldozing ◆ Frequent compulsive speaking to help decrease anxiety

diate peer supervision and use of a coleader for firsthand feedback.

◆ Provide privacy by arranging for sessions to be held in an enclosed area that isn't visually accessible to others and in which comments can't be overheard by nonparticipants.

Many individuals feel threatened by therapeutic groups designed to examine their own behavior. To protect themselves, these individuals may respond by exhibiting problem behaviors or signs of resistance. (See *Problem behaviors in a group.*)

Common signs of resistance include:

- ◆ missing sessions
- ◆ showing up late
- ◆ rescuing others
- ◆ projecting blame
- ◆ engaging in small-talk
- ◆ changing the subject
- ◆ forming cliques
- ◆ verbally attacking other members or the leader
- ◆ becoming overinvolved or focused on social behaviors.

Interventions for resistant behaviors

◆ Acknowledge a member's absence or chronic lateness, seek clarification about the meaning of the behavior, and assist the member to formulate theories and solutions for being consistently late.

◆ When one member "rescues" another, point out the behavior and ask the rescuer what prompted it; also ask the one "rescued" to provide feedback about the rescuer's behavior.

◆ If members project blame, ask them to identify the parts of the situation for which they're responsible and to focus on the actions under their control.

◆ Observe patterns of engaging in small-talk or changing the subject; comment on the observations made, and ask if the group members have any ideas about what's happening or what the group is trying to avoid.

◆ If cliques form, state specific indicative behaviors among group members and ask both clique and nonclique members to analyze what's happening in the group.

◆ Intervene immediately if one group member makes a verbal attack on the group leader or another member. Have the attacker nonabrasively state the issue and ask those attacked to provide feedback; help the attacker analyze the intent of the behavior, and assist all group members in identifying boundary issues.

◆ Redirect the group member who's doing things for others, such as providing food or setting up the room. These tasks distract members from thinking and talking about their issues and needs.

CRISIS INTERVENTION

An event that disrupts a person's usual manner of coping with stress can precipitate a crisis. Such an event may be situational (such as divorce), maturational (occurring when a person enters a new developmental phase of his life or career), or adventitious (caused by uncontrolled events, such as flood, war, or assault). An event that triggers a crisis in one person may not do so in another.

According to some practitioners, three balancing factors offset a crisis:

- ◆ Realistic perception of the event
- ◆ Adequate emotional support
- ◆ Adequate coping mechanisms.

Absence of any of these factors predisposes a person to crisis. This section reviews the key phases of a crisis, and then provides an in-depth look at an adventitious crisis, namely *rape-trauma syndrome.*

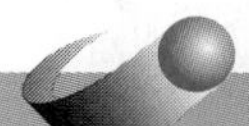

FAST FACT

The types of crisis are:

- adventitious (precipitated by uncontrolled events)
- maturational (associated with developmental phases of life or career)
- situational (related to situations or events).

PHASES OF A CRISIS

A crisis develops in four phases:

◆ *Phase 1* — The person responds with increased anxiety and tries to problem-solve to decrease anxiety.

◆ *Phase 2* — The person's problem solving is unsuccessful and anxiety increases. The person becomes very distressed and may use a trial-and-error approach to handle the situation.

◆ *Phase 3* — The person's attempts to cope fail and he must find behaviors that bring relief. He may flee from the situation or redefine the event to make it understandable and prevent maladaptive responses such as violence to self or others.

◆ *Phase 4* — As the crisis resolves, work begins to return to one of three levels of functioning (precrisis level, higher level, or lower level). The person can learn adaptive coping skills and sets goals to recover from the event.

Crisis intervention aims to restore at least a precrisis level of functioning and prevent untoward emotional sequelae. (See *Caring for the client who has been raped,* pages 138 and 139.)

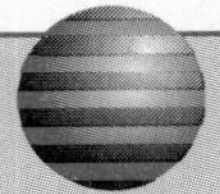

CLINICAL SITUATION

Caring for the client who has been raped

Evaluate the clinical situation described here. See if you're able to answer the questions as you go.

A deeply religious 24-year-old woman is brought into the emergency department by the police. During triage, she sits stiffly, clutching her coat tightly around her and keeping her head down. "I'm so ashamed," she says in a barely audible voice. "It's all my fault." She doesn't raise her head to answer questions. She repeatedly says, "I don't know what to do." The nurse finds out that the client lives alone, that her parents live in a nearby city, and that she has a married sister who lives within 5 miles of the hospital. She has few friends.

During the medical examination (performed using the hospital's rape protocol), the client tries to maintain her composure, but she can't help crying at times. The examination reveals small lacerations of the external genitalia and vagina as well as scratches on her face, throat, breasts, arms, and legs.

Following completion of the rape-protocol examination, the client tells the nurse she's afraid to leave the hospital and return to her apartment because the rapist has her purse containing identification and house keys. After much persuasion on the nurse's part, the client agrees to contact her sister.

While waiting for her sister to arrive, the client sits in her cubicle crying softly. She says she can't understand how God could let this happen to her, that she was a virgin, and now she's "nothing more than a dirty rag that no one would ever want."

"I guess it doesn't make any difference what happens now," she says. "No one will ever want me."

What key elements should be established during assessment?

- The client's physical condition – When a client has a physical condition and a psychological one, the physical condition (more basic need) must be assessed before psychological intervention can take place.
- The client's level of anxiety – Identifying the client's anxiety level will help establish which nursing interventions are required. Nursing interventions will change as the client's anxiety level fluctuates.
- The presence of balancing factors – Absence of any of these balancing factors will prolong the crisis:
  - realistic perception of the event
  - adequate social supports
  - adequate coping skills.
- The availability of a rape counselor and survivor group referrals for continued support while back in the community – Nurses in the emergency department don't provide support after the client leaves the hospital. Follow-up counseling will help the client put the rape into perspective and allow her to move along with her life.

What are appropriate interventions for the initial treatment of this client?

- Don't leave the client alone *to allow the client to feel safe.* A calming influence can prevent the client from becoming more overwhelmed by the rape experience.
- Ask the client where she's experiencing pain *to help the client focus on something specific;* it also communicates the nurse's caring and concern.
- Assist the client with completing the hospital's rape protocol *to allow her to concentrate on the tasks at hand.* Because of her traumatic experience, the client's anxiety level will fluctuate. The client will need assistance with completing the hospital's rape protocol, which includes documenting her condition and obtaining laboratory specimens and potential legal evidence.
- Offer the client a cleansing shower, mouthwash, and other supplies only after all evidence has been gathered (remember that it's necessary to preserve the chain of evidence in rape cases); help her clean up if she can't care for herself *to help decrease her level of anxiety.* The client may feel the need to wash away the traumatic experience. Symbolically, this cleaning can help the client decrease her high level of anxiety. The nurse's assistance conveys caring and concern.
- When her anxiety level is at or below the moderate level, ask the client to tell you about the rape, letting her set the pace. Phrase your questions and comments with care and sensitivity. *This approach promotes the client's eventual cognitive mastery over the rape experience, decreasing her tendency to withdraw and to feel guilt and shame.* Thoughtlessly worded comments and questions ("Were you really raped?") convey doubt and project blame. In contrast, a carefully worded statement ("I'd like to hear about what happened.") conveys the nurse's desire to understand the client's experience.
- Help the client to identify her most immediate concern, *which provides a concrete focus to her thoughts and allows the client to begin regaining control of her life.*
- Ask the client to name someone who can stay with her for the next 24 to 48 hours, *which may ease her anxiety, help her feel safe, and help her cope with periodic waves of anxiety and fear.*
- Provide the names and telephone numbers of appropriate community resources. If possible, introduce the client to a rape counselor *before* she leaves the emergency department. *Explaining*

Caring for the client who has been raped *(continued)*

about community resources lets the client know that she won't be abandoned. Giving her the information in writing increases the probability that she'll contact someone for rape counseling. Establishing contact with the rape counselor before leaving the emergency department will decrease the client's sense of aloneness and better ensure that she'll seek follow-up rape counseling.

If the client accepts rape counseling in the weeks after the rape, the event will be explored and the client's coping skills will be strengthened, as appropriate.

What interventions would be appropriate during the counseling sessions?

◆ Encourage the client to recall how she has dealt with past traumatic events *to help demonstrate to the client that she'll be able to cope with this unwanted experience just as she has coped with others.*

◆ Help the client talk about the rape and vent her feelings, *which can decrease her sense of helplessness, powerlessness, and self-doubt. Talking about the rape helps the client put the traumatic experience into perspective, permitting self-growth and healing.* Unexpressed feelings may lead to depression and other symptoms in the future.

◆ Help the client examine differences in her lifestyle that have resulted from the rape *to help the client determine whether she's giving this experience more power in her life than she would like,* which helps her gain a realistic perception of the rape.

◆ Allow the client to express negative thoughts and feelings. Encouraging her to sort out thoughts and feelings *enables her to determine the reality of the situation.*

◆ Talk with the client about her spiritual beliefs. If appropriate, consider seeking pastoral assistance for her *because the client's spiritual condition shouldn't be ignored. For the deeply religious client, restoration of her faith in God may enhance healing.*

◆ Discuss the client's thoughts and feelings about prosecuting her attacker. *This discussion conveys that the client has the option to take direct action against her attacker.* Under no circumstances, however, should the nurse coerce the client into filing charges.

◆ Encourage the client to participate in group therapy, individual therapy, or a support group. *Group or individual therapy can assist the client in developing coping skills and promote an optimal level of functioning. Support groups can enable the person to decrease anxiety and increase feelings of well-being.*

◆ Encourage the client to engage in problem solving. *Use of problem-solving skills decreases anxiety levels and promotes the client's sense of control.*

Questions for further thought

◆ What would be appropriate nursing diagnoses for this client?

◆ What assessment findings would indicate that the client is able to function with minimal posttraumatic stress symptoms?

DOMESTIC ABUSE

Physical, emotional, and sexual abuse are common in families and constitute an urgent mental health issue. Recipients of abuse are primarily women (battered wives), children, elderly persons, the infirm, and the physically or mentally disabled.

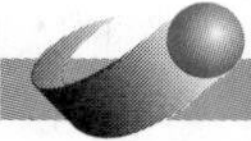

FAST FACT

Domestic abuse can take many forms, including physical, sexual, psychological, and economic abuse and neglect. No one is immune.

Violence in the family is a serious misuse of a person's power over another. In our society, tolerance of violent behavior must be stopped to decrease the incidence of family violence. Physical, emotional, and sexual abuse are major health issues. Family abuse may continue for years without detection. The secondary consequences of family violence, such as anxiety, depression, posttraumatic stress disorder, and other health problems, can cause a lifetime of difficulty. In abusive families, seemingly mild stressors can precipitate abusive episodes.

Persons unfamiliar with abuse may be overwhelmed when they must assist recipients of abuse. Thus, nurses must be aware of their own feelings about abuse so that they can assist the abuser and the abused. The nurse must also be able to identify possible situations in which abuse may be present.

CHILD ABUSE

◆ Major types of child abuse include:
- physical abuse
- emotional abuse

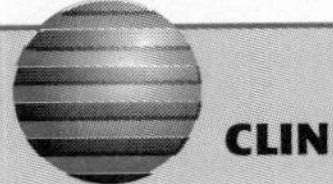

CLINICAL SITUATION

Caring for the child who has been abused

Evaluate the clinical situation described here. See if you're able to answer the questions as you go.

A child, age 2, is admitted to the pediatric unit at 4:30 p.m. from the emergency department (ED). She has bruises on her back and a spiral fracture of her left upper arm, which has been put in a cast. The ED report indicates that the client's father, who has been unemployed for 6 months, became upset with her when she wet her pants while playing. According to him, he placed the child firmly on her potty chair and told her not to move. When she got off the potty chair in "direct defiance" of his authority, he grabbed her arm and put her back on the chair to show her that he was the boss. When she screamed, he spanked her. The child's screaming was so persistent, and her arm looked so reddened and swollen, that her mother (8 months pregnant with twins) convinced the child's father that they should bring her to the ED.

In the pediatric unit, both parents express their concern about the child to the nursing staff. They say that the father didn't intend to hurt her and that he was only trying to teach her to be obedient. However, when the nurse-manager indicates a desire to talk more about the child's broken arm, the parents become angry and quickly leave the hospital, saying they'll be back later. The child cries and calls after her departing parents, "Come back! Me be good. Me be good girl."

What are some key steps the nurse should include as part of the child's assessment?

- Perform a physical assessment of the child: Is she well nourished? Does she have unexplained marks or bruises on her body? Are her height and weight appropriate for her age? *This provides baseline data about the abused child's condition; subsequent progress is measured against baseline findings.*
- Assess the child's response to her broken arm. *An abused child may react passively to pain from a broken arm.*
- Assess the child's response to being hospitalized and separated from her parents. *The child's response provides information about her developmental level and current care needs.* The child probably has never been away from her parents overnight. From her perspective, she has been abandoned.
- When her parents return later in the evening, assess the child's usual routine. Have the parents describe the child's bedtime and toileting habits, and ask them to identify her favorite foods, toys, and play activities. *The abused child's adjustment to hospitalization will be enhanced if her normal routine is followed as closely as possible. Furthermore, this information facilitates individualized nursing care.*
- Assess the child's response to her parents: Does she flinch when either parent reaches out to touch her? Does she avoid eye contact with either parent? *This assessment provides further information about the existence of abuse. A nurse who suspects child abuse is expected to follow the reporting protocol mandated by agency and state laws.*
- Assess the parents' willingness to help the staff care for the child. *If the parents are willing to help with care of the abused child, they and the nursing staff have an opportunity to form a working relationship. In addition, increased familiarity will help everyone feel more at ease during the child's hospitalization.*
- Assess the underlying needs of each family member, keeping in mind that their needs will probably differ. *This will allow the nurse to plan appropriate care and help the child feel safe in this new environment.*
- Assess the child's parents for predisposing factors of child abuse. *Referral to a social service agency may bring help to the abused child's family.*

What are some of the predisposing factors of child abuse?

- Abuse of drugs (including alcohol)
- Unemployment
- Debt
- Lack of knowledge about child behavior
- Lack of social supports
- Inadequate housing
- Limited coping abilities
- Marital strife

What is a key intervention that must be included when monitoring the child's physical progress?

Any physical injury must be attended to first. Lower-level needs must be met before higher-level needs. The nurse should check the child's cast for tightness every hour for the next 24 hours.

Questions for further thought

- How can the nurse get the parents involved in the child's care?
- How would anticipatory planning help the parents when caring for their child?

- sexual abuse
- neglect
- exploitation.

◆ Signs of child abuse include:
- avoidance of eye contact with parent or caregiver
- flinching when approached by parent or caregiver
- inappropriate height and weight for age
- withdrawn, passive response to injuries (conversely, may also be aggressive)
- injuries in various states of healing (fractures, burns, marks, or bruises on the body)
- signs of irritation, bruising, infection, or bleeding in the genital area. (See *Caring for the child who has been abused.*)

ELDER ABUSE

◆ Major types of elder abuse include physical, psychological, and economic abuse; neglect; and exploitation.

◆ Signs of elder abuse include:
- dehydration
- injuries in various stages of healing
- malnutrition
- overuse of medications
- pressure sores
- rub burns
- self-protective reactions
- severe anxiety.

SPOUSAL ABUSE

◆ Major types of spousal abuse include mental, physical, sexual, or economic abuse.

◆ Some indicators of spousal abuse include:
- injuries in various states of healing (fractures, burns, marks, or bruises on the body)
- withdrawal, depression, fear, anxiety.

ANXIETY AND MOOD DISORDERS

The client with an anxiety disorder experiences overwhelming anxiety, which interferes with his quality of life. To relieve the anxiety, the client develops a variety of symptoms, which may or may not control the anxiety. Defenses used in anxiety disorders include:

◆ displacement
◆ reaction formation
◆ intellectualization
◆ undoing
◆ repression.

(See *Comparing anxiety disorders,* page 142.)

Types of anxiety and mood disorders include:

◆ bipolar disorder
◆ generalized anxiety disorder
◆ major depressive disorder
◆ obsessive-compulsive disorder
◆ panic disorder
◆ phobias
◆ posttraumatic stress disorder.

BIPOLAR DISORDER

BIPOLAR DISORDER, also known as *manic-depression,* is a severe disturbance in affect, manifested by episodes of extreme sadness alternating with episodes of euphoria. Severity and duration of episodes vary. The exact biological basis of bipolar disorder remains unknown.

Three major types of bipolar disorder are:

◆ bipolar I, in which depressive episodes alternate with full manic episodes (hyperactive behavior, delusional thinking, grandiosity and, commonly, hostility)
◆ bipolar II, characterized by depressive episodes and milder hypomanic episodes
◆ cyclothymic disorder, characterized by a history of numerous hypomanic episodes intermingled with numerous depressive episodes that don't meet the criteria for major depressive episodes.

During the manic phase, the client commonly exhibits excessive motor activity and may become highly irritable if caregivers place limits on behavior. The client also demonstrates disturbed thought processes that lead to socially inappropriate behavior. Because the client lacks self-pacing and problem-solving abilities, care and treatment focus on slowing the client's movements and activities. Otherwise, a manic client can die of self-induced exhaustion or injury. The potential for suicide increases when the client's mood is changing from mania to depression or from depression to mania; suicide precautions may be needed.

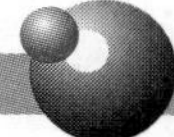

SPOT CHECK

Which bipolar pattern is characterized by depressive episodes alternating with full manic episodes?

Answer: Bipolar 1 is characterized this way.

Comparing anxiety disorders

Anxiety disorders are described briefly in the chart here. A combination of drug therapy and behavioral or cognitive approaches is used to treat these disorders.

DISORDER	DESCRIPTION	TREATMENT
Generalized anxiety disorder	Excessive worry about many life circumstances with persistant anxiety during most waking hours	◆ Benzodiazepines ◆ Cognitive reframing ◆ Relaxation exercises
Obsessive-compulsive disorder	Overwhelming need to carry out a stereotypical act to relieve anxiety precipitated by an obsessive thought	◆ Antidepressant drugs ◆ Behavioral techniques, such as response prevention and thought stopping
Panic disorder	Unpredictable attacks of intense anxiety lasting a few minutes to several hours	◆ Antidepressant drugs ◆ Benzodiazepines ◆ Relaxation exercises
Posttraumatic stress disorder	Re-experiencing the original traumatic event; may be acute, delayed, or chronic	◆ Antidepressant drugs ◆ Benzodiazepines ◆ Cognitive therapy ◆ Group therapy ◆ Hypnosis
Simple phobia	Disproportionate fear and avoidance of something that, in reality, is harmless	◆ Benzodiazepines ◆ Desensitization ◆ Distraction
Social phobia	Disproportionate fear and avoidance of social situations that, in reality, aren't life-threatening	◆ Benzodiazepines ◆ Social skills training

Contributing factors

- Concurrent major illness
- Environment
- Genetics
- History of psychiatric illnesses
- Seasons and circadian rhythms that affect mood
- Sleep deprivation
- Stressful events (may produce limbic system dysfunction)

Assessment findings

During periods of mania

- Bizarre, eccentric appearance
- Cognitive manifestations, such as difficulty concentrating, flight of ideas, delusions of grandeur, and impaired judgment
- Motor agitation
- Decreased sleep
- Deteriorated physical appearance
- Dry mouth
- Euphoria, hostility
- Feelings of grandiosity
- Increased libido
- Increased social contacts
- Inflated sense of self-worth
- Lack of inhibition, recklessness
- Rapid, jumbled speech
- Tremors, tachycardia, labored respirations

During periods of depression

- Altered sleep patterns
- Amenorrhea
- Anorexia and weight loss
- Confusion and indecisiveness
- Constipation

- Decreased alertness
- Delusions, hallucinations
- Difficulty thinking logically
- Guilt, helplessness, sadness, and crying
- Impotence and lack of interest in sex
- Inability to experience pleasure
- Irritability, pessimism
- Lack of motivation, low self-esteem
- Poor hygiene
- Poor posture

Diagnostic evaluation

- Diagnostic testing rules out organic causes of disorder.

Nursing diagnoses

- Disturbed thought processes
- Risk for injury
- Disturbed sleep pattern
- Impaired social interaction

Treatment

- Electroconvulsive (ECT) therapy, if drug therapy fails
- Individual therapy and family therapy

Drug therapy options

- Anticonvulsant agents: carbamazepine (Tegretol), valproic acid (Depakote)
- Antimanic agent: lithium carbonate (Eskalith)
- Antidepressant agent: fluoxetine (Prozac)
- Antipsychotic agents: olanzapine (Zyprexa), quetiapine (Seroquel), risperidone (Risperdal), ziprasidone (Geodon)

Planning and goals

- The client won't harm himself.
- The client will control thought processes.
- The client will demonstrate a stable mood and a normal sleep pattern and will practice self-care activities such as eating.
- The client will interact appropriately with others.

Implementation

During the manic phase

- Decrease environmental stimuli by behaving consistently and supplying external controls *to promote relaxation and enable sleep.*
- Ensure a safe environment *to protect the client from himself.*
- Channel the client's energy in one direction and pace activities, *which may decrease the client's energy expenditure, prevent overstimulation and, sometimes, have a soothing effect.*
- Define and explain acceptable behaviors and then set limits *to begin a process in which the client will eventually define and set his own limits.*
- Monitor drug levels, especially lithium, *to keep dosages within the therapeutic range.*
- If a mood swing to depression seems imminent, implement suicide precautions. *The client is at increased risk for suicide during mood swings.*

During the depressive phase

- Assess the level and intensity of the client's depression *to obtain baseline information essential for effective nursing care.*
- Ensure a safe environment for the client *to protect him from self-inflicted harm.*
- Assess the risk for suicide and formulate a safety contract with the client, as appropriate, *to ensure the client's well-being and to open lines of communication.*
- Observe the client for medication compliance and adverse effects; *without compliance, there's little hope for progress.*
- Encourage the client to identify current problems and stressors *so that he can begin therapeutic treatment.*
- Promote opportunities for increased involvement in activities through a structured, daily program *to help the client feel comfortable with himself and others.*
- Select activities that ensure success and accomplishment *to increase self-esteem.*
- Help the client to modify negative expectations and think more positively *because positive thinking will help him to begin healing.*
- Spend time with the client, even if he's too depressed to talk, *to enhance the therapeutic relationship.*

Evaluation

- The client engages in goal-directed activity and no longer exhibits disturbed thinking.
- The client sleeps through the night.
- The client doesn't harm himself or others.
- The client is adequately maintained on medication, expresses a desire to follow the medication regimen, understands why he must take the drug, knows its side effects and how to manage them, and has a plan for getting serum drug levels analyzed once per month.
- The client maintains adequate nutrition.
- The client expresses understanding of the illness and states how to obtain assistance or support from others.

GENERALIZED ANXIETY DISORDER

A client with GENERALIZED ANXIETY DISORDER worries excessively and experiences tremendous anxiety almost daily. The client experiences moderate to severe levels of anxiety during most waking hours. He can't feel calm or relaxed in situations that most persons don't perceive as particularly stressful. The worry lasts for longer than 6 months and is usually disproportionate to the situation. Both adults and children can be diagnosed with generalized anxiety disorder, although the content of the worry may differ. Because the anxiety is so pervasive, it affects most areas of the client's life.

Contributing factors

- Genetics
- Biochemical abnormalities (imbalance in serotonin and gamma-aminobutyric acid)
- Stress, unresolved conflicts

Assessment findings

- Excessive worry and anxiety
- Excessive attention to surroundings
- Distractibility
- Fatigue, sleep disorder
- Motor and muscle tension
- Pounding heart
- Repetitive thoughts
- Strained expression
- Tingling of hands or feet
- Easy startle reflex
- Fears of grave misfortune or death
- Autonomic hyperactivity

Diagnostic evaluation

- Diagnostic testing rules out organic causes of the disorder.

Nursing diagnoses

- Anxiety
- Ineffective coping
- Deficient knowledge: Disease process and treatment

Treatment

- Cognitive therapy focusing on coping skills
- Biofeedback training

Drug therapy options

- Antianxiety agents: diazepam (Valium), venlafaxine (Effexor), alprazolam (Xanax), lorazepam (Ativan), clonazepam (Klonopin), buspirone (BuSpar)
- Selective serotonin reuptake inhibitors: paroxetine (Paxil), sertraline (Zoloft)
- Tricyclic antidepressant: imipramine (Tofranil)

Planning and goals

- The client will verbalize signs and symptoms of increasing anxiety.
- The client will identify coping mechanisms to manage the physical, emotional, and behavioral signs and symptoms of anxiety.

Implementation

- Help the client identify and explore coping mechanisms used in the past. *Establishing a baseline for the level of current functioning will enable the nurse to build on the client's knowledge.*
- Observe for signs of mounting anxiety *to direct measures for moderating it.*
- Negotiate a contract to work on goals *to give the client control of his situation.*
- Alter the environment *to reduce the client's anxiety or meet his needs.*
- Monitor the client's diet and nutrition, and reduce his caffeine intake *to reduce anxiety.*
- Review key teaching topics with the client and his family members *to ensure adequate knowledge about the condition and treatment,* including:
  - recognizing signs of anxiety
  - altering diet (Caffeine can cause arrhythmias. Foods containing tyramine, such as fava beans, yeast-containing and fermented foods, and avocados, can cause a hypertensive crisis.)
  - reviewing coping behaviors.

Evaluation

- The client exhibits decreased signs and symptoms of anxiety.
- The client verbalizes coping strategies for use in managing increased anxiety levels.

MAJOR DEPRESSIVE DISORDER

MAJOR DEPRESSIVE DISORDER is a syndrome of depressed mood that's present for most of the day, nearly every day for at least 2 weeks.

Major depressive disorder can profoundly alter social functioning, but the most severe complication is the potential for suicide. (See *Forms of depression and nursing implications.*)

Effective emergency intervention should be based on an assessment of the client's lethality. For this, the nurse uses a lethality scale, which considers such factors as the client's age, employment status, availability of support

Forms of depression and nursing implications

Use this chart to review commonly observed forms of depression and related nursing implications.

FORM	CHARACTERISTICS	NURSING IMPLICATIONS
Dysthymic disorder	◆ Depressed mood that occurs for more days than not over a period of 2 years ◆ Poor appetite ◆ Low energy level or fatigue ◆ Feelings of hopelessness ◆ Poor concentration ◆ Sleep pattern disturbances ◆ Low self-esteem ◆ Difficulty making decisions	◆ Help the client identify activities that promote well-being. ◆ Help the client establish a healthy daily routine. ◆ Assist the client in setting realistic goals.
Major depressive disorder	◆ Depressed mood that occurs for most of the day, nearly every day for a period of 2 weeks ◆ Limited ability to perform life-sustaining activities ◆ Severe anhedonia ◆ Feelings of worthlessness ◆ Excessive guilt ◆ Morbid thoughts, preoccupation with death	◆ Provide a structured daily routine. ◆ Don't give the client choices. ◆ Make the client engage in activities. ◆ Use compliments sparingly. Ill-timed compliments indicate insensitivity to the client's inner pain and may precipitate regression or a suicide attempt. ◆ Assist the client with self-care activities until energy returns. ◆ Make decisions for the client until energy returns.
Major depressive disorder with psychosis	◆ Characteristics of major depressive disorder, plus hallucinations, delusions, or both	◆ Intervene as for a severely depressed client. ◆ Orient a hallucinatory or delusional client to reality, as needed. ◆ Provide a consistent environment.
Seasonal affective disorder	◆ Onset between mid-October and mid-November ◆ Remission between mid-February and mid-April ◆ Signs and symptoms of dysthymic disorder	◆ Advise the client to use bright lights and go outdoors as much as possible. ◆ If possible, advise the client to purchase full-spectrum lights designed specifically to treat this disorder. ◆ Suggest that the client vacation in the winter, rather than the summer, in a place with longer daylight hours.

systems, and intended manner of committing suicide. Nearly 15% of those with severe major depressive disorder commit suicide. (For indicators of suicidal behavior, see *Identifying a suicidal client,* page 146.)

Contributing factors

◆ Current substance abuse
◆ Deficiencies in the receptor sites for some neurotransmitters: norepinephrine, serotonin, dopamine, and acetylcholine
◆ Family history of depressive disorders
◆ Hormonal imbalances
◆ Lack of social support
◆ Nutritional deficiencies
◆ Previous episode of depression
◆ Significant medical problems
◆ Stressful life events

Assessment findings

◆ Sadness and crying
◆ Lack of motivation, low self-esteem
◆ Inability to experience pleasure
◆ Guilt, helplessness, pessimism
◆ Confusion and indecisiveness

Identifying a suicidal client

A client with a mood disorder may be at risk for attempting suicide. Stay alert for:

- overwhelming anxiety
- withdrawal and social isolation
- saying farewell to family and friends
- putting affairs in order
- giving away prized possessions
- sending covert suicidal messages and death wishes
- expressing obvious suicidal thoughts
- describing a suicide plan
- hoarding medications
- talking about death and a feeling of futility
- behavior changes, especially as depression begins to subside.

If you think your client is at risk for suicide, take these steps:

- Keep communication lines open, and help him maintain emotional ties to others.
- Ensure a safe environment by checking for dangerous conditions.
- Remove belts, sharp objects (such as razors, knives, nail files, and clippers), suspenders, light and window-blind cords, and glass from the client's room.
- Make sure the acutely suicidal client is observed around the clock.

- Altered sleep patterns
- Anorexia and weight loss
- Decreased alertness
- Difficulty thinking logically
- Amenorrhea
- Irritability
- Poor hygiene
- Poor posture
- Impotence or lack of interest in sex
- Constipation or diarrhea
- Delusions, hallucinations (major depressive disorder with psychosis)

Diagnostic test results

- Diagnostic testing rules out organic causes of the disorder.

Nursing diagnoses

- Hopelessness
- Impaired social interaction
- Chronic low self-esteem

Treatment

- ECT
- Individual therapy
- Family therapy
- Group therapy
- Phototherapy (seasonal affective disorder)

Drug therapy options

- Monoamine oxidase inhibitors: phenelzine (Nardil), tranylcypromine (Parnate)
- Selective serotonin reuptake inhibitors: paroxetine (Paxil), fluoxetine (Prozac), sertraline (Zoloft)
- Serotonin-norepinephrine reuptake inhibitor: venlafaxine (Effexor)
- Tricyclic antidepressants: amitriptyline (Elavil), desipramine (Norpramin), imipramine (Tofranil)
- Atypical antidepressants: bupropion (Wellbutrin), trazodone (Desyrel)

Planning and goals

- The client will remain safe from suicidal impulses.
- The client will develop a positive attitude about himself, other people, and the future by the time of discharge.
- The client will initiate interactions with peers, staff, and family members by the time of discharge.
- The client will learn to cope with problems, stressors, and losses.

Implementation

- Assess the level and intensity of the client's depression *because baseline information is essential for effective nursing care.*
- Ensure a safe environment for the client *to protect him from self-inflicted harm.*
- Assess the risk for suicide and formulate a safety (no-suicide) contract with the client, as appropriate, *to ensure the client's well-being and to open lines of communication.* A NO-SUICIDE CONTRACT is an agreement stating that the client will seek out a person with whom to talk out suicidal feelings, rather than acting on them.

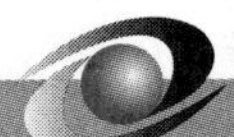

QUICK STUDY

When assessing different aspects of a suicide plan, remember **SLAP**:

Specific details of a plan
Lethality of method
Availability of method
Proximity of help

◆ Reorient the client undergoing ECT as needed; *clients commonly have temporary memory loss after ECT.*
◆ Observe the client for medication compliance and adverse reactions; *without compliance, there's little hope of progress.*
◆ Encourage the client to identify current problems and stressors *so that therapeutic treatment can begin.*
◆ Promote opportunities for increased involvement in activities through a structured, daily program *to help the client feel comfortable with himself and others.*
◆ Select activities that ensure success and accomplishment *to increase self-esteem.*
◆ Help the client modify negative expectations and think more positively *because positive thinking will help him to begin healing.*
◆ Spend time with the client, even if he's too depressed to talk, *to enhance the therapeutic relationship.*
◆ Review key teaching topics with the client and family members *to ensure adequate knowledge about the condition and treatment,* including:
– learning relaxation and sleep methods
– complying with therapy
– avoiding tyramine-containing foods (such as wine, beer, cheeses, preserved fruits, meats, and vegetables) for the client taking monoamine oxidase inhibitors.

Evaluation

◆ The client remains safe.
◆ The client demonstrates positive attitude and interacts spontaneously with staff, peers, and visitors.
◆ The client practices positive coping skills.

OBSESSIVE-COMPULSIVE DISORDER

OBSESSIVE-COMPULSIVE DISORDER is characterized by recurrent OBSESSIONS (intrusive thoughts, images, and impulses) and COMPULSIONS (repetitive behaviors in response to an obsession). The obsessions and compulsions cause intense stress and impair the client's functioning. The client spends a great deal of emotional energy containing his underlying anxiety and maintaining control of himself and life situations. He frequently uses the defense mechanisms of denial, isolation, reaction formation, and undoing. Some clients have simultaneous symptoms of depression.

Fear of losing control and fear of losing the esteem of others are central issues for persons with obsessions and compulsions. Perfectionistic, overly conscientious, and filled with self-doubt, they have trouble being spontaneously emotional because of their intense underlying need to stay "in control" and not make waves. They have intense needs for love, affection, and belonging. (See *Caring for the client with obsessive-compulsive disorder,* page 148.)

Contributing factors

◆ Genetics
◆ Anatomic-physiologic disturbances in brain areas involved with learning or maintaining and acquiring habits
◆ Anxiety-provoking events

Assessment findings

◆ Obsessive thoughts (which may include thoughts of contamination, repeated worries about impending tragedy, and repeating and counting images or words)
◆ Compulsive behavior (which may include repetitive touching or counting, doing and undoing, or any other repetitive activity)
◆ Social impairment
◆ Perceived need to achieve perfection

Diagnostic evaluation

Diagnostic testing rules out organic causes of the disorder.

Nursing diagnoses

◆ Anxiety
◆ Ineffective coping
◆ Chronic low self-esteem

Treatment

◆ Behavioral therapy
◆ Relaxation techniques
◆ Support groups
◆ Partial hospitalization and day treatment programs

Drug therapy options

◆ Benzodiazepines: alprazolam (Xanax), clonazepam (Klonopin), lorazepam (Ativan)
◆ Monoamine oxidase inhibitors: phenelzine (Nardil), tranylcypromine (Parnate)
◆ Selective serotonin reuptake inhibitors: paroxetine (Paxil), fluoxetine (Prozac), fluvoxamine (Luvox), sertraline (Zoloft)
◆ Tricyclic antidepressants: desipramine (Norpramin), imipramine (Tofranil)

Planning and goals

◆ The client will verbalize signs and symptoms of increasing anxiety.

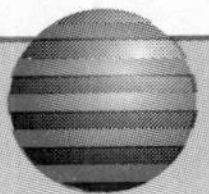

CLINICAL SITUATION

Caring for the client with obsessive-compulsive disorder

Evaluate the clinical situation described here. See if you're able to answer the questions as you go.

A 40-year-old female client is seeing a nurse on an outpatient basis at a community mental health center. Although her colleagues consider her a top-notch travel agent, she seldom feels she has done her job well enough.

For the past 6 weeks, the resulting anxiety has greatly interfered with her ability to eat and sleep. She sleeps only 3 hours at a time and can't eat more than a few bites of food at each meal. She also spends a great deal of time thinking and talking about what she should have done or should be doing. An exceptionally neat person, she spends about 1½ hours each morning dressing and applying makeup. She calls her husband at work throughout the day to make sure he's all right, and she calls the children when they get home from school to check on them. She says she becomes tense when things don't go well or when she has to make spur-of-the-moment changes.

The client tells the nurse she's a super-organized person who easily becomes upset if the house is messy or if her three high-school–age children fail to follow the daily schedule she establishes for them. She came to the mental health clinic because she felt exhausted and believed her life was getting out of control.

The following nursing diagnoses have been established:

- *Anxiety related to fear of losing control of the environment*
- *Disturbed sleep pattern related to the client's underlying anxiety.*

What key points should be established during the client assessment?

- The client's anxiety level and underlying needs, *which allow the nurse to plan appropriate care*
- Identifying obsessive-compulsive behaviors and the types of events in the client's environment that precipitate her obsessive-compulsive behavior, *which will enable the nurse to engage in anticipatory planning with the client to manage her anxiety*
- The client's eating and sleeping patterns, *which indicate the amount of anxiety she's experiencing*
- The client's expectations of her meetings with the nurse and what goals should be set, *which enable the nurse and the client to monitor the client's progress and provide clues about the appropriateness of the client's expectations of herself and others*
- The client's expectations of her family: Does she see family members as autonomous individuals? How does she feel when family members don't behave as she expects? *Answers to these questions help evaluate whether there are inappropriate expectations of others, which can reflect an individual's problems with autonomy and feelings of self-worth.* The obsessive-compulsive client typically feels a great need to control everyone around her and derives her sense of worth from being perfect. For example, she may not be satisfied with the way others do their jobs.

What are appropriate goals to include when planning this client's care?

- The client will verbalize her feelings of anxiety and distress and how they influence her ability to function.
- The client will discuss the unhealthy consequences of her thoughts and actions.
- The client will discuss self-esteem issues or feelings she has about herself.
- The client will develop new coping skills.
- The client will identify factors that precipitate her obsessive--compulsive behavior and plan accordingly.
- The client will relinquish her need to control others.
- The client will sleep for at least 6 hours at a time and feel rested on arising.

- The client will learn coping strategies to decrease obsessive thinking and compulsions.
- The client will develop and maintain enhanced self-esteem and an increased sense of competency.

Implementation

- Encourage the client to express his feelings *to decrease the client's level of stress.*
- Help the client assess how his compulsive behaviors affect his functioning. *The client needs to realistically evaluate the consequences of his behavior.*
- Instruct the client to keep a daily journal of thoughts, feelings, and actions *to identify those that immediately precede the onset of his obsessive-compulsive behavior. A journal helps the obsessive-compulsive client identify anxiety-precipitating factors and can provide a sense of being in control.*

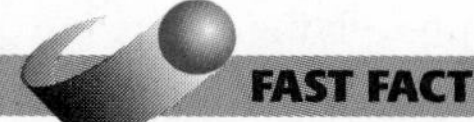

FAST FACT

When caring for a client diagnosed with obsessive-compulsive disorder, remember that compulsions shouldn't be forbidden or interrupted because doing so escalates the client's anxiety.

- Help the client engage in anticipatory planning, *which helps the obsessive-compulsive client feel in control of potentially anxiety-producing situations.*
- Help the client identify expectations of self and others *to avoid unrealistic expectations.* Obsessive-compulsive people typically set themselves up for failure because their unrealistically high expectations make it impossible to accept anything less than perfection in themselves or others.
- Encourage the client to identify situations that produce anxiety and precipitate obsessive-compulsive behavior *to help the client evaluate and cope with his own condition.*
- Work with the client to develop appropriate coping skills, such as response prevention and thought stopping, *to reduce anxiety and interrupt automatic obsessive-compulsive behavior.*
- Review key teaching topics with the client and family members *to ensure adequate knowledge about the condition and treatment,* including understanding anxiety and obsessive-compulsive disorder.

Evaluation

- The client identifies situations and activities that may precipitate obsessive-compulsive behavior.
- The client demonstrates a decreased reliance on negative coping mechanisms, such as rituals, and demonstrates new coping strategies.
- The client is able to verbalize thoughts openly and has realistic expectations of self and others.

PANIC DISORDER

While everyone experiences some level of anxiety, clients with PANIC DISORDER experience a nonspecific feeling of terror and dread, accompanied by symptoms of physiologic stress. Attacks can be unpredictable and paralyzing. Many can't identify trigger events and live in constant fear of having an attack. To avoid public embarrassment, they may refuse to leave home, and may then concurrently develop agoraphobia (fear of public and open places). This level of anxiety makes it difficult, if not impossible, for the client to carry out the normal functions of everyday life.

Contributing factors

- AGORAPHOBIA (fear of being alone or in public places)
- Medical conditions, such as obsructive sleep apnea, mitral valve prolapse, irritable bowel syndrome, chronic fatigue, premenstrual syndrome
- Familial pattern
- Cognitive and behavioral factors
- Autonomic factors
- Failure to resolve childhood conflicts
- Biochemical abnormalities
- Stressful lifestyle

Assessment findings

- Chest pain or pressure
- Sensation of smothering, a lump in the throat, or choking
- Diminished ability to focus, even with direction from others
- Fidgeting or pacing
- Chills, flushing, or pallor
- Generalized weakness or trembling
- Palpitations and tachycardia
- Abdominal discomfort or pain, nausea, heartburn, or diarrhea
- Dizziness, tingling sensation, or lighheadedness
- Rapid, shallow breathing or shortness of breath
- Rapid speech, startle reaction
- Sweating

Diagnostic evaluation

- Diagnostic testing rules out organic causes of the disorder.
- Urine and blood tests are used to check for presence of psychoactive agents.

Nursing diagnoses

- Anxiety
- Ineffective coping
- Powerlessness

Treatment

- Patient teaching
- Cognitive therapy
- Behavioral therapy
- Relaxation techniques

Drug therapy options

- Tricyclic antidepressants: desipramine (Norpramin), imipramine (Tofranil)

◆ Selective serotonin reuptake inhibitors: paroxetine (Paxil), fluoxetine (Prozac), sertraline (Zoloft)
◆ Triazolopyridine derivative: trazodone (Desyrel)
◆ Benzodiazepines: alprazolam (Xanax), lorazepam (Ativan), clonazepam (Klonopin)

Planning and goals

◆ The client will identify life stressors — specific situations, events, or activities that initiate a panic attack — and will be able to identify signs and symptoms of a panic attack.
◆ The client will recognize which situations can and can't be changed and will demonstrate coping skills that can decrease anxiety.

Implementation

◆ During panic attacks, distract the client from the attack *to alleviate the effects of panic.*
◆ Discuss other methods of coping with stress *to make the client aware of alternatives.*
◆ Approach the client calmly and unemotionally *to reduce the risk of further stressing the client.*
◆ Use short, simple sentences *because the client's ability to focus and relate to others is diminished.*
◆ Administer medications as needed *to ensure a therapeutic response.*
◆ Review key teaching topics with the client and family members *to ensure adequate knowledge about the condition and treatment,* including:
– learning decision-making and problem-solving skills
– learning relaxation techniques.

Evaluation

◆ The client can identify situations and activities that initiate a sense of panic.
◆ The client verbalizes the steps needed to manage a panic attack.
◆ The client has less anxiety and verbalizes a feeling of increased control.

PHOBIAS

A PHOBIA is an irrational fear of something that, in reality, can cause little, if any, harm. It's a fear that persists, even though the client recognizes its irrationality. Phobias may be social, such as performance-related phobias, or simple, such as a fear of dogs, water, or blood.

A phobia develops when anxiety about an entity or a situation compels the client to avoid it. Forced contact with the phobic object or situation may precipitate panic. Persons experiencing phobias have underlying needs for love, affection, and belonging.

Phobias become problems if they expand or if the object can't be successfully avoided. When expansion or contact occurs, the person's ability to meet daily commitments is impaired. Phobias are resistant to insight-oriented therapies. Behavioral techniques, such as desensitization and distraction, have provided relief for clients with phobias.

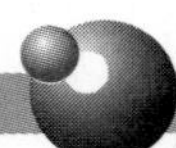

SPOT CHECK

Name two types of behavioral therapy that are effective in the treatment of phobias.

Two types of behavioral therapy that are effective in the treatment of phobias are:
- desensitization
- distraction.

Contributing factors

◆ Biochemical imbalance involving neurotransmitters
◆ Familial patterns
◆ Environmental factors

Assessment findings

◆ Panic when confronted with the feared situation or entity
◆ Persistent fear of specific things, places, or situations
◆ Displacement (shifting of emotions from their original object) and symbolization
◆ Disruption of social life or work life

Diagnostic evaluation

◆ No specific test is used to diagnose phobias.

Nursing diagnoses

◆ Anxiety
◆ Fear
◆ Powerlessness

Treatment

◆ Distraction techniques
◆ Relaxation techniques
◆ Systematic desensitization

Drug therapy options

◆ Benzodiazepines: alprazolam (Xanax), clonazepam (Klonopin), lorazepam (Ativan)
◆ Selective serotonin reuptake inhibitor: paroxetine (Paxil)
◆ Tricyclic antidepressant: amitriptyline (Elavil)

Planning and goals
◆ The client will become desensitized to the phobic entity or situation.
◆ The client will discuss fears and anxiety related to the phobic entity or situation.

Implementation
◆ Collaborate with the client to identify the feared entity or situation *to develop an effective treatment plan.*
◆ Assist in desensitizing the client *to diminish the client's fear.*
◆ Remind the client about resources and personal strengths *to build self-esteem.*
◆ Review key teaching topics with the client and family members *to ensure adequate knowledge about the condition and treatment,* including:
– learning assertiveness techniques
– learning relaxation techniques
– participating in the desensitizing process.

Evaluation
◆ The client identifies situations, activities, or entities that increase his anxiety level.
◆ The client verbalizes signs and symptoms of increasing anxiety.
◆ The client engages in desensitization activities and exhibits decreased symptoms of anxiety.

POSTTRAUMATIC STRESS DISORDER
POSTTRAUMATIC STRESS DISORDER (PTSD) is a group of symptoms that develop after a traumatic event. This traumatic event may involve death, injury, witnessing an event that results in serious injury or death of another person, or a threat to physical integrity. In PTSD, ordinary coping behaviors fail to relieve the anxiety. The client may experience reactions that are acute, chronic, or delayed.

Acute PTSD resolves spontaneously; chronic or delayed PTSD requires intervention. The nurse plays an essential role in assessing the client with PTSD and in making appropriate referrals. Regardless of the cause, a crucial component of intervention is encouraging the client to express and share emotions associated with the trauma.

Contributing factors
◆ Biochemical predisposition
◆ High anxiety
◆ History of psychiatric disorder
◆ Limited social support
◆ Low self-esteem
◆ Neurotic and extraverted characteristics
◆ Traumatic event

Assessment findings
◆ Anger, self-hatred
◆ Anxiety, depression
◆ Avoidance of people involved in the trauma
◆ Avoidance of places where the trauma occurred
◆ Chronic tension, intrusive thoughts
◆ Detachment, emotional numbness
◆ Difficulty concentrating, hyperalertness
◆ Difficulty falling or staying asleep
◆ Flashbacks of the traumatic experience
◆ Hopelessness
◆ Inability to recall details of the traumatic event
◆ Labile affect (rapid, easily changing expression)
◆ Nightmares about the traumatic experience
◆ Poor impulse control
◆ Relationship problems
◆ Social withdrawal
◆ Survivor guilt

Diagnostic evaluation
◆ No specific tests identify or confirm PTSD.

Nursing diagnoses
◆ Posttrauma syndrome
◆ Powerlessness
◆ Chronic low self-esteem

Treatment
◆ Alcohol and drug rehabilitation, when indicated
◆ Individual therapy
◆ Interoceptive exposure
◆ Group therapy
◆ Progressive relaxation
◆ Systematic desensitization

Drug treatment options
◆ Benzodiazepines: alprazolam (Xanax), clonazepam (Klonopin), lorazepam (Ativan)
◆ Beta-adrenergic blocker: propranolol (Inderal)
◆ Monoamine oxidase inhibitors: phenelzine (Nardil), tranylcypromine (Parnate)
◆ Selective serotonin reuptake inhibitors: paroxetine (Paxil), sertraline (Zoloft)
◆ Tricyclic antidepressants: amitriptyline (Elavil), imipramine (Tofranil)

Planning and goals
◆ The client will discuss the traumatic event and feelings related to it.

◆ The client will experience less anxiety with intrusive thoughts and memories.
◆ The client will regain control over feelings, behaviors, and symptoms related to PTSD.
◆ The client will have enhanced self-esteem and an increased ability to handle frustrations and problems.

Implementation

◆ Work with the client to identify stressors *to initiate effective coping.*
◆ Provide for client safety *because the client's ineffective coping, coupled with the intensity of the reaction and poor impulse control, increases the client's risk of injury.*
◆ Encourage the client to explore the traumatic event and the meaning of the event *to promote effective coping.*

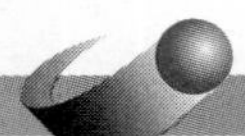

FAST FACT

The client with PTSD must acknowledge the experience and his feelings or he won't be able to gain cognitive mastery over them. Through active listening, the nurse can help the client gain objectivity.

◆ Assist the client with problem solving and resolving guilt to help the client understand that chance probably played a larger part in the trauma than his personal actions, decisions, or inactions.
◆ Review key teaching topics with the client and family members *to ensure adequate knowledge about the condition and treatment,* including:
- information about PTSD
- joining support groups
- learning relaxation techniques
- promoting social interaction.

Evaluation

◆ The client acknowledges his experience and feelings and verbalizes less anxiety regarding intrusive thoughts and memories.
◆ The client reports a sense of control over feelings and behaviors and exhibits the ability to manage emotional reactions.
◆ The client verbalizes positive statements regarding self.

COGNITIVE DISORDERS

COGNITIVE DISORDERS result from any condition that alters or destroys brain tissue and, in turn, impairs cerebral functioning. Symptoms include cognitive impairment, behavioral dysfunction, and personality changes.

Cognitive mental disorders are characterized by the disruption of cognitive functioning. Clinically, they manifest as mental deficits in clients who had not previously exhibited such deficits.

Cognitive disorders are difficult to identify and treat. The key to diagnosis lies in the discovery of an organic problem with the brain's tissue. They may result from:
◆ primary brain disease
◆ brain's response to a systemic disturbance such as a medical condition
◆ brain tissue's reaction to a toxic substance (as in substance abuse).

The most common symptomatology identified by the *Diagnostic and Statistical Manual of Mental Disorder,* 4th edition, Text Revision are delirium and dementia disorders.

ALZHEIMER'S TYPE DEMENTIA

A client with ALZHEIMER'S TYPE DEMENTIA suffers a global impairment of cognitive functioning, memory, and personality. The dementia occurs gradually, but with continuous decline. Damage from Alzheimer's type dementia is irreversible. Because it's difficult to obtain direct pathological evidence of Alzheimer's disease, the diagnosis can be made only when other causes of the dementia have been eliminated.

Contributing factors

◆ Genetics
◆ Altered immune function, with autoantibody production in the brain
◆ Increased brain atrophy, with wider sulci and cerebral ventricles than that seen in normal aging
◆ Neurofibrillary tangles and beta-amyloid neuritic plaques, mainly in the frontal and temporal lobes

Assessment findings

Alzheimer's type dementia has three identifiable stages. In stage I, look for:
◆ decline in recent memory, inability to retain new memories
◆ decreased concentration
◆ disorientation regarding time
◆ decline in personal appearance
◆ agitated or apathetic mood
◆ depression
◆ attempts to cover up symptoms
◆ disturbed sleep
◆ susceptibility to falls

Key nursing considerations in Alzheimer's disease

Alzheimer's disease has an insidious onset. At first, changes are barely perceptible, but they gradually lead to serious problems. This table provides some key interventions the nurse can perform to assist the client and caregiver as the symptoms of this disease progress.

SIGNS AND SYMPTOMS	NURSING CONSIDERATIONS
◆ Forgetfulness	◆ Provide support for the client concerned about forgetfulness to reduce stress and promote independence. ◆ Encourage the client to discuss feelings with family members to reduce stress.
◆ Noticeable changes in mental status and personal appearance ◆ Attempts to hide symptoms ◆ Decreased recall of current events ◆ Difficulty performing job ◆ History of wandering, getting lost	◆ Encourage the client to verbalize feelings about deteriorating status to promote coping skills. ◆ Discuss ways to help the client function at work and at home, such as writing notes to herself to promote independence. ◆ As condition progresses, encourage the client's caregiver to allow the client to perform simple household tasks, as tolerated, as her condition declines to promote independence.
◆ Decreasing ability to understand or use language ◆ Inability to complete activities of daily living ◆ Difficulty recognizing family members, gaps in memory ◆ Socially unacceptable behavior	◆ Instruct the caregiver to keep the demands on the client to a minimum to decrease stress. ◆ Encourage the caregiver to set up a daily routine that meets the caregiver's and the client's needs to promote continuity and reduce anxiety. ◆ Discuss the need to provide observation with the caregiver to promote client safety and decrease wandering episodes. ◆ Discuss the availability of local support groups with the client's caregiver and ways for the caregiver to get some relief (such as consulting a home health care agency and family members) to assist in family coping. ◆ Support the caregiver's decisions regarding the care and placement of the client to promote coping.
◆ Decreased response to stimuli ◆ Deterioration in motor ability ◆ Nonresponsiveness	◆ Perform skin care and range-of-motion exercises if the client is bedridden to prevent complications. ◆ Assist with other aspects of the client's care (such as elimination), as the client's condition warrants to promote self-worth. ◆ Allow the caregiver to verbalize feelings and grieve for the client to enable coping.

◆ wandering
◆ transitory delusions of persecution.

In stage II, look for:

◆ inability to retain new information
◆ diminishing ability to understand or use language
◆ disorientation to person, place, and time
◆ confabulation (unconscious filling of gaps in memory with fabricated facts and experiences)
◆ inability to recognize family members
◆ continuous, repetitive behaviors
◆ socially unacceptable behavior
◆ tantrums
◆ increased appetite with no weight gain
◆ requiring assistance with activities of daily living
◆ hoarding
◆ bowel and bladder incontinence.

In stage III, look for:

◆ severe decline in cognitive functioning
◆ compulsive touching and examination of objects
◆ deterioration in motor ability
◆ emaciation
◆ decreased response to stimuli
◆ nonresponsiveness.

(See *Key nursing considerations in Alzheimer's disease.*)

Diagnostic evaluation

◆ Cognitive assessment scale demonstrates cognitive impairment.
◆ Functional dementia scale shows degree of dementia.

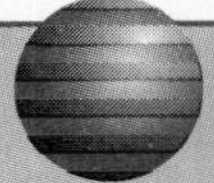

CLINICAL SITUATION

Caring for the client with Alzheimer's disease

Evaluate the clinical situation described here. See if you're able to answer the questions as you go.

A 65-year-old female lives at home with her husband; their four children are grown. A florist, the client owns her business. During the past year, her husband relates, she has become forgetful and absent-minded and has had occasional outbursts of anger, which are atypical for her.

One month ago, the client started withdrawing from social activities and began refusing to go to the florist shop. She said she was tired and didn't need to waste her time in meaningless activities. Her husband has noticed that she frequently misidentifies people, doesn't remember simple things unless prompted, makes up stories about events, and rarely uses people's names. Sometimes at night the client becomes agitated and wanders around the house. If the client's husband asks what she's doing, the client tells him it's none of his business. The client has been diagnosed with Alzheimer's type dementia.

The client's husband has decided that his wife will remain at home until he can no longer care for her, but he confided to the office nurse that he feels inadequate to care for his wife because he knows so little about her illness. A referral to a visiting nurse association has been made.

After the initial assessment, these nursing diagnoses were established:

- Risk for injury related to impaired cognition
- Anticipatory grieving related to loss of ability to function
- Interrupted family processes related to role changes necessitated by the client's condition

What are appropriate interventions the nurse can implement for this client and caregiver?

- Initiate health assessments by the visiting nurse every 3 weeks. A 3-week interval between home visits is long enough *to allow observable changes to develop yet short enough to prevent the client and her husband from feeling abandoned.*
- Have the client's husband establish a daily routine for the client, *which can help preserve the client's memory function so she stays reality-oriented and functional.*
- Label and color-code any objects that the client has difficulty identifying, *which can help the client use it appropriately and avoid confusion.*
- Ensure that someone is available to help the client with grocery lists, cleaning, and other home tasks *to promote healthy functioning and enhance the client's self-esteem.*
- Write down the client's routines and procedures, put a large clock in a prominent spot, and hang signs showing the day and date to help the client stay reality-oriented and functional.
- Give the client's husband the name and telephone number of an Alzheimer's support group. *A support group can help the client's husband mourn his loss and decrease his burden and sense of loneliness. The group will also provide him with valuable information about Alzheimer's disease and suggestions for managing his wife's care.*
- Teach the client's husband the predictable progression of Alzheimer's disease *to allow him to make sound decisions about disease management.*
- Help the client's husband identify areas where he needs assistance in managing his wife at home, such as respite care, meal preparation, and toileting, *to reduce the husband's anxiety and enhance his ability to remain in control of the situation.*
- Write down at least three options for each problem identified that gives the client's spouse a sense of being in control rather than feeling trapped or limited.
- Give the client's husband information about community resources available to help him, such as weekend respite care, day care for persons with Alzheimer's disease, and home health aide services. *Community resources can help the client's spouse manage care so that the client need not enter an extended-care facility until the late stage of her illness.*

Questions for further thought

- What type of communication skills would be helpful when the nurse makes her home visits?
- How can the nurse evaluate whether the client's husband is engaging in anticipatory problem-solving to meet the client's needs?

- Magnetic resonance imaging (MRI) shows apparent structural and neurologic changes.
- Mini–Mental Status Examination reveals disorientation and cognitive impairment.
- Spinal fluid contains increased beta amyloid.

Nursing diagnoses

- Impaired memory
- Bathing or hygiene self-care deficit
- Caregiver role strain (See *Caring for the client with Alzheimer's disease.*)

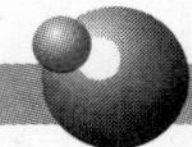

SPOT CHECK

During what stage of Alzheimer's type dementia does confabulation occur?

Answer: Confabulation occurs during stage 2.

During what stage does a decrease in recent memory occur?

Answer: Decrease in recent memory occurs during stage 1.

Treatment

- Psychotherapy
- Hyperbaric oxygen treatment
- Palliative medical treatment
- Tissue transplantation (currently being studied)

Drug therapy options

- Anticholinesterase agents: donepezil (Aricept), tacrine (Cognex), rivastigmine (Exelon), galantamine (Reminyl)
- Antipsychotic agents: haloperidol (Haldol), risperidone (Risperdal) in low doses
- Benzodiazepine: alprazolam (Xanax)
- N-methyl-D-aspartate inhibitor: memantine (Namenda)

Planning and goals

- The client will maintain the ability to engage in familiar activities and to meet personal safety needs and hygiene and grooming needs as long as possible.
- The caregiver will take steps to help preserve the client's memory as long as possible.
- The caregiver will seek out information about Alzheimer's type dementia and engage in healthy grieving about the significant other's illness.

Implementation

- Remove any hazardous items or potential obstacles from the client's environment *to maintain a safe environment for the client.*
- Monitor food and fluid intake *because the client may not take in enough nutrition.*
- Provide verbal and nonverbal communication that's consistent and structured *to prevent added confusion.*
- State expectations simply and completely *to orient the client.*
- Increase social interaction *to provide stimuli for the client.*
- Encourage the use of community resources; make appropriate referrals as necessary *to find outside support for caregivers.*
- Promote physical activity and sensory stimulation *to alleviate symptoms of the disorder.*
- Review key teaching topics with the client and family members *to ensure adequate knowledge about the condition and treatment,* including:
  - finding support and education (for caregivers)
  - learning stress-relief techniques (for caregivers).

Evaluation

- The client demonstrates ability to meet physical, safety, and hygiene needs with minimal assistance.
- The caregiver relates steps taken to help promote the client's memory.
- The caregiver joins an Alzheimer's disease support group.
- The caregiver maintains his social network and uses family and community resources for help when needed.
- The caregiver copes with the client's ongoing deterioration of health and loss of self-care ability.

DELIRIUM

DELIRIUM is a disturbance of consciousness accompanied by a change in cognition that can't be attributed to preexisting dementia. It's characterized by an acute onset and may last from hours to a number of days. It's potentially reversible but can be life-threatening if not treated.

Contributing factors

- Cerebral hypoxia
- Effects of medication
- Fever
- Fluid and electrolyte imbalances
- Infection (especially of the urinary tract and upper respiratory system)
- Metabolic disorders
- Multiple drug use, especially anticholinergics
- Neurotransmitter imbalance
- Pain
- Sensory overload or deprivation
- Sleep deprivation
- Stress
- Substance intoxication

Assessment findings

- Attention disturbance, distractibility
- Impaired decision making
- Disorganized thinking
- Disorientation (especially to time and place)
- Visual and auditory illusions
- Inability to complete tasks or recall events
- Insomnia or daytime sleepiness

◆ Altered psychomotor activity, such as apathy, withdrawal, and agitation
◆ Altered respiratory depth or rhythm
◆ Poor impulse control
◆ Rambling or incoherent speech
◆ Bizarre behavior, worsening at night

Diagnostic evaluation

◆ Laboratory results indicate that the delirium is a result of a physiologic condition, intoxication, substance withdrawal, toxic exposure, prescribed medicines, or a combination of these factors.

Nursing diagnoses

◆ Risk for injury
◆ Impaired verbal communication
◆ Sensory or perceptual alterations

Treatment

◆ Correction of underlying physiologic problem
◆ Individual therapy

Drug therapy options

◆ Benzodiazepine: low-dose lorazepam (Ativan)
◆ Antipsychotic agent: haloperidol (Haldol)

Planning and goals

◆ The client will remain free from injury and have a safe environment.
◆ The client will have minimal anxiety over misperceptions about care and environment.

Implementation

◆ Determine the degree of cognitive impairment *to understand and treat the client.*
◆ Create a structured and safe environment *to prevent self-harm.*
◆ Institute measures to help the client relax and fall asleep *to comfort the client.*
◆ Keep room lit to allay the client's fears and prevent visual hallucinations.
◆ Monitor effects of medications *to prevent exacerbating symptoms.*

Evaluation

◆ The client remains free from injury.
◆ The client demonstrates calm behavior regardless of cognitive impairment.

VASCULAR DEMENTIA

Also called *multi-infarct dementia,* VASCULAR DEMENTIA impairs the client's cognitive functioning, memory, and personality but doesn't affect the client's level of consciousness. It's caused by an irreversible alteration in brain function that damages or destroys brain tissue.

Contributing factors

◆ Cerebral emboli or thrombosis
◆ Diabetes
◆ Heart disease
◆ High cholesterol level
◆ Hypertension (leading to stroke)
◆ Transient ischemic attacks

Assessment findings

◆ Confusion
◆ Depression
◆ Difficulty following instructions
◆ Dizziness
◆ Emotional lability
◆ Inappropriate emotional reactions
◆ Less of bowel or bladder control
◆ Neurologic symptoms that last only a few days
◆ Problems handling money
◆ Problems with recent memory
◆ Rapid onset of symptoms
◆ Slurred speech
◆ Wandering and getting lost in familiar places
◆ Weakness in an extremity

Diagnostic evaluation

◆ Cognitive assessment scale shows deterioration in cognitive ability.
◆ Global deterioration scale signifies degenerative dementia.
◆ Mini–Mental Status Examination reveals disorientation and recall difficulty.
◆ Structural and neurologic changes can be seen on MRI or computed tomography scans.

Nursing diagnoses

◆ Disturbed thought processes
◆ Impaired memory
◆ Risk for injury

Treatment

◆ Carotid endarterectomy to remove blockages in the carotid artery
◆ Dietary interventions
◆ Smoking cessation

◆ Treatment for the underlying condition (hypertension, high cholesterol, or diabetes)

Drug therapy options

◆ Aspirin or ticlodipine (Ticlid) to decrease platelet aggregation and prevent clots

Planning and goals

◆ The client will have decreased deterioration in thought processes after treatment is initiated.
◆ The client will remain free from injury.
◆ The client will establish realistic goals to deal with memory loss.

Implementation

◆ Orient the client to his surroundings *to alleviate anxiety.*
◆ Monitor the environment *to prevent overstimulation.*
◆ Encourage the client to express feelings of sadness and loss *to foster a healthy therapeutic environment.*

Evaluation

◆ The client's health and safety status is maintained.
◆ The client describes plans to modify lifestyle and mechanisms for coping with memory loss.

ATTENTION DEFICIT AND DISRUPTIVE BEHAVIOR DISORDERS

Attention deficit and disruptive behavior disorders can manifest in various settings, such as in the home, school, work, and social settings. One of the major neurologic disorders in pediatric patients is ATTENTION DEFICIT HYPERACTIVITY DISORDER (ADHD).

ATTENTION DEFICIT HYPERACTIVITY DISORDER

ADHD was previously called *attention deficit disorder.* The child with ADHD displays long-term behaviors of hyperactivity, impulsiveness, and inattention. These behaviors occur in all facets of the child's life and frequently worsen when sustained attention is required. When a child is involved in an activity for a long time or one in which sustained attention is required, the symptoms are exacerbated. Males are affected by this disorder more commonly than females.

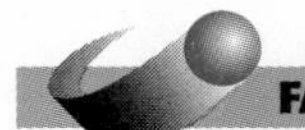

FAST FACT

The symptoms of ADHD are commonly determined when the child has difficulty adjusting to elementary school, a time when symptoms are likely to manifest.

Unless identified and treated properly, ADHD may progress to conduct disorder, academic and job failure, depression, relationship problems, and substance abuse.

Chaotic family life and parents who struggle with their parenting skills are factors that accentuate the difficulties of a child with ADHD.

Contributing factors

◆ Genetics
◆ Drug exposure in utero
◆ Birth complications (toxemia, hypoxia, head trauma)
◆ Low birth weight
◆ Preexisting neurologic conditions (cerebral palsy, epilepsy)
◆ Lead poisoning
◆ Multiple stressful events
◆ Child abuse

Assessment findings

◆ Inattention
- short attention span
- seeming not to listen
- difficulty keeping mind on one thing
- bored easily
- failure to finish tasks or instructions
- difficulty organizing tasks

◆ Impulsiveness
- acting before thinking
- interrupting others
- difficulty waiting in line for turn

◆ Hyperactivity
- inability to sit still
- trying to do several things at once
- in school, fidgeting, roaming around room, or talking excessively
- difficulty engaging in quiet activity and sitting through a class
- tapping pencil incessantly, wiggling feet, or touching everything

Diagnostic evaluation

◆ Complete psychological, medical, and neurologic evaluations rule out other problems, such as epilepsy, lead poisoning, and preexisting conditions such as child abuse.
◆ To diagnose ADHD, the findings are combined with data from several sources, including parents, teachers, and the child.

Nursing diagnoses

◆ Impaired social interaction
◆ Ineffective coping
◆ Risk for injury
◆ Risk for impaired parenting

Treatment

◆ Behavioral modifications
◆ Individual and family therapy
◆ Interdisciplinary interventions, including individualized educational plan

Drug therapy options

◆ Amphetamine: methylphenidate (Ritalin), to ease inattention, impulsiveness, and hyperactivity
◆ Selective norepinephrine reuptake inhibitor: atomoxetine (Strattera)

Planning and goals

◆ The client will learn new coping skills, acknowledge strengths, and demonstrate beginning social skills.
◆ The client and family members will learn strategies to assist the child in coping with the condition.

Implementation

◆ Monitor growth. *If the child is receiving methylphenidate, growth may be slowed.*
◆ Give one simple instruction at a time so the child can successfully complete the task, *which promotes self-esteem.*
◆ Give medications in the morning and at lunch *to avoid interfering with sleep.*
◆ Ensure adequate nutrition; *medications and hyperactivity may cause increased nutrient needs.*
◆ Reduce environmental stimuli *to decrease distraction.*
◆ Formulate a schedule for the child *to provide consistency and routine.*
◆ Develop situations and assist the child in performing all the steps necessary to complete a task without getting distracted *to allow the child to feel good and to set the stage for continued successful behaviors.*
◆ Teach the child strategies to get along with other children without taking on the role of class clown. *By knowing the correct ways of behaving and interacting with peers, the client doesn't have to resort to attention-seeking behaviors.*
◆ Encourage the child to identify strengths *to enhance self-esteem.*
◆ Give positive reinforcement for the child's attempts to change negative behavior, *which contributes to the child's desire and motivation to change disruptive behaviors.*
◆ Teach family members how to avoid overstimulation of the child to handle disruptive behaviors, *which permits the family to cope and handle problematic situations in an effective manner.*
◆ Discuss the family's method of disciplining the child *to establish a framework for reinforcing positive strategies already being used and to teach additional disciplinary techniques.*
◆ Review key teaching topics with the client and family members *to ensure adequate knowledge about the condition and treatment,* including:
– allowing the child to expend energy after being in restrictive environments such as school
– monitoring for adverse reactions to medications
– structuring learning to minimize distractions
– taking breaks from caregiving to avoid strain
– teaching important material in the morning (when medication levels peak).

Evaluation

◆ The client participates in healthy interactions with peers.
◆ The client practices effective coping skills.
◆ The client's family members verbalize understanding of the child's diagnosis and the child's strengths and learn how to effectively handle their child.

PERSONALITY DISORDERS

Clients with personality disorders control anxiety by adopting behavior patterns that interfere with their ability to adapt to daily stressors and establish healthy relationships. Personality disorders fall into three major groups:
◆ Cluster A — odd or eccentric behavior
◆ Cluster B — dramatic, emotional, or erratic behavior
◆ Cluster C — anxious or fearful behavior.

In this section, you'll find an overview of the disorders that fall within each cluster as well as an example from each group. (See *Personality disorders.*)

Personality disorders

Personality disorders fall into three groups, or clusters, as shown in this chart. Clients with cluster A personality disorders are characteristically aloof and restrained in relationships; others may describe them as odd or strange. Clients with cluster B disorders typically are dramatic, unrestrained, and unpredictable. Those with cluster C disorders are overly apprehensive about the present and future, and worry about failing.

PERSONALITY DISORDER	CLIENT DESCRIPTION
Cluster A	
Paranoid personality disorder	◆ Uses projection ◆ Is extremely suspicious of others' motives ◆ Is very guarded in relationships and finds hidden meanings ◆ Is very private ◆ Expects to be exploited or harmed by others ◆ Questions others' loyalty ◆ Reads hidden meaning into harmless remarks or events ◆ Doesn't forgive slights, insults, or injuries
Schizoid personality disorder	◆ Is emotionally cold and detached ◆ Is withdrawn and controlled ◆ Can't form warm, spontaneous relationships ◆ Usually lives alone or in parents' home ◆ Has little need for friendships or intimacy ◆ Has a solitary lifestyle ◆ Seems indifferent to praise or criticism
Schizotypal personality disorder	◆ Has some cognitive and perceptual distortion ◆ May be viewed as odd or eccentric in speech and behavior ◆ Has poorly developed social skills ◆ Has strained and uncomfortable relationships ◆ Is easily overwhelmed by too much social or interpersonal stimuli
Cluster B	
Antisocial personality disorder	◆ Is aggressive and impulsive ◆ Acts out conflicts within social contexts ◆ Has no regard for rules and norms ◆ Lacks remorse ◆ Takes no responsibility for outcomes of own behavior ◆ Blames others when things go wrong ◆ Believes others are unreliable ◆ Must have immediate gratification ◆ Disregards the truth ◆ Has a poor work history ◆ Can't sustain a monogamous relationship
Borderline personality disorder	◆ Has a poorly developed sense of self and is easily influenced by other people ◆ Struggles with overwhelming feelings of anger and anxiety ◆ Views situations in extremes (all good or all bad) ◆ Has intense fear of abandonment ◆ Feels empty and devoid of substance ◆ Needs others around to maintain a sense of self (you + me = self)

(continued)

Personality disorders *(continued)*

PERSONALITY DISORDER	CLIENT DESCRIPTION
Histrionic personality disorder	◆ Controls anxiety through dramatic presentation of self ◆ Uses attention-seeking behaviors and flattery to get others to meet needs ◆ Is overly concerned with physical attractiveness ◆ Can't tolerate delayed gratification ◆ Has a seductive appearance or engages in seductive behavior ◆ Becomes anxious when limits are placed on attention-seeking behaviors
Narcissistic personality disorder	◆ Can't empathize with others because of intense need for love and admiration ◆ Demands much time and attention from others ◆ Feels entitled or special ◆ Is arrogant, haughty, and envious ◆ Expects to be recognized as superior without commensurate achievements
Cluster C	
Avoidant personality disorder	◆ Remains aloof in relationships ◆ Wants friendships but can form them only if assured of not getting hurt or shamed ◆ Doesn't like surprises ◆ Is preoccupied with fear of being criticized or rejected in social situations ◆ Feels inferior to others
Dependent personality disorder	◆ Is unable to be assertive ◆ Remains in abusive situations ◆ Falls apart if significant other leaves or dies ◆ Doesn't trust own judgment ◆ Feels incapable of managing on own ◆ Needs excessive reassurance and advice ◆ Lacks self-confidence ◆ Will go to extremes to get nurturing from others
Obsessive-compulsive personality disorder	◆ Controls anxiety through extreme orderliness, cleanliness, and punctuality ◆ Needs to be in control ◆ Is excessively devoted to work and productivity ◆ Is overly conscientious ◆ Is unable to discard worn or useless objects ◆ Is reluctant to delegate tasks to others ◆ Hoards supplies for future catastrophes

BORDERLINE PERSONALITY DISORDER

BORDERLINE PERSONALITY DISORDER results in a pattern of instability in a person's mood, interpersonal relationships, self-esteem, self-identity, behavior, and cognition. Impulsiveness is the most prominent characteristic of this disorder, and the disorder appears to originate in early childhood.

Most clients with personality disorders are treated as outpatients. However, those with borderline personality disorder may be hospitalized after a self-destructive act, such as a suicide attempt. Typically, clients with borderline personality disorder attempt suicide when feeling abandoned; their goal is to get others to take care of them.

Contributing factors

◆ Abuse, neglect, or separation
◆ Chronic trauma or long-term stressors
◆ Deficiencies in the ego and superego development
◆ Developmental challenges of adolescence
◆ Genetics: biologic basis of brain function and personality structure affected

Assessment findings

◆ Inability to maintain relationships
◆ Inability to develop a healthy sense of self
◆ Compulsive behavior
◆ Destructive behavior
◆ Emotional reactions, with few coping skills
◆ Dissociation (separating objects from their emotional significance)
◆ Dysfunctional lifestyle
◆ High self-expectations
◆ Impulsive behavior
◆ Extreme fear of abandonment
◆ Moodiness
◆ Self-directed anger
◆ Paranoid ideation
◆ Self-mutilation
◆ Shame
◆ Suicidal behavior
◆ View of others as extremely good or bad

Diagnostic evaluation

◆ Standard psychological tests reveal a high degree of dissociation.

Nursing diagnoses

◆ Impaired social interaction
◆ Risk for self-directed violence
◆ Chronic low self-esteem

Treatment

◆ Alcohol and drug rehabilitation, as indicated
◆ Milieu therapy
◆ Group therapy
◆ Family therapy
◆ Individual therapy

Drug therapy options

◆ Antianxiety agent: buspirone (BuSpar)
◆ Antimanic agents: carbamazepine (Tegretol), lithium carbonate (Eskalith)
◆ Antipsychotic agent: haloperidol (Haldol)
◆ Monoamine oxidase inhibitor: phenelzine (Nardil)
◆ Selective serotonin reuptake inhibitors: paroxetine (Paxil), sertraline (Zoloft)

Planning and goals

◆ The client will learn how to process experiences before and after taking action.
◆ The client will refrain from self-destructive behaviors or destructive behavior toward others.
◆ The client will learn new coping skills.

Implementation

◆ Recognize behaviors that the client uses to manipulate others *to avoid unconsciously reinforcing these behaviors.*
◆ Set appropriate expectations for social interaction, and praise the client when these expectations are met *to create a healthy therapeutic environment.*
◆ Teach the client how to engage in anticipatory planning *to aid in the development of new coping skills.*
◆ Respect the client's sense of personal space *to increase trust.*
◆ Review key teaching topics with the client and family members *to ensure adequate knowledge about the condition and treatment,* including:
– developing problem-solving skills
– developing therapeutic communication skills
– implementing relaxation techniques.

Evaluation

◆ The client exhibits the ability to see how his behavior affects others.
◆ The client develops new coping skills, which can provide a sense of empowerment and improve self-esteem.
◆ The client exhibits the ability to identify and plan for situations that precipitate acting out.
◆ The client doesn't exhibit behavior that's harmful to himself or others.

DEPENDENT PERSONALITY DISORDER

The client with DEPENDENT PERSONALITY DISORDER experiences an extreme need to be taken care of that leads to submissive, clinging behavior and fear of separation. This pattern begins by early adulthood, when behaviors designed to elicit caring from others become predominant. These behaviors arise from the client's perception that he's unable to function adequately without others.

Contributing factors

◆ Childhood physical or sexual abuse

◆ Childhood traumas
◆ Closed family system that discourages relationships with others
◆ Genetic predisposition
◆ Social isolation

Assessment findings
◆ Clinging, demanding behavior
◆ Exaggerated fear of losing support and approval
◆ Fear and anxiety about losing the people he's dependent upon
◆ Hypersensitivity to criticism, potential rejection, and decision making
◆ Indirect resistance to occupational and social performance
◆ Low self-esteem
◆ Tendency to be passive (lack of initiative) and submissive

Diagnostic evaluation
◆ Laboratory tests rule out underlying medical conditions.

Nursing diagnoses
◆ Interrupted family processes
◆ Ineffective coping
◆ Chronic low self-esteem

Treatment
◆ Behavior modification through assertiveness training
◆ Individual therapy
◆ Self-help support groups

Drug therapy options
◆ Benzodiazepines: alprazolam (Xanax), lorazepam (Ativan), clonazepam (Klonopin)
◆ Monoamine oxidase inhibitor: phenelzine (Nardil)
◆ Selective serotonin reuptake inhibitor: paroxetine (Paxil)
◆ Tricyclic antidepressants: desipramine (Norpramin), imipramine (Tofranil)

Planning and goals
◆ The client and family members will learn strategies to promote growth, role flexibility, and healthy relationships.
◆ The client will learn new adaptive coping strategies.

Implementation
◆ Encourage activities that require decision making (balancing a checkbook, planning meals, paying bills) *to promote independence.*
◆ Help the client establish and work toward goals *to foster a sense of independence.*
◆ Help the client identify manipulative behaviors, focusing on specific examples, *to decrease the perception that others are an extension of the self.*
◆ Limit interactions with the client to a few consistent staff members *to increase the client's sense of security.*
◆ Help the client and family members identify role and function changes *to help develop healthier family relationships by promoting cooperation among members while allowing for individualization.*
◆ Review key teaching topics with the client and family members *to ensure adequate knowledge about the condition and treatment,* including:
– expressing ideas and feelings assertively
– improving social skills and promoting social interaction.

Evaluation
◆ The client is able to demonstrate problem-solving and decision-making skills to manage anxiety and promote feelings of self-worth.
◆ The client and family members specify areas requiring change.
◆ The client verbalizes decreased anxiety when involved in a social gathering.

PARANOID PERSONALITY DISORDER
PARANOID PERSONALITY DISORDER is characterized by extreme distrust of others. Paranoid people avoid relationships in which they aren't in control or have the potential of losing control.

Contributing factors
◆ Genetic predisposition
◆ Negative childhood experiences
◆ Threatening domestic atmosphere

Assessment findings
◆ Bad temper, hyperactivity, and irritability
◆ Hypersensitivity
◆ Hypervigilance
◆ Inability to collaborate with others
◆ Jealousy, anger, or envy
◆ Lack of humor
◆ Lack of social support systems
◆ Need to be in control
◆ Poor self-image
◆ Refusal to confide in others
◆ Self-righteousness

◆ Social isolation
◆ Sullen attitude, hostility, coldness, and detachment

Diagnostic evaluation

◆ There are no specific diagnostic tests for paranoid personality disorder.

Nursing diagnoses

◆ Anxiety
◆ Ineffective coping
◆ Chronic low self-esteem
◆ Social isolation

Treatment

◆ Individual therapy

Drug therapy options

◆ Antipsychotic agents: olanzapine (Zyprexa), risperidone (Risperdal)
◆ Selected serotonin reuptake inhibitor: sertraline (Zoloft)

Planning and goals

◆ The client will identify feelings that impede social interaction.
◆ The client will learn new coping skills to decrease anxiety during social interactions.
◆ The client will feel safe about changing behaviors when coping with situations.

Implementation

◆ Establish a therapeutic relationship by listening and responding to the client *to initiate therapeutic communication.*
◆ Encourage the client to take part in social interactions *to introduce other people's perceptions and realities to the client.*
◆ Help the client identify negative behaviors that interfere with relationships *so the client can see how his behavior impacts others.*
◆ Instruct and help the client practice strategies that facilitate the development of social skills *so the client can gain confidence and practice interacting with others.*
◆ Review key teaching topics with the client and family members *to ensure adequate knowledge about the condition and treatment,* including:
- learning coping strategies
- understanding the disorder.

Evaluation

◆ The client verbalizes what factors cause impaired social interactions.
◆ The client identifies strategies for improving behaviors during social interactions.
◆ The client verbalizes decreased anxiety when socializing with others and participates in group or social interactions.

EATING DISORDERS

Anorexia nervosa and bulimia nervosa, two major forms of eating disorder, result in death for 5% to 15% of the persons they affect. The incidence of eating disorders is particularly high among adolescent girls from highly competitive, upwardly mobile families.

These two eating disorders share many characteristics, including:
◆ excessive concern about food and weight control
◆ use of extreme measures to control weight (starvation, purging)
◆ perfectionist self-expectations
◆ concern about how one is viewed by others
◆ eagerness to please and make a good impression
◆ underdeveloped sense of personal identity
◆ discomfort in social situations
◆ unresolved issues of autonomy
◆ underlying needs for love, affection, and belonging.

The anorexic client and the bulimic client also display distinct behavioral differences. For example, when the client is finally hospitalized for treatment of anorexia nervosa, malnutrition is apparent. (See *Anorexia nervosa and bulimia nervosa: Client behaviors,* page 164.) It isn't unusual for a client with anorexia nervosa to weigh as little as 70 or 80 lb (31.8 or 36.3 kg). In most cases, the client must weigh at least 90 lb (40.8 kg) before psychotherapy can be initiated successfully.

ANOREXIA NERVOSA

In ANOREXIA NERVOSA, the client deliberately starves herself or engages in binge eating and purging. A client with anorexia nervosa wants to become as thin as possible and refuses to maintain an appropriate weight. There are two categories of anorexia nervosa — the restricting type (where the amount of food intake is restricted) and the binge-eating–purging type.

Anorexia nervosa and bulimia nervosa: Client behaviors

This chart compares typical behaviors of clients with anorexia nervosa with those of clients with bulimia nervosa.

ANOREXIA NERVOSA	BULIMIA NERVOSA
◆ Denies that the eating pattern is abnormal	◆ Recognizes that the eating pattern is abnormal
◆ Loses significant amounts of body weight	◆ Keeps weight within a normal range; preoccupied with weight gain
◆ Is introverted and perfectionistic	◆ Appears extroverted with poor impulse control
◆ Copes with stress by starving self	◆ Copes with stress by bingeing
◆ Denies feeling fatigued	◆ Admits feeling fatigued
◆ Exercises compulsively	◆ May or may not exercise strenuously
◆ Tightly controls food intake	◆ Is unable to control food intake
◆ Is unlikely to abuse alcohol	◆ May abuse alcohol
◆ Feels powerful after abstaining from food	◆ May be suicidal after bingeing
◆ Is secretive and self-absorbed	◆ Is secretive with food
◆ Is overwhelmed by fear of losing control	◆ Feels overwhelmed and out of control
◆ Is a high achiever	◆ Has low self-esteem that can prevent achievement

A key clinical finding is a refusal to sustain weight at or above minimum requirements for age and height. If left untreated, anorexia nervosa can cause the client's death.

Contributing factors

- Age (most prominent in adolescents)
- Below-normal levels of neurotransmitters
- Distorted body image
- Gender (primarily affects females)
- Genetic predisposition
- Low self-esteem
- Poor family relationships
- Preoccupation with weight and dieting
- Sexual abuse

Assessment findings

- A decrease in a person's body weight to less than 85% of the weight considered normal for the person's age and height
- Amenorrhea, fatigue, loss of libido, infertility
- Body image disturbance
- Cognitive distortions, such as overgeneralization, dichotomous thinking, or ideas of reference
- Compulsive behavior
- Decreased blood volume, evidenced by lowered blood pressure and postural hypertension
- Dependency on others for self-worth
- Electrolyte imbalance, evidenced by muscle weakness, seizures, or arrhythmias
- Emaciated appearance
- Denial of hunger, guilt associated with eating
- Exercising to excess despite fatigue
- GI complications, such as constipation or laxative dependence
- Impaired decision making
- Need to achieve and please others
- Obsessive rituals concerning food
- Overly compliant attitude
- Perfectionist attitude
- Refusal to eat, severe curtailment of intake, fear of gaining weight

Diagnostic evaluation

- Electrocardiogram reveals nonspecific ST interval, prolonged PR interval, and T-wave changes.
- Laboratory test results show elevated blood urea nitrogen and electrolyte imbalances.
- Female clients exhibit low estrogen levels.
- Male clients exhibit low serum testosterone levels.
- Leukopenia and mild anemia are apparent.
- Thyroid study findings are low.

Nursing diagnoses

- Imbalanced nutrition: Less than body requirements
- Disturbed body image
- Chronic low self-esteem

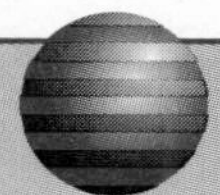

CLINICAL SITUATION

Caring for the client with anorexia nervosa

Evaluate the clinical situation described here. See if you're able to answer the questions as you go.

A 17-year-old female client has been admitted to your unit in the hospital for treatment of severe weight loss. The client is 5′6″ (167.6 cm) tall and weighs 85 lb (38.6 kg). She has been in counseling at a community mental health center for the past 2 months but was hospitalized when her weight dropped below 90 lb (40.8 kg).

The client, who lives with her parents and three younger siblings, is an honor student and president of the student council. She works hard to please her teachers and her parents.

According to her history, 6 months ago the client decided to lose 25 lb (11.3 kg) so others would find her more attractive and she would look slimmer in her graduation pictures. When she attained her goal of 110 lb (49.9 kg), she decided to continue dieting in the firm belief that her ability to lose weight and remain thin would demonstrate her self-discipline and ability to succeed.

On your unit, the client becomes extremely upset when anyone tries to get her to eat, saying that the sight of food nauseates her. When she does eat, she complains of feeling bloated and needs to go to the bathroom immediately. The client says she doesn't understand why everyone is so concerned about her weight. She just feels fat and doesn't want to be any heavier. The client rarely socializes with the other teenagers on the unit, preferring to spend time in solitary activity. When she does socialize, she appears uncomfortable and sometimes makes tactless remarks.

What are appropriate nursing diagnoses for this situation?

◆ Ineffective denial related to uncertainty about the future

◆ Imbalanced nutrition: Less than body requirements related to fear of becoming fat

◆ Disturbed body image related to distorted perception of body size

What interventions are appropriate to promote intake of nutritious foods?

◆ Offer highly nutritious foods every 3 hours in small amounts *because the client isn't able to ingest large quantities of food at one time.*

◆ Observe the client for at least 90 minutes after she eats a meal or snack *to prevent unobserved actions, such as vomiting, to keep her weight down.*

Questions for further thought

◆ How would a therapy group consisting of clients with similar problems help the client?

◆ How would assertiveness skills assist this client?

Treatment

◆ Behavioral modification

◆ Group therapy

◆ Individual therapy

◆ Nutritional therapy

◆ Activity curtailment as needed

Drug therapy options

◆ There are no specific drug therapy options for this disorder.

Planning and goals

◆ The client will increase weight according to established goals.

◆ The client will formulate a healthy self-concept and engage in independent behaviors.

◆ The client's physiologic processes will be within normal limits.

◆ The client will learn coping techniques to deal with anxiety.

Implementation

◆ Obtain a complete physical assessment *to identify complications of anorexia nervosa.*

◆ Establish a contract for amounts to be eaten *to avoid arguments and conflicts between staff and client.*

◆ Provide one-on-one support before, during, and after meals *to foster a strong nurse-client relationship and ensure that the client is eating.* (See *Caring for the client with anorexia nervosa.*)

◆ Prevent the client from using the bathroom for 90 minutes after eating *to break the purging cycle.*

◆ Encourage verbal expression of feelings *to foster open communication about body image.*

◆ Help the client identify coping mechanisms for dealing with anxiety *to promote healthy coping techniques.*

◆ Help the client learn ways to satisfy personal, unmet needs *to facilitate developing a healthy lifestyle. The client needs to learn the coping skills and strategies to meet both physiologic and emotional needs.*
◆ Weigh the client once or twice a week at the same time of day using the same scale *to accurately monitor weight gains.*
◆ Help the client to understand the anorectic cycle *to prevent future anorectic behavior.*
◆ Discuss the client's perception of her appearance. Help her understand how arbitrary social standards for beauty have affected her self-perception. Point out that she doesn't have to accept society's equation of thinness and beauty. Explain that she has a right to think of herself as beautiful regardless of how she compares with others *to build self-esteem.*
◆ Discuss the client's progress with her *to increase awareness of achievements and promote continued effort.*
◆ Review key teaching topics with the client and family members *to ensure adequate knowledge about the condition and treatment,* including:
– need for gradual weight gain
– nutritional support measures
– treatment options
– support services and community resources.

Evaluation
◆ The client's vital signs, electrolyte levels, and fluid intake and output are within reference limits.
◆ The client verbalizes that she's pleased with her appearance and expresses self-confidence.
◆ The client is able to maintain healthy food intake and weight has reached the established goal.
◆ The client relates the coping strategies that can be used when anxiety level is increased.

BULIMIA NERVOSA
BULIMIA NERVOSA is characterized by episodic bingeing on food, followed by purging in the form of vomiting. The client's weight may remain normal or close to normal. The severity of the disorder depends on the frequency of the binge and purge cycle as well as physical complications. The client commonly views food as a source of comfort.

Contributing factors
◆ Biologic factors
◆ Family disturbance or conflict
◆ Genetics
◆ History of sexual abuse
◆ Low self-esteem

Assessment findings
◆ Alternating periods of binge eating and purging
◆ Anxiety
◆ Avoidance of conflict
◆ Cognitive distortions, such as those with anorexia nervosa
◆ Constant preoccupation with food
◆ Disruptions in interpersonal relationships
◆ Dissatisfaction with body image
◆ Extreme need for acceptance and approval
◆ Feelings of helplessness
◆ Focus on changing a specific body part
◆ Frequent lies and excuses to explain behavior
◆ Guilt and self-disgust
◆ Irregular menses
◆ Perfectionist attitude
◆ Parotid and salivary gland swelling
◆ Pharyngitis
◆ Physiologic problems as in anorexia nervosa (amenorrhea, fatigue, loss of libido, infertility, electrolyte imbalance, GI complications)
◆ Possible use of amphetamines or other drugs to control hunger
◆ Problems caused by frequent vomiting
◆ Repression of anger and frustration
◆ Russell sign (bruised knuckles or abrasions on the back of the hand due to induced vomiting)
◆ Sporadic, excessive exercise

Diagnostic evaluation
◆ Beck Depression Inventory may reveal depression.
◆ Metabolic acidosis may occur from diarrhea caused by enemas and excessive laxative use.
◆ Metabolic alkalosis (the most common metabolic complication) may occur from frequent vomiting.
◆ Cardiac arrhythmias may occur from electrolyte imbalance.
◆ Electrolyte imbalance may occur from frequent vomiting.
◆ Hypoglycemia may occur from inadequate nutritional intake.

Nursing diagnoses
◆ Imbalanced nutrition: Less than body requirements
◆ Anxiety
◆ Powerlessness

Treatment

◆ Cognitive therapy (to identify triggers for bingeing and purging)
◆ Individual, group, and family therapy

Drug therapy options

◆ Selective serotonin reuptake inhibitors: fluoxetine (Prozac), paroxetine (Paxil); sertraline (Zoloft).

Planning and goals

◆ The client will learn coping techniques to deal with increased anxiety.
◆ The client will increase weight according to established goals and maintain normal eating habits.
◆ The client will formulate a healthy self-concept.
◆ The client's physiologic processes will be within normal limits.

Implementation

◆ Perform a complete physical assessment *to identify complications associated with bulimia nervosa.*
◆ Explain the purpose of a nutritional contract *to encourage a dietary change without initiating argument or struggle.*
◆ Avoid power struggles around food *to keep the focus on establishing and maintaining a positive self-image and self-esteem.*
◆ Prevent the client from using the bathroom for 2 hours after eating *to help the client avoid purging behavior.*
◆ Provide one-on-one support before, during, and after meals *to monitor and assist the client with eating.*
◆ Encourage the client to express her feelings *to facilitate conversations and promote understanding.*
◆ Weigh the client once or twice per week at the same time of day using the same scale *to accurately monitor weight.*
◆ Help the client identify the cause of the disorder *to help her gain understanding and work toward wellness.*
◆ Point out cognitive distortions *to help identify sources of the problem.*
◆ Discuss the client's perception of her appearance. Help her understand how arbitrary social standards for beauty have affected her self-perception. Point out that she doesn't have to accept society's equation of thinness with beauty. Explain that she has a right to think of herself as beautiful regardless of how she compares herself with others *to build self-esteem.*
◆ Discuss the client's progress with her *to increase awareness of achievements and promote continued effort.*
◆ Review key teaching topics with the client and family members *to ensure adequate knowledge about the condition and treatment,* including:
- need to gain weight gradually
- treatment options
- support services and community resources.

Evaluation

◆ The client's vital signs, electrolyte levels, and fluid intake and output are within reference limits.
◆ The client can maintain a healthy food intake, and her weight has reached the established goal.
◆ The client relates the coping strategies that can be used when anxiety level is increased.

SCHIZOPHRENIC AND DELUSIONAL DISORDERS

People with major distortions in ego functioning experience serious disturbances in all areas of their lives, having impaired reality testing and a compromised ability to relate with others. Common signs of impairment in reality testing include bizarre behaviors, inability to assume responsibility for oneself, and misinterpretation of environmental stimuli.

Major disturbances in ego functioning can result from functional causes, such as acute psychosis, or from underlying organic causes related to drug ingestion, high fever, an accumulation of toxins in the body, or dementia.

SCHIZOPHRENIA is a brain disease characterized by neurotransmitter imbalances and structural changes within the brain. Distorted thought processes make living with this disease a challenge. Symptoms from schizophrenia may be characterized as positive or negative. Positive symptoms focus on a distortion of normal functions; negative symptoms focus on a loss of normal functions. (See *Symptom classification of schizophrenia,* page 168.)

CATATONIC SCHIZOPHRENIA

Clients with CATATONIC SCHIZOPHRENIA show little reaction to their environments. Catatonic behavior involves remaining completely motionless or continuously repeating one motion. This behavior can last for hours. Catatonic schizophrenia is the least common type of schizophrenia.

Symptom classification of schizophrenia

Here are examples of positive, negative, and disorganized symptoms of schizophrenia.

POSITIVE SYMPTOMS	NEGATIVE SYMPTOMS	DISORGANIZED SYMPTOMS
◆ Delusions ◆ Hallucinations	◆ Apathy ◆ Blunted affect ◆ Inability to have pleasure (anhedonia) ◆ Lack of motivation ◆ Lack of self-initiated behaviors (avolition) ◆ Poverty of speech (alogia) ◆ Asociality, or avoidance of relationships	◆ Thought disorder (confused thinking and speech) ◆ Bizarre behavior, such as silliness, agitation, and inappropriate appearance or conduct

Contributing factors

◆ Biochemical abnormalities — involving dopamine
◆ Developmental abnormalities
◆ Fragile ego, which can't withstand the demands of reality
◆ Genetics
◆ Infectious agent or autoimmune response (unproven cause)
◆ Social or environmental stress, interacting with the person's inherited biological makeup
◆ Structural brain abnormalities
◆ Underlying physical conditions (birth trauma, head injury, epilepsy, stroke, parkinsonism, alcohol abuse)

Assessment findings

◆ Bizarre postures, waxy flexibility (posture held in odd or unusual fixed positions for extended periods), resistance to being moved
◆ Diminished sensitivity to painful stimuli
◆ Echolalia (repetition of another's words)
◆ Echopraxia (involuntary imitation of another person's movements and gestures)
◆ Resisting instructions, such as staying in a rigid posture and mutism (failure to speak)
◆ Rapid swings between stupor and excitement

Diagnostic evaluation

◆ Testing aims to rule out other possible causes of symptoms.

Nursing diagnoses

◆ Disturbed thought processes
◆ Ineffective coping
◆ Bathing or hygiene self-care deficit

Treatment

◆ Electroconvulsive therapy
◆ Family therapy
◆ Milieu therapy
◆ Outpatient group therapy
◆ Psychoeducational programs
◆ Supportive psychotherapy
◆ Vocational counseling

Drug therapy options

◆ Benzodiazepines: diazepam (Valium), lorazepam (Ativan)
◆ Atypical antipsychotic agents: ziprasidone (Geodon), aripiprazole (Abilify)

Planning and goals

◆ The client will regain control of thought processes.
◆ The client will perform self-care without assistance.
◆ The client won't experience physical harm.
◆ The client will establish a relationship with the primary nurse, refer to other clients by name, and make eye contact when talking with others.
◆ The client will develop healthy ways to handle anxiety, fears, and other threats to self.

Implementation

◆ Provide skin care *to prevent skin breakdown.*
◆ Monitor intake and output. *Body weight may decrease as a result of inadequate intake.*
◆ Monitor the client for adverse effects of antipsychotic drugs, such as dystonic reactions and tardive dyskinesia. *Early identification of extrapyramidal effects can help diminish or eliminate the client's anxiety about these symptoms.*

◆ Be aware of the client's personal space; use gestures and touch judiciously. *Invading the client's personal space can increase his anxiety.*
◆ When discussing care, give short, simple explanations at the client's level of understanding *to increase cooperation.*
◆ Provide appropriate measures to ensure client safety and explain to the client why you're doing so. *Implementing and explaining safety measures can promote trust and decrease anxiety while increasing the client's sense of security.*
◆ Promote a trusting relationship *to create a safe environment in which the client can practice social interaction skills and prepare for social interaction.*
◆ Briefly explain procedures, routines, and tests *to allay the client's anxiety.*
◆ Collaborate with the client to identify anxious behavior as well as probable causes. *Involving the client in examination of behavior can increase his sense of control.*
◆ Provide opportunities for the client to learn adaptive social skills in a nonthreatening environment. *Learning new social skills can enhance the client's adjustment after discharge.*
◆ Review key teaching topics with the client and family members *to ensure adequate knowledge about the condition and treatment,* including:
– accepting that feelings are valid
– recognizing extrapyramidal effects of antipsychotic medications
– preventing photosensitivity reactions to drugs by avoiding exposure to sunlight.

Evaluation

◆ The client experiences less confusion in thinking or thought processes.
◆ The client talks about situations and issues that reinforce reality.
◆ The client independently manages daily care.
◆ The client doesn't place self at risk for harm.
◆ The client interacts appropriately with staff, selected peers, and visitors.

DELUSIONAL DISORDER

A delusion is a false belief to which a person adheres despite contradictory evidence. Clients with DELUSIONAL DISORDER (also called *psychotic depression* or *delusional depression*) hold firmly to false beliefs despite contradictory information. The client with delusional disorder tends to be intelligent and can have a high level of competence but has impaired social and personal relationships. One indication of delusional disorder is an absence of hallucinations.

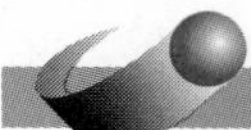

FAST FACT

The most common types of delusions include:
- *delusions of grandeur* – belief that one is highly important, famous, or powerful
- *delusions of persecution* – belief that one is being persecuted or harmed by others
- *delusions of reference* – belief that one is connected to events unrelated to himself.

Contributing factors

◆ Family history of depression or psychotic illness
◆ Social or environmental stress, interacting with the person's inherited biological makeup

Assessment findings

◆ Antagonism
◆ Delusions that are visual, auditory, or tactile
◆ Denial
◆ Harming self or others
◆ Ideas of reference (where everything in the environment takes on a personal significance)
◆ Inability to trust
◆ Irritable or depressed mood
◆ Marked anger and violence
◆ Projection

Diagnostic evaluation

◆ Blood and urine testing eliminates an organic or chemical cause.
◆ Endocrine function tests rule out hyperadrenalism, pernicious anemia, and thyroid disorders.
◆ Neurologic evaluations rule out an organic cause.

Nursing diagnoses

◆ Impaired social interaction
◆ Ineffective coping

Treatment

◆ Family therapy
◆ Group therapy
◆ Milieu therapy
◆ Stress management
◆ Supportive psychotherapy

Drug therapy options

◆ Antiparkinsonian agent: benztropine (Cogentin), for adverse effects of antipsychotic medications

◆ Antipsychotic agents: chlorpromazine (Thorazine), fluphenazine (Prolixin), haloperidol (Haldol), olanzapine (Zyprexa), risperidone (Risperdal), thioridazine (Mellaril)
◆ Atypical antipsychotic agents: aripiprazole (Abilify), ziprasidone (Geodon)

Planning and goals

◆ The client won't harm himself or others.
◆ The client will learn alternative coping strategies.
◆ The client will regain his normal level of functioning.

Implementation

◆ Formulate realistic, modest goals with the client *to help diminish suspicion while increasing the client's self-esteem and sense of control.*
◆ Establish a therapeutic relationship *to foster trust.*
◆ Designate one nurse to communicate with the client and supervise other staff members regarding the client's care *to build trust and minimize opportunities for the client to exhibit hostility.*
◆ Explore events that trigger delusions *to help you understand the dynamics of the client's delusional system.* Discuss anxiety associated with triggering events.
◆ Don't directly attack the delusion *to avoid increasing the client's anxiety.* Instead, be patient in formulating a trusting relationship.
◆ When the dynamics of the delusions are understood, discourage repetitious talk about delusions and refocus the conversation on the client's underlying feelings. *As the client identifies and explores feelings, he'll decrease reliance on delusional thought.*
◆ Recognize delusion as the client's perception of the environment. Avoid arguing with the client regarding the content of delusions *to foster trust.*
◆ Teach the client alternative coping mechanisms *to handle periods of increased anxiety and enhance the client's self-esteem and self-control.*
◆ Review key teaching topics with the client and family members *to ensure adequate knowledge about the condition and treatment,* including:
– learning decision-making, problem-solving, and negotiating skills
– understanding potential adverse effects of medication.

Evaluation

◆ The client doesn't harm himself or others.
◆ The client demonstrates less suspicious behavior.
◆ The client can identify signs and symptoms of anxiety.
◆ The client identifies factors that precipitate delusions and alternative coping mechanisms to handle anxiety.

DISORGANIZED SCHIZOPHRENIA

Clients with DISORGANIZED SCHIZOPHRENIA have a flat or inappropriate affect and incoherent thoughts, and exhibit loose associations and disorganized speech and behaviors.

Contributing factors

◆ Biochemical abnormalities involving dopamine
◆ Fragile ego, which can't withstand the demands of external reality
◆ Genetics
◆ Social or environmental stress, interacting with the person's inherited biological makeup
◆ Structural brain abnormalities
◆ Underlying physical conditions (birth trauma, head injury, epilepsy, stroke, parkinsonism, alcohol abuse)

Assessment findings

◆ Blunted, silly, superficial, flat, or inappropriate affect
◆ Extreme social withdrawal
◆ Grimacing
◆ Grossly disorganized behavior
◆ Hypochondriacle complaints
◆ Incoherent, disorganized speech with markedly loose associations

Diagnostic evaluation

◆ Testing rules out other possible causes of behavior.

Nursing diagnoses

◆ Disturbed thought processes
◆ Social isolation
◆ Disturbed sensory perception (auditory)

Treatment

◆ Family therapy
◆ Milieu therapy
◆ Psychoeducational programs
◆ Social skills training
◆ Supportive psychotherapy

Drug therapy options

◆ Antipsychotic agents: chlorpromazine (Thorazine), fluphenazine (Prolixin), haloperidol (Haldol), olanzapine (Zyprexa), risperidone (Risperdal), thioridazine (Mellaril)
◆ Atypical antipsychotic agents: aripiprazole (Abilify), ziprasidone (Geodon)

Helping a client cope with hallucinations

This table details the progression of behaviors and sensations that a schizophrenic client may experience just before and during a hallucination, and describes nursing interventions that may help the client cope with these occurrences. After a hallucination, the client may be exhausted. Be sure to allow time for the client to rest or sleep.

BEHAVIORS AND SENSATIONS	NURSING INTERVENTIONS
The client feels anxious or lonely and attempts to cope by daydreaming or seeking out a trusted person.	◆ Provide the client with a highly structured daily routine and engage the client in a structured activity to dissipate anxiety and feelings of loneliness. Lack of structure and feelings of loneliness may precipitate hallucinations. ◆ *Don't* allow the client hours of free time.
The client experiences increasing anxiety, which leads to a state of alertness. The client becomes preoccupied with internal sensations (such as voices and images) and starts to respond to them. Aware that the sensations are internal, the client attempts to control them.	◆ Help the client compare internal sensations with external reality. ◆ Engage the client in a structured activity. ◆ Teach the client to hum, whistle, or talk out loud to "crowd out" internal sensations. ◆ Ask the client to identify concrete things in the external environment.
As internal sensations become increasingly dominant, the client has trouble controlling them and eventually yields to them.	◆ Talk to the client about external reality. ◆ Ask the client to compare the hallucination with external reality. ◆ Use self as a focal point to get the client's attention and the client to focus on what you're doing and saying. ◆ Instruct the client to firmly tell the hallucination to go away. ◆ Engage the client in a large-muscle activity.
The client becomes immersed in internal sensations and feels powerless over them. Depending on the nature of the hallucination, the client may become very frightened.	◆ Have the client focus on external reality. ◆ Do whatever is necessary to get the client's attention. ◆ Maintain a firm but kindly tone of voice.

Planning and goals

◆ The client will no longer hear voices or will learn to control them.
◆ The client will begin to regain control of thought processes.
◆ The client will establish a relationship with the primary nurse, refer to other clients by name, and make eye contact when talking with others.

Implementation

◆ Help the client meet basic needs for food, comfort, and a sense of safety *to ensure the client's well-being and build trust.*
◆ During an acute psychotic episode, remove potentially hazardous items from the client's environment *to promote safety.*
◆ Briefly explain procedures, routines, and tests *to decrease the client's anxiety.*
◆ Protect the client from self-destructive tendencies or aggressive impulses *to ensure safety.*
◆ Convey sincerity and understanding when communicating *to promote a trusting relationship.*
◆ Formulate realistic goals with the client. *Including the client in formulating goals can help diminish suspicion while increasing self-esteem and sense of control.*
◆ If the client experiences hallucinations, don't attempt to reason with him or challenge his perception of hallucinations. Instead, ensure the client's safety and provide comfort and support. *Attempts to reason with the client will increase anxiety, possibly making hallucinations worse.* (See *Helping a client cope with hallucinations.*)

◆ Encourage the client with auditory hallucinations to reveal what voices are telling him *to help prevent harm to the client and others.*
◆ First, encourage the client to participate in one-on-one interactions, and then progress to small groups *to enable the client to practice newly acquired social skills.*
◆ Provide positive reinforcement for socially acceptable behavior, such as efforts to improve hygiene and table manners, *to foster improved social relationships and acceptance from others.*
◆ Encourage the client to express feelings related to experiencing hallucinations *to promote better understanding of the client's experiences and to allow the client to vent emotions, thereby reducing anxiety.*
◆ Review key teaching topics with the client and family members *to ensure adequate knowledge about the condition and treatment,* including learning to use distraction techniques.

Evaluation
◆ The client no longer hears voices or learns to control them.
◆ The client regains control of thought processes.
◆ The client establishes a relationship with the primary nurse, refers to other clients by name, and makes eye contact when talking with others.

PARANOID SCHIZOPHRENIA
Clients with PARANOID SCHIZOPHRENIA have delusions unrelated to reality. Clients commonly display bizarre behavior, are easily angered, and are at high risk for violence. The prognosis for independent functioning is often better than for other types of schizophrenia.

Contributing factors
◆ Biochemical abnormalities involving dopamine
◆ Fragile ego, which can't withstand the demands of external reality
◆ Genetics
◆ Social or environmental stress, interacting with the person's inherited biological makeup
◆ Structural brain abnormalities
◆ Underlying physical condition (birth trauma, head injury, epilepsy, stroke, parkinsonism, substance abuse)

Assessment findings
◆ Anger
◆ Argumentativeness
◆ Auditory hallucinations
◆ Persecutory or grandiose delusional thoughts
◆ Potential for violence
◆ Stilted formality or intensity when interacting with others
◆ Unfocused anxiety

Diagnostic evaluation
Diagnostic testing rules out organic causes of the disorder.

Nursing diagnoses
◆ Disturbed thought processes
◆ Social isolation
◆ Disturbed sensory perception (auditory)

Treatment
◆ Family therapy
◆ Group therapy
◆ Milieu therapy
◆ Psychoeducational programs
◆ Social skills training
◆ Supportive psychotherapy

Drug therapy options
◆ Antiparkinsonian agent: benztropine (Cogentin), for adverse effects of antipsychotic drugs
◆ Antipsychotic agents: chlorpromazine (Thorazine), clozapine (Clozaril), fluphenazine (Prolixin), haloperidol (Haldol), olanzapine (Zyprexa), risperidone (Risperdal), thioridazine (Mellaril)
◆ Atypical antipsychotic agents: aripiprazole (Abilify), ziprasidone (Geodon)

Planning and goals
◆ The client will be regain control of thought processes.
◆ The client will establish a relationship with the primary nurse, refer to other clients by name, and make eye contact when talking with others.
◆ The client will no longer experience delusions.

Implementation
◆ Inform the client that you'll help him control his behavior *to promote feelings of safety.*
◆ Set limits on aggressive behavior, and communicate your expectations to the client *to prevent injury to the client and others.*
◆ Designate one nurse to communicate with the client and direct other staff members who care for the client *to foster trust and a stable environment and minimize opportunities for the client to exhibit hostility.*

◆ Maintain a low level of stimuli *to minimize the client's anxiety, agitation, and suspiciousness.*
◆ Be flexible — allow the client some control. Approach him in a calm, unhurried manner. Let the client talk about anything he wishes, but keep the conversation light and social *to avoid entering into power struggles.*
◆ Don't let the client put you on the defensive, and don't take his remarks personally. If he tells you to leave him alone, do so but return soon. *Brief contacts with the client may be most useful at first.*
◆ Don't make attempts to combat the client's delusions with logic. Instead, respond to feelings, themes, or underlying needs — for example, "It seems you feel you've been treated unfairly." *Combating delusions may increase feelings of persecution or hostility.*
◆ If the client is taking clozapine, stress the importance of returning weekly to the facility or an outpatient setting to have his blood checked *to monitor for adverse effects and prevent toxicity.*
◆ Teach the client the importance of complying with the medication regimen. Tell him to report any adverse reactions instead of discontinuing the drug *to maintain therapeutic drug levels.*
◆ If he takes a slow-release formulation, make sure that he understands when to return for his next dose *to promote compliance.*
◆ Review key teaching topics with the client and family members *to ensure adequate knowledge about the condition and treatment,* including:
- avoiding exposure to sunlight (to prevent photosensitive reactions to antipsychotic drugs)
- reporting any adverse affects of antipsychotic medication
- visiting the hospital weekly to have blood chemistry monitored.

Evaluation

◆ The client regains control of thought processes.
◆ The client establishes a relationship with the primary nurse, refers to other clients by name, and makes eye contact when talking with others.
◆ The client no longer has delusions or can take action to control delusions.

SOMATOFORM DISORDERS

A SOMATOFORM DISORDER is the literal transference of inner conflict onto a body part, commonly resulting in crippling. Individuals with somatoform disorders channel anxiety through a body system. Channeling anxiety in this manner usually succeeds because the person is unaware of uncomfortable amounts of anxiety.

Symptoms of a somatoform disorder aren't under voluntary control and suggest a physical disorder with a psychogenic origin. Physical symptoms aren't consistent with the presence of or degree of underlying pathophysiology. At an affective level, persons with somatoform disorders don't experience emotional distress over life events, but are keenly aware of uncomfortable somatic sensations, for which they seek treatment.

Two examples of somatoform disorders, conversion reaction and hypochondriasis are presented in this section.

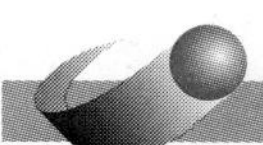

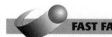

FAST FACT

Forcing a client with a somatoform disorder to renounce his symptoms heightens his anxiety and prolongs the condition.

CONVERSION DISORDER

The client with CONVERSION DISORDER exhibits symptoms that suggest a physical disorder, but evaluation and observation can't determine a physiologic cause. The onset of symptoms is preceded by psychological trauma or conflict, and the physical symptoms are a manifestation of the conflict. Most people who experience conversion reactions accept their condition with a complacency known as *la belle indifference.*

Contributing factors

◆ Biological factors involving the brain's left hemisphere
◆ Overwhelming stress
◆ Physical or sexual abuse
◆ Psychological conflict

Assessment findings

◆ Aphonia (inability to produce sound)
◆ Dysphagia
◆ Impaired balance and impaired coordination
◆ La belle indifference (a lack of concern about the symptoms or limitation on functioning)
◆ Loss of a special sense, such as vision (blindness or double vision), hearing (deafness), or touch
◆ Lump in the throat
◆ Pseudoseizures (seizurelike attacks that are thought to be psychogenically produced)
◆ Urinary retention

Diagnostic evaluation

◆ Test results are inconsistent with physical findings.
◆ The absence of expected diagnostic findings can confirm the disorder.

Nursing diagnoses

◆ Ineffective coping
◆ Anxiety

Treatment

◆ Behavior modification
◆ Biofeedback training
◆ Family therapy
◆ Hypnosis
◆ Individual therapy
◆ Relaxation training

Drug therapy options

◆ Benzodiazepines: alprazolam (Xanax), lorazepam (Ativan)

Planning and goals

◆ The client will demonstrate new coping skills.
◆ The client will identify signs and symptoms of anxiety.

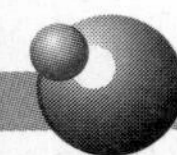

SPOT CHECK

What precedes the onset of symptoms in a conversion disorder?
Answer: Psychological trauma or conflict precedes the onset of symptoms in a conversion disorder.

Implementation

◆ Ensure and maintain a safe environment *to protect the client.*
◆ Establish a supportive relationship that communicates acceptance of the client but keeps the focus away from symptoms *to help the client learn to recognize and express anxiety.*
◆ Review all laboratory and diagnostic study results *to ascertain whether any physical problems are present.*
◆ Encourage the client to identify any emotional conflicts occurring before the onset of physical symptoms *to make the relationship between the conflict and the symptoms more clear.*
◆ Promote social interaction *to decrease the client's level of self-involvement.*
◆ Identify constructive coping mechanisms *to encourage the client to use practical coping skills and relinquish the role of being sick.*
◆ Review key teaching topics with the client and family members *to ensure adequate knowledge about the condition and treatment,* including:
– setting limits on the client's sick role behavior while continuing to provide support
– stress-reduction methods
– the importance of REM and NREM sleep; some individuals may have increased amounts of slow-wave sleep.

Evaluation

◆ The client identifies signs and symptoms of increased anxiety.
◆ The client demonstrates acquired coping strategies when dealing with increased anxiety.
◆ The client focuses less attention on sick role and physical symptoms.

HYPOCHONDRIASIS

In HYPOCHONDRIASIS, the client is preoccupied by fear of a serious illness, despite medical assurance of good health. The client with hypochondriasis interprets all physical sensations as indications of illness, impairing his ability to function normally.

Contributing factors

◆ Death of someone close to the individual
◆ Family member with a serious illness
◆ Previous serious illness

Assessment findings

◆ Abnormal focus on bodily functions and sensations
◆ Anger, frustration, depression
◆ Frequent visits to doctors and specialists despite assurance from health care providers that the client is healthy
◆ Intensified physical symptoms around sympathetic people
◆ Rejection of the idea that the symptoms are stress-related
◆ Use of symptoms to avoid difficult situations
◆ Vague physical symptoms

Diagnostic evaluation

◆ Test results are inconsistent with client's complaint and physical findings.
◆ Projective psychological tests may show preoccupation with somatic concerns.

Nursing diagnoses

- Deficient knowledge
- Ineffective coping
- Ineffective health maintenance

Treatment

- Cognitive and behavioral therapy
- Family therapy
- Group therapy
- Individual therapy

Drug therapy options

- Benzodiazepines: alprazolam (Xanax), lorazepam (Ativan)
- Tricyclic antidepressants: amitriptyline (Elavil), imipramine (Tofranil)
- Selective serotonin reuptake inhibitors: paroxetine (Paxil), sertraline (Zoloft)

Planning and goals

- The client will become aware of how emotional issues affect physiologic functioning.
- The client will learn coping strategies for emotional issues.
- The client will demonstrate a decreased focus on symptoms.

Implementation

- Assess the client's level of knowledge about how emotional issues can impact physiologic functioning *to promote understanding of the condition.*
- Encourage emotional expression *to discourage emotional repression, which can have physical consequences.*
- Respond to the client's symptoms in a matter-of-fact way *to reduce secondary gain the client achieves from talking about symptoms.*
- Review key teaching topics with the client and family members *to ensure adequate knowledge about the condition and treatment,* including:
  - relaxation and assertiveness techniques
  - initiating conversations that focus on something other than physical maladies.

Evaluation

- The client verbalizes an understanding of his condition.
- The client identifies coping strategies to use when dealing with emotional issues.
- The client initiates conversations unrelated to physical complaints.

SUBSTANCE ABUSE DISORDERS

Some people discover that certain chemical substances appear to relieve their anxiety, boredom, depression, or feelings of inadequacy. Over time, continual intake of a chosen substance becomes abusive, tolerance develops, and the person must ingest increasingly larger quantities to obtain the desired effects. (See *Selected substances of abuse,* pages 176 and 177.)

Continued substance abuse leads to physiologic and psychological changes. Some family members, friends, and coworkers may notice these changes and protect the abuser, either by excusing poor behavior at home or by taking on extra work to make up for the abuser's decreased productivity on the job. Others may be slow to recognize that substance abuse is adversely affecting the abuser as well as family members, friends, and associates.

Health professionals typically see a substance abuser for the first time when the client seeks treatment for a related health problem, such as gastric ulcers, malnutrition, or hepatitis. The abuser may be admitted to a general hospital directly or through the emergency department — for example, following an accident or overdose.

Lack of cause-and-effect insight makes treating such a client a challenge for nurses. Because most substance abusers don't view themselves as having a problem, they don't initiate treatment for their abusive behavior. Furthermore, they overuse the defense mechanisms of denial, rationalization, and projection, and they make considerable use of negative manipulation.

ALCOHOL ABUSE DISORDER

Although alcohol abuse is considered a substance abuse disorder, assessment findings and treatment differ somewhat from those for other substances. Alcohol is a sedative but creates a feeling of euphoria. Sedation increases with the amount ingested.

Possible causes

- Allergic response
- Biochemical abnormalities
- Endocrine imbalances
- Genetic tendency
- Influence of nationality and ethnicity
- Nutritional deficiencies
- Psychological factors

(Text continues on page 178.)

Selected substances of abuse

This chart lists various substances of abuse, signs of withdrawal, and corresponding nursing interventions. During the acute withdrawal stage (detoxification), the nurse may administer medications intended to prevent or minimize the severe consequences of withdrawal, such as seizure or delirium.

SUBSTANCE	WITHDRAWAL SIGNS	NURSING INTERVENTIONS
Alcohol (beer, wine, liquor)		
	◆ Diaphoresis ◆ Increased blood pressure ◆ Increased heart rate ◆ Mild tremors ◆ Nervousness	◆ Monitor the client's vital signs. ◆ Obtain order for benzodiazepines to relieve withdrawal symptoms. ◆ Remain with the client and monitor behavior. ◆ Promote sleep and rest.
	◆ Appetite loss ◆ Delusions ◆ Disorientation ◆ Hallucinations ◆ Moderate to severe tremors	◆ Monitor the client's vital signs. ◆ Administer benzodiazepines, as ordered. ◆ Maintain a quiet environment. ◆ Remain with the client.
	◆ Grand mal seizures ◆ Persistent hallucinations	◆ Monitor the client's vital signs. ◆ Remain with the client. ◆ Administer anticonvulsants, as ordered. ◆ Take seizure precautions. ◆ Minimize environmental stimulation. ◆ Offer foods and fluids when the client is lucid.
	◆ Delirium tremens ◆ Hallucinations ◆ Sleeplessness ◆ Tachycardia	◆ Monitor the client's vital signs. ◆ Remain with the client. ◆ Minimize environmental stimulation. ◆ Offer foods and fluids, as tolerated.
Central nervous system stimulants		
Amphetamines	◆ Agitation ◆ Depression ◆ Disorientation ◆ Fatigue ◆ Insomnia or hypersomnia ◆ Paranoia ◆ Suicidal thoughts	◆ Monitor the client's vital signs. ◆ Monitor the client for suicidal ideation. ◆ Promote sleep and rest. ◆ Administer antidepressants, if ordered. ◆ Remain with a disoriented or frightened client; orient the client to reality.
Cocaine, crack cocaine	◆ Agitation ◆ Craving for drug ◆ Depression ◆ Fatigue ◆ Increased appetite ◆ Insomnia or hypersomnia ◆ Paranoia ◆ Suicidal thoughts	◆ Monitor the client's vital signs. ◆ Monitor the client for suicidal ideation. ◆ Promote sleep and rest. ◆ Administer antidepressants, if ordered. ◆ Remain with a disoriented or frightened client; orient the client to reality.

Selected substances of abuse *(continued)*

SUBSTANCE	WITHDRAWAL SIGNS	NURSING INTERVENTIONS
Hallucinogens		
LSD	◆ Apprehension ◆ Flashbacks ◆ Panic	◆ Monitor the client's vital signs and safety. ◆ Administer diazepam, as ordered, if the client has severe anxiety during flashbacks.
Phencyclidine (PCP)	◆ Bizarre behavior ◆ Craving for drug ◆ Depression ◆ Hypertension ◆ Lethargy ◆ Seizures	◆ Monitor the client's vital signs and safety. ◆ Monitor the client for suicidal ideation. ◆ Promote sleep and rest. ◆ Administer antidepressants, if ordered. ◆ Remain with a disoriented or frightened client; orient the client to reality.
Marijuana (cannabis)	◆ Agitation ◆ Anorexia ◆ Chronic respiratory problems ◆ Depression ◆ Insomnia ◆ Irritability ◆ Restlessness ◆ Tremors	◆ Monitor the client for respiratory problems. ◆ If the client is depressed, attend to his physiologic and safety needs. ◆ Be aware that physicians rarely order medication to ease withdrawal.
Inhalants		
	◆ Anxiety, hallucinations ◆ Tremors ◆ Chills, sweats ◆ Cramps, nausea ◆ Sleep problems ◆ Characteristic withdrawal syndrome varies with sustance abused	◆ Monitor the client's vital signs. ◆ Evaluate and monitor the client's physiologic condition. ◆ Promote rest. ◆ Minimize environmental stimuli. ◆ Administer antipsychotic agents, as ordered.
Opiates (such as morphine and heroin)		
	◆ Chills ◆ Diaphoresis ◆ Dilated pupils ◆ Drug craving ◆ Fever ◆ Insomnia ◆ Lacrimation ◆ Muscle aches ◆ Nausea and vomiting ◆ Runny nose ◆ Tachycardia ◆ Yawning	◆ Monitor the client's vital signs. ◆ Remain with the client. ◆ Offer foods and fluids, as tolerated. ◆ Provide a soothing environment. ◆ If ordered, wean the client by offering small doses of opiate. ◆ If ordered, administer methadone.
Sedatives (such as benzodiazepines and barbiturates)		
	◆ Anxiety ◆ Diaphoresis ◆ Hallucinations ◆ Seizures ◆ Tachycardia	◆ Monitor the client's vital signs. ◆ Attend to the client's physiologic and safety needs, especially if seizures occur. ◆ Promote rest and a calm environment.

Assessment findings

- ◆ Adrenocortical insufficiency
- ◆ Alcoholic cardiomyopathy
- ◆ Alcoholic cirrhosis
- ◆ Alcoholic hepatitis
- ◆ Alcoholic paranoia
- ◆ Blackouts
- ◆ Erection problems
- ◆ Esophageal varices
- ◆ Gastritis or gastric ulcers
- ◆ Hallucinations
- ◆ Korsakoff's psychosis
- ◆ Liver damage
- ◆ Muscular myopathy
- ◆ Pancreatitis
- ◆ Pathologic intoxication
- ◆ Peripheral neuropathy
- ◆ Wernicke's encephalopathy

Diagnostic evaluation

◆ Positive blood and urine drug screenings confirm the diagnosis.

◆ Diagnostic testing supports assessment findings.

◆ Standard alcoholism screening tools indicate alcoholism.

Nursing diagnoses

- ◆ Ineffective coping
- ◆ Ineffective denial
- ◆ Risk for injury

Treatment

◆ Counseling and ongoing support groups

◆ Individual therapy

◆ Symptomatic treatment for acute intoxication or withdrawal

Drug therapy options

◆ Alcohol abuse deterrent: disulfiram (Antabuse) to prevent relapse into alcohol abuse (The client must be alcohol-free for 12 hours before receiving this drug.)

◆ Opioid antagonist: naltrexone (Trexan) to prevent relapse into alcohol abuse

Planning and goals

◆ The client will recognize that alcohol is creating problems in his life.

◆ The client will develop specific plans for abstaining from alcohol use and managing stress.

◆ The client will experience an uncomplicated recovery from alcohol withdrawal.

Implementation

◆ Monitor the client for signs of alcohol withdrawal *so that protective nursing measures, such as one-on-one care, can be implemented if the client's symptoms progress beyond mild tremors, diaphoresis, nausea, nervousness, tachycardia, and increased blood pressure.* (See *Recognizing alcohol withdrawal syndrome.*)

◆ Assess the client's use of denial as a coping mechanism *to promote healthy coping behaviors.*

◆ Encourage the verbalization of anger, fear, inadequacy, grief, and guilt *to begin a therapeutic relationship.*

◆ Set limits on denial and rationalization *to help the client gain control and perspective.*

◆ Have the client formulate goals for maintaining a drug-free lifestyle *to help avoid relapses.*

◆ Review key teaching topics with the client and family members *to ensure adequate knowledge about the condition and treatment,* including:
– understanding substance abuse and relapse prevention
– maintaining good nutrition.

Evaluation

◆ The client freely acknowledges the problems created by alcohol ingestion and makes plans for restitution.

◆ The client participates in stress-management group sessions and identifies specific strategies for managing stress.

◆ The client exhibits no signs of adverse effects from alcohol withdrawal.

◆ The client identifies and takes care of physical health problems.

COCAINE-USE DISORDER

COCAINE-USE DISORDER results from the potent euphoric effects of the drug. Individuals exposed to cocaine develop dependence after a very short time. Maladaptive behavior follows, resulting in social dysfunction. Toxic amounts may cause acute cardiovascular problems, stroke, seizures, respiratory failure, bowel gangrene, and sudden death.

Contributing factors

◆ Genetic predisposition or family history of substance abuse

◆ History of abuse, depression, or anxiety

Assessment findings

◆ Apprehension, inability to sit still, teeth grinding

◆ Chest pain, tachycardia, ventricular fibrillation, or cardiac arrest

◆ Cocaine psychosis (resembling paranoid schizophrenia)

Recognizing alcohol withdrawal syndrome

Use this chart to review alcohol withdrawal syndrome, keeping in mind that the client should have one-on-one care as symptoms worsen. For nursing management, use restraints only as a last resort; restraining the client will heighten anxiety and increase agitation.

SIGNS AND SYMPTOMS	ONSET	NURSING MANAGEMENT
Mild tremors, diaphoresis, nausea, nervousness, tachycardia, increased blood pressure	May occur within 4 to 6 hours after the last drink	◆ Carefully monitor the client's behavior. ◆ Obtain a physician's order for medication to relieve withdrawal symptoms. ◆ Talk to the client about symptoms, and remain with the client when withdrawal begins. ◆ Monitor the client's vital signs.
Increased tremors, hyperactivity, insomnia, anorexia, disorientation, delusions, transient visual hallucinations, tachycardia	Commonly occur 8 to 10 hours after the last drink	◆ Administer medications, as ordered, to relieve withdrawal symptoms. ◆ Remain with the client and orient him to reality. ◆ Keep the room free from distractions and unnecessary noise. ◆ Monitor the client's vital signs as able.
Same as those listed above plus persistent hallucinations, nausea and vomiting as well as withdrawal seizures possible	Occur 12 to 48 hours after the last drink; withdrawal seizures, 7 to 48 hours after the last drink	◆ Remain with the client. ◆ Monitor the client's vital signs as able. ◆ Institute seizure precautions. ◆ Administer anticonvulsant medications as ordered. ◆ Offer fluids and light foods, as tolerated, during periods of lucidity. ◆ Maintain a peaceful environment.
Delirium tremens (withdrawal delirium, which lasts 2 to 3 days), disorientation, fluctuating consciousness, hallucinations, agitation, and low-grade fever	Most commonly occur 48 to 72 hours after the last drink, but may not arise until 7 days after	◆ Remain with the client. ◆ Monitor the client's vital signs as able. ◆ Maintain a peaceful environment. ◆ Offer fluids and light foods, as tolerated, during periods of lucidity. ◆ Administer medications, as ordered.

- Cold sweats, tremors, muscle twitching, seizures
- Decreased sensation of pain
- Dilated pupils
- Euphoria; increased energy, excitement, and sociability
- Flightiness, emotional instability, restlessness, and irritability
- Good humor and laughing
- Grandiosity, sense of increased physical and mental strength
- Reduced hunger, nausea, vomiting, headache
- Runny nose, nasal congestion
- Tachypnea or respiratory arrest
- Talkativeness, pressured speech
- Vertigo
- Violent or bizarre behavior, hallucinations
- Withdrawal symptoms

Diagnostic evaluation

- Drug screening is positive for cocaine.

Nursing diagnoses

- Imbalanced nutrition: Less than body requirements
- Ineffective health maintenance
- Risk for self-directed violence

Treatment

- Detoxification
- Individual therapy
- Narcotics Anonymous or similar self-help group
- Rehabilitation (inpatient or outpatient)
- Supportive and symptomatic treatment for cocaine intoxication

Drug therapy options

- Selective serotonin reuptake inhibitor: paroxetine (Paxil)

Planning and goals

- The client will learn the adverse effects of cocaine on the body.
- The client will have adequate nutritional intake.
- The client won't harm himself or others.

Implementation

- Establish a trusting relationship with the client *to alleviate anxiety or paranoia.*
- Provide the client with well-balanced meals *to compensate for nutritional deficits.*
- Provide a safe environment *to prevent the client from injuring himself or others.*
- Set limits on the client's attempts to rationalize behavior *to reduce inappropriate behavior.*
- Review key teaching topics with the client and family members *to ensure adequate knowledge about the condition and treatment,* including:
  - contacting Narcotics Anonymous
  - coping strategies
  - managing stress.

Evaluation

- The client relates the adverse effects of cocaine and verbalizes plans for lifestyle changes and follow-up support.
- The client has sufficient nutritional intake.
- The client doesn't harm himself or others during hospitalization.

SUBSTANCE ABUSE DISORDER

SUBSTANCE ABUSE DISORDER includes all patterns of abuse excluding alcohol and cocaine. Abuse disorders have a great deal in common, although symptoms vary depending on the abused substance.

Contributing factors

- Familial tendency
- History of abuse, depression, or anxiety
- Personality disorders

Assessment findings

- Attempts to avoid anxiety and other emotions, such as conscious feelings of guilt and anger
- Attempts to meet needs by influencing others
- Development of biological or psychological need for a substance
- Dysfunctional anger
- Feelings of grandiosity
- Impulsiveness
- Manipulation and deceit
- Need for immediate gratification
- Pattern of negative interactions
- Possible malnutrition
- Symptoms of intoxication or withdrawal
- Use of denial and rationalization to explain consequences of behavior

Diagnostic evaluation

- Positive blood and urine drug screening results confirm the diagnosis.

Nursing diagnoses

- Imbalanced nutrition: Less than body requirements
- Ineffective health maintenance
- Risk for self-directed violence

Treatment

- Behavior modification
- Employee assistance programs
- Family counseling
- Group therapy
- Halfway houses
- Individual therapy
- Informal social support
- Self-help groups

Drug therapy options

- Opioid withdrawal syndrome suppressant: clonidine (Catapres) for opiate withdrawal symptoms
- Suppressant, narcotic abstinence syndrome: methadone maintenance (Roxanol, OxyContin) for opiate addiction detoxification

Planning and goals

◆ The client will learn the adverse effects of substance abuse on the body.
◆ The client will have adequate nutritional intake.
◆ The client won't harm himself or others.
◆ The client will commit to a recovery program and get assistance to maintain abstinence and develop effective coping skills.

Implementation

◆ Ensure a safe, quiet environment free from stimuli *to provide a therapeutic setting and alleviate withdrawal symptoms.*
◆ Monitor for withdrawal symptoms, such as delirium, tremors, seizures, or anxiety *to provide the most comfortable environment possible.*
◆ Assess the client for polysubstance abuse *to plan appropriate interventions.*
◆ Help the client understand the ultimate consequences of substance abuse *to assist recovery.*
◆ Provide measures to induce sleep *to help the client manage the discomfort of withdrawal.*
◆ Encourage the client to vent fear and anger *so that he can begin the healing process.*
◆ Review key teaching topics with the client and family members *to ensure adequate knowledge about the condition and treatment,* including:
– contacting addiction support agencies
– learning healthy coping mechanisms.

Evaluation

◆ The client relates the adverse effects of substance abuse and verbalizes plans for lifestyle changes and getting follow-up support.
◆ The client has sufficient nutritional intake.
◆ The client doesn't harm himself or others during hospitalization.

Maternal-neonatal nursing

10

INTRODUCTION

Maternal and neonatal nursing care involves application of the nursing process during family planning as well as during the antepartum, intrapartum, postpartum, and neonatal periods.

FAMILY PLANNING

Family planning involves exercising choices to prevent or achieve pregnancy and to control the timing and number of pregnancies, lifestyle, and partner support. Effectiveness, cost, contraindications, and adverse reactions for all contraceptives should be presented to the client.

Information from the client's menstrual and obstetric history is used for determining the safety of using hormonal contraceptives and which contraceptive method is best for the client. (See *Comparing contraceptives,* pages 184 to 187.)

The nurse uses information obtained during the interview to plan appropriate teaching. The effectiveness and safety of hormonal contraceptives depend greatly on the client's knowledge of and compliance with the chosen method. Inability to understand the proper use of the contraceptive method or unwillingness to use it correctly or consistently may result in pregnancy.

FAMILY PLANNING ASSESSMENT

An assessment for family planning involves collecting a reproductive history, including:

- interval between periods (See *Menstrual cycle.*)
- duration and amount of flow
- problems occurring during menstruation
- number of pregnancies
- number of births (date of each)
- duration of each pregnancy
- type of each delivery
- gender and weight of neonates when delivered
- problems occurring during pregnancy
- problems occurring after delivery.

Complications

Information obtained from the client's health history may identify the client as being at risk for complications:

- Contraindications for hormonal contraceptives include malignancies of the reproductive system, hypertension, pregnancy, and liver dysfunction. A client older than age 35 is at increased risk for a fatal heart attack if she smokes more than 15 cigarettes per day and takes hormonal contraceptives.
- Hormonal contraceptive use affects the reproductive system. Use of hormonal contraceptives is contraindicated in the presence of malignant cell growth. A Papanicolaou (Pap) test may be performed to detect cellular abnormalities.
- If the client's sexual partner is infected with human immunodeficiency virus, acquired immunodeficiency syndrome, or hepatitis B, ideally abstinence should be exercised. If this isn't an option, the client must use the condom method of contraception to prevent transmitting the infection.
- For a breast-feeding client, the physician may prescribe progesterone alone or a low-dose combination of hormonal contraceptives. This may cause the client's milk supply to decrease.
- Low-dose hormonal contraceptives may be prescribed for a client who has diabetes with no vascular complications.
- The Food and Drug Administration recently revised its position on hormonal contraceptives, stating that for healthy, nonsmoking women older than age 40, the benefits (such as decreased menstrual cramps and increased cycle regularity) may outweigh the risks.

Nursing diagnoses

- Imbalanced nutrition: Less than body requirements
- Noncompliance with family planning

Menstrual cycle

The menstrual cycle (female reproductive cycle) typically lasts 28 days. Throughout the cycle, hormones influence the release of a mature ovum from a graafian follicle in the ovary. Hormones also stimulate changes in the endometrial layer of the uterus, preparing it for ovum implantation.

Hormones involved in this cycle are estrogen, progesterone, follicle-stimulating hormone (FSH), and luteinizing hormone (LH). The diagram below illustrates how hormones relate to various phases of the menstrual cycle.

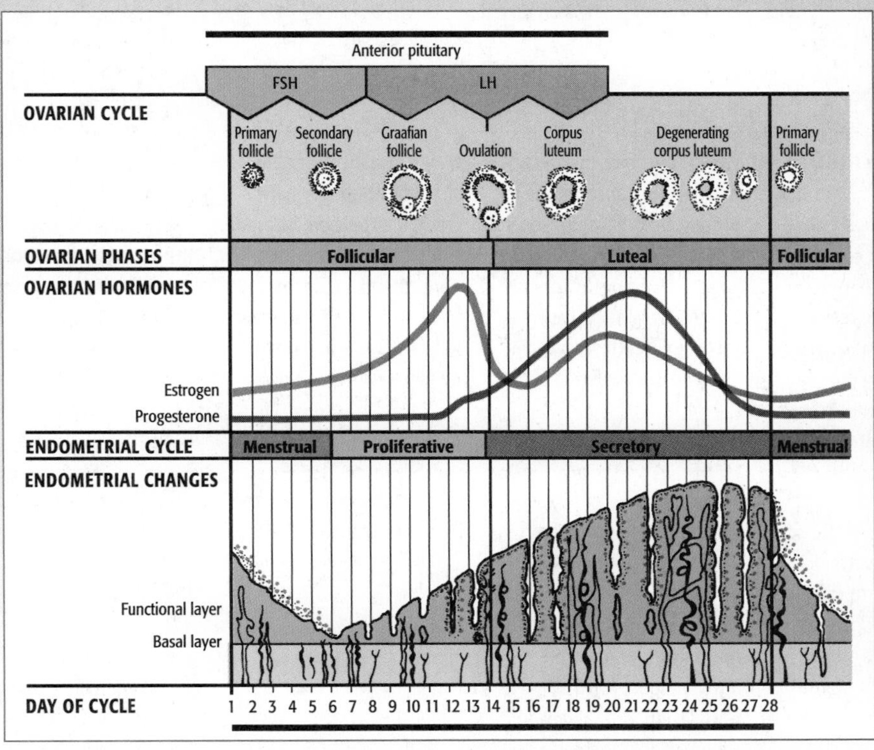

◆ Deficient knowledge regarding family planning
◆ Risk for injury

Planning and goals

◆ All questions will be answered in a manner understood by the client, and the procedure for the chosen contraceptive method will be described accurately by the client.
◆ The client will describe possible adverse reactions to the selected contraceptive.
◆ The client will keep follow-up appointments.
◆ The client will express satisfaction and success with the chosen contraceptive method.

Implementation

◆ Teach the proper use of the selected contraceptive method *to obtain desired effects of contraception and minimize adverse effects.*
◆ Inform the client about possible adverse reactions to contraceptives, especially hormonal contraceptives (fluid retention, weight gain, breast tenderness, headache, breakthrough bleeding, chloasma, acne, yeast infection, nausea, and fatigue), and direct the client to report any of these to the physician. *It may be necessary to change the type of contraceptive or the dosage of a hormonal contraceptive to relieve adverse reactions.*

(Text continues on page 187.)

Comparing contraceptives

When discussing contraception with clients, emphasize the importance of medical history, physical examination, diagnostic tests, and follow-up examinations. Use this chart to review the methods and proper use of contraception, their effectiveness against sexually transmitted diseases (STDs), and the possible adverse reactions that can occur.

METHOD AND ACTIONS	CONTRAINDICATIONS	POTENTIAL PROBLEMS	CLIENT TEACHING
Abstinence 100% effective against pregnancy and STDs	No contraindications	Partners and peers may have negative reaction to it	◆ Teach that refraining from having sexual intercourse has a 0% failure rate. Abstinence should always be presented as an option.
Intrauterine device (IUD) 99% effective ParaGard-T: a T-shaped polyethylene device with copper; interferes with sperm mobility Progestasert: a T-shaped device made of ethylene vinyl acetate copolymer with progesterone in an oil base; prevents endometrium proliferation	Pelvic infections, uterine abnormalities, cancer of the reproductive organs, Wilson's disease, STDs, unexplained vaginal bleeding, history of ectopic pregnancy, severe vasovagal reactivity, valvular heart disease, anemia	May cause increased menstrual flow, abdominal cramps, expulsion, infection, ectopic pregnancy, uterine perforation, and increased incidence of pelvic inflammatory disease (PID); no protection against STDs	◆ Teach the client to check string placement after each menstrual period and before coitus. ◆ Advise her to follow the manufacturer's timetable for replacement (12 years for ParaGard; 12 months for the Progestasert)
Diaphragm Mechanical barrier; 80% to 93% effective in new users when used with spermicidal jelly; 97% effective in long-term users; helps protect against STDs when used with spermicide	Cervicitis; history of cystocele, rectocele, toxic shock syndrome, repeated urinary tract infections (UTIs), vaginal stenosis, pelvic abnormalities, and uterine retroversion, prolapse, retroflexion, or anteflexion; allergy to spermicidal jellies or rubber; unwillingness to learn proper insertion technique; first 6 weeks postpartum	May be allergenic; causes higher incidence of UTIs	◆ Teach the client to keep the diaphragm clean and dry, and to check it for holes. ◆ Advise her to use a spermicidal agent along with the diaphragm. ◆ Tell her to insert it up to 2 hours before intercourse and leave it in place for at least 6 hours after coitus. It may be left in place up to 24 hours. If intercourse is repeated before 6 hours, tell her to insert more spermicidal jelly. ◆ Caution her that she must have the diaphragm refitted after significant weight gain or loss, cervical surgery, miscarriage, dilatation and curettage, therapeutic abortion, and childbirth.
Spermicidal agent (jelly, cream, foam, film, suppository) Chemical barrier; 82% effective	Cervicitis	May be allergenic; possible discomfort with vaginal leakage that occurs, especially with cocoa- and glycerine-based suppositories	◆ Instruct the client to insert the agent high into the vagina not more than 1 hour before coitus and to remain supine after insertion. ◆ Advise her to use the agent with a condom. ◆ Tell her to avoid douching for up to 6 hours after intercourse.

Comparing contraceptives *(continued)*

METHOD AND ACTIONS	CONTRAINDICATIONS	POTENTIAL PROBLEMS	CLIENT TEACHING
Male condom Mechanical barrier; 90% effective	Known allergy to latex products	May be allergenic; may tear; must be applied before any vulval contact; may affect sexual pleasure	◆ Advise the client to make sure her partner leaves a small space in the tip of the condom when applying. ◆ Instruct her on proper condom use to avoid tears. ◆ Emphasize that the condom must be held in place during withdrawal to prevent spillage.
Female condom Mechanical barrier; 95% effective	Known allergy to latex products	May break or become dislodged; difficult to use; expensive	◆ Teach about insertion procedure (inner ring covers cervix, second ring remains outside the vagina). ◆ Tell her the condom may be inserted 8 hours before intercourse. ◆ Advise her that the female condom shouldn't be used with a male condom.
Cervical cap 84% to 91% effective for women who never gave birth; 68% to 74% for those who have; mechanical barrier (similar to diaphragm but smaller, fitting over just the cervix and held in place by suction); chemical barrier when used with spermicide	Known allergy to latex products	Ineffectiveness common due to failure to use the device or inappropriate use of the device	◆ Explain that those who aren't suited for a diaphragm may use a cervical cap. ◆ Instruct to fill cervical cap only to ⅓ full with spermicides. ◆ Teach insertion procedure (squeeze rim of cervical cap and insert far inside the vagina; use finger to push cap over cervix and make sure cervix is covered; test suction by gently pulling on dome – you should feel resistance); wait 8 hours after intercourse to remove it. ◆ Instruct on proper care and storage.
Natural family planning Abstinence during the fertile period, determined by one or more methods (calendar method, basal body temperature graph, and cervical mucus test); 80% to 90% effective	None	Requires meticulous record keeping and ability to monitor body changes; only reliable in those with regular menstrual cycles; may be unreliable during illness, infection, or stress; may reduce spontaneity	◆ Calendar (rhythm) method: Tell the client to document the duration of her periods and to presume that ovulation occurs 14 days before menses. ◆ Basal body temperature graph: Tell the client to document her body temperature over time and to presume that a drop in temperature followed by a sustained increase indicates ovulation. ◆ Cervical mucus test: Teach the client that the spinnbarkeit is high at ovulation. The client must be self-disciplined, keep accurate records, and be prepared to cope with unexpected pregnancy.

(continued)

Comparing contraceptives *(continued)*

METHOD AND ACTIONS	CONTRAINDICATIONS	POTENTIAL PROBLEMS	CLIENT TEACHING
Hormonal contraceptives (such as estrogen and progestin combination) Prevents ovulation; 99.5% effective	Reproductive system cancers, hypertension, pregnancy, breast-feeding, liver dysfunction, history of stroke or coronary artery disease (CAD), undiagnosed vaginal bleeding	May cause spotting, nausea, headache, weight gain, monilial vaginal infections, breast tenderness; no protection against STDs	◆ Inform the client of benefits, such as the reduced risk of endometrial and ovarian cancer, ectopic pregnancy, ovarian cyst, noncancerous breast tumors, PID, dysmenorrhea, and premenstrual tension. ◆ Clients older than age 35 who smoke 15 or more cigarettes per day are at increased risk for fatal heart attack. ◆ If she wants to become pregnant, the client may be advised to wait 2 months after stopping the drug before attempting pregnancy. Conception may not occur until 8 months after stopping contraceptives.
Transdermal contraceptive patches Worn for 1 week and replaced on the same day each week for 3 weeks, then no patch on the 4th week; prevents ovulation; 99% effective	Breast-feeding; family history of stroke, CAD, thrombohemolytic disease or liver disease; undiagnosed vaginal bleeding; sensitivities to the patch	No protection against STDs	◆ Teach the client to change the patch on the same day every week, then leave it off for the fourth week.
Medroxyprogesterone acetate (Depo-Provera; 150 mg administered I.M. every 3 months) Suppresses release of gonadotropic hormones and prevents ovulation; 99% effective	Pregnancy, liver disease, undiagnosed vaginal bleeding, breast cancer, blood clotting disorders, cardiovascular disease	May cause changes in menstrual cycle, weight gain, headache, nervousness, fatigue; no protection against STDs	◆ Teach the client that this drug prevents pregnancy for 3 months. ◆ Inform her that it may take up to 10 months to conceive after the last dose. ◆ Counsel the client about adverse effects to promote long-term compliance.
Levonorgestrel (subdermal implant consisting of six capsules) Prevents ovulation and stimulates production of thick cervical mucus, which inhibits sperm penetration; 99% effective	Pregnancy, liver disease, undiagnosed vaginal bleeding, breast cancer, blood clotting disorders, cardiovascular disease	May cause irregular menstruation, spotting, amenorrhea, weight gain, headache; no protection against STDs	◆ Inform the client that capsules must be replaced every 5 years. ◆ Counsel the client about potential adverse effects, such as menstrual irregularities.

Comparing contraceptives *(continued)*

METHOD AND ACTIONS	CONTRAINDICATIONS	POTENTIAL PROBLEMS	CLIENT TEACHING
Tubal ligation Interruption of fallopian tube passageways; 99.6% effective (40% to 75% reversible)	Client-specific surgical risks; umbilical hernia; obesity	May cause menstrual disorders; discomfort from CO_2 during laparoscopy; problems in laparotomy, such as infection, hemorrhage, small-bowel perforation, and anesthesia complications; no protection against STDs	◆ Advise the client to approach the procedure as irreversible. ◆ Demonstrate aseptic incision care. ◆ Instruct the client to refrain from unprotected sex prior to the procedure.
Vasectomy Interruption of vas deferens passageways; 99.6% effective (95% reversible)	Client-specific surgical risks; uncertainty about desire for permanent sterilization	May be associated with development of kidney stones; surgical complications; no protection against STDs	◆ Advise the client to approach the procedure as irreversible (although reversal may be possible). ◆ Suggest an alternative contraceptive method for the first 6 months after surgery until a sperm count confirms the procedure's effectiveness. ◆ Teach incision care.

◆ Instruct the client about her dietary needs while taking a hormonal contraceptive. Tell her to increase her intake of foods high in vitamin B_6 (wheat, corn, liver, meat) and folic acid (liver and green, leafy vegetables). *About 20% to 30% of hormonal contraceptive users have dietary deficiencies of vitamin B_6 (pyridoxine) and folic acid. Moreover, health care professionals increasingly speculate that hormonal contraceptive users should increase their intake of vitamins A, B_2, B_{12}, C, and niacin.*

◆ Encourage compliance with follow-up appointments, and explain their importance. *Follow-up visits may include evaluation of contraceptive use and adverse reactions as well as repeating a Pap test and addressing the client's questions.*

Evaluation

◆ The client cooperates in providing health history information.

◆ The client correctly describes the use of the selected contraceptive.

◆ The client describes adverse reactions to the selected contraceptive and states her responsibility to report any that occur.

◆ The client makes an appointment for her next visit (if indicated).

◆ The client states that the current method of birth control is acceptable.

ANTEPARTUM PERIOD

The antepartum period extends from conception to the onset of labor. During this time, care of the mother (client) and the fetus focuses on health maintenance and the prevention of complications. Nursing care during the normal antepartum period includes taking a thorough maternal history, performing a complete physical examination, and educating the client about antepartum health.

GAMETOGENESIS AND CONCEPTION

GAMETOGENESIS is the production of specialized sex cells called *gametes:*

◆ The male gamete (spermatozoon) is produced in the seminiferous tubules of the testes during spermatogenesis.

◆ The female gamete (ovum) is produced in the graafian follicle of the ovary during oogenesis.

◆ As gametes mature, the number of chromosomes they contain is halved (through meiosis), from 46 to 23.

Conception, or fertilization, occurs with the fusion of a spermatozoon and an ovum (oocyte) in the ampulla of the fallopian tube.
- The fertilized egg is called a *zygote.*
- The diploid number of chromosomes (a pair of each chromosome; 44 autosomes and 2 sex chromosomes) is restored when the zygote is formed.
- A male zygote is formed if the ovum is fertilized by a spermatozoon carrying a Y chromosome.
- A female zygote is formed if the ovum is fertilized by a spermatozoon carrying an X chromosome.

IMPLANTATION AND FETAL DEVELOPMENT

Implantation occurs when the cellular wall of the blastocyst (trophoblast) implants itself in the endometrium of the anterior or posterior fundal region about 7 to 9 days after fertilization.
- Primary villi appear within weeks after implantation.
- After implantation, the endometrium is called the *decidua.*

Fetal structures

Structures unique to the fetus include fetal membranes, the umbilical cord, the placenta, and amniotic fluid. During placentation, chorionic villi invade the decidua and become the fetal portion of the future placenta. By the 4th week of gestation, a normal fetus begins to show noticeable signs of growth.

Fetal membranes

Two fetal membranes are unique to the fetus:
- The CHORION is the fetal membrane closest to the uterine wall; it gives rise to the placenta.
- The AMNION is the thin, tough, inner fetal membrane that lines the amniotic sac.

Three different embryonic germ layers generate fetal tissues:
- The ECTODERM generates the epidermis, nervous system, pituitary gland, salivary glands, optic lens, lining of the lower portion of the anal canal, hair, and tooth enamel.
- The ENDODERM generates the epithelial lining of the larynx, trachea, bladder, urethra, prostate gland, auditory canal, liver, pancreas, and alimentary canal.
- The MESODERM generates the connective and sclerous tissues; the blood and vascular system; the musculature; teeth (except enamel); mesothelial lining of the pericardial, pleural, and peritoneal cavities; kidneys; and ureters.

Umbilical cord

The umbilical cord serves as the lifeline from the embryo to the placenta. At term, it measures 20″ to 22″ (51 to 56 cm) in length and about 0.8″ (2 cm) in diameter. The umbilical cord contains two arteries, one vein, and Wharton's jelly (which prevents kinking of the cord in utero). Blood flows through the cord at about 400 ml/minute.

Fetal circulation

Fetal circulation structures include the:
- umbilical vein, which carries oxygenated blood to the fetus from the placenta
- umbilical arteries, which carry deoxygenated blood from the fetus to the placenta
- foramen ovale, which serves as the septal opening between the atria of the fetal heart
- ductus arteriosus, which connects the pulmonary artery to the aorta, allowing blood to shunt around the fetal lungs
- ductus venosus, which carries oxygenated blood from the umbilical vein to the inferior vena cava, bypassing the liver.

Placenta

The placenta weighs about 1 to 1 lb, 5 oz (455 to 590 g), measures 6″ to 10″ (15 to 25 cm) in diameter and, at term, is 1″ to 1¼″ (2.5 to 3.2 cm) thick. It contains 15 to 20 subdivisions called *cotyledons.* Rough in texture, the placenta appears red on the maternal surface and shiny and gray on the fetal surface. The placenta:
- functions as a transport mechanism between the mother and the fetus
- has a life span and function that depend on oxygen consumption and maternal circulation (circulation to the fetus and placenta improves when the mother lies on her left side)
- receives maternal oxygen by way of diffusion
- produces hormones, including human chorionic gonadotropin, human placental lactogen, gonadotropin-releasing hormone, thyrotropin-releasing factor, corticotropin, estrogen, and progesterone
- supplies the fetus with carbohydrates, water, fat, protein, minerals, and inorganic salts
- carries end products of fetal metabolism to the maternal circulation for excretion
- transfers passive immunity by way of maternal antibodies.

Amniotic fluid

The amniotic fluid prevents heat loss, preserves constant fetal body temperature, cushions the fetus, and facilitates fetal growth and development. Amniotic fluid is replaced every 3 hours.

At term, the uterus contains 800 to 1,200 ml of amniotic fluid, which is clear and yellowish and has a specific gravity of 1.007 to 1.025 and a pH of 7.0 to 7.25. Maternal serum provides amniotic fluid in early gestation, with increasing amounts derived from fetal urine late in gestation. Amniotic fluid contains:

- albumin
- bilirubin
- creatinine
- enzymes
- fat
- lanugo
- lecithin
- leukocytes
- sphingomyelin
- urea.

ASSESSMENT

The client's general health history and family health history may identify abnormal conditions that place the client at high risk for pregnancy-related complications. The client's menstrual history may be used to identify potential problems and determine the client's expected date of delivery. (See *Estimating delivery dates and gestational age.*)

The client's obstetrical history may reveal potential problems. Useful information from previous pregnancies includes *gravida* (the number of pregnancies, including the current one; also the term used for a pregnant woman) and *para* (the number of past pregnancies of at least 20 weeks' gestation; also the term used for a woman who has given birth to a viable fetus or infant). For each pregnancy, identify the type of delivery, the length of gestation, the length of labor, the size of the neonate, and information about problems that occurred. Many hospitals use the GTPAL or GTPALM system to document previous pregnancies:

- G stands for the number of pregnancies (gravida).
- T stands for the number of term infants born.
- P stands for the number of preterm infants born (para).
- A stands for the number of pregnancies ending in spontaneous or elective abortion.
- L stands for the number of living children. Multiple gestation doesn't change G (gravida) or P (para).
- M stands for the total number of multiple pregnancies the client has experienced.

Estimating delivery dates and gestational age

- Nägele's rule is used to determine the estimated date of delivery by subtracting 3 months from the first day of the last menstrual period and adding 7 days; for example:
  October 5 – 3 months = July 5; + 7 days = July 12.
- Quickening is described as light fluttering and usually is felt between 16 and 22 weeks' gestation.
- Fetal heart sounds can be detected at 12 weeks' gestation with a Doppler ultrasound and can be auscultated with a fetoscope at 16 to 20 weeks' gestation.
- Fetal crown-to-rump measurements, determined by ultrasonography, can be used to assess the fetus's age until the head can be defined.
- Biparietal diameter is the widest transverse diameter of the fetal head. Measurements can be made by about 12 to 13 weeks' gestation.
- McDonald's rule uses fundal height to determine the duration of pregnancy in either lunar months or weeks. To use this rule, place a tape measure at the symphysis pubis and measure up and over the fundus. Fundal height in centimeters $\times \frac{2}{7}$ = duration of pregnancy in lunar months; fundal height in centimeters $\times \frac{8}{7}$ = duration of pregnancy in weeks.

Family assessment

Health status and risk behaviors of the client's family members may reveal potential transmission of disease to the pregnant client and her fetus. Genetically transmitted diseases should be identified and considered in the care plan for the pregnant client.

Psychosocial assessment of the client and her partner discloses the couple's needs. The client's learning needs disclose deficient knowledge of changes that will occur in the upcoming months. Evaluation of the client's support systems discloses the degree of emotional support available to the client. Assessment of the client's economic status may reveal potential problems in meeting basic needs for a healthy pregnancy and delivery. Assessment of the family's ethnic and cultural values, beliefs, and practices reveals variations in family members' understanding of adaptations to pregnancy.

Maternal assessment

The client experiences changes in all body systems, occuring due to pregnancy. Systemic highlights of changes are addressed in the following sections.

Cardiovascular changes

- Cardiac hypertrophy from increased blood volume and cardiac output
- Displacement of the heart upward and to the left from pressure on the diaphragm
- Progressive increase in blood volume, peaking in the third trimester at 30% to 50% of prepregnancy levels
- Resting pulse rate fluctuations, with increases ranging from 0 to 15 beats/minute at term
- Pulmonic systolic and apical systolic murmurs resulting from decreased blood viscosity and increased blood flow
- Increased femhormonal venous pressure caused by impaired circulation in the lower extremities (from pressure of the enlarged uterus on the pelvic veins and inferior vena cava)
- Decreased cerebrospinal fluid space from enlargement of the vessels surrounding the spinal cord's dura mater
- Increased fibrinogen levels (up to 50% at term) from hormonal influences
- Increased levels of blood coagulation factors VII, IX, and X, leading to a hypercoagulable state
- Increase of approximately 33% in total red blood cell (RBC) volume, despite hemodilution and decreasing erythrocyte count
- Decrease in hematocrit (HCT) of about 7%
- Increase in total hemoglobin (Hb) level of 12% to 15%, which is less than the overall plasma volume increase, thus reducing Hb concentration and leading to physiologic anemia of pregnancy
- Leukocyte production equal to or slightly greater than blood volume increase (average leukocyte count is 10,000 to 11,000/µl; this peaks at 25,000/µl during labor, possibly through an estrogen-related mechanism)

GI changes

- Gum swelling from increased estrogen levels (gums may be spongy and hyperemic)
- Lateral and posterior displacement of the intestines
- Superior and lateral displacement of the stomach
- Delayed intestinal motility and gastric and gallbladder emptying time from smooth-muscle relaxation caused by high placental progesterone levels
- Nausea and vomiting, which usually subside after the first trimester
- Hemorrhoids late in pregnancy from venous pressure
- Constipation from increased progesterone levels, resulting in increased water absorption from the colon
- Displacement of the appendix from McBurney's point (making diagnosis of appendicitis difficult)

Hormonal changes (endocrine system)

- Increased basal metabolic rate (up 25% at term) caused by demands of the fetus and uterus and increased oxygen consumption
- Increased iodine metabolism from slight hyperplasia of the thyroid caused by increased estrogen levels
- Slight hyperparathyroidism from increased requirement for calcium and vitamin D
- Elevated plasma parathyroid hormone levels, peaking between 15 and 35 weeks' gestation
- Slightly enlarged pituitary gland
- Increased production of prolactin by the pituitary gland late in pregnancy
- Increased estrogen levels and hypertrophy of the adrenal cortex
- Increased cortisol levels to regulate protein and carbohydrate metabolism
- Possibly decreased maternal blood glucose levels
- Decreased insulin production early in pregnancy
- Increased production of estrogen, progesterone, and human chorionic somatomammotropin by the placenta and increased levels of maternal cortisol, which reduce the mother's ability to use insulin, thus ensuring an adequate glucose supply for the fetus and placenta

Respiratory changes

- Increased vascularization of the respiratory tract caused by increased estrogen levels
- Shortening of the lungs caused by the enlarged uterus
- Upward displacement of the diaphragm by the uterus
- Increased tidal volume, causing slight hyperventilation
- Increased chest circumference (by about 2⅜" [6 cm])
- Altered breathing, with abdominal breathing replacing thoracic breathing as pregnancy progresses
- Slight increase (2 breaths/minute) in respiratory rate
- Lowered threshold for carbon dioxide due to increased levels of progesterone

Metabolic changes

- Increased water retention caused by higher levels of steroidal sex hormones, decreased serum protein levels and increased intracapillary pressure and permeability
- Increased levels of serum lipids, lipoproteins, and cholesterol

◆ Increased iron requirements caused by fetal demands
◆ Increased carbohydrate needs
◆ Increased protein retention from hyperplasia and hypertrophy of maternal tissues
◆ Weight gain of 25 to 30 lb (11.5 to 13.5 kg)

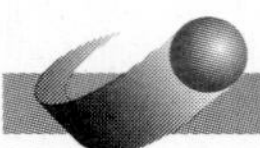

FAST FACT

Maternal weight gain is commonly estimated at 3 lb (1.4 kg) in the first trimester, 12 lb (5.4 kg) in the second trimester, and 12 lb (5.4 kg) in the third trimester.

Musculoskeletal changes

◆ Forward-tilting pelvis, shifting the center of gravity
◆ Increased lumbosacral curve and weight of larger breasts, which pulls shoulders forward
◆ Relaxing of sacroiliac, sacrococcygeal, and pelvic joints, which affects gait, posture, and comfort
◆ Hypocalcemia and muscle cramps if insufficient calcium is ingested (due to greater need for calcium from increased maternal metabolism)
◆ Separation of abdominal muscles and stretching of umbilicus

Immune system changes

◆ Decreased immunologic competency, which prevents rejection of the fetus

Neurologic changes

◆ Entrapment neuropathies may occur in the peripheral nervous system as a result of mechanical pressure

Skin changes

◆ Hyperactive sweat and sebaceous glands
◆ Changing pigmentation from the increase of melanocyte-stimulating hormone caused by increased estrogen and progesterone levels (darkened line from symphysis pubis to umbilicus known as linea nigra)
◆ Darkening of the nipples, areola, cervix, vagina, and vulva
◆ Pigmentary changes, known as *facial chloasma,* on the nose, cheeks, and forehead

Genitourinary changes

◆ Dilated ureters and renal pelvis caused by progesterone and pressure from the enlarged uterus
◆ Increased glomerular filtration rate (GFR) and renal plasma flow (RPF) early in pregnancy; elevated GFR until delivery, but a near-normal RPF level by term
◆ Increased clearance of urea and creatinine due to increased renal function
◆ Decreased blood urea and nonprotein nitrogen values due to increased renal function
◆ Glucosuria due to increased glomerular filtration without an increase in tubular reabsorptive capacity
◆ Decreased bladder tone
◆ Increased sodium retention due to hormonal influences
◆ Increases in dimensions of the uterus from approximately 2½″ to 12½″ (6.5 to 32 cm) in length; 1½″ to 9½″ (4 to 24 cm) in width; 8⅝″ to 10″ (22 to 25 cm) in depth; 2 to 42 oz (57 to 1,191 g) in weight; and ⅛ to 170 oz (3.5 to 5,028 ml) in volume (see *Typical uterine changes during pregnancy,* page 192)
– Hypertrophied uterine muscle cells (5 to 10 times normal size)
– Increased vascularity, edema, hypertrophy, and hyperplasia of the cervical glands
– Increased vaginal secretions with a pH of 3.5 to 6
– Discontinued ovulation and maturation of new follicles
– Thickening of vaginal mucosa, loosening of vaginal connective tissue, and hypertrophy of small muscle cells

Signs and symptoms of pregnancy

Presumptive (early) signs and symptoms

◆ AMENORRHEA or slight, painless spotting of unknown cause in early gestation
◆ Breast enlargement and tenderness
◆ Fatigue
◆ Increased skin pigmentation
◆ Nausea and vomiting
◆ Quickening (the first recognizable movement of the fetus)
◆ Linea nigra (dark line pigment on abdomen)
◆ Chloasma (pigmentary skin change on the face)
◆ Striae gravidarum (red streaks on abdomen)
◆ Urinary frequency and urgency

Signs and symptoms of a probable pregnancy

◆ Ballottement (passive fetal movement in response to tapping of the lower portion of the uterus or cervix)
◆ BRAXTON HICKS CONTRACTIONS (painless uterine contractions that occur throughout pregnancy)
◆ CHADWICK'S SIGN (change in color of the vaginal walls from normal light pink to deep violet)

Typical uterine changes during pregnancy

Beginning at the 20th week, fundal height equals gestational age, plus or minus 2 cm.

UTERUS	NONPREGNANT	PREGNANT (AT TERM)
Length	6.5 cm	32 cm
Width	4 cm	24 cm
Depth	2.5 cm	22 cm
Weight	50 g	1,000 g

FUNDAL HEIGHT RELATED TO GESTATIONAL WEEKS

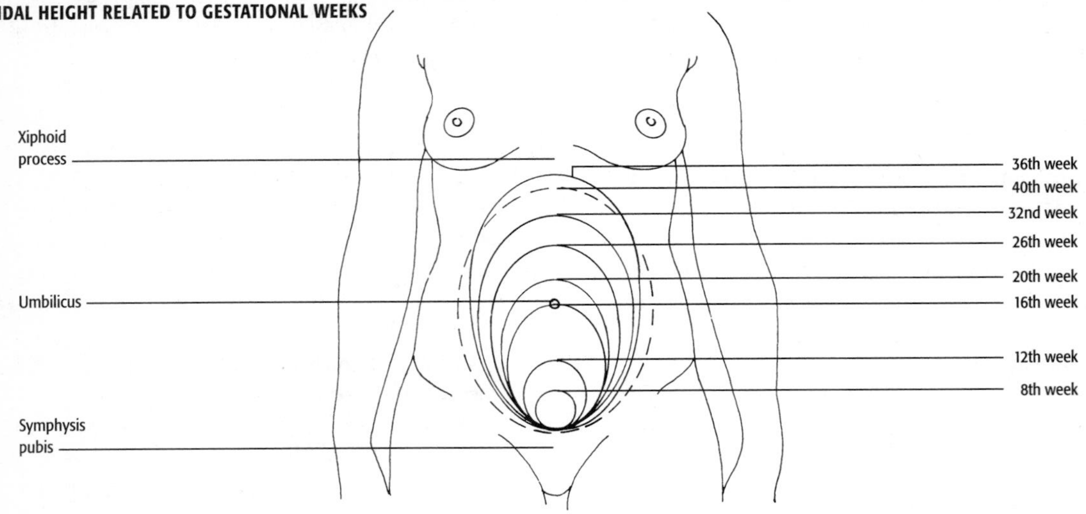

◆ GOODELL'S SIGN (softening of the cervix)
◆ HEGAR'S SIGN (softening of the lower uterine segment that may be present at 6 to 8 weeks' gestation)
◆ Palpation of fetal outline

Signs and symptoms of a definite pregnancy

◆ Detection of fetal heartbeat by Doppler ultrasound (by 10 to 12 weeks' gestation)
◆ Palpation of fetal movements (after 20 weeks' gestation)
◆ Ultrasonography evidence of fetal outline (as early as 8 weeks' gestation)

Diagnostic evaluation

Numerous tests are performed as part of antepartum care. The results can be used to confirm pregnancy and reveal maternal and fetal complications:

◆ Blood type, Rh, and abnormal antibodies identify whether the fetus is at risk for erythroblastosis fetalis or hyperbilirubinemia.
◆ Immunologic tests, such as rubella antibodies, detect the presence of rubella; rapid plasma reagin detects untreated syphilis; and hepatitis B surface antigen detects hepatitis B.
◆ Maternal serum assays, such as estrogens, human placental lactogen (hPL), and human chorionic gonadotropin (HCG), are used in addition to urinalysis to monitor the pregnant patient for problems. Premature labor risk may be identified by presence of estriol levels, which tend to

Maternal and neonatal laboratory values

TEST	NONPREGNANT WOMEN	PREGNANT WOMEN	POSTPARTUM WOMEN	TERM NEONATES
Hemoglobin (Hb)	12 to 16 g/dl	11 to 15 g/dl	11 to 15 g/dl	15 to 20 g/dl
Hematocrit	37% to 48%	36% to 46% (32% to 35% indicates physiologic anemia)	32% to 46%	43% to 61%
Red blood cells	4 to 5 million/µl	5 to 6.25 million/µl	5 to 6.25 million/µl	5 to 6 million/µl
White blood cells	5,000 to 10,000/µl	5,000 to 12,000/µl	5,000 to 16,000/µl (possibly up to 25,000/µl)	10,000 to 30,000/µl
Platelets	150,000 to 400,000/mm^3	150,000 to 400,000/mm^3	150,000 to 400,000/mm^3	100,000 to 280,000/mm^3
Serum glucose	65 to 100 mg/dl	≤ 100 mg/dl	≤ 100 mg/dl	*First 24 hours:* 40 to 100 mg/dl
2-hour glucose tolerance test	below 140 mg/dl	below 140 mg/dl	(Not performed)	(Not performed)
Hb A_1C	6% to 8%	6% to 8%	(Not performed)	(Not performed)
Serum bilirubin (total)	(Not performed)	(Not performed)	(Not performed)	*Cord blood:* Below 2.8 mg/dl *At 24 hours:* 2 to 6 mg/dl *At 3 to 5 days:* 4 to 6 mg/dl
Urine protein	Negative	Negative or trace	Negative to +1 False positive may occur due to lochia	Negative
Urine glucose	Negative	Negative or 1+	Negative to +1 False positive may occur due to lochia	Negative

increase prior to delivery. Low hPL concentrates are associated with postmaturity syndrome, intrauterine growth retardation, preeclampsia, and eclampsia. Serum HCG is used to detect pregnancy; significantly high levels indicate multiple pregnancy or a baby with Down syndrome; low levels can occur with ectopic pregnancy or pregnancy less than 9 days.

◆ Urine tests measure HCG to confirm pregnancy.

◆ Hematologic studies involve the use of blood samples to analyze and measure RBCs, white blood cells (WBCs), erythrocyte sedimentation rate, prothrombin time (PT), partial thromboplastin time (PTT), platelets, Hb level, and HCT. (See *Maternal and neonatal laboratory values.*)

◆ Genital cultures, such as a gonorrhea smear and chlamydia test, are used to detect sexually transmitted diseases.
◆ Triple screen between 15 and 20 weeks' gestation is used to identify a fetus at increased risk for Down syndrome, trisomy 18, spina bifida, anencephaly, omphalocele, and gastroschisis.
◆ High maternal serum alpha-fetoprotein levels may suggest fetal neural tube defects, such as spina bifida and anencephaly. Low levels may suggest Down syndrome.
◆ AMNIOCENTESIS is usually performed after the 14th week of gestation, when amniotic fluid is sufficient and the uterus has moved into the abdominal cavity. This procedure involves transabdominal insertion of a spinal needle into the uterus to aspirate amniotic fluid. This procedure is used to:
- determine gestational age and fetal lung maturity by analyzing the lecithin-sphingomyelin ratio, two key components of surfactant
- measure creatinine levels
- detect hemolytic disease of the fetus
- diagnose metabolic disorders, amino acid disorders, and mucopolysaccharidosis
- measure ammniotic levels of estriol and fetal thyroid hormone
- identify fetal gender
- diagnose genetic disorders, such as chromosomal aberrations, sex-linked disorders, inborn errors of metabolism, and neural tube defect
- diagnose and evaluate isoimmune disease, including Rh sensitization and ABO blood type incompatibility.
◆ Chorionic villi sampling can be performed as early as 8 weeks' gestation. It involves removal and analysis of a small tissue specimen from the fetal portion of the placenta. This test helps determine the genetic makeup of the fetus, providing earlier diagnosis of genetic disorders. The test also identifies sex, allowing early detection of X-linked conditions in male fetuses.
◆ Ultrasonography, a noninvasive and painless procedure, uses ultrasonic waves reflected by tissues of different densities to visualize deep structures of the body. Reflected signals are then amplified and processed to produce a visual display, providing immediate results without harm to the fetus or mother. Ultrasound can be used to detect:
- overall fetal condition
- possible fetal complications (malformation, malpresentation, placental abnormalities, multiple gestation, hydramnios or oligohydramnios)
- pregnancy status (pregnancy detected by 7th gestational week; may be necessary if pregnancy test results are questionable)
- fetal size to correlate with estimated due date
- location of fetus prior to amniocentesis
- an IUD that was left in place at time of pregnancy.
◆ The nonstress test (NST) is used to detect fetal heart accelerations in response to fetal movement. This noninvasive test provides simple, inexpensive, immediate results without contraindications or complications. It may be indicated for a client at risk for uteroplacental insufficiency or fetal distress. The NST can be performed between 32 and 34 weeks' gestation. A nonreactive test result indicates the possibility of fetal hypoxia, fetal sleep cycle, or the effects of drugs. The results may be inconclusive if the client is extremely obese.
◆ The contraction stress test, also called the *oxytocin challenge test* (OCT), is used to evaluate fetal ability to withstand the stress of labor. This test requires monitoring the fetus's response to natural contractions or I.V. administration of oxytocin. The contraction stress test is performed on a client at risk for uteroplacental insufficiency or fetal compromise from diabetes, heart disease, hypertension, or renal disease or a client with a history of stillbirth. The contraction stress test isn't indicated for those with previous classic cesarean delivery or third-trimester bleeding or for those at high risk for preterm labor.
◆ The nipple stimulation stress test induces contractions by activating sensory receptors in the areola, triggering the release of oxytocin by the posterior pituitary gland. The receptors are activated by rolling the nipple manually or applying a warm washcloth. This test has the same reactive pattern as the reactive NST result.
◆ The biophysical profile assesses four to six parameters — fetal breathing movements, body movements, muscle tone, amniotic fluid volume, heart rate reactivity, and placental grade — using real-time ultrasound. This test is noninvasive and quick and can detect central nervous system (CNS) depression.
◆ Fetal blood flow studies use umbilical or uterine Doppler velocimetry to evaluate vascular resistance, especially in clients with hypertension, diabetes, isoimmunization, and lupus. These studies are useful when congenital anomalies or cardiac arrhythmias are suspected.
◆ Percutaneous umbilical blood sampling (PUBS) is an invasive procedure that involves inserting a spinal needle into the umbilical cord to obtain fetal blood samples or transfuse the fetus in utero. Usually performed during the second or third trimester, PUBS is indicated when the fetus is at risk for congenital and chromosomal abnormalities, congenital infection, or anemia. It's also useful in assessing the fetus's acid-base status and fetal karyotyping. It carries a 1% to 2% risk of fetal loss.

◆ Fetoscopy is a procedure in which a fetoscope, a telescoping instrument with lights and lenses, is inserted into the amniotic sac where it can view and photograph the fetus. It's used to diagnose, through blood and tissue sampling, several blood and skin diseases that amniocentesis can't detect. It carries a 3% to 5% risk of fetal loss, but can help treat or correct a defect in the fetus.

Nursing diagnoses

◆ Ineffective health maintenance
◆ Risk for deficient fluid volume

Planning and goals

◆ The results of the client's health history and physical and diagnostic examinations will be within normal limits.
◆ The client will be able to describe the warning signs of pregnancy complications.
◆ The client will verbalize acceptance of the body changes of early pregnancy.
◆ The client will discuss concerns about her pregnancy related to personal and family psychosocial needs.
◆ The client will return for routine follow-up visits.

Implementation

◆ Teach the warning signs of pregnancy-related complications: vaginal bleeding, gush of fluid from the vagina, persistent vomiting, chills and fever, abdominal pain, visual disturbances, severe headache, and swelling of the face and hands. *These warning signs indicate complications, such as spontaneous abortion, fluid and electrolyte imbalance, gestational hypertension, and infection.*
◆ Explain that only prescribed medication should be taken. *Many medications are teratogenic, especially in the first trimester when the fetal organs are developing.*
◆ Explain the suggested treatment for nausea and vomiting (morning sickness). *Nausea and vomiting can be managed by eating dry crackers before rising; eating small, frequent, high-protein meals; and avoiding spicy and fried foods.*
◆ Stress the importance of regular health supervision during pregnancy. *The quality of prenatal care has a great impact on the well-being of the mother and fetus. In addition to enabling the physician to detect and treat problems promptly, prenatal visits provide an opportunity for teaching the client about pregnancy, labor and delivery, and postpartum and neonatal care.*
◆ Provide the opportunity for the client to ask questions and talk about expectations. *Listening to the client helps establish a communicative, positive, caring nurse-client relationship. It also provides an opportunity to evaluate individual needs and provide appropriate care.*

Evaluation

◆ The results of the client's health history and physical and diagnostic examinations are within normal limits.
◆ The client describes the warning signs of pregnancy complications and the importance of reporting them.
◆ The client verbalizes gradual acceptance of the body changes of early pregnancy.
◆ The client identifies sources of emotional and material support that will adequately meet personal and family needs during this pregnancy.
◆ The client has made an appointment for her next visit.

ANTEPARTUM COMPLICATIONS

During the antepartum period, the client must be monitored carefully for complications, some of which can be life threatening for the mother and fetus. The following entries focus on nursing care of the antepartum client with complications.

ABORTION, SPONTANEOUS

SPONTANEOUS ABORTION, or simply *abortion,* is the term used to describe termination of a pregnancy when gestation is less than 20 weeks. (See *Care during threatened or inevitable abortion,* page 196; *Complications of early pregnancy,* page 197; and *Preterm labor,* page 198.)

Possible causes

Fetal factors

◆ Defective embryonic development from abnormal chromosome division (most common cause of fetal death)
◆ Faulty implantation of the fertilized ovum
◆ Failure of the endometrium to accept the fertilized ovum

Placental factors

◆ Premature separation of the normally implanted placenta
◆ Abnormal placental implantation
◆ Abnormal platelet function

Maternal factors

◆ Infection
◆ Severe malnutrition

Care during threatened or inevitable abortion

TYPE	SYMPTOMS	NURSING CONSIDERATIONS
Threatened abortion	Vaginal bleeding, cramping, cervix remains closed	◆ Maintain the client on bed rest with a light diet. ◆ Instruct the client to avoid any kind of straining. ◆ Administer a mild sedative as ordered. ◆ Keep a perineal pad count to determine blood loss. ◆ Tell the client to restrict sexual intercourse.
Inevitable abortion	Vaginal bleeding, cramping, cervical dilation	*Complete abortion* ◆ Keep a complete perineal pad count and save all tissue samples. ◆ Replace blood or fluid loss as necessary. *Incomplete abortion* ◆ Use the same considerations as for complete abortion. ◆ Assist with dilatation and curettage.

- ◆ Abnormalities of the reproductive organs
- ◆ Endocrine problems
- ◆ Trauma
- ◆ ABO blood group incompatibility and Rh isoimmunization
- ◆ Drug ingestion

Assessment findings

- ◆ Bleeding, abdominal cramps or pain, cervical dilation, rupture of membranes, and expulsion of uterine contents
- ◆ Alteration in vital signs, which may indicate shock or infection
- ◆ Change in emotional status that may reflect fear, guilt, and anxiety

Diagnostic evaluation

- ◆ The amount of bleeding can be assessed through a pad count.
- ◆ Examination of tissue expelled vaginally may reveal products of conception and can be used to determine if the abortion was complete or incomplete.
- ◆ Ultrasound confirms presence or absence of fetal heart sounds or an empty amniotic sac.

Nursing diagnoses

- ◆ Risk for injury
- ◆ Dysfunctional grieving

Treatment

- ◆ Bed rest until bleeding is controlled
- ◆ Transfusion with packed RBCs in severe bleeding
- ◆ I.V. administration of oxytocin (Pitocin) to stimulate uterine contractions
- ◆ Dilatation and curettage (D&C) if incomplete abortion occurs

Planning and goals

- ◆ The client won't develop complications, such as infection or shock.
- ◆ The client will express knowledge of her condition and the procedures being performed.
- ◆ The client won't exhibit signs of extreme anxiety and fear.
- ◆ The client will have an opportunity to begin grieving.
- ◆ The client will identify her support system and available resources.

Implementation

- ◆ Explain all procedures *to promote client trust and help reduce anxiety.*
- ◆ Estimate blood loss, recording the number of perineal pads used, the degree of pad saturation, and a description of pad contents *to estimate the client's blood loss and risk for hemorrhagic shock.*
- ◆ Evaluate pad contents *to determine whether an abortion has occurred and to determine whether all the products of conception were expelled (complete abortion) or only a portion (incomplete abortion).*
- ◆ Obtain a type and cross-match blood specimen *in preparation for replacement of blood or blood products, if necessary.*

Complications of early pregnancy

CONDITION	DEFINITION	SIGNS AND SYMPTOMS	TREATMENT	NURSING CONSIDERATIONS
Ectopic pregnancy	Pregnancy outside the uterine cavity (most commonly in the fallopian tube)	◆ Signs and symptoms of pregnancy ◆ Rupture at 6 to 12 weeks' gestation (usually) ◆ Possible vaginal bleeding ◆ Severe pain in lower abdomen ◆ Vaginal tenderness ◆ Shock	◆ Salpingectomy ◆ Salpingostomy and tubal repair	◆ Assess the client for bleeding and pain. ◆ Prepare the client for abdominal surgery. ◆ Provide emotional support to the client.
Hydatidiform mole	Abnormal pregnancy that results in a grapelike cluster of vesicles; also called *gestational trophoblastic disease* or *molar pregnancy;* highest incidence is among clients younger than age 20 and older than age 40	◆ Rapid uterine growth ◆ Nausea and vomiting ◆ Elevated levels of chorionic gonadotropin ◆ Uterine bleeding in first and second trimesters ◆ Symptoms of preeclampsia	◆ Hysterotomy ◆ Hysterectomy ◆ Dilatation and curettage	◆ Prepare the client for the procedures. ◆ Allow the client to verbalize her feelings. ◆ Stress the importance of follow-up care. (A high incidence of choriocarcinoma is associated with hydatidiform mole.) ◆ Plan birth control for at least 1 year.
Hyperemesis gravidarum	Persistent vomiting during pregnancy, thought to be caused by high chorionic gonadotropin levels or psychological problem	◆ Nausea and vomiting ◆ Weight loss ◆ Fatigue ◆ Signs of dehydration ◆ Signs of starvation	◆ Antiemetics ◆ I.V. fluids (vitamins and electrolytes) ◆ Quiet environment ◆ Sedation ◆ Counseling	◆ Provide treatment as ordered. ◆ Allow the client to verbalize her feelings.
Incompetent cervix	Failure of the cervix to remain closed, resulting in abortion at 18 to 20 weeks' gestation	◆ Signs and symptoms of inevitable abortion	◆ Cerclage or surgical reinforcement of the cervix for future pregnancies	◆ Assist with the procedure. ◆ Provide emotional support to the client. ◆ Maintain bed rest for 24 hours after cerclage.

◆ Monitor vital signs frequently *to detect complications, such as infection and hemorrhage.*

◆ If the abortion is incomplete, prepare the client for D&C *to remove the risk for hemorrhage and infection.*

◆ Provide emotional support and counseling during the grieving process. Allow verbalization *to assist with acceptance of the loss of pregnancy.*

Evaluation

◆ The client doesn't develop complications.

◆ The client verbalizes understanding of what happened with her pregnancy.

◆ The client begins to use positive coping strategies to deal with her anxiety and grief and begins to express her feelings about the loss of her pregnancy.

Preterm labor

Preterm labor begins between 20 and 37 weeks' gestation. This quick-reference overview of preterm labor outlines its incidence and etiology, symptoms, risk factors, treatments, and associated nursing care.

Incidence and etiology

- Occurs in 8% to 19% of all births
- Associated with 75% to 80% of all neonatal mortality and morbidity
- Pathophysiology related to increased estrogen, fetal stress, increased stretch of uterine muscle, increased prostaglandins, increased maternal oxygen

Symptoms

- Palpable uterine contractions, more than 4 per hour, greater than 30 seconds in duration
- Effaced and dilated cervix
- Increased vaginal drainage

Risk factors

- Medical and pregnancy history factors (such as previous preterm delivery, diethylstilbestrol [DES] exposure and cervical shortening)
- Current pregnancy problems (such as multiple gestation, gestational hypertension, infection and premature rupture of membranes)
- Socioeconomic factors (such as age extremes, insufficient prenatal care, and education)
- Lifestyle habits (such as poor nutrition and substance abuse)

Treatments

- Tocolytics (such as magnesium sulfate, ritodrine, and terbutaline)
- Glucocorticoids (such as betamethasone)
- Medical therapy (such as cervical cerclage and bed rest)

Nursing care

- Discuss risks related to preterm delivery with client and her support system.
- Teach self-care measures:
  - Increase fluid intake to 2 to 3 qt (2 to 3 L)/day.
  - Empty bladder every 2 hours while awake.
  - Follow activity restrictions (such as bed rest and laying on left side).
  - Avoid nipple stimulation.
  - Use home monitoring techniques.

ABRUPTIO PLACENTAE

ABRUPTIO PLACENTAE is premature separation of the placenta from the uterine wall after 20 to 24 weeks' gestation. It may occur as late as the first or second stage of labor. Placental separation is measured by degree (from grades 0 to 3) to determine the fetal and maternal outcome. (See *Grading abruptio placentae.*)

Perinatal mortality depends on the degree of placental separation and the fetal level of maturity. Most serious complications stem from hypoxia, prematurity, and anemia. The maternal mortality rate is about 6% and depends on the severity of the bleeding, the presence of coagulation defects, hypofibrinogenemia, and the time lapse between placental separation and delivery.

Possible causes

- Abdominal trauma
- Decreased blood flow to the placenta
- Dietary deficiency
- Multifetal pregnancy
- Placental bleeding caused by needle puncture during amniocentesis
- Pressure on vena cava from enlarged uterus
- Other risk factors (low serum folic acid levels, vascular or renal disease, gestational hypertension, chronic hypertension)
- Short umbilical cord
- Smoking

Assessment findings

- Acute abdominal pain, which may indicate placental abruption
- Hemorrhage, either concealed or apparent, with dark red vaginal bleeding, which indicates intrauterine bleeding
- Rigid abdomen, which indicates high uterine tonicity resulting from hemorrhage
- Altered vital signs, which may indicate shock
- Frequent, low-amplitude contractions (noted with external fetal monitor), which may occur as the uterus at-

Grading abruptio placentae

Separation of the placenta from the uterine wall is classified as minimal, moderate, or extreme. Hemorrhaging may or may not be apparent, even with complete separation.

GRADE	CRITERIA
0	Maternal and fetal signs don't indicate difficulty. Premature separation isn't apparent until the placenta is examined after delivery.
1	Minimal separation causes vaginal bleeding and alterations in maternal vital signs, but hemorrhagic shock and fetal distress don't appear.
2	Moderate separation produces signs of fetal distress. The uterus is tense and painful when palpated.
3	Extreme separation occurs, possibly causing maternal shock and fetal death without immediate intervention.

tempts to contract or constrict blood vessels and control bleeding
- ◆ Uteroplacental insufficiency as evidenced by fetal distress

Diagnostic evaluation
- ◆ Ultrasonography locates the placenta, and a clot or hematoma may be apparent.
- ◆ Hematology may show disseminated intravascular coagulation (DIC) as indicated by increased PTT and PT, elevated level of fibrinogen degradation products, decreased fibrinogen level, or decreased platelet count.

Nursing diagnoses
- ◆ Ineffective tissue perfusion (cardiopulmonary)
- ◆ Risk for deficient fluid volume
- ◆ Acute pain
- ◆ Anxiety

Treatment
- ◆ I.V. infusion of lactated Ringer's solution to combat hypovolemia
- ◆ Transfusion of packed RBCs, platelets, and fresh frozen plasma, if necessary
- ◆ Cesarean delivery

Planning and goals
- ◆ The client will remain hemodynamically stable.
- ◆ The fetus will maintain an adequate heart rate and perfusion until delivery.
- ◆ The client won't exhibit signs of extreme anxiety and fear.
- ◆ The client will indicate a decrease in pain.

Implementation
- ◆ Monitor maternal vital signs, fetal heart rate (FHR), uterine contractions, and vaginal bleeding *to assess maternal and fetal well-being.*
- ◆ Assess fluid and electrolyte balance *to assess kidney function.*
- ◆ Avoid pelvic or vaginal examinations and enemas *to prevent further placental disruption.*
- ◆ Administer fresh whole blood, packed RBCs, platelets, or plasma *to replace blood volume.*
- ◆ Provide oxygen by mask *to minimize fetal hypoxia.*
- ◆ Evaluate maternal laboratory values *to assess for DIC.*
- ◆ Maintain the client in a left lateral recumbent position *to help relieve pressure on the vena cava from an enlarged uterus, which could further compromise fetal circulation, and to promote comfort.*
- ◆ Provide emotional support *to allay client anxiety.*

Evaluation
- ◆ The client has stable vital signs.
- ◆ The fetus maintains a strong heartbeat until delivery and is adequately perfused.
- ◆ The client remains calm.
- ◆ The client is more comfortable.

ADOLESCENT PREGNANCY

A teenage mother is at risk for such complications as gestational hypertension, cephalopelvic disproportion, anemia, and nutritional deficiencies. Teenagers also have a high incidence of sexually transmitted diseases (STDs), posing a concern for the mother and the neonate.

Infants born to teenage mothers are at risk for such complications as prematurity and low birth weight.

Possible causes

- Desire to gain love, adulthood, and independence through pregnancy
- Fear of reporting sexual activity to parents
- High level of adolescent sexual activity
- Lack of appropriate role models
- Limited access to contraceptives
- Low level of education correlated with incorrect use of contraceptives
- Lack of knowledge about ability to become pregnant
- Sporadic use of contraception

Assessment findings

- Amenorrhea
- Denial of pregnancy, which may delay the client from seeking medical attention early in pregnancy

Diagnostic evaluation

- Pregnancy test is positive.
- Ultrasound confirms the presence of a fetus.

Nursing diagnoses

- Deficient knowledge (maternal) about pregnancy and related responsibilities
- Imbalanced nutrition: Less than body requirements
- Interrupted family processes

Treatment

- Diet with calorie intake sufficient to support the growing adolescent and her developing fetus
- Educating client about proper prenatal care and signs of potential problems to report to health care providers

Drug therapy options

- Antibiotic for STDs (if necessary)

Planning and goals

- The client will increase her knowledge concerning pregnancy and related responsibilities concerning the fetus.
- The client will follow a nutritious diet.
- The client will receive support from family members.

Implementation

- Monitor the client's weight gain *to assess for nutritional deficiencies.*
- Monitor urine protein *to detect possible gestational hypertension* and glucose levels *to detect possible gestational diabetes.*
- Assess fundal height *to detect how the pregnancy is progressing.*
- Assess fetal heart sounds *to monitor fetal well-being.*
- Assess the client's knowledge of her pregnancy *to determine the need for further teaching.*
- Assess the client's family and available support *to determine the need for referrals.*
- Provide nutritional support and encouragement *to promote the well-being of the mother and fetus.*
- Stress the importance of attending scheduled prenatal appointments *to promote the well-being of the mother and fetus.*
- Advise the client of her options, including terminating the pregnancy, continuing the pregnancy and giving up the infant for adoption, and continuing the pregnancy and keeping the infant *to promote informed decision making.*
- Allow the client to express her feelings about her pregnancy and herself *to promote mental and emotional well-being.*

Evaluation

- The client participates in prenatal care.
- The client follows a nutritious diet and has appropriate weight gain.
- The client receives support during pregnancy.

ECTOPIC PREGNANCY

ECTOPIC PREGNANCY is implantation of the fertilized ovum outside the uterine cavity. Most commonly, ectopic pregnancy occurs in a fallopian tube; other sites include the cervix, ovary, and abdominal cavity. It's the second most common cause of vaginal bleeding in early pregnancy.

Possible causes

- Congenital defects of reproductive tract
- Diverticular disease
- Endosalpingitis
- Progestin-only hormonal contraceptives
- Sexually transmitted tubal infection
- Transmigration of the ovum from one ovary to the opposite tube resulting in delayed implantation
- Tubal atony or spasms

◆ Tubal damage from pelvic inflammatory disease
◆ Previous pelvic or tubal surgery
◆ Tumors pressing against the tube
◆ Use of intrauterine devices

Assessment findings

◆ Irregular vaginal bleeding and dull abdominal pain on the affected side early in pregnancy
◆ Rupture of tubes, causing sudden and severe abdominal pain, syncope, and referred shoulder pain as the abdomen fills with blood
◆ Unstable blood pressure and rapid, thready pulse, possibly indicating shock secondary to hemorrhage

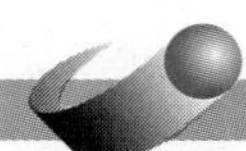

FAST FACT

Signs of possible early ectopic pregnancy are irregular vaginal bleeding and dull abdominal pain. Signs of possible ruptured ectopic pregnancy are severe abdominal pain, orthostatic hypotension, tachycardia, and dizziness.

Diagnostic evaluation

◆ HCG titers are abnormally low.
◆ Ultrasonography is positive for ruptured tube and collection of fluid in the pelvis
◆ Culdocentesis (aspiration of fluid from the vaginal cul-de-sac) detects free blood in the peritoneum; performed if ultrasonography detects the absence of a gestational sac in the uterus.
◆ Laparoscopy is performed if culdocentesis is positive and may reveal pregnancy outside the uterus.

Nursing diagnoses

◆ Deficient fluid volume
◆ Risk for infection
◆ Acute pain

Treatment

◆ Laparotomy to ligate the bleeding vessels and remove or repair damaged fallopian tube (oophorectomy in ovarian pregnancy and hysterectomy in interstitial pregnancy)
◆ Transfusion therapy, including packed RBCs (if bleeding is uncontrolled)

Drug therapy options

◆ Antimetabolite methotrexate (Folex) followed by antineoplastic leucovorin (Wellcovorin) to stop the trophoblastic cells from growing (continous therapy until negative HCG levels are achieved), if the fallopian tube hasn't ruptured
◆ Antibiotics for sepsis specific to the organism
◆ Supplemental oral or I.M. iron

Planning and goals

◆ The client will remain hemodynamically stable.
◆ The client's ectopic pregnancy will resolve safely.
◆ The client will verbalize understanding the possible cause and required treatment of the ectopic pregnancy.
◆ The client will verbalize feelings over the termination of the pregnancy.

Implementation

◆ Monitor vital signs and intake and output *to assess for intense blood loss and shock.*
◆ Monitor for severe abdominal pain, orthostatic hypotension, tachycardia, and dizziness, *which may indicate rupturing ectopic pregnancy.*
◆ Monitor WBC count and erythrocyte sedimentation rate *for signs of infection.*
◆ Administer I.V. fluid replacement *to accommodate for blood loss.*
◆ Administer blood products *to replace volume loss.*
◆ Administer $Rh_{O}D$ immune globulin *to combat isoimmunization in the client who is Rh-negative.*
◆ Provide routine postoperative care if surgical intervention is necessary.
◆ Provide emotional support for parents grieving over the loss of the pregnancy.

Evaluation

◆ The client maintains stable vital signs.
◆ The ectopic pregnancy was resolved without injury to the client.
◆ The client verbalizes understanding of the ectopic pregnancy.
◆ The client demonstrates appropriate coping mechanisms in dealing with the loss of the pregnancy.

GESTATIONAL DIABETES MELLITUS

In GESTATIONAL DIABETES MELLITUS, the client's pancreas, stressed by the normal adaptations to pregnancy, can't meet the increased demands for insulin. A client may have preexisting diabetes or may develop gestational diabetes while she's pregnant. Gestational diabetes is associated with an increased risk of congenital anomalies, hydramnios, macrosomia, gestational hypertension, spontaneous abortion, and fetal death. Additionally, the infant of a client with diabetes is at risk for developing sacral agenesis, a congenital anomaly characterized by incomplete formation of the vertebral column. The client with gestational diabetes has an increased risk of developing diabetes mellitus.

Possible causes

- Environment (infection, diet, exposure to toxins, and stress)
- Family history of diabetes
- Gestational diabetes in previous pregnancies
- Lifestyle in genetically susceptible persons

Assessment findings

- Dizziness and confusion
- Microvascular changes (peripheral vascular disease, retinopathy, nephropathy, neuropathy)
- Polyuria
- Possible monilial infection (vaginal yeast infection)

Diagnostic evaluation

- One-hour glucose tolerance test reveals:
  - a glucose level greater than 180 mg/dl.
- Three-hour glucose tolerance test reveals:
  - a fasting serum glucose level of 95 mg/dl or greater
  - a 1-hour serum glucose level of 180 mg/dl or greater
  - a 2-hour serum glucose level of 155 mg/dl or greater
  - a 3-hour serum glucose level of 140 mg/dl or greater.

Nursing diagnoses

- Imbalanced nutrition: More than body requirements
- Risk for deficient fluid volume
- Ineffective coping

Treatment

- 1,800- to 2,200-calorie diet, divided into three meals and three snacks that should also be low in fat and cholesterol and high in fiber
- Oral antidiabetic agents contraindicated because of adverse effects on the fetus

Drug therapy options

- Administration of insulin

Planning and goals

- The client will describe the responsibility related to insulin administration and blood glucose regulation.
- The client will understand the recommended diet and the importance of following it.
- The client will demonstrate coping mechanisms to adequately deal with the complications of gestational diabetes mellitus.
- The client will verbalize understanding the potential effects diabetes mellitus may have on her fetus.

Implementation

- Teach the client to use the glucose monitoring system and administer insulin correctly *to adequately control blood glucose.*
- Encourage adherence to dietary regulations *to maintain euglycemia.*
- Encourage the client to exercise moderately *to reduce blood glucose levels and decrease the need for insulin.*
- Prepare the client for antepartum fetal surveillance testing, including oxytocin challenge testing, nipple stimulation stress testing, amniotic fluid index, biophysical profile, and NST *to assess fetal well-being.*
- Encourage the client to verbalize her feelings *to allay her fears.*
- Provide emotional support *to reduce anxiety.*

Evaluation

- The client appropriately performs serum glucose monitoring and insulin regulation and administration.
- The client follows the recommended diet appropriately.
- The client demonstrates coping mechanisms that address the occurrence of diabetes mellitus.
- The client asks appropriate questions about the diagnostic assessments of the fetus's well-being.

GESTATIONAL HYPERTENSION

GESTATIONAL HYPERTENSION is characterized by hypertension, proteinuria, and edema. The client is at risk for cerebral hemorrhage, circulatory collapse, heart failure, hepatic rupture, or renal failure. If delivery occurs before term, fetal prognosis is poor because of hypoxia, acidosis, and immaturity. (See *Caring for the pregnant client with a cardiovascular disorder* and *Nursing care during fetal distress*, age 204.)

Uncontrolled gestational hypertension may progress to seizures (ECLAMPSIA). The maternal mortality from eclampsia is 10% to 15%, usually resulting from intracranial hemorrhage and heart failure.

Risk factors

- Geographic, ethnic, and racial factors
- Nutritional factors

Caring for the pregnant client with a cardiovascular disorder

This chart lists cardiovascular disorders and their implications for the pregnant patient.

CONDITION	IMPLICATIONS
Vena cava syndrome (supine hypotensive syndrome)	Vena cava syndrome occurs when something interferes with blood flow to the right atrium. This interference may occur if the near-term or full-term pregnant woman lies on her back, with the weight of the uterus compressing the inferior vena cava. The symptoms are dizziness, tingling of the extremities, circumoral pallor, and faintness. The client should lie on her side to relieve pressure on the inferior vena cava and restore circulation.
Chronic hypertension	Although a client with chronic hypertension develops the condition before pregnancy, her blood pressure will rise with each pregnancy and won't return to the prepregnancy level. Because it interferes with oxygen supply, chronic hypertension poses a danger to the mother and fetus.
Anemia ◆ First trimester: Hemoglobin (Hb) level below 12 g/dl Hematocrit (HCT) below 37% ◆ Second and third trimesters: Hb below 11 g/dl HCT below 35%	Maternal problems associated with anemia include abortion, infection, preeclampsia, premature labor, and heart failure. Fetal problems associated with anemia include growth retardation, morbidity, and mortality. Treatment includes an iron-rich diet, vitamin C, and folic acid. Additionally, the physician may prescribe an iron supplement (for example, ferrous sulfate). If so, teach the client to take the supplement between meals with a source of vitamin C and to include roughage and fluids in her diet because iron may cause constipation. Also caution the client that iron will make her stools black.
Heart disease	The normal physiologic changes of pregnancy are stressful to the client with heart disease. Periods of increased risk typically occur: ◆ around 28 weeks' gestation, when the blood volume increase peaks, resulting in additional stress on the heart ◆ during the second trimester, when an elevated basal metabolic rate increases maternal-fetal oxygen requirements ◆ during labor and delivery, at which time epidural or caudal anesthesia is recommended (Forceps may be used to prevent pushing.) ◆ during the first postpartum week as body fluid levels return to normal. Care focuses on adequate rest, prevention of infection, dietary management, and controlled, cautious weight loss.

- Familial factors
- Immunologic factors
- Adolescents and primiparas older than age 35
- Toxic sources (autolysis of placental infarcts)
- Autointoxication
- Uremia
- Maternal sensitization to proteins
- Pyelonephritis

Assessment findings

Gestational hypertension usually appears between 20 and 24 weeks' gestation and disappears within 42 days after delivery. It's classified as *gestational hypertension, mild eclampsia, severe preeclampsia,* or *eclampsia,* depending on the degree of hypertension and other symptoms. (See *Caring for the client with preeclampsia,* page 205.)

Gestational hypertension

- Blood pressure 140/90 mm Hg or a systolic pressure elevated 30 mm Hg above the prepregnancy level
- No proteinuria

Mild eclampsia

- Blood pressure of 140/90 mm Hg, systolic pressure elevated more than 30 mm Hg above prepregnancy level, or

Nursing care during fetal distress

Fetal distress is caused primarily by decreased oxygen supply to the fetus. The decrease may be maternal or fetal in origin.

MATERNAL-RELATED CAUSES

- Anemia
- Hypertension or hypotension
- Preeclampsia
- Abruptio placentae
- Placenta previa
- Medication
- Prolonged contraction
- Pressure on the placenta

FETAL-RELATED CAUSES

- Prolapsed cord
- Knotted cord
- Nuchal cord

FETAL DISTRESS SIGNS

- Fetal hyperactivity
- Meconium-stained amniotic fluid, except in a known breech presentation
- Persistent fetal bradycardia (below 100 beats/minute) or tachycardia (above 180 beats/minute) or loss of beat-to-beat variability

FETAL DISTRESS PATTERN GRAPHS

Continuous electronic monitoring can identify fetal heart rate patterns that indicate fetal distress and its possible cause.

EARLY DECELERATION (RELATED TO HEAD COMPRESSION)

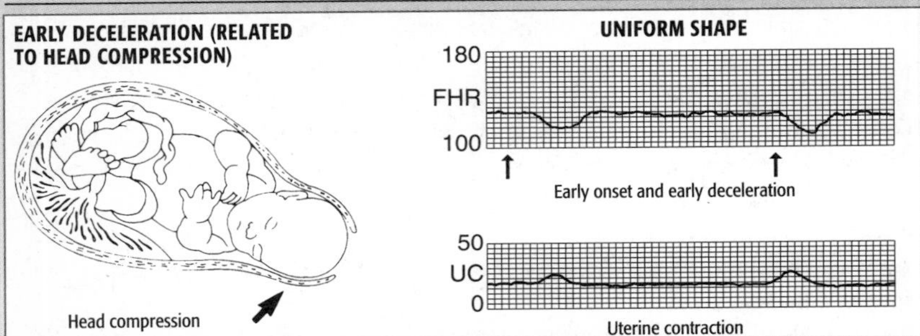

Nursing interventions

- Continue observation. This pattern usually indicates head compression as the fetal head passes through the birth canal.

LATE DECELERATION (RELATED TO UTEROPLACENTAL INSUFFICIENCY)

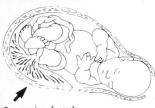

Compression of vessels

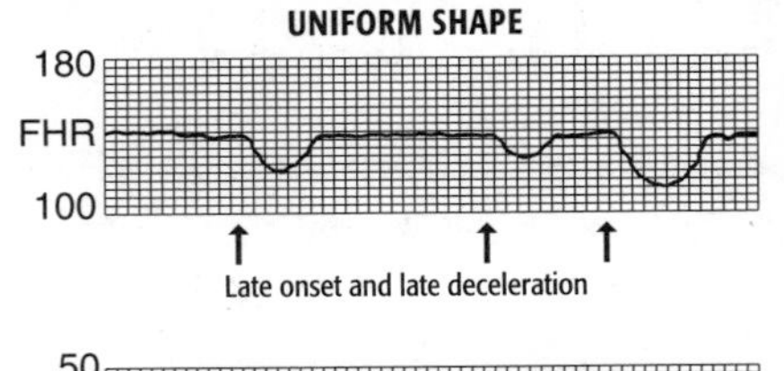

Nursing interventions

- Stop oxytocin if in progress, and replace I.V. fluid.
- Change the client's position to the preferred left-side-lying position.
- Check blood pressure and pulse rate.
- Administer oxygen.
- Notify the physician.

VARIABLE DECELERATION (RELATED TO UMBILICAL CORD COMPRESSION)

The first deceleration is V-shaped; the second, U-shaped. Transitory acceleration precedes or follows the deceleration. The fetal heart rate may fall below 100 beats/minute.

VARIABLE SHAPE

180 FHR 100

Variable onset and variable deceleration

50 UC 0

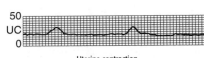

Uterine contraction

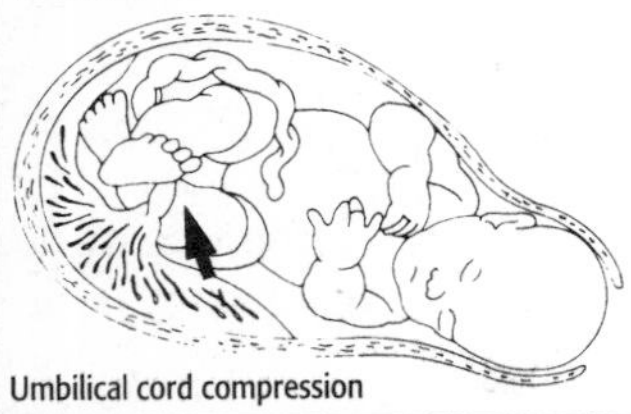

Nursing interventions

- Stop oxytocin if in progress, and replace I.V. fluid.
- Change the mother's position.
- Check for a prolapsed cord.
- Check blood pressure and pulse rate.
- Administer oxygen.
- Notify the physician.
- Prepare to assist with drawing a blood sample from the fetal scalp.

diastolic pressure elevated 15 mm Hg above prepregnancy level
- ◆ Weight gain of more than 2 lb (0.9 kg) per week in the second trimester and 1 lb (0.5 kg) per week in the third trimester
- ◆ Mild edema in the upper extremities or face
- ◆ Frontal headaches, blurred vision, hyperreflexia, nausea, vomiting, irritability, cerebral disturbances, and epigastric pain

Severe preeclampsia
- ◆ Blood pressure of 160/110 mm Hg (noted on two readings taken 6 hours apart while on bed rest)
- ◆ Oliguria (500 ml or less in 24 hours)
- ◆ Ophthalmoscopic examnation reveals vascular spasm, papilledema, retinal edema or detachment, and arteriovenous nicking or hemorrhage
- ◆ Pulmonary edema with shortness of breath
- ◆ Peripheral edema or severe facial edema

Eclampsia
- ◆ Blood pressure higher than 160/100 mm Hg
- ◆ Tonic-clonic seizures

Diagnostic evaluation
- ◆ Blood chemistry reveals increased blood urea nitrogen, creatinine, and uric acid levels and elevated liver function studies.
- ◆ Hematology reveals thrombocytopenia (HELLP syndrome).
- ◆ Proteinuria (more than 300 mg/24 hours or 1+ with preclampsia and 5 g/24 hours or 5+ or more with severe eclampsia)

Nursing diagnoses
- ◆ Excess fluid volume
- ◆ Risk for injury
- ◆ Activity intolerance
- ◆ Ineffective coping

Treatment
- ◆ Bed rest in a lateral position
- ◆ Delivery (in mild preeclampsia, once the fetus is mature and safe induction is possible; in severe preeclampsia, regardless of gestational age)
- ◆ High-protein diet with restriction of excessively salty foods
- ◆ Restriction of I.V. fluid administration during labor

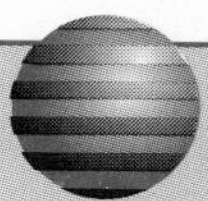

CLINICAL SITUATION

Caring for the client with preeclampsia

A 38-year-old primigravida is in her 8th month of pregnancy. During a routine checkup, the nurse notes a weight gain of 8 lb (3.6 kg) since the client's last visit. The client remarks that she has had to remove her rings because her fingers are swollen. Her blood pressure is 144/92 mm Hg.

What should be included in the client assessment?
- ◆ Blood pressure evaluation – Elevated blood pressure to 140/90, systolic measurement 30 mm Hg above normal, or diastolic measurement 15 mm Hg above normal indicates a problem; a blood pressure of 160/110 indicates a more severe problem.
- ◆ Testing for protein in urine – Protein is a sign of preeclampsia.
- ◆ Weight measurement – Weight gain greater than 1 lb (0.45 kg) per week may indicate fluid weight gain.
- ◆ Review of client's diet – Excessive sodium intake can cause fluid weight gain
- ◆ Evaluation of serum electrolytes – Serum electrolytes help assess nutritional and hydration status as well as renal function.
- ◆ Monitoring fetal heart tones – Fetal heart tones indicate fetal well-being.

What initial interventions are appropriate to prevent preeclampsia from progressing?
- ◆ Recommend bed rest in the left side-lying position to promote better circulation.
- ◆ Provide a quiet environment to enhance relaxation.
- ◆ Provide a high-protein and moderate-salt diet to replace protein loss and control fluid retention.
- ◆ Measure weight daily to evaluate fluid retention.
- ◆ Report signs and symptoms of possible progression to severe preeclampsia: generalized edema, decreased urine output, headache, visual disturbances, nausea, vomiting, epigastric pain, and hyperreflexia.
- ◆ Schedule follow-up visits as recommended, usually twice weekly.

Questions for further thought
- ◆ What evaluation findings would indicate that this client is compliant with recommended interventions?
- ◆ What support measures would assist this client in maintaining maternal and fetal safety?

Drug therapy options

- Antihypertensives (in severe preeclampsia): betamethasone (Celestone) to accelerate fetal lung maturation, diazoxide (Hyperstat), hydralazine (Apresoline)
- Magnesium sulfate to reduce the amount of acetylcholine produced by motor nerves, thereby preventing seizures

Planning and goals

- The client will describe the warning signs that indicate the need for immediate medical attention.
- The client will describe the required alterations to diet and activity.
- The client will exhibit decreased severity of signs and symptoms of preeclampsia.
- The client will verbalize concerns and fears over blood pressure problems.

Implementation

All clients

- Assess the client for edema and proteinuria, *which may indicate impending eclampsia.*
- Monitor daily weight *to identify sodium and water retention.*
- Maintain a high-protein diet with moderate sodium restriction *as a measure against gestational hypertension.*
- Maintain seizure precautions *to ensure client safety.*
- Encourage bed rest in a left lateral recumbent position *to improve uterine and renal perfusion.*
- Monitor FHR continuously during labor *to assess fetal well-being.*

Severe preeclampsia

- Assess maternal blood pressure every 4 hours, or more frequently if unstable, *to assess for abnormalities.*
- Monitor FHR *to assess for decreased variability after magnesium sulfate administration.*
- Monitor serum magnesium levels *to assess for toxicity.*
- If necessary, prepare the client for amniocentesis *to assess fetal maturity.*
- Administer I.V. fluids, as prescribed. Restrict fluids to 60 to 150 ml/hour in the client with preeclampsia who's in labor.
- Obtain blood samples for complete blood count, platelet count, liver function studies, blood urea nitrogen (BUN), creatinine, PTT, PT, and fibrin degradation products *to detect signs of complications such as renal failure, HELLP syndrome or DIC.*
- Be prepared to obtain a blood sample for typing and crossmatching *because the client is at risk for developing placenta previa.*
- Obtain urine specimens to determine urine protein levels and specific gravity, and perform 24-hour urine collection for protein and creatinine, as ordered, *to evaluate renal function.*
- Be prepared to administer I.V. magnesium sulfate *to evaluate for toxicity evidenced by deep tendon reflexes.*
- Monitor serum blood levels while the client is receiving I.V. magnesium sulfate *to assess for magnesium sulfate toxicity.*
- Monitor urine output *to assess for complications.*
- Be prepared to administer calcium gluconate at the first sign of magnesium sulfate toxicity (elevated serum levels, decreased deep tendon reflexes, muscle flaccidity, central nervous system depression, and decreased respiratory rate and renal function) as antidote to magnesium sulfate toxicity.
- Promote relaxation *to reduce fatigue.*
- Encourage the client to verbalize her feelings *to allay anxiety.*

Evaluation

- The client appropriately identifies situations requiring immediate medical attention.
- The client effectively manages her diet and activity as recommended.
- The client maintains a stable blood pressure, edema decreases, and renal function is stable.
- The client demonstrates effective coping mechanisms in dealing with gestational hypertension.

HYDATIDIFORM MOLE

HYDATIDIFORM MOLE (also known as *gestational trophoblastic disease* or *molar pregnancy*) is a developmental anomaly of the placenta that converts the chorionic villi into a mass of clear vesicles (hydatid vesicles). There are two types:

- Complete mole, in which there's neither an embryo nor an amniotic sac
- Partial mole, in which there's an embryo (usually with multiple abnormalities) and an amniotic sac.

Possible causes

- Chromosomal abnormalities
- Hormonal imbalances
- Protein and folic acid deficiency

◆ Previous molar, ectopic, or normal pregnancy or sponatenous or induced abortion

Assessment findings

◆ Intermittent or continuous bright red or brownish vaginal bleeding by 12 weeks' gestation
◆ Passage of clear fluid-filled vesicles along with vaginal bleeding
◆ Lower abdominal cramps
◆ Disproportionate enlargement of the uterus
◆ Absence of fetal heart tones
◆ Excessive nausea and vomiting
◆ Symptoms of gestational hypertension before 20 weeks' gestation

Diagnostic evaluation

◆ HCG levels are extremely high for early pregnancy.
◆ Ultrasonography shows grapelike clusters and fails to reveal a fetal skeleton.
◆ Histologic examination confirms the presence of vesicles.
◆ Amniography reveals the absence of a fetus.
◆ Doppler ultrasonography shows the absence of fetal heart tones.
◆ Hemoglobin, hematocrit, and coagulation studies and hepatic and renal function findings are abnormal.
◆ WBC and ESR are increased.

Nursing diagnoses

◆ Risk for deficient fluid volume
◆ Anticipatory grieving
◆ Deficient knowledge (client and partner)

Treatment

◆ Therapeutic abortion (suction and curettage) if a spontaneous abortion doesn't occur
◆ Pelvic examinations and chest X-rays at regular intervals
◆ Weekly monitoring of HCG levels until they remain normal for 3 consecutive weeks
◆ Periodic follow-up for 1 to 2 years because of the increased risk of neoplasm

Drug therapy options

◆ Antimetabolite methotrexate (Rheumatrex) prophylactically (the drug of choice for choriocarcinoma)
◆ Chemotherapy and irradiation for metastatic choriocarcinoma

Planning and goals

◆ The client will remain stable, and the molar pregnancy will be resolved safely.
◆ The client will verbalize feelings over the loss of the pregnancy.
◆ The client will express knowledge about the cause and treatment of molar pregnancy.

Implementation

◆ Monitor and record vital signs and intake and output *to assess for changes that may indicate complications.*
◆ Provide emotional support for the grieving couple *to assist in coping with pregnancy loss.*
◆ Monitor vaginal bleeding *to assess for hemorrhage.*
◆ Send the contents of the uterine evacuation to the laboratory for analysis *to assess for the presence of hydatid vesicles.*
◆ Advise the client to avoid pregnancy until HCG levels are normal (may take up to 2 years) *to avoid future complications.*

Evaluation

◆ The client's condition is stable and the pregnancy is resolved safely.
◆ The client demonstrates appropriate coping mechanisms in dealing with pregnancy loss.
◆ The client verbalizes understanding the cause of and treatment for hydatidiform mole.

HYPEREMESIS GRAVIDARUM

HYPEREMESIS GRAVIDARUM is persistent, uncontrolled vomiting that begins in the first weeks of pregnancy and may continue throughout pregnancy. Unlike "morning sickness," hyperemesis can have serious complications, including severe weight loss, dehydration, and electrolyte imbalance. (See *Comparing morning sickness to hyperemesis gravidarum,* page 208.)

Possible causes

◆ Pancreatitis
◆ Biliary tract disease
◆ Decreased secretion of free hydrochloric acid in the stomach
◆ Decreased gastric motility
◆ Drug toxicity
◆ Inflammatory obstructive bowel disease
◆ Vitamin deficiency (especially B_6)
◆ Psychological factors

Comparing morning sickness to hyperemesis gravidarum

MORNING SICKNESS	HYPEREMESIS GRAVIDARUM
◆ Onset occurs in first trimester and resolves in second trimester.	◆ Onset occurs in first trimester and continues throughout pregnancy.
◆ Weight is maintained or increased.	◆ Weight loss occurs.
◆ Serum electrolytes remain normal.	◆ Serum electrolytes are abnormal.
◆ Ketosis doesn't develop.	◆ Ketosis occurs.
◆ Skin turgor remains hydrated.	◆ Skin turgor is dehydrated.
◆ Serum thyroid levels remain normal.	◆ Serum thyroid levels are abnormal.
◆ Skin color remains normal.	◆ Jaundice may occur.

Assessment findings

◆ Continuous, severe nausea and vomiting
◆ Confusion or delirium, lassitude, stupor, and, possibly, coma
◆ Jaundice
◆ Dry, coated tongue
◆ Fetid, fruity breath
◆ Dry skin and mucous membranes
◆ Nonelastic skin turgor
◆ Oliguria
◆ Metabolic acidosis
◆ Rapid pulse
◆ Vertigo
◆ Weight loss

Diagnostic evaluation

◆ Arterial blood gas analysis reveals alkalosis.
◆ Hb level, hematocrit, and WBC are elevated.
◆ Serum potassium level reveals hypokalemia.
◆ Decreased protein, chloride, and sodium levels
◆ Increased BUN
◆ Urine ketone levels are elevated.
◆ Urine specific gravity is increased.

Nursing diagnoses

◆ Imbalanced nutrition: Less than body requirements
◆ Deficient fluid volume
◆ Risk for injury
◆ Anxiety

Treatment

◆ Removal of potential triggers to vomiting
◆ Total parenteral nutrition (TPN)
◆ Restoration of fluid and electrolyte balance through diet strategies or supplements

Drug therapy options

◆ Antiemetics for vomiting
◆ Continuous I.V. infusion of metoclopramide

Planning and goals

◆ The client will maintain proper hydration and nutrition.
◆ The client will have decreased episodes of vomiting.
◆ The client will verbalize feelings regarding potential fetal injury.

Implementation

◆ Monitor vital signs and fluid intake and output *to assess for fluid volume deficit.*
◆ Obtain blood samples and urine specimens for laboratory tests *to evaluate nutritional and hydration status.*
◆ Provide small, frequent meals *to maintain adequate nutrition.*
◆ Encourage liquids between meals instead of with meals *to maintain adequate hydration.*
◆ Recommend the client maintain an upright position for 1 to 2 hours after eating *to decrease gastric reflux.*
◆ Maintain I.V. fluid replacement and TPN *to reduce fluid deficit and pH imbalance.*
◆ Provide emotional support *to help the client cope with her condition.*

Evaluation

◆ The client increases her weight during pregnancy.
◆ The client remains adequately hydrated.
◆ The client and fetus maintain stable conditions throughout the pregnancy.

PLACENTA PREVIA

In PLACENTA PREVIA, the placenta is implanted in the lower uterine segment (low implantation). The placenta can occlude the cervix partially or totally.

Risk factors

- Defective vascularization of the decidua
- Maternal age older than 35
- Multiple pregnancy
- Multiparity
- Previous uterine fibroid tumors
- Previous uterine surgery

Assessment findings

- Painless, bright red vaginal bleeding, usually beginning after the 20th week of pregnancy

Diagnostic evaluation

- Early ultrasound evaluation reveals the placenta implanted in the lower uterine segment.

Nursing diagnoses

- Risk for injury
- Risk for deficient fluid volume
- Anxiety

Treatment

Treatment depends on the gestational age, when the first episode occurs, and the amount of bleeding:

- Surgical intervention (by cesarean delivery), depending on the placental placement and maternal and fetal stability (treatment of choice)
- If gestational age is less than 34 weeks, hospitalization of the client and restriction to bed rest to avoid preterm labor
- Administration of supplemental iron if anemia is present
- Restriction of maternal activities (for example, avoiding lifting heavy objects, long-distance travel, and sexual intercourse)
- Transfusion of packed RBCs if Hb level and HCT are low.

Drug therapy options

- Betamethasone to increase fetal lung maturity if preterm labor can't be halted

Planning and goals

- The client and fetus will remain hemodynamically stable.
- The client will verbalize anxiety related to potential pregnancy loss.

Implementation

- Monitor maternal vital signs, including uterine activity *to assess for maternal well-being.*
- Monitor for vaginal bleeding *to estimate blood loss.*
- Monitor FHR, using electronic fetal monitoring, *to assess for complications.*
- Don't perform rectal or vaginal examinations unless equipment is available for vaginal and cesarean delivery *to avoid stimulating the uterine activity.*
- Obtain blood samples for HCT, Hb level, PT, PTT, fibrinogen level, platelet count, and typing and crossmatching *to assess for complications.*
- Provide routine postoperative care if cesarean delivery is performed *to ensure the client's well-being.*
- Monitor for postpartum hemorrhage *because a client with placenta previa is more prone to hemorrhage.*
- Provide emotional support *to reduce anxiety.*
- Provide I.V. fluids as ordered *to reduce fluid loss.*

Evaluation

- The client and fetus maintain stable vital signs; the fetus is delivered safely.
- The client demonstrates appropriate coping mechanisms in dealing with anxiety over fetal injury.

INTRAPARTUM PERIOD

The intrapartum period includes labor and delivery. During the intrapartum period, the stages of labor as well as fetal posture and positioning are monitored.

INTRAPARTUM ASSESSMENT

Nursing care in the intrapartum period depends on which signs and symptoms are present at the onset of labor and the client's physiologic and psychosocial responses to labor. Care may involve basic obstetric procedures and methods of monitoring the client and fetus. To intervene effectively during the birthing process (considered a normal process), the nurse must understand not only the physiology of labor and delivery but also the impact of sociocultural and personal factors on the client's childbearing experience.

Fetal posture and positioning

The posture and positioning of the fetus may be monitored during labor and delivery.

Fetal head diameters

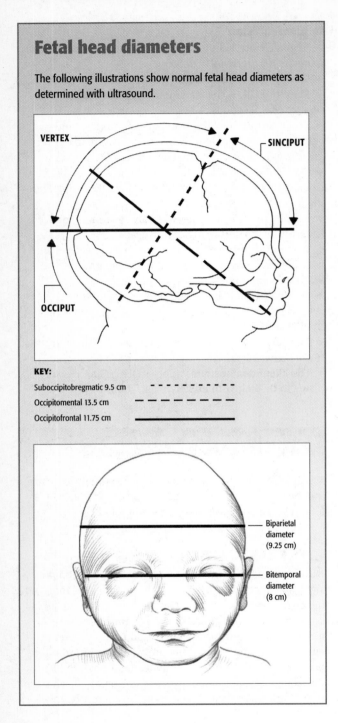

The following illustrations show normal fetal head diameters as determined with ultrasound.

VERTEX
SINCIPUT
OCCIPUT

KEY:

Suboccipitobregmatic 9.5 cm
Occipitomental 13.5 cm
Occipitofrontal 11.75 cm

Biparietal diameter (9.25 cm)
Bitemporal diameter (8 cm)

Fetal habitus

The term *fetal habitus,* or *fetal attitude,* is used to describe the relationship of fetal parts. The relationship is usually one of flexion, that is, legs flexed against the trunk, arms flexed across the chest, and so on. Any extended part presents a potential problem for labor and delivery.

The fetal head is the most significant body part because it's the least malleable. (See *Fetal head diameters.*) Suture lines enable molding of the fetal head during labor and delivery. They meet to form the anterior and posterior fontanels; the location of the fontanels is helpful in assessing fetal position. Suture lines also enable rapid growth during the infant's first year.

Fetal lie

Fetal lie is the relationship of the long axis (spine) of the fetus to the long axis of the mother. That is, whether the fetus is lying in a horizontal (transverse) or vertical (longitudinal) position. Approximately 99% of fetuses assume a longitudinal lie (long axis parallel to the long axis of the mother).

Fetal presentation and presenting part

Fetal presentation refers to the part of the fetus closest to the internal os of the mother's cervix, or portion of the fetus that enters the pelvic passageway first. Various fetal presentations are possible. (See *Fetal positions and variations in presentation.*)

- ◆ In a cephalic presentation, any part of the head can present, including the occiput or vertex, brow, or face.
- ◆ In a transverse presentation, the back or shoulders present, and vaginal delivery isn't possible.
- ◆ In a breech presentation, the buttocks (frank breech), one or both feet (footling breech), or both the buttocks and feet (complete breech) are the presenting parts.

Fetal position

Fetal position describes the relationship of the presenting part of the fetus to the four quadrants of the mother's pelvis (front, back, and sides).

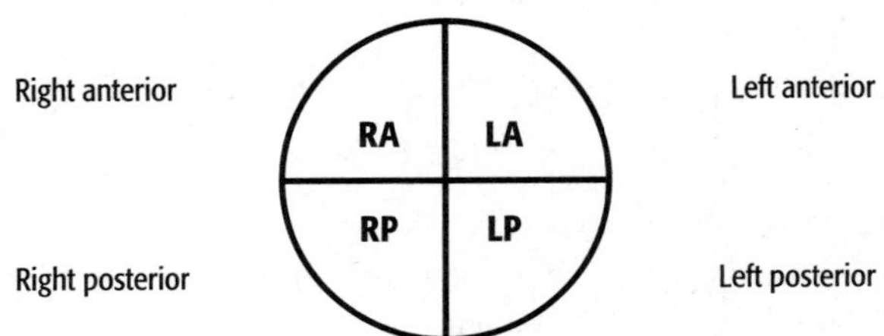

The examiner can determine fetal position through vaginal examination, location of fetal heart tones, Leopold's maneuvers, and ultrasonography or X-ray. During a vaginal

Fetal positions and variations in presentation

These illustrations depict the four fetal positions and the variations in presentation as the fetus enters the pelvic passageway.

Fetal positions

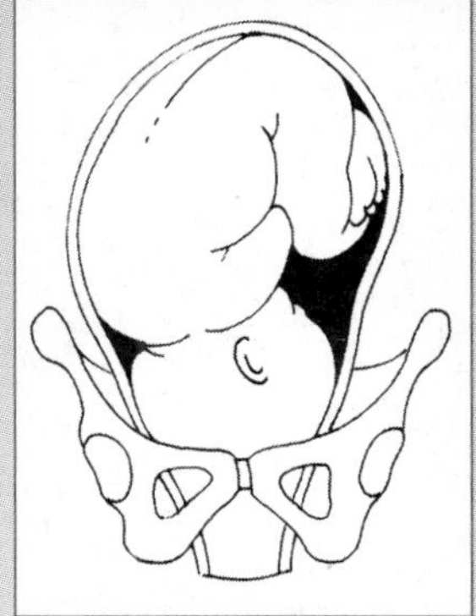

RIGHT OCCIPITOANTERIOR

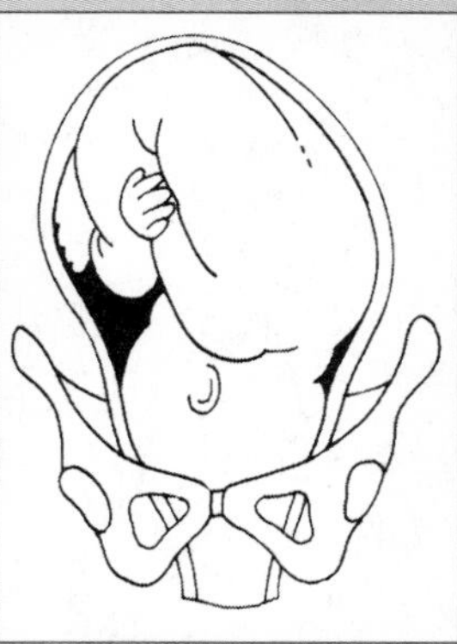

LEFT OCCIPITOANTERIOR

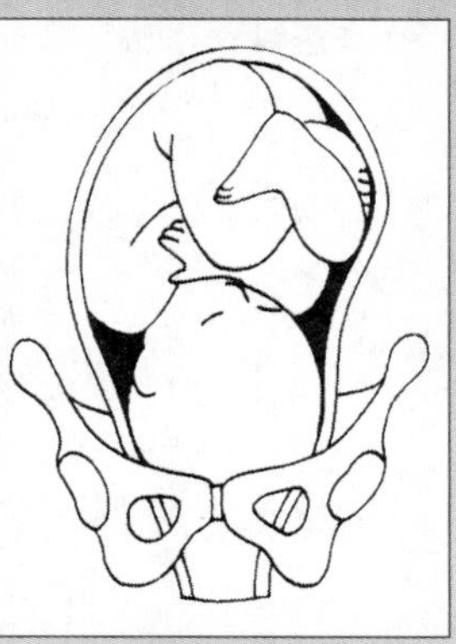

RIGHT OCCIPITOPOSTERIOR

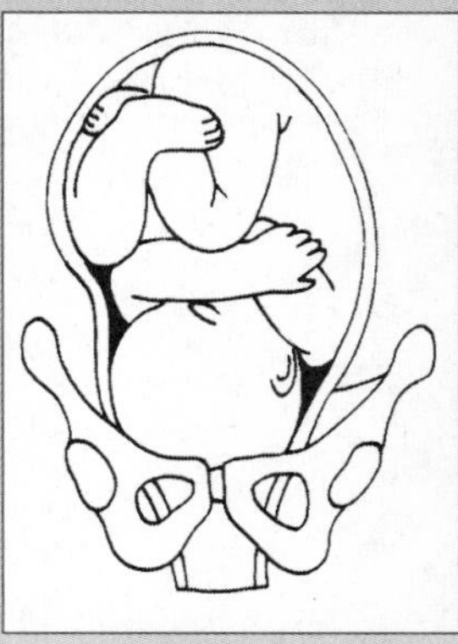

LEFT OCCIPITOPOSTERIOR

Variations in presentation

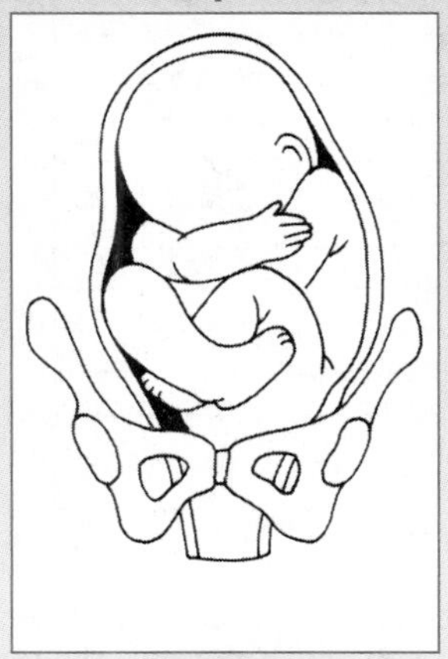

COMPLETE BREECH

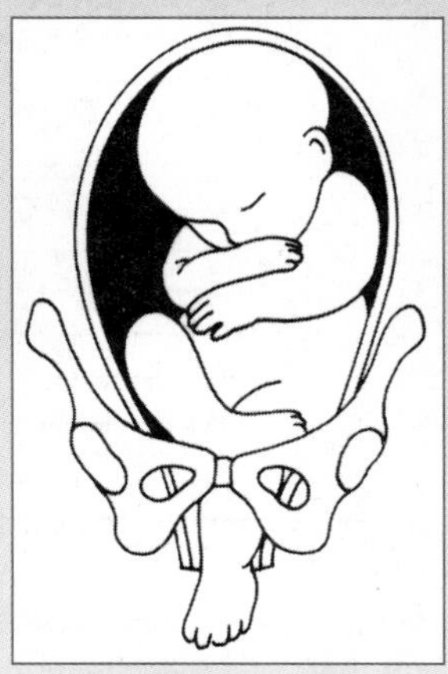

FOOTLING BREECH

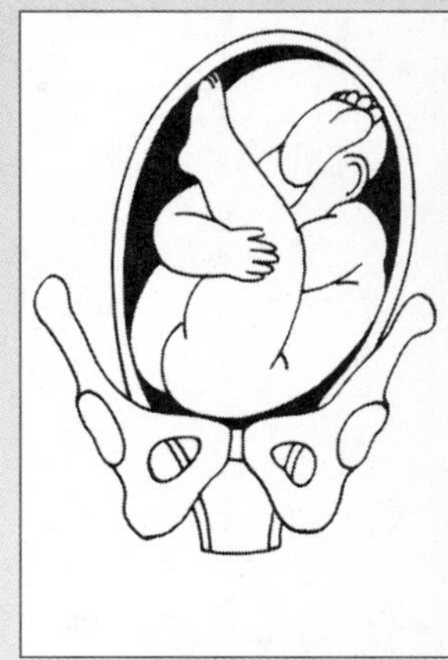

FRANK BREECH

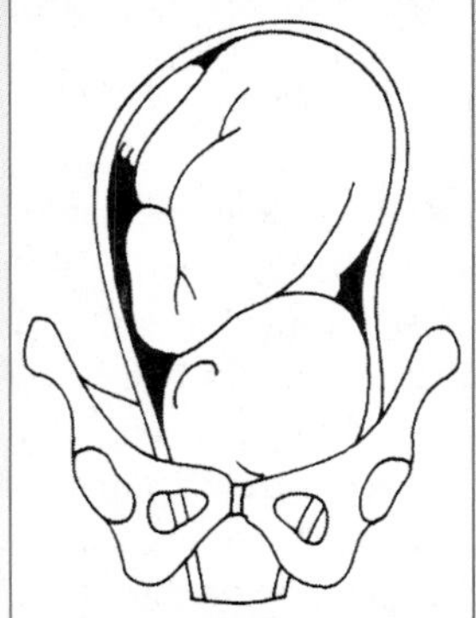

FACE OR BROW CEPHALIC

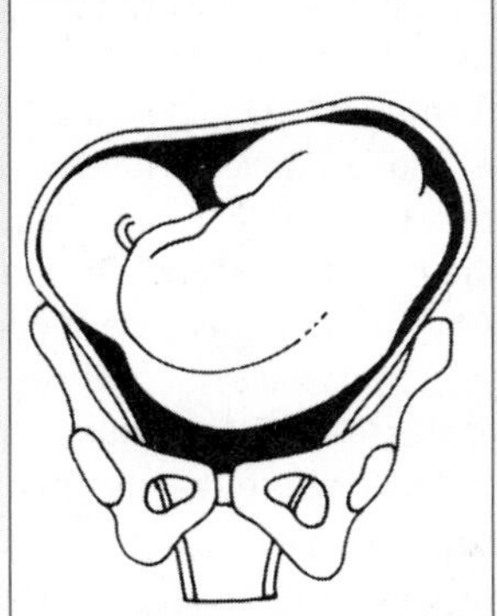

SHOULDER OR TRANSVERSE

Measuring fetal station

Fetal station (also called *degree of engagement*) describes where the presenting part lies in relation to the level of the ischial spines. Measured in centimeters, fetal station advances from -5 cm to 0 (ischial spine level) to +5 cm. The head is considered engaged when it reaches 0.

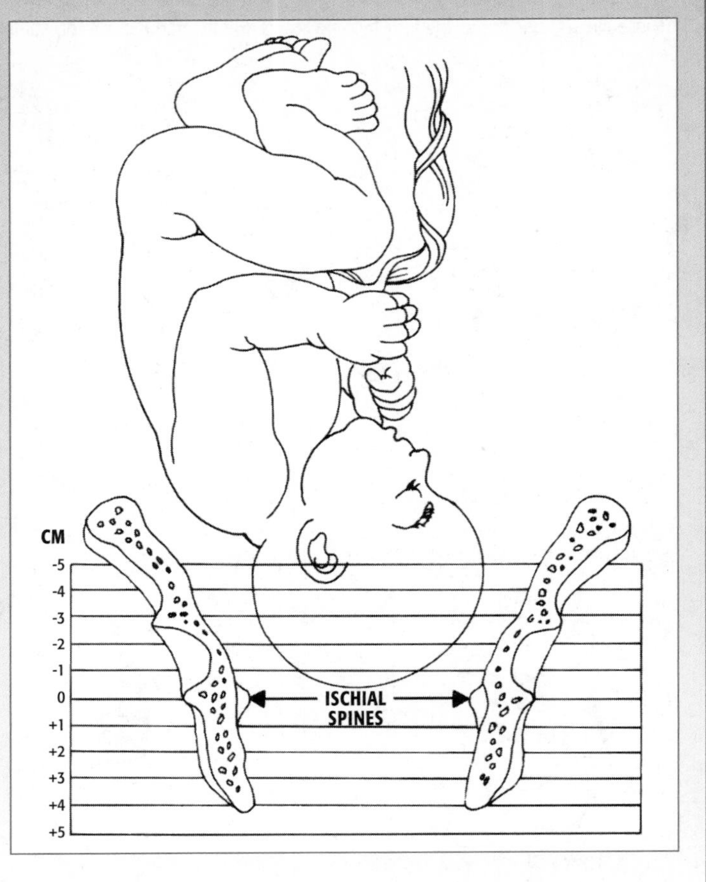

examination, the examiner first determines the presenting part (location of the suture lines and fontanels) and then determines whether the presenting part is directed toward the right or left side of the mother and toward the symphysis pubis (anterior) or the sacral area (posterior). For example, in the left occipital anterior (LOA) position, the presenting part is the occiput, and it's directed toward the left side of the pelvis and toward the symphysis pubis. (The middle initial represents the presenting part.) Occipital anterior is the preferred delivery position because the fetal head can extend under the arch of the symphysis pubis; LOA is the ideal position because, with the fetus lying on the mother's left side, oxygen supply to the client and the fetus is maximized. With occipital posterior, the occiput attempts to extend into the sacral area.

Fetal station

Fetal station, also called *degree of engagement,* is the location of the presenting part in relation to the mother's ischial spines. (See *Measuring fetal station.*) Fetal station can be determined by vaginal examination.

LABOR AND DELIVERY

Preliminary signs that indicate the onset of labor include:

◆ lightening, or fetal descent into the pelvis, which usually occurs 2 to 3 weeks before term in a primiparous client and later or during labor in a multiparous client

◆ Braxton Hicks contractions, which can occur irregularly and intermittently throughout pregnancy and may become uncomfortable and produce false labor

◆ cervical changes, including softening, effacement, and slight dilation several days before the initiation of labor
◆ bloody show as the mucous plug is expelled from the cervix
◆ membrane rupture, occurring before the onset of labor in about 12% of clients and within 24 hours for about 80% of clients
◆ sudden burst of energy before the onset of labor, commonly demonstrated by house cleaning activities and called the *nesting instinct.*

Passage, passenger, and power

Three important components of labor are the passage, passenger, and power. These components must work together for labor to progress normally.

Passage

Passage refers to the maternal pelvis and soft tissues, the passageway through which the fetus exits the body. This area is affected by the shape of the inlet, structure of the pelvis, and pelvic diameters.

Passenger

Passenger refers to the fetus and its ability to move through the passage. This ability is affected by such fetal features as:
◆ fetal skull
◆ lie
◆ presentation
◆ position.

The fetal head can flex or extend 45 degrees and rotate 180 degrees, allowing its smallest diameters to move down the birth canal and pass through the maternal pelvis. Pressure exerted by the maternal pelvis and birth canal during labor and delivery causes the sutures of the skull to allow the cranial bones to shift, resulting in molding of the fetal head.

Power

Power refers to uterine contractions, which cause complete cervical effacement and dilation.

Other factors

Other factors that affect labor are:
◆ accomplishment of the tasks of pregnancy
◆ coping mechanisms
◆ the mother's ability to bear down (voluntary use of abdominal muscles to push during the second stage of labor)
◆ past experiences
◆ placental positioning
◆ preparation for childbirth
◆ psychological readiness
◆ support systems.

Stages of labor

The labor process is divided into four stages, ranging from the onset of true labor, through delivery of the fetus and placenta, to the first hour after delivery. (See *Stages of labor,* pages 214 and 215.) Nursing care may be specific to the stage of labor that the client is experiencing. (See *Nursing care during labor and delivery,* page 216.)

First stage

The first stage is measured from the onset of true labor to complete dilation of the cervix. This period lasts from 6 to 18 hours in a primiparous client and from 2 to 10 hours in a multiparous client. There are three phases of this dilation stage:
◆ During the latent phase, the cervix is dilated 0 to 3 cm, contractions are irregular, and the client may experience anticipation, excitement, or apprehension.
◆ During the active phase, the cervix is dilated 4 to 7 cm. Contractions are about 5 to 8 minutes apart and last 45 to 60 seconds with moderate to strong intensity. During this phase, the client becomes serious and concerned about the progress of labor; she may ask for pain medication or use breathing techniques. If the membranes haven't ruptured spontaneously, amniotomy may be performed.
◆ During the transitional phase, the cervix is dilated 8 to 10 cm. Contractions are about 1 to 2 minutes apart and last 60 to 90 seconds with strong intensity. During this phase, the client may lose control, thrash in bed, groan, or cry out.

Second stage

The second stage of labor extends from complete dilation to delivery. This stage lasts an average of 40 minutes (20 contractions) for the primiparous client and 20 minutes (10 contractions) for the multiparous client. It may last longer if the client has had epidural anesthesia.

The client may become exhausted and dehydrated as she moves from coping with contractions to actively pushing. During this stage, the fetus is moved along the birth canal by the mechanisms of labor listed below:
◆ The fetus's head is considered to be engaged when the biparietal diameter passes the pelvic inlet.
◆ The movement of the presenting part through the pelvis is called *descent.*

Stages of labor

This chart lists the stages of labor along with a description , contraction characteristics, physical changes in the mother, fetal position changes, and appropriate nursing care for each.

STAGE	CONTRACTION CHARACTERISTICS	MATERNAL PHYSICAL CHANGES	FETAL POSITION CHANGES	NURSING CARE
First: Dilation				
Starts with the first true labor contraction; ends with complete cervical effacement and dilation	See contraction characteristics for individual stage 1 phases below.	◆ Percent of effacement (0% to 100%) ◆ Dilation (1 to 10 cm)	◆ Engagement ◆ Descent ◆ Flexion ◆ Internal rotation	
Phases *Early (latent, inactive)*: Cervix dilates 1 to 4 cm; longest, least uncomfortable phase	◆ Every 5 to 20 minutes for 15 to 40 seconds ◆ Mild to moderate, increasing in frequency, duration, and intensity		◆ Descent ◆ Flexion ◆ Internal rotation	◆ Collect assessment data. ◆ Orient the client to the environment and equipment. ◆ Establish a nurse-client relationship. ◆ Welcome the support person. ◆ Provide comfort measures. ◆ Encourage ambulation. ◆ Measure vital signs and fetal heart rate per protocol. ◆ Teach or review breathing methods.
Active: Cervix dilates 4 to 8 cm; most effacement and dilation occurring in shortest period during this phase	◆ Every 2 to 4 minutes for 60 seconds ◆ Moderate to strong			◆ Reinforce breathing techniques. ◆ Keep the client informed of her progress. ◆ Change the client's position frequently. ◆ Encourage the client to void every 2 hours. ◆ Provide ice chips and lip moisturizer.
Transitional: Cervix dilates 8 to 10 cm; shortest, most uncomfortable phase	◆ Every 2 minutes for up to 60 seconds ◆ Increase in strength and duration; may decrease in frequency			◆ Provide positive reinforcement to the support person. ◆ Encourage the client to rest between contractions. ◆ Keep emesis basin nearby.
Second: Expulsion				
Starts with complete cervical effacement and dilation and ends with delivery	◆ Strong ◆ Upper part of uterus is active; lower part is passive	◆ Perineal bulging ◆ Crowning of fetal head ◆ Delivery of fetus	◆ Extension ◆ External rotation ◆ Expulsion	◆ Assist the client to push. ◆ Praise the client, and keep her informed of her progress. ◆ Maintain the client's privacy.

Stages of labor *(continued)*

STAGE	CONTRACTION CHARACTERISTICS	MATERNAL PHYSICAL CHANGES	FETAL POSITION CHANGES	NURSING CARE
Third: Placental stage				
Starts with delivery of neonate and ends with delivery of placenta and membranes	◆ Strong ◆ Every 3 minutes	◆ Placental separation 5 minutes after delivery ◆ Gush of blood ◆ Descent of umbilical cord ◆ Uterus rises in the abdomen and becomes globular ◆ Placental expulsion		◆ Measure the client's blood pressure. ◆ Assess estimated blood loss. ◆ Assess neonate. ◆ Praise the client, and provide information about the client's and neonate's status. ◆ Administer oxytocin, as ordered.
Fourth: 1st hour postdelivery				
	Not applicable	◆ Uterus contracted and usually midway between umbilicus and symphysis pubis ◆ Lochia present		◆ Monitor the client's vital signs, lochia, and fundus every 15 minutes. ◆ Provide comfort measures, including warm blankets and perineal ice. ◆ Introduce the neonate to the family, and encourage attachment behaviors.

◆ During flexion, the head flexes so that the chin moves closer to the chest.
◆ Internal rotation is the rotation of the head in order to pass through the ischial spines.
◆ Extension is when the head extends as it passes under the symphysis pubis.
◆ External rotation involves the external rotation of the head as the shoulders rotate to the anteroposterior position in the pelvis.

Third stage

The third stage of labor extends from delivery of the neonate to expulsion of the placenta and lasts from 5 to 30 minutes. During this period, the client typically focuses on the neonate's condition. The client may experience discomfort from uterine contractions before expelling the placenta.

Fourth stage

The fourth stage of labor is the first hour after delivery, when the primary activity is the promotion of maternal-neonatal bonding.

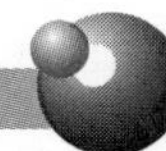

SPOT CHECK

A client is admitted to the hospital with contractions that are about 1 to 2 minutes apart and last for 60 seconds. Vaginal examination reveals that her cervix is dilated 8 cm. The client is in what phase of labor?

A. Latent phase
B. Active phase
C. Early phase
D. Transitional phase

Answer: D. The client is in the transitional phase of labor, characterized by cervical dilation of 8 to 10 cm and contractions that are about 1 to 2 minutes apart and last for 60 to 90 seconds with strong intensity.

Evaluating the fetus during labor

Evaluation of uterine contractions and FHR during labor involves external and internal monitoring:
◆ FHR can be monitored intermittently with a handheld device or continuously with a large fetal monitor. (See *Fetal heart rate patterns,* page 217.)

Nursing care during labor and delivery

Nursing actions include interventions that correspond to all stages of labor as well as those that apply only to certain stages.

Care during all stages of labor

- Monitor and record vital signs, I.V. fluid intake, and urine output.
- Provide emotional support to the client and her coach.
- Assess the need for pain medication, and evaluate the effectiveness of pain-relief measures.
- Maintain aseptic technique and standard precautions.
- Maintain the client's comfort by offering mouth care, ice chips, and a change of bed linen.
- Explain the purpose of all nursing actions and medical equipment.

Care during first and second stages

- Inform the client of labor progress, such as dilation, station, effacement, and fetal well-being.
- Monitor the frequency, duration, and intensity of contractions.
- Monitor fetal heart rate (FHR) during and between contractions, noting rate, accelerations, decelerations, and variability.
- Observe for rupture of membranes, noting the time, color, odor, amount, and consistency of amniotic fluid.
- Observe for prolapsed cord and check FHR immediately after rupture of membranes.
- Assess for signs of hypotensive supine syndrome; if blood pressure falls, position the client on the left side, increase the I.V. flow rate, and administer oxygen through a face mask at 6 to 10 L/minute.
- During the second stage, observe the perineum for show and bulging.

Care during first, second, and third stages

- Assist with breathing techniques.
- Encourage rest between contractions.

Care during the fourth stage

- Assess lochia and the location and consistency of the fundus.
- Encourage bonding.
- Initiate breast-feeding.

◆ Contraction frequency and intensity is monitored externally with a transducer. This pressure-sensitive device records uterine motion during contractions.

◆ Internal electronic fetal monitoring can evaluate fetal status during labor more accurately than external methods. A spiral electrode attached to the presenting fetal part provides the baseline FHR and allows evaluation of FHR variability.

◆ To determine the true intensity of contractions, a pressure-sensitive catheter is inserted into the uterine cavity alongside the fetus.

Evaluating the mother during labor

Review the methods and techniques used to monitor the progress of labor and the mother's condition:

◆ Observe dilation. The external os opening should increase from 0 to 10 cm.

◆ Observe effacement, cervical thinning and shortening, which is measured from 0% (thick) to 100% (paper thin).

◆ Using abdominal palpation (Leopold's maneuvers), determine fetal position and presentation. The process consists of four maneuvers:

1. Palpate the fundus to identify the occupying fetal part. The fetus's head is firm and rounded and moves freely; the breech is softer and less regular and moves with the trunk.
2. Palpate the abdomen to locate the fetus's back. The back should feel firm, smooth, and convex, whereas the front is soft, irregular, and concave.
3. Determine the level of descent of the head by grasping the lower portion of the abdomen above the symphysis pubis to identify the fetal part presenting over the inlet. The head feels firm; a breech fetus feels soft; an unengaged head can be rocked from side to side.
4. Determine head flexion by moving fingers down both sides of the uterus to assess the descent of the presenting part into the pelvis. Greater resistance is met as the fingers move downward on the cephalic prominence (brow) side.

◆ Check the station, the relationship of the presenting part to the pelvic ischial spines:

- The presenting part is even with the ischial spines at 0 station.
- The presenting part is above the ischial spines at –3, –2, or –1.
- The presenting part is below the ischial spines at +1, +2, or +3.

◆ Monitor the client for signs of dehydration, such as poor skin turgor, decreased urine output, and dry mucous membranes.

◆ Use an external pressure transducer to monitor the client for tetanic contractions (sustained prolonged contractions with little rest between).

Fetal heart rate patterns

Here's a quick review of fetal heart rate (FHR) patterns.

Decelerations of FHR

Decelerations of FHR can be a reassuring sign but may also indicate complications.

Early decelerations

Early decelerations are caused by head compression in the fetus. They're smooth, uniformly shaped waveforms that inversely mirror the corresponding contractions. Early decelerations:

- normally range from 120 to 160 beats/minute
- are a reassuring pattern not associated with fetal difficulties
- reassure the client that labor is progressing as expected.

Later decelerations

Later decelerations are caused by uteroplacental insufficiency. They are smooth, uniformly shaped waveforms that inversely mirror the contractions but are late in onset and may remain after the contraction is over. Later decelerations:

- are usually within the normal range with a high baseline but may drop to below 100 beats/minute when severe
- are considered an ominous sign if they are persistent and uncorrected; the pattern is associated with decreased Apgar scores, fetal hypoxia, and acidosis
- may require emergency cesareandelivery if persistent.

Variable decelerations

Variable decelerations of FHR occur in about half of all labors and are due to umbilical cord compression. They vary in onset, occurrence, and waveform.

- Variable decelerations are characterized by a heart rate that may (in severe cases) decelerate below 70 beats/minute for more than 30 seconds with a slow return to baseline
- usually are transient and correctable
- aren't associated with low Apgar scores.

Accelerations of FHR

Accelerations of FHR are normally caused by fetal movements but can also occur with contractions. Accelerations of FHR:

- can be uniformly or variably shaped
- are usually above 150 beats/minute.

Variability of FHR

Normal cardiac irregularity is caused by continuous interplay of the parasympathetic and sympathetic nervous systems. This normal variability can be long-term (rhythmic fluctuations and waves occurring three to five times/minute) or short-term (beat-to-beat changes between 6 and 10 beats/minute).

Increased variability

Increased variability can be caused by early, mild hypoxia and fetal stimulation. It's the earliest sign of mild fetal hypoxia that accompanies fetal vein compression. Carefully evaluate the FHR tracing for signs of fetal distress.

Decreased variability

Decreased variability can be caused by hypoxia, acidosis, central nervous system depressants, or medications and may require fetal blood sampling or internal monitoring. Decreased variability is:

- benign when associated with analgesics
- ominous if caused by hypoxia or associated with late decelerations.

Measuring contractions

Phases of uterine contractions include increment (buildup and longest phase), acme (peak of the contraction), and decrement (letting-down phase). Contractions are measured by duration, frequency, and intensity. Here's how to measure each:

- Duration is measured from the beginning of the increment to the end of the decrement and averages 30 seconds early in labor and 60 seconds later in labor.
- Frequency is measured from the beginning of one contraction to the beginning of the next and averages 5 to 30 minutes apart early in labor and 2 to 3 minutes apart later in labor.
- Intensity is assessed during the acme phase and can be measured with an intrauterine catheter or by palpation. (Normal resting pressure when using an intrauterine catheter is 5 to 15 mm Hg; pressure increases to 30 to 50 mm Hg during the acme.)

Maternal responses to labor

During labor, the mother undergoes various physiologic changes. Monitor changes in fluid and electrolyte balance as well as the cardiovascular, respiratory, hematopoietic, GI, and renal systems to avoid serious complications.

Fluid and electrolyte balance

- Increased water loss from diaphoresis and hyperventilation
- Increased evaporative water volume from increased respiratory rate

Cardiovascular system

- Increased intrathoracic pressure during pushing in the second stage
- Increased peripheral resistance during contractions, which elevates blood pressure and decreases pulse rate
- Increased cardiac output

Respiratory system

- Increased oxygen consumption
- Increased respiratory rate

Hematopoietic system

- Increased plasma fibrinogen level and leukocyte count
- Decreased blood coagulation time and blood glucose levels

GI system

- Decreased gastric motility and absorption
- Prolonged gastric emptying time

Renal system

- Forward and upward displacement of the bladder base at engagement
- Possibly proteinuria from muscle breakdown
- Possibly impaired blood and lymph drainage from the bladder base, resulting from edema caused by the presenting fetal part
- Decreased bladder sensation if epidural anesthetic has been administered

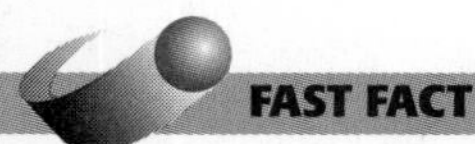

FAST FACT

Key terms related to contractions include *increment, acme, decrement, duration, frequency,* and *intensity*.

Labor also prompts a series of responses throughout the mother's body, including changes in the cardiovascular, respiratory, and GI systems. (See *Maternal responses to labor.*)

Pain relief during labor and delivery

Pain relief is an important element of client care during labor and delivery. Pain relief during labor includes nonpharmacologic methods, analgesics, and general and regional anesthetics.

Nonpharmacologic

- Effleurage, a light abdominal stroking with the fingertips in a circular motion, is effective for mild to moderate discomfort.
- Distraction can divert attention from mild discomfort early in labor.
- Patterns of controlled chest breathing are used primarily during the active and transitional phases of labor.
- Relaxation techniques include positioning, focusing and imagery, therapeutic touch and massage, music therapy, and support of a birthing partner.
- The stimulation of key trigger points with needles (acupuncture) or finger pressure (acupressure) can reduce pain and enhance energy flow.
- Other methods include heat and cold application, transcutaneous stimulation (TENS), hypnosis, and yoga to help reduce pain and promote comfort.

Analgesic

- An opioid such as meperidine (Demerol) can be used to relieve pain. If medication is given within 2 hours of delivery, it can cause neonatal respiratory depression, hypotonia, and lethargy.

Anesthetic

- Lumbar epidural anesthesia requires an injection of medication into the epidural space in the lumbar region, leaving the client awake and cooperative. An epidural provides analgesia for the first and second stages of labor and anesthesia for delivery without adverse fetal effects. Hypotension is uncommon, but its incidence increases if the client doesn't receive a proper fluid load before the procedure. Epidural anesthesia may decrease the client's urge to push.
- Spinal anesthesia involves an injection of medication into the cerebrospinal fluid in the spinal canal. Because of its rapid onset, spinal anesthesia is useful for urgent cesarean deliveries.

◆ Local infiltration involves an injection of an anesthetic into the perineal nerves. It offers no relief from discomfort during labor but relieves pain during delivery.
◆ A pudendal block involves blockage of the pudendal nerve. This procedure is used only for delivery.
◆ A paracervical block involves the blockage of nerves in the peridural space at the sacral hiatus, which provides analgesia for the first and second stages of labor and anesthesia for delivery. This procedure increases the risk of forceps delivery.
◆ General anesthetics can be administered I.V. or through inhalation, resulting in loss of consciousness (LOC). General anesthetics should be used only if regional anesthetics are contraindicated or in a rapidly developing emergency.

INTRAPARTUM COMPLICATIONS

During the intrapartum period the client must be monitored carefully for complications, some of which can be life-threatening for the mother or fetus.

DYSTOCIA

Dystocia is a difficult or abnormal labor. In many cases, surgical intervention is required to safely deliver the fetus.

Possible causes

◆ Contracted pelvis
◆ Obstructive tumors
◆ Malpresentation of the fetus
◆ Malformation of the fetus
◆ Hypertonic uterine patterns
◆ Hypotonic uterine patterns

Assessment findings

◆ Arrested descent
◆ Hypertonic contractions
◆ Hypotonic contractions
◆ Prolonged active phase
◆ Prolonged deceleration phase
◆ Protracted latent phase
◆ Uncoordinated contractions

Diagnostic evaluation

◆ Contraction monitoring reveals hypotonic or hypertonic contractions and progression of labor.
◆ Abdominal and vaginal examinations are used to determine fetal presentation.
◆ Ultrasonography confirms fetal presentation.

Nursing diagnoses

◆ Risk for injury
◆ Anxiety
◆ Deficient knowledge (client and family members)

Treatment

◆ Amniotomy (artificial rupture of membranes)
◆ Fluid hydration
◆ Cesarean delivery

Drug therapy options

◆ Analgesic (or to relax hypertonic contractions): morphine sulfate
◆ Labor augmentation: oxytocin

Planning and goals

◆ The client will have decreased fear during labor because of health care and personal support.
◆ The client and her fetus will remain hemodynamically stable during labor and delivery.
◆ The client will have increased knowledge of all circumstances of labor and delivery.

Implementation

◆ Administer I.V. fluids *to maintain adequate hydration of the client and her fetus.*
◆ Monitor fetal heart tones and vital signs *to evaluate hemodynamic status.*
◆ Tell the client to remain in a side-lying position *to provide increased perfusion to the fetus.*
◆ Answer all questions and keep the client informed about all procedures and findings *to decrease anxiety and assist her and her family members in understanding the status of labor and planned treatment.* (See *Caring for the client with dystocia,* page 220.)
◆ Be supportive of the client and her family *to decrease fear of complications.*

Evaluation

◆ The client experiences less fear.
◆ The client and fetus remain hemodynamically stable.
◆ The client has increased knowledge regarding her labor.

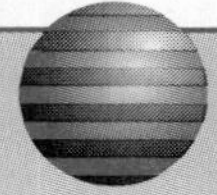

CLINICAL SITUATION

Caring for the client with dystocia

A client in your care is gravida 3, para 2, and has been in labor for 14 hours. Her membranes ruptured 6 hours ago. A pelvic examination reveals the same findings as those from an examination 2 hours earlier: Her cervix is dilated 6 cm and 100% effaced, and the presenting part is at -2 station. An I.V. infusion has been started. The fetal heart rate (FHR) is 152 beats/minute; variability is minimal to average, with intermittent decelerations. Her contractions have become less frequent and less intense (a hypotonic pattern), and the client and her husband sense that something is wrong. The physician orders ultrasonographic studies and considers a cesarean delivery.

What signs and symptoms should the nurse be looking for?

The nurse should assess the client for signs and symptoms associated with dystocia: abnormal uterine contraction patterns, delayed cervical progress, and delayed descent of the presenting part.

Normal labor contractions increase in frequency, duration, and intensity. Dystocia is diagnosed in a primigravida if the latent phase lasts more than 20 hours or if cervical dilation doesn't progress more than 1.2 cm/hour in the active phase; in a multigravida, if the latent phase lasts more than 14 hours or if cervical dilation doesn't progress more than 1.5 cm/hour in the active phase. Delay in descent of the presenting part also indicates dystocia.

What should the nurse assess regarding the fetus?

The nurse should assess fetal heart tones, fetal activity, and amniotic fluid to detect possible fetal distress. Prolonged labor compromising the fetal oxygen supply may cause fetal distress, indicated by abnormal fetal heart tones, fetal hyperactivity, and meconium-stained amniotic fluid. Fetal scalp pH indicates the acid-base balance of the fetus.

Question for further thought

◆ What is the appropriate treatment for the client if it's discovered that the fetus is in distress?

EMERGENCY BIRTH

Emergency delivery of the fetus may become necessary when the well-being of the client or fetus is in jeopardy.

Possible causes

◆ Contributing factors vary for each emergency birth situation.

Prolapsed umbilical cord

A prolapsed umbilical cord occurs when the umbilical cord descends into the vagina before the presenting part. It may be caused by:
◆ fetus at high fetal station
◆ hydramnios (excess of amniotic fluid)
◆ multifetal pregnancy
◆ small fetus or breech presentation
◆ transverse lie.

Uterine rupture

A uterine rupture occurs when the uterus undergoes more strain than it can bear. It can be caused by:
◆ prolonged labor
◆ faulty presentation
◆ obstructed labor
◆ blunt abdominal trauma
◆ high parity with thin uterine wall
◆ intense uterine contractions (natural or oxytocin-induced), especially with fetopelvic disproportion
◆ previous uterine surgery
◆ traumatic manuevers involving forceps or traction.

Amniotic fluid embolism

In amniotic fluid embolism, amniotic fluid escapes into the maternal circulation. During labor (or during the postpartum period), solid particles such as skin cells enter the maternal circulation and reach the lungs as small emboli, forcing a massive pulmonary embolism. It may be caused by:
◆ defect in the membranes after rupture
◆ partial abruptio placentae
◆ fetal particulate matter (skin, hair, vernix, cells, meconium) in the fluid that obstructs the maternal pulmonary vessels
◆ polyhydramonios
◆ oxytocin administration.

Assessment findings

Assessment findings vary for each emergency birth situation.

Prolapsed umbilical cord

◆ Cord palpable during vaginal examination
◆ Cord visible at the vaginal opening
◆ Variable decelerations or bradycardia noted on fetal monitor strip

Uterine rupture

◆ Appearance of a pathologic retraction ring, an indentation that appears across the abdomen over the uterus, just before rupture
◆ Abdominal pain and tenderness especially at the peak of a contraction or the feeling that "something ripped"
◆ Excessive external bleeding
◆ Late decelerations, reduced FHR variability, tachycardia and bradycardia, cessation of FHR
◆ Hypovolemic shock caused by hemorrhage
◆ Chest pain or pain on inspiration
◆ Cessation of uterine contractions
◆ Palpation of the fetus outside the uterus

Amniotic fluid embolism

◆ Chest pain
◆ Sudden dyspnea
◆ Tachypnea
◆ Coughing with pink, frothy sputum
◆ Increasing restlessness and anxiety
◆ Hemorrhage
◆ Shock disproportionate to blood loss
◆ Cyanosis

Diagnostic evaluation

Prolapsed umbilical cord

◆ Ultrasonography confirms that the cord is prolapsed.

Uterine rupture

◆ Urinalysis can detect gross hematuria.
◆ Ultrasonography may reveal the absence of the amniotic cavity within the uterus.

Amniotic fluid embolism

◆ Arterial blood gas analysis reveals hypoxemia.
◆ Hematology reveals thrombocytopenia, decreased fibrinogen level and platelet count, prolonged PT, and a PTT consistent with disseminated intravascular coagulation.

Cesarean delivery

Cesarean delivery is the planned or emergency removal of the neonate from the uterus through an abdominal incision. The surgical incision may be midline and vertical (classic), allowing easy access to the fetus, and is usually the approach of choice in emergency situations. A low-segment, transverse, or Pfannenstiel's (bikini) incision is usually chosen in a planned cesarean birth.

Nursing actions

During a cesarean birth, you should:
◆ provide emotional support and reassurance to the client and her family, including reassurance about the well-being of the fetus
◆ assess fetal heart rate, maternal vital signs, and intake and output
◆ monitor uterine contractions and labor progress, when appropriate
◆ obtain blood samples for hematocrit, hemoglobin level, prothrombin and partial thromboplastin times, fibrinogen level, platelet count, and typing and crossmatching
◆ initiate and maintain I.V. fluid replacement, as necessary
◆ prepare the client for surgery, including shaving of the abdomen and perineal area as necessary
◆ insert an indwelling urinary catheter as ordered
◆ provide preoperative teaching as necessary
◆ administer preoperative sedation as ordered
◆ provide immediate postoperative care after surgery.

Nursing diagnoses

◆ Ineffective tissue perfusion (fetal cardiopulmonary)
◆ Acute pain
◆ Risk for infection
◆ Ineffective coping

Treatment

◆ Administration of I.V. fluid
◆ Administration of oxygen by nasal cannula or mask (Endotracheal intubation and mechanical ventilation may be necessary in the case of amniotic fluid embolism.)
◆ Emergency cesarean delivery (see *Cesarean delivery*)
◆ Emergency hysterectomy (with uterine rupture)
◆ Possible transfusion of packed RBCs, fresh frozen plasma, or platelets

Planning and goals

- The fetus will maintain adequate cardiopulmonary perfusion.
- The client will remain free from infection.
- The client will verbalize understanding of the complication, its treatment, and potential outcomes.
- The client will demonstrate decreased anxiety.
- The client will experience decreased pain.

Implementation

- Position the client in the knee-chest or Trendelenburg position *to decrease pressure on the umbilical cord and promote fetal cardiopulmonary perfusion.*
- Monitor maternal vital signs, pulse oximetry, intake and output, and FHR *to assess for complications.*
- Administer maternal oxygen by cannula or mask at 8 to 10 L/minute *to maintain uteroplacental oxygenation.*
- Initiate and maintain I.V. fluid replacement *to replace volume loss.*
- Provide emotional support and reassurance to the client *to allay fears and reduce anxiety.*
- Obtain blood samples to determine HCT, Hb level, PT, PTT, fibrinogen level, and platelet count, type and crossmatch blood *to establish baseline values.*
- Administer blood products as necessary *to replace volume loss.*
- Prepare the client and her family for the possibility of cesarean delivery *to reduce anxiety.*

Evaluation

- The neonate is delivered safely.
- The client is free from infection.
- The client has decreased pain and anxiety.

LACERATION

Laceration refers to tears in the perineum, vagina, or cervix from the stretching of tissues during delivery. A laceration is classified as first, second, third, or fourth degree:

- A first-degree laceration involves the vaginal mucosa and the skin of the perineum and fourchette.
- A second-degree laceration involves the vagina, perineal skin, fasciae, levator ani muscle, and perineal body.
- A third-degree laceration involves the entire perineum and the external anal sphincter.
- A fourth-degree laceration involves the entire perineum, rectal sphincter, and portions of the rectal mucosa.

Possible causes

- Delivery of a large fetus
- Rapid delivery
- Use of forceps or vacuum extractor during delivery

Assessment findings

- Increased vaginal bleeding after delivery of placenta
- Visualization of the tear

Diagnostic evaluation

- Inspection of the affected area will reveal the extent of laceration.

Nursing diagnoses

- Risk for deficient fluid volume
- Acute pain

Treatment

- Surgical repair
- Administration of appropriate pain medication

Planning and goals

- The client will remain hemodynamically stable.
- The client will have relief from pain.

Implementation

- Monitor vital signs after delivery *to evaluate signs of shock.*
- Evaluate the amount of vaginal bleeding *to determine if surgical repair is warranted (if not done) or if the client needs blood replacement.*
- Administer appropriate pain medication *to make the client more comfortable.*

Evaluation

- The client remains hemodynamically stable.
- The client has an expected amount of postdelivery vaginal bleeding.
- The client verbalizes relief from pain.

PREMATURE RUPTURE OF MEMBRANES

In premature rupture of membranes (PROM), rupture occurs 1 or more hours before the onset of labor. Chorioamnionitis may occur if the time between rupture of membranes and onset of labor is longer than 24 hours.

Possible causes

- Infection
- Fetal distress
- Malpresentation of the fetus
- Incompetent cervix

Assessment findings
◆ Fetal tachycardia
◆ Foul-smelling amniotic fluid
◆ Maternal fever
◆ Uterine tenderness

Diagnostic evaluation
◆ Vaginal examination reveals fluid leakage from the cervical os when the client bears down.
◆ Amniotic fluid testing, which is obtained by vaginal examination, confirms nonintact membranes.

Nursing diagnoses
◆ Risk for infection
◆ Anxiety
◆ Deficient knowledge (maternal and family members)

Treatment
◆ Bed rest
◆ Administration of I.V. fluids
◆ Emergency cesarean delivery

Planning and goals
◆ The client will remain hemodynamically stable and free from infection.
◆ The client will demonstrate decreased anxiety.
◆ The client will verbalize understanding of procedures and findings related to premature rupture of membranes.

Implementation
◆ Monitor vital signs *to evaluate signs of infection and fetal distress.*
◆ Evaluate WBC count *to determine the presence of infection.*
◆ Evaluate amniotic fluid for color and meconium *to detect fetal infection or distress.*
◆ Provide education about treatment and potential complications *to promote client understanding.*
◆ Provide emotional support *to decrease anxiety regarding unexpected complications.*

Evaluation
◆ The client and fetus remain infection-free.
◆ The client verbalizes understanding the procedure and treatment.
◆ The client demonstrates decreased anxiety over unexpected events of pregnancy.

PRETERM LABOR
Preterm labor, also known as *premature labor,* occurs before the end of the 37th week of gestation. Preterm labor can place the client and fetus at high risk for complications.

Possible causes
◆ Causes of preterm labor can be maternal or fetal.

Maternal causes
◆ Abdominal surgery or trauma
◆ Cardiovascular or renal disease
◆ Chronic hypertension
◆ Dehydration
◆ Diabetes mellitus
◆ Genetic defect in the mother
◆ Incompetent cervix
◆ Infection
◆ Placental abnormalities
◆ Gestational hypertension
◆ PROM
◆ Structural abnormalities of the uterus

Fetal causes
◆ Fetal death
◆ Hydramnios
◆ Infection
◆ PROM

Assessment findings
◆ Feeling of pelvic pressure or abdominal tightening
◆ Menstrual-like cramps
◆ Persistent, low, dull backache
◆ Vaginal spotting
◆ Intestinal cramping
◆ Increased vaginal discharge
◆ Uterine contractions that result in cervical dilation and effacement

Diagnostic evaluation
◆ Electronic fetal monitoring confirms uterine contractions.
◆ Vaginal examination confirms cervical effacement and dilation.

Nursing diagnoses
◆ Risk for injury
◆ Anxiety
◆ Deficient knowledge (maternal and family members)

Treatment

◆ Suppression of preterm labor (if fetal membranes are intact, there's no evidence of bleeding, the well-being of the fetus and mother isn't in jeopardy, cervical effacement is no more than 50%, and cervical dilation is less than 4 cm)

Drug therapy options

◆ Magnesium supplement: magnesium sulfate to prevent reflux of calcium into the myometrial cells, thereby maintaining a relaxed uterus
◆ Tocolytic agent: terbutaline sulfate (Brethine) to inhibit uterine contractions

Planning and goals

◆ Preterm contractions will cease or the fetus will be delivered safely.
◆ The client will verbalize understanding of the treatment and potential outcomes of preterm labor.
◆ The client will demonstrate decreased anxiety over the unexpected complication of preterm labor.

Implementation

◆ Monitor maternal vital signs, contractions, and FHR every 15 minutes during tocolytic therapy (otherwise, provide continuous fetal monitoring) *to assess maternal and fetal well-being.*
◆ Assess the client's respiratory status *to assess for pulmonary edema, an adverse effect associated with tocolytic therapy.*
◆ Monitor for maternal adverse reactions to terbutaline *to detect possible tachycardia, diarrhea, nervousness, tremors, nausea, vomiting, headache, hyperglycemia, hypoglycemia, hypokalemia, or pulmonary edema.*
◆ Notify the physician if the maternal pulse rate exceeds 120 beats/minute or the FHR exceeds 180 beats/minute *to expedite medical evaluation of maternal and fetal status.*
◆ Provide emotional support to the client *to ease anxiety and establish a therapeutic relationship.*
◆ Monitor laboratory results *to detect abnormalities and initiate early intervention.*
◆ Place the client in the lateral position *to increase placental perfusion.*
◆ Monitor for magnesium sulfate toxicity, which causes central nervous system depression in the mother and fetus; make sure calcium gluconate is available *to reverse these effects.*

Evaluation

◆ Preterm labor subsides.
◆ The neonate is delivered safely.
◆ The client verbalizes decreased anxiety.
◆ The client verbalizes understanding of treatments and follows all medical advice appropriately.

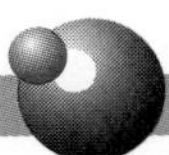

SPOT CHECK

A client in the 28th week of gestation comes to the emergency department because she thinks that she's in labor. To confirm a diagnosis of preterm labor, the nurse would expect physical examination to reveal:

A. irregular uterine contractions with no cervical dilation.
B. painful contractions with no cervical dilation.
C. regular uterine contractions with cervical dilation.
D. regular uterine contractions with no cervical dilation.

Answer: C. Regular uterine contractions (every 10 minutes or more) along with cervical dilation before 36 weeks' gestation or rupture of fluids indicates preterm labor. Uterine contractions without cervical change don't indicate preterm labor.

POSTPARTUM PERIOD

The postpartum period, or *puerperium,* begins with the fourth stage of labor and lasts approximately 6 weeks. During this period, the client's reproductive organs return to their nonpregnant state. Knowledge of normal physiologic and psychological changes during the postpartum period enables the nurse to recognize deviations and intervene early.

PHYSIOLOGIC CHANGES AFTER DELIVERY

In the vascular system, blood volume decreases and HCT increases after vaginal delivery. Excessive activation of blood-clotting factors also occurs. Blood volume returns to prenatal levels within 3 weeks.

In the reproductive system, uterine involution occurs rapidly immediately after delivery. Progesterone production ceases until the client's first ovulation. Endometrial regeneration begins after 6 weeks. The cervical opening is permanently altered from a circle to a jagged slit.

GI system changes

- ◆ Increased hunger after labor and delivery
- ◆ Delayed bowel movement from decreased intestinal muscle tone and perineal discomfort
- ◆ Increased thirst from fluids lost during labor and delivery

Genitourinary system changes

- ◆ Increased urine output during the first 24 hours after delivery due to increased glomerular filtration rate and a drop in progesterone levels
- ◆ Increased bladder capacity
- ◆ Proteinuria caused by the catalytic process of involution (in 50% of women)
- ◆ Decreased bladder-filling sensation caused by swollen and bruised tissues
- ◆ Return of dilated ureters and renal pelvis to prepregnancy size after 6 weeks

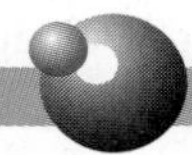

SPOT CHECK

Which of the following is a normal physiologic response in the early postpartum period?

A. Urinary urgency and dysuria
B. Rapid diuresis
C. Decrease in blood pressure
D. Increased motility of the GI system

Answer: B. In the early postpartum period there's an increase in the glomerular filtration rate and a drop in progesterone levels, which result in rapid diuresis. There should be no urinary urgency, although the client may be anxious about voiding. There's minimal change in blood pressure following childbirth and a residual decrease in GI motility.

Endocrine system

- ◆ Increased thyroid function and production of anterior pituitary gonadotropic hormones
- ◆ Decreased production of other hormones, including estrogen, aldosterone, progesterone, HCG, corticoids, and ketosteroids

PSYCHOLOGIC CHANGES AFTER DELIVERY

More than 50% of women experience transient mood alterations immediately after delivery. This mood change is called *postpartum depression,* or the "baby blues." Signs and symptoms include sadness, crying, fatigue, and low self-esteem. Possible causes include hormonal changes, genetic predisposition, and adjustment to an altered role and self-concept.

Teach the client that mood swings and bouts of depression are normal postpartum responses; they typically occur during the first 3 weeks after delivery and subside within 1 to 10 days.

Postdelivery phases

Maternal behavior after delivery is divided into three phases:

- ◆ Taking-in phase
- ◆ Taking-hold phase
- ◆ Letting-go phase.

During the taking-in phase (1 to 2 days after delivery), the mother is passive and dependent, directing energy toward herself instead of toward her infant. She may relive her labor and delivery experience to integrate the process into her life and may have difficulty making decisions.

During the taking-hold phase (about 2 to 7 days after delivery), the mother has more energy and begins to act independently and initiate self-care activities. Although she may express a lack of confidence in her abilities, she accepts responsibility for her neonate and becomes receptive to infant care and teaching about self-care activities.

During the letting-go phase (about 7 days after delivery), the mother begins to readjust to family members, assuming the mother role and the responsibility that comes with it. She relinquishes the infant she has imagined during her pregnancy and accepts her real infant as an entity separate from herself.

POSTPARTUM ASSESSMENT

The period immediately after labor and delivery is crucial to good postpartum nursing care. An understanding of normal and abnormal assessment findings is essential.

Vital signs

- ◆ The client's respiratory rate should return to normal after delivery.
- ◆ The client's temperature may be elevated to 100.4° F (38° C) from dehydration and the exertion of labor.
- ◆ Blood pressure is usually normal within 24 hours after delivery.
- ◆ Bradycardia of 50 to 70 beats/minute is common during the first 6 to 10 days after delivery because of reductions in cardiac strain, stroke volume, and the vascular bed.

Nursing actions

◆ Monitor vital signs every 15 minutes for the first 1 to 2 hours, then every 4 hours for the first 24 hours, and then during every shift.

Uterus

Check the tone and location of the fundus (the uppermost portion of the uterus) every 15 minutes for the first 1 to 2 hours after delivery and then during every shift. The involuting uterus should be at the midline. The fundus is usually:

◆ midway between the umbilicus and symphysis 1 to 2 hours after delivery
◆ 1 cm above or at the level of the umbilicus 12 hours after delivery
◆ 3 cm below the umbilicus by the 3rd day after delivery
◆ firm to the touch.

The fundus will continue to descend about 1 cm per day until it isn't palpable above the symphysis (about 9 days after delivery). The uterus shrinks to its prepregnancy size 5 to 6 weeks after delivery.

A firm uterus helps control postpartum hemorrhage by clamping down on uterine blood vessels. The physician may prescribe oxytocin (Pitocin), ergonovine maleate (Ergotrate), or methylergonovine (Methergine) to maintain uterine firmness.

Nursing actions

◆ Massage a boggy (soft) fundus gently; if the fundus doesn't respond, use a firmer touch.
◆ Be aware that the uterus may relax if overstimulated by massage or medications.
◆ Suspect a distended bladder if the uterus isn't firm at the midline. A distended bladder can impede the downward descent of the uterus by pushing it upward and, possibly, to the side.
◆ Assess for excessive vaginal bleeding.

Lochia

Lochia is discharge from the sloughing of the uterine decidua. There are different types of lochia:

◆ Lochia rubra is the vaginal discharge that occurs for the first 2 to 3 days after delivery; it has a fleshy odor and is bloody with small clots.
◆ Lochia serosa refers to the vaginal discharge that occurs during days 3 through 9; it's pinkish or brown with a serosanguineous consistency and fleshy odor.
◆ Lochia alba is a yellow to white discharge that usually begins about 10 days after delivery; it may last from 2 to 6 weeks.

Lochia may be scant but should never be absent; absence may indicate postpartum infection. Some lochia characteristics may indicate the need for further intervention, for example:

◆ foul-smelling lochia may indicate an infection
◆ continuous seepage of bright red blood may indicate a cervical or vaginal laceration
◆ numerous large clots may interfere with involution and should be evaluated further
◆ lochia that saturates a sanitary pad within 45 minutes usually indicates an abnormally heavy flow.

Nursing actions

◆ Assess the lochia during every shift, and note its color, amount, odor, and consistency.

Breasts

Assess the size and shape of the client's breasts every shift, noting reddened areas, tenderness, and engorgement. Check the nipples for cracking, fissures, and soreness.

Nursing actions

◆ Tell the client that she can relieve discomfort from engorged breasts by wearing a support bra, applying ice packs, and taking prescribed medications.
◆ If the client is breast-feeding, advise her that she can relieve breast engorgement by eating frequent meals, applying warm compresses, and expressing milk manually.

Elimination

Assess the client's elimination patterns. The client should void within the first 6 to 8 hours after delivery. Assess for a distended bladder, which can interfere with elimination, within the first few hours after delivery.

Nursing actions

◆ Tell the client that she may use pain medication before urination. Pour warm water over the perineum to eliminate the fear of pain.
◆ Be prepared to insert a catheter if the client can't void.
◆ Encourage the client to have a bowel movement within 1 to 2 days after delivery to avoid constipation.
◆ Provide the client with hemorrhoids with ice packs or analgesic preparations, if needed.
◆ Encourage the client to increase her fluid and roughage intake.
◆ Alleviate maternal anxieties regarding pain from or damage to the site of episiotomy (surgical incision into the perineum and vagina).

◆ Provide the client with laxatives, stool softeners, suppositories, or enemas, if needed.
◆ When caring for a client with a fourth-degree laceration, never take a rectal temperature reading or administer an enema.

Perineum and rectum
The site of episiotomy should be assessed every shift to evaluate healing, noting erythema, intactness of stitches, edema, and odor or drainage. Twenty-four hours after delivery, the edges of an episiotomy are usually sealed.

Nursing actions
◆ Assist in performing perineal care to promote cleanliness and comfort. Cold therapy helps reduce edema and prevents hematoma formation and is used in the first 24 hours.
◆ Administer medications to relieve discomfort from the episiotomy, uterine contractions, incisional pain, or engorged breasts, as prescribed. Medications may include analgesics, stool softeners and laxatives, or oxytocic agents.

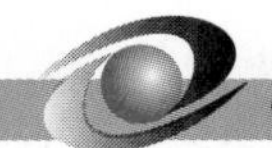
QUICK STUDY

To remember what to assess in the postpartum patient, remember **BE BLUE**:

Bladder
Elimination

Breasts
Lochia
Uterus
Episiotomy

POSTPARTUM COMPLICATIONS

Common postpartum complications include mastitis, postpartum hemorrhage, psychological maladaptation, and puerperal infection.

MASTITIS
Mastitis is an infection of the lactating breast. It most commonly occurs during weeks 2 and 3 after birth but can occur at any time.

Possible causes
◆ *Staphylococcus aureus* (the most common causative pathogen)
◆ Altered immune response
◆ Constriction from a bra that's too tight (may interfere with complete emptying of the breast)
◆ Engorgement and stasis of milk (usually precede mastitis)
◆ Injury to nipple, which may allow a causative organism to enter through an injured area of the nipple, such as a crack or blister

Assessment findings
◆ Localized area of redness and inflammation
◆ Temperature of 101.1° F (38.4° C) or higher
◆ Purulent drainage
◆ Chills
◆ Fatigue
◆ Headache
◆ Aching muscles
◆ Malaise

Diagnostic evaluation
◆ Culture of the purulent discharge may test positive for *S. aureus.*

Nursing diagnoses
◆ Acute pain
◆ Ineffective coping
◆ Risk for situational low self-esteem

Treatment
◆ Incision and drainage if abscess occurs
◆ Moist heat application
◆ Breast pumping to preserve breast-feeding ability

Drug therapy options
◆ Analgesics: acetaminophen (Tylenol), ibuprofen (Advil)
◆ Antibiotics: oral cephalosporins, dicloxacillin (Dynapen)

Planning and goals
◆ The client will positively respond to treatment, with resolution of the infection.
◆ The client will report relief from pain.
◆ The client will have her self-esteem restored.

Implementation
◆ Monitor vital signs *to assess for complications.*
◆ Administer antibiotic therapy *to treat infection.*

◆ Apply moist heat *to increase circulation and reduce inflammation and edema.*
◆ Be supportive of alternate feeding for the infant and include other family members in infant care *to foster improved client self-esteem.*

Evaluation

◆ The client is free from infection.
◆ The client verbalizes relief from pain.
◆ The client demonstrates improved self-esteem.

POSTPARTUM HEMORRHAGE

Postpartum hemorrhage is maternal blood loss from the uterus greater than 500 ml within a 24-hour period. It can occur immediately after delivery (within the first 24 hours) or later (during the remaining days of the 6-week puerperium). (See *Caring for the client with postpartum hemorrhage.*)

Possible causes

◆ Administration of magnesium sulfate
◆ Cesarean birth
◆ Clotting disorders
◆ DIC
◆ General anesthesia
◆ Low implantation of placenta or placenta previa
◆ Multiparity
◆ Overdistention of uterus (multifetal pregnancy, hydramnios, large infant)
◆ Perineal laceration
◆ Precipitate labor or delivery
◆ Previous postpartum hemorrhage
◆ Previous uterine surgery
◆ Prolonged labor
◆ Retained placental fragments
◆ Soft, boggy uterus, indicating relaxed uterine tone
◆ Use of tocolytic drugs

Assessment findings

◆ Blood loss greater than 500 ml within the first 24 hours after delivery
◆ Uterine atony
◆ Signs of shock (tachycardia, hypotension, oliguria)
◆ Perineal lacerations
◆ Retained placental fragments

Diagnostic evaluation

◆ Hematology studies show a low fibrinogen level and decreased Hb level, HCT, and PTT.

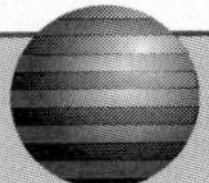

CLINICAL SITUATION

Caring for the client with postpartum hemorrhage

You're assigned to care for a 24-year-old primigravida client who delivered an 8-lb, 9-oz male infant 12 hours ago by spontaneous vaginal delivery over a midline episiotomy. In the client's room 4 hours later, you notice a large amount of blood on her peripad.

What further assessment should be done?
Assess vital signs for signs of shock related to hemorrhage (tachycardia, hypotension), inspect the episiotomy incision for signs of a tear, palpate the fundus for uterine atony, and assess the bladder for fullness and establish when the client last voided. Assess hemoglobin level and hematocrit if excessive bleeding persists.

Which of the following circumstances is the most likely cause of uterine atony, leading to postpartum hemorrhage?
A. Hypertension
B. Cervical and vaginal tears
C. Urine retention
D. Endometritis

Answer: C. Urine retention is the most likely cause of uterine atony and subsequent postpartum hemorrhage. Urine retention causes a distended bladder to displace the uterus above the umbilicus and to the side, which prevents the uterus from contracting. The uterus needs to remain contracted if bleeding is to stay within normal limits. Cervical and vaginal tears can cause postpartum hemorrhage but, in the postpartum period, a full bladder is the most common cause of uterine bleeding. Endometritis, an infection of the inner lining of the endometrium, and maternal hypertension don't cause postpartum hemorrhage.

Question for further thought
◆ What nursing action is appropriate if the uterus is boggy (soft) on assessment?

Nursing diagnoses

◆ Ineffective tissue perfusion (cardiopulmonary)
◆ Risk for deficient fluid volume
◆ Anxiety

Treatment

- Bimanual compression of the uterus and D&C to remove clots
- I.V. replacement of fluids and blood
- Abdominal hysterectomy if other interventions fail to control blood loss

Drug therapy options

- Parenteral administration of methylergonovine (Methergine), oxytocin (Pitocin), prostaglandins (carboprost thromethamine)
- Rapid I.V. infusion of dilute oxytocin

Planning and goals

- The client will remain hemodynamically stable.
- The client will maintain adequate circulating blood volume.
- The client will verbalize anxiety concerning bleeding.

Implementation

- Monitor vital signs *to assess for complications.*
- Massage the fundus, and express clots from the uterus *to increase uterine contraction and tone.*
- Perform a pad count *to assess the amount of vaginal bleeding.*
- Monitor lochia, including amount, color, and odor, *to assess for infection.*
- Monitor the fundus for location *to assess for uterine displacement.*
- Administer parenteral agents such as oxytocin as ordered *to increase uterine contraction and tone.*
- Administer methylergonovine as ordered *to increase uterine contraction and tone.*
- Administer blood products and I.V. fluids as prescribed *to replace volume loss.*
- Provide emotional support *to help alleviate fear and anxiety.*

Evaluation

- The client has stable vital signs.
- The client has blood volume restored as appropriate.
- The client's anxiety over the unexpected complication has decreased.

PSYCHOLOGICAL MALADAPTATION

Psychological maladaptation is depression of a significant depth and duration after childbirth. Many postpartum clients experience some level of mood swings; psychological maladaptation refers to depression that lasts longer than 2 days, indicating a serious problem.

Possible causes

Possible causes and risk factors include:

- history of depression
- hormonal shifts as estrogen and progesterone levels decline
- lack of support from family and friends
- lack of self-esteem
- stress in the home or work
- troubled childhood.

Assessment findings

- Extreme fatigue
- Inability to make decisions
- Inability to stop crying
- Increased anxiety about self and infant's health
- Overall feeling of sadness
- Postpartum psychosis (hallucinations, delusions, potential for suicide or homicide)
- Psychosomatic symptoms (nausea, vomiting, diarrhea)
- Unwillingness to be left alone

Nursing diagnoses

- Fatigue
- Ineffective coping
- Interrupted family processes

Treatment

- Counseling for the client and family at risk
- Group therapy
- Psychotherapy

Drug therapy options

- Antidepressants: imipramine (Tofranil), nortriptyline (Pamelor)

Planning and goals

- The client will verbalize feelings over life changes and begin to adapt to maternal role.
- The client will demonstrate coping skills to successfully interact with others as well as the infant.

Implementation

- Obtain a health history during the antepartum period *to assess whether the client is at risk for postpartum depression.*
- Assess the client's support systems *to determine the need for additional help.*

◆ Assess maternal-infant bonding *to evaluate for signs of depression.*
◆ Provide emotional support and encouragement *to reduce anxiety.*
◆ Notify a skilled professional if you observe psychotic symptoms in the client *to promote appropriate care and treatment if these symptoms develop.*

Evaluation
◆ The client interacts with infant and family appropriately.
◆ The client verbalizes decreased anxiety in maternal role.
◆ The client demonstrates increased energy in everyday activities.

PUERPERAL INFECTION
Puerperal infection occurs after childbirth in 2% to 5% of all women who have vaginal deliveries and in 15% to 20% of those who have cesarean deliveries. Puerperal infection is one of the leading causes of maternal death.

Possible causes
◆ Catheterization
◆ Cesarean delivery
◆ Colonization of lower genital tract with pathogenic organisms, such as group B streptococcus, *Chlamydia trachomatis, Staphylococcus aureus, Escherichia coli,* and *Gardnerella vaginalis*
◆ Excessive number of vaginal examinations
◆ History of previous infection
◆ Low socioeconomic status
◆ Medical conditions such as diabetes mellitus
◆ Poor general health
◆ Poor nutrition
◆ Prolonged labor
◆ Prolonged rupture of membranes
◆ Retained placental fragments
◆ Trauma

Assessment findings
◆ Abdominal pain and tenderness
◆ Purulent, foul-smelling lochia
◆ Fever
◆ Tachycardia
◆ Chills
◆ Uterine cramping
◆ Subinvolution
◆ Anorexia
◆ Lethargy
◆ Malaise

Diagnostic evaluation
◆ A catheterized urine specimen may reveal the causative organism.
◆ A complete blood count may show an elevated WBC count in the upper ranges of normal (more than 30,000/µl) for the postpartum period.
◆ Cultures of the blood or of the endocervical and uterine cavities may reveal the causative organism.

Nursing diagnoses
◆ Risk for infection
◆ Acute pain

Treatment
◆ Administration of I.V. fluids (if hydration is needed)

Drug therapy options
◆ Appropriate drug therapy: broad-spectrum I.V. antibiotics, until a causative organism is identified

Planning and goals
◆ The client will remain hemodynamically stable.
◆ The client will have decreased pain.

Implementation
◆ Monitor vital signs every 4 hours *to assess for complications.*
◆ Place the client in Fowler's position *to facilitate lochia drainage.*
◆ Administer pain medication as ordered *to relieve pain and discomfort.*
◆ Provide emotional support and reassurance *to ease anxiety.*
◆ Initiate and maintain I.V. fluid administration as ordered *to replace volume loss.*
◆ Administer antibiotics as prescribed *to fight infection.*

Evaluation
◆ The client has stable vital signs.
◆ The client reports relief of pain.

NEONATAL CARE

A neonate experiences many changes as he adapts to life outside the uterus. Knowledge of these changes and of the normal physiologic characteristics of the neonate provides the basis for normal neonatal care.

NEONATAL CHANGES

This is how the neonate's body systems change:

◆ The cardiovascular system changes from the very first breath, which expands the neonate's lungs and decreases pulmonary vascular resistance. Clamping the umbilical cord increases systemic vascular resistance and left atrial pressure, which functionally closes the foramen ovale (fibrosis may take from several weeks to a year).

◆ The respiratory system also begins to change with the first breath. The neonate's breathing is a reflex triggered in response to noise, light, and temperature and pressure changes. Air immediately replaces the fluid that filled the lungs before birth.

◆ Renal system function doesn't fully mature until after the first year of life; as a result, the neonate has a minimal range of chemical balance and safety. The neonate's limited ability to excrete drugs, coupled with excessive neonatal fluid loss, can rapidly lead to acidosis and fluid imbalances.

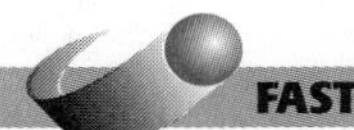

FAST FACT

Because the neonate's renal system hasn't fully matured yet, he can easily develop acidosis and fluid imbalances.

◆ The GI system also isn't fully developed because normal bacteria aren't present in the neonate's GI tract. The lower intestine contains meconium at birth; the first meconium (sterile, greenish black, and viscous) usually passes within 24 hours. Some aspects of GI development include:

- audible bowel sounds 1 hour after birth
- uncoordinated peristaltic activity in the esophagus for the first few days of life
- limited ability to digest fats because amylase and lipase are absent at birth
- frequent regurgitation because of an immature cardiac sphincter.

◆ Changes in neonatal thermogenesis depend on the environment. In an optimal environment, the neonate can produce sufficient heat, but rapid heat loss may occur in a suboptimal thermal environment.

◆ The neonatal immune system depends largely on three immunoglobulins: immunoglobulin G (IgG), IgM, and IgA. IgG (detected in the fetus at the 3rd month of gestation) is a placentally transferred immunoglobulin, providing antibodies to bacterial and viral agents. The infant synthesizes its own IgG during the first 3 months of life, thus compensating for concurrent catabolism of maternal antibodies. By 20 weeks' gestation, the fetus synthesizes IgM, which is undetectable at birth because it doesn't cross the placenta.

High levels of IgM in the neonate indicate a nonspecific infection. Secretory IgA (which limits bacterial growth in the GI tract) is found in colostrum and breast milk.

In the neonatal hematopoietic system, blood volume accounts for 80 to 85 ml/kg of body weight. The neonate experiences prolonged coagulation time because of decreased levels of vitamin K.

◆ The full-term neonate's neurologic system should produce equal strength and symmetry in responses and reflexes. Diminished or absent reflexes may indicate a serious neurologic problem, and asymmetrical responses may indicate trauma during birth, including nerve damage, paralysis, or fracture. Some neonatal reflexes gradually weaken and disappear during the early months.

◆ Jaundice is a major concern in the neonatal hepatic system because of increased serum levels of unconjugated bilirubin from increased RBC lysis, altered bilirubin conjugation, or increased bilirubin reabsorption from the GI tract. Physiologic jaundice appears after the first 24 hours of extrauterine life, pathologic jaundice is evident at birth or within the first 24 hours of extrauterine life, and breast milk jaundice appears after the 1st week of extrauterine life when physiologic jaundice is declining.

NEONATAL ASSESSMENT

Neonatal assessment includes initial and ongoing assessment as well as a thorough physical examination.

Initial assessment

Initial neonatal assessment involves draining secretions, assessing abnormalities, and keeping accurate records.

Nursing actions

◆ Ensure a proper airway by suctioning, and administer oxygen as needed.

◆ Dry the neonate under the warmer while keeping the head lower than the trunk (to promote drainage of secretions).

◆ Apply a cord clamp and monitor the neonate for abnormal bleeding from the cord; check the number of cord vessels.

◆ Observe the neonate for voiding and meconium; document the first void and stools.

◆ Assess the neonate for gross abnormalities and clinical manifestations of suspected abnormalities.

Apgar scoring

The Apgar scoring system provides a way to evaluate the neonate's cardiopulmonary and neurologic status. The assessment is performed at 1 and 5 minutes after birth and is repeated every 5 minutes until the infant stabilizes. A score of 8 to 10 indicates that the neonate is in no apparent distress; a score below 8 indicates that resuscitative measures may be needed.

SIGN	0	1	2
Heart rate	Absent	Less than 100 beats/minute	Greater than 100 beats/minute
Respiratory effort	Absent	Slow, irregular	Good crying
Muscle tone	Flaccid	Some flexion of extremities	Active motion
Reflex irritability	None	Grimace	Vigorous cry
Color	Pale, blue	Body pink, blue extremities	Completely pink

- ◆ Continue to assess the neonate by using the Apgar score criteria even after the 5-minute score is received. (See *Apgar scoring.*)
- ◆ Obtain clear footprints and fingerprints (the neonate's footprints are kept on a record that includes the mother's fingerprints).
- ◆ Apply identification bands with matching numbers to the mother (one band) and her neonate (two bands) before they leave the delivery room.
- ◆ Promote bonding between the mother and her neonate.

Ongoing assessment

Ongoing neonatal physical assessment includes observing and recording vital signs and administering prescribed medications.

Nursing actions

- ◆ Assess the neonate's vital signs.
- ◆ Take the first temperature by the axillary route (rectal route isn't recommended because of possible rectal mucosa damage).
- ◆ Take the apical pulse for 60 seconds (normal rate is 120 to 160 beats/minute).
- ◆ Count respirations with a stethoscope for 60 seconds (normal rate is 30 to 60 breaths/minute).
- ◆ Measure and record blood pressure. (Normal reading ranges from 60/40 mm Hg to 90/45 mm Hg.)
- ◆ Measure and record the neonate's vital statistics.
- ◆ Complete a gestational age assessment.
- ◆ Administer prescribed medications such as vitamin K (AquaMEPHYTON), which is a prophylactic against transient deficiency of coagulation factors II, VII, IX, and X.
- ◆ Administer erythromycin ointment (Ilotycin), the drug of choice for neonatal eye prophylaxis, to prevent damage and blindness from conjunctivitis caused by *Neisseria gonorrhoeae* and chlamydia; treatment is required by law.
- ◆ Administer the first hepatitis B vaccine within 12 hours after birth.
- ◆ Perform laboratory tests.
- ◆ Monitor glucose levels and HCT. (Test results aid in assessing for hypoglycemia and anemia.)

Neonatal physical examination

The neonate should receive a thorough visual and physical examination of each body part. The following is a brief review of normal and abnormal neonatal physiology.

Head

The neonate's head is about one-fourth of its body size. The term *molding* refers to asymmetry of the cranial sutures due to difficulties during labor and delivery. Cranial abnormalities include:

- ◆ cephalhematoma — a collection of blood between a skull bone and the periosteum that doesn't cross suture lines
- ◆ caput succedaneum — localized swelling over the presenting part that can cross suture lines.

The neonatal skull has two fontanels: a diamond-shaped anterior fontanel and a triangular-shaped posterior fontanel. The anterior fontanel is located at the juncture of the frontal and parietal bones, measures 1 1/8″ to 1 5/8″ (3 to 4 cm) long and 3/4″ to 1 1/8″ (2 to 3 cm) wide, and closes in about 18 months. The posterior fontanel is located at the juncture of the occipital and parietal bones, measures about 3/4″ across, and closes in 8 to 12 weeks. The fontanels:

- should feel soft to the touch
- shouldn't be depressed — a depressed fontanel indicates dehydration
- shouldn't bulge — bulging fontanels require immediate attention because they may indicate increased intracranial pressure.

Eyes

The neonate's eyes are usually blue or gray because of scleral thinness; permanent eye color is established within 3 to 12 months. Lacrimal glands are immature at birth, resulting in tearless crying for up to 2 months. The neonate may demonstrate transient strabismus. Doll's eye reflex (when the head is rotated laterally, the eyes deviate in the opposite direction) may persist for about 10 days. Subconjunctival hemorrhages may appear from vascular tension changes during birth.

Nose

Because infants are obligatory nose breathers for the first few months of life, nasal passages must be kept clear to ensure adequate respiration. Neonates instinctively sneeze to remove obstruction.

Mouth

The neonate's mouth usually has scant saliva and pink lips. Epstein's pearls may be found on the gums or hard palate, and precocious teeth may also be apparent.

Ears

The neonate's ears are characterized by incurving of the pinna and cartilage deposition. The top of the ear should be above or parallel to an imaginary line from the inner to the outer canthus of the eye. Low-set ears are associated with several syndromes, including chromosomal abnormalities.

Neck

The neonate's neck is typically short and weak with deep folds of skin.

Chest

The neonate's chest is characterized by a cylindrical thorax and flexible ribs. Breast engorgement from maternal hormones may be apparent, and supernumerary nipples may be located below and medially to the true nipples.

Abdomen

The neonatal abdomen is usually cylindrical with some protrusion; a scaphoid appearance indicates diaphragmatic hernia. The umbilical cord is white and gelatinous with two arteries and one vein and begins to dry within 1 to 2 hours after delivery.

Genitalia

Characteristics of a male neonate's genitalia include rugae on the scrotum and testes descended into the scrotum. The urinary meatus is located in one of three places:

- at the penile tip (normal)
- on the dorsal surface (epispadias)
- on the ventral surface (hypospadias).

In the female neonate, the labia majora cover the labia minora and clitoris, vaginal discharge from maternal hormones appears, and the hymenal tag is present.

Extremities

All neonates are bowlegged and have flat feet. Some neonates may have abnormal extremities. For example, neonates may be polydactyly (more than five digits on an extremity) or syndactyly (two or more digits fused together).

Spine

The neonatal spine should be straight and flat, and the anus should be patent without any fissure. Dimpling at the base of the spine is commonly associated with spina bifida.

Skin

The skin of a neonate can indicate many conditions — some normal and others requiring more serious attention. Make general obsevations in relationship to the neonate's activity. Assessment findings include:

- acrocyanosis (cyanosis of the hands and feet resulting from adjustments to extrauterine circulation) for the first 24 hours after birth
- milia (clogged sebaceous glands) on the nose or chin
- lanugo (fine, downy hair) appearing after 20 weeks' gestation on the entire body except the palms and soles
- vernix caseosa (a white, cheesy protective coating composed of desquamated epithelial cells and sebum)

- erythema toxicum neonatorum (a transient, maculopapular rash)
- telangiectasia (flat, reddened vascular areas) appearing on the neck, upper eyelid, or upper lip
- port-wine stain (nevus flammeus), a capillary angioma located below the dermis and commonly found on the face
- strawberry hemangioma (nevus vasculosus), a capillary angioma located in the dermal and subdermal skin layers indicated by a rough, raised, sharply demarcated birthmark.

Reflexes

Normal neonates display a number of reflexes, which include:

- Babinski's — when the sole on the side of the small toe is stroked, the neonate's toes fan upward
- grasping — when a finger is placed in each of the neonate's hands, the neonate's fingers grasp tightly enough to be pulled to a sitting position
- Moro's — when lifted above the crib and suddenly lowered, the arms and legs symmetrically extend and then abduct while the fingers spread to form a "C"
- rooting — when the cheek is stroked, the neonate turns his head in the direction of the stroke
- startle — a loud noise such as a hand clap elicits neonatal arm abduction and elbow flexion and the neonate's hands stay clenched
- stepping — when held upright with the feet touching a flat surface, the neonate exhibits dancing or stepping movements
- sucking — sucking motion begins when a nipple is placed in the neonate's mouth
- tonic neck (fencing position) — when the neonate's head is turned while he is lying in a supine position, the extremities on the same side straighten while those on the opposite side flex
- trunk incurvature — when a finger is run laterally down the neonate's spine, the trunk flexes and the pelvis swings toward the stimulated side.

NEONATAL COMPLICATIONS

Common neonatal complications and disorders include drug dependency, fetal alcohol syndrome, human immunodeficiency virus, hypothermia, infections, jaundice, and respiratory distress syndrome.

DRUG DEPENDENCY, NEONATAL

Infants born to drug-addicted mothers are at risk for preterm birth, aspiration pneumonia, meconium-stained fluid, and meconium aspiration. Drug-dependent infants may also experience withdrawal from such substances as heroin and cocaine. Methadone shouldn't be given to neonates because of its addictive nature. (See *Caring for the client with neonatal drug dependency.*)

Possible causes

- Drug addiction in the mother

Assessment findings

- Diarrhea
- Frequent sneezing and yawning
- High-pitched cry
- Hyperactive reflexes
- Increased tendon reflexes
- Irritability
- Jitteriness
- Poor feeding habits
- Poor sleeping pattern
- Tremors
- Vigorous sucking on hands
- Withdrawal symptoms (depend on the length of maternal addiction, the drug ingested, and the time of last ingestion before delivery; usually appear within 24 hours after delivery)

Diagnostic evaluation

- Drug screen reveals agent abused by mother.

Nursing diagnoses

- Ineffective infant feeding pattern
- Deficient fluid volume
- Risk for disorganized infant behavior

Treatment

- Gavage feedings, if necessary
- I.V. therapy to maintain hydration

Drug therapy options

- Suppressant, opioids (abstinence syndrome), phenobarbital (Solfonton), chlorpromazine (Thorazine), clonidine (Catapres), diazepam (Valium), morphine, tincture of opium to treat withdrawal symptoms

Planning and goals

- The infant will maintain nutrition and demonstrate appropriate weight gain.

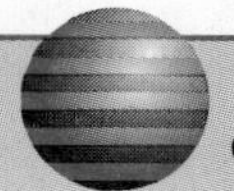

CLINICAL SITUATION

Caring for the client with neonatal drug dependency

The client, who is 1 day old, was born at 28 weeks' gestation to a 16-year-old single mother. You're caring for the client in the neonatal high-risk nursery. She had an Apgar score of 5 at 1 minute after delivery and 8 after 5 minutes. The neonate now demonstrates signs of substance withdrawal, and it's discovered that her mother has a history of cocaine abuse.

What behavior patterns do you expect to see?

The neonate may demonstrate irritability, jitteriness, poor sleep patterns, poor eating pattern, hyperactive reflexes, and vigorous sucking of her hands. She may also have diarrhea, tremors, and frequent yawning. These classic signs and symptoms of drug dependency usually appear within the first 24 hours after birth.

What are appropriate nursing diagnoses for the neonate?

Appropriate nursing diagnoses include:

- *Ineffective infant feeding pattern*
- *Deficient fluid volume*
- *Risk for disorganized infant behavior.*

Questions for further thought

- What are appropriate goals for the mother and neonate?
- How can you support parental adaptation to the neonate?

- The infant will maintain adequate hydration.
- The infant will develop an improved sleep pattern and more organized behavior.

Implementation

- Monitor cardiovascular, respiratory, and neurologic status *to detect cardiovascular compromise.*
- Monitor vital signs and fluid intake and output *to assess for complications.*
- Encourage the mother to hold the infant *to promote maternal-infant bonding.*
- Use tight swaddling *for comfort.*
- Place the neonate in a darkened, quiet room *to provide a stimulus-free environment.*
- Encourage the use of a pacifier *to meet sucking needs (in cases of heroin withdrawal).*
- Be prepared to administer gavage feeding *because of the neonate's poor sucking reflex (in cases of methadone withdrawal).*
- Maintain fluid and electrolyte balance *to replace fluid loss.*
- Monitor bilirubin levels and assess for jaundice (in cases of methadone withdrawal) *to assess for liver damage.*

Evaluation

- The infant has appropriate weight gain.
- The infant is well hydrated.
- The infant has an established sleep pattern and improved behavior.

FETAL ALCOHOL SYNDROME

Fetal alcohol syndrome (FAS) results from a mother's chronic or periodic intake of alcohol during pregnancy. The degree of alcohol consumption necessary to cause the syndrome varies. Because alcohol crosses the placenta in the same concentration as is present in the maternal bloodstream, alcohol consumption (particularly binge drinking) is especially dangerous during critical periods of organogenesis. The fetal liver isn't mature enough to detoxify alcohol.

Possible causes

- Risk of teratogenic effects increases proportionally with daily alcohol intake. (FAS has been detected in neonates of even moderate drinkers [1 to 2 oz of alcohol daily].)

Assessment findings

- Prenatal and postnatal growth retardation
- Facial anomalies (microcephaly, microphthalmia, maxillary hypoplasia, short palpebral fissures)
- Weak sucking reflex
- Sleep disturbances (either always awake or always asleep, depending on the mother's alcohol level close to birth)
- CNS dysfunction (decreased IQ, developmental delays, neurologic abnormalities)

Diagnostic evaluation

- Chest X-ray may reveal congenital heart defect.

Nursing diagnoses

- Imbalanced nutrition: Less than body requirements
- Delayed growth and development
- Impaired parenting

Treatment
◆ Swaddling

Drug therapy options
◆ I.V. phenobarbital (to control hyperactivity and irritability)

Planning and goals
◆ The infant will obtain adequate nutrition.
◆ The infant will maintain a steady growth pattern.
◆ The infant will receive adequate care.

Implementation
◆ Monitor cardiovascular, respiratory, and neurologic status *to detect compromise.*
◆ Refer the mother to an alcohol treatment center *for ongoing support and rehabilitation.*
◆ Provide a stimulus-free environment for the neonate; darken the room, if necessary, *to minimize stimuli.*
◆ Provide gavage feedings as necessary *to provide adequate nutrition for the infant.*
◆ Encourage the mother to spend time with her infant *to promote maternal-infant attachment.*

Evaluation
◆ The infant maintains a steady growth pattern related to adequate nutrition.
◆ The infant demonstrates contentment as a result of receiving adequate care.

HUMAN IMMUNODEFICIENCY VIRUS
A mother can transmit HUMAN IMMUNODEFICIENCY VIRUS (HIV) to her infant transplacentally at various gestational ages — perinatally, through maternal blood and bodily fluids, and postnatally, through breast milk. Administration of zidovudine (AZT) to HIV-positive pregnant women significantly reduces the risk of transmission to the neonate.

Possible causes
◆ Transmission of the virus to the fetus or neonate from an HIV-positive mother

Assessment findings
◆ Neonate is asymptomatic at birth
◆ Opportunistic infections may appear by age 3 to 6 months

Diagnostic evaluation
◆ HIV-deoxyribonucleic acid polymerase chain reaction or viral cultures for HIV should be performed within 48 hours of birth, and again at 3 to 6 months. Two positive tests at different ages are required for a positive diagnosis.

Nursing diagnoses
◆ Risk for infection
◆ Imbalanced nutrition: Less than body requirements
◆ Ineffective protection

Treatment
◆ I.V. fluid administration
◆ Nutritional supplements to prevent weight loss

Drug therapy options
◆ Prophylactic antibiotic: co-trimoxazole (Bactrim) for infants age 4 weeks or older
◆ Antiviral: zidovudine (Retrovir) administration to the HIV-positive mother during the second and third trimesters and during labor and delivery, and to neonates during the first 6 weeks of life.

Planning and goals
◆ The infant will receive adequate nutrition.
◆ The infant will be protected from opportunistic infection.

Implementation
◆ Assess the neonate's cardiovascular and respiratory status *to detect complications.*
◆ Monitor vital signs and fluid intake and output *to assess for dehydration.*
◆ Monitor fluid and electrolyte status *to guide fluid and electrolyte replacement therapy.*
◆ Maintain standard precautions *to prevent the spread of infection.*
◆ Keep the umbilical stump meticulously clean *to prevent opportunistic infection.*
◆ Assist with blood sample and urine specimen collection *to prevent the spread of infection.*
◆ Administer medications, as indicated, *to treat infection and improve immune function.*
◆ Provide emotional support to the family *to allay anxiety.*
◆ Explain that breast-feeding isn't recommended *because HIV is transmitted in breast milk.*

Evaluation
◆ The infant has appropriate weight gain related to adequate nutrition.
◆ The infant remains free from infection.

HYPOTHERMIA

A neonate's temperature is about 99° F (37.2° C) at birth. Inside the womb, the fetus is confined in an environment where the temperature is constant. At birth, this temperature can decrease rapidly.

Possible causes

- Cold temperature in delivery environment
- Heat loss due to evaporation, conduction, or convection
- Immature temperature-regulating system
- Inability to conserve heat due to little subcutaneous fat

Assessment findings

- Core body temperature lower than 97.7° F (36.5° C)
- Kicking and crying (a mechanism to increase the metabolic rate to produce body heat)

Diagnostic evaluation

- Arterial blood gas analysis shows hypoxemia.
- Blood glucose level reveals hypoglycemia.

Nursing diagnoses

- Hypothermia
- Ineffective thermoregulation
- Risk for impaired parent-infant attachment

Treatment

- Radiant warmer

Planning and goals

- The infant will maintain an adequate body temperature.
- The infant will have appropriate interaction with parents.

Implementation

- Dry the neonate immediately *to prevent heat loss.*
- Allow the mother to hold the neonate *to provide warmth.*
- Monitor vital signs every 15 to 30 minutes *to assess temperature fluctuations and complications.*
- Provide a knitted cap for the neonate *to prevent heat loss through the head.*
- Place the neonate in a radiant warmer *to maintain thermoregulation.*

Evaluation

- The infant is able to maintain a normal body temperature.
- Parent-infant bonding is evident.

INFECTIONS

A neonate may contract an infection before, during, or after delivery. Maternal IgM doesn't cross the placenta and IgA requires time to reach optimum levels after birth, limiting the neonate's immune response. Dysmaturity caused by intrauterine growth retardation, preterm birth, or postterm birth can further compromise the neonate's immune system and predispose him to infection.

Sepsis is one of the most significant causes of neonatal morbidity and mortality. Toxoplasmosis, syphilis, rubella, cytomegalovirus, and herpes are common perinatal infections known to affect infants.

Possible causes

- Chorioamnionitis
- Low birth weight or premature birth
- Maternal substance abuse
- Maternal urinary tract infections
- Meconium aspiration
- Nosocomial infection
- Premature labor
- Prolonged maternal rupture of membranes

Assessment findings

- Subtle, nonspecific behavioral changes, such as lethargy or hypotonia
- Feeding pattern changes, such as poor sucking or decreased intake
- Temperature instability
- Sternal retractions
- Apnea
- Abdominal distention
- Vomiting
- Diarrhea
- Pallor
- Petechiae
- Hyperbilirubinemia
- Poor weight gain

Diagnostic evaluation

- Blood and urine cultures are positive for the causative organism, most commonly gram-positive beta-hemolytic streptococci and gram-negative *Escherichia coli, Aerobacter, Proteus,* and *Klebsiella.*
- Blood chemistry shows increased direct bilirubin levels.
- Complete blood count shows an increased WBC count.
- Lumbar puncture is positive for causative organisms.

Nursing diagnoses

- Hypothermia

- Risk for deficient fluid volume
- Imbalanced nutrition: Less than body requirements

Treatment

- Gastric aspiration
- I.V. therapy to provide adequate hydration
- Temperature regulation

Drug therapy options

- Broad-spectrum antibiotic therapy until the causative organism is identified; then specific antibiotic

Planning and goals

- The infant will have adequate intake to maintain hydration and nutrition.
- The infant will maintain normal temperature.
- The infant's infection will resolve.

Implementation

- Assess cardiovascular and respiratory status *to assess for complications.*
- Monitor vital signs and transcutaneous blood oxygen tension *to assess for complications.*
- Monitor fluid and electrolyte status *to assess the need for fluid replacement.*
- Initiate and maintain respiratory support as needed *to maintain respiratory filtration.*
- Administer broad-spectrum antibiotics before culture results are received and specific antibiotic therapy after results are received *to treat infection.*
- Provide the family with reassurance and support *to reduce anxiety.*
- Provide the neonate with physiologic supportive care *to maintain a neutral thermal environment.*
- Initiate and maintain I.V. therapy as ordered *to replace fluid loss.*
- Obtain blood samples and urine specimens *to assess the efficacy of antibiotic therapy.*

Evaluation

- The infant is hydrated with oral and I.V. fluids.
- The infant maintains a normal temperature.
- The infant is free from infection.

JAUNDICE

Also called *hyperbilirubinemia,* neonatal jaundice is characterized by a bilirubin level that:

- is elevated after delivery
- remains elevated beyond 7 days (in a full-term neonate)
- remains elevated for 10 days (in a premature neonate).

The neonate's bilirubin levels rise as bilirubin production exceeds the liver's capacity to metabolize it. Unbound, unconjugated bilirubin can easily cross the blood-brain barrier, leading to kernicterus (an encephalopathy).

Possible causes

- Absence of intestinal flora needed for bilirubin passage in the bowel
- Enclosed hemorrhage
- Erythroblastosis fetalis (hemolytic disease of the neonate)
- Hypoglycemia
- Hypothermia
- Impaired hepatic functioning
- Neonatal asphyxia (respiratory failure in the neonate)
- Polycythemia
- Prematurity
- Reduced bowel motility and delayed meconium passage
- Sepsis

Assessment findings

- Jaundice
- Lethargy
- High-pitched crying
- Decreased reflexes
- Opisthotonos
- Seizures

Diagnostic evaluation

- Bilirubin levels exceed 12 mg/dl in premature or term neonates.
- Bilirubin level rises by more than 5 mg/day.

Nursing diagnoses

- Deficient fluid volume
- Risk for injury
- Risk for impaired parent-infant attachment

Treatment

- Albumin infusion
- Exchange transfusion to remove maternal antibodies and sensitized RBCs if phototherapy fails
- Increased fluid intake
- Phototherapy (preferred treatment)

Planning and goals

- The infant will be nurtured by the parents as much as possible.
- The infant will have decreased bilirubin levels.

◆ The infant will have adequate intake to maintain hydration.

Implementation

◆ Assess neurologic status *to assess for signs of encephalopathy, which indicates the potential for permanent damage.*
◆ Maintain a neutral thermal environment *to prevent hypothermia.*
◆ Monitor serum bilirubin levels *to assess for reduction of bilirubin.*
◆ Initiate and maintain phototherapy (provide eye protection while the neonate is under phototherapy lights and remove eye shields promptly when he's removed from the phototherapy lights) *to prevent complications.*
◆ Allow time for maternal-infant bonding and interaction during phototherapy *to promote bonding.*
◆ Keep the neonate's anal area clean and dry. *Frequent, greenish stools result from bilirubin excretion and can lead to skin irritations.*
◆ Provide the parents with support, reassurance, and encouragement *to reduce anxiety.*

Evaluation

◆ The infant is adequately hydrated.
◆ The infant has decreased jaundice and bilirubin levels.
◆ The parents are able to care for the infant.

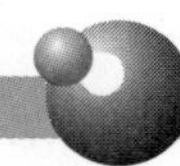

SPOT CHECK

Which intervention is a preferred treatment for neonatal jaundice?

A. Exchange transfusion
B. Phototherapy
C. Observing and monitoring bilirubin levels
D. Stool softener

Answer: B. The preferred treatment for neonatal jaundice is phototherapy. Exchange transfusion is performed when the bilirubin level rises rapidly despite the use of phototherapy or hydration. Neonates with high bilirubin levels shouldn't just be observed; intervention is necessary. Stool softeners aren't part of medical management for neonatal jaundice.

RESPIRATORY DISTRESS SYNDROME

Respiratory distress syndrome occurs most commonly in preterm infants, infants of diabetic mothers, and infants delivered by cesarean section. In respiratory distress syndrome, a hyaline-like membrane lines the terminal bronchioles, alveolar ducts, and alveoli, preventing the exchange of oxygen and carbon dioxide.

Possible causes

◆ Inability to maintain alveolar stability
◆ Low level or absence of surfactant

Assessment findings

◆ Nasal flaring
◆ Expiratory grunting
◆ Tachypnea (more than 60 breaths/minute)
◆ Sternal and substernal retractions
◆ Fine rales and diminished breath sounds
◆ Apneic episodes
◆ Cyanosis
◆ Unresponsiveness
◆ Flaccidity

Diagnostic evaluation

◆ Arterial blood gas analysis reveals respiratory acidosis.
◆ Chest X-rays reveal alveolar atelectasis and dilated bronchioles.
◆ Analysis of amniotic fluid for lecithin-sphingomyelin ratio reveals level of fetal lung maturity.

Nursing diagnoses

◆ Impaired gas exchange
◆ Ineffective tissue perfusion (cardiopulmonary)
◆ Ineffective infant feeding pattern
◆ Risk for impaired parent/infant attachment

Treatment

◆ Maintenance of acid-base balance.
◆ Endotracheal intubation and mechanical ventilation
◆ Nutrition supplements (TPN or enteral feedings, if possible)
◆ Surfactant replacement by way of endotracheal tube
◆ Temperature regulation with a radiant warmer

Drug therapy options

◆ Corticosteroids to mother prenatally
◆ Antiinflammatory, nonsteroidal indomethacin (Indocin) to promote closure of ductus arteriosus (a fetal blood vessel connecting the left pulmonary artery to the descending aorta)

Planning and goals

◆ The infant will achieve adequate oxygenation.
◆ The infant will have adequate nutritional intake.

◆ The parents will participate in infant care as much as possible.

Implementation

◆ Assess cardiovascular, respiratory, and neurologic status *to detect respiratory distress.*
◆ Monitor continuous electrocardiography and vital signs *to detect changes.*
◆ Provide mechanical ventilation, if indicated, *to maintain adequate oxygenation.*
◆ Administer medications, including endotracheal surfactant, as prescribed, *to improve respiratory function.*
◆ Assess hydration status *to assess fluid loss.*
◆ Initiate and maintain I.V. therapy *to achieve adequate fluid levels.*
◆ Provide nutrition through enteral feedings, if possible, or TPN *to ensure adequate nutrition.*
◆ Maintain thermoregulation *to reduce cold stress.*
◆ Obtain blood samples as necessary *to assess for complications.*

Evaluation

◆ The infant has improved oxygenation and increased lung function.
◆ The infant demonstrates adequate nutritional intake through appropriate weight gain.
◆ The parents participate in caring for the infant.

Pediatric nursing

INTRODUCTION

This chapter focuses on children's health problems from birth through adolescence, especially conditions and disorders that are common to these age-groups:

- Infant (birth to age 12 months)
- Toddler (ages 1 to 3 years)
- Preschooler (ages 4 to 5 years)
- School-age child (ages 6 to 12 years)
- Adolescent (ages 13 to 19 years).

The health problems that follow are commonly covered in test questions on the NCLEX-RN examination. The nursing diagnoses specified for each disorder aren't exhaustive; other diagnoses may also be appropriate, depending on the clinical situation. To enhance your understanding, review the section on growth and development in chapter 3, Nursing concepts and skills, pages 31 to 44, and the general information on body systems at the beginning of each adult clinical nursing section.

INFANT DISORDERS

BRONCHIOLITIS

BRONCHIOLITIS, an infection of the lower respiratory tract, produces inflammation and obstruction by thick mucus and edema. In some areas of the lungs, mucus plugs and bronchiolar edema completely obstruct the small bronchioles, resulting in atelectasis. Some of these obstructed bronchioles trap air in the alveoli, producing hyperinflation. Overall, the infant experiences generalized hypoxia and progressive respiratory distress. (See *Pediatric respiratory facts.*)

The infection is viral; RESPIRATORY SYNCYTIAL VIRUS (RSV) is the most common causative agent. Bronchiolitis is most prevalent during winter and spring. It occurs in infants from birth to age 2; peak incidence is between the ages of 2 and 5 months. Reinfection is common. (See *Pediatric respiratory infections,* pages 242 and 243.)

> **Pediatric respiratory facts**
>
> A child's respiratory tract differs anatomically from an adult's in ways that predispose the child to many respiratory problems. Here's how a child's respiratory tract differs from an adult's:
>
> - Lungs aren't fully developed at birth.
> - Alveoli continue to grow and increase in number through age 8.
> - A child's respiratory tract has a narrower lumen than an adult's until age 5; the narrow airway makes the young child prone to airway obstruction and respiratory distress from inflammation, mucus secretion, or a foreign body.
> - Elastic connective tissue becomes more abundant with age in the peripheral part of the lung.
> - A child's respiratory rate decreases as body size increases.

Possible causes

- RSV
- Other viruses such as some adenoviruses

Assessment findings

- Anorexia
- Apnea spells
- Dyspnea
- Low-grade fever for several days
- Possible air trapping and atelectasis
- Retractions
- Signs of a mild upper respiratory infection, such as nasal drainage or pharyngitis
- Tachypnea
- Thick mucus
- Wheezing and a prolonged expiratory phase

(Text continues on page 244.)

Pediatric respiratory infections

This chart lists common pediatric respiratory infections along with a description of each, age at peak incidence, manifestations, and nursing management steps. In order to meet the emotional needs, remember to provide support to the child as well as the family.

CONDITION (ETIOLOGY) AND PATHOLOGY	AGE AT PEAK INCIDENCE	MANIFESTATIONS	MANAGEMENT
Acute epiglottiditis *(Haemophilus influenzae* type B [Hib]) Infection of epiglottis; can be severe, rapidly progressive, and fatal if untreated	2 to 7 years	◆ Abrupt onset ◆ Sore throat, inability to swallow ◆ Tripod positioning (the child remains upright, resting weight on the hands; the chin is thrust out, with the mouth open and drooling) ◆ Froglike sound on inspiration ◆ Marked restlessness and anxiety ◆ High fever	◆ Don't try to visualize the epiglottis with a tongue blade. ◆ Prepare for intubation or tracheostomy. ◆ Provide high humidity with oxygen and I.V. hydration. ◆ Withhold food and fluids. ◆ Administer antibiotics as ordered. ◆ Prevention: Encourage Hib vaccine.
Acute laryngo-tracheo-bronchitis (viral) Inflammation and edema of the larynx, trachea, and bronchi with exudate	1 to 3 years	◆ Possible marked temperature elevation ◆ Marked dyspnea, tachypnea, bilateral wheezing, diminished breath sounds, prolonged expiration ◆ Tachycardia ◆ Complications: secondary pneumonia, septicemia, cardiac failure	◆ To maintain an open airway, keep intubation equipment and a tracheostomy set at the bedside; provide cool humidity with oxygen; suction as needed; and administer ordered medication (possibly epinephrine by aerosol or intermittent positive-pressure breathing) ◆ Maintain hydration by giving I.V. fluids. ◆ Take measures to reduce temperature.
Acute spasmodic laryngitis–spasmodic croup (viral) Inflammation of the larynx, leading to laryngeal muscle spasms and partial obstruction of the upper airway	3 months to 4 years	◆ Predominantly nighttime attacks that last 1 to 3 hours ◆ Inspiratory stridor with barklike, nonproductive cough ◆ Restlessness, dyspnea, anxiety ◆ Slight, if any, temperature elevation	◆ Provide cool mist.
Atypical primary pneumonia *(Mycoplasma pneumoniae)* Interstitial pneumonitis, bronchitis, bronchiolitis	5 years to adulthood	◆ Fever, chills, headache, malaise, anorexia, myalgia, rhinitis, sore throat	◆ Treat symptomatically.
Bronchiolitis (usually respiratory syncytial virus)	Infancy and early childhood	◆ Rapid or insidious onset after upper respiratory tract infection ◆ Mild to marked temperature elevation ◆ Slight to severe cough	◆ Treat symptomatically.

Pediatric respiratory infections *(continued)*

CONDITION (ETIOLOGY) AND PATHOLOGY	AGE AT PEAK INCIDENCE	MANIFESTATIONS	MANAGEMENT
Bronchiolitis *(continued)*		◆ Possible signs of obstructive emphysema ◆ Symptoms similar to bronchiolitis	
Bronchitis (secondary to cystic fibrosis, asthma, or bronchiolitis) Inflammation of the mucous membrane that lines the bronchi	Late infancy and early childhood	◆ Wheezing if underlying asthma is present ◆ Dry cough, progressing to productive cough with purulent sputum ◆ Moderate emphysema	◆ Provide high humidity and maintain adequate hydration. ◆ Administer sympathomimetic bronchodilators (subcutaneous epinephrine or oral ephedrine), if ordered.
Chlamydial pneumonia (bacterial) Acquired as ascending infection before or during birth; nonspecific pathology, but severe disease is thought to be responsible for one-third of reported pneumonia cases in infants under age 6 months	Less than 6 months	◆ Persistent cough, tachypnea ◆ Normal or mildly elevated temperature ◆ Feeding difficulty ◆ Failure to thrive ◆ Possible accompanying condition: conjunctivitis, chlamydial otitis	◆ Treat symptomatically. ◆ Administer erythromycin and sulfa drugs, as ordered. (Penicillin isn't effective.)
Pneumococcal pneumonia (bacterial) Involves all or almost all of one or more pulmonary lobes; transmitted by droplet spread	1 to 4 years	◆ Fever (102° to 105° F [38.9° to 40.6° C]) ◆ Shaking, chills, headache ◆ Tachycardia ◆ Rapid, shallow respirations; hacking, nonproductive cough; pleuritic chest pain ◆ Complications: otitis media, pleural effusion, empyema	◆ Administer penicillin G and antipyretics, as ordered. ◆ Provide high humidity with oxygen and increased hydration. Suction as needed. ◆ Percuss lung segments with postural drainage. ◆ Use thoracentesis or closed chest drainage (or both) to treat pulmonary complications, if needed.
Staphylococcal pneumonia (bacterial) Bronchopneumonia (begins in bronchioles; exudate consolidates in neighboring lobules)	Infancy (70% of cases) to 2 years	◆ Mild symptoms of upper respiratory infection, which may progress to tachypnea and anxiety ◆ Fever, shocklike state ◆ Progressive dyspnea ◆ Complications: empyema, tension pneumothorax, pyopneumothorax	◆ Treat symptomatically. ◆ Administer semisynthetic penicillins (such as methicillin or nafcillin) because many staphylococcal organisms are penicillin-resistant.
Streptococcal pneumonia (bacterial) Interstitial pneumonitic pneumonia with disseminated infiltration; caused by strep throat, upper respiratory tract infection, or contagious disease	Not age-specific	◆ Similar to those of pneumococcal pneumonia in most cases, but sometimes only mild symptoms ◆ Complications: pleural effusion, empyema	◆ Treat symptomatically. ◆ Administer penicillin G (I.V. or I.M.).

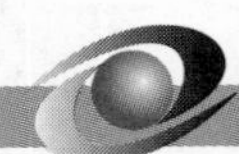

QUICK STUDY

To remember early RSV symptoms, remember the word **WIPERS.**

Wheezing
Intermittent fever
Pharyngitis
Ear infection
Rhinorrhea
Sneezing and coughing

Diagnostic evaluation

◆ Diagnostic evaluation of bronchial mucus culture shows RSV.

Nursing diagnoses

◆ Impaired gas exchange
◆ Ineffective breathing pattern
◆ Ineffective airway clearance

Treatment

◆ Cool mist vaporizer
◆ Humidified oxygen
◆ I.V. fluids

Drug therapy options

◆ Bronchodilator: albuterol (Proventil)
◆ Immune globulin: RSV immune globulin
◆ Antiviral agent: ribavirin (Virazole) for high-risk infants

Planning and goals

◆ The infant will have a respiratory rate less than 40 breaths/minute and be free from physical signs of respiratory distress within 24 hours.
◆ The infant will have clear breath sounds and exhibit no accessory muscle use.

Implementation

◆ Monitor vital signs and pulse oximetry *to determine oxygenation needs and detect deterioration or improvement in the infant's condition.*
◆ Assess respiratory and cardiovascular status *to identify signs of respiratory distress or adverse reactions to medications. Tachycardia may result from hypoxia or the effects of bronchodilator use.*

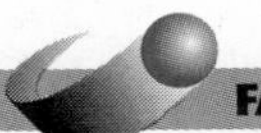

FAST FACT

Early signs of respiratory distress include:
- anxiety
- dyspnea
- restlessness
- tachycardia
- tachypnea.

◆ Use gloves, gowns, and aseptic hand washing as secretion precautions *to prevent the spread of infection.*
◆ Administer chest physiotherapy after edema has abated *to loosen mucus that may be blocking small airways.*
◆ Administer humidified oxygen therapy *to liquefy secretions and reduce bronchial edema.*
◆ Administer and maintain I.V. therapy *to promote hydration and replace electrolytes.*

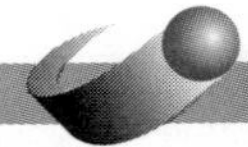

FAST FACT

The best indicator of fluid balance is found by weighing the patient – 2.2 lb (1 kg) of weight loss could indicate 1 L (1.1 qt) of fluid loss.

◆ Review key teaching topics with family members *to ensure adequate knowledge about the condition and treatments,* including:
– medications, dosages, and adverse reactions
– adequate nutrition and hydration
– importance of humidified environment
– importance of avoiding people with cold symptoms. (See *Caring for an infant with RSV.*)

Evaluation

◆ The infant has a normal respiratory rate and shows no signs of respiratory distress.
◆ The infant has clear breath sounds on auscultation.
◆ The infant doesn't use accessory muscles when breathing.

CEREBRAL PALSY

CEREBRAL PALSY is a neuromuscular disorder resulting from damage to or a defect in the part of the brain that controls motor function. It's a group of disorders arising from a malfunction of motor centers and neural pathways in the brain. The disorder is commonly seen in children born prematurely. Cerebral treatment includes interventions that encourage optimum DEVELOPMENT. Defects are common, including musculoskeletal, neurologic, GI, and

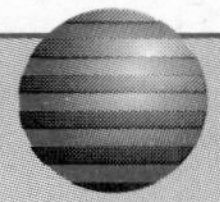

CLINICAL SITUATION

Caring for an infant with RSV

A 5-month-old infant weighing 15.2 lb (6.9 kg) has just been admitted with a diagnosis of respiratory syncytial virus (RSV). His temperature is 101.5° F (38.6° C); respiratory rate, 56 breaths/minute; and apical pulse, 166 beats/minute. His respirations are accompanied by nasal flaring, retractions, and expiratory grunting. The infant is in a high-humidity tent with 30% oxygen and is receiving dextrose 5% in normal saline 0.45% solution I.V. at 25 ml/hour. He may have clear liquids by bottle as tolerated. His parents are present.

What are appropriate nursing diagnoses for this infant?

- Ineffective airway clearance *related to increased tracheobronchial secretions and bronchial edema*
- Ineffective breathing pattern *related to mucus accumulation and respiratory tract edema*
- Risk for deficient fluid volume *related to increased insensible fluid loss and decreased intake*
- Compromised family coping *related to parents' anxiety over infant's illness*

What measures can the nurse take to ease the infant's respirations?

- Suction the nose and mouth as necessary, but avoid suctioning the upper respiratory tract if secretions aren't apparent. *Suctioning irritates the mucous membrane, resulting in edema and mucus secretion. This, in turn, can narrow and obstruct the upper airway, further complicating the infant's respiratory problems.*
- Place the infant upright in an infant seat, and closely observe to ensure that he doesn't slump down. *Sitting upright in an infant seat facilitates respirations. If the infant slumps down, his tongue can obstruct the posterior pharynx, interfering with adequate lung expansion.*
- Administer nothing by mouth during an acute phase of dyspnea *to reduce the infant's risk of aspirating secretions and keep him from overtiring.*

Questions for further thought

- Why is adequate hydration required for this infant?
- How can you help relieve the parents' anxiety?

nutritional defects as well as other systemic complications (such as abnormal reflexes, fatigue, GROWTH failure, genitourinary complaints, and respiratory infections). Some defects may be corrected surgically, optimizing the child's potential.

Possible causes

- Anoxia before, during, or after giving birth
- Infection
- Trauma (hemorrhage)

Risk factors

- Low birth weight
- Low Apgar scores at 5 minutes
- Metabolic disturbances
- Seizures

Assessment findings

All types

- Abnormal muscle tone and coordination (the most common associated problem)
- Dental anomalies
- Mental retardation of varying degrees in 18% to 50% of cases (Most children with cerebral palsy have at least a normal IQ but can't demonstrate it on standardized tests.)
- Seizures
- Speech, vision, or hearing disturbances
- Difficulty sucking or keeping the nipple or food in his mouth
- Rare voluntary movement or arm or leg tremors with voluntary movement
- Crossed legs when lifted from behind (rather than pulled up or "bicycling" like a normal infant)
- Difficulty separating legs, making diaper changing difficult
- Persistent use of only one hand or, as he gets older, use of both hands but not legs

Ataxic cerebral palsy

- Poor balance and muscle coordination
- Unsteady, wide-based gait

Athetoid cerebral palsy

- Slow state of writhing muscle contractions whenever voluntary movement is attempted
- Facial grimacing
- Poor swallowing
- Drooling
- Poor speech articulation

Rigid cerebral palsy
- Rigid posture
- Lack of active movement

Spastic cerebral palsy
- Hyperactive stretch reflex in associated muscle groups
- Hyperactive deep-tendon reflexes
- Rapid involuntary muscle contraction and relaxation
- Contractures affecting the extensor muscles
- Scissoring

Mixed cerebral palsy
- Signs of more than one type of cerebral palsy
- Severe disability

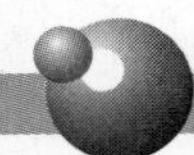

SPOT CHECK

What are the most common problems associated with cerebral palsy?

Answer: The most common problems are abnormal muscle tone and coordination, which are seen in all types of cerebral palsy.

Diagnostic evaluation
- Neuroimaging studies determine the site of brain impairment.
- Cytogenic studies (genetic evaluation of the child and other family members) rule out other potential causes.
- Metabolic studies rule out other causes.

Nursing diagnoses
- Impaired physical mobility
- Imbalanced nutrition: Less than body requirements
- Delayed growth and development
- Impaired verbal communication
- Impaired parenting
- Deficient knowledge (child care and development)
- Compromised family coping

Treatment
- High-calorie diet, if appropriate
- Artificial urinary sphincter for the incontinent child who can use hand controls
- Braces or splints and special appliances, such as adapted eating utensils and a low toilet seat with arms, to help child perform activities independently
- Neurosurgery to decrease spasticity, if appropriate
- Orthopedic surgery to correct contractures
- Range-of-motion (ROM) exercises to minimize contractures

Drug therapy options
- Muscle relaxant: tizanidine (Sirdalud) to decrease spasticity, if appropriate
- Anticonvulsants: phenytoin (Dilantin), phenobarbital (Luminal), or another anticonvulsant to control seizures

Planning and goals
- The infant will consume adequate daily calories as required.
- The infant will maintain joint mobility and ROM.
- The infant's parents will develop adequate coping mechanisms.
- The infant's parents will demonstrate knowledge of the condition.

Implementation
- Assist with locomotion, communication, and educational opportunities *to enable the child to attain optimal developmental level.*
- Increase caloric intake for the child with increased motor function *to keep up with increased metabolic needs.*
- Make food easy to manage *to decrease stress during mealtimes.*
- Provide a safe environment — for example by using protective headgear or bed pads — *to prevent injury.*
- Provide rest periods *to promote rest and reduce metabolic needs.*
- Perform ROM exercises if the child is spastic *to maintain proper body alignment and mobility of joints.*
- Promote age-appropriate mental activities and incentives for motor development *to promote growth and development.*
- Divide tasks into small steps *to promote self-care and activity and increase self-esteem.*
- Refer the child for speech therapy, nutrition counseling, and physical therapy *to maintain or improve functioning.*
- Use assistive communication devices if the child can't speak *to enable communication and promote a positive self-concept.*

Evaluation
- The infant is maintaining joint mobility and ROM to the best degree possible.
- The infant continues to grow and meet developmental milestones.
- The infant's parents express an understanding of their infant's disorder and associated conditions.
- The infant's parents are providing opportunities for the infant to be stimulated and learn.

CLEFT LIP AND CLEFT PALATE

Cleft lip and cleft palate are developmental defects. CLEFT LIP is a facial malformation resulting from failure of the premaxillary process to merge during gestational weeks 7 and 8. The malformation may be unilateral or bilateral and range from a notch in the vermilion border of the lip to a separation extending to the floor of the nose. CLEFT PALATE results from failure of the palatal process to fuse from the 7th to the 12th week of gestation.

Long-term problems with cleft palate include impaired speech, malpositioned teeth and maxillary arches, impaired hearing from repeated otitis media, and recurring respiratory infections — all of which can result in impaired growth. Long-term problems with cleft lip include speech and language problems.

Possible causes

- CONGENITAL defects (in some cases, inheritance plays a role)
- Part of another chromosomal or Mendelian abnormality
- Prenatal exposure to TERATOGENS

Assessment findings

- Appearance ranging from a simple notch on the upper lip to complete cleft from the lip edge to the floor of the nostril on either side of the midline but rarely along the midline itself
- Cleft lip with or without cleft palate obvious at birth (cleft palate without cleft lip may not be detected until a mouth examination is done or until feeding difficulties develop)
- Partial or complete cleft palate
- Difficulty swallowing
- Signs of upper or lower respiratory infections and otitis media, common in infants with cleft palate, resulting from difficulty in sucking and swallowing
- Abdominal distention from swallowed air
- Changes in weight and growth pattern since birth
- Altered parent-infant attachment (Parents may exhibit anxiety and lack of understanding regarding preoperative and postoperative care routines for cleft lip repair.)

Diagnostic evaluation

- Prenatal ultrasonography may indicate severe defects.
- Complete blood count (CBC) shows alterations.
- Serum electrolyte levels are abnormal.
- Urine specific gravity is high due to alterations in oxygenation and nutrition.

Nursing diagnoses

- Impaired swallowing
- Imbalanced nutrition: Less than body requirements
- Risk for aspiration
- Ineffective airway clearance
- Risk for infection
- Risk for impaired parent-infant attachment
- Deficient knowledge (child care, growth and development)

Treatment

- Cleft lip repair surgery (CHEILOPLASTY) immediately after birth or in early infancy (ages 6 to 12 weeks) to unite the lip and gum edges in anticipation of teeth eruption, providing a route for adequate nutrition and sucking; done after a steady growth rate has been established
- Cleft palate repair surgery (staphylorrhaphy) usually between ages 1 and 2 years to allow for growth of the palate but before speech patterns develop (The infant must be free from ear and respiratory infections and may require several stages of repair over a period of years.)

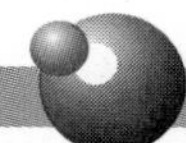

SPOT CHECK

At what age is cleft palate repair surgery scheduled and why?

Answer: The surgery is typically scheduled between ages 1 and 2 years – before the infant develops speech patterns – to allow for growth of the palate.

- Long-term, team-oriented care to address speech defects, dental and orthodontic problems, nasal defects, and possible alterations in hearing
- Possible fetal repair if cleft lip is detected on sonogram while the infant is in utero

Planning and goals

- The infant will maintain satisfactory respiratory and nutritional status.
- The infant's suture line will remain intact and free from infection.
- The parents will understand preoperative and postoperative procedures used in the infant's care.
- The parents will participate in the infant's care to the extent they feel comfortable.
- The parents will help plan home care after cheiloplasty and ongoing care of cleft palate.

Implementation

◆ Monitor vital signs and intake and output *to determine fluid volume status.*

◆ Assess respiratory status *to detect signs of aspiration.*

◆ Assess the quality of the infant's suck by determining if he can form an airtight seal around a finger or nipple placed in his mouth *to determine an effective feeding method.*

◆ Be alert for respiratory distress when feeding *to avoid aspiration.*

◆ As the infant grows older, explore his feelings *to assess actual and potential coping problems.*

Preoperative interventions for cleft lip repair

◆ Feed the infant slowly and in an upright position *to decrease the risk of aspiration.*

◆ Burp the infant frequently during feeding *to eliminate swallowed air and decrease the risk of emesis.*

◆ Use gavage feedings if oral feedings are unsuccessful *to maintain adequate nutrition.*

◆ Administer a small amount of water after feedings *to prevent formula from accumulating and becoming a medium for bacterial growth.*

◆ Give small, frequent feedings *to promote adequate nutrition and prevent tiring the infant.*

◆ Hold the infant while feeding and promote sucking between meals. *Sucking is important to speech development.*

◆ Provide support as the child's appearance may be upsetting to the parents. Counseling may be necessary, especially if surgery is delayed.

Postoperative interventions for cleft lip repair

◆ Observe for cyanosis as the infant begins to breathe through the nose *to detect signs of respiratory compromise.*

◆ Keep the infant's hands away from his mouth by using restraints or pinning the sleeves to his shirt; Steri-Strips are used to hold the suture line in place *to prevent tension and to maintain an intact suture line.*

◆ Anticipate the infant's needs *to prevent crying and avoid stress on the suture line;* don't position him prone *to help prevent direct contact with the suture line.*

◆ Give extra care and support *because the infant can't meet emotional needs by sucking.*

◆ Use a syringe with tubing to administer foods at the side of his mouth *to prevent trauma to the suture line.*

◆ Feed the infant in an upright position, burping after every 1 to 2 oz (29.6 to 59.1 ml) *to decrease the amount of air swallowed and to make it easier to manage coughing or gagging.* Rinse his mouth with clear water after formula feeding *to prevent infection of the suture line and decrease the risk of ear infections.* Place the infant in an infant seat after feeding *to decrease the risk of aspiration.*

◆ When lying the infant down, place him on his right side *to prevent aspiration.*

◆ Clean the suture line after each feeding by dabbing it with half-strength hydrogen peroxide or saline solution *to prevent crusts and scarring.*

◆ Encourage the parents to participate in feeding if they feel comfortable doing this. Demonstrate if the parents are hesitant. *These measures can assist the parents if they have fear of traumatizing the suture line.*

◆ Monitor for pain and administer pain medication as prescribed; note the effectiveness of pain medication *to ensure adequate pain relief.*

◆ Cleft palate repair is usually done between the ages of 1 and 2 years. Ask the parents to explain their understanding of how to care for the infant's cleft palate *to ensure adequate knowledge.*

◆ Discuss with family members available resources, such as children's medical services, social services, public health associations, and a local cleft palate parent group, *so the parents can receive support and guidance from health care professionals and other parents.*

Preoperative interventions for cleft palate repair

◆ Feed the infant with a cleft palate nipple or a Teflon implant *to enhance nutritional intake.*

◆ Wean the infant from the bottle or breast before cleft palate surgery; *the infant must be able to drink from a cup.*

Postoperative interventions for cleft palate repair

◆ Position the toddler in semi-Fowler's position *to promote a patent airway.*

◆ Anticipate edema and a decreased airway from the palate closure; this may cause the toddler to appear temporarily dyspneic; assess for signs of altered oxygenation *to promote good respiration.*

◆ Assess breath sounds and monitor vital signs every 4 hours *to detect signs of respiratory infection from aspiration.*

◆ Keep hard or pointed objects (such as utensils, straws, and frozen dessert sticks) away from the toddler's mouth *to prevent trauma to the suture line.*

◆ Use a cup to feed; don't use a nipple or pacifier *to prevent injury to the suture line.*

◆ Maintain an upright position for 30 minutes after feeding *to prevent aspiration.*

◆ After each feeding, rinse the toddler's mouth and suture line with at least 1 oz of water *to decrease irritation and sloughing of the incision.*

◆ Use elbow restraints *to keep the toddler's hands out of his mouth.*
◆ Provide soft toys *to prevent injury.*
◆ Start the toddler on clear liquids and progress to a soft diet; rinse the suture line by giving the toddler a sip of water after each feeding *to prevent infection.*
◆ Distract or hold the toddler *to keep his tongue away from the roof of his mouth.*
◆ Review key teaching topics with family members *to ensure adequate knowledge about the condition and treatment,* including:
– the importance of parental involvement (Because it results in facial disfigurement, the condition may cause shock, guilt, and grief for the parents and may block parental bonding with the infant.)
– the need for follow-up speech therapy
– understanding of the infant's susceptibility to pathogens and otitis media because of the altered position of the eustachian tubes.

Evaluation

◆ The infant remains afebrile, has clear breath sounds bilaterally, feeds without aspiration, and maintains admission weight.
◆ The infant's suture line remains intact and free from inflammation and sloughing.
◆ The infant has no skin irritation or breakdown under elbow restraints.
◆ The infant responds well to cuddling and stops crying quickly after being held.
◆ The infant's parents participate in feeding and caring for the suture line before discharge.
◆ The infant's parents verbalize an understanding of long-term cleft palate care and the potential problems with respiratory infection, dentition, and speech development.
◆ The infant's parents verbalize plans to continue follow-up care with an interdisciplinary cleft lip and cleft palate team.

CLUBFOOT

CLUBFOOT, also known as *talipes,* is a congenital disorder in which the foot and ankle are twisted and can't be manipulated into the correct position. Clubfoot occurs in these five forms:
◆ Equinovarus — combination of positions
◆ Talipes calcaneus — dorsiflexion, as if walking on one's heels
◆ Talipes equinus — plantar flexion, as if pointing one's toes
◆ Talipes valgus — eversion of the ankles, with the feet turning out
◆ Talipes varus — inversion of the ankles, with the soles of the feet facing each other.

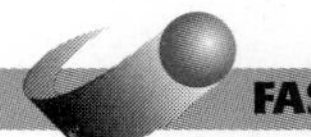

FAST FACT

Nearly all cases of talipes are equinovarus, involving a combination of abnormal positions.

Possible causes

◆ Arrested development during the 9th and 10th weeks of gestation, when the feet are formed
◆ Deformed talus and shortened Achilles tendon
◆ Possible genetic predisposition

Assessment findings

◆ Deformity usually obvious at birth
◆ Disorder can't be corrected manually (distinguishes true clubfoot from apparent clubfoot)

Diagnostic evaluation

◆ X-rays show superimposition of the talus and calcaneus and a ladderlike appearance of the metatarsals.

Nursing diagnoses

◆ Impaired physical mobility
◆ Delayed growth and development
◆ Risk for peripheral neurovascular dysfunction
◆ Risk for impaired skin integrity
◆ Risk for impaired parent-infant attachment
◆ Deficient knowledge (child care, growth and development)

Treatment

Treatment is administered in three stages:
◆ Correcting the deformity surgically or with a series of casts to gradually stretch and realign the angle of the foot and, after cast removal, application of a splint at night until age 1
◆ Maintaining the correction until the foot gains normal muscle balance
◆ Observing the foot closely for several years to prevent the deformity from recurring.

Planning and goals

◆ The infant will maintain joint mobility and ROM.
◆ The infant will maintain muscle strength.

◆ The infant will show no evidence of complications, such as contractures, venous stasis, thrombus formulation, or skin breakdown.
◆ The infant's parents verbalize an understanding of the condition and treatment options.

Implementation

◆ Assess neurovascular status *to ensure circulation to the foot with the cast in place.*
◆ Ensure that shoes fit correctly *to promote comfort and prevent skin breakdown.*
◆ Prepare the child and parents for surgery, if necessary, *to maintain or promote the healing process and decrease anxiety.*
◆ Provide emotional support and education to the parents *to help optimize the child's outcome.*

Evaluation

◆ The infant shows improved joint mobility and ROM.
◆ The infant shows no sign of circulatory impairment to the legs and maintains skin integrity.
◆ The infant's parents demonstrate an understanding of care once the infant is home with a clubfoot cast, including cast care and checking for signs of circulatory impairment.
◆ The infant's parents understand the importance of doing exercises to help maintain the correction.
◆ The infant's parents exhibit bonding with their infant and appropriate coping skills.

DEVELOPMENTAL DYSPLASIA OF THE HIP

DEVELOPMENTAL DYSPLASIA OF THE HIP (DDH), also known as *dislocated hip,* results from an abnormal development of the hip socket. It occurs when the head of the femur is still cartilaginous and the acetabulum (socket) is shallow; as a result, the head of the femur comes out of the hip socket. DDH can affect one or both hips and occurs in varying degrees of dislocation, from partial (subluxation) to complete. (See *Pediatric musculoskeletal facts.*)

DDH is seven times more common in girls than in boys. It's usually diagnosed during the initial pediatric assessment, but screening for DDH should be done at all visits for the first year of life. (See *Assessing DDH.*)

Possible causes

◆ Breech delivery
◆ Fetal position in utero
◆ Genetic predisposition
◆ Laxity of the ligaments
◆ Swaddling infants with hip adduction and extension

Assessment findings

◆ Restricted abduction of the hips
◆ Appearance of a shortened limb on the affected side
◆ On the affected side, an increased number of folds on the posterior thigh when the infant is supine with knees bent

Diagnostic evaluation

◆ BARLOW'S SIGN is present. A click is felt when the infant is placed supine with hips flexed 90 degrees, knees fully flexed, and the hip brought into midabduction.
◆ ORTOLANI'S SIGN is present. A click can be felt by the examiner's fingers at the hip area as the femur head snaps out of and back into the acetabulum. It's also palpable during examination with the infant's legs flexed and abducted.
◆ Ultrasonography and magnetic resonance imaging may be used to assess reduction.
◆ TRENDELENBURG'S TEST is positive. When the infant or child stands on the affected leg, the opposite pelvis dips to maintain erect posture.

Pediatric musculoskeletal facts

Bones and muscles

◆ Bones and muscles grow and develop throughout childhood.
◆ Bone lengthening occurs in the epiphyseal plates at the ends of bones; when the epiphyses close, growth stops.
◆ Bone healing occurs much faster in a child than in an adult because the child's bones are still growing.
◆ The younger the child, the faster a bone heals.
◆ Bone healing takes approximately 1 week for every year of life up to age 10.

Fractures

The most common fractures in children are clavicular fractures and greenstick fractures:
◆ Clavicular fractures may occur during vaginal birth because the shoulders are the widest part of the body.
◆ Greenstick fractures of the long bones are related to the increased flexibility of a young child's bones. (The compressed side of the bone bends while the side under tension fractures.)

Assessing DDH

The following illustrations demonstrate what signs would be found in an infant with developmental dysplasia of the hip.

ASYMMETRIC THIGH AND GLUTEAL FOLDS

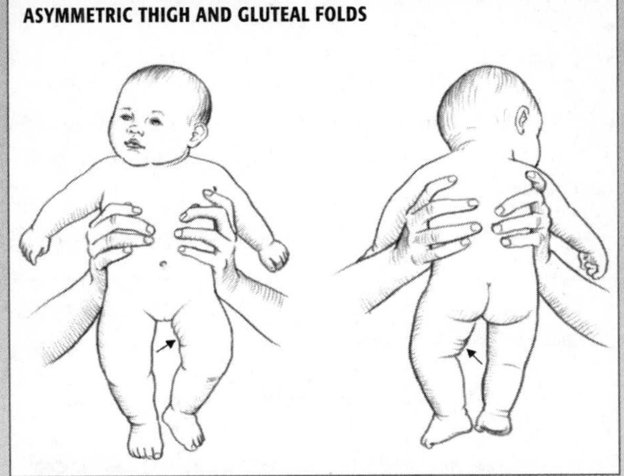

ORTOLANI'S SIGN (HIP CLICK FELT DURING EXTERNAL ROTATION)

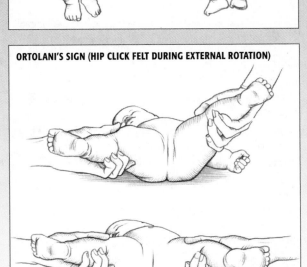

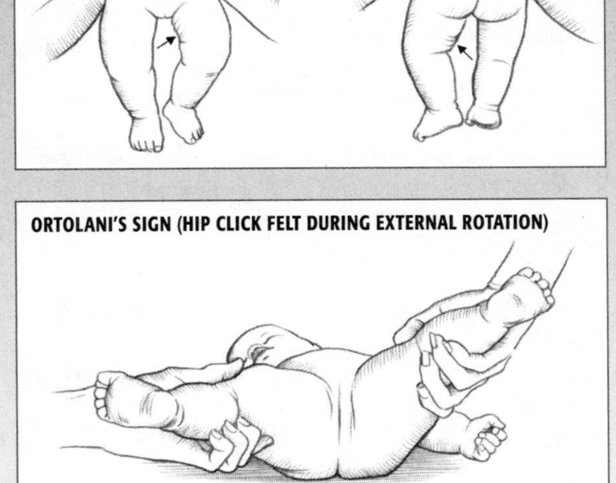

LIMITED HIP ABDUCTION

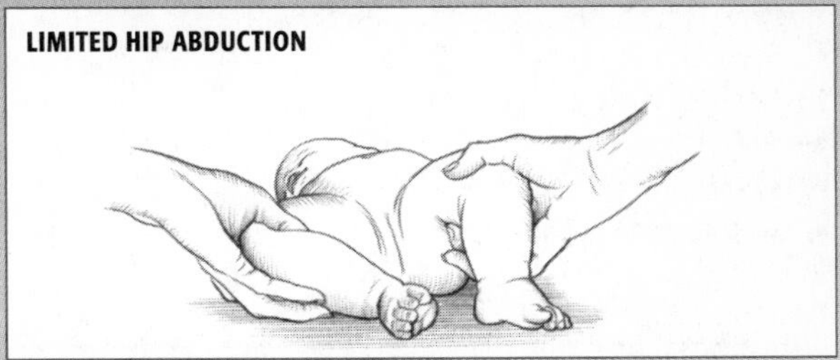

ALLIS' SIGN (ONE KNEE LOWER THAN THE OTHER)

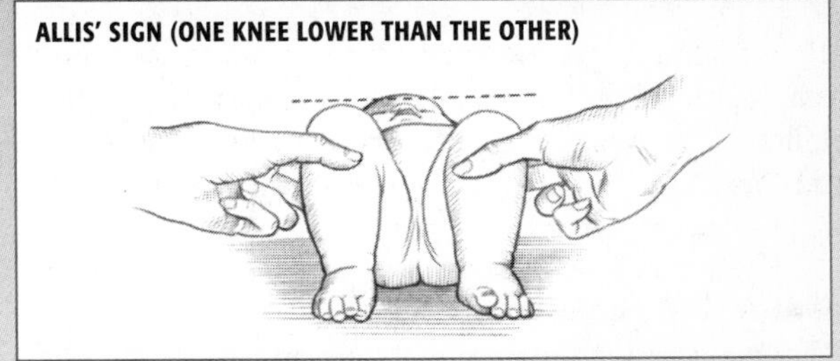

TRENDELENBURG'S SIGN (IN A CHILD OF WEIGHT-BEARING AGE)

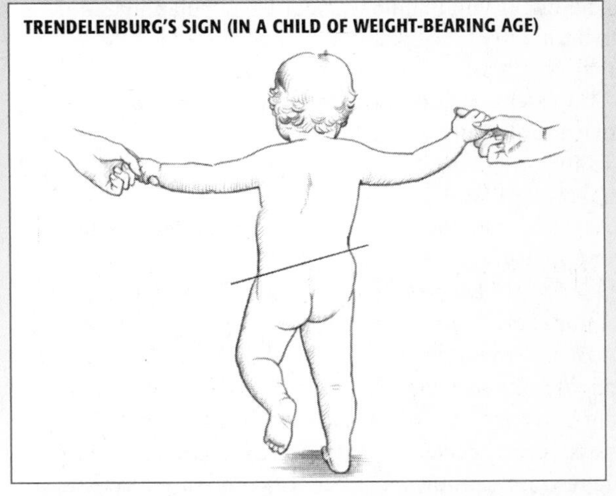

- X-rays show the location of the femur head and a shallow acetabulum. X-rays can also be used to monitor progression of the disorder.

Nursing diagnoses

- Impaired physical mobility
- Risk for peripheral neurovascular dysfunction
- Risk for impaired skin integrity
- Delayed growth and development

Treatment

Treatment varies according to the infant's or child's age. It's most successful when begun when the child is younger than age 2 months, becomes difficult after age 4 years, and is inadvisable after age 6 years. The goal, regardless of age, is to maintain abduction and prevent deformity. Treatment may include:

- hip-spica casting or corrective surgery for older children
- Bryant's traction, if the acetabulum doesn't deepen

Comparing plaster and synthetic casts

PLASTER CAST	SYNTHETIC CAST
◆ Heavy	◆ Lightweight
◆ Takes 10 to 72 hours to dry	◆ Takes 5 to 30 minutes to dry
◆ Molds easily to body parts	◆ Doesn't mold easily (not useful for small children)
◆ Smooth exterior	◆ Rough exterior (can abrade adjacent body parts)
◆ Inexpensive	◆ Expensive (three to seven times more costly than a plaster cast)
◆ Must be protected around water	◆ Can be immersed in water (observe for macerated skin if dried inadequately)

◆ triple-cloth diapering, casting, or a harness to keep the hips and knees flexed and the hips abducted for at least 3 months. (If this method is unsuccessful, corrective surgery is needed.) (See *Comparing plaster and synthetic casts.*)

Planning and goals

◆ The infant will maintain hip abduction.
◆ The infant will maintain adequate circulation and innervation of the legs while in a cast.
◆ The infant's skin integrity won't be impaired.
◆ The parents will demonstrate cast care and be able to provide it at home.

Implementation

◆ Assess circulation before application of a cast or traction; after application, ask the infant to wiggle his toes *to detect signs of impaired circulation.* You should be able to place one finger between the skin and the cast. (See *Cast care.*)
◆ Assess for pain that's unrelieved by analgesia *to identify signs of compartment syndrome.*
◆ Provide skin care *to prevent skin breakdown.*
◆ Give reassurance that early, prompt treatment will probably result in complete correction *to decrease anxiety.*
◆ Assure the parents that the infant will adjust to restricted movement and return to normal sleeping, eating, and play in a few days *to ease anxiety.*
◆ Inspect the skin, especially around bony prominences, *to detect cast complications and skin breakdown.*
◆ Review key teaching topics with family members *to ensure adequate knowledge about the condition and treatment,* including:
– correctly splinting or bracing the hips
– receiving frequent checkups
– coping with restricted movement

Cast care

1. Maintain hip abduction by applying a hip-spica cast; abduction holds the femoral head in the acetabulum.
2. Neurovascular checks are vital because infants can indicate discomfort only through crying, fretfulness, and not eating. Observe for circulatory and nerve impairment:
◆ Feel the cast for tightness.
◆ Blanch toes or toenails every 1 to 2 hours initially.
◆ Feel the toes for coldness; observe for swelling, cyanosis, pain.
◆ Feel the cast for warm spots, especially over bony prominences.
◆ Smell the cast for odors from pressure areas under the cast.
◆ Observe respirations carefully for signs of impairment.
3. Maintain skin integrity under the cast:
◆ Inspect the skin and cast regularly for crumbs.
◆ Inspect cast edges.
◆ Petal raw cast edges as soon as the cast is dry.
◆ Keep exposed skin clean and dry.
◆ Keep small objects and toys away from the infant because they may be put inside the cast.
4. Maintain cast integrity:
◆ Turn the infant every 2 hours until the cast is dry; then change the infant's position frequently for comfort.
◆ Handle a wet cast with the palms. Finger indentation can cause pressure sores.
◆ Check the infant's temperature while the cast is drying.
◆ Position the infant with hips lower than shoulders for toileting; use a plastic-backed disposable diaper under the cast rim to prevent soiling.
◆ Clean the cast with only a damp cloth and a small amount of cleanser; apply the cleanser only to soiled areas.
5. Teach the parents how to care for the cast and ways to perform routine activities.
6. Refer the family to an agency for disabled children.

– removing braces and splints while bathing the infant and replacing them immediately afterward
– stressing good hygiene.

Evaluation

◆ The infant maintains adequate circulation and innervation of the legs while in the cast.
◆ The infant is interested in his environment and shows age-appropriate developmental behaviors.
◆ The infant's parents can describe the cast-care procedures they must follow when they bring the infant home from the hospital.

DIARRHEA

Diarrhea is an increase in the frequency, volume, and liquidity of stools. Acute diarrhea is the sudden onset of frequent loose or watery stools. Chronic diarrhea begins more slowly, with a gradual increase in the number of stools; consistency becomes loose and unformed.

Diarrhea becomes a problem for infants and children because water and electrolyte loss from the bowel can cause dehydration. Dehydration is classified as isotonic, hypertonic, or hypotonic, based on the relationship of electrolyte loss to fluid loss or the percentage of body weight loss (mild: 2% to 4% weight loss; moderate: 5% to 9% weight loss; or severe: 10% or greater weight loss).

Possible causes

◆ Acute — inflammatory response to an intestinal tract infection
◆ Chronic — usually results from inflammatory reaction and allergic response or malabsorption syndrome

Assessment findings

◆ Stool evaluation:
– stools tinged with blood, mucus, or pus
– foul-smelling stools
– change in stool color (light or dark)
– change in stool consistency or frequency
◆ Signs of abdominal cramping:
– crying
– clutching the abdomen
– flexing the knees to the abdomen
◆ Signs of dehydration:
– dry mucus membranes
– sunken anterior fontanel
– crying without tears
– decreased number of wet diapers
◆ Dietary intake (food and fluid) for the 24 hours before the diarrhea started
◆ Environmental issues, such as source of water, presence of family pets, travel to another country; other family members with similar symptoms (or others in the child's environment, such as daycare and school)

Diagnostic evaluation

◆ Stool cultures may reveal the presence of bacteria or other infectious agents.
◆ Microscopic examination of stool may reveal the presence of ova or parasites.
◆ Stool guaiac test can reveal occult blood.
◆ Serum electrolytes may reveal signs of dehydration and metabolic acidosis.

Nursing diagnoses

◆ Risk for infection
◆ Risk for deficient fluid volume
◆ Risk for impaired skin integrity
◆ Delayed growth and development

Treatment

◆ Replacement of fluids and electrolytes
◆ Treatment of infection if present
◆ Prevention of spread of infection (if applicable)
◆ Hospitalization, depending on the length of illness, extent of dehydration, serum electrolyte levels, and age

Drug therapy options

◆ Antibiotics: specific to infecting organism

Planning and goals

◆ The infant's infection won't be transmitted to others.
◆ The infant will regain fluid and electrolyte balance.
◆ The infant will have fewer stools per day.
◆ The infant's skin will remain intact in the perianal area.
◆ Members of the infant's family will demonstrate understanding of current treatments and the anticipated approach to the diet when oral intake is resumed.
◆ The infant will maintain or regain his pre-illness developmental level.

Implementation

◆ Weigh the infant daily using the same scale and at the same time of day *to assist with fluid status evaluation.*
◆ Maintain hourly intake and output; monitor hydration status (for dehydration and overhydration) every 4 hours *to identify signs of increase or decrease in hydration.*

◆ Weigh diapers on a gram scale *to help determine fluid loss.* (If stools are watery, apply a pediatric urine collector *to differentiate urine and stool amounts.*)
◆ Send stools to the laboratory for ordered cultures. Place in double containers *to prevent personnel contamination during the transport.*
◆ Record amount, consistency, and frequency of stools and perform stool testing for the presence of blood, as ordered, *to determine the infant's elimination patterns and response to therapy.*
◆ Clean perianal skin thoroughly. Apply protective ointment as needed and report alterations in skin integrity *to help prevent skin irritation and breakdown, which can lead to secondary infection.*
◆ Administer I.V. fluids at maintenance and greater levels, as ordered, *to provide hydration.*
◆ Monitor the I.V. administration insertion site and surrounding areas for signs of infiltration *to quickly identify any disruption in the administration of I.V. fluids.*
◆ Administer oral fluids as ordered when stools decrease in frequency and liquid content. Give foods high in sodium content (broth, salted crackers) sparingly *to avoid hypernatremia.*
◆ Ensure that hospital personnel and visitors wash hands carefully and follow hospital policies regarding isolation precautions *to prevent the spread of infection to personnel and visitors.*
◆ Offer the infant a pacifier as desired *to provide for intensified oral needs in response to regression and food and fluid restrictions.*
◆ Provide age-appropriate sensorimotor stimulation; include auditory (musical toys, verbal conversation), visual (colorful toys, pictures, mobiles), and tactile (age-appropriate toys, stroking, books) stimuli *to provide appropriate stimulation and activities for maintaining the infant's developmental stage.*
◆ Encourage parents to remain with the infant as much as possible *to help prevent separation anxiety (fear of abandonment).* The infant needs repeated reassurance of the parents' love and presence.
◆ Discuss the treatment regimen with family members. Prepare family members for possible follow-up and discharge planning. If the disease is communicable, they should receive written instructions for careful hand washing, disposing of the infant's excretions, and cleaning toilet facilities. Family members should also be taught how to avoid transmitting enteropathologic organisms, with an emphasis on proper hand washing and food handling. If stool specimens are needed from family members, provide written instructions for proper collection and delivery. *These steps help to ensure effectiveness of the planned treatment regimen and prevent the transmission of the infection to others.*

Evaluation

◆ The infant's I.V. infusion remained patent, fluids were administered as ordered, and there was no further weight loss. Urine output increased by day 2.
◆ The number of stools has decreased.
◆ No open lesions or rash has developed on the infant's perianal area.
◆ The infant played peek-a-boo with parents and staff members.
◆ The infant's parents express an understanding of verbal instructions regarding the hospital treatment regimen and receive, discuss, and express an understanding of written discharge instructions.
◆ Members of the infant's family are free from symptoms and remain so after the infant's discharge from the hospital.

FAILURE TO THRIVE

FAILURE TO THRIVE is a chronic, potentially life-threatening condition characterized by failure to maintain weight and height above the 5th percentile on age-appropriate growth charts. Most children are diagnosed before age 2. It can result from physical, emotional, or psychological causes.

Possible causes

◆ Organic — acute or chronic illness (GI reflux, malabsorption syndrome, congenital heart defect, or cystic fibrosis)
◆ Nonorganic — psychological problem between infant and typically the primary caregiver (parent), such as failure to bond
◆ Mixed — combination of organic and nonorganic

Assessment findings

◆ Altered body posture; infant is stiff or floppy; doesn't cuddle
◆ Disparities between chronologic age and height and weight
◆ History of insufficient stimulation and inadequate parental knowledge of child development
◆ Delayed psychosocial behavior; for example, reluctance to smile or talk
◆ History of inadequate feeding techniques, such as bottle propping or insufficient burping
◆ History of medical problems

◆ History of sleep disturbances
◆ Psychosocial family problems
◆ REGURGITATION of food after almost every feeding, part being vomited and the remainder swallowed (rumination of food)

Diagnostic evaluation

◆ Negative nitrogen balance indicates inadequate intake of protein or calories.
◆ Associated physiologic causes may be detected.
◆ Reduced creatinine-height index reflects muscle mass and estimates muscle protein depletion.

Nursing diagnoses

◆ Delayed growth and development
◆ Imbalanced nutrition: Less than body requirements
◆ Impaired parenting

Treatment

◆ High-calorie diet
◆ Parent counseling
◆ Respite care for the infant

Drug therapy options

◆ Vitamin and mineral supplements

Planning and goals

◆ The infant will have improved growth and development as evidenced by maintaining body weight and meeting age-appropriate milestones.
◆ The infant's parents will demonstrate improved parenting skills as evidenced by asking appropriate questions about the infant's condition and participating in the infant's care.

Implementation

◆ Weigh the infant on admission and measure head circumference and length and height *to determine baseline weight.*

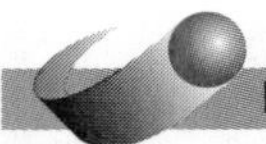

FAST FACT

In general, adequate growth in an infant is considered to be a weight gain of 15 to 30 grams per day. With decreased caloric intake, weight will decrease first, then linear growth will slow down, followed by stunted growth of the head. However, the head circumference will be normal in most infants with failure to thrive.

◆ Assess growth and development using an appropriate tool, such as the Denver Developmental Screening Test, *to determine the infant's developmental level.*
◆ Properly feed and interact with the infant *to promote nutrition and growth and development.*

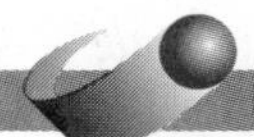

FAST FACT

For a breast-fed infant, the mother should be doing approximately 8 feedings (every 3 hours) in a 24-hour period for adequate nutrition. Formula fed infants typically will have 6 feedings per day, or about every 4 hours.

◆ Establish specific times for feeding, bathing, and sleeping *to establish and maintain a structured routine.*
◆ Provide the infant with visual and auditory stimulation *to promote normal sensory development.*
◆ Assess interaction of the caregiver with the infant *to determine if failure to thrive is due to the caregiver's inability to form an emotional attachment to the infant.*
◆ When caring for the infant in the parent's presence, act as a role model for effective parenting skills. Demonstrate comfort measures such as rocking the infant, and show the caregiver how to hold the infant *to enhance knowledge of routine infant care practices.*
◆ Teach the caregiver about normal growth and development and identify ages at which the infant should be able to master developmental tasks, such as rolling over, crawling, and walking. This will assist in monitoring the infant's growth and development. Also, discuss problem behaviors associated with specific ages, such as colic, temper tantrums, and sleeping difficulties, *to further enhance the parents' understanding of developmental norms.*
◆ Discuss the infant's need for tactile and sensory stimulation. Demonstrate play activities that promote developmental skills, such as shaking a rattle in front of the infant *to build eye-and-hand coordination* or placing a mobile above the infant *to encourage visual tracking and trunk and head control. Sensory experiences promote* COGNITIVE DEVELOPMENT.

Evaluation

◆ The infant is maintaining or increasing in body weight and achieving age-appropriate developmental milestones.
◆ The infant's parents express an understanding of his feeding requirements and of age-appropriate growth and development.
◆ The infant's parents maintain a loving and supportive relationship with him.

MYELOMENINGOCELE

MYELOMENINGOCELE, the most severe SPINA BIFIDA defect, is a protruding, saclike cyst, usually in the lumbosacral area, that contains meninges, spinal fluid, and a portion of the spinal cord with its nerves. This congenital neural tube defect is readily apparent at birth. The myelomeningocele is commonly encased in a thin membrane that's prone to tears and leakage of cerebrospinal fluid (CSF). The extent of neurologic dysfunction depends on the level of the vertebral column at which the defect occurs. Lumbosacral lesions tend to be associated with flaccid paralysis of the legs; NEUROGENIC BLADDER and fecal incontinence; musculoskeletal deformities, including flexion or extension contractures; talipes varus or valgus; and hip dislocation or subluxation.

HYDROCEPHALUS associated with Arnold-Chiari malformation (downward displacement of the cerebellar tonsils through the foramen magnum into the cervical spinal canal) occurs in approximately 90% of those with lumbosacral myelomeningocele.

Possible causes

- ◆ Combination of genetic and environmental factors
- ◆ Exposure to a teratogen
- ◆ Part of a multiple-malformation syndrome (for example, chromosomal abnormalities, such as trisomy 13 or 18 syndrome)

Assessment findings

- ◆ Saclike structure protruding over the spine with evidence of solid matter on TRANSILLUMINATION (light passed through the side of the sac); translucent sac may indicate MENINGOCELE rather than myelomeningocele
- ◆ Permanent neurologic dysfunction (paralysis, bowel and bladder incontinence)
- ◆ Increased head circumference or unusual disproportion between the head and chest circumferences; may indicate hydrocephalus before other neurologic symptoms appear (A neonate's head circumference is normally about 1" [2.5 cm] larger than the chest circumference.)
- ◆ Hydrocephalus
- ◆ Increased intracranial pressure (ICP)
- ◆ Arnold-Chiari syndrome
- ◆ Curvature of the spine
- ◆ Clubfoot
- ◆ Possible mental retardation
- ◆ Knee contractures

Diagnostic evaluation

- ◆ Amniocentesis reveals elevated alpha-fetoprotein (AFP) levels, indicating a neural tube defect. (Maternal serum AFP levels aren't as specific.)
- ◆ Acetylcholinesterase measurement can be used to confirm the diagnosis.
- ◆ After birth, spinal X-ray can be used to show the bone defect.
- ◆ Chromosomal abnormalities associated with neural tube defects may be revealed by fetal karyotype and biochemical test results.
- ◆ Myelography can be used to differentiate spina bifida from other spinal abnormalities, particularly spinal cord tumors.
- ◆ Ultrasound may be used to identify the open neural tube or ventral wall defect.

Nursing diagnoses

- ◆ Impaired physical mobility
- ◆ Risk for infection
- ◆ Impaired skin integrity
- ◆ Delayed growth and development
- ◆ Risk for impaired parent-infant attachment

Treatment

- ◆ Surgical closure of the sac by skin grafts 24 to 48 hours after birth or after the infant can more easily tolerate the procedure (doesn't reverse neurologic deficits)
- ◆ Supportive measures to promote independence and prevent further complications
- ◆ Placement of VENTRICULOPERITONEAL SHUNT to treat hydrocephalus (see *Ventriculoperitoneal shunt*)

Planning and goals

◆ During hospitalization, the infant will:
- maintain an intact myelomeningocele sac before surgery
- maintain stable vital signs and neurologic status
- show no symptoms of increased ICP (indicating shunt malfunction or infection)
- maintain ROM and corrective positioning
- maintain skin integrity
- maintain urinary elimination without bladder distention and no sign of urinary tract infection (UTI) due to catheterization.

◆ The infant's parents will:
- demonstrate at least three positive signs of attachment within 72 hours
- verbalize an understanding of operative procedures, the need to report signs of increased ICP and infection promptly, and the need for long-term follow-up of problems related to myelomeningocele and hydrocephalus

Ventriculoperitoneal shunt

This illustration shows the placement of the ventriculoperitoneal shunt. Note that the end in the peritoneal cavity is coiled to allow room for growth of the infant.

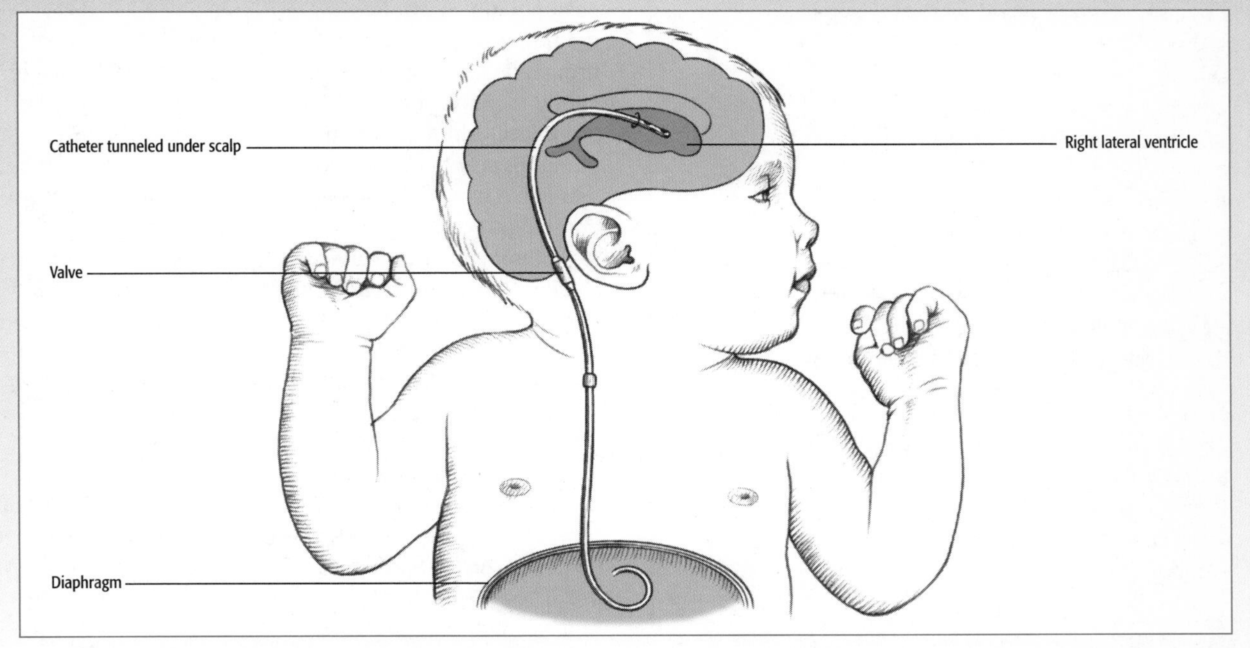

– demonstrate appropriate care techniques (for example, monitoring neurologic status for increased ICP, monitoring for infection, and performing intermittent catheterization and ROM exercises), which they will continue after discharge.

Implementation

Before surgery to correct myelomeningocele

◆ Hold and cuddle the infant on your lap and position him on his abdomen; handle the infant carefully, and don't apply pressure to the defect *to prevent injury at the site of the defect.*

◆ Clean the defect, inspect it often, and cover it with sterile dressings moistened with sterile saline solution *to prevent infection.*

◆ Keep the infant warm in an infant Isolette *to prevent hypothermia.* Usually, the infant can't wear a diaper or a shirt until after surgical correction *because it will irritate the sac.*

◆ Watch for signs of hydrocephalus. Measure head circumference daily. Be sure to mark the spot where the measurement was made *to ensure accurate readings.*

◆ Watch for signs of meningeal irritation, such as fever and nuchal rigidity, *to detect signs of meningitis.*

◆ Contractures can be minimized by passive ROM exercises and casting. *To prevent hip dislocation, moderately abduct hips with a pad between the knees or with sandbags and ankle rolls to prevent hip dislocation.*

◆ Monitor intake and output. Watch for decreased skin turgor and dryness *to detect dehydration.*

◆ Provide a diet high in calories and protein *to ensure adequate nutrition.*

After surgery to correct myelomeningocele

◆ Watch for hydrocephalus, which follows surgery in many cases. Measure the infant's head circumference, as ordered, *to detect signs of hydrocephalus and prevent associated complications.*

◆ Monitor vital signs often *to detect early signs of shock, infection, and increased ICP.* (See *Signs and symptoms of increased ICP,* page 258.)

◆ Change the dressing regularly, as ordered, and check and report signs of drainage, wound rupture, and infection *to promote early treatment and prevent complications.*

Signs and symptoms of increased ICP

The lists below include signs and symptoms of increased intracranial pressure (ICP) in an infant and a child.

Infant

- Refusal of feedings or difficulty feeding
- Irritability, altered level of consciousness (LOC)
- Vomiting
- Bulging fontanel
- Increased frontal occipital circumference
- High-pitched cry
- Setting-sun sign (eyes are rotated downward and the sclera are visible above the pupil)
- Cries when picked up but settles when lying still

Child

- Headache in the morning (with or without vomiting)
- Altered LOC
- Ataxia
- Irritability
- Lethargy

◆ Place the infant in the prone position *to protect and assess the site.*

◆ If leg casts have been applied to treat deformities, watch for signs that the infant is outgrowing the cast. Regularly check distal pulses *to ensure adequate circulation.*

After placement of ventriculoperitoneal shunt to treat hydrocephalus

◆ Place the infant flat, with hips abducted, or on the nonsurgical side; change his position every hour *to help prevent excessively rapid decompression of the intracranial fluid.* Hip abduction continues to be necessary because of the neurologic deficit to the lower body. A side-lying position must be on the nonsurgical side *to avoid putting pressure on the shunt valve. Changing the infant's position reduces the risk of hypostatic pneumonia and pressure sores.*

◆ Document head circumference every shift; assess and document vital signs and neurologic status (anterior fontanel and pupils, blood pressure, level of irritability, sucking reflex, listlessness, and seizure activity) every 4 hours *to identify complications.* The valve opens at a certain intraventricular pressure and closes when the pressure is sufficiently reduced by fluid drainage. A depressed fontanel may indicate a successful shunt if unaccompanied by other signs of dehydration (such as increased heart rate or respirations, decreased urine output, and irritability). A tense, bulging fontanel indicates a nonfunctioning shunt and increased ICP. Signs of increased ICP may indicate infection or shunt malfunction, the greatest postoperative hazards.

◆ Pump the shunt, if ordered, by depressing the valve firmly and quickly with the index finger; leave the finger lightly in place to check for refill. Teach the parents this procedure. Although not performed routinely, shunt pumping may be needed *to maintain valve patency or assess valve function.* The physician orders the desired pumping frequency.

◆ Maintain strict intake and output records, monitoring I.V. fluid intake every hour *to reduce the risk of cerebral edema and increased ICP.* The physician may restrict fluids for the first 24 to 48 hours.

◆ Observe for abdominal distention *to assess for signs of an ileus or peritonitis, which can be caused by CSF drainage.*

◆ Have the parents assume more responsibility for the infant's care, including feeding, passive ROM exercises, skin care, and hygiene. Provide positive reinforcement and guidance. *Active participation and feedback enhance learning. The parents must become more involved with the infant's care during hospitalization if they're to provide adequate care after the infant is discharged.*

◆ Give the parents a list of signs of infection and increased ICP; include the physician's telephone number. *A written list reminds the parents of signs that require medical treatment.*

◆ Have the parents demonstrate their understanding of long-term follow-up care that the infant will need, including continuous medical evaluation of hydrocephalus and myelomeningocele; orthopedic evaluation and possible appliances; and urologic evaluation to prevent complications. *The shunt will require periodic readjustment to compensate for growth or malfunction.*

◆ Tell the parents what to expect regarding the infant's future development and refer them to an early childhood development program and support group *so they have a general idea of what to expect and how best to help the infant at each stage of development.*

◆ When spina bifida is diagnosed prenatally, refer the parents to a genetic counselor, *who can provide information and support the couple's decisions on how to manage the pregnancy.*

◆ Review key teaching topics with the parents *to ensure adequate knowledge about the condition and treatment,* including:

– handling the infant without applying pressure to the defect
– coping with the infant's physical problems
– recognizing early signs of complications, such as hydrocephalus, pressure ulcers, and urinary tract infections
– recognizing signs of shunt blockage, such as morning headache, vomiting, or irritability
– maintaining a positive attitude and working through feelings of guilt, anger, and helplessness
– conducting intermittent catheterization and conduit hygiene
– emptying the child's bowel by administering a glycerin suppository, as needed
– recognizing developmental lags (a possible result of hydrocephalus)
– ensuring maximum mental development
– planning activities appropriate to their infant's age and abilities.

Evaluation

◆ The infant's vital signs remain stable; his fontanel remains soft to slightly depressed; and he's alert with a lusty cry.
◆ The infant is free from infection.
◆ The infant's skin remains intact.
◆ The infant's parents assume more responsibility for his care; they demonstrate an understanding of procedures, complication signs, and the need for long-term follow-up evaluation and treatment.

PYLORIC STENOSIS

In PYLORIC STENOSIS, hyperplasia and hypertrophy of the circular muscle at the pylorus narrow the pyloric canal, thereby preventing the stomach from emptying normally. The defect is most common in male infants younger than 4 months old.

Infants with pyloric stenosis are usually well for the first few weeks after birth. As the hypertrophy and hyperplasia progress, pyloric obstruction becomes apparent. Typically, the infant initially regurgitates occasionally after feeding, then after every feeding. Vomiting quickly progresses to projectile vomiting, usually within 1 to 2 weeks. Moderate to severe dehydration occurs as vomiting increases.

Possible causes

◆ Exact cause unknown

Assessment findings

◆ Projectile emesis during or shortly after feedings, preceded by reverse peristaltic waves (going left to right); infant resumes eating after vomiting
◆ Olive-size bulge palpated below the right costal margin
◆ Poor weight gain
◆ Tetany
◆ Symptoms of malnutrition and dehydration despite the infant's apparent adequate intake of food
◆ Symptoms appearing at about 4 weeks in formula-fed infants and at about 6 weeks in breast-fed infants

Diagnostic evaluation

◆ Arterial blood gas (ABG) analysis reveals metabolic alkalosis.
◆ Blood chemistry tests may reveal hypocalcemia, hypokalemia, and hypochloremia.
◆ Hematest reveals blood in emesis.
◆ Ultrasonography shows a hypertrophied sphincter.
◆ Endoscopy reveals a hypertrophied sphincter.

Nursing diagnoses

◆ Risk for deficient fluid volume
◆ Imbalanced nutrition: Less than body requirements
◆ Risk for infection

Treatment

◆ Nothing-by-mouth status maintained before surgery
◆ I.V. therapy to correct fluid and electrolyte imbalances
◆ Possible insertion of a nasogastric (NG) tube, kept open and elevated for gastric decompression
◆ Surgical intervention (pyloromyotomy performed by laparoscopy)

Drug therapy options

◆ Potassium supplements (only after proper kidney function is confirmed)
◆ Calcium I.V.

Planning and goals

Before surgery, the infant will:
◆ regain fluid and electrolyte balance
◆ not vomit after feeding
◆ be free from infection
◆ gain depleted body fat and protein stores
◆ develop at the appropriate level.

After surgery, the infant will:
◆ regain fluid and electrolyte balance
◆ not vomit after feeding
◆ be free from infection
◆ gain depleted body fat and protein stores

◆ develop at the appropriate level
◆ gain weight.

The infant's parents will understand care to be continued at home, including:
◆ feeding and positioning techniques
◆ incision care
◆ behaviors to expect and which behaviors to report
◆ providing warm, loving care.

Implementation

◆ Weigh the infant daily *to assess growth.*
◆ Monitor vital signs and intake and output *to assess renal function and check for signs of dehydration.*
◆ Assess for metabolic alkalosis and dehydration from frequent emesis *to detect early complications.*
◆ Assess abdominal and cardiovascular status *to detect early signs of compromise.*
◆ Provide small, frequent, thickened feedings with the head of the bed elevated; burp the infant frequently (preoperatively) *to promote nutrition and prevent aspiration.*
◆ Position the infant on his right side *to prevent the aspiration of vomitus.*

After surgery:
◆ Feed the infant small amounts of oral electrolyte solution at first; then increase the amount and concentration of food until normal feeding is achieved *to meet nutritional needs and prevent vomiting.*
◆ Provide a pacifier *to meet nonnutritive sucking needs and maintain comfort.*
◆ Provide routine postoperative care *to maintain and improve the infant's condition and detect early complications.* Position the infant on his side *to prevent aspiration if vomiting occurs. Lying the infant on his right side possibly aids the flow of fluid through the pyloric valve by gravity.*
◆ Keep the incision area clean. *The infant is at an increased risk for infection because the incision is near the diaper area.*
◆ Review key teaching topics with family members *to ensure adequate knowledge about the condition and treatment,* including:
– feeding the infant, including specific formula, volume, and technique
– preventing infection.
◆ Assess need for home care and support of caregivers. Obtain referrals as needed.

Evaluation

◆ The infant ingests appropriate amounts of formula without regurgitating or vomiting and shows appropriate weight gain.
◆ The infant's parents can:
– explain feeding and positioning techniques
– describe incision care
– list signs and symptoms of incision infection.
◆ The parents demonstrate a warm, caring relationship with the infant.

SUDDEN INFANT DEATH SYNDROME

SUDDEN INFANT DEATH SYNDROME (SIDS) is the sudden death of an infant in which a postmortem examination fails to confirm the cause of death. The peak age is 3 months; 90% of cases occur before age 6 months, especially during the winter and early spring months.

Infants who are diagnosed with SIDS are typically described as healthy with no previous medical problems. Death commonly occurs sometime after the infant has been put down to sleep.

Possible causes

◆ Abnormality in the control of ventilation, causing prolonged apneic periods with profound hypoxia and cardiac arrhythmias
◆ Undetected abnormalities, such as an immature respiratory system and respiratory dysfunction

Assessment findings

◆ Death occurring during sleep without noise or struggle
◆ History of low birth weight
◆ History of siblings with SIDS (see *Recommendations for decreasing SIDS*)

Diagnostic evaluation

◆ Autopsy is the only way to diagnose SIDS. Autopsy findings indicate pulmonary edema, intrathoracic petechiae, and other minor changes suggesting chronic hypoxia.

Nursing diagnoses

◆ Ineffective coping
◆ Dysfunctional grieving
◆ Fear
◆ Hopelessness
◆ Spiritual distress

Treatment

◆ If the parents bring the infant to the emergency department, the physician decides whether to try to resuscitate.
◆ If successfully resuscitated, the infant is temporarily placed on mechanical ventilation. After he's extubated,

Recommendations for decreasing SIDS

The American Academy of Pediatrics has set forth the following recommendations to decrease the incidence of sudden infant death syndrome (SIDS):

◆ Place the infant on his back to sleep.

◆ Don't place the infant on a waterbed, sofa, soft mattress, or other soft surface to sleep.

◆ Avoid soft materials in the infant's sleeping area, such as a pillow, stuffed toy, loose blanket, quilt, or comforter.

◆ Make sure that the infant's crib meets the safety standards of the Consumer Product Safety Commission and the ASTM (formerly the American Society for Testing and Materials).

the infant is tested for infantile apnea and the parents are given a home apnea monitor.

Drug therapy options

◆ Epinephrine, atropine, sodium bicarbonate (after ABG analysis), if appropriate (according to Pediatric Advanced Life Support protocols)

Planning and goals

◆ Family members will use available support systems to assist in coping with fear.

◆ Family members will share feelings about the event.

◆ Family members will identify feelings of hopelessness regarding the current situation.

◆ Family members will use effective coping strategies to ease spiritual discomfort.

◆ Family members will seek appropriate support persons for assistance.

Implementation

◆ Because most infants can't be resuscitated, focus your interventions on providing emotional support for the family. Keep in mind that their grief may be coupled with guilt. Also, the parents may express anger at emergency department personnel, each other, or anyone involved with the infant's care. Stay calm and let them express their feelings. Parents need to express feelings *to prevent dysfunctional grieving.*

◆ Let the parents touch, hold, and rock the infant if desired, and allow them to say goodbye to the infant *to facilitate the grieving process.*

◆ Provide momentos and keepsakes to the parents. Express sympathy sincerely regarding their loss *to facilitate the grieving process.*

◆ Provide literature on SIDS and support groups; suggest psychological support for the surviving children *to help prevent maladaptive emotional responses to loss and promote coping and a realistic perspective on the tragedy.*

Evaluation

◆ Family members are coping with their grief, as demonstrated by sharing their feelings, using support systems, and having a realistic perspective about the tragedy.

◆ Family members are coping with feelings of hopelessness, fear, and guilt.

TRACHEOESOPHAGEAL FISTULA AND ESOPHAGEAL ATRESIA

TRACHEOESOPHAGEAL FISTULA is an abnormal passage between the esophagus and the trachea. A reflux of gastric juice after feeding can allow acidic stomach contents to cross the fistula, irritating the trachea.

ESOPHAGEAL ATRESIA occurs when the proximal end of the esophagus ends in a blind pouch; food from the esophagus can't enter the stomach.

Tracheoesophageal fistula and esophageal atresia occur in many combinations and may be associated with other defects. Esophageal atresia with tracheoesophageal fistula is the most common of these conditions. Esophageal atresia alone is the second most common of these conditions. (See *Common types of tracheoesophageal fistula and atresia,* page 262, and *Caring for an infant with tracheoesophageal fistula,* page 263.)

Esophageal atresia with tracheoesophageal fistula occurs when:

◆ the distal end of the esophagus ends in a blind pouch and the proximal end of the esophagus is linked to the trachea by a fistula.

◆ the proximal end of the esophagus ends in a blind pouch and the distal portion of the esophagus is connected to the trachea by a fistula.

Possible causes

◆ Prematurity (contributing factor)

Assessment findings

Esophageal atresia

◆ Excessive salivation and drooling due to an inability to pass food through the esophagus

Common types of tracheoesophageal fistula and atresia

These illustrations depict two common types of tracheoesophageal fistula and atresia.

ESOPHAGEAL ATRESIA WITH FISTULA TO THE DISTAL SEGMENT
(Occurrence: approximately 85% to 88%)

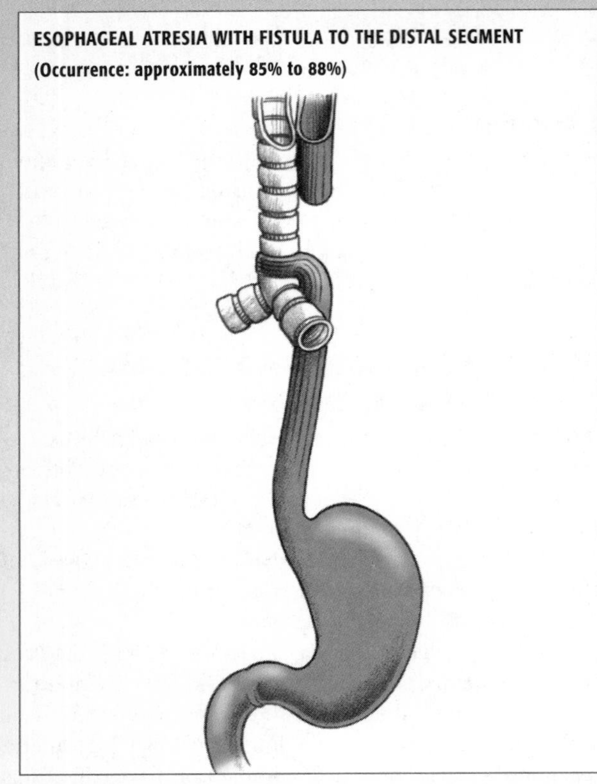

ESOPHAGEAL ATRESIA WITHOUT FISTULA
(Occurrence: approximately 6% to 8%)

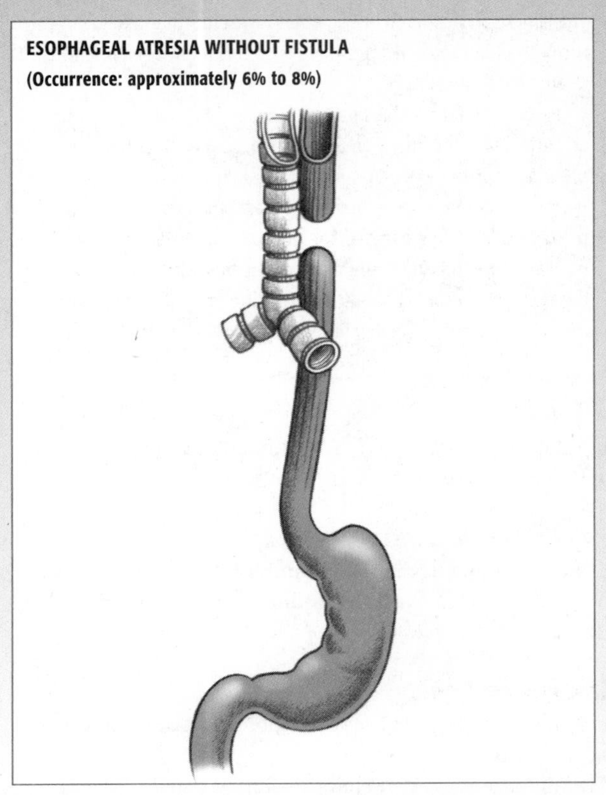

- ◆ Regurgitation of undigested formula immediately after feeding; possible respiratory distress and cyanosis if secretions are aspirated
- ◆ Inability to insert an NG tube

Tracheoesophageal fistula

- ◆ Excessive drooling of saliva (possibly the first symptom)
- ◆ Choking, coughing, and intermittent cyanosis during feeding due to food going into the trachea through the fistula
- ◆ Tracheal irritation from gastric acids that reflux across the fistula
- ◆ Abdominal distention from air going into the stomach through the fistula

Esophageal atresia with tracheoesophageal fistula

- ◆ Excessive salivation and drooling due to an inability to pass food through the esophagus
- ◆ Regurgitation of undigested formula immediately after feeding; possible respiratory distress and cyanosis if secretions are aspirated
- ◆ Signs of respiratory distress (coughing, choking, and intermittent cyanosis) because the infant has difficulty tolerating oral foods and handling oral secretions or refluxed gastric contents
- ◆ Inability to insert an NG tube

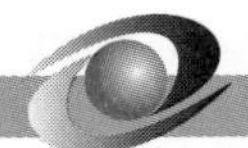

QUICK STUDY

Remember the 3 C's when assessing for tracheoesophageal fistula:

Coughing
Choking
Cyanosis

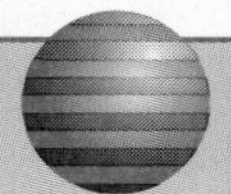

CLINICAL SITUATION

Caring for an infant with tracheoesophageal fistula

An infant has been in the newborn nursery for about 3½ hours when he suddenly becomes cyanotic and begins coughing and choking. The nurse notices that he has excessive mucus in his mouth and that he has been drooling. The infant is scheduled to be fed the first bottle of glucose water in about 2 hours. A diagnosis of a tracheoesophageal fistula with esophageal atresia has been made. The infant receives an esophagostomy and a gastrostomy (PEG) tube is placed.

What are appropriate interventions following surgery?

◆ Observe and care for wounds, and apply and change sterile dressings, as needed. If the infant has undergone a cervical esophagostomy, perform special skin care to prevent breakdown from continuous moisture. *The nurse must carefully observe all incision sites for signs of infection and take appropriate measures to prevent it.*

◆ Maintain adequate respiratory exchange and prevent pneumonia, as follows:

– Maintain a patent airway by carefully suctioning the infant's trachea, nose, and mouth as needed. Use the specially marked suction catheter as a guide *to prevent trauma to the anastomosis site.* During surgery, the surgeon measures and marks a suction catheter at a distance slightly above the anastomosis site; the catheter's length is communicated to all caregivers.

– Keep a laryngoscope and endotracheal tube at bedside *in case extreme edema causes obstruction.*

– Periodically check the chest tubes by auscultating both lungs for breath sounds, checking for loose connections and kinking and checking the drainage system for proper functioning every 4 to 8 hours based on the infant's condition *to ensure that his lungs are fully expanded.*

– Place the infant in an Isolette with humidity and oxygen *to reduce tracheal drying and irritation.*

– Keep the infant on his back or left side, and elevate the head of the bed 30 degrees *to help prevent aspiration of secretions and make breathing easier.*

◆ On the second or third postoperative day, begin PEG tube feedings. Continue the feedings, if tolerated, for 10 to 14 days. *This delay helps avoid postoperative vomiting.* Tube feedings maintain the infant's nutrition while bypassing the operative site to promote healing. Within 10 to 14 days, the anastomosis should heal completely; the surgeon may order an upper GI series to confirm healing.

◆ Begin oral feedings with sterile water or expressed breast milk, observing the infant carefully *to ensure that he can swallow without choking.* Progress to small, frequent formula feedings; supplement these with PEG tube feedings if the infant can't consume enough orally to meet nutritional needs. *Sterile water or expressed breast milk is given initially because it causes fewer problems than other solutions if the infant aspirates it or can't swallow.* Small, frequent formula feedings are gradually increased until they're sufficient to meet the infant's needs. The stomach will expand as the amount of food increases.

How can the nurse prepare the parents for home care?

◆ Teach proper care of the PEG tube and an esophagostomy if the infant has had a staged palliative procedure. *If a staged repair is performed and anastomosis is delayed until age 18 to 24 months, the infant will be sent home with a PEG tube and an esophagostomy.*

◆ Teach the parents to recognize signs of wound infection, including swelling, redness, foul or oozing drainage, or elevated temperature. *The infant typically is discharged 2 or 3 weeks after surgery; infection is possible even after discharge.*

◆ Teach the parents to recognize signs of esophageal stenosis: choking or coughing with feeding, refusal to eat, and painful swallowing. *Recurring esophageal stenosis and dysphagia are common complications of scarring, which may develop at the anastomosis site.*

◆ Teach correct positioning of the infant after feeding (on his back or right side, with the head of the bed slightly elevated), *which helps prevent regurgitation into the esophagus. (Begin oral feedings after day 14, as advised.)*

◆ Teach the parents to recognize signs of respiratory distress, including nasal flaring, retractions, and grunting, *to allow promt treatment. Respiratory distress may accompany dysphagia, or a fistula may develop at the operative site where the esophagus is separated from the trachea.*

Question for further thought

◆ How could the nurse provide mild sensorimotor stimulation to the infant?

Diagnostic evaluation

- Neonates are fed first with a few sips of sterile water to detect anomalies and to avoid aspiration of formula or breast milk into the lungs.
- Abdominal X-rays reveal air in the stomach.
- Fluoroscopy, using radiopaque fluid carefully introduced into the esophagus, reveals atresia.
- Bronchoscopy shows a blind pouch.

Nursing diagnoses

- Imbalanced nutrition: Less than body requirements
- Risk for infection
- Risk for impaired parent-infant attachment

Treatment

- Percutaneous endoscopic gastrostomy (PEG) tube insertion (infant not fed orally)
- Surgical correction by ligating the tracheoesophageal fistula and reanastomosing the esophageal ends (In many cases, repair is done in stages.)

Planning and goals

- The infant will have adequate nutritional intake.
- The infant will be afebrile and demonstrate no symptoms of infection.
- The parents will participate in the infant's care.

Implementation

- Monitor vital signs *to detect tachycardia and tachypnea,* which could indicate hypoxemia.
- Assess respiratory status *to detect poor respiratory status,* which may result in hypoxemia.
- Position the infant with his head elevated 30 degrees *to decrease reflux at the distal esophagus.*
- Suction as needed *to stimulate coughing and clear airways.*
- Keep the PEG tube open and suspended above the infant *to release gas.*
- Administer gastrostomy feedings only by gravity flow — not a feeding pump — *to help meet nutritional and metabolic requirements.*
- Allow parents to hold and touch their child *to allow bonding with the child.*

After surgery

- Maintain chest tube and respiratory support *to prevent respiratory compromise.*
- Keep a suction catheter ready *to eliminate secretions and prevent aspiration.*
- Mark the catheter to indicate the distance from the infant's nose to the point just above the anastomosis *to avoid causing trauma to the anastomosis site.*
- If feeding the infant through a PEG tube, anticipate abdominal distention from air; keep the infant upright during feedings *to reduce the chance of refluxed stomach contents and aspiration pneumonia* and keep the tube open and elevated before and after feedings.
- Make sure the PEG tube is secure and handle it with extreme caution *to avoid displacement.*
- Administer antibiotics as prescribed *to prevent infection.*
- Administer TPN *to maintain nutritional support.*
- Review key teaching topics with the parents, such as proper care of the infant at home (for example, feeding and bathing techniques), *to ensure adequate knowledge about the condition and treatment.*

Evaluation

- The infant receives sufficient nutrition — either in formula or breast milk — to maintain growth without choking, coughing, or aspirating.
- The infant remains afebrile and infection-free.
- The parents demonstrate the ability to provide care without anxiety.
- The parents demonstrate caring behaviors toward the infant.

TODDLER DISORDERS

ACUTE ACETAMINOPHEN POISONING

Because toddlers and preschoolers are mobile, active, and curious, they're especially vulnerable to accidental ingestion. Among drugs that children ingest most commonly, acetaminophen (Tylenol) ranks number one. Although aspirin poisoning has decreased, it still occurs in young children. Like acetaminophen, aspirin is readily available in most homes and taken freely by adults, whom children imitate. Also, children's aspirin and acetaminophen are brightly colored, with an appealing flavor. (See *Common poisoning agents.*)

In acetaminophen poisoning, hepatic damage results from a metabolite of acetaminophen. Usually, the liver enzyme glutathione combines with and neutralizes the metabolite, which is then excreted in the urine. With ingestion of large acetaminophen doses, the metabolite overwhelms glutathione, causing hepatic necrosis. (Administration of acetylcysteine [Mucomyst] provides a sub-

Common poisoning agents

This chart lists common poisoning agents in young children, along with assessment steps and treatments for each.

SUBSTANCE INGESTED	ASSESSMENT	TREATMENT
Corrosives (oven and drain cleaners, dishwasher detergents, and other strong detergents and cleaning agents)	◆ Observe for signs of toxicity: severe, burning pain of the mouth, lips, tongue, throat, and stomach; white, swollen oral mucous membranes; swollen tongue and pharynx; violent vomiting with blood; shock; anxiety; and agitation.	◆ Maintain a patent airway. ◆ Don't give emetics; vomiting will redamage tissue. ◆ Administer steroids as ordered. ◆ Give nothing by mouth except as ordered. ◆ Give analgesics as needed. ◆ Call the poison control center.
Hydrocarbons (petroleum distillates, such as kerosene, gasoline, turpentine, lighter fluid, furniture polish, metal polish, cleaning fluid, and insecticides)	◆ Recognize early signs of toxicity: gagging, choking, coughing, nausea, vomiting, lethargy, drowsiness, weakness, and respiratory symptoms (from inhalation of vapors), including cyanosis, retractions, grunting, and tachypnea.	◆ Maintain a patent airway. ◆ Give nothing by mouth. ◆ Call the poison control center. ◆ Take the child to the emergency department for immediate treatment. ◆ Don't give emetics.
Lead	◆ Risk assessment for lead exposure begins prenatally and continues through childhood to age 6. Identify high-risk groups by screening for pica (an abnormal desire to eat substances, such as lead paint and hair) and an environment high in lead. (Universal blood screening is recommended for infants and children ages 6 months to 6 years.) ◆ Observe for signs of encephalopathy: hyperactivity, aggression, impulsiveness, lethargy, irritability, clumsiness, learning difficulties, short attention span, convulsions, mental retardation, and coma. ◆ Observe for signs of anemia: fatigability, irritability, decreased hemoglobin level, and exercise intolerance. ◆ Observe for signs of renal damage: excretion of glucose, protein, amino acids, and phosphate.	◆ Administer chelating agents (recommended for levels of 45 mcg/dl or more), such as ethylenediamine tetra-acetic acid (EDTA) and dimercaprol (BAL in Oil), which cause lead to be removed from blood and soft tissues, deposited in bone, and excreted in urine. ◆ Give EDTA and dimercaprol in a series of deep I.M. injections in rotating sites; multiple injections may result in painful fibrotic tissues. ◆ Wath for EDTA adverse reactions, including hypocalcemia (resulting in tetany and seizures) and nephrotoxicity (resulting in decreased urine output). ◆ Eliminate lead from the environment; a few chips of paint the size of a thumbnail contain 100 mg of lead (200 times the safe daily dose). Other sources of lead are unglazed pottery, colored newsprint, and painted food wrappers.
Salicylates (such as aspirin)	◆ Determine if ingestion is acute or chronic. ◆ Assess for signs and symptoms of salicylate poisoning, including deep respirations, decreased level of consciousness, dehydration, metabolic acidosis, blood loss, and tinnitus. ◆ Assess the parents' knowledge of proper aspirin administration. ◆ Assess the child's serum salicylate levels; peak levels may vary with enteric coated aspirin.	◆ Maintain a patent airway. ◆ Remove aspirin from the child's stomach by giving ipecac syrup or administering gastric lavage, as ordered. ◆ Administer activated charcoal as ordered to absorb drug in the stomach. ◆ Administer electrolyte solutions and sodium bicarbonate as ordered to correct metabolic acidosis. ◆ Administer diazepam for seizure control. ◆ Offer adequate calories and fluids to meet the child's increased metabolic demands. ◆ Administer vitamin K for bleeding.

stitute for glutathione.) Hepatotoxicity occurs at plasma levels greater than 200 mg/ml at 4 hours after ingestion and greater than 50 mg/ml by 12 hours after ingestion.

Possible causes

Acetaminophen poisoning is caused by acetaminophen overdose. Other substances children commonly ingest include soap, plants, cleaning agents, detergents, vitamins, and other drugs with an appealing flavor.

Assessment findings

- Anorexia
- Nausea
- Diaphoresis
- Liver dysfunction
- Right upper quadrant tenderness and jaundice evident 72 to 96 hours after ingestion
- Shock
- Oliguria
- Pallor
- Hypothermia
- Severe hypoglycemia
- Encephalopathy
- Hepatic failure, death, or resolution of symptoms 7 to 8 days after ingestion

Diagnostic evaluation

- Blood glucose levels are decreased.
- Serum aspartate aminotransferase and serum alanine aminotransferase levels become elevated soon after ingestion.
- Prothrombin time is prolonged.

Nursing diagnoses

- Risk for poisoning
- Risk for imbalanced fluid volume
- Deficient knowledge (childhood growth and development)

Treatment

- Gastric lavage or emesis induction with Ipecac syrup
- Hyperthermia blanket
- I.V. fluid
- Oxygen therapy (intubation and mechanical ventilation may be required)

Drug therapy options

- Mucolytic: acetylcysteine (Mucomyst) in one loading dose and 17 maintenance doses
- Emetic: Ipecac syrup

Planning and goals

- The child will regain normal liver function.
- The child will regain fluid and electrolyte balance.
- The child will regain a normal energy level.
- The child's parents will verbalize understanding of emergency measures to take for a child with acute acetaminophen poisoning.
- The child's parents will learn how to childproof their home to prevent accidental poisonings.

Implementation

- Monitor liver function studies immediately and 3 and 6 months after the incident *to detect signs of liver damage and monitor the treatment's effectiveness.*
- Monitor vital signs and intake and output every 1 to 4 hours. *Tachycardia and decreased urine output may signify dehydration.*
- Assess cardiovascular and GI status *to detect the treatment's effectiveness.*
- Administer hyperthermia therapy by using a warming blanket, limiting exposure during routine nursing care, and covering the child with warm blankets *to help the child become normothermic.*
- Administer acetylcysteine in a juice. *Acetylcysteine has an offensive odor and taste. Administering this drug in juice will help the child swallow it. For young children, administer it directly into an NG tube to avoid this difficulty.*
- Record fluid intake and output. *Monitoring the child's fluid balance helps evaluate for signs of fluid retention and decreased urine output, which can be caused by hepatic failure. Vomiting and anorexia may also decrease urine output, further complicating fluid balance assessment.*
- Monitor the child's activity level and LOC *to assess for signs of hepatic coma (the most severe stage of hepatic toxicity), indicated by reduced activity level and altered LOC.*

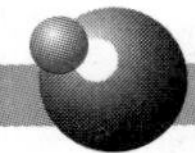

SPOT CHECK

What's the best way to administer acetylcysteine?

Answer: Acetylcysteine has an offensive odor and taste so administering it in juice helps a child to swallow it. For a young child, you may need to use an NG tube.

- Encourage the parents to express their feelings about circumstances surrounding the poisoning *to help them resolve feelings of guilt and refocus their attention on promoting the child's recovery and health.*
- Teach the child's parents about poison control measures, such as keeping ipecac syrup in the home, placing the telephone number for the poison control center near

the telephone, and viewing the home from a toddler's eye level to find hazards. *Poisoning is an emergency. Advance preparation can lead to earlier intervention, resulting in milder toxicity.*
– Teach the parents to store all medications and drugs out of the child's reach and sight. List several examples of over-the-counter medications, such as aspirin and cold remedies, *because many people don't realize these products contain potent drugs.*
– Caution the parents not to store drugs in containers without safety caps if small children are part of the household.
– Instruct the parents to teach their children not to take nonfood items without supervision.
– Instruct the parents to read the labels of cold remedies for ingredients, recommended dosages, and contraindications.

◆ Explain all procedures and treatments to the parents *to reduce anxiety.*
◆ Consult with social service workers *to evaluate the home environment.*

Evaluation

◆ The child regains fluid and electrolyte balance and normal liver function and returns home free from complications.
◆ The child's parents have made their home childproof.
◆ The family doesn't experience another accidental poisoning.

ANEMIA, IRON DEFICIENCY

ANEMIA is a reduction in the volume of red blood cells (RBCs) in the body usually measured as a decrease in hemoglobin concentration. Because hemoglobin is the red pigment in RBCs that transports oxygen, any decrease diminishes the blood's capacity to carry oxygen to tissues and vital organs throughout the body. Anemia is the most common hematologic disorder in infants and children. Symptoms of anemia result from tissue hypoxia and the body's compensatory response.

Iron deficiency anemia, the most prevalent nutritional disorder in the United States, occurs most commonly in children between ages 6 months and 2 years (iron stores are depleted between the 5th and 6th month) and again during adolescence. Iron deficiency anemia is characterized by poor RBC production. Insufficient body stores of iron lead to:

◆ depleted RBC mass
◆ decreased hemoglobin concentration (hypochromia)
◆ decreased oxygen-carrying capacity of the blood.

In the early stages of iron deficiency anemia, the child may be asymptomatic. Compensatory mechanisms effectively prevent most overt symptoms at that point. Blood viscosity is reduced because the number of RBCs is reduced. Such hemodilution results in decreased peripheral resistance, which increases the volume of blood returned to the heart. The cardiac workload increases as the heart pumps faster to circulate the thinned blood. If the condition persists, the heart may enlarge and have a functional systolic murmur. Increased cardiac output (from tachycardia and cardiac dilatation) compensates for the decreased number of RBCs. However, with exercise, infection, emotional stress, or circulatory overload, cardiac failure may occur.

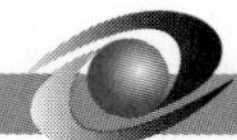

QUICK STUDY

Think **PLATE** to remember key blood components:

Plasma
Leukocytes
AB antigens
Thrombocytes
Erythrocytes

Possible causes

◆ Blood loss secondary to drug-induced GI bleeding (from anticoagulants, aspirin, steroids) or due to heavy menses, hemorrhage from trauma, GI ulcers, or cancer
◆ Inadequate dietary intake of iron, which may occur following prolonged nonsupplemented breast-feeding or bottle-feeding of infants, or during periods of stress such as rapid growth in children and adolescents
◆ Iron malabsorption, as in chronic diarrhea, partial or total gastrectomy, and malabsorption syndromes, such as celiac disease and pernicious anemia
◆ Intravascular hemolysis-induced hemoglobinuria or paroxysmal nocturnal hemoglobinuria
◆ Fad diets and poor nutritional choices and eating habits in adolescents
◆ Mechanical erythrocyte trauma caused by a prosthetic heart valve or vena cava filters
◆ Lead poisoning

Assessment findings

Anemia progresses gradually, and many children are initially asymptomatic, except for symptoms of an underlying condition. Symptoms can be vague and insidious. Children with advanced anemia display:

◆ pallor
◆ irritability
◆ fatigue
◆ dyspnea on exertion
◆ inability to concentrate

- listlessness
- headache
- susceptibility to infection
- tachycardia
- growth retardation
- edema.

With chronic iron deficiency anemia, children may also display:

- numbness and tingling of the extremities
- vasomotor disturbances
- neuralgic pain
- cracks in corners of the mouth
- smooth tongue
- spoon-shaped, brittle nails
- dysphagia
- signs of infection, such as tugging at the ear (otitis media), runny nose, reluctance to swallow (sore throat), coughing, sneezing, and elevated temperature.

Diagnostic evaluation

- Bone marrow studies reveal depleted or absent iron stores and normoblastic hyperplasia.
- Hemoglobin level, hematocrit, and serum ferritin level are low.
- Mean corpuscular hemoglobin level is decreased in severe anemia.
- RBC count is low, with microcytic and hypochromic cells. In early stages, RBC count may be normal, except in infants and children.
- Serum iron levels are low, with high binding capacity.
- Positive fecal occult blood test (Hemoccult) results can indicate chronic hidden blood loss, which is a cause of anemia.

Nursing diagnoses

- Imbalanced nutrition: Less than body requirements
- Impaired gas exchange
- Risk for infection
- Delayed growth and development
- Activity intolerance

Treatment

For children and adolescents, treatment consists of increasing iron intake by adding iron-rich foods to the diet. For infants, iron supplements are added.

Drug therapy options

- Oral iron preparation or a combination of iron and ascorbic acid (which enhances iron absorption); iron dextran (InFeD), if additional therapy is needed
- Vitamin B_{12} (cyanocobalamin), if intrinsic factor is lacking

Infant iron needs

An infant should receive only breast milk or commercial formula with iron until age 6 months. From age 6 months to 1 year, the infant receives breast milk or iron-fortified formula and cereal with a gradual introduction of other baby foods.

As a rule, an infant should receive no more than 32 oz of milk per day. One quart of milk provides only 0.5 mg of iron, whereas 1 tbs of fortified baby cereal provides 2.5 to 5 mg of iron. Infants with iron deficiency anemia should receive no more than 16 oz of milk per day, because it's deficient in iron, zinc, and vitamin C and has a high renal solute load.

Planning and goals

- The child won't develop cardiac complications from the anemia.
- The child's iron intake will increase sufficiently to replace depleted stores and to maintain RBC production.
- The child will remain free from infection.
- The child's parents will verbalize understanding of a nutritionally balanced diet that has recommended amounts of iron.
- The child will return to physical activity levels that are appropriate to his developmental age.

Implementation

- Carefully assess a child's drug history. *Certain drugs, such as pancreatic enzymes and vitamin E, may interfere with iron metabolism and absorption; other drugs, such as aspirin and steroids, can cause GI bleeding.*
- Provide passive stimulation; allow frequent rest; give small, frequent feedings; and elevate the head of the bed *to decrease oxygen demands.*
- Implement proper hand washing *to decrease the risk of infection.*
- Provide foods high in iron (liver; dark, leafy vegetables; and whole grains) *to replenish iron stores.* (See *Infant iron needs.*)
- Monitor the infant for signs of infection *to identify complications from inadequate nutrition.*
- Administer iron before meals with citrus juice. *Iron is best absorbed in an acidic environment.*
- Give liquid iron through a straw *to prevent staining the child's skin and teeth.* For infants, administer by oral syringe toward the back of the mouth.

◆ Don't give iron with milk products. *Milk products may interfere with iron absorption.*
◆ Monitor the child's cardiac function *to identify signs of increased cardiac workload, such as tachycardia or tachypnea, which may lead to cardiac failure.*
◆ Monitor reticulocyte count *to evaluate the child's response to treatment.* The reticulocyte count should begin to increase approximately 1 week after beginning iron supplements.
◆ Be supportive of family members and keep them informed of the child's status *to decrease anxiety.*
◆ Review key teaching topics with family members *to ensure adequate knowledge about the condition and treatment,* including:
– keeping iron supplements safely stored out of the child's reach at home
– brushing teeth after iron administration
– reporting reactions to iron supplementation, such as nausea, vomiting, diarrhea, constipation, fever, or severe stomach pain, which may require a dosage adjustment
– providing a nutritionally balanced diet with adequate amounts of iron.
◆ Consult with a registered dietician to assist parents with understanding nutritional needs and providing an adequate diet.

Evaluation

◆ The child doesn't develop cardiac decompensation.
◆ The child's reticulocyte count indicates rapid RBC proliferation; RBC and hemoglobin levels are within the normal range.
◆ The child demonstrates appropriate physical and emotional development for his age.
◆ The child's parents verbalize understanding that they must provide a balanced, iron-rich diet.
◆ The child is free from infection at discharge.

CONGENITAL HEART DISEASE, ACYANOTIC

Congenital heart disease occurs in approximately 8 to 10 of every 1,000 live births and — like prematurity — is a major cause of death in the first year. There are two types of congenital heart defects (based on alteration in blood flow): acyanotic, in which deoxygenated blood isn't mixed in the systemic circulation (the child doesn't appear blue), and cyanotic, in which deoxygenated blood is mixed in the systemic circulation (the child usually appears blue or dusky). Congenital heart defects may be further categorized by normal, decreased, or increased pulmonary blood flow. (See *Common congenital heart defects,* page 270.)

In an acyanotic defect, blood is usually shunted from the left (oxygenated) side of the heart to the right (unoxygenated) side. Acyanotic defects include:
◆ AORTIC STENOSIS — a narrowing or fusion of the aortic valves, interfering with left ventricular outflow
◆ ATRIAL SEPTAL DEFECT — a defect stemming from a patent foramen ovale or the failure of a septum to develop completely between the atria (an abnormal opening between the right and left atria)
◆ COARCTATION OF THE AORTA — a narrowing of the aortic arch, usually distal to the ductus arteriosus beyond the left subclavian artery
◆ PATENT DUCTUS ARTERIOSUS — a defect resulting from the failure of the ductus to close, causing shunting of blood to the pulmonary artery
◆ PULMONARY ARTERY STENOSIS — a narrowing or fusing of valve leaflets at the entrance of the pulmonary artery, interfering with right ventricular outflow
◆ VENTRICULAR SEPTAL DEFECT — a defect occurring when the ventricular septum fails to complete its formation between the ventricles, resulting in a left-to-right shunt.

Possible causes

◆ Defects between structures that inhibit blood flow to the system or alter pulmonary resistance
◆ Defects in the septa that lead to left-to-right shunt

Assessment findings

◆ Congested cough
◆ Diaphoresis
◆ Fatigue
◆ Frequent respiratory infections
◆ Hepatomegaly
◆ Machinelike heart murmur (in patent ductus arteriosus)
◆ Mild cyanosis (if the condition leads to right-sided heart failure)
◆ Poor growth and development due to increased energy expenditure for breathing
◆ Respiratory distress
◆ Tachycardia
◆ Tachypnea

Diagnostic evaluation

◆ Chest X-ray results and cardiac catheterization are used to confirm the type of acyanotic heart defect:
– In *aortic stenosis,* chest X-ray shows left ventricular hypertrophy and prominent pulmonary vasculature. Cardiac catheterization is used to determine the degree of shunting and extent of pulmonary vascular disease.

Common congenital heart defects

The illustrations below show common congenital heart defects along with a description of each.

Major acyanotic defects

Atrial septal defect

An abnormal opening between the right and left atria

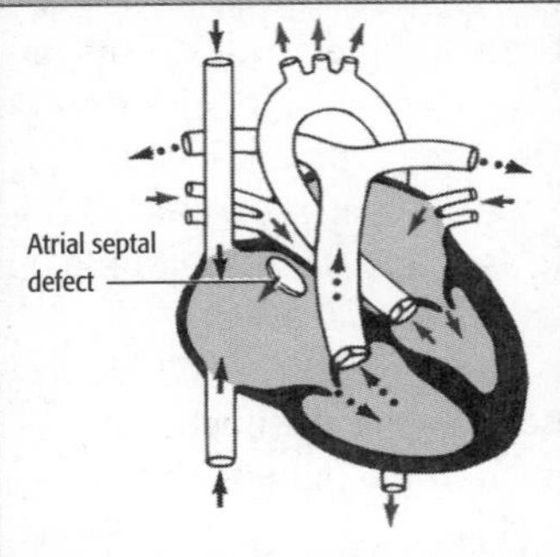

Coarctation of the aorta

A narrowing of the aortic lumen that results in a preductal or postductal obstruction

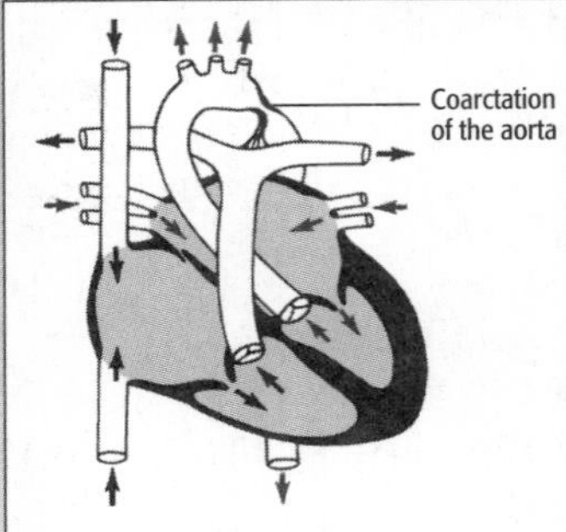

Patent ductus arteriosus

A defect resulting from the failure of the ductus to close, causing shunting of blood to the pulmonary artery

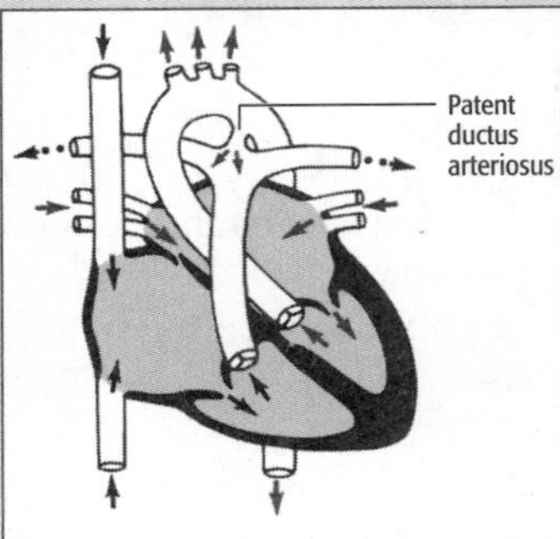

Ventricular septal defect

An abnormal opening between the right and left ventricles

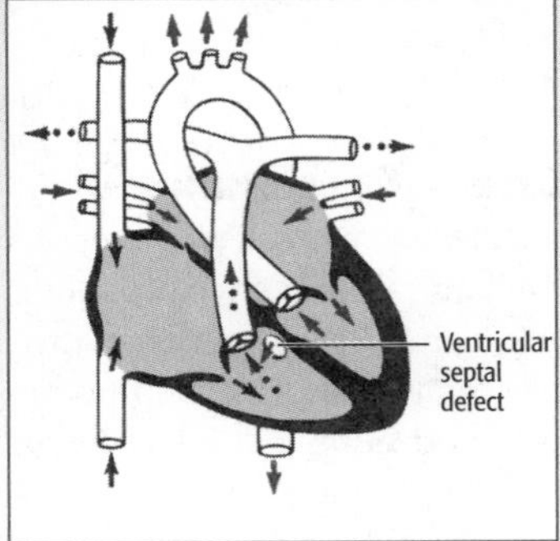

Major cyanotic defects

Complete transposition of great vessels

A defect in which the aorta arises from the right ventricle and the pulmonary artery arises from the left ventricle

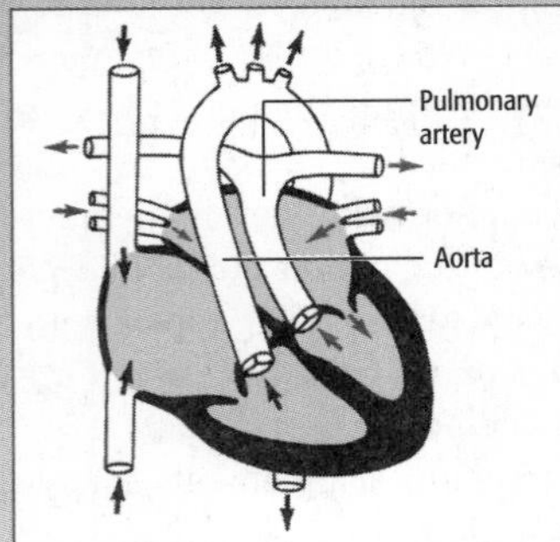

Tetralogy of Fallot

A combination of four defects: pulmonic stenosis, ventricular septal defect, overriding aorta, and hypertrophy of the right ventricle

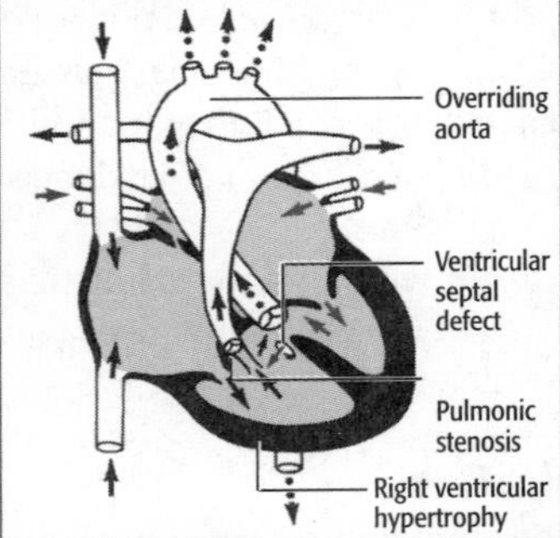

Tricuspid atresia

Characterized by absence of tricuspid valve and no blood flow between the right atrium and right ventricle, a small right ventricle a large left ventricle, and, usually, diminished pulmonary circulation

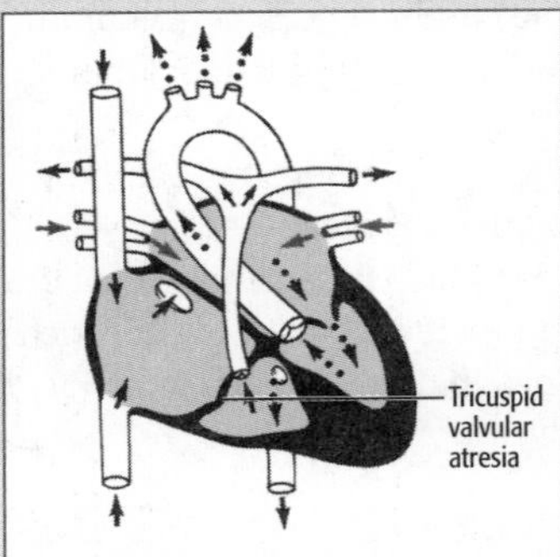

Truncus arteriosus

Normal septation of the embryologic bulbar trunk into an aorta and pulmonary artery doesn't occur. A single arterial trunk overrides the ventricles and receives blood from them through a ventricular septal defect.

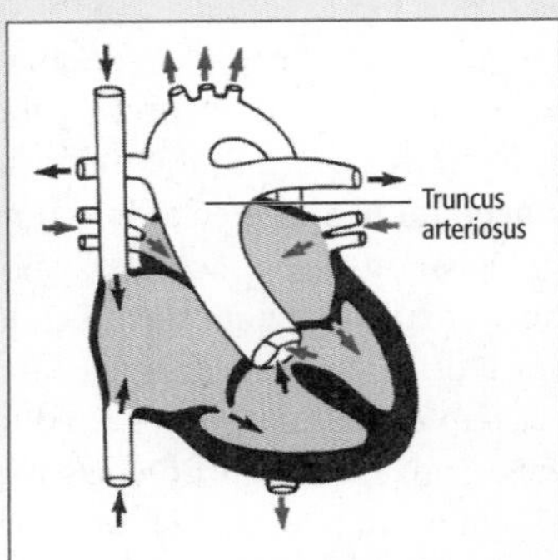

– In *atrial septal defect,* chest X-ray shows an enlarged right atrium and ventricle and prominent pulmonary vasculature. Cardiac catheterization shows right atrial blood that's more oxygenated than superior vena cava blood. It's also used to determine the degree of shunting and extent of pulmonary vascular disease.
– In *coarctation of the aorta,* chest X-ray shows left ventricular hypertrophy, wide ascending and descending aorta, and prominent collateral circulation. Cardiac catheterization shows affected collateral circulation and pressures in the right and left ventricles.
– In *patent ductus arteriosus,* chest X-ray shows prominent pulmonary vasculature and enlargement of the left ventricle and aorta. Cardiac catheterization is used to determine the extent of pulmonary vascular disease and shows an oxygen content higher in the pulmonary artery than in the right ventricle.
– In *pulmonary artery stenosis,* chest X-ray shows right ventricular hypertrophy. Cardiac catheterization is used to gather evidence about the degree of shunting.
– In *ventricular septal defect,* chest X-ray may be normal for small defects or show cardiomegaly with a large left atrium and ventricle. In a large defect, chest X-ray may show prominent pulmonary vasculature. Cardiac catheterization is used to determine the size and exact location of the ventricular septal defect and the degree of shunting.

Nursing diagnoses

◆ Decreased cardiac output
◆ Impaired gas exchange
◆ Risk for infection
◆ Anxiety
◆ Deficient knowledge (childhood growth and development)

Treatment

◆ For *aortic stenosis:* surgery (valvulotomy or commissurotomy)
◆ For *atrial septal defect:* surgery to patch the hole (Mild defects may close spontaneously.)
◆ For *coarctation of the aorta:* inoperable if coarctation is proximal to the ductus arteriosus; closed heart resection if coarctation is distal to the ductus arteriosus
◆ For *patent ductus arteriosus:* ligation of the patent ductus arteriosus in closed-heart operation
◆ For *pulmonary artery stenosis:* open-heart surgery to separate the pulmonary valve leaflets
◆ For *ventricular septal defect:* pulmonary artery banding to prevent heart failure and permanent correction with a patch, later, when heart is larger (Spontaneous closure of the ventricular septal defect occurs in some children by age 3.)

Drug therapy options

◆ Antiarrhythmic: digoxin (Lanoxin)
◆ Diuretic: furosemide (Lasix)
◆ Non-steroidal anti-inflammatory drug: indomethacin (Indocin) to achieve pharmacologic closure in patent ductus arteriosus
◆ Prophylactic antibiotics to prevent endocarditis

Planning and goals

◆ The child will remain free from infection.
◆ The child will exhibit signs of improved gas exchange and cardiac output.
◆ The child and family members will exhibit decreased anxiety.
◆ The child will maintain age-appropriate activities.
◆ Members of the child's family will verbalize knowledge about the disorder, treatment, home care, and how to contact appropriate community resources.

Implementation

◆ Explain the heart defect and answer questions *to prepare the child for cardiac catheterization.*
◆ Monitor vital signs, pulse oximetry, and intake and output *to assess renal function and detect change.*
◆ Assess cardiovascular and respiratory status *to detect early signs of decompensation.*
◆ Take apical pulse for 1 minute before giving digoxin and withhold the drug if the heart rate is less than 100 beats/minute (which indicates bradycardia in an infant) *to prevent toxicity.*
◆ Monitor fluid status, enforcing fluid restrictions as appropriate *to prevent fluid overload.*
◆ Weigh the child daily *to determine fluid overload or deficit.*
◆ Organize physical care and anticipate the child's needs *to reduce the child's oxygen demands.*
◆ Give the child high-calorie, easy-to-chew, and easy-to-digest foods *to maintain adequate nutrition and decrease oxygen demands.*
◆ Maintain normal body temperature *to prevent cold stress.*
◆ Raise the head of the bed or place the child in an infant car seat *to ease breathing.*
◆ Prepare the child and parents for the sights and sounds of the intensive care unit (ICU) *to reduce anxiety.*

Evaluation

- The child's incision site remains free from infection.
- The child remains free from respiratory infections and endocarditis.
- The child exhibits normal respirations and adequate oxygen saturation.
- The child exhibits no signs of heart failure, no evidence of severe skin mottling, adequate urine output, and a normal liver on palpation.
- The child and family members exhibit decreased anxiety.
- The child takes part in age-appropriate activities.
- Family members express concerns, ask appropriate questions about the child's condition, and participate in the child's care.
- The parents demonstrate knowledge and understanding of management of the child's cardiac condition.

CONGENITAL HEART DISEASE, CYANOTIC

Cyanotic heart defects include:

- TRANSPOSITION OF THE GREAT VESSELS or arteries — a defect in which the aorta arises from the right ventricle and the pulmonary artery arises from the left ventricle
- TETRALOGY OF FALLOT — a defect consisting of pulmonary artery stenosis, ventricular septal defect, hypertrophy of the right ventricle, and an overriding aorta
- hypoplastic left heart syndrome (HLHS) — a defect consisting of aortic valve atresia, mitral atresia or stenosis, diminutive or absent left ventricle, and severe hypoplasia of the ascending aorta and aortic arch
- TRICUSPID VALVULAR ATRESIA — a defect characterized by absence of the tricuspid valve and no blood flow between the right atrium and right ventricle, a small right ventricle, and a large left ventricle and, usually, diminished pulmonary circulation.

The skin of a child with a cyanotic heart disease usually appears blue or dusky because unoxygenated blood or a mixture of oxygenated and unoxygenated blood is shunted through the cardiovascular system. This shunting can lead to left-sided heart failure, decreased oxygen supply to the body, and the development of collateral circulation. (See *Common congenital heart defects,* page 270.)

Possible causes

- Any condition that increases pulmonary vascular resistance
- Structural defects

Assessment findings

- Cyanosis
- Crouching position assumed frequently
- History of inadequate feeding
- Clubbing
- Increasing cyanosis as the foramen ovale or ductus arteriosus closes (in transposition of the great vessels), leading to loss of consciousness, also known as a *tet spell* (in tetralogy of Fallot)
- Increasing dyspnea, cyanosis, and tachypnea during the first few days after birth; without treatment, heart failure after closure of the ductus (in HLHS).
- Irritability
- Tachycardia
- Tachypnea

Diagnostic evaluation

- ABG analysis shows diminished arterial oxygen saturation.
- Cardiac catheterization results confirm the diagnosis by allowing visualization of defects and measurement of oxygen saturation level. (See *Caring for a child with cardiac catheterization.*)
- Complete blood count (CBC) shows polycythemia. (Hypoxia stimulates the body to increase RBC production.)

Nursing diagnoses

- Decreased cardiac output
- Impaired gas exchange
- Risk for infection
- Anxiety
- Deficient knowledge (childhood growth and development)

Treatment

For transposition of the great vessels or arteries

- Corrective surgery to redirect blood flow by switching the position of the major blood vessels (performed around age 1)
- Palliative surgery to provide communication between the chambers

For tetralogy of Fallot

- Complete repair or palliative treatment during the first year to increase blood flow to the lungs by bypassing pulmonic stenosis (Blalock-Taussig shunt to connect the right pulmonary artery to the right subclavian artery)
- Oxygen therapy
- Repair of ventricular septal defect and stenosis (possibly done in stages)

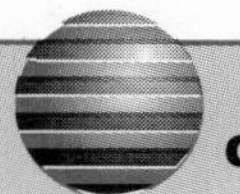

CLINICAL SITUATION

Caring for a child with cardiac catheterization

A 2½-year-old child is admitted to the hospital for cardiac catheterization. He was diagnosed in infancy as having tetralogy of Fallot, the most common cyanotic heart defect, and underwent his first catheterization at that time. This procedure is performed to determine pressure readings and the degree of oxygen saturation in the chambers and major vessels and to release a radiopaque contrast medium that allows fluoroscopic visualization of the heart.

The child is being reevaluated and will have corrective surgery as soon as it can be scheduled. He's small for his age and appears dusky, with cyanotic lips and nail beds, although he isn't in acute distress.

What are appropriate nursing interventions after catheterization?

◆ Measure and record the child's vital signs every 15 minutes until stable or as ordered. Monitor for arrhythmias. The immediate post-catheterization period can be precarious, with complications developing rapidly. *Early detection of unstable vital signs can prevent more serious complications.*

◆ Examine pressure dressings *to check for bleeding* every time you measure and record vital signs. Check the sheets for blood and wetness under the limb used in catheterization *because the pressure dressing can cause blood to flow under the body part used.* Keep the limb straight *because movement can disrupt the arterial closure and initiate bleeding.*

◆ Measure and record pulse quality in *all* distal extremities, and compare with that of the limb used in catheterization. Mark the location of pedal pulses with a ballpoint or felt-tipped pen. *Comparing pulse quality helps detect diminished circulation in the affected extremity.* The circulation may be impaired by thrombosis, hematoma, or vessel reaction to the contrast medium or the catheter. *The pen mark helps locate the pedal pulses for consistency between caregivers.*

◆ Assess the child's overall skin color as well as the color and temperature of extremities, *which helps to detect diminished circulation in the affected extremity.* This decrease may indicate arterial obstruction. Monitor oxygen saturation levels *to identify abnormalities.*

◆ Provide the child with small sips of water, gradually increasing the amount as tolerated. *Large sips or gulping may produce vomiting and aspiration if the child isn't fully awake.*

◆ Maintain I.V. intake as ordered, monitoring closely for dehydration. *The contrast medium has a diuretic effect that, combined with the child's nothing-by-mouth status and blood loss during catheterization, puts him at risk for hypovolemia and dehydration.*

◆ Keep the child in bed for 3 to 4 hours after catheterization. Immobilize the affected leg or arm, keeping it as straight as possible. Provide a calm, quiet environment. *Immobility reduces the likelihood of bleeding at the catheterization site. A calm, quiet environment prevents undue excitement and promotes rest and recovery.* The parents may hold the child, keeping the affected limb in the correct position.

◆ Keep the child comfortably warm; avoid overheating or chilling. *Overheating causes peripheral vasodilation, and chilling may cause vasoconstriction. Either of these conditions can precipitate bleeding at the catheter insertion site.*

◆ Prepare the parents and child for discharge. Teach them to keep the catheterization insertion site clean and dry and to cover it with a bandage *to help prevent infection at the site.*

Questions for further thought

◆ What are appropriate nursing diagnoses for this child on admission?

◆ What are appropriate goals and outcomes for treatment?

For HLHS

◆ Heart transplantation

◆ Surgical restructuring of the heart (two-step procedure) (Without surgery, death occurs in early infancy.)

For tricuspid valvular atresia

◆ Systemic to pulmonary shunt or pulmonary artery banding

◆ Surgery to join the superior vena cava and right pulmonary artery

◆ Conduit surgical procedure to bypass the right ventricle, thus diverting systemic venous blood to the main pulmonary artery

Drug therapy options

◆ Analgesic: morphine during tet spell

◆ Beta-adrenergic blocking agent: propranolol (Inderal) as prophylactic

◆ Vasodilator prostaglandin E1 inhibitor (Indomethacin) to keep the ductus arteriosus patent

Planning and goals

- The child will remain free from infection.
- The child will exhibit signs of improved gas exchange and cardiac output.
- The child and family members will exhibit decreased anxiety.
- The child will maintain age-appropriate activities.
- Members of the child's family will verbalize knowledge about the disorder, treatment, home care, and how to contact appropriate community resources.

Implementation

- Assess cardiovascular and respiratory status *to detect early signs of compromise.*
- Monitor vital signs and pulse oximetry *to detect hypoxia.*
- Monitor intake and output *to assess renal status.*
- Provide oxygen when necessary *to compensate for impaired oxygen exchange.*
- Anticipate needs and prevent distress *to decrease oxygen demands on the child.*
- Use a nipple designed for premature infants *to decrease the energy needed for sucking.*
- Provide adequate hydration *to prevent sequelae of polycythemia.*
- Administer prophylactic antibiotics *to prevent endocarditis.*
- Provide thorough skin care *to prevent skin breakdown.*
- Prepare the child for cardiac catheterization *to decrease anxiety.*
- Prepare the child and his parents for the sights and sounds of the ICU *to decrease anxiety.*
- Explain the difference between palliative and corrective procedures to the child's parents *to improve knowledge regarding diagnosis and treatment.*
- Consult with the case manager *to ensure support services are available when the child goes home.*

Evaluation

- The child's incision site remains free from infection.
- The child remains free from respiratory infections and endocarditis.
- The child exhibits normal respirations and adequate oxygen saturation.
- The child exhibits no signs of heart failure, no evidence of severe skin mottling, adequate urine output, and a normal liver on palpation.
- The child and family members exhibit decreased anxiety.
- The child takes part in age-appropriate activities.
- Family members express concerns, ask appropriate questions about the child's condition, and participate in the child's care.
- The child's parents demonstrate knowledge of and ability to provide care for their child.

CROUP

CROUP is a group of related upper airway respiratory conditions that commonly affect toddlers. It includes acute spasmodic laryngitis, acute obstructive laryngitis, and acute laryngotracheobronchitis.

Possible causes

- Virus-induced edema around the larynx

Assessment findings

- Barking, brassy cough or hoarseness, sometimes described as a "seal bark" cough
- Inspiratory stridor with varying degrees of respiratory distress
- Condition usually begins at night and during cold weather and frequently recurs
- Crackles and decreased breath sounds (indicate the condition has progressed to bronchi)
- Increased dyspnea and lower accessory muscle use
- Onset may be sudden or gradual

Diagnostic evaluation

- If bacterial infection is the cause, throat cultures may identify the organisms and their sensitivity to antibiotics as well as rule out diphtheria.
- Laryngoscopy may reveal inflammation and obstruction in epiglottal and laryngeal areas.
- Neck X-ray shows areas of upper airway narrowing and edema in subglottic folds and rules out the possibility of foreign body obstruction as well as masses and cysts.

Nursing diagnoses

- Impaired gas exchange
- Ineffective breathing pattern
- Ineffective airway clearance
- Risk for imbalanced fluid volume
- Anxiety

Treatment

- Clear liquid diet to keep mucus thin
- Cool humidification during sleep with a cool mist tent or a room humidifier
- Rest from activity
- Tracheostomy and oxygen administration

Drug therapy options

- Antipyretic: acetaminophen (Tylenol)
- Inhaled racemic epinephrine
- Corticosteroid: nebulizer or parenteral glucocorticoids for respiratory distress

Planning and goals

- The child will maintain adequate ventilation as evidenced by relief of respiratory distress.
- The child's temperature will be within normal range.
- The child will maintain a patent airway.
- The child's parents will demonstrate an understanding of the illness and treatment.
- The child's parents will use available support systems to assist with coping.

Implementation

- Assess respiratory and cardiovascular status *to detect indications that obstruction is worsening.*
- Monitor vital signs and pulse oximetry *to detect early signs of respiratory compromise.*
- Administer oxygen therapy and provide cool mist, if needed. *Cool mist helps liquefy secretions.*
- Administer medications, as ordered, and note effectiveness *to maintain or improve the child's condition.*
- Provide emotional support to the parents *to decrease anxiety.*
- Provide age-appropriate activities for the child *to ease anxiety.*
- Monitor for rebound obstruction when administering racemic epinephrine; *the drug's effects are short-term and may result in rebound obstruction.*

Evaluation

- The child's respirations return to normal with no further signs of respiratory distress.
- The child's vital signs are within normal range.
- The child's parents verbalize an understanding of methods to decrease laryngeal spasm, such as taking the child into the bathroom, turning on the shower, and letting the room fill with steam.
- The child's parents demonstrate appropriate coping.

DOWN SYNDROME

The first disorder researchers attributed to a chromosomal aberration, DOWN SYNDROME is characterized by:

- mental retardation
- dysmorphic facial features
- other distinctive physical abnormalities (60% of clients have congenital heart defects, respiratory infections, chronic myelogenous leukemia, and a weak immune response to infection).

Possible causes

- Genetic nondisjunction, with three chromosomes on the 21st pair (total of 47 chromosomes)

Risk factors

- Maternal age (the older the mother, the greater the risk of genetic nondisjunction)

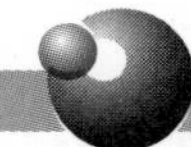

SPOT CHECK

What's the most probable cause of Down syndrome?

Answer: Down syndrome usually results from trisomy 21, in which chromosome 21 has three copies instead of two (normal), resulting in a karyotype of 47 chromosomes, instead of the normal 46.

Assessment findings

- Brushfield's spots (marbling and speckling of the iris)
- Flat nose and low-set ears
- Hypotonia
- Mild to moderate retardation
- Protruding tongue (because of a small oral cavity)
- Short stature with pudgy hands
- Simian crease (a single crease across the palm)
- Small skull
- Upward-slanting eyes

Diagnostic evaluation

- Amniocentesis allows prenatal diagnosis. It's recommended for women older than age 34 regardless of a negative family history, or a woman of any age if she or the father carries a translocated chromosome.
- Karyotyping shows the specific chromosomal abnormality.

Nursing diagnoses

- Delayed growth and development
- Risk for injury
- Risk for aspiration
- Ineffective coping

Treatment

- Treatments for skeletal, immunologic, metabolic, biochemical, and oncologic disorders, depending on specific problem
- Treatment for coexisting conditions — congenital heart problems, visual defects, or hypothyroidism
- Therapies to optimize child's growth and development

Drug therapy options

◆ Megavitamin therapy: promotes growth and development potential (controversial)

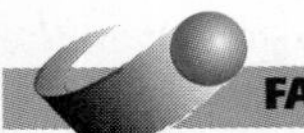

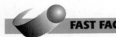

FAST FACT

Special education programs, available in most communities, permit the child with Down syndrome to maximize his potential and promote self-esteem. His physical condition and self-image can also benefit from special athletic programs.

Planning and goals

◆ The child will demonstrate age-appropriate skills and behaviors to the extent possible.
◆ The child will participate in developmental stimulation programs to increase skill levels.
◆ The child's parents will express an understanding of norms for growth and development.
◆ The child's parents will express an understanding of the condition and demonstrate appropriate coping.

Implementation

◆ Provide activities appropriate for the child *to support optimal development.*
◆ Set realistic, reachable, short-term goals; break tasks into small steps *to encourage their successful accomplishment.*
◆ Use behavior modification, if applicable, *to promote safety and prevent injury to the child and others.*
◆ Provide stimulation and communicate at a level appropriate to the child's mental age rather than chronological age *to promote a healthy emotional environment.*
◆ Provide a safe environment *to prevent injury.*
◆ Mainstream daily routines *to promote normalcy.*
◆ Consult with social services to provide services t*o optimize outcome for the child,* such as physical therapy, occupational therapy, speech therapy, early intervention, and home care.

Evaluation

◆ The child's potential is maximized through stimulation and learning.
◆ The child's parents express knowledge of the condition and seek treatment for any coexisting conditions.
◆ The child's parents demonstrate appropriate coping, such as using support groups and contacting early intervention programs.

DUCHENNE'S MUSCULAR DYSTROPHY

A genetic disorder that occurs only in males, DUCHENNE'S MUSCULAR DYSTROPHY (also called pseudohypertrophic dystrophy) is marked by muscular deterioration that progresses throughout childhood. It generally results in death from cardiac or respiratory failure in the late teens or early 20s due to a defect on the X chromosome, resulting in a lack of production of dystrophin. The absence of dystrophin results in breakdown of muscle fibers. Muscle fibers are replaced with fatty deposits and collagen in muscles. There's no known cure.

Possible causes

◆ Sex-linked recessive trait

Assessment findings

◆ Begins with pelvic girdle weakness, indicated by waddling gait and falling
◆ GOWERS' SIGN (use of hands to push self up from floor)
◆ Eventual muscle weakness and wasting
◆ Cardiac or pulmonary failure
◆ Decreased ability to perform self-care activities
◆ Delayed motor development
◆ Eventual contractures and muscle hypertrophy

Diagnostic evaluation

◆ Electromyography typically demonstrates short, weak bursts of electrical activity in affected muscles.
◆ Muscle biopsy shows variations in the size of muscle fibers and, in later stages, fat and connective tissue deposits with no dystrophin.

Nursing diagnoses

◆ Impaired physical mobility
◆ Impaired walking
◆ Impaired gas exchange
◆ Compromised family coping

Treatment

◆ High-fiber, high-protein, low-calorie diet
◆ Physical therapy
◆ Surgery to correct contractures
◆ Use of devices, such as splints, braces, trapeze bars, overhead slings, and a wheelchair to help preserve mobility

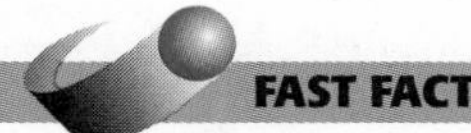

FAST FACT

The primary focus of treatment in Duchenne's muscular dystrophy is to help the child remain as active and independent as possible.

Planning and goals

- ◆ The child will maintain muscle strength.
- ◆ The child will maintain joint mobility and ROM.
- ◆ The child will show no evidence of complications.
- ◆ The child will achieve the highest level of mobility possible within the confines of the disease.
- ◆ The child will remain as active and independent as possible.
- ◆ The child will maintain normal cardiorespiratory status for as long as possible.
- ◆ The child's parents will recognize the early signs of respiratory complications, such as tachypnea and use of accessory muscles to breathe.

Implementation

- ◆ Perform ROM exercises *to promote joint mobility.*
- ◆ Provide age-appropriate activities *to promote growth and development.*
- ◆ Provide emotional support to the child and parents *to decrease anxiety and promote coping mechanisms.*
- ◆ Initiate genetic counseling *to inform the child and family about passing the disorder on to future children.*
- ◆ Allow the child to perform activities of daily living as able *to promote independence.*
- ◆ If respiratory involvement occurs, encourage coughing and deep-breathing exercises, and diaphragmatic breathing *to maintain a patent airway and mobilize secretions to prevent complications associated with retained secretions.*
- ◆ Encourage use of a footboard or high-topped sneakers and a foot cradle *to increase comfort and prevent footdrop.*
- ◆ Encourage adequate fluid intake, increase dietary fiber, and obtain an order for a stool softener *to prevent constipation associated with inactivity.*
- ◆ Consult social services *to assist in discharge planning and to meet the needs of the child.*

Evaluation

- ◆ The child maintains muscle strength, joint mobility, and ROM to the fullest degree possible.
- ◆ The child's parents verbalize an understanding of the disease and keep the child as active and involved as possible.
- ◆ The child's parents verbalize an understanding of possible respiratory complications and how to handle a respiratory infection. Urge the parents to report signs of infection to the physician immediately.

HIRSCHSPRUNG'S DISEASE

In HIRSCHSPRUNG'S DISEASE, also known as *congenital aganglionic megacolon,* a portion of the colon lacks ganglionic cells and the peristaltic waves needed to pass feces through that segment of the colon. The result is chronic constipation as stool accumulates proximal to the aganglionic segment, which is narrowed. However, the child may pass small ribbonlike stools through the narrow segment despite the internal sphincter's failure to relax. Hirschsprung's disease is four times more common in boys than girls and it occurs in 1 out of 5,000 births. (See *Causes of lower bowel obstruction,* pages 278 and 279.)

Possible causes

- ◆ Lack of ganglionic cells (which normally form along the digestive tract of the fetus between the 5th and 12th week of gestation) beyond a certain point in the intestine (See *Pediatric GI facts.*)

Pediatric GI facts

Characteristics of the pediatric GI system include the following:

- ◆ Peristalsis occurs within 2¼ to 3 hours in the neonate and 3 to 6 hours in older infants and children.
- ◆ Gastric stomach capacity of the neonate is 30 to 60 ml, which gradually increases to 200 to 350 ml by age 12 months and to 1,500 ml as an adolescent.
- ◆ The neonatal abdomen is larger than the chest up to ages 4 to 8 weeks, and the musculature is poorly developed.
- ◆ The sucking and extrusion reflex persists to age 3 to 4 months (extrusion reflex protects the infant from food substances that his system is too immature to digest).
- ◆ At age 4 months, saliva production begins and aids in the digestion process.
- ◆ Neonates frequently spit up due to the immature muscle tone of the lower esophageal sphincter and the small volume capacity of the stomach.
- ◆ Increased myelination of nerves to the anal sphincter allows for physiologic control of bowel function, usually around age 2 years.
- ◆ The liver's slow development of glycogen storage capacity makes the infant prone to hypoglycemia.
- ◆ From ages 1 to 3 years, composition of intestinal flora becomes more adultlike and stomach acidity increases, reducing the number of GI infections.

Causes of lower bowel obstruction

This chart lists common causes of lower bowel obstruction along with a description as well as characteristics, diagnosis and treatment, and nursing care for each.

CONDITION	CHARACTERISTICS	MEDICAL DIAGNOSIS AND TREATMENT	NURSING CARE
Appendicitis (inflammation of the appendix; the most common cause of abdominal surgery in children)	◆ Abdominal pain, localized tenderness, and fever ◆ Initially, generalized pain around the umbilicus, then localized pain in the right lower quadrant ◆ Changes in behavior, anorexia, or vomiting (common early signs) ◆ White blood cell (WBC) count of 15,000 to 20,000/µl ◆ Constipation or diarrhea ◆ Possible perforation (indicated by sudden pain relief) or peritonitis (indicated by increased pain, rigid abdomen, obvious guarding of the abdomen, high fever, and elevated WBC count) if untreated	◆ Chest X-ray to differentiate appendicitis from pneumonia (Pneumonia may cause referred pain in the right lower quadrant and, thus, may be misdiagnosed as appendicitis.) ◆ Barium GI series and ultrasonography to differentiate appendicitis from other abdominal problems ◆ Surgical removal of the appendix ◆ Management of peritonitis, shock, dehydration, and infection	◆ Don't administer enemas or laxatives or apply heat to the abdomen. ◆ When the appendix isn't perforated, perform the same postoperative care as for any abdominal surgery. ◆ When the appendix is perforated (and Penrose drains are in place), place the child in semi-Fowler's position or on his right side after surgery. ◆ Change dressings frequently, and provide meticulous skin care at the operative site.
Hirschsprung's disease (congenital aganglionic megacolon)	◆ Four times more common in boys than in girls ◆ Incidence: 1 in 5,000 births ◆ Failure to pass meconium within 48 hours after birth ◆ Food refusal, vomiting, and abdominal distention ◆ Inadequate weight gain, constipation, abdominal distention, episodes of vomiting, and diarrhea in older infant ◆ Chronic symptoms of constipation; ribbonlike, foul-smelling stools; abdominal distention; and impaction in older child	◆ Diagnosis in early infancy based on signs of intestinal obstruction ◆ Dilated proximal colon and aganglionic segment indicated by barium enema ◆ Diagnosis confirmed by rectal biopsy ◆ Anorectal manometry (pressure-sensitive catheter and balloon placed in the rectum and pressures of the internal and external sphincters recorded) ◆ Two-stage bowel resection performed surgically, with a temporary colostomy for 4 to 6 weeks	◆ Observe for signs of complications, such as fever, bloody diarrhea, and vomiting, and notify the physician if these occur. ◆ Keep the infant in an upright position, for example, in an infant seat. ◆ After colostomy, keep the area around the stoma clean and dry and cover with dressings or a colostomy or ileostomy appliance to absorb drainage. Watch for prolapse, discoloration, or excessive bleeding (slight bleeding is common). ◆ After the final corrective surgery, keep the wound clean and dry. Don't use a rectal thermometer. The infant will have a bowel movement in 3 to 4 days, which may create discomfort. Watch for signs of anastomic leaks (sudden development of abdominal distention, temperature spike, or extreme irritability). ◆ Because an infant with Hirschsprung's disease needs surgery and hospitalization so early in life, provide emotional support to the family.

Causes of lower bowel obstruction *(continued)*

CONDITION	CHARACTERISTICS	MEDICAL DIAGNOSIS AND TREATMENT	NURSING CARE
Imperforate anus (absent anal opening or opening obliterated by thin, translucent membrane)	◆ One of the most common congenital anomalies caused by abnormal development ◆ Absence of anus noted when taking the first rectal temperature in the neonatal unit ◆ Absence of meconium ◆ Possible meconium in urine, indicating an associated rectourinary fistula	◆ Digital and endoscopic examination ◆ Abdominal X-ray with opaque marker at the anal dimple and with the infant in the inverted position (The air outlines a blind rectal pouch.) ◆ Surgery to reconstruct the anus and perform a colon pull-through or sigmoid colostomy with anastomosis and pull-through 1 year later	◆ After anorectal repair, place the infant in a side-lying or prone position, with the hips elevated to keep pressure off the sutures. ◆ Feed the infant when peristalsis returns. ◆ Help the parents adjust to the infant's congenital disorder. ◆ Conduct a thorough assessment and history, particularly concerning diet and bowel habits. ◆ Preoperatively, teach parents colostomy care and what to expect postoperatively. ◆ Monitor abdominal distention: Measure girth every 8 hours. ◆ Provide resources for parents before discharge.
Intussusception (telescoping of the intestine into an adjacent portion)	◆ Incidence: rare in first month after birth; most common between ages 3 and 12 months ◆ Paroxysmal abdominal pain ◆ Currant-jelly stools (mixture of blood and mucus) ◆ Vomiting ◆ Abdominal distention, tenderness, and a palpable mass ◆ Dehydration and fever progressing to shock	◆ Air enema (may reduce intussusception; also used in diagnosis) ◆ Surgery to remove hypoxic bowel section and reconnect remaining healthy bowel sections	◆ Restore and maintain fluid and electrolyte balance. ◆ Prevent vomiting and aspiration. ◆ Carefully assess progression of the infant's stools (Normal brown indicates resolved intussusception.) ◆ After surgery, maintain stomach decompression until the infant passes the first stool.

Assessment findings

◆ Absence or delayed passing of meconium stool within 48 hours after birth
◆ Distended abdomen
◆ Lack of stool in the rectum
◆ Episodes of vomiting and diarrhea
◆ Foul-smelling stool
◆ Presence of ribbonlike or pellet-shaped stools
◆ Constipation
◆ Anemia
◆ Refusal of food, inadequate weight gain
◆ Thin, undernourished appearance

Diagnostic evaluation

◆ Rectal examination reveals absence of stool in the rectum.
◆ Barium enema films show a dilated colon segment proximal to the narrowed aganglionic segment of colon.
◆ Rectal biopsy confirms the diagnosis.

Nursing diagnoses

◆ Imbalanced nutrition: Less than body requirements
◆ Risk for deficient fluid volume
◆ Risk for infection
◆ Deficient knowledge
◆ Disturbed sleep pattern

Treatment

◆ Surgical treatment involves a two-stage bowel resection with a temporary colostomy for 4 to 6 weeks.

Planning and goals

◆ The child's bowel will be emptied preoperatively and prepared for a colostomy.
◆ The child's parents will verbalize understanding of the procedures involved in preoperative bowel preparation, the surgical procedure and desired outcome, and changes in body function.
◆ The child will regain and maintain fluid and electrolyte balance.
◆ The child will heal without infection postoperatively.
◆ The child will maintain adequate nutrition to promote growth and weight gain.
◆ The child will participate in appropriate age-related activities.
◆ The child's colostomy will function normally.
◆ The child's parents will understand and participate in colostomy care.
◆ The child and parents will return home able to cope with the child's altered body functions.

Implementation

Before surgery

◆ Prepare the child's bowel for surgery by administering antibiotics and saline colonic enemas until the bowel is clear *to reduce bacterial flora.* This preparation isn't necessary in the neonate, whose bowel is sterile.
◆ Teach the child's parents about the surgical procedure (temporary colostomy with or without pull-through anastomosis to anus) and about required preoperative care *to reduce anxiety.* Space the explanations *to prevent anxiety and confusion from too much information.*

After surgery

◆ Weigh the child at the same time each day, using the same scale *to obtain accurate weight measurements, which can help in monitoring the child's fluid balance and nutritional state.*
◆ Monitor and record abdominal circumference at least once every shift *to evaluate for abdominal distention, which can crowd the diaphragm and interfere with respirations.* Use a pen to mark where the measurement is taken.
◆ Withhold food and fluids until bowel sounds return, the nasogastric tube is removed, and the colostomy or anastomosed bowel can tolerate feedings; begin with small, frequent meals. *Bowel decompression continues postoperatively until bowel sounds return.*
◆ Change the child's diaper frequently, especially immediately after each bowel movement *to prevent contamination of the surgical site and promote healing.* The stoma is typically placed low on the abdomen *to eliminate the need for stoma bags when possible and to prevent the abrasion of the skin surrounding the stoma.*
◆ If stoma bags are necessary, change stomal dressings with each bowel movement. Keep the diaper below the stoma. Use appropriate-sized ostomy supplies. *Changing dressings prevents contamination of the surgical site and promotes healing. Keeping the diaper below the stoma avoids contaminating the stoma with urine. Appropriate-sized ostomy supplies can help prevent skin breakdown.*
◆ Involve the parents early in dressing changes and irrigations, if ordered, *to help them gradually accept their child's altered body functions.*
◆ Evaluate the child's pain level; include the parents' assessment of the child's behavior *because parents know their child's behavior and commonly can assess their child's pain level.* Provide pain relief measures, such as medications, distraction, and relaxation techniques *to relieve pain.*
◆ Consult a registered dietician *to help meet the child's nutritional needs.*
◆ Consult a skin care specialist or stomal therapist *to help meet the child's ostomy needs.*

Evaluation

◆ The child returns home free from stomal infection.
◆ The child's discomfort is relieved by non-opioid analgesia.
◆ The child has an average of at least one bowel movement each day and is free from abdominal distention.
◆ The child is beginning to enjoy mealtimes and eats without discomfort.
◆ The child is gaining weight and continues to develop at the appropriate developmental rate.
◆ The child's parents are performing stoma care and irrigations as instructed.

NEPHROTIC SYNDROME

NEPHROTIC SYNDROME (also known as *idiopathic nephrotic syndrome* or *minimal change nephrotic syndrome)* develops when large amounts of plasma protein are lost in urine because of increased glomerular permeability. The syndrome occurs most commonly in preschool-age children. About 80% of those affected display no other signs of systemic or renal disease; about 60% are boys. The pathogenesis of nephrotic syndrome isn't clearly understood. The increased glomerular permeability to plasma protein results in massive proteinuria, hypoproteinemia, hypovolemia, edema, and hyperlipidemia. (See *Pediatric genitourinary facts.*)

Possible causes

- ◆ Unknown (in about 75% of cases)
- ◆ Infection, particularly streptococcal infection
- ◆ Metabolic diseases
- ◆ Circulatory diseases
- ◆ Nephrotoxins
- ◆ Allergic reactions
- ◆ Tuberculosis or hepatitis B
- ◆ Preeclampsia toxemia
- ◆ hereditary nephritis
- ◆ Multiple myeloma or other neoplastic diseases

Assessment findings

- ◆ Anorexia
- ◆ Ascites
- ◆ Diminished urine volume; urine dark in color, opalescent, and frothy; urine specific gravity greatly increased; high protein level; and low RBC level
- ◆ Generalized edema, starting as facial puffiness and progressing over a period of weeks to abdominal swelling, respiratory difficulty, and labial or scrotal swelling
- ◆ Lethargy, irritability, decreased activity tolerance, and fatigability
- ◆ Regression in developmental level in response to illness and hospitalization

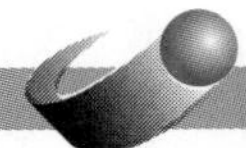

FAST FACT

The nephrotic syndrome symptom triad includes:

- proteinuria
- hypoalbuminemia
- edema.

Diagnostic evaluation

- ◆ Urinalysis reveals increased number of hyaline, granular, and waxy, fatty casts as well as oval fat bodies and consistent, heavy proteinuria.
- ◆ Blood values reveal increased levels of cholesterol, phospholipids, and triglycerides and decreased albumin levels.
- ◆ Renal biopsy provides histologic identification.

Nursing diagnoses

- ◆ Risk for imbalanced fluid volume
- ◆ Imbalanced nutrition: Less than body requirements
- ◆ Impaired skin integrity
- ◆ Risk for infection

Pediatric genitourinary facts

- ◆ An infant has a much greater percentage of total body water in extracellular fluid (42% to 45%) than an adult does (20%).
- ◆ Because of the increased percentage of water in a child's extracellular fluid, the child's water turnover rate is two to three times greater than an adult's. Every day, 50% of an infant's extracellular fluid is exchanged, compared with only 20% of an adult's; a child is therefore more susceptible than an adult to dehydration.
- ◆ A neonate also has a greater ratio of body-surface area to body weight than an adult; this greater ratio results in greater fluid loss through the skin.
- ◆ A neonate's kidneys attain the adult number of nephrons (about 1 million in each kidney) shortly after birth. The nephrons, which form urine, continue to mature throughout early childhood.
- ◆ A neonate's renal system can maintain a healthy fluid and electrolyte status. However, it doesn't function as efficiently during stress as an adult's renal system.
- ◆ An infant's kidneys don't concentrate urine at an adult level (average specific gravity less than 1.010 for an infant, compared with 1.010 to 1.030 for an adult).
- ◆ An infant usually voids 5 to 10 ml/hour, a 10-year-old child usually voids 10 to 25 ml/hour, and an adult usually voids 35 ml/hour.
- ◆ A child also has a short urethra; therefore, organisms can be easily transmitted into the bladder, increasing the risk of bladder infection.

Treatment

Treatment is usually symptomatic and supportive and inclues treating the underlying cause. Supportive treatment may consist of providing protein replacement with a nutritional diet of 1 g protein/kg of body weight with restricted salt.

Drug therapy options

- ◆ Immunosuppressant therapy: including cyclophosphamide (Cytoxan) for 2 to 3 months
- ◆ Diuretics for edema
- ◆ Steroid therapy until urine is free from protein
- ◆ Antibiotics for infection

- Angiotensin-converting enzyme inhibitors to decrease protein loss in urine
- Vitamin D replacement for chronic nephrotic syndrome

Planning and goals

- The child will remain free from secondary infection.
- The child will have increased urine output, decreased proteinuria, decreased body weight, decreased edema, decreased respiratory effort, and increased appetite within 7 to 21 days.
- The child will maintain or regain age-appropriate development.

Implementation

- Monitor the child's vital signs (including blood pressure) every 4 hours *to identify increased blood pressure, which, although rare, may indicate renal failure. Increased temperature and pulse rate could be related to a secondary infection.*
- Prevent visitors and staff members with respiratory symptoms or other infections from coming in close contact with the child. *Children with nephrotic syndrome are susceptible to secondary infection because the plasma proteins lost in the urine are immunoglobulins.*
- Maintain the child on complete bed rest in semi-Fowler's position until edema subsides. *Bed rest decreases tissue oxygen demands. Semi-Fowler's position decreases upward pressure of the ascitic abdomen on the diaphragm.*
- Turn the child every 2 hours and provide support (sheepskin pad, special skin care) to extremely edematous areas, such as the scrotum, *to help prevent infection and skin breakdown.* Taut, edematous skin breaks down quickly. Skin surfaces should be cleaned and separated by clothing or padding.
- Keep strict intake and output records. Document voiding times and the volume, color, and specific gravity of urine. Test urine after each voiding, and document the presence or absence of proteins and RBCs. Corticosteroids are used in the primary treatment of a patient with nephrosis. Within 7 to 21 days of starting treatment, urine excretion should increase and proteinuria should disappear. *Careful monitoring helps evaluate the child's response to therapy.*
- Assess and document edema status at least every shift. Accurately measure body weight and abdominal girth daily, and assess the periorbital area, abdomen, sacrum, pretibial area, and extremities *to identify the degree of fluid accumulation or fluid shift.*
- Offer the child small amounts of a no-salt-added regular diet at frequent intervals *to promote adequate nutrition.* Severe salt and fluid restrictions are usually unnecessary unless the child shows signs of renal failure. Consult a registered dietician to assit in meeting the child's protein and other nutritional needs.
- As the child's energy level permits, offer age-appropriate toys, such as large blocks, crayons and coloring books, illustrated books, music boxes, and large puzzles *to enhance normal growth and development and prevent boredom.*
- Before discharge, prepare the parents for providing home care, as follows, *to promote careful monitoring because the syndrome is marked by remissions and exacerbations:*
  - Tell parents to report weight gain, headaches, nausea, fever, and other signs of infection, which may signal a relapse.
  - Teach parents how to test urine for protein to identify early signs of an exacerbation. (Parents should participate in urine testing in the hospital and continue testing at least twice weekly at home.) The child should receive medical attention before extensive edema occurs.
- Teach parents to identify degrees of edema and what to report.
  - Inform parents of adverse reactions to corticosteroids, including cushingoid response and masking of usual infection signs. Warn them not to stop therapy suddenly; if the drug is stopped suddenly, the child will develop signs of shock and vascular collapse, requiring emergency care.
  - Tell parents what kind of behaviors to expect in response to illness and hospitalization. Regressive behaviors, especially increased dependence and clinging behaviors, may persist for several weeks. Discuss limit-setting to maintain normalcy for the child.

Evaluation

- The child remains free from secondary infection, skin breakdown, and skin irritation.
- The child responds positively to steroid therapy.
- The child shows more interest in his surroundings and participates willingly in age-appropriate activities before discharge.
- The parents demonstrate knowledge and assessment skills to manage care.

OTITIS MEDIA

OTITIS MEDIA is inflammation of the middle ear that may or may not be accompanied by infection. Fluid presses on the tympanic membrane, causing pain and leading to possible rupture or perforation. This condition may be acute or chronic and secretory or suppurative.

Acute otitis media is common in children. Its incidence increases during the winter months, paralleling the seasonal increase in nonbacterial respiratory tract infections. With prompt treatment, the prognosis for a client with acute otitis media is excellent; however, prolonged accumulation of fluid in the middle ear cavity causes chronic otitis media and, possibly, perforation of the tympanic membrane.

Possible causes

All types of otitis media

- Obstructed eustachian tube
- Wider, shorter, more horizontal eustachian tubes and increased lymphoid tissue in children as well as other anatomic anomalies

Acute secretory otitis media

- Barotrauma (pressure injury caused by inability to equalize pressure between the environment and the middle ear), as occurs during rapid aircraft descent in a person with upper respiratory tract infection or during rapid underwater ascent in scuba diving (barotitis media)
- Obstruction of the eustachian tube secondary to eustachian tube dysfunction from viral infection or allergy, which causes a buildup of negative pressure in the middle ear that promotes transudation of sterile serous fluid from blood vessels in the membrane of the middle ear

Acute suppurative otitis media

- Bacterial infection with pneumococci, *Haemophilus influenzae* (the most common cause in children under age 6), *Moraxella (Branhamella) catarrhalis,* beta-hemolytic group A streptococci, staphylococci (most common cause in children age 6 or older), or gram-negative bacteria
- Respiratory tract infection, allergic reaction, nasotracheal intubation, or position changes that allow nasopharyngeal flora to reflux through the eustachian tube and colonize the middle ear

Chronic secretory otitis media

- Persistent eustachian tube dysfunction from mechanical obstruction (adenoidal tissue overgrowth or tumors), edema (allergic rhinitis or chronic sinus infection), or inadequate treatment of acute suppurative otitis media

Chronic suppurative otitis media

- Inadequate treatment of acute otitis episodes
- Infection by resistant strains of bacteria
- Tuberculosis (rarely)

Assessment findings

Acute secretory otitis media

- Echo heard by child when speaking; vague feeling of top-heaviness (caused by accumulation of fluid)
- Popping, crackling, or clicking sounds on swallowing or with jaw movement
- Sensation of fullness in the ear
- Severe conductive hearing loss

Acute suppurative otitis media

- Bulging and erythema of tympanic membrane
- Dizziness
- Fever (mild to very high)
- Hearing loss (usually mild and conductive)
- Nausea and vomiting
- Pain pattern (Pulling the pinna doesn't exacerbate pain.)
- Pain that suddenly stops (which occurs if tympanic membrane ruptures)
- Purulent drainage in the ear canal from tympanic membrane rupture
- Severe, deep, throbbing pain (from pressure behind the tympanic membrane)
- Signs of upper respiratory tract infection (sneezing and coughing)
- Tinnitus

Chronic otitis media

- Cholesteatoma (cystlike mass in the middle ear)
- Decreased or absent tympanic membrane mobility
- Painless, purulent discharge in chronic suppurative otitis media
- Thickening and scarring of the tympanic membrane

Diagnostic evaluation

Acute secretory otitis media

- Otoscopy reveals clear or amber fluid behind the tympanic membrane and tympanic membrane retraction, which causes the bony landmarks to appear more prominent. If hemorrhage into the middle ear has occurred, as in barotrauma, the tympanic membrane appears blue-black.

Acute suppurative otitis media

- Culture of the ear drainage identifies the causative organism.

◆ Otoscopy reveals obscured or distorted bony landmarks of the tympanic membrane.
◆ Pneumatoscopy may show decreased tympanic membrane mobility, but this procedure is painful with an obviously bulging, erythematous tympanic membrane.

Chronic otitis media
◆ Otoscopy shows thickening, sometimes scarring, and decreased mobility of the tympanic membrane.
◆ Pneumatoscopy shows decreased or absent tympanic membrane movement.

Nursing diagnoses
◆ Acute pain
◆ Ineffective thermoregulation
◆ Deficient knowledge regarding childhood growth and development

Treatment
Acute secretory otitis media
◆ Concomitant treatment of the underlying cause, such as elimination of allergens or adenoidectomy for hypertrophied adenoids
◆ Inflation of the eustachian tube by performing Valsalva's maneuver several times per day (which may be the only treatment required)
◆ Myringotomy and aspiration of middle ear fluid if decongestant therapy fails, followed by insertion of a polyethylene tube into the tympanic membrane for immediate and prolonged equalization of pressure (The tube falls out spontaneously after 9 to 12 months.)

Acute suppurative otitis media
◆ Myringotomy for children with severe, painful bulging of the tympanic membrane

Chronic otitis media
◆ Elimination of eustachian tube obstruction
◆ Excision of cholesteatoma
◆ Mastoidectomy
◆ Treatment of otitis externa; myringoplasty and tympanoplasty to reconstruct middle ear structures when thickening and scarring are present

Drug therapy options
Acute secretory otitis media
◆ Nasopharyngeal decongestant therapy for at least 2 weeks and sometimes indefinitely with periodic evaluation (Current research questions the benefits of this practice but it's still done.)

Acute suppurative otitis media
◆ Antibiotic therapy if the disease is bacterial in origin (used with discretion to prevent development of resistant strains of bacteria)
◆ Nasal spray, nose drops, decongestants, antihistamines to promote drainage of fluid through the eustachian tube
◆ Eardrops to relieve pain, analgesics such as acetaminophen
◆ Oral corticosteroids to reduce inflammation

Chronic otitis media
◆ Broad-spectrum antibiotics for exacerbations of otitis media

Planning and goals
◆ The child will be afebrile and demonstrate no signs of secondary infection.
◆ The child will verbalize or demonstrate pain relief by showing signs of increased comfort
◆ The parents will verbalize knowledge about the condition, treatment, postoperative care (if applicable), and preventive measures.

Implementation
◆ Monitor vital signs *to determine baseline values and detect early signs of worsening infection.*
◆ Watch for and report headache, fever, severe pain, or disorientation *to detect early signs of complications.*
◆ Administer analgesics, as needed, or recommend applying heat to the ear *to relieve pain.*
◆ Identify and treat allergies *to prevent recurrences of otitis media.*
◆ Encourage the child and parents to complete the prescribed course of antibiotic treatment *to prevent reinfection.*
◆ For children with acute secretory otitis media, watch for and immediately report pain and fever *to detect early signs of secondary infection.*
◆ Tell the parents to avoid feeding an infant in a supine position or putting him to bed with a bottle *to prevent reflux of nasopharyngeal flora.*
◆ Encourage the child to perform Valsalva's maneuver several times daily *to promote eustachian tube patency.*
◆ After myringotomy, maintain drainage flow; place sterile cotton loosely in the external ear *to absorb drainage,* and change the cotton frequently *to prevent infection.*
◆ After tympanoplasty, reinforce dressings and observe for excessive bleeding from the ear canal *to assess for fluid volume deficit.*

◆ Review key teaching topics with the child and family members *to ensure adequate knowledge about the condition and treatment,* including:
- avoiding blowing the nose or getting the ear wet when bathing
- instilling nasopharyngeal decongestants properly, if prescribed
- recognizing upper respiratory tract infections and getting treatment early
- reporting complications, such as increasing fever, severe pain, or altered LOC.

Evaluation

◆ The child demonstrates a body temperature within normal range.
◆ The child exhibits pain relief from analgesics.
◆ The parents express an understanding of discharge instructions if a surgical procedure has been performed.
◆ The parents state interventions appropriate for preventing future infections.

PRESCHOOL-AGE CHILD DISORDERS

ASTHMA

ASTHMA is a reversible respiratory disorder of bronchial obstruction and irritation after exposure to stimuli. It's the leading cause of acute and chronic illness in children. Attacks may be triggered by many stimuli, including:
◆ allergens, such as wool, animals, and foods
◆ environmental pollutants
◆ exercise
◆ weather change
◆ infections
◆ medications
◆ emotions.

Most patients with asthma have extrinsic (immunoglobulin E–mediated) disease, although exercise- or infection-induced (non-IgE-mediated) disease isn't uncommon. Most asthmatic patients experience a first attack before age 4. Asthma produces:
◆ inflammation of the mucous membranes
◆ smooth-muscle bronchospasm
◆ increased mucus secretion leading to airway obstruction and air trapping.

Possible causes

◆ Hyperresponsiveness of the lower airway (may be idiopathic or intrinsic hyperresponsive reaction to an allergen, exercise, or environmental change)

Assessment findings

◆ Diaphoresis and rapid pulse
◆ Dyspnea
◆ Exercise intolerance
◆ Fatigue, apprehension, restlessness
◆ Prolonged expiration with an expiratory wheeze; in severe distress, may hear an inspiratory wheeze
◆ Recent exposure to attack triggers
◆ Tachypnea, along with use of accessory muscles
◆ Unequal or decreased breath sounds

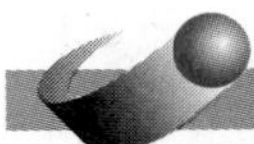

FAST FACT

Stay observant. Decreased wheezing – caused by decreased air movement in the airways – can indicate deterioration in a child's condition.

Diagnostic evaluation

◆ Pulmonary function studies reveal signs of airway obstruction (decreased peak expiratory flow and decreased expiratory volume in 1 minute).
◆ Oxygen saturation levels measured by pulse oximetry may show decreased oxygen saturation.
◆ ABG measurement may show increased partial pressure of arterial carbon dioxide from respiratory acidosis.
◆ Skin test is used to identify the source of the allergy.
◆ Sputum analysis is used to rule out respiratory infection.
◆ Chest X-rays may demonstrate hyperinflation, pulmonary infiltrates, and atelectasis.

Nursing diagnoses

◆ Impaired gas exchange
◆ Ineffective airway clearance
◆ Anxiety
◆ Risk for deficient fluid volume
◆ Caregiver role strain

Treatment

◆ Chest physiotherapy (after edema has abated)
◆ Hyposensitization through the use of allergy shots, if appropriate
◆ Parenteral fluids to thin mucus secretions
◆ Oxygen therapy, as tolerated
◆ Mechanical ventilation for respiratory failure

Drug therapy options

◆ Bronchodilating therapy: combination therapy with beta$_2$-adrenergic agonist (albuterol [Proventil]), methylxanthine (Theophylline, Aminophylline)
◆ Mast cell stabilizer: cromolyn (Intal) to prevent the release of mast cell products after an antigen-antibody union has taken place and to treat seasonal asthma
◆ Corticosteroids (inhaled) to decrease edema of the mucous membranes; for chronic asthma, daily doses to control chronic inflammation
◆ Leukotriene modifier: montelukast (Singulair) to inhibit bronchoconstriction and inflammatory effects of leukotrienes

Planning and goals

◆ The child's respiratory rate will be within the age-appropriate normal range and normal breath sounds will be present throughout all lung fields by discharge.
◆ The child will maintain adequate hydration.
◆ The child will attain normal respiratory oxygenation on room air.
◆ The child will respond positively to the nursing staff in non-threatening situations and receive comfort and support from the parents during invasive procedures.
◆ The parents will express understanding of current treatment and planned diagnostic workup.
◆ The parents will discuss concerns about caring for a child with asthma and demonstrate understanding of how to allergy-proof their home.
◆ The parents will provide a smoke-free environment.

Implementation

◆ Assess respiratory and cardiovascular status. *Tachycardia, tachypnea, and quiet breath sounds signal worsening respiratory status.*
◆ Monitor vital signs *to detect changes and prevent complications.*
◆ Assess the nature of the child's cough (hacking, unproductive progressing to productive), especially at night in the absence of infection. *Early detection and treatment reduces respiratory distress.*
◆ Modify the environment to avoid an allergic reaction; remove the offending allergen. *Allergens can trigger an asthma attack.*
◆ Rinse the child's mouth after he inhales medication *to promote comfort and prevent irritation to the oral mucosa.*
◆ For exercise-induced asthma, give prophylactic treatments of cromolyn or beta-adrenergic blockers 10 to 15 minutes before the child exercises. *Premedication before exercise may prevent an asthma attack.*
◆ Position the child upright *to assist with breathing and instruct on use of a spacer.*
◆ Assist the child with the use of inhaled medications. Monitor the child's respiratory status *to evaluate the response to medications,* as follows:
– Auscultate the lungs for rate, depth, and adventitious sounds.
– Assess for changes in the amount and quality of cough and sputum.
– Assess the use of accessory muscles and energy expended on breathing.
◆ Monitor the child's level of oxygenation through oxygen saturation *to evaluate for stable oxygen saturation levels.*
◆ Offer the child small sips of fluids, but avoid cold beverages. Record intake and output. *Promoting adequate fluid intake is important, but cold beverages should be avoided because they can trigger bronchospasm. Recording intake and output helps evaluate the effectiveness of treatment.*
◆ Have the parents stay with the child during invasive procedures *to reduce anxiety.* Family-centered care should be maintained. Offer simple explanations of all procedures to be done.
◆ Teach parents the purpose and use of a peak expiratory flow meter (PEFM). *The PEFM has color zones that aid in guiding the treatment of asthma at home and aid in early identification of respiratory infections.*
◆ Teach allergen control measures in the home *to reduce the risk of attacks.* Specific allergens identified by skin tests must be removed, if possible, or minimized. Humidity should be kept below 50% to remove dust mites. Exposure to animals should be limited.
◆ Help parents plan activities *to encourage normal child development.* Asthmatic children should be encouraged to participate in all age-appropriate activities, including sports, particularly those that require an even-level expenditure of energy, such as distance running or swimming.

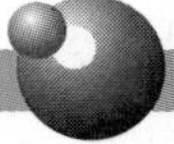

SPOT CHECK

What prophylactic action can be taken for a child who has exercise-induced asthma?

Answer: Prophylactic treatments of cromolyn or beta-adrenergic blockers taken 10 to 15 minutes before exercise may prevent an asthma attack.

◆ Prohibit smoking in the child's environment. *Second-hand smoke can trigger an asthma attack.*

◆ Review key teaching topics with family members *to ensure adequate knowledge about the condition and treatment,* including:
- use of breathing exercises to increase ventilatory capacity
- proper use of inhalers
- ways to avoid allergens.

During an acute attack:

◆ Provide moist oxygen, if necessary, *to promote mobilization of secretions.*

◆ Allow the child to sit upright *to ease breathing. This position promotes chest expansion.*

◆ Monitor for alterations in vital signs (especially cardiac stimulation and hypotension) *to detect signs of impending respiratory arrest and cardiac decompensation.*

◆ Monitor urine for glucose if the child is receiving corticosteroids *to detect early signs of hyperglycemia.*

◆ Administer inhaled medications by metered-dose inhaler and monitor peak flow rates. *Peak flow rates indicate the degree of lung impairment.*

◆ Maintain a calm environment; provide emotional support and reassurance *to decrease anxiety and decrease oxygen demands.*

◆ Monitor the effectiveness of drug therapy. *Failure to respond to drugs during an acute attack can result in status asthmaticus.*

Evaluation

◆ The child breathes easily and with normal breath sounds.

◆ The child breathes room air and has normal oxygen saturation levels.

◆ The child takes fluids freely and has a normal hydration status.

◆ The parents outline a plan for coping with upcoming tests and measures to decrease the child's exposure to allergens.

◆ The parents correctly describe asthma and the treatment the child needs.

HEMOPHILIA

HEMOPHILIA results from a deficiency in one of the coagulation factors. Hemophilia affects 1 in 5,000 males. The types of hemophilia are:

◆ hemophilia A (also called *factor VIII deficiency* or *classic hemophilia*), the most common type (75% of all cases)

◆ hemophilia B (also called *factor IX deficiency* or *Christmas disease*)

◆ hemophilia C (also called *factor XI deficiency*).

Hemophilia is an X-linked recessive disorder. The inheritance pattern is described below:

◆ If the father has the disorder and the mother doesn't, all the daughters will be carriers but the sons won't have the disease.

◆ If the mother is a carrier and the father doesn't have hemophilia, each son has a 50% chance of getting hemophilia and each daughter has a 50% chance of being a carrier.

Possible causes

◆ Genetic inheritance

Assessment findings

◆ Multiple bruises without petechiae

◆ Prolonged bleeding after circumcision, immunizations, or minor injuries

◆ Bleeding into the throat, mouth, and thorax

◆ Hemarthrosis

◆ Peripheral neuropathies from bleeding near peripheral nerves

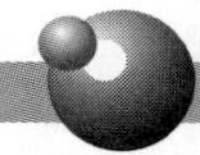

SPOT CHECK

What's a classic sign of hemophilia?

Answer: A classic sign of hemophilia is prolonged bleeding after minor injuries.

Diagnostic evaluation

◆ Prolonged partial thromboplastin time (PTT)

Nursing diagnoses

◆ Risk for fluid volume deficit

◆ Risk for injury

◆ Acute pain

◆ Anxiety

◆ Powerlessness

Treatment

◆ Avoid aspirin, sutures, and cauterization, which may aggravate bleeding.

◆ Administer blood transfusion, if necessary.

◆ Administer cryoprecipitate (in hemophilia A) to maintain an acceptable serum level of the clotting factor (usually done by the family at home).

◆ Administer factor IX concentrate for bleeding (in hemophilia B)

◆ Assess human immunodeficiency virus (HIV) status. (Child is at increased risk for acquiring HIV through blood product transfusions.)
◆ Administer fresh frozen plasma to restore deficient coagulation factors.
◆ Promote vasoconstriction during bleeding episodes by applying ice, pressure, and hemostatic agents.

Drug therapy options
◆ Antihemorrhagic: desmopressin acetate (DDAVP) to promote the release of factor VIII in individuals with mild or moderate hemophilia A
◆ Antihemorrhagic: aminocaproic acid (Amicar) for oral bleeding

Planning and goals
◆ The child will show evidence of hemodynamic stability.
◆ The child's fluid volume will remain within normal range.
◆ The child will express feelings of comfort and decreased pain.
◆ The parents will demonstrate adequate coping skills.
◆ The parents will demonstrate knowledge related to the treatment and management of the disease.
◆ The parents will identify strategies to prevent injuries.

Implementation
◆ Monitor vital signs and intake and output *to assess renal status and monitor for fluid overload or dehydration.*
◆ Assess cardiovascular status and check for signs of bleeding; *fever, tachycardia, or hypotension may indicate hypovolemia.*
◆ Measure the joint's circumference and compare it to that of the unaffected joint *to assess for bleeding into the joint, which may lead to hypovolemia.*
◆ Note swelling, pain, or limited joint mobility. *Changes may indicate progressive decline in function.*
◆ Assess for joint degeneration from repeated hemarthroses *to detect extent of damage.*
◆ Pad toys and other objects in the child's environment *to promote child safety and prevent bleeding.*
◆ Recommend protective headgear, soft foam Toothettes (instead of bristle toothbrushes), and stool softeners as appropriate *to prevent bleeding.*
◆ Discourage abnormal weight gain, *which increases the load on joints.*
◆ Teach the parents how *to manage the disease, prevent injuries, and treat bleeding in the home environment.*
◆ Consult social services *to ensure that resources are available to meet the child's home health care needs.*

When bleeding occurs
◆ Elevate the affected extremity above the heart *to decrease circulation to the affected area and promote venous return.*
◆ Immobilize the site *to prevent clots from dislodging.*
◆ Take appropriate measures to decrease the child's anxiety *to lower the heart rate.*

Treating hemarthrosis
◆ Immobilize the affected extremity; elevate it in a slightly flexed position *to prevent further injury.*
◆ Decrease pain and anxiety *to lower the child's heart rate and minimize blood loss.*
◆ Avoid excessive handling or having the child bear weight for 48 hours *to prevent bleeding and to rest the site.*
◆ Begin mild ROM exercises after 48 hours *to facilitate absorption and prevent contractures.*

Evaluation
◆ The child is hemodynamically stable with minimal complications.
◆ The parents demonstrate an understanding of how to respond during a bleeding episode.
◆ The parents recognize signs of further bleeding, such as increased pain and swelling, fever, and symptoms of shock.
◆ The parents verbalize an understanding of the need to protect their child from injury while avoiding unnecessary restrictions that impair his normal development. For instance, the knees and elbows of a child's pants can be padded to protect these joints during falls.

HYPOSPADIAS
HYPOSPADIAS (opening of the urethra on the ventral surface of the penis) occurs in approximately 8 of every 1,000 male neonates. The defect may be accompanied by a downward curvature of the penis (chordee) resulting from penile constriction by a fibrous band of tissue. Circumcision should be avoided in a neonate with hypospadias; the foreskin can be used in reconstructive surgery.

Possible causes
◆ Genetic factors (most likely)

Assessment findings
◆ Meatus terminating at some point along lateral fusion line, ranging from the perineum to the distal penile shaft
◆ Normal urination with penis elevated impossible
◆ Altered angle of urination

Diagnostic evaluation

◆ Observation confirms aberrant placement of the opening; therefore, diagnostic testing isn't necessary.

Nursing diagnoses

◆ Impaired urinary elimination
◆ Risk for infection
◆ Anxiety

Treatment

◆ No treatment (in mild disorder)
◆ Surgical treatment (if repair is to be extensive, surgical repair may be delayed until age 4), including:
– meatotomy, in which the urethra is extended into a normal position, possibly performed initially to restore normal urinary function
– surgery to release the adherent chordee performed when the child is age 12 to 18 months
◆ Indwelling urinary catheter or suprapubic urinary catheter postoperatively.

The objectives of surgical correction are to enable voiding while standing, provide a more normal physical appearance of the male genitalia, and facilitate reproductive capability later. The timing of hypospadias repair depends on the site of the defective urethral opening. The trend is to carry out the repair in one surgical procedure before age 18 months. Repair can be a relatively simple procedure if the urethral opening is near the glans penis and chordee is absent. If the urethral opening is nearer the middle of the shaft, more than one surgical procedure may be necessary to lengthen the urethra progressively.

Drug therapy options

◆ Analgesics: morphine sulfate, acetaminophen (Tylenol), acetaminophen with codeine (Tylenol #3) for postoperative pain relief
◆ Antispasmodic agent: propantheline (Pro-Banthine) to treat bladder spasms postoperatively

Planning and goals

◆ The parents will demonstrate a basic understanding of postoperative procedures and catheter drainage and will participate in the care of the child.
◆ Postoperatively, the child will remain free from infection, and any bladder or urethral catheter will remain patent.
◆ Postoperatively, the child will maintain adequate urine output.

Implementation

◆ Monitor urine output *to ensure the child maintains a normal urine output of 1ml/kg/hour.*
◆ Keep the genital area clean *to prevent bacteria invasion and infection.*
◆ Encourage parents to express feelings and concerns about changes in the child's body appearance or function. Provide accurate information and answer questions thoroughly. *Encouraging open discussion enables the nurse to provide emotional support and may help ease the parents' anxiety.*

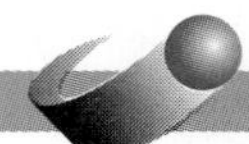

FAST FACT

The key intervention in hypospadias is scrupulous cleaning to deter bacteria.

After surgery

◆ After the procedure, a pressure dressing is typically used to reduce bleeding and tissue swelling; keep the child's hands away from the penis *so that the dressing isn't dislodged, causing trauma to the site.*
◆ Check the tip of the penis frequently *to make sure it's pink and viable.*
◆ Leave the dressing in place for several days *to encourage healing of the grafted skin flap.*
◆ Avoid putting pressure on the child's catheter *to prevent trauma to the incision site.* Avoid kinking of the catheter *to ensure urine flow.*
◆ Encourage early ambulation *to prevent complications of immobility.*
◆ Administer prophylactic antibiotics *to prevent infection.*

Evaluation

◆ Postoperatively, the child experiences no adverse temperature elevation.
◆ Postoperatively, the child voids sufficient quantities of clear, yellow urine and has no unusual drainage or inflammation of the operative site.
◆ The parents verbalize understanding of the diagnosis, the treatment needed, and the need for them to participate in the child's care.

LEUKEMIA

LEUKEMIA a is the most common form of cancer in children, with peak onset between ages 3 and 5. The 5-year survival rate varies from 50% to 90%, depending on the type of leukemia. Leukemia's main feature is a rapid in-

Signs and symptoms of leukemia

Acute leukemia is a rapidly progressing disease that affects bone marrow, the reticuloendothelial and central nervous systems, and metabolism. This flowchart outlines these changes.

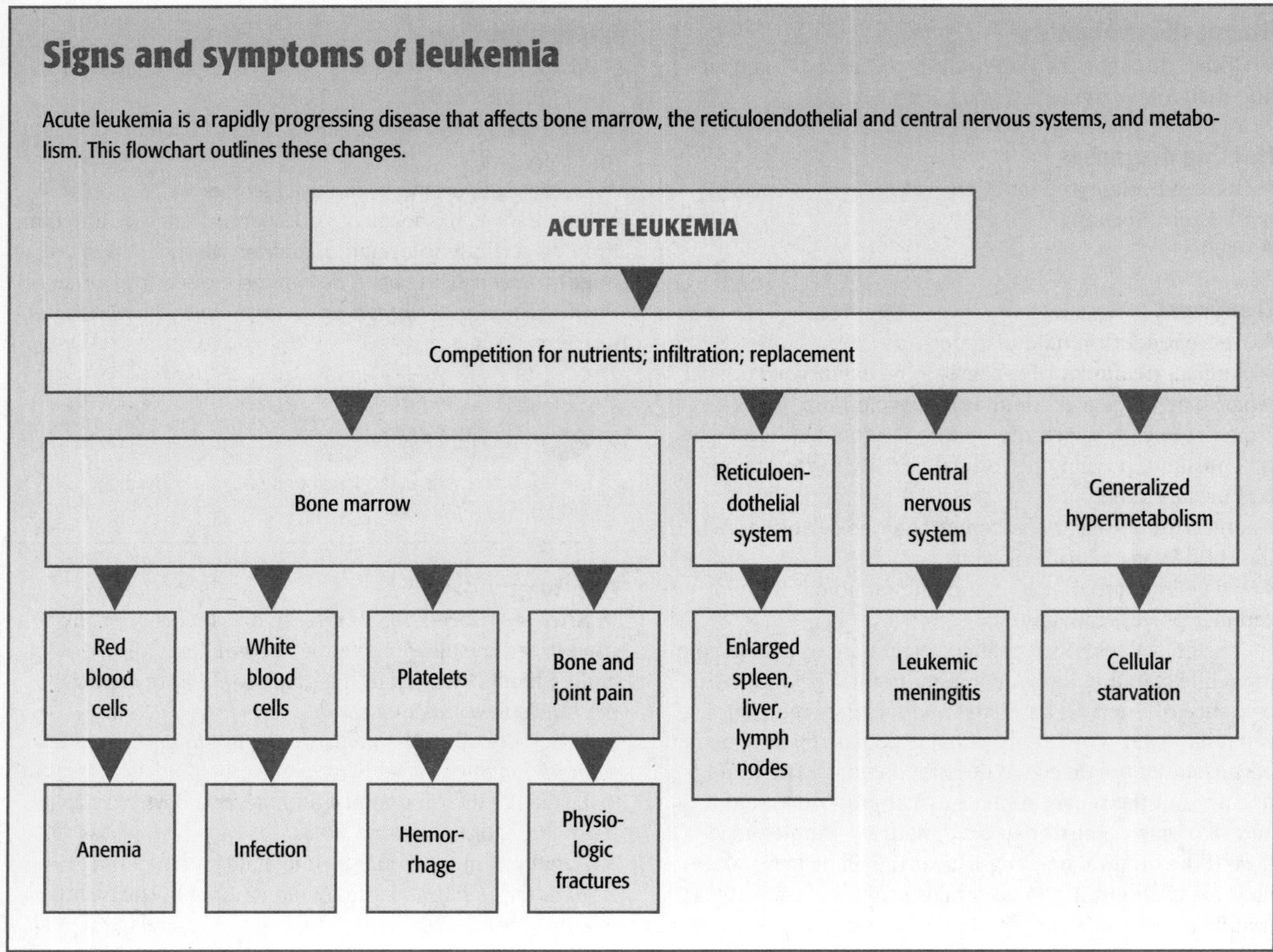

crease in the number of immature white blood cells (WBCs).

Leukemic cells have the same properties as malignant cells of solid tumors, including:

- high metabolic rate
- infiltration of surrounding tissue
- migration to other body parts.

Because leukemic cells proliferate rapidly in the bone marrow, other blood components are deprived of nutrients and crowded out. The result is progressive anemia from decreased erythrocyte levels and bleeding problems from decreased thrombocyte levels. Though increased in number, the leukemic WBCs can't fight infection.

The leukemic cells tend to migrate first to the highly vascular organs of the reticuloendothelial system (the spleen, liver, and lymph glands). Infiltration of the central nervous system (CNS) results in signs of increased ICP and meningeal irritation. Finally, all organs are involved, and the child is deprived of metabolic nutrients, resulting in generalized wasting.

In children, the most common type of leukemia is ACUTE LYMPHOCYTIC LEUKEMIA (ALL). This type of leukemia is marked by extreme proliferation of immature lymphocytes (blast cells). In adolescents, acute myelogenous leukemia is more common and is believed to result from a malignant transformation of a single stem cell.

Clinical findings for leukemia may appear with surprising abruptness in children with few, if any warning signs. (See *Signs and symptoms of leukemia.*)

Possible causes

- Chemical exposure and viruses
- Chromosomal disorders
- Down syndrome
- Ionizing radiation

Assessment findings

- Blood in urine, stool, or emesis
- Bone and joint pain
- Decrease in all blood cells when bone marrow undergoes atrophy (leading to anemia, bleeding disorders, and immunosuppression)
- Enlarged spleen, liver, and lymph nodes
- History of infections
- Lassitude
- Leukemic meningitis
- Low-grade fever
- Lymphadenopathy
- Pallor
- Pathologic fractures (when bone marrow undergoes hypertrophy)
- Petechiae and ecchymosis
- Poor wound healing and oral lesions

Diagnostic evaluation

- Blast cells appear in the peripheral blood (where they normally don't appear).
- Blast cells may be as high as 95% in the bone marrow (normally less than 5%) as measured by marrow aspiration in the posterior iliac crest. (The sternum can't be used in children.)
- Initial WBC count may be less than 10,000/µl at the time of diagnosis in a child with ALL between ages 3 and 7. (This child has the best prognosis.)
- Lumbar puncture indicates if leukemic cells have crossed the blood-brain barrier.

Nursing diagnoses

- Risk for infection
- Acute pain
- Chronic pain
- Interrupted family processes
- Ineffective protection

Treatment

- Bone marrow or stem cell transplantation
- High-protein, high-calorie, bland diet
- I.V. fluids as necessary
- Oxygen therapy if needed
- Radiation therapy
- Transfusion therapy as needed

Drug therapy options

- Analgesics: acetaminophen (Tylenol), acetaminophen with codeine, ibuprofen (Motrin), morphine sulfate for pain relief
- Antiemetics: hydroxyzine (Atarax), ondansetron (Zofran)
- Chemotherapy, which varies with the type of leukemia
- Corticosteroid: prednisone (Deltasone)
- Antibiotic, antiviral, antifungal to control infections

Planning and goals

- The child will have a normal temperature and be free from signs of infection at the time of discharge.
- The child will experience pain control through medication and alternative comfort measures.
- The child and family members will demonstrate appropriate coping skills to deal with the problems of the disease.
- The parents will demonstrate an understanding of the disease process and management.

Implementation

- Monitor vital signs and intake and output *to determine fluid volume deficit and renal status.*
- Give special attention to mouth care *to prevent infection and bleeding.*
- Inspect the skin frequently *to assess for skin breakdown.*
- Give increased amounts of fluids *to flush chemotherapeutic drugs through the kidneys.*
- Provide a high-protein, high-calorie, bland diet with no raw fruits or vegetables. *Eliminating raw fruits and vegetables helps prevent infection. A diet meeting the child's caloric requirements helps ensure that the child's maintenance and growth needs are met.*
- Provide pain relief as ordered and document effectiveness and adverse reactions. *Analgesics depress the CNS, thereby reducing pain.*
- Monitor the CNS *to assess for such changes as confusion that may result from cerebral damage.*
- Provide nursing measures to ease adverse reactions to radiation and chemotherapy *to promote comfort and encourage adequate nutritional intake.* (See *Implementation for adverse reactions to radiation therapy and chemotherapy,* page 292.)
- Review key teaching topics with the child and his family *to ensure adequate knowledge about the condition and treatment,* including:
  - avoiding infection
  - adjusting to changes in body image
  - contacting support groups
  - recognizing signs and symptoms of infection and the need to seek immediate medical attention. (See *Caring for a child with ALL,* page 293.)
- Consult with social services to ensure resources are available to meet the child's home health care needs.

Implementation for adverse reactions to radiation therapy and chemotherapy

This table describes key nursing care measures to use when caring for a child receiving radiation therapy and chemotherapy.

ADVERSE REACTION	NURSING IMPLICATIONS
Alopecia	◆ Keep the scalp clean and dry to prevent infection. ◆ Obtain a baseball cap or favorite hat for the child to wear. ◆ Tell the child's parents to keep his head covered when exposed to the sun, wind, or cold.
Anorexia	◆ Allow the child to select his own food. ◆ Give the child any food he wants. ◆ Take advantage of hungry periods by providing snacks. ◆ Add nutritious supplements (such as custards, puddings, and milk shakes) to the child's diet.
Hemorrhagic cystitis	◆ Maintain fluid intake above maintenance level, usually 3,000 ml/m²/day. (Use the West Nomogram to estimate body surface area.) ◆ Monitor the child for burning pain on urination. ◆ Encourage frequent voiding; arouse the child at night to void. ◆ An empty bladder reduces the amount of time that the bladder is exposed to the alkylating agent in urine.
Mouth ulcers	◆ Have the child use a soft-bristle, infant-size toothbrush. ◆ Provide frequent mouthwash with normal saline solution ◆ Provide a bland, moist, soft diet; avoid hot and cold foods and beverages. ◆ Administer local anesthesia such as lidocaine hydrochloride (Xylocaine Viscous Solution) before meals or as needed for comfort. (Don't use with a very young child because it may depress the gag reflex and result in aspiration.)
Nausea and vomiting	◆ When possible, administer chemotherapeutic drugs when the child's stomach is empty; administer an antiemetic 20 minutes before chemotherapy begins and continue at regular intervals as ordered.
Rectal ulcers	◆ Don't use rectal thermometers or suppositories. ◆ Give sitz baths or tub baths as often as necessary for comfort. Use no additives in the water. ◆ Expose the affected area to air or moist heat. ◆ Apply A and D Ointment before a bowel movement. ◆ Provide dietary fiber, fluids, and stool softeners, as ordered.

Evaluation

◆ The child is free from infection at the time of discharge.
◆ The child verbalizes or exhibits pain relief with the measures being used.
◆ The child and his parents verbalize understanding of the disease, treatment measures, and when to seek medical attention.
◆ The child and his parents express understanding of various coping strategies.

NEPHRITIS

NEPHRITIS, also known as *acute infective tubulointerstitial nephritis, pyelonephritis,* or *glomerular nephritis,* is a sudden inflammation that primarily affects the interstitial area and the renal pelvis or, less commonly, the renal tubules. One of the most common renal diseases, nephritis occurs more commonly in females, probably because of a shorter urethra and the proximity of the urinary meatus to the vagina and rectum.

With treatment and continued follow-up care, the prognosis is good, and extensive permanent damage is rare.

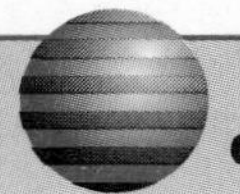

CLINICAL SITUATION

Caring for a child with ALL

The nurse is reviewing discharge instructions with the parents of a 4-year-old boy diagnosed with acute lymphocytic leukemia (ALL) during his admission. The child has a recent history of a bad cold and several sore throats, bruises and petechiae over his body without a history of injuries, anorexia, weight loss, or fatigue.

What key points should be included in the discharge instructions?

◆ Teach the parents how to assess and care for the child, including how to observe for signs of chronic and acute blood loss. (See "Shock disorders," page 76.) Tell them to take necessary measures to prevent hemorrhage, such as padding the child's crib and living area and keeping sharp objects out of the child's reach.

◆ Instruct the parents to monitor the child for infection and to take measures to prevent it, such as:

– removing broken toys and other sharp objects from the child's environment
– screening visitors for signs of infection
– advising visitors to use good hand-washing technique.

◆ Instruct the parents to make sure the child maintains a well-balanced diet.

◆ Schedule analgesia to get maximum pain relief and optimal mental functioning.

◆ Support the child and parents through the grief process. (See "Grieving," page 38.) The child and his parents will experience differing levels of anticipatory grief and loss. They'll profit from support during this time.

◆ Inform the parents of expected adverse effects of medication, as follows:

– Give the parents specific instructions on which adverse effects need medical attention (mouth and rectal ulcers, hemorrhagic cystitis, peripheral neuropathy, infection, and dehydration).
– Inform the parents that adverse effects of drugs don't indicate a return of leukemia.

Questions for further thought

◆ How can the nurse evaluate the parents' understanding of the instructions provided?

◆ What indicates a need for further instruction?

Possible causes

◆ Bacterial infection of the kidneys (the most common cause); bacteria are usually from normal intestinal and fecal flora growing readily in urine (most commonly *Escherichia coli,* but also *Proteus, Pseudomonas, Staphylococcus aureus,* and *Enterococcus faecalis* [formerly *Streptococcus faecalis*])

◆ Hematogenic infection (as in septicemia or endocarditis)

◆ Inability to empty the bladder (for example, in patients with neurogenic bladder), urinary stasis, or urinary obstruction due to tumors or strictures

◆ Contamination from instruments used in diagnostic testing, surgery, and routine patient care (such as catheterization, cystoscopy, or urologic surgery)

◆ Lymphatic infection

Assessment findings

◆ Anorexia
◆ Burning during urination
◆ Dysuria
◆ Flank pain
◆ General fatigue
◆ Hematuria (usually microscopic but may be gross)
◆ Nocturia
◆ Shaking chills
◆ Temperature of 102° F (38.9° C) or higher
◆ Urinary frequency
◆ Urinary urgency
◆ Urine that's cloudy and has an ammonia-like or fishy odor

Diagnostic evaluation

◆ Excretory urography may show asymmetrical kidneys.

◆ Pyuria (pus in urine) is present. Urine sediment reveals the presence of leukocytes singly, in clumps, and in casts and, possibly, a few RBCs.

◆ Urine culture reveals significant bacteriuria — more than 100,000/µl of urine. Proteinuria, glycosuria, and ketonuria are less common.

◆ Urine specific gravity and osmolality are low, resulting from a temporarily decreased ability to concentrate urine.

◆ Urine pH is slightly alkaline.

◆ Kidney, ureter, and bladder radiography may reveal calculi, tumors, or cysts in the kidneys and the urinary tract.

Nursing diagnoses

◆ Ineffective tissue perfusion (renal)
◆ Impaired urinary elimination
◆ Risk for infection
◆ Acute pain

Treatment

◆ Follow-up treatment for antibiotic therapy: reculturing urine 1 week after drug therapy stops, then periodically for the next year to detect residual or recurring infection
◆ Surgery to relieve obstruction or correct the anomaly responsible for obstruction or vesicoureteral reflux (Antibiotics aren't always effective.)

Drug therapy options

◆ Antibiotics to target the specific infecting organism, (10- to 14-day course); therapy for specific organism:
- *Enterococcus* — ampicillin, penicillin G, or vancomycin
- *E. coli* — sulfisoxazole (Gantrisin), nitrofurantoin (Macrobiol)
- *Proteus* — ampicillin, cephalosporins
- *Pseudomonas* — gentamicin, tobramycin, and carbenicillin
- *Staphylococcus* — penicillin G; if resistance develops, a semisynthetic penicillin, such as nafcillin or a cephalosporin (Keflex)

◆ Broad-spectrum antibiotics: ampicillin or cephalexin (Keflex) (when the infecting organism can't be identified)
◆ Urinary analgesic: phenazopyridine (Pyridium)

Planning and goals

◆ The child will remain afebrile.
◆ The child will maintain adequate calcium intake.
◆ The child will remain free from renal calculi.
◆ The child will maintain fluid balance and adequate urine elimination as evidenced by a urine output of 1 to 2 ml/kg/hour.
◆ The child will maintain a urine specific gravity within the designated limits.
◆ The child will exhibit increased comfort.
◆ The parents will verbalize an understanding of the child's condition and methods to prevent infection (such as proper toileting).

Implementation

◆ Monitor urine specific gravity *to detect dehydration.*
◆ Monitor vital signs *to detect fever and hypertension.*
◆ Assess renal status *to determine baseline renal function and detect changes from baseline.*
◆ Administer antipyretics *to reduce fever.*
◆ Force fluids *to achieve urine output of more than 2 L/day.* However, discourage intake greater than 3 L/day. *Excessive fluid intake may decrease the effectiveness of the antibiotics.*
◆ Provide a diet that contains 500 mg of calcium for children up to age 3 years, 800 mg for school-age children, and 1,300 mg for adolescents; moderate restriction of sodium; moderate intake of animal protein; and avoidance of high doses of vitamin C. *These measures will help prevent formation of renal calculi.*

Evaluation

◆ The child maintains normal fluid balance and adequate urine output.
◆ The child is relieved of symptoms, such as pain, urinary frequency, and burning on urination.
◆ The parents demonstrate an understanding of the need to complete the full antibiotic course to decrease the chance of reinfection and to help prevent the growth of antibiotic-resistant organisms.
◆ The parents demonstrate an understanding of methods to prevent infection such as, for a female, teaching her to wipe from front to back after voiding or having a bowel movement.

REYE'S SYNDROME

REYE'S SYNDROME is an acute illness that causes fatty infiltration of the liver, kidneys, brain, and myocardium. It can lead to hyperammonemia, encephalopathy, and increased ICP.

Possible causes

◆ Acute viral infection, such as upper respiratory tract, type B influenza, or varicella (Reye's syndrome almost always follows within 1 to 3 days of infection.)
◆ Concurrent aspirin use (high incidence)

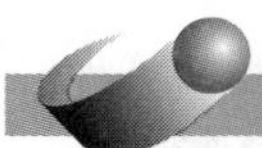

FAST FACT

To prevent Reye's syndrome, use nonsalicylate analgesics and antipyretics.

Assessment findings

Reye's syndrome develops in five stages. The severity of signs and symptoms varies with the degree of encephalopathy and cerebral edema:
◆ Stage 1 — vomiting, lethargy, hepatic dysfunction
◆ Stage 2 — hyperventilation, delirium, hyperactive reflexes, hepatic dysfunction
◆ Stage 3 — coma, hyperventilation, decorticate rigidity, hepatic dysfunction
◆ Stage 4 — deepening coma; decerebrate rigidity; large, fixed pupils; minimal hepatic dysfunction
◆ Stage 5 — seizures, loss of deep tendon reflexes, flaccidity, respiratory arrest. (Death is usually a result of cerebral edema or cardiac arrest.)

Diagnostic evaluation

◆ Blood test results show elevated serum ammonia levels; serum fatty acid and lactate levels are also increased.
◆ CSF analysis shows a WBC count less than 10/µl; with coma, there's increased CSF pressure.
◆ Coagulation studies reveal prolonged PT and PTT.
◆ Liver biopsy shows fatty droplets uniformly distributed throughout cells.
◆ Liver function studies show aspartate aminotransferase and alanine aminotransferase are elevated to twice their normal levels.

Nursing diagnoses

◆ Decreased intracranial adaptive capacity
◆ Ineffective thermoregulation
◆ Impaired gas exchange
◆ Risk for fluid volume deficit
◆ Impaired physical mobility
◆ Risk for impaired skin integrity

Treatment

◆ Decompressive craniotomy
◆ Endotracheal intubation and mechanical ventilation to control partial pressure of arterial carbon dioxide levels
◆ Enteral or parenteral nutrition as needed
◆ Exchange transfusion
◆ Induced hypothermia
◆ Transfusion of fresh frozen plasma

Drug therapy options

◆ Osmotic diuretic: mannitol (Osmitrol)
◆ Vitamin: phytonadione (AquaMEPHYTON)

Planning and goals

◆ The child will maintain normal oxygenation, as evidenced by ABG levels within normal parameters and adequate oxygen saturation
◆ The child will maintain adequate ventilation.
◆ The child will maintain blood glucose levels within normal parameters.
◆ The child will be free from seizure activity.
◆ The child will maintain orientation to environment without evidence of deficit.
◆ The child will maintain joint mobility and range of motion.
◆ The child will maintain skin integrity.
◆ The parents will verbalize understanding of Reye's syndrome and how to prevent it.

Implementation

◆ Monitor ICP with a subarachnoid screw or other invasive device *to closely assess for increased ICP.*
◆ Monitor vital signs and pulse oximetry *to determine oxygenation status.*
◆ Assess cardiac, respiratory, and neurologic status *to evaluate the effectiveness of interventions and monitor for complications such as seizures.*
◆ Monitor fluid intake and output *to prevent fluid overload.*
◆ Monitor blood glucose levels *to detect hyperglycemia or hypoglycemia and prevent complications.*
◆ Maintain seizure precautions *to prevent injury.*
◆ Keep the head of the bed at a 30-degree angle *to decrease ICP and promote venous return.*
◆ Assess pulmonary artery catheter pressures *to assess cardiopulmonary status.*
◆ Maintain oxygen therapy, which may include intubation and mechanical ventilation, *to promote oxygenation and maintain thermoregulation.*
◆ Administer blood products as necessary *to increase oxygen-carrying capacity of blood and prevent hypovolemia.*
◆ Administer medications, as ordered, and monitor for adverse effects *to detect complications.*
◆ Provide a hypothermia blanket as needed, and monitor the client's temperature every 15 to 30 minutes while the blanket is in use *to prevent injury and maintain thermoregulation.*
◆ Check for loss of reflexes and signs of flaccidity *to determine degree of neurologic involvement.*
◆ Provide good skin and mouth care and perform ROM exercises *to prevent alteration in skin integrity and promote joint motility.*
◆ Provide postoperative craniotomy care if necessary *to promote wound healing and prevent complications.*
◆ Be supportive of the family and keep them informed of the child's status *to decrease anxiety.*
◆ Teach the parents about Reye's syndrome and how to prevent it by using nonsalicylate analgesics and antipyretics.
◆ Consult social services *to provide the parents with resources to make sure the child's home health care needs are met.*

Evaluation

◆ The child returns to a normal respiratory state without signs of respiratory distress.
◆ The child has minimal neurologic complications as ICP decreases, as evidenced by reflexes, LOC, and orientation.

◆ The child maintains joint mobility, ROM, and skin integrity during hospital course.
◆ The parents verbalize an understanding of avoiding this syndrome by using nonsalicylate analgesics and antipyretics.
◆ The child remains free from skin breakdown.

SCHOOL-AGE CHILD DISORDERS

HEAD LICE

HEAD LICE (pediculosis capitis) is a contagious infestation. In an infected child, lice eggs, which look like white flecks, are firmly attached near the base of hair shafts. The cause of this disorder isn't related to the hygiene of a child or family members; however, head lice is easily transmitted among children and family members.

Possible causes

◆ Sharing of clothing and combs; close physical contact with peers — for example, in gym class (common in school-age children)

Assessment findings

◆ Excoriation (with severe itching)
◆ Pruritus of the scalp
◆ White flecks attached to the hair shafts
◆ Matted, foul-smelling, lusterless hair
◆ Occiptal and cervical adenopathy

Diagnostic evaluation

◆ Examination reveals lice eggs, which look like white flecks, firmly attached near the base of hair shafts.

Nursing diagnoses

◆ Impaired skin integrity
◆ Disturbed body image
◆ Social isolation

Treatment

◆ Removal of lice and eggs using a fine-toothed comb

Drug therapy options

◆ Pyrethrins (RID) or permethrin (NIX) shampoos (for other family members and classmates)
◆ Lindane (Kwell) in resistant cases

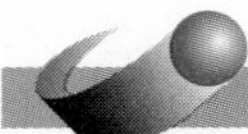

FAST FACT

When applying insecticidal treatments, carefully follow the manufacturer's directions to avoid neurotoxicity.

Planning and goals

◆ The child will exhibit improved or healing wounds, if any.
◆ The child will report feelings of increased comfort.
◆ The child will verbalize feelings about changed body image or social isolation.
◆ The child and his parents will demonstrate appropriate treatment application.

Implementation

◆ Instruct the parents to carefully follow the manufacturer's directions when applying medicated shampoo *to avoid neurotoxicity.*
◆ Confine the child to home for 24 hours *to reduce the risk of transmission.*
◆ Repeat treatment in 7 to 12 days *to ensure that all the eggs have been killed.*

Evaluation

◆ The child is free from infestation.
◆ The child exhibits or verbalizes a sense of well-being.
◆ The child and his parents demonstrate an understanding of methods to avoid reinfestation, including washing bed linens, hats, combs, and brushes, and refraining from exchanging combs, brushes, headgear, or clothing with other children.

HYPOTHYROIDISM

HYPOTHYROIDISM occurs when the body doesn't produce enough thyroid gland hormone, the hormone necessary for normal growth and development. (See *Understanding thyroid gland hormones.*)

Two types of hypothyroidism exist. Congenital hypothyroidism is present at birth. Acquired hypothyroidism is commonly due to thyroiditis, an inflammation of the thyroid gland that results in injury or damage to thyroid tissue. Hypothyroidism is three times more common in girls than in boys.

Early diagnosis and treatment offers the best hope. Infants treated before age 3 months usually grow and develop normally. Children who remain untreated beyond age 3 months and children with acquired hypothyroidism who remain untreated beyond age 2 years suffer irreversible cognitive impairment. Skeletal abnormalities, however, may be reversible with treatment.

Possible causes

- ◆ Antithyroid drugs taken during pregnancy (in infants)
- ◆ Chromosomal abnormalities
- ◆ Chronic autoimmune thyroiditis (in children older than age 2 years)
- ◆ Defective embryonic development that causes congenital absence or underdevelopment of the thyroid gland (most common cause in infants)
- ◆ Inherited enzymatic defect in the synthesis of thyroxine (T_4) caused by an autosomal recessive gene (in infants)

Understanding thyroid gland hormones

The thyroid gland secretes the iodinated hormones thyroxine and triiodothyronine. These hormones:

- ◆ act on many tissues to increase metabolic activity and protein synthesis
- ◆ are necessary for normal growth and development
- ◆ may lead to varying degrees of hypothyroidism (from a mild, clinically insignificant form to life-threatening myxedema coma) if deficient.

Assessment findings

General

- ◆ Cognitive impairment (develops as the disorder progresses)
- ◆ Delayed dentition
- ◆ Enlarged tongue
- ◆ Hypotonia
- ◆ Legs shorter in relation to trunk size
- ◆ Short stature with the persistence of infant proportions
- ◆ Short, thick neck

With slow basal metabolic rate

- ◆ Cool body and skin temperature
- ◆ Decreased perspiration
- ◆ Dry, scaly skin
- ◆ Easy weight gain
- ◆ Slow pulse

Untreated hypothyroidism in infants

- ◆ Hoarse crying
- ◆ Persistent jaundice
- ◆ Respiratory difficulties

Untreated hypothyroidism in older children

- ◆ Bone and muscle dystrophy
- ◆ Cognitive impairment
- ◆ Stunted growth (dwarfism)

Diagnostic evaluation

- ◆ Electrocardiography shows bradycardia and flat or inverted T waves in untreated infants.
- ◆ Hip, knee, and thigh X-rays reveal absence of the femoral or tibial epiphyseal line and delayed skeletal development that's markedly inappropriate for the child's chronological age.
- ◆ In myxedema coma, laboratory tests may also show low serum sodium levels, decreased pH, and increased partial pressure of arterial carbon dioxide, indicating respiratory acidosis.
- ◆ Increased gonadotropin levels accompany sexual precocity in older children and may coexist with hypothyroidism.
- ◆ Serum cholesterol, alkaline phosphatase, and triglyceride levels are elevated.
- ◆ Normocytic normochromic anemia is present.
- ◆ Radioimmunoassay confirms hypothyroidism with low triiodothyronine and T_4 levels.
- ◆ Thyroid scanning and ^{131}I uptake tests show decreased uptake levels and confirm the absence of thyroid tissue in athyroid children.
- ◆ Thyroid-stimulating hormone (TSH) level is decreased when hypothyroidism is due to hypothalamic or pituitary insufficiency.
- ◆ TSH level is increased when hypothyroidism is due to thyroid insufficiency.

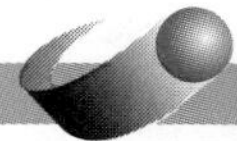

FAST FACT

Newborn screens are blood tests performed on every neonate to determine the presence of certain congenital disorders. Hypothyroidism and phenylketonuria are the only two disorders screened in every state of the United States. However, a positive result should always be confirmed with further testing, such as the radioimmunoassay for T_4, TSH, or both.

Nursing diagnoses

- ◆ Delayed growth and development
- ◆ Disturbed body image
- ◆ Constipation

- Compromised family coping
- Deficient knowledge regarding childhood growth and development

Treatment

- Routine monitoring of T_4 and TSH levels.
- Periodic evaluation of growth to ensure thyroid replacement is adequate

Drug therapy options

- Oral thyroid hormone: levothyroxine (Synthroid)
- Supplemental vitamin D (to prevent rickets resulting from rapid bone growth)

Planning and goals

- The child will suffer minimally from the disease as evidenced by maintaining normal T_4 and TSH levels and meeting age-appropriate developmental milestones.
- The child and his parents will demonstrate an understanding of the disease and its long-term effects.
- The child and his parents will understand and appropriately administer the treatment regimen.
- The child and his parents will state adverse reactions of thyroid replacement medication.
- The child and his parents will effectively cope with this chronic illness.

Implementation

- During early management of infantile hypothyroidism, monitor blood pressure and pulse rate; report hypertension and tachycardia immediately. (Normal infant heart rate is approximately 120 beats/minute.) *These signs of hyperthyroidism indicate that the dose of thyroid replacement medication is too high.*
- Check rectal temperature every 2 to 4 hours. Keep the infant warm and his skin moist *to promote normothermia and reduce metabolic demands.*
- If the infant's tongue is unusually large, position him on his side and observe him frequently *to prevent airway obstruction.*
- Provide the parents with support, referrals, and counseling as necessary *to help them cope with the possibility of caring for a physically and cognitively impaired child.*
- Teach the parents and the child (as appropriate) about management of hypothyroidism.
- Teach the parents about medication administration and which adverse reactions to report.
- Provide the parents with information about appropriate child care services and activities *to assist with growth and development.*
- Ensure that adolescent girls receive future-oriented counseling that stresses the importance of adequate thyroid replacement during pregnancy. Ideally, females should have excellent control before conception *to prevent congenital hypothyroidism in their children.*

Evaluation

- The child maintains normal thyroid hormone levels, thus experiencing minimal effects of the disease.
- The child and parents appropriately administer thyroid replacement medication and return for thyroid hormone level monitoring.
- The parents help the child to engage in stimulating activities to help him reach maximum potential.

RHEUMATIC FEVER

RHEUMATIC FEVER, an autoimmune disease affecting connective tissue, primarily affects people between ages 5 and 20. It occurs most commonly during cold, humid weather. The disease, which declined in the United States during most of the 20th century, has recently increased in the western part of the country and remains a major problem in developing countries.

Evidence suggests that rheumatic fever is preceded by a group A beta-hemolytic streptococcal infection. Antibodies against the streptococci develop and remain after the organism is eradicated.

Possible causes

- Production of antibodies against group A beta-hemolytic *Streptococcus*
- Untreated group A beta-hemolytic *Streptococcus* infection, such as scarlet fever, strep throat, otitis media, impetigo, and tonsillitis. About 2 to 6 weeks later, the antibodies mistake the child's connective tissue for the streptococci and begin to attack it. (Of children infected with *Streptococcus,* 1% to 5% develop rheumatic fever.)

Assessment findings

The Jones criteria for assessing major rheumatic fever include:

- carditis, which damages the heart valves
- chorea (involuntary movement of extremities and face)
- erythema marginatum (temporary, disk-shaped, nonpruritic, reddened macules that fade in the center, leaving raised margins)
- polyarthritis
- subcutaneous nodules.

The Jones criteria for assessing minor rheumatic fever include:

- arthralgia
- evidence of a *Streptococcus* infection
- fever
- history of rheumatic fever.

Diagnostic evaluation

- Antistreptolysin-O titer is elevated.
- Erythrocyte sedimentation rate (ESR) is increased.
- Electrocardiography shows a prolonged PR interval.

Nursing diagnoses

- Acute pain
- Imbalanced nutrition: Less than body requirements
- Deficient diversional activity
- Deficient knowledge regarding growth and development

Treatment

- Bed rest during the acute febrile stage until the ESR returns to normal

Drug therapy options

- Antibiotic: penicillin, erythromycin (for patients with penicillin hypersensitivity) even if cultures are negative; prophylactic treatment with penicillin to prevent additional damage from future attacks (taken until age 20 or for 5 years after the attack, whichever is longer)
- Anti-inflammatory medications: ibuprofen (Children's Motrin) for inflammation

Planning and goals

- The child will maintain vital signs within normal parameters.
- The child will be free from joint pain.
- The child will regain and maintain nutrition that's adequate for growth needs.
- The child will continue to perform age-appropriate developmental tasks.
- The child and his parents will verbalize an understanding of the condition and treatment.

Implementation

- Monitor vital signs and intake and output *to detect fluid volume overload or deficit.*
- Monitor and record vital signs and assess for signs of carditis. Teach the parents to monitor temperature, pulse, and respirations *to help them recognize the signs of carditis. Typically, the child has a low-grade fever (100° to 102° F [37.8° to 38.9° C]) in the late afternoon and early evening. Symptoms of carditis include a sudden high fever (104° F [40° C]), tachycardia, pallor, and a feeling of severe illness.*
- Institute safety measures for chorea; maintain a calm environment, reduce stimulation, avoid the use of forks or glass, and assist in walking *to prevent injury.*
- Provide appropriate passive stimulation *to maintain growth and development.*
- Provide emotional support for long-term convalescence *to relieve anxiety.*
- Use sterile technique in dressing changes and standard precautions *to prevent reinfection.*
- Review key teaching topics with the parents *to ensure adequate knowledge about the condition and treatment,* including:
  - understanding the need to inform health care providers of existing medical conditions
  - notifying health care providers at the first signs of streptococcal infection (scarlet fever, strep throat, otitis media, impetigo, or tonsillitis)
  - understanding that, throughout life, penicillin should be taken before dental work, certain medical procedures, and oral surgery to prevent bacterial endocarditis.

Evaluation

- The child's parents demonstrate strategies to decrease boredom, such as involving siblings and friends in quiet play and schoolwork, *to relieve the boredom of bed rest.*
- The child maintains normal growth patterns without becoming overweight.
- The child verbalizes pain relief with the measures being used.
- The child and his parents verbalize understanding of the disease, treatments, and the need to seek medical attention at the first signs of streptococcal infection.

SICKLE CELL ANEMIA

SICKLE CELL ANEMIA, also called *sickle cell disease,* occurs in about 1 out of 400 African Americans and rarely in whites. In sickle cell anemia, hemoglobin, in the presence of low oxygen tension (caused by hypoxia, acidosis, dehydration, or fever), crystallizes quickly, causing RBCs to bend into a crescent (or sickle) shape. The sickle cells accumulate, obstructing capillary flow throughout the body. The thickened blood results in capillary stasis, obstructed blood flow, and thrombosis. Ischemia occurs distal to the thrombosis, causing further oxygen depletion and sickling, which can lead to necrosis. The body hemolyzes the fragile sickle cells, quickly producing severe anemia (sickle cell crisis). (See *Sickling phenomenon,* page 300.)

Sickling phenomenon

This diagram shows the cycle of the sickling phenomenon in sickle cell anemia.

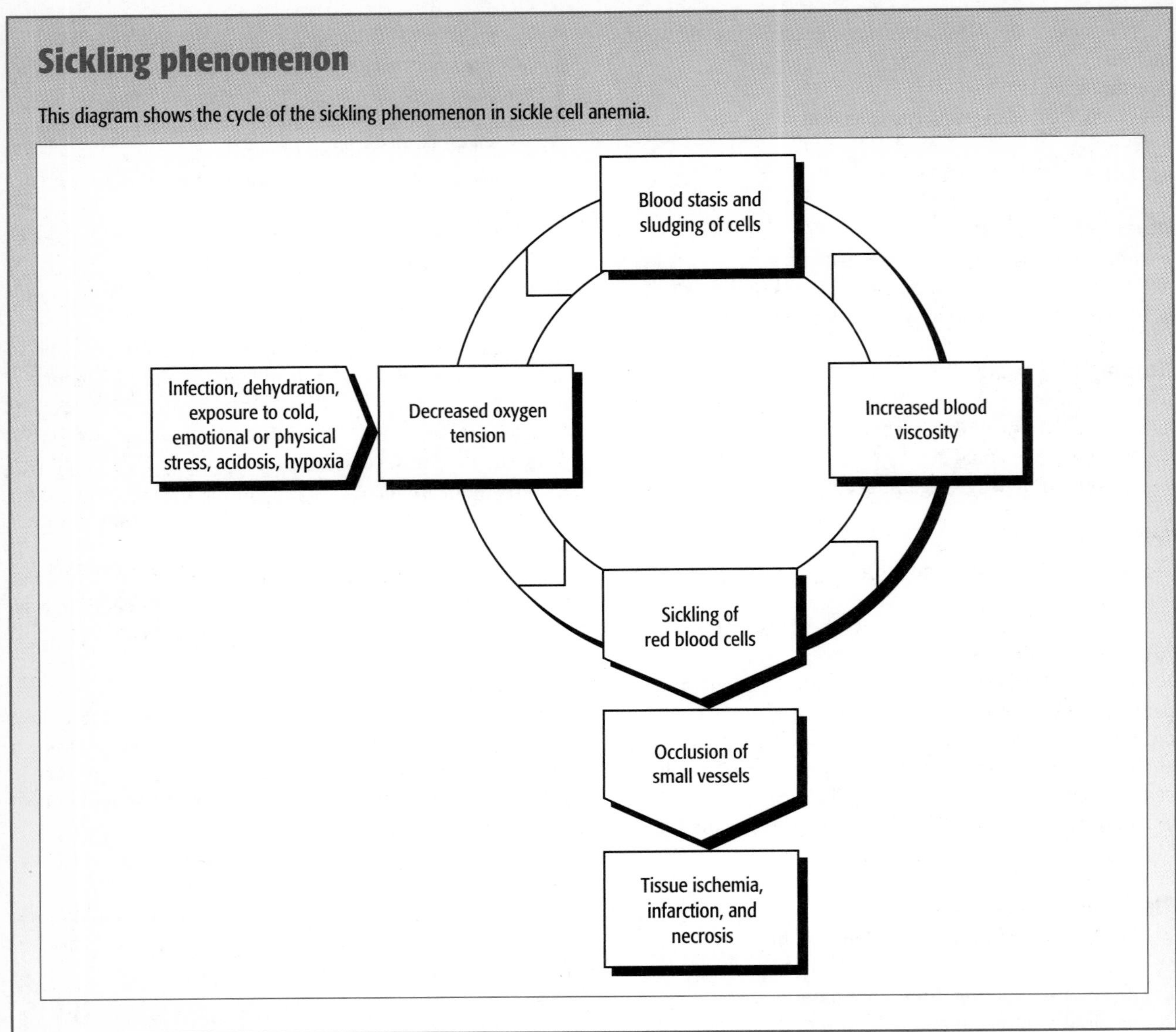

Possible causes

- Genetic inheritance (Sickle cell anemia is an autosomal recessive trait; the child inherits the gene that produces hemoglobin S from two healthy parents who carry the defective gene.)

Assessment findings

Assessment findings vary with the child's age. Before age 4 months, symptoms are rare (because fetal hemoglobin prevents excessive sickling).

Infants

- Colic from pain caused by an abdominal infarction
- Dactylitis or hand-foot syndrome from infarction of the small bones of the hands and feet
- Splenomegaly from sequestered RBCs

Toddlers and preschoolers

- Pain at the site of vaso-occlusive crisis
- Hypovolemia and shock from sequestration of large amounts of blood in the spleen

School-age children and adolescents

- Extreme pain at the crisis site
- Poor healing of leg wounds from inadequate peripheral circulation of oxygenated blood
- History of pneumococcal pneumonia and other infections due to atrophied spleen
- Enuresis
- Priapism
- Delayed growth and development and delayed sexual maturity

Diagnostic evaluation

- Laboratory studies show a hemoglobin level of 6 to 9 g/dl (in a toddler).
- More than 50% hemoglobin S indicates sickle cell disease; a lower level of hemoglobin S indicates sickle cell trait.
- RBCs are crescent-shaped and prone to agglutination.

Nursing diagnoses

- Ineffective tissue perfusion (peripheral)
- Acute pain
- Risk for infection
- Ineffective coping
- Compromised family coping
- Deficient knowledge regarding child growth and development

Treatment

- Bed rest
- Hydration with I.V. fluids (which may be increased to 3 L [2.8 qt] per day during crisis)
- Pain relief (analgesics)
- Short-term oxygen therapy (Long-term oxygen decreases bone marrow activity, further aggravating anemia.)
- Transfusion therapy as necessary
- Treatment of acidosis as necessary
- Bone marrow transplants

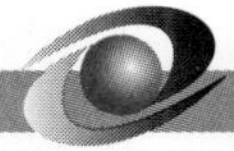

QUICK STUDY

To remember treatment priorities for clients with sickle cell disease, remember the word **HOP.**

Hydration
Oxygenation
Pain relief

Drug therapy options

- Analgesic: morphine
- Antineoplastic: hydroxyurea (Droxia)
- Pneumococcal vaccine
- Prophylactic antibiotic: penicillin (Ampicillin) before certain treatments

Planning and goals

- The child's progressive sickling process will be halted.
- The child will maintain adequate levels of blood oxygen concentration.
- The child will be free from infection.
- The child will receive pain relief.
- The child will maintain adequate renal function and urine output.
- The parents and the child will verbalize knowledge about the condition, treatment, and options for genetic counseling.
- The parents will verbalize understanding of methods to reduce the child's stress.

Implementation

- Administer sufficient pain medication *to promote comfort.* (Concerns about addiction are clinically unfounded.) A narcotic may be administered using a patient-controlled analgesia pump at a continuous base rate with periodic rescue boluses available. *Lack of pain relief can cause further sickling.*

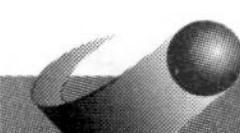

FAST FACT

Meperidine (Demerol) is *not* recommended for children due to production of the metabolite nor-meperidine, which causes anxiety, tremors, myoclonus, and seizures.

- Assess cardiovascular, respiratory, and neurologic status. *Tachycardia, dyspnea, or hypotension may indicate fluid volume deficit or electrolyte imbalance. Change in LOC may signal neurologic involvement.*
- Assess for symptoms of acute chest syndrome from a pulmonary infarction *to identify early complications.*
- Assess vision *to monitor for retinal infarction.*
- Encourage the parents to have their child receive the pneumococcal vaccine *to prevent infection.*
- Give large amounts of oral or I.V. fluids *to prevent fluid volume deficit, induce hemodilution, and prevent further sickling and additional complications.*
- Teach the child relaxation techniques *to decrease his stress level.*
- Maintain the child's normal body temperature *to prevent stress and maintain an adequate metabolic state.*

◆ Monitor vital signs and intake and output *to assess renal function and hydration status.*
◆ Provide proper skin care *to prevent skin breakdown.*
◆ Reduce the child's energy expenditure *to improve oxygenation.*
◆ Remove tight clothing *to prevent inadequate circulation.*
◆ Suggest family screening and initiate genetic counseling *to identify possible carriers of the disease.*
◆ Review key teaching topics with the child and family members *to ensure adequate knowledge about the condition and treatment,* including:
– avoiding activities that promote a crisis, such as excessive exercise, mountain climbing, and deep-sea diving
– avoiding high altitudes
– recognizing signs of infection and actions to take to help prevent infection
– seeking early treatment of illness to prevent dehydration
– avoiding aspirin use, which enhances acidosis and promotes sickling.

Evaluation

◆ The child will return home with an improved hemoglobin level and without signs or symptoms of sickle cell crisis.
◆ The child will continue to perform age-appropriate developmental tasks.
◆ The parents will monitor the child's health status, avoid situations that precipitate a crisis, and seek early, aggressive medical care for infections or signs of crisis.
◆ The child will be infection-free at discharge.
◆ The parents relate an awareness of the child's condition and how to avoid a crisis, the importance of early treatment, and options for genetic counseling.

TYPE 1 DIABETES MELLITUS

DIABETES MELLITUS is a disorder of carbohydrate metabolism characterized by insufficient insulin to allow glucose to cross the cell membrane. Type 1 diabetes (formerly called *juvenile diabetes* or *insulin-dependent diabetes*) most commonly occurs in childhood. A child with this type of diabetes must take insulin to replace what his pancreas can no longer produce.

Type 1 diabetes is most commonly diagnosed during childhood or adolescence but can occur at any time from infancy to about age 30. The psychological and emotional demands of growth and development and the generally increased but unpredictable activity levels of children complicate management, making them at risk for such complications as hyperglycemia and hypoglycemia. (See *Age-related considerations with type 1 diabetes mellitus.*)

Possible causes

◆ Autoimmune mechanisms
◆ Genetic predisposition
◆ Viral infection

Assessment findings

◆ Abdominal cramping
◆ Dry, flushed skin
◆ Fatigue
◆ Fruity breath odor
◆ Headache
◆ Nausea
◆ Polydipsia
◆ Polyphagia
◆ Polyuria
◆ Vomiting
◆ Weakness
◆ Thin appearance and possible malnourishment

Diagnostic evaluation

◆ Fasting plasma glucose level (no caloric intake for at least 8 hours) is greater than or equal to 126 mg/dl.
◆ Plasma glucose value in the 2-hour sample of the oral glucose tolerance test is greater than or equal to 200 mg/dl. This test should be performed after a loading dose of 75 g (2.6 oz) of anhydrous glucose.
◆ A random plasma glucose value (obtained without regard to the time of the child's last food intake) greater than or equal to 200 mg/dl and accompanied by symptoms of diabetes indicates diabetes mellitus.
◆ Testing for glycosuria and ketonuria using dipstick, Clinitest, Acetest, Keto-Diastix, or glucose enzymatic test strip is positive.

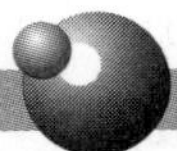

SPOT CHECK

What are the key signs and symptoms of diabetes mellitus?
Answer: Polydipsia, polyuria, and polyphagia

Nursing diagnoses

◆ Imbalanced nutrition: Less than body requirements
◆ Risk for deficient fluid volume
◆ Disturbed body image

Treatment

◆ Exercise
◆ Strict diet planned to meet nutritional needs, control blood glucose levels, and reach and maintain appropriate body weight

Age-related considerations with type 1 diabetes mellitus

Considerations about type 1 diabetes mellitus change throughout childhood. Here are some common issues listed by age-group.

Infants
- Careful monitoring of insulin needs secondary to rapid metabolism and growth and an infant's potential for acute illnesses
- Frequent infections and, in late infancy, food preferences that make management difficult
- Difficulty of recognizing hypoglycemia and ketoacidosis in infants

Toddlers
- Erratic activity patterns, decreased growth rate, and finicky eating behaviors that affect insulin needs
- Toddlers who have difficulty understanding why their parents purposely hurt them with finger sticks and injections
- Difficulty of recognizing hypoglycemia and ketoacidosis in toddlers

Preschoolers
- Readiness to learn about the disease and participate in care
- Resistance to daily injections (Management of resistant behavior may be more difficult at this age than any other.)

School-age children
- Adequate cognitive and motor ability for participating actively in managing diabetes (that is, injecting insulin, planning diet and exercise, and blood testing)
- Use of disease to achieve secondary gain such as pretending to be ill to stay home from school
- Increased participation in active sports (can present problems in balancing diet, insulin, and activity)

Adolescents
- Should be capable of self-management. (However, rapid growth and metabolic changes make management complex.)
- Effect of chronic disease on identity formation
- Need to express grief and anger regarding the burden of disease (Group discussions, health clinics for diabetic adolescents, and juvenile diabetes camps can help.)

Drug therapy options
- Antidiabetic agent: insulin replacement (Humulin, Lente, Novolin, NPH)

Planning and goals
Outcomes relate to the school-age child. Age-appropriate modifications — such as increased parental involvement with insulin administration — should be made, depending on the child's age:
- The child and his parents will state the onset, peak, and duration of action for the insulin form being taken.
- The child will accurately and safely draw up and administer insulin daily during the hospital stay.
- The child and his parents will demonstrate an understanding of appropriate body sites for insulin administration and rotation scheduling.
- The child and his parents will accurately test the child's blood for glucose at least four times per day.
- The child and his parents will state appropriate actions to take in case of illness or change in normal activity schedule.
- The child and his parents will state at least three signs or symptoms of hyperglycemia and hypoglycemia.
- The child and his parents will describe appropriate action to take during an insulin reaction.
- The child and his parents will be able to discuss the principles and rationales of the required diet.
- The child will maintain a positive self-image and will demonstrate the ability to deal with peer pressure.

Implementation
- Monitor vital signs and fluid intake and output. *High urine output may signify hyperglycemia. A weak, thready pulse may indicate hypoglycemia.*
- Monitor the child for signs of hypoglycemia, such as diaphoresis, tremors, palpitations, tachycardia, and behavioral changes (belligerence, confusion, slurred speech) *to prevent treatment delay.*
- Monitor blood glucose level and electrolytes *to detect early signs of electrolyte imbalance.*
- If you aren't sure whether the child is hypoglycemic or hyperglycemic and the child is stuporous or unconscious, treat him for hypoglycemia. *If he's hypoglycemic, he'll respond quickly; if he's hyperglycemic, this action won't significantly worsen his condition.*
- Evaluate the child's understanding of type 1 diabetes and his attitude about the need to manage it. *This will help you plan teaching.*
- Correct any misconception the child or adolescent has regarding type 1 diabetes and the therapeutic regimen. Use age-appropriate teaching materials *to increase knowledge of the condition and instill confidence in the child's ability to manage it.*

◆ Provide an opportunity for the child to interact with peers who have experienced diabetes *to decrease feelings of isolation and the sense of being different from others.*
◆ Discuss issues surrounding peer pressure. Ask the adolescent if he feels that social pressure causes him to ignore his diet or avoid self-administering insulin. Ask if he feels embarrassed by his disorder. Explore ways of dealing with peer pressure. *Peer pressure is a reality that each adolescent must learn to deal with.*
◆ Consult with a diabetes educator and assist the parents and the child with disease management.

Hyperglycemia

◆ Administer regular insulin for fast action *to promote euglycemia and prevent complications.*
◆ Administer I.V. fluids without dextrose *to flush out acetone and maintain hydration.*
◆ Monitor electrolytes and ABG levels; administer bicarbonate as needed *to combat acidosis.*
◆ Monitor blood glucose level *to detect early changes and prevent complications such as diabetic ketoacidosis.*

Hypoglycemia

◆ Give a fast-acting carbohydrate, such as honey, orange juice, or sugar cubes, followed later by a protein source *to establish normal glucose levels, thereby preventing complications of hypoglycemia.*
◆ If the child is stuporous or unconscious, administer glucagon (subcutaneously, I.V., or I.M.) or dextrose I.V. *to prevent complications of hypoglycemia.*
◆ Review key teaching topics with the child and his family members *to ensure adequate knowledge about the condition and treatment,* including:
- complying with the prescribed treatment program (see *Teaching about insulin administration*)
- monitoring blood glucose levels
- understanding the importance of good hygiene
- preventing, recognizing, and treating hypoglycemia and hyperglycemia
- understanding the effect of blood glucose control on long-term health
- managing diabetes during minor illness (such as a cold, the flu, and an upset stomach) including testing urine for ketones
- providing the child and his parents with written materials that cover the teaching topic
- providing the parents with information about the Juvenile Diabetes Foundation.

Teaching about insulin administration

Here are some important elements to teach children, adolescents, and parents about insulin administration:
◆ When both types of insulin are used, clear insulin should be drawn up first to prevent contamination.
◆ The vial shouldn't be shaken; intermediate forms are suspensions and should be gently rotated to prevent air bubbles.
◆ Injection sites should be rotated to prevent lipodystrophy.
◆ The infant, child, or adolescent should eat when the insulin peaks (for example, in mid-afternoon and at bedtime).
◆ Insulin requirements may be altered with illness, stress, growth, food intake, and exercise; blood glucose measurements are the best way to determine insulin adjustments.

Evaluation

◆ The child and his parents accurately monitor blood glucose levels.
◆ The child and his parents verbalize knowledge about the disease, treatment required, and dietary needs.
◆ The child and his parents can state the signs of hyperglycemia and hypoglycemia and know how to intervene appropriately.
◆ The child verbalizes strategies to cope with peer pressure and shows verbal evidence of a positive self-image.
◆ The parents can identify support services in the community.

URINARY TRACT INFECTION

URINARY TRACT INFECTION is a microbial invasion of the kidneys, ureters, bladder, or urethra.

The risk of UTIs varies depending on the child's age and the presence of obstructive uropathy or voiding dysfunction. In the neonatal period, UTIs occur most commonly in males, possibly because of the higher incidence of congenital abnormalities in male neonates. By age 4 months, UTIs are much more common in girls than in boys. The increased incidence in girls continues throughout childhood.

After infancy, nearly all UTIs occur when bacteria enter the urethra and ascend the urinary tract. Females are especially at risk for infection because the female urethra is much shorter than the male urethra. Also, the female urethra is subject to direct contamination because of its proximity to the anal opening. *Escherichia coli* causes approximately 75% to 90% of all UTIs in females.

Possible causes

- Incomplete bladder emptying
- Irritation by bubble baths
- Poor hygiene
- Reflux
- Sexual abuse

Assessment findings

- Abdominal pain
- Enuresis
- Frequent urges to void with pain or burning on urination
- Hematuria
- Lethargy
- Low-grade fever
- Poor feeding patterns
- Urine that's cloudy and foul-smelling

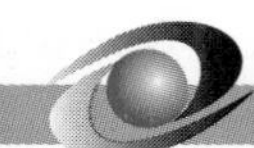

QUICK STUDY

To remember the clinical findings associated with urinary tract infection, think, "The urinary tract is **FULL** of infection."

Frequent urges to void
Urine that's foul-smelling and cloudy
Low-grade fever
Lethargy

Diagnostic evaluation

- Clean-catch urine culture yields large amounts of bacteria.
- Urine pH is increased.

Nursing diagnoses

- Impaired urinary elimination
- Acute pain
- Risk for infection
- Deficient knowledge regarding child growth and development.

Treatment

- Cranberry juice (acidifies urine)
- Forced fluids (flushes infection from the urinary tract)

Drug therapy options

- Antibiotic: co-trimoxazole (Bactrim), ampicillin (to prevent glomerulonephritis)

Planning and goals

- The child will report increased comfort.
- The child will have minimal complications.
- The child and his parents will verbalize an understanding of the condition and methods to reduce recurrence (perineal cleaning, increasing fluids, avoiding bubble baths, and more frequent voiding).
- The parents will verbalize an understanding of the treatment and medication administration.

Implementation

- Monitor input and output *to determine if fluid replacement therapy is adequate.*
- Assess toileting habits for proper front-to-back wiping and proper hand washing *to prevent recurrent infection.*
- Encourage increased intake of fluids and cranberry juice *to flush the infection from the urinary tract and acidify the urine.*
- Assist the child when necessary *to ensure that the perineal area is clean after elimination. Cleaning the perineal area by wiping from the area of least contamination (urinary meatus) to the area of greatest contamination (anus) helps prevent UTIs.*
- Assess family interaction for signs of sexual abuse, as appropriate; follow protocol for reporting if necessary *to promote child safety.*

Evaluation

- The child expresses relief from symptoms, such as pain, urinary frequency, and burning on urination.
- The child has no complications resulting from the infection.
- The child and his parents verbalize an understanding of the need to complete the full course of antibiotics.
- The child and his parents demonstrate an understanding of the methods of preventing a UTI, such as avoiding bubble baths, using the toilet every 2 hours, and performing proper toilet hygiene (wiping from front to back).

ADOLESCENT DISORDERS

ACNE VULGARIS

An inflammatory disease of the sebaceous follicles, ACNE VULGARIS primarily affects adolescents, although lesions can appear as early as age 8. Although acne strikes boys more commonly and more severely, it usually occurs in girls at an earlier age and tends to last longer, sometimes into adulthood. The prognosis is good with treatment.

Possible causes

- Androgen-stimulated sebum production
- Follicular occlusion
- *Propionibacterium acnes,* a normal skin flora

Risk factors

- Androgen stimulation
- Certain drugs, including corticosteroids, corticotropin, androgens, iodides, bromides, phenytoin (Dilantin), isoniazid (Liniazid), lithium (Lithobid), halothane (Fluothane); cobalt irradiation; total parenteral nutrition
- Cosmetics
- Emotional stress
- Exposure to heavy oils, greases, or tars
- Heredity
- Hormonal contraceptives (Many females experience an acne flare-up during their first few menses after starting or discontinuing hormonal contraceptives.)
- Trauma or rubbing from tight clothing
- Unfavorable climate

Assessment findings

- Closed comedo, or whitehead (acne plug not protruding from the follicle and covered by the epidermis)
- Open comedo, or blackhead (acne plug protruding and not covered by the epidermis)
- Inflammation and characteristic acne pustules, papules or, in severe forms, acne cysts or abscesses (caused by rupture or leakage of an enlarged plug into the dermis)
- Acne scars from chronic, recurring lesions

Diagnostic evaluation

- Diagnostic testing isn't necessary. The appearance of characteristic acne lesions, especially in an adolescent, confirms the presence of acne vulgaris.

Nursing diagnoses

- Impaired skin integrity
- Disturbed body image
- Risk for infection
- Risk for situational low self-esteem

Treatment

- Acne surgery (in severe cases)
- Cryotherapy
- Exposure to ultraviolet light (but never when a photosensitizing agent such as tretinoin [Retinoic acid, Retin-A] is being used)

Drug therapy options

- Intralesional corticosteroid injection
- Oral isotretinoin (Accutane) (limited to those with severe papulopustular or cystic acne that doesn't respond to conventional therapy)
- Systemic therapy: usually tetracycline (Achromycin), which decreases bacterial growth but, alternatively, erythromycin (tetracycline is contraindicated during pregnancy and childhood because it discolors developing teeth.)
- Topical medications: benzoyl peroxide (Benzac), clindamycin (Cleocin), erythromycin (Benzamycin)
- Antibacterial agent: alone or in combination with tretinoin (retinoic acid, Retin-A) or a keratolytic
- Antiandrogenic agents: estrogens, spironolactone (Aldactazide)

Planning and goals

- The adolescent will exhibit improved or healed wounds or lesions.
- The adolescent and his parents will demonstrate an understanding of the skin-care regimen.
- The adolescent will maintain a positive self-image.
- The adolescent will voice feelings about changed body image.
- The adolescent will maintain a positive self-image.

Implementation

- Try to identify predisposing factors *to determine if any may be eliminated or modified.*
- Explain the causes of acne to the adolescent and his parents. Make sure they understand the prescribed treatment is more likely to improve acne than a strict diet and fanatic scrubbing with soap and water. Provide written instructions regarding treatment *to eliminate misconceptions.*
- Instruct the adolescent receiving tretinoin to apply it at least 30 minutes after washing the face and at least 1 hour before bedtime. Warn against using it around the eyes or lips to prevent damage. After treatments, the skin should look pink and dry. If it appears red or starts to peel, the preparation may have to be weakened or applied less often.
- Advise the adolescent to avoid exposure to sunlight or to use a sunscreen *to prevent photosensitivity reaction.* If the prescribed regimen includes tretinoin and benzoyl peroxide, tell the adolescent to use one preparation in the morning and the other at night *to avoid skin irritation.*
- Instruct the adolescent to take tetracycline on an empty stomach and not to take it with antacids or milk *because it interacts with their metallic ions and is then poorly absorbed.*

◆ Tell the adolescent who's taking isotretinoin to avoid vitamin A supplements, which can worsen adverse effects. Also, discuss how to deal with the dry skin and mucous membranes that usually occur during treatment. Warn the female adolescent about the severe risk of teratogenesis and recommend effective contraception during treatment if she's sexually active. Monitor liver function and lipid levels *to avoid toxicity.*
◆ Inform the adolescent that acne takes a long time to clear — even years for complete resolution. Encourage continued local skin care even after acne clears. Explain the adverse effects of all drugs *to promote compliance.*
◆ Pay special attention to the adolescent's perception of his physical appearance, and offer emotional support *to help the adolescent cope with the effects of his illness.*

Evaluation

◆ The adolescent has improved skin integrity and acne diminishes.
◆ The adolescent expresses positive feelings about his body image.
◆ The adolescent and his parents understand predisposing factors for acne, such as cosmetic use or emotional stress.

CYSTIC FIBROSIS

CYSTIC FIBROSIS of the pancreas (also known as *fibrocystic disease of the pancreas* and *mucoviscidosis*) is a generalized dysfunction of the exocrine glands characterized by thickened tenacious secretions that occlude glandular ducts, causing dysfunction in many organ systems. It's a chronic, life-shortening disease that occurs in 1 out of every 2,500 to 3,000 live births and primarily affects white children.

Possible causes

◆ Cystic fibrosis is an autosomal recessive disease resulting from mutations in a gene located on chromosome 7. Research suggests that there may be as many as 800 genes that code for cystic fibrosis.

Assessment findings

Overall

◆ Failure to thrive; malnutrition

Respiratory

◆ Dry, nonproductive cough and wheezey respirations
◆ Excess mucus plugs in the airways leading to chronic obstructive pulmonary disease
◆ History of chronic, productive cough and recurrent respiratory infections, typically due to *Pseudomonas* infections

GI

◆ Bulky, greasy, foul-smelling stools that contain undigested food
◆ Distal intestinal obstruction syndrome (a partial or complete intestinal obstruction due to thick intestinal secretions)
◆ Increased appetite from undigested food lost in stools
◆ Meconium ileus at birth (the earliest symptom)
◆ Obstruction of pancreatic ducts preventing digestive enzymes from being released, resulting in decreased absorption of nutrients, especially fat-soluble vitamins (A, D, E, and K)
◆ Rectal prolapse due to large, bulky stools
◆ Thickened bile, which obstructs the ducts and results in eventual liver cirrhosis

Reproductive

◆ Blockage of the vas deferens by secretions, resulting in sterility in males
◆ Delayed puberty
◆ Viscous cervical secretions, which can lead to decreased fertility in females

Integumentary

◆ Channel defect in sweat glands, preventing sodium and chloride reabsorption, which places the child or adolescent at risk for abnormal salt loss and dehydration
◆ Salty taste of skin

Diagnostic evaluation

◆ Chest X-ray indicates early signs of obstructive lung disease.
◆ Sweat test using pilocarpine iontophoresis is positive.
◆ Stool specimen analysis indicates the absence of trypsin.

Nursing diagnoses

◆ Ineffective airway clearance
◆ Risk for infection
◆ Imbalanced nutrition: Less than body requirements
◆ Activity intolerance

Treatment

◆ Chest physiotherapy, postural drainage, and breathing exercises
◆ Multivitamins twice per day, especially fat-soluble vitamins

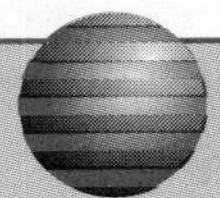

CLINICAL SITUATION

Caring for an adolescent with cystic fibrosis

A 16-year-old boy was diagnosed with cystic fibrosis at age 16 months and has been hospitalized many times for the condition. This time, he's in acute respiratory distress, with an upper and lower respiratory tract infection. He has a fever of 101.8° F (38.8° C), a respiratory rate of 38 breaths/minute, and a pulse rate of 128 beats/minute. His skin is dusky, and the nail beds are cyanotic. He has a barrel chest and supraclavicular and intercostal retractions. He's orthopneic, highly anxious, and restless. He's receiving oxygen by face mask.

What are appropriate steps to take when assessing the adolescent?

◆ Assess the level of the adolescent's respiratory distress and infection, noting respiratory rate and depth; skin color; breath sounds; amount, color, and consistency of sputum; temperature; and clubbing of fingers and toes. Clubbing of fingers and toes stems from chronic hypoxia.

◆ Assess the adolescent's cardiac status, noting blood pressure and apical pulse rate, rhythm, and quality. Chronic obstructive pulmonary disease can progress to cor pulmonale (right-sided heart failure), which can be a cause of death in cystic fibrosis.

◆ Assess the adolescent's nutritional status, estimating the thickness of subcutaneous tissue and comparing his weight and height with growth chart measurements. Diminished amounts of pancreatic enzymes result in malnutrition and malabsorption. The adolescent appears small for his age, thin and wasted, with little, if any, subcutaneous fat. He has a distended abdomen, a voracious appetite, and pale, transparent skin and is easily fatigued, displaying malaise, irritability, and lethargy.

◆ Assess the adolescent's fluid and electrolyte balance. *Prevention of dehydration is important because dehydration thickens mucoid secretions.*

◆ Assess the family's ability to cope with the acute episode and their continuing ability to cope with chronic cystic fibrosis. This clarifies their need for support or counseling.

◆ Assess the adolescent's developmental level. (See the section on Growth and development, page 21.) *This assessment helps the nurse to determine whether the adolescent is meeting age-appropriate developmental expectations.*

How can the nurse assist the adolescent in maintaining an age-appropriate developmental level?

◆ The adolescent is different from his peers and needs guidance in identifying ways in which he's the same to help him through the teen years when peer relationships are most important.

◆ Encourage independence within the limits imposed by his condition. Independence promotes a feeling of control over his situation and helps him regain and maintain self-esteem.

◆ Allow the adolescent to participate in decisions about care. Explain procedures, treatments, and routines directly and candidly. Approach him as an adult – avoid condescending or berating him – to help him regain a sense of control.

Questions for further thought

◆ What referrals are appropriate for the adolescent and family members?

◆ What adverse reactions would occur if the adolescent became dehydrated?

◆ High-protein formula and high-calorie supplement such as Pediasure

◆ Sodium supplementation, especially during hot weather

◆ Lung transplantation

Drug therapy options

◆ Antibiotics (I.V.): gentamycin (Garamycin) for *Pseudomonas* infection when infection interferes with daily functioning

◆ Mucolytic: dornase alfa (Pulmozyme), bronchodilator (Albuterol), antibiotic nebulizer inhalation treatment before chest physiotherapy

◆ Pancreatic enzyme: pancrelipase (Pancrease) for oral pancreatic enzyme replacement

Planning and goals

◆ The child will maintain adequate ventilation.

◆ The child will be free from acute respiratory infection.

◆ The child's nutrition will be adequate to meet his needs for growth and development.

◆ The child will continue to achieve age-appropriate developmental tasks. (See *Caring for an adolescent with cystic fibrosis.*)

◆ The child and parents will cope with chronic cystic fibrosis.

◆ The child and parents will verbalize understanding of treatment regimen.
◆ The child will maintain positive self-esteem.

Implementation

◆ Assess respiratory and cardiovascular status *for early detection of hypoxia.*
◆ Monitor vital signs and intake and output *to detect dehydration, which may worsen respiratory status. Dehydration can cause even thicker mucus secretions in the respiratory tract as well as constipation in children with cystic fibrosis.*
◆ Monitor pulse oximetry *to detect early signs of hypoxia.*
◆ Administer pancreatic enzymes with meals and snacks *to aid digestion and absorption of nutrients.*

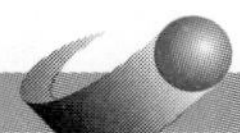

FAST FACT

When administering pancreatic enzymes, open the capsule and add the powder to a small amount of cold applesauce if the child can't swallow the capsule.

◆ Provide high-calorie, high-protein foods with added salt *to replace sodium loss and promote normal growth.*
◆ Encourage breathing exercises, verify that the child receives ordered respiratory treatments, and perform chest physiotherapy two to four times per day *to mobilize secretions, maintain lung capacity, and increase oxygenation.*
◆ Encourage physical activity *to promote normal development.*
◆ Review key teaching topics with the child and family members *to ensure adequate knowledge about the condition and treatment,* including:
– avoiding cough suppressants and antihistamines because the child must be able to cough and expectorate
– genetic counseling for the family
– promoting as normal a life as possible for the child.
◆ Consult with social services to assist with discharge planning and meeting home care needs to optimize outcomes.

Evaluation

◆ The child is afebrile and doesn't exhibit signs of respiratory infection.
◆ The child's nutritional intake results in slow, steady weight gain and meets his growth needs.
◆ The child and family members perform aerosol therapy (if ordered) and chest physiotherapy accurately and as frequently as necessary to prevent respiratory infection.
◆ The parents state that they'll seek medical care for respiratory infections or weight loss and have the child see the physician routinely for preventive care.
◆ The child engages in age-appropriate behaviors.
◆ The parents verbalize understanding of the treatment regimen and support services in the community.

MENINGITIS

MENINGITIS is an inflammation of the brain and spinal cord meninges. It's most common in infants and toddlers. The incidence of meningitis is greatly reduced with routine *Haemophilus influenzae* type B vaccine.

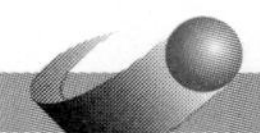

FAST FACT

About 70% of cases occur in children younger than age 5. Also, incidence increases among college students who reside in dormatories.

Possible causes

◆ Viral or bacterial agents, transmitted by the spread of droplets (organisms enter the blood from nasopharynx or middle ear)
◆ Complication of another bacterial infection
◆ Skull fracture, head wound, lumbar puncture, ventricular shunt

Assessment findings

◆ Coma
◆ Delirium
◆ Fever
◆ Headache
◆ High-pitched cry
◆ Irritability
◆ Nuchal rigidity that may progress to opisthotonos (arching of the back)
◆ Onset gradual or abrupt following an upper respiratory infection
◆ Petechial or purpuric lesions possibly present in bacterial meningitis
◆ Positive Brudzinski's sign (The child flexes the knees and hips in response to passive neck flexion.)
◆ Positive Kernig's sign (inability to extend leg when hip and knee are flexed)
◆ Projectile vomiting
◆ Seizures

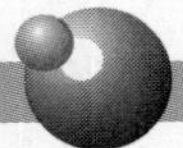

SPOT CHECK

A positive response to which tests help establish a diagnosis of meningitis?

Answer: A positive Brudzinski's sign and positive Kernig's sign help establish a diagnosis of meningitis.

Diagnostic evaluation

- Lumbar puncture shows increased CSF pressure, cloudy color, increased WBC count and protein level, and a decreased glucose level if the meningitis is caused by bacteria.
- Cultures of blood, urine, nose and throat secretions, chest X-ray, and ECG detect primary site.

Nursing diagnoses

- Decreased intracranial adaptive capacity
- Ineffective breathing pattern
- Risk for injury
- Hyperthermia
- Anxiety

Treatment

- Burr holes to evacuate subdural effusion, if present
- Droplet precautions, which should be maintained until at least 24 hours of effective antibiotic therapy have elapsed, with continued precautions recommended for meningitis caused by *H. influenzae* or *Neisseria meningitidis*
- Hypothermia blanket
- Oxygen therapy (which may require intubation and mechanical ventilation) to induce hyperventilation to decrease ICP
- Seizure precautions
- Treatment for coexisting conditions

Drug therapy options

- Analgesic: acetaminophen (Tylenol) (treats pain of meningeal irritation)
- Corticosteroid: dexamethasone (Decadron)
- Parenteral antibiotics: ceftazidime (Fortaz), ceftriaxone (Rocephin); possibly intraventricular administration of antibiotics

Planning and goals

- The child will maintain normal vital signs, including adequate ventilation and temperature within the normal range.
- The child will express feelings of comfort and relief from pain.
- The child will maintain fluid volume within normal range.
- The child and his parents will verbalize an understanding of the condition and its treatment.

Implementation

- Monitor vital signs and intake and output *to assess for fluid volume excess.*
- Assess the child's neurologic status frequently *to monitor for signs of increased ICP.*
- Provide a dark, quiet environment. Environmental stimuli can increase ICP or stimulate seizure activity.
- Maintain seizure precautions *to prevent injury.*
- Administer medications as ordered *to combat infection and decrease ICP.*
- Move the child gently *to prevent a rise in ICP.*
- Maintain isolation precautions, as ordered, *to prevent the spread of infection.*
- Provide emotional support for the family *to decrease anxiety.*
- Examine the infant for bulging fontanels and measure head circumference; *hydrocephalus is a complication that can result from meningitis.*

Evaluation

- The child expresses relief from symptoms and has no complications.
- The child's vital signs are normal.
- The child and his parents express an understanding of methods to prevent meningitis, including seeking proper medical treatment for chronic sinusitis or other chronic infections.

SCOLIOSIS

SCOLIOSIS, a lateral curvature of the spine, occurs more commonly in girls than in boys. About 10% of preadolescent children have some degree of scoliosis. The curvature progresses insidiously and may be prominent before the condition is diagnosed. It becomes more obvious at prepuberty, a time of rapid growth. The curve progression stops when bone growth stops. (See *Defects of the spinal column.*)

Possible causes

- Nonstructural, functional, or postural scoliosis — a nonprogressive C curve from some other condition, such as poor posture, unequal leg length, and poor vision

Defects of the spinal column

The illustrations below show degrees of spinal column curvature.

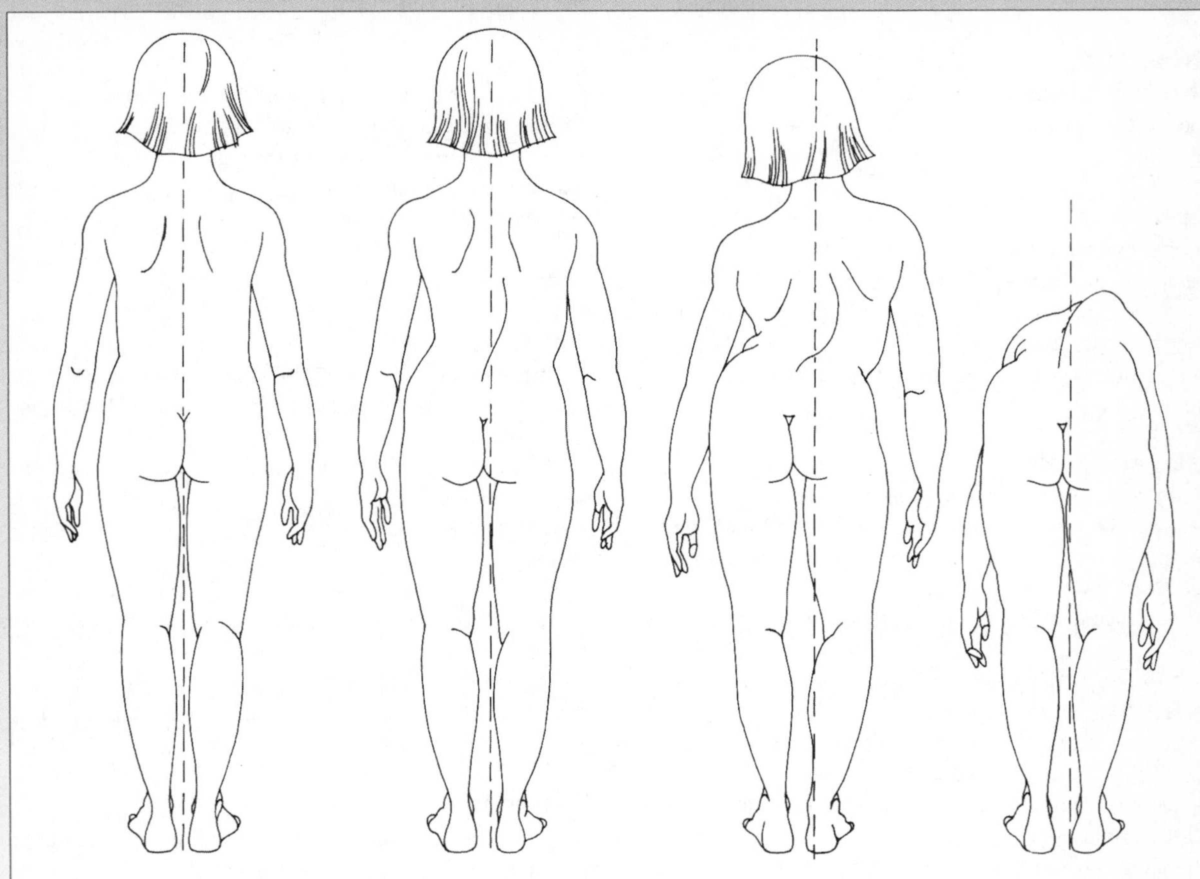

The normal spine in the upright position is vertically aligned, not twisted.

A child with mild to moderate spinal curvature (the upright spine has a marked serpentine twist) may benefit from corrective bracing or surgery.

The rib hump, a hallmark of severe scoliosis, is accentuated when the child bends forward. A child with severe curvature is generally treated with surgery.

◆ Structural or progressive scoliosis — a progressive S curve with a primary and compensatory curvature resulting in spinal and rib changes

Assessment findings

Nonstructural scoliosis

◆ Disappearing curve in the spinal column when the child bends at the waist to touch the toes

Structural scoliosis

◆ Failure of the spinal curve to straighten when the child bends forward with the knees straight and the arms hanging down toward the feet (The hips, ribs, shoulders, and shoulder blades are asymmetrical.)

Diagnostic evaluation

◆ X-rays may aid the diagnosis.

Nursing diagnoses

- ◆ Chronic pain
- ◆ Disturbed body image
- ◆ Delayed growth and development
- ◆ Powerlessness

Treatment

Nonstructural scoliosis

- ◆ Postural exercises
- ◆ Shoe lifts

Structural scoliosis

- ◆ Surgical placement of rods for curves greater than 40 degrees (to realign the spine or when curves fail to respond to orthotic treatment) along with spinal fusion with a bone graft from the iliac crest
- ◆ Possible prolonged bracing to slow progression of the condition

Planning and goals

- ◆ The adolescent's scoliosis will be arrested.
- ◆ The adolescent's skin will remain free from breakdown.
- ◆ The adolescent and his parents will comply with bracing and traction recommendations.
- ◆ The adolescent will adapt to brace and activity restrictions.
- ◆ The adolescent will physically adjust to the brace and help select clothing to wear with it.
- ◆ The adolescent will develop a positive self-image and continue with developmental tasks of adolescence.
- ◆ The parents will demonstrate understanding and support of the adolescent's independence.
- ◆ If the spinal fusion and rods are inserted, the adolescent and his parents will verbalize an understanding of the treatment, ongoing medical regimen and care, and injury prevention.
- ◆ If the adolescent undergoes surgery, he'll experience minimal complications (fluid volume deficit, infection, neurologic deficit).

Implementation

◆ Review key teaching topics with the adolescent and his parents *to ensure adequate knowledge about the condition and treatment,* including:
- performing stretching exercises for the spine
- taking steps to help the child maintain self-esteem.

◆ Consult with physical therapy to help develop a home care plan for the adolescent.

Adolescent with bracing

- ◆ Instruct the adolescent and his parents on proper application and wearing of the brace and inform them that the brace must be worn 16 to 23 hours each day *to slow progression of the condition.*
- ◆ Advise the adolescent to wear a cotton T-shirt under the brace *to protect the skin.*
- ◆ Examine the skin daily, especially over bony prominences, *to evaluate for signs of skin breakdown.*
- ◆ Instruct the adolescent on strategies to protect the skin (padding bony prominences, lubrication, proper nutrition) *to prevent skin breakdown.*

After spinal fusion and insertion of rods

- ◆ Monitor vital signs and intake and output *to prevent fluid volume deficit.*
- ◆ Turn the adolescent only by logrolling for the first 24 to 48 hours, depending on the type of instrumentation used, *to prevent injury.*
- ◆ Maintain correct body alignment *to promote joint mobility and prevent injury.*
- ◆ Maintain the bed in a flat position *to prevent injury and complications.*
- ◆ Help the adolescent adjust to the increase in height and altered self-perception *to promote self-esteem and decrease anxiety.*
- ◆ Perform neurologic assessment of lower extremities *to detect any change in condition* and report abnormalities to the physician immediately.

Evaluation

- ◆ The adolescent and his parents comply with the bracing regimen, and the scoliosis is arrested.
- ◆ The adolescent demonstrates a positive self-image.
- ◆ The adolescent demonstrates independence.
- ◆ The parents support the need for independence while allowing the adolescent to be dependent when appropriate.
- ◆ The adolescent maintains friendships with peers, who accept him in a brace.
- ◆ The adolescent returns for scheduled follow-up visits.
- ◆ The adolescent maintains skin integrity and complications are minimized.
- ◆ The adolescent and his parents are able to identify community and home resources.

Adult nursing

12

INTRODUCTION

This chapter reviews nursing care of adult clients with physiologic health problems, which are organized by body system for easy reference. As in other chapters of this book, the text follows the nursing process format to help you solve the nursing problems presented. Selected clinical situations (case studies) represent their high incidence among hospitalized clients or demonstrate nursing care principles essential to safe practice.

Before you being reading this chapter, consider reviewing entries on the nursing process, acid-base balance, fluid and electrolyte balance, shock, immobility, and perioperative nursing.

CARDIOVASCULAR SYSTEM

The cardiovascular system is made up of the heart and a network of arteries, veins, and smaller blood vessels that transport blood to and from all body organs and tissues.

CARDIOVASCULAR STRUCTURE AND FUNCTION

The cardiovascular system serves several vital functions, including:

◆ transporting life-supporting oxygen and nutrients to cells

◆ removing metabolic waste products

◆ carrying hormones from one part of the body to another.

Heart

The central organ of the cardiovascular system is the heart, which propels blood through the body by continuous rhythmic contractions. Review these other characteristics of the heart:

◆ It's a muscular organ composed of two atria (left and right) and two ventricles (left and right).

◆ The heart is surrounded by a pericardial sac that consists of two layers:

– visceral (inner) layer

– parietal (outer) layer.

◆ The heart wall has three layers:

– epicardium (visceral pericardium), the outer layer

– myocardium, the thick, muscular middle layer

– endocardium, the inner layer.

◆ Inside the heart are four valves:

– The tricuspid valve and mitral valve lie between the atria and ventricles; because of their location, they're also called *atrioventricular (AV) valves.* These valves prevent backflow of blood during systole.

– The pulmonic semilunar valve lies between the right ventricle and the pulmonary artery. The aortic semilunar valve lies between the left ventricle and the aorta. These valves prevent backflow of blood during diastole.

Coronary arteries

The heart is nourished by blood from two main arteries, the left coronary artery and the right coronary artery:

◆ As the left coronary artery branches off the aorta, it branches into the left anterior descending (LAD) artery and the circumflex artery. The LAD artery then supplies blood to the anterior wall of the left ventricle, the anterior ventricular septum, and the apex of the left ventricle. The circumflex artery supplies blood to the left atrium, the lateral and posterior portions of the left ventricle.

◆ The right coronary artery (RCA) fills the groove between the atria and ventricles and gives rise to the acute marginal artery, which becomes the posterior descending artery. The RCA sends blood to the sinoatrial (SA) and AV nodes and to the right atrium. The posterior descending artery supplies the posterior and inferior wall of the left ventricle and the posterior portion of the right ventricle.

Cardiac circulation

Blood circulates through the heart along the following pathway:

◆ from the inferior and superior venae cavae to the right atrium
◆ through the tricuspid valve to the right ventricle
◆ through the pulmonic valve to the pulmonary artery
◆ to the lungs, where blood is oxygenated
◆ through the pulmonary veins to the left atrium
◆ through the mitral valve to the left ventricle
◆ through the aortic valve to the aorta and throughout the body.

Conduction

The system that conducts electrical impulses and coördinates the heart's contractions consists of the SA node, internodal tracts, AV node, bundle of His, right and left bundle branches, and Purkinje fibers.

A normal electrical impulse is initiated at the SA node, the heart's intrinsic pacemaker, which results in the following chain of events:

◆ atrial depolarization
◆ atrial contraction
◆ impulse transmission to the AV node
◆ impulse transmission to the bundle of His, bundle branches, and Purkinje fibers
◆ ventricular depolarization
◆ ventricular contraction
◆ ventricular repolarization.

Cardiac function

Cardiac function is assessed by measuring these parameters:

◆ Cardiac output is the total amount of blood ejected from a ventricle per minute. Cardiac output equals stroke volume multiplied by heart rate ($CO = SV \times HR$).
◆ Stroke volume is the amount of blood ejected from a ventricle with each beat.
◆ Ejection fraction is the percent of left ventricular end-diastolic volume ejected during systole (normally 60% to 70%).

Systemic circulation

Blood is carried throughout the body in arteries and veins and through smaller vessels, such as arterioles, capillaries, and venules. Think of them as a series of large and small canals forming an interlocking system of blood flow.

◆ Arteries carry oxygenated blood from the heart to the tissues. They consist of three layers: the intima, media, and adventitia.
◆ Arterioles are small-resistance vessels that feed into capillaries.
◆ Capillaries join arterioles to venules (larger, lower-pressured vessels than arterioles), where nutrients and wastes are exchanged.
◆ Venules join capillaries to veins.
◆ Veins are large-capacity, low-pressure vessels that return unoxygenated blood to the heart.

CARDIOVASCULAR DISORDERS

Major cardiovascular disorders include angina, aortic aneurysm (abdominal and thoracic), arrhythmias, arterial occlusive disease, cardiac tamponade, cardiomyopathy, chronic venous insufficiency, coronary artery disease (CAD), endocarditis, heart failure, hypertension, myocardial infarction (MI), myocarditis, pericarditis, pulmonary edema, Raynaud's disease, rheumatic fever and rheumatic heart disease, thrombophlebitis, and valvular heart disease.

For all major cardiovascular disorders, the goal of nursing management is to decrease cardiac workload and increase myocardial blood supply so that tissue oxygenation increases and overall damage to the heart is reduced.

ANGINA

ANGINA — chest pain that results from myocardial ischemia — is the most common symptom of CAD, the term for cardiac conditions that result from myocardial ischemia, usually secondary to atherosclerosis. Angina is an imbalance between myocardial oxygen supply and demand.

Angina is generally categorized as one of three main forms:

◆ With stable angina, symptoms are consistent and pain is relieved by rest.
◆ With unstable angina, pain is marked by increasing severity, duration, and frequency. Pain from unstable angina responds slowly to nitroglycerin.
◆ With variant angina, pain is unpredictable and may occur at rest.

Possible causes

◆ Activity or disease that increases metabolic demands
◆ Aortic stenosis
◆ Atherosclerosis
◆ Pulmonary stenosis
◆ Small-vessel disease (associated with rheumatoid arthritis, radiation injury, or lupus erythematosus)
◆ Thromboembolism
◆ Vasospasm

Ischemic pain patterns

Ischemic pain experienced during a myocardial infarction radiates in various directions, as illustrated here.

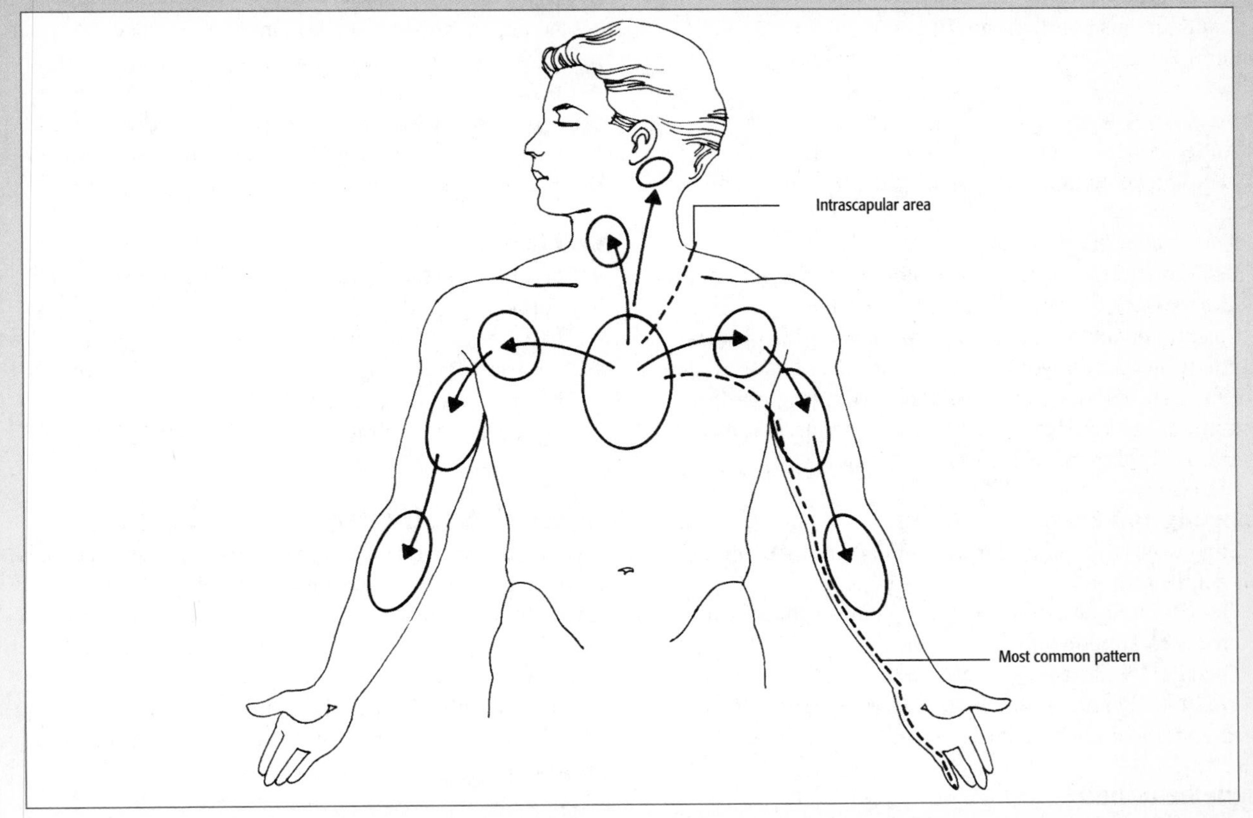

Assessment findings

- Pain: may be substernal, crushing, or compressing; may radiate to the arms, jaw, or back; usually lasts 3 to 5 minutes; it usually occurs after exertion, emotional excitement, or exposure to cold but can also develop when the client is at rest (see *Ischemic pain patterns*)
- Anxiety
- Diaphoresis
- Dyspnea
- Tachycardia
- Palpitations
- Epigastric distress

Diagnostic evaluation

- Blood chemistry test results may show increased cholesterol and low-density lipoprotein (LDL) levels, low high-density lipoprotein (HDL) levels, and elevated triglycerides.
- Cardiac enzyme levels are within normal limits.
- Coronary arteriography shows narrowing of coronary arteries.
- Electrocardiography (ECG) may show ST-segment depression and T-wave inversion during angina.
- Holter monitoring may reveal ST-segment depression and T-wave inversion during angina.
- Stress testing results include abnormal ECG results and chest pain.

Nursing diagnoses

- Acute pain
- Anxiety
- Activity intolerance
- Deficient knowledge (disorder and treatment)

Treatment

- Low-fat and low-cholesterol (and low-calorie, if necessary) diet
- Coronary artery bypass grafting
- Oxygen therapy
- Percutaneous coronary intervention
- Semi-Fowler's position

Drug therapy options

- Anticoagulant: heparin, warfarin (Coumadin)
- Antiplatelet aggregates: clopidogrel (Plavix), ticlopidine (Ticlid)
- Antiplatelet drug: aspirin
- Beta-adrenergic blockers: atenolol (Tenormin), metoprolol (Lopressor), nadolol (Corgard), propranolol (Inderal)
- Calcium channel blockers: diltiazem (Cardizem), nicardipine (Cardene), nifedipine (Procardia), verapamil (Calan)
- Nitrates: isosorbide dinitrate (Isordil), nitroglycerin (Nitrostat), topical nitroglycerin (Nitrol), transdermal nitroglycerin (Transderm-Nitro)

Planning and goals

- The client will reduce cardiovascular events by modifying risk factors.
- The client will increase activity tolerance through appropriate treatment.
- The client will have decreased anxiety by increasing his knowledge of cardiovascular status and experiencing fewer episodes of ischemic pain.

Implementation

- Assess cardiovascular status, hemodynamic variables, and vital signs *to detect evidence of cardiac compromise and response to treatment.*
- Monitor and record intake and output *to monitor fluid balance.*
- Administer medications, as prescribed, *to increase oxygenation and reduce cardiac workload.* If systolic blood pressure is less than 90 mm Hg, withhold the nitrate and beta-adrenergic blocker and notify the physician. If heart rate is less than 60 beats/minute, withhold the beta-adrenergic blocker and notify the physician *to prevent complications that can occur as a result of therapy.*
- Assess the client for chest pain, and evaluate its characteristics. *Assessment allows for modification of the care plan, as necessary.*
- Advise the client to rest when pain begins *to reduce cardiac workload.*
- Obtain a 12-lead ECG during an acute attack *to check for ischemic changes.*
- Keep the client in semi-Fowler's position *to promote chest expansion and ventilation.*
- Maintain the client's prescribed diet (low fat, low cholesterol and, if necessary, low calorie) *to reduce the risk of CAD.*
- Encourage weight reduction and smoking cessation, if necessary, *to reduce the risk of CAD.*
- Encourage the client to express anxiety, fears, or concerns *because anxiety can increase oxygen demands.*
- Administer oxygen therapy as needed *to increase oxygen supply during the anginal attack.*

Evaluation

- The client describes appropriate lifestyle changes to help prevent anginal episodes.
- The client understands and complies with the prescribed treatment plan.
- The client has fewer anginal episodes.
- The client demonstrates increased activity tolerance.

AORTIC ANEURYSM, ABDOMINAL

An ABDOMINAL AORTIC ANEURYSM results from damage to the medial layer of the abdominal portion of the aorta. Aneurysm commonly results from atherosclerosis which, over time, causes weakening in the medial layer of the artery. Continued weakening from the force of blood flow results in outpouching of the artery and formation of the aneurysm. The aneurysm may then rupture, leading to hemorrhage, hypovolemic shock, and even death.

An abdominal aneurysm can be one of five types:

- dissecting (rupture in the intimal layer, resulting in dissection of the vessel)
- false (bilateral outpouching in which layers of the vessel wall separate, forming a cavity)
- fusiform (bilateral outpouching)
- mycotic (caused by local infection)
- saccular (unilateral outpouching).

Possible causes

- Atherosclerosis
- Congenital defect
- Hypertension
- Infection
- Marfan syndrome
- Syphilis
- Trauma

Assessment findings

- Commonly asymptomatic

◆ Diminished femoral pulses
◆ Lower abdominal pain and lower back pain
◆ Abdominal pulsations
◆ Pulsatile abdominal mass to the left of the midline
◆ Systolic blood pressure in the legs lower than that in the arms
◆ Bruits over the site of the aneurysm
◆ Severe back or abdominal pain with hypotension indicates rupture

Diagnostic evaluation

◆ Abdominal computed tomography (CT) scanning shows an aneurysm.
◆ Abdominal ultrasound shows an aneurysm.
◆ Arteriography shows an aneurysm.
◆ ECG differentiates an aneurysm from an MI.

Nursing diagnoses

◆ Ineffective tissue perfusion (peripheral)
◆ Acute pain
◆ Death anxiety
◆ Risk for deficient fluid volume

Treatment

◆ Abdominal aortic aneurysm resection if greater than 5 cm or dissecting
◆ Bed rest
◆ Measures to control hypertension

Drug therapy options

◆ Analgesics: oxycodone (OxyContin), morphine sulfate
◆ Antihypertensives: hydralazine (Apresoline), nitroprusside (Nitropress)
◆ Vasodilator: nitroglycerin (Tridil)
◆ Beta-adrenergic blockers: propranolol (Inderal), metoprolol (Lopressor)

Planning and goals

◆ The client will be hemodynamically stable.
◆ The client will have pain relief.
◆ The client will maintain adequate peripheral tissue perfusion.

Implementation

◆ Assess cardiovascular status, and monitor and record vital signs. *Tachycardia, dyspnea, or hypotension may indicate fluid volume deficit caused by rupture of the aneurysm.*
◆ Monitor intake and output and the results of laboratory studies. *Low urine output and high specific gravity indicate hypovolemia.*
◆ Observe the client for signs and symptoms of hypovolemic shock, (such as anxiety, restlessness, severe back pain, decreased pulse pressure, increased thready pulse, and pale, cool, moist, clammy skin) *to detect aneurysm rupture.*
◆ Gently palpate the abdomen *to check for distention and pulsation. Increasing distention may signify impending rupture.*
◆ Check peripheral circulation — including pulses, temperature, color, and any sites where the client is experiencing abnormal sensations — *to detect poor arterial blood flow.*
◆ Assess pain *to detect enlarging aneurysm or rupture.*
◆ Administer medications, as prescribed, *to reduce hypertension and control pain.*
◆ Encourage the client to express feelings, such as a fear of dying, *to reduce anxiety.*
◆ Maintain a quiet environment *to control blood pressure and reduce the risk of rupture.*
◆ If the client has had surgery, perform postoperative care *to minimize complications.*

Evaluation

◆ The client maintains stable vital signs and doesn't exhibit signs of bleeding.
◆ The client verbalizes pain relief.
◆ The client verbalizes decreased fear after treatment.
◆ The client has palpable peripheral pulses.

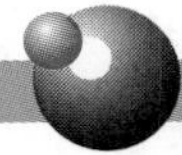

SPOT CHECK

A client comes into the emergency department with a dissecting aortic aneurysm. Is he at greatest risk for septic shock, anaphylactic shock, cardiogenic shock, or hypovolemic shock?
Answer: A dissecting aortic aneurysm is a precursor to aortic rupture, which leads to hemorrhage and hypovolemic shock.

AORTIC ANEURYSM, THORACIC

THORACIC AORTIC ANEURYSM is characterized by an abnormal widening of the ascending, transverse, or descending part of the aorta. Aneurysm of the ascending aorta is most common and most commonly fatal.

The aneurysm may be dissecting (hemorrhagic separation in the aortic wall, usually within the medial layer), saccular (outpouching of the arterial wall, with a narrow neck), or fusiform (spindle-shaped enlargement encompassing the entire circumference of the aorta).

Some aneurysms progress to serious and, eventually, lethal complications, such as rupture of an untreated thoracic dissecting aneurysm into the pericardium, with resulting tamponade.

Possible causes

- Atherosclerosis
- Congenital disorders such as coarctation of the aorta
- Fungal infection (infected aneurysm) of the aortic arch and descending segments
- Hypertension
- Syphilis, usually of the ascending aorta (uncommon because of antibiotics)
- Trauma, usually of the descending thoracic aorta, from an accident that shears the aorta transversely (acceleration-deceleration injuries)

Assessment findings

Ascending aneurysm

- Pain (described as severe, boring, and ripping and extending to the neck, shoulders, lower back, or abdomen)
- Unequal intensities of the right carotid and left radial pulses
- Bradycardia
- Pericardial friction rub caused by a hemopericardium

Descending aneurysm

- Pain (described as sharp and tearing, usually starting suddenly between the shoulder blades and possibly radiating to the chest)

Transverse aneurysm

- Pain (described as sharp and tearing and radiating to the shoulders)
- Dyspnea
- Dry cough
- Dysphagia
- Hoarseness

Diagnostic evaluation

- Aortography, the definitive test, shows the lumen of the aneurysm, its size and location, and the false lumen in a dissecting aneurysm.
- Blood chemistry test results may show low hemoglobin level because of blood loss from a leaking aneurysm.
- Chest X-ray shows widening of the aorta.
- CT scanning can be used to confirm and locate the aneurysm and may be used to monitor its progression.
- Echocardiography may be used to identify a dissecting aneurysm of the aortic root.
- ECG is used to distinguish a thoracic aneurysm from MI.
- Transesophageal echocardiography can be used to detect and measure the aneurysm in the ascending or descending aorta.

Nursing diagnoses

- Acute pain
- Anxiety
- Decreased cardiac output

Treatment

- Surgery (resection of the aneurysm through a Dacron or Teflon graft replacement and, possibly replacement of, the aortic valve)

Drug therapy options

- Analgesic: morphine sulfate
- Antihypertensives: nitroprusside (Nitropress), hydralazine (Apresoline)
- Vasodilator: nitroglycerin (Tridil)
- Negative inotropics: propranolol (Inderal), metoprolol (Lopressor)

Planning and goals

- The client will remain hemodynamically stable.
- The client will have pain relief.
- The client will verbalize understanding of the illness and treatment.

Implementation

- Monitor the client's blood pressure, pulmonary artery wedge pressure (PAWP), and central venous pressure (CVP) *to detect fluid volume deficit.* Also, evaluate pain, breathing, and carotid, radial, and femoral pulses *to detect early signs of aneurysm rupture.*
- Review laboratory test results, which must include a complete blood count (CBC) with differential, electrolyte levels, typing and crossmatching for whole blood, arterial blood gas (ABG) analysis, and urinalysis, *to assess hemoglobin levels and ensure that the client can tolerate surgery.*
- Insert an indwelling urinary catheter *to closely monitor urine output.*
- Administer dextrose 5% in water or lactated Ringer's solution and an antibiotic, if needed. Carefully monitor the nitroprusside I.V. infusion rate; use a separate I.V. line for infusion. Adjust the dose by slowly increasing the infusion rate. Meanwhile, check blood pressure every 5 minutes until it stabilizes *to note the effectiveness of treatment*

and prevent hypotension caused by a large dose of nitroprusside.

◆ With suspected bleeding from an aneurysm, give a whole-blood transfusion *to adequately replace the fluid volume deficit.*

◆ Explain diagnostic tests. If surgery is scheduled, explain the procedure and the expected postoperative care (I.V. lines, endotracheal (ET) and drainage tubes, cardiac monitoring, ventilation) *to alleviate the client's anxiety.*

After repair of thoracic aneurysm

◆ Evaluate the client's level of consciousness (LOC). Monitor vital signs; pulmonary artery pressure (PAP), PAWP, and CVP; pulse rate; urine output; and pain *to guide the treatment regimen and evaluate its effectiveness.*

◆ Check respiratory function. Carefully observe it and record the type and amount of chest tube drainage and frequently assess heart and breath sounds *to detect early signs of compromise.*

◆ Monitor I.V. therapy *to prevent fluid excess, which may occur with rapid fluid replacement.*

◆ Give medications, as appropriate, *to improve the client's condition.*

◆ Watch for signs of infection, especially fever, and excessive wound drainage *to initiate treatment promptly and prevent complications such as sepsis.*

◆ Assist with range-of-motion (ROM) exercises of legs *to prevent thromboembolism due to venostasis during prolonged bed rest.*

◆ After the client's vital signs have been stabilized, encourage him to turn, cough, and deep-breathe; assist if needed. If necessary, provide intermittent positive pressure breathing *to promote lung expansion.*

◆ Help the client walk as soon as he's able *to prevent complications of immobility, such as pneumonia and thromboembolism formation.*

◆ Throughout hospitalization, offer the client and his family members psychological support *to relieve anxiety and feelings of helplessness.*

◆ Before discharge, ensure adherence to antihypertensive therapy by explaining the need for such drugs and the expected adverse reactions. Teach the client how to monitor his blood pressure *to prevent complications associated with ineffective blood pressure management such as stroke.*

Evaluation

◆ The client has stable vital signs.

◆ The client verbalizes pain relief.

◆ The client cooperates with the treatment regimen and states understanding of the illness.

ARRHYTHMIAS

With cardiac ARRHYTHMIAS, abnormal electrical conduction or automaticity changes heart rate and rhythm. Arrhythmias vary in severity, from mild and asymptomatic ones that require no treatment (such as sinus arrhythmia, in which heart rate increases and decreases with respirations) to catastrophic ventricular fibrillation (VF), which necessitates immediate resuscitation.

Arrhythmias are generally classified according to origin (atrial or ventricular). The effect on cardiac output and blood pressure, partially influenced by the site of origin, determines the clinical significance. The most common arrhythmias include atrial fibrillation (AF), asystole, VF, and ventricular tachycardia (VT).

Possible causes

◆ Congenital
◆ Degeneration of conductive tissue
◆ Drug toxicity
◆ Electrolyte imbalance
◆ Heart disease
◆ MI
◆ Myocardial ischemia

Assessment findings

AF

◆ Complaints of feeling faint (with new onset)
◆ Irregular pulse with no pattern to the irregularity
◆ Palpitations
◆ Possibly asymptomatic (especially with chronic AF)

Asystole

◆ No pulse
◆ No palpable blood pressure
◆ Apnea
◆ Cyanosis

VF

◆ No pulse
◆ No palpable blood pressure
◆ Apnea

VT

◆ Chest pain
◆ Diaphoresis
◆ Dizziness
◆ Hypotension
◆ Possible loss of consciousness
◆ Weak pulse or pulselessness

Diagnostic evaluation

AF

◆ ECG shows irregular atrial rhythm, atrial rate greater than 400 beats/minute, irregular ventricular rhythm, QRS complexes of uniform configuration and duration, indiscernible PR interval, and no P waves or P waves that appear as erratic, irregular baseline fibrillation waves.

Asystole

◆ ECG shows no atrial or ventricular rate or rhythm and no discernible P waves, QRS complexes, or T waves.

VF

◆ ECG shows rapid and chaotic ventricular rhythm, wide and irregular QRS complexes, and no visible P waves.

VT

◆ ECG shows ventricular rate of 140 to 220 beats/minute, wide and bizarre QRS complexes, and no discernible P waves. VT may start or stop suddenly.

Nursing diagnoses

◆ Decreased cardiac output
◆ Ineffective tissue perfusion (cardiopulmonary)
◆ Impaired gas exchange
◆ Anxiety
◆ Deficient knowledge (disorder and treatment)

Treatment

AF

◆ Radiofrequency catheter ablation
◆ Synchronized cardioversion

Asystole

◆ Advanced cardiac life support (ACLS) protocol for treatment of arrhythmia and possible transcutaneous pacing
◆ Cardiopulmonary resuscitation (CPR)

VF

◆ ACLS protocol
◆ CPR
◆ Defibrillation
◆ Implantable cardioverter-defibrillator

VT

◆ ACLS protocol
◆ CPR, if pulseless
◆ Implantable cardioverter-defibrillator
◆ Synchronized cardioversion, if symptomatic

Drug therapy options

AF

◆ Antiarrhythmics (if client's condition is stable): amiodarone (Cordarone), digoxin (Lanoxin), diltiazem (Cardizem), procainamide (Pronestyl), verapamil (Calan)

Asystole

◆ Antiarrhythmics: atropine, epinephrine (Adrenalin), vasopressin (Pitressin) per ACLS protocol

VF

◆ Antiarrhythmics: amiodarone (Cordarone), epinephrine (Adrenalin), lidocaine (Xylocaine), magnesium sulfate, procainamide (Pronestyl), vasopressin (Pitressin) per ACLS protocol

VT

◆ Antiarrhythmics (if pulseless): amiodarone (Cordarone), epinephrine (Adrenalin), lidocaine (Xylocaine), vasopressin (Pitressin) per ACLS protocol if pulseless
◆ Antiarrhythmics (if VT with pulse): amiodarone (Cordarone), lidocaine (Xylocaine), procainamide (Pronestyl), sotalol (Betapace) per ACLS protocol
◆ Antiarrhythmics (if polymorphic VT): beta-adrenergic blockers, lidocaine (Xylocaine), amiodarone (Cordarone), procainamide (Pronestyl), sotalol (Betapace) per ACLS protocol
◆ Antiarrhythmics (if torsades de pointes): isoproterenol (Isuprel), lidocaine (Xylocaine), magnesium per ACLS protocol

Planning and goals

◆ The client will have improved cardiac circulation.
◆ The client will have adequate cardiac output.
◆ The client will have adequate oxygenation.

Implementation

◆ Assess an unmonitored client for rhythm disturbances *to promptly identify and treat life-threatening arrhythmias.*
◆ If the client's pulse is abnormally rapid, slow, or irregular, watch for signs of hypoperfusion, such as hypotension and diminished urine output, *to prevent such complications as renal failure and cerebral anoxia.*
◆ Document any arrhythmias in a monitored client *to create a record of their occurrence.* Assess the client for possible causes and effects *so proper treatment can be instituted.*
◆ When life-threatening arrhythmias develop, rapidly assess LOC, respirations, and pulse *to avoid crisis.*

◆ Initiate CPR, if indicated, *to maintain cerebral perfusion until other ACLS measures are successful.*
◆ Evaluate the client for altered cardiac output resulting from arrhythmias. *Decreased cardiac output may cause inadequate perfusion of major organs, leading to irreversible damage.*
◆ If trained, perform defibrillation early for VT and VF. *Studies show that early intervention with defibrillation improves the client's chance of survival.*
◆ Administer medications as needed, and prepare for medical procedures (for example, cardioversion) if indicated *to ensure prompt treatment of life-threatening arrhythmias.*
◆ Monitor the client for predisposing factors — such as fluid and electrolyte imbalance — and signs of toxic reaction to his drug therapy, especially if he's taking digoxin. If he has such a reaction, his next dose may need to be withheld. *Alleviating predisposing factors decreases the risk of arrhythmias.*
◆ Provide adequate oxygen, and reduce the heart's workload, while carefully maintaining metabolic, neurologic, respiratory, and hemodynamic status *to prevent arrhythmias in a cardiac client.*
◆ Install a fresh pacemaker battery before use. Carefully secure the external catheter wires and the pacemaker box. Assess the threshold daily. Watch closely for premature contractions, a sign of myocardial irritation. *These measures are necessary to avoid temporary pacemaker malfunction.*
◆ Restrict the client's activity after permanent pacemaker insertion. Monitor the pulse rate regularly, and watch for signs of decreased cardiac output. *These measures avert permanent pacemaker malfunction.*
◆ Caution if the client with a permanent pacemaker about environmental hazards, as indicated by the pacemaker manufacturer, *to avoid pacemaker malfunction.*

Evaluation

◆ The client has stable vital signs and a controlled cardiac rhythm.
◆ The client maintains optimal oxygenation.

ARTERIAL OCCLUSIVE DISEASE

With ARTERIAL OCCLUSIVE DISEASE, the obstruction or narrowing of the lumen of the aorta and its major branches causes an interruption of blood flow, usually to the legs and feet. Arterial occlusive disease may affect the carotid, vertebral, innominate, subclavian, mesenteric, and celiac arteries. Occlusions may be acute or chronic, and commonly cause severe ischemia, skin ulceration, and gangrene.

Arterial occlusive disease is more common in males than in females. The prognosis depends on the location of the occlusion, the development of collateral circulation to counteract reduced blood flow and, in acute disease, the time elapsed between the onset of the occlusion and its removal.

Possible causes

◆ Atherosclerosis
◆ Emboli formation
◆ Thrombosis
◆ Trauma or fracture

Risk factors

◆ Age
◆ Diabetes
◆ Family history of vascular disorders, MI, or stroke
◆ Hyperlipemia
◆ Hypertension
◆ Smoking

Assessment findings

Femoral, popliteal, or innominate arteries

◆ Mottling of the extremity
◆ Pallor
◆ Paralysis and paresthesia in the affected arm or leg
◆ Pulselessness distal to the occlusion
◆ Sudden and localized pain in the affected arm or leg (most common symptom)
◆ Temperature change that occurs distal to the occlusion

Internal and external carotid arteries

◆ Diminished pulses with an auscultatory bruit over affected vessels
◆ Transient ischemic attacks (TIAs), which produce transient monocular blindness, dysarthria, hemiparesis, possible aphasia, confusion, decreased mentation, headache
◆ Stroke

Subclavian artery

◆ Subclavian steal syndrome (characterized by the backflow of blood from the brain through the vertebral artery on the same side as the occlusion, into the subclavian artery distal to the occlusion; clinical effects of vertebrobasilar occlusion and exercise-induced arm claudication)

Vertebral and basilar arteries

◆ TIAs, which produce binocular vision disturbances, vertigo, dysarthria, and falling down without loss of consciousness

Diagnostic evaluation

◆ Arteriography demonstrates the type (thrombus or embolus), location, and degree of obstruction and collateral circulation.
◆ Doppler ultrasonography shows decreased blood flow distal to the occlusion.
◆ EEG and a CT scan may be necessary to rule out brain lesions.
◆ Ophthalmodynamometry helps determine the degree of obstruction in the internal carotid artery by comparing ophthalmic artery pressure to brachial artery pressure on the affected side. A more than 20% difference between pressures suggests insufficiency.

Nursing diagnoses

◆ Ineffective tissue perfusion (type depends on the location of the occlusion)
◆ Acute pain
◆ Fear

Treatment

◆ Exercise such as walking
◆ Smoking cessation
◆ Surgery (for acute arterial occlusive disease), including atherectomy, balloon angioplasty, bypass grafting, embolectomy, laser angioplasty, patch grafting, stent placement, thromboendarterectomy, or amputation

Drug therapy options

◆ Anticoagulants: heparin, warfarin (Coumadin)
◆ Antiplatelet drugs: aspirin, pentoxifylline (Trental), cilostazol (Pletal)
◆ Thrombolytics: alteplase (Activase), streptokinase (Streptase)

Planning and goals

◆ The client will have increased perfusion to the affected area.
◆ The client will report decreased pain in the affected area.
◆ The client will verbalize decreased fear regarding occlusion and treatment.

Implementation

◆ Advise the client to stop smoking and to follow the prescribed medical regimen *to modify risk factors and promote adherence.*

Preoperative (during an acute episode)

◆ Check for the most distal pulses, and inspect skin color and temperature *to assess the client's circulatory status. Decreased tissue perfusion causes mottling; skin also becomes cooler, and skin texture changes.*
◆ Provide pain relief as needed *to help decrease ischemic pain.*
◆ Administer heparin by continuous I.V. drip as needed *to prevent thrombi.* Use an infusion monitor or pump *to ensure the proper flow rate.*
◆ Wrap the client's affected foot in soft cotton batting, and reposition it frequently *to prevent pressure on any one area.* Strictly avoid elevating or applying heat to the affected leg. *Directly heating extremities causes increased tissue metabolism; if arteries don't dilate normally, tissue perfusion decreases and ischemia may occur.*
◆ Watch for signs of fluid and electrolyte imbalance, and monitor intake and output for signs of renal failure (urine output less than 30 ml/hour). *Electrolyte imbalances and renal failure are complications that may occur as a result of arterial occlusion and tissue damage.*
◆ If the client has a carotid, innominate, vertebral, or subclavian artery occlusion, monitor him for signs of stroke, such as numbness in an arm or leg and intermittent blindness, *to detect early signs of decreased cerebral perfusion.*

Postoperative

◆ Monitor the client's vital signs *to assess for changes in condition.* Continuously assess his circulatory function by inspecting skin color and temperature and by checking for distal pulses. In charting, compare earlier assessments and observations. Watch closely for signs of hemorrhage (such as tachycardia and hypotension), and check dressings for excessive bleeding *to prevent or detect postoperative complications.*
◆ If the client has carotid, innominate, vertebral, or subclavian artery occlusion, assess neurologic status frequently for changes in LOC or muscle strength and pupil size *to ensure prompt treatment of deteriorating neurologic status.*
◆ If the client has mesenteric artery occlusion, connect a nasogastric (NG) tube to low, intermittent suction. Monitor intake and output. *Low urine output may indicate damage to renal arteries during surgery.* Assess abdominal status. *Increasing abdominal distention and tenderness*

may indicate extension of bowel ischemia with resulting gangrene, (necessitating further excision) or peritonitis.

◆ If the client has saddle block occlusion, check distal pulses *to assess for adequate circulation.* Watch for signs of renal failure and mesenteric artery occlusion (such as severe abdominal pain) and cardiac arrhythmias, which may precipitate embolus formation, *to ensure prompt recognition and treatment of complications.*

◆ If the client has iliac artery occlusion, monitor urine output *to assess for signs of renal failure from decreased perfusion to the kidneys as a result of surgery.* Provide meticulous catheter care *to prevent complications.*

◆ If the client has femoral or popliteal artery occlusion, assist with early ambulation and discourage prolonged sitting *to encourage circulation to the extremities.*

◆ After amputation, check the client's stump carefully for drainage and record its color and amount and the time *to detect hemorrhage.* Elevate the stump, and administer adequate analgesic *to treat edema and pain.* Because phantom limb pain is common, explain this phenomenon to the client *to reduce his anxiety.*

◆ When preparing the client for discharge, instruct him to watch for signs of recurrence (pain, pallor, numbness, paralysis, coldness, absence of pulse) that can result from graft occlusion or occlusion at another site. Warn him against wearing constrictive clothing. *These measures enable the client to participate in his care, and allow him to make more informed decisions about his health status.*

Evaluation

◆ The client discusses lifestyle adjustments to reduce the risk of occlusion.

◆ The client has a decreased level of pain.

◆ The client demonstrates decreased fear after being treated for occlusion.

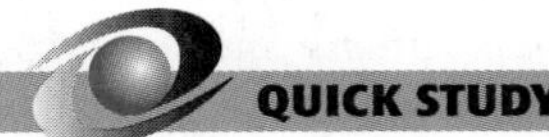

QUICK STUDY

Remember the signs and symptoms of acute occlusion by the six P's.

Pain
Pallor
Paralysis
Paresthesia
Polar (coldness)
Pulselessness

CARDIAC TAMPONADE

In CARDIAC TAMPONADE, a rapid, unchecked rise in intrapericardial pressure impairs diastolic filling of the heart. The rise in pressure usually results from blood or fluid accumulation in the pericardial sac.

If fluid rapidly accumulates, this condition is commonly fatal and necessitates emergency lifesaving measures. (See *Caring for the client with cardiac tamponade,* page 324.) Slow accumulation and rise in pressure, as in pericardial effusion associated with cancer, may not produce immediate symptoms because the fibrous wall of the pericardial sac can gradually stretch to accommodate as much as 1 to 2 L of fluid.

Possible causes

◆ Dressler's syndrome

◆ Effusion (in cancer, bacterial infections, tuberculosis and, rarely, acute rheumatic fever)

◆ Hemorrhage from nontraumatic causes (such as rupture of the heart or great vessels or anticoagulant therapy in a client with pericarditis)

◆ Hemorrhage from trauma (such as gunshot or stab wounds of the chest and perforation by a catheter during cardiac or central venous catheterization or after cardiac surgery)

◆ MI

◆ Uremia

Assessment findings

◆ Anxiety

◆ Diaphoresis

◆ Dyspnea

◆ Reduced arterial blood pressure

◆ Restlessness

◆ Tachycardia

◆ Muffled heart sounds on auscultation

◆ Narrow pulse pressure

◆ Neck vein distention

◆ Pallor or cyanosis

◆ Hepatomegaly

◆ Increased venous pressure

◆ Pulsus paradoxus (an abnormal inspiratory drop in systemic blood pressure greater than 15 mm Hg)

◆ Upright, leaning forward posture

Diagnostic evaluation

◆ Chest X-ray shows slightly widened mediastinum and cardiomegaly.

◆ Echocardiography records pericardial effusion with collapse of the cardiac chambers during diastole.

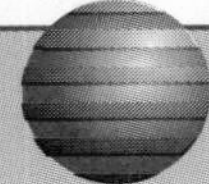

CLINICAL SITUATION

Caring for the client with cardiac tamponade

A 40-year-old male client is admitted to the telemetry unit after being involved in a motor vehicle crash during which he forcefully struck the steering wheel. Slight bruising is evident over the sternal area. On admission, the client's electrocardiogram (ECG) is normal and he denies chest discomfort. Six hours after admission, the client suddenly complains of chest discomfort and difficulty breathing. He's diaphoretic and anxious.

What emergency measures should be instituted?

A. Notify the physician, administer oxygen, assess vital signs, obtain an ECG, and have an emergency cart nearby containing a pericardiocentesis needle.

B. Assess vital signs, obtain an ECG, and administer nitroglycerin and morphine sulfate.

C. Notify the family, make the client comfortable, and administer a sedative.

D. Notify the physician, obtain blood work, administer oxygen, and obtain an ECG.

Answer: A. Trauma to the chest can result in cardiac tamponade. Because this is a life-threatening situation, notify the physician immediately, administer oxygen to improve cardiac perfusion, assess vital signs to evaluate hemodynamic status, obtain an ECG to detect arrhythmias or ischemia, and have emergency equipment available in case the client's condition deteriorates and pericardiocentesis is necessary.

Questions for further thought

◆ What further measures could be taken to relieve cardiac tamponade, other than pericardiocentesis?

◆ What nursing diagnoses apply to the client complaining of chest discomfort and exhibiting signs of anxiety?

◆ ECG may reveal changes produced by acute pericarditis. This test is useful to rule out other cardiac disorders.

◆ Pulmonary artery catheterization detects increased right atrial pressure, right ventricular diastolic pressure, and CVP.

Nursing diagnoses

◆ Decreased cardiac output

◆ Ineffective tissue perfusion (cardiopulmonary)

◆ Anxiety

Treatment

◆ PERICARDIOCENTESIS (needle aspiration of the pericardial sac), surgical creation of an opening to drain fluid, or thoracotomy

Drug therapy options

◆ Heparin antagonist: protamine sulfate in heparin-induced tamponade

◆ Inotropic agents: dopamine (Intropin), isoproterenol (Isuprel)

◆ Vitamin: vitamin K (AquaMEPHYTON) in warfarin-induced cardiac tamponade

Planning and goals

◆ The client will maintain hemodynamic stability.

◆ The client will have adequate tissue perfusion.

◆ The client will have decreased anxiety after appropriate treatment.

Implementation

If the client needs pericardiocentesis

◆ Explain the procedure to the client *to alleviate anxiety.*

◆ Keep a pericardial aspiration needle attached to a 50-ml syringe by a three-way stopcock, an ECG machine, and an emergency cart with a defibrillator at the bedside. Make sure the equipment is turned on and ready for immediate use *to avoid treatment delay.*

◆ Position the client at a 45- to 60-degree angle. Connect the precordial ECG lead to the hub of the aspiration needle with an alligator clamp and connecting wire. When the needle touches the myocardium during fluid aspiration, ST-segment elevation or premature ventricular contractions will be seen. *Monitoring the client's ECG ensures the accuracy of the procedure and helps prevent complications.*

◆ Monitor blood pressure and CVP during and after pericardiocentesis *to monitor for complications, such as hypotension, which may indicate cardiac chamber puncture.*

◆ Infuse I.V. solutions *to maintain blood pressure.* Watch for a decrease in CVP and a concomitant rise in blood pressure, *which indicate relief of cardiac compression.*

◆ Watch for complications of pericardiocentesis, such as VF, vasovagal response, and coronary artery or cardiac chamber puncture *to prevent crisis.*

◆ Closely monitor ECG changes, blood pressure, pulse rate, LOC, and urine output *to detect signs of decreased cardiac output.*

If the client needs thoracotomy

◆ Explain the procedure to the client. Tell him what to expect postoperatively (chest tubes, drainage bottles, administration of oxygen) *to decrease anxiety.* Teach him how to turn, deep-breathe, and cough *to prevent postoperative complications and relieve his anxiety.*
◆ Give antibiotics *to prevent or treat infection,* and protamine sulfate or vitamin K (AquaMEPHYTON) as needed *to prevent hemorrhage.*
◆ Postoperatively, monitor critical parameters, such as vital signs and ABG levels, and assess heart and breath sounds *to detect early signs of complications such as reaccumulation of fluid.*
◆ Give pain medication as needed *to alleviate pain and promote comfort.*
◆ Maintain the chest drainage system and be alert for complications, such as hemorrhage and arrhythmias, *to prevent further decompensation.*

Evaluation

◆ The client has stable vital signs and adequate oxygenation.
◆ The client verbalizes an understanding of the condition and its treatment.

CARDIOMYOPATHY

In CARDIOMYOPATHY, the myocardium (middle muscular layer) around the left ventricle becomes hypertrophic, altering cardiac function and resulting in decreased cardiac output. Increased heart rate and increased muscle mass compensate in early stages, but in later stages heart failure develops.

The three types of cardiomyopathy are:
◆ dilated (congestive), the most common form, in which dilated heart chambers contract poorly, causing blood to pool and reducing cardiac output
◆ hypertrophic (obstructive), in which a hypertrophied left ventricle can't relax and fill properly
◆ restrictive (obliterative), a rare form, characterized by stiff ventricles resistant to ventricular filling.

Possible causes

Dilated cardiomyopathy

◆ Chronic alcoholism
◆ Infection
◆ Metabolic and immunologic disorders
◆ Pregnancy and postpartum disorders

Hypertrophic cardiomyopathy

◆ Congenital
◆ Chronic hypertension

Restrictive cardiomyopathy

◆ Amyloidosis
◆ Cancer and other infiltrative diseases
◆ Postradiation treatment
◆ Diabetes mellitus

Assessment findings

◆ Chest pain
◆ Cough
◆ Crackles on lung auscultation
◆ Enlarged heart
◆ Dependent pitting edema
◆ Dyspnea, paroxysmal nocturnal dyspnea
◆ Enlarged liver
◆ Fatigue
◆ Jugular vein distention
◆ Murmur, S_3 or S_4 heart sounds
◆ Syncope

Diagnostic evaluation

◆ Cardiac catheterization excludes the diagnosis of coronary artery disease.
◆ Chest X-ray shows cardiomegaly and pulmonary congestion.
◆ ECG findings indicate left ventricular hypertrophy, nonspecific changes, or low voltage.
◆ Echocardiography shows decreased myocardial function and enlarged chamber sizes.
◆ Exercise thallium-201 scintigraphy detects underlying coronary artery disease.

Nursing diagnoses

◆ Decreased cardiac output
◆ Impaired gas exchange
◆ Activity intolerance

Treatment

◆ Dietary changes: establishing a low-sodium diet with vitamin supplements
◆ Dual-chamber pacing (for hypertrophic cardiomyopathy)
◆ Surgery (when medication fails): heart transplantation or cardiomyoplasty (for dilated cardiomyopathy); ventricular myotomy (for hypertrophic cardiomyopathy); cardiomyostimulator (for dilated cardiomyopathy)

Drug therapy options

- Beta-adrenergic blockers: propranolol (Inderal), nadolol (Corgard), metoprolol (Lopressor) for hypertrophic cardiomyopathy
- Calcium channel blockers: particularly, verapamil (Calan), and diltiazem (Cardizem) for hypertrophic cardiomyopathy
- Diuretics: furosemide (Lasix), bumetanide (Bumex), metolazone (Zaroxolyn) for dilated cardiomyopathy
- Inotropic drugs: dobutamine (Dobutrex), milrinone (Primacor), digoxin for dilated cardiomyopathy
- Oral anticoagulant: warfarin (Coumadin) for dilated cardiomyopathy
- Vasodilators: nitroprusside (Nitropress), nitroglycerin (Tridil) to reduce preload and afterload in dilated cardiomyopathy

Planning and goals

- The client will remain hemodynamically stable.
- The client will have adequate oxygenation.
- The client will have increased activity tolerance.

Implementation

- Monitor ECG *to detect arrhythmias and ischemia.*
- Monitor laboratory results *to detect abnormalities such as hypokalemia from the use of diuretics.*
- Monitor respiratory status *to detect evidence of heart failure, such as dyspnea and crackles.*
- Assess cardiovascular status, vital signs, and hemodynamic variables *to detect heart failure.*
- Monitor and record intake and output *to detect fluid volume overload.*
- Keep the client in semi-Fowler's position *to enhance gas exchange.*
- Maintain bed rest *to reduce oxygen demands on the heart.*
- Administer oxygen therapy and medications, as prescribed, *to improve oxygenation and cardiac output.*
- Maintain the client's prescribed diet. *A low-sodium diet reduces fluid retention.*
- If the client requires surgery, explain the procedure and tell him what to expect postoperatively *to decrease anxiety.*

Evaluation

- The client has stable vital signs.
- The client has a stable respiratory status.
- The client has safely increased his activity level.

CORONARY ARTERY DISEASE

CORONARY ARTERY DISEASE (CAD) results from the buildup of atherosclerotic plaque in the arteries of the heart. This buildup causes a narrowing of the arterial lumen and reduces blood flow to the myocardium.

Possible causes

- Arteriosclerosis
- Atherosclerosis

Risk factors

- Aging
- Depletion of estrogen after menopause
- Diabetes
- Genetics
- High-fat, high-cholesterol diet
- Hyperlipidemia
- Hypertension
- Obesity
- Sedentary lifestyle
- Smoking
- Stress

Assessment findings

- Angina (manifests as substernal pain or compression or pressure; may radiate to the arms, jaw, or back; usually lasts 3 to 5 minutes; usually occurs after exertion, emotional excitement, or exposure to cold but can also develop at rest)

Diagnostic evaluation

- Blood chemistry test results may show increased cholesterol levels; specifically, decreased HDL levels and increased LDL levels.
- Coronary arteriography shows narrowing of the coronary arteries.
- ECG or Holter monitoring shows ST-segment depression and T-wave inversion during an anginal episode.
- Stress testing reveals ST-segment changes and provokes chest discomfort.

Nursing diagnoses

- Acute pain
- Impaired gas exchange
- Activity intolerance

Treatment

- Activity changes, including weight loss (if necessary)
- Low-cholesterol, low-fat and, if appropriate, low-calorie and low-sodium diet with more dietary fiber

- Percutaneous coronary intervention, such as atherectomy, percutaneous transluminal coronary angioplasty, or coronary artery stenting
- Coronary artery bypass grafting surgery

Drug therapy options

- Analgesic: morphine sulfate
- Anticoagulant: heparin
- Antilipemics: atorvastatin (Lipitor), gemfibrozil (Lopid), lovastatin (Mevacor), nicotinic acid (Niaspan), pravastatin (Pravachol), simvastatin (Zocor)
- Antiplatelet aggregate: aspirin
- Beta-adrenergic blockers: metoprolol (Lopressor), nadolol (Corgard), propranolol (Inderal)
- Calcium channel blockers: nifedipine (Procardia), diltiazem (Cardizem), verapamil (Calan)
- Nitrates: isosorbide dinitrate (Isordil), nitroglycerin (Nitro-Bid)

Planning and goals

- The client will demonstrate increased activity tolerance.
- The client will have adequate oxygenation.
- The client will report pain relief.
- The client will verbalize understanding of treatment and comply with the regimen.

Implementation

- Obtain an ECG during anginal episodes *to detect evidence of ischemia.*
- Monitor laboratory studies. Evaluate cardiac enzyme levels *to rule out an MI.* Obtain a lipid panel *to determine the need for diet changes and antilipemics.*
- Assess cardiovascular status, vital signs, and hemodynamic variables *to detect evidence of compromise.*
- Monitor intake and output *to detect changes in fluid status.*
- Encourage the client to express anxiety, fears, or concerns *to help cope with illness.*
- Administer nitroglycerin sublingually *to provide pain relief from anginal episodes.*
- Consult with a registered dietitian *to help meet the client's nutritional or dietary needs.*

Evaluation

- The client demonstrates increased activity tolerance.
- The client maintains a stable respiratory status.
- The client remains free from pain.
- The client verbalizes understanding of the treatment modality and complies with the regimen.

ENDOCARDITIS, INFECTIVE

INFECTIVE ENDOCARDITIS is a bacterial or fungal infection of the endocardium, heart valves, or a cardiac prosthesis. This invasion produces vegetative growths on the heart valves, the endocardial lining of a heart chamber, or the endothelium of a blood vessel that may embolize to the spleen, kidneys, central nervous system, and lungs. This disorder is also called *endocarditis* or *bacterial endocarditis.*

In infective endocarditis, fibrin and platelets aggregate on the valve tissue and engulf circulating bacteria or fungi that flourish and produce friable verrucous vegetations. Such vegetations may cover the valve surfaces, causing ulceration and necrosis; they may also extend to the chordae tendineae, leading to their rupture and subsequent valvular insufficiency.

Untreated infective endocarditis is usually fatal but, with proper treatment, about 70% of clients recover. The prognosis is worse when infective endocarditis causes severe valvular damage, leading to insufficiency and heart failure, or when it involves a prosthetic valve.

Possible causes

- Enterococci
- I.V. drug abuse
- Staphylococci (especially *Staphylococcus aureus*)
- Streptococci (especially *Streptococcus viridans*)

Risk factors

- Coarctation of the aorta
- Degenerative heart disease
- Marfan syndrome
- Patent ductus arteriosus
- Pulmonary stenosis
- Subaortic and valvular aortic stenosis
- Tetralogy of Fallot
- Ventricular septal defects

Assessment findings

- Intermittent, recurring fever
- Night sweats
- Malaise
- Arthralgia
- Chills
- Fatigue
- Weakness
- Anorexia
- Weight loss
- Petechiae
- Roth spots (hemorrhagic areas with white centers on retina)

- Osler nodes (tender, raised subcutaneous lesions on fingers or toes)
- Janeway lesions (purplish macules on palms or soles)
- Signs of cerebral, pulmonary, renal, or splenic infarction
- Valvular insufficiency
- Heart murmur
- Sublingual splinter hemorrhage
- Splenomegaly

Diagnostic evaluation

- Blood chemistry test results may include normal or elevated white blood cell (WBC) count, abnormal histiocytes (macrophages), elevated erythrocyte sedimentation rate (ESR), normocytic normochromic anemia (in 70% to 90% of endocarditis cases), and positive serum rheumatoid factor (in about one-half of all clients with endocarditis after the disease is present for 3 to 6 weeks).
- Echocardiography may reveal valvular damage.
- ECG may show AF and other arrhythmias that accompany valvular disease.
- Three blood cultures taken at 1-hour intervals enable identification of the causative organism in up to 90% of clients.

Nursing diagnoses

- Decreased cardiac output
- Activity intolerance
- Risk for injury

Treatment

- Bed rest
- Sufficient fluid intake
- Surgery (in cases of severe valvular damage) to replace defective valve

Drug therapy options

- Antibiotic: infecting organism determines which drug is used
- Antipyretic: aspirin
- Anticoagulant: heparin

Planning and goals

- The client will have increased activity tolerance as the infection is resolved.
- The client will remain hemodynamically stable.
- The client will remain free from complications of infective endocarditis.

Implementation

- Before giving an antibiotic, obtain blood cultures and a client history of allergies *to prevent anaphylaxis.*
- Observe the client for signs of infiltration and inflammation, possible complications of long-term I.V. drug administration, at the venipuncture site. Rotate venous access sites *to reduce the risk of these complications.*
- Watch for signs and symptoms of embolization (such as petechiae, hematuria, pleuritic chest pain, left upper quadrant pain, and paresis), a common occurrence during the first 3 months of treatment. *These signs and symptoms may indicate impending peripheral vascular occlusion or splenic, renal, cerebral, or pulmonary infarction.*
- Monitor the client's renal status (blood urea nitrogen [BUN] levels, creatinine clearance, and urine output) *to check for signs of renal emboli or evidence of toxic reaction to the drug therapy.*
- Observe the client for signs of heart failure, such as dyspnea, tachypnea, tachycardia, crackles, neck vein distention, edema, and weight gain. *Detecting heart failure early ensures prompt intervention and treatment and decreases the risk of heart failure progressing to pulmonary edema.*
- Provide reassurance by teaching the client and his family members about infective endocarditis and the need for prolonged treatment. Tell them to watch closely for fever, anorexia, and other signs and symptoms of relapse about 2 weeks after treatment stops. Suggest quiet diversionary activities to prevent excessive physical exertion. *Having the client and his family involved in care gives them a feeling of control and promotes compliance with long-term therapy.*
- Make sure a susceptible client understands the need for prophylactic antibiotics before, during, and after dental work, childbirth, and genitourinary, GI, or gynecologic procedures *to prevent further episodes of endocarditis.*

Evaluation

- The client demonstrates increased activity tolerance.
- The client has stable vital signs.
- The client is free from infection and without complications.

HEART FAILURE

HEART FAILURE occurs when the heart can't pump enough blood to meet the body's metabolic needs. It can occur on the left or right side of the heart:

- Left-sided heart failure causes mostly pulmonary signs and symptoms, such as shortness of breath, dyspnea on exertion, a moist cough, and crackles on inspiration

◆ Right-sided heart failure causes systemic signs, such as peripheral edema and swelling, jugular vein distention, and hepatomegaly.

Possible causes

- Atherosclerosis
- Cardiac conduction defects
- Cardiomyopathy
- Chronic obstructive pulmonary disease
- Fluid overload
- Hypertension
- MI
- Pulmonary hypertension
- Valvular insufficiency
- Valvular stenosis

Assessment findings

Left-sided heart failure

- Dyspnea
- Crackles
- Orthopnea
- Wheezing
- Cyanosis or pallor
- Paroxysmal nocturnal dyspnea
- Tachypnea
- Tachycardia
- Gallop rhythm, third (S_3) or fourth (S_4) heart sound
- Fatigue
- Anxiety
- Arrhythmias
- Cough

Right-sided heart failure

- Dependent edema
- Weight gain
- Fatigue
- Jugular vein distention
- Tachycardia
- Gallop rhythm, S_3 or S_4
- Nausea
- Anorexia
- Hepatomegaly
- Splenomegaly
- Ascites

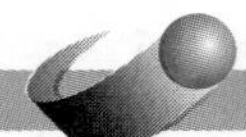

FAST FACT

Left-sided heart failure causes pulmonary symptoms. Right-sided heart failure causes systemic symptoms.

Diagnostic evaluation

Left-sided heart failure

- ABG levels indicate hypoxemia and hypercapnia.
- Blood chemistry test results reveal decreased potassium and sodium levels and increased BUN and creatinine levels.
- Chest X-ray shows increased pulmonary congestion and left ventricular hypertrophy.
- ECG may show left ventricular hypertrophy or acute ST-T wave changes.
- Echocardiography shows increased size of cardiac chambers and decreased wall motion.
- Hemodynamic monitoring reveals increased PAP and PAWP and decreased cardiac output.
- Brain natruiretic peptide (BNP) assay detects abnormal hormone levels produced by failing ventricles.

Right-sided heart failure

- ABG levels indicate hypoxemia.
- Blood chemistry test results show decreased sodium and potassium levels and increased BUN and creatinine levels.
- Chest X-ray reveals pulmonary congestion, cardiomegaly, and pleural effusions.
- ECG may show left and right ventricular hypertrophy or acute ST-T wave changes.
- Echocardiogram shows increased size of chambers and decreased wall motion.
- Hemodynamic monitoring shows increased right atrial pressure, CVP, and right ventricular pressure and decreased cardiac output.
- BNP assay detects abnormal hormone levels by failing ventricles.

Nursing diagnoses

- Excess fluid volume
- Activity intolerance
- Ineffective health maintenance
- Impaired gas exchange
- Anxiety

Treatment

- Low-sodium diet and limited intake of fluids
- Intra-aortic balloon pump (IABP)
- Oxygen therapy (possibly intubation and mechanical ventilation)
- Biventricular pacemaker to control ventricular dysynchrony
- Cellular cardiomyoblasty (transplanted muscle cells) to promote heart regeneration
- Left ventricular assist device (for left-sided heart failure)

- Paracentesis (for right-sided heart failure)
- Thoracentesis (for right-sided heart failure)

Drug therapy options
- Analgesic: morphine sulfate
- Angiotensin-converting enzyme (ACE) inhibitors: captopril (Capoten), enalapril (Vasotec), lisinopril (Prinivil)
- Beta-adrenergic blockers: carvedilol (Coreg), metoprolol (Lopressor)
- Cardiac glycoside: digoxin (Lanoxin)
- Diuretics: bumetanide (Bumex), furosemide (Lasix), metolazone (Zaroxolyn), spironolactone (Aldactone)
- Human B-type natriuretic peptide: nesiritide (Natrecor)
- Inotropic agents: inamrinone lactate (Inocor), dobutamine hydrochloride (Dobutrex), dopamine hydrochloride (Intropin)
- Nitrates: isosorbide dinitrate (Isordil), nitroglycerin (Nitro-Bid)
- Vasodilator: nitroprusside (Nitropress), isosorbide dinitrate and hydralazine hydrochloride (BiDil) (new drug approved for blacks only)

Planning and goals
- The client will understand how to cope with necessary lifestyle changes.
- The client won't develop preventable complications.
- The client will verbalize the need to continue therapy at home and comply with the regimen.

Implementation
- Assess cardiovascular status, vital signs, and hemodynamic variables *to detect signs of reduced cardiac output.*
- Assess respiratory status *to detect increasing fluid in the lungs and respiratory failure.*
- Keep the client in semi-Fowler's position *to increase chest expansion and improve ventilation.*
- Administer medications, as prescribed, *to enhance cardiac performance and reduce excess fluids.*
- Administer oxygen *to enhance arterial oxygenation.*
- Measure and record intake and output. *Intake greater than output may indicate fluid retention.*
- Monitor laboratory test results *to detect electrolyte imbalances, renal failure, and impaired cardiac circulation.*
- Provide suctioning, if necessary; assist with turning, and encourage coughing and deep breathing *to prevent pulmonary complications.*
- Restrict oral fluids *to avoid worsening the client's condition.*

Low-salt diet

Many medical conditions, such as heart failure and high blood pressure, necessitate decreased salt intake. Reduced salt intake can also reduce the risk of high blood pressure. Include the following tips when instructing your client about a low-salt diet:
- Avoid salty foods.
- Read food labels. Look for sodium on the labels of medicines and foods. Pay close attention to the amount of sodium per serving.
- Use reduced sodium or no-salt-added products.
- Use herbs and spices instead of salt. Be aware that some seasonings, such as horseradish, and additives, such as monosodium glutamate (MSG), are high in sodium.
- Prepare food by baking, broiling, steaming, roasting, or poaching without salt. Order food prepared this way in restaurants. Skip gravies, soups, and salad dressings, unless you can get low-salt varieties.
- Eat fresh fruits and vegetables. If you must use canned foods, get low-salt types and rinse them.
- Get permission before using a salt substitute. Many contain potassium or ammonium. These can cause harm if the client has kidney, liver, or heart disease.

- Weigh the client daily *to detect fluid retention. A weight gain of 2 lb (0.9 kg) in 1 day or 5 lb (2.3 kg) in 1 week indicates fluid gain.*
- Measure and record the client's abdominal girth. *An increase in abdominal girth suggests worsening fluid retention and right-sided heart failure.*
- Make sure the client maintains a low-sodium diet *to reduce fluid accumulation.* (See *Low-salt diet.*)
- Consult a registered dietitian to help meet the client's nutritional needs at home.
- Encourage the client to express feelings, such as a fear of dying, *to reduce anxiety.*

Evaluation
- The client accurately describes recommended dietary restrictions and medication regimens.
- The client experiences minimal complications.
- The client verbalizes important signs and symptoms to report.
- The client complies with the therapy upon discharge at home.

HYPERTENSION

A serious condition marked by persistently elevated blood pressure, HYPERTENSION is defined as a sustained systolic pressure of 140 mm Hg or higher or a sustained diastolic pressure of 90 mm Hg or higher. It results when blood pumped through the arteries meets increased peripheral resistance (due to arteriolar narrowing), necessitating increased force to circulate throughout the body. Prehypertension, a new classification characterized by persistent systolic pressure of 120 to 130 mm Hg or a diastolic pressure of 80 to 89 mm Hg, places the client at increased risk for developing hypertension and other problems, such as heart disease, kidney disease, and stroke.

There are two major types of hypertension:

- Essential or primary hypertension, the most common type, has no known cause, but many factors play a role in its development.
- Secondary hypertension is caused by an identifiable cause, such as renal disease or other systemic disease, or another cause.

Possible causes

- Atherosclerosis
- Coarctation of the aorta
- Cushing's disease
- Hyperlipidemia
- Neurologic disorders
- No known cause (essential hypertension)
- Oral contraceptive use
- Pheochromocytoma
- Pregnancy
- Primary hyperaldosteronism
- Renovascular disease
- Thyroid, pituitary, or parathyroid disease
- Use of drugs such as cocaine, epoetin alfa, and cyclosporine

Risk factors

- Aging
- Atherosclerosis
- Diet (high intake of sodium, fat, cholesterol, and caffeine)
- Family history
- Obesity
- Race (incidence is higher in blacks)
- Sex (incidence is higher in males older than age 40)
- Smoking
- Stress

Assessment findings

- Possibly asymptomatic (commonly termed the "silent" killer)
- Elevated blood pressure
- Dizziness
- Headache
- Left ventricular hypertrophy
- Heart failure
- Cerebral ischemia
- Renal failure
- Papilledema
- Visual disturbances, including blindness

Diagnostic evaluation

- Blood chemistry test results may show elevated sodium, BUN, creatinine, and cholesterol levels.
- Blood pressure measurements result in sustained readings higher than 119/79 mm Hg for prehypertension and 140/90 mm Hg or higher for hypertension.
- Chest X-ray reveals cardiomegaly.
- ECG shows left ventricular hypertrophy.
- Echocardiogram may show left ventricular hypertrophy.
- Ophthalmoscopic examination shows retinal changes, such as severe arteriolar narrowing, papilledema, and hemorrhage.
- Urinalysis discloses proteinuria, red blood cells (RBCs), and WBCs.

Nursing diagnoses

- Ineffective health maintenance
- Imbalanced nutrition: More than body requirements
- Deficient knowledge (regarding disorder and treatment)

Treatment

- Regular exercise to reduce weight, if appropriate
- Dietary Approaches to Stop Hypertension (DASH) eating plan
- Lifestyle modifications, such as quitting smoking and reducing alcohol intake

Drug therapy options

- ACE inhibitors: captopril (Capoten), enalapril (Vasotec), lisinopril (Prinivil)
- Angiotensin receptor blockers: candesartan (Atacand), irbasartan (Avapro), losartan (Cozaar)
- Antihypertensives: doxazosin mesylate (Cardura), methyldopa (Aldomet), hydralazine (Apresoline), prazosin (Minipress)

◆ Beta-adrenergic blockers: carteolol hydrochloride (Cartrol), metoprolol (Lopressor), penbutolol sulfate (Levatol), propranolol (Inderal)
◆ Calcium channel blockers: diltiazem (Cardizem), nicardipine (Cardene), nifedipine (Procardia), verapamil (Calan)
◆ Diuretics: bumetanide (Bumex), furosemide (Lasix), spironolactone (Aldactone), hydrochlorothiazide (HydroDIURIL)
◆ Vasodilators: nitroprusside (Nitropress)

Planning and goals

◆ The client will exhibit a reduction in blood pressure.
◆ The client will express understanding and acceptance of necessary lifestyle changes and comply with treatment.

Implementation

◆ Assess cardiovascular status, including vital signs, *to detect cardiac compromise.*
◆ Take an average of two or more blood pressure readings *to establish hypertension.*
◆ Check the client's blood pressure in lying, sitting, and standing positions *to determine if orthostatic hypotension is present.* Also check for pallor, diaphoresis, and vertigo.
◆ Assess neurologic status, and observe the client for changes *that may indicate an alteration in cerebral perfusion* (stroke or hemorrhage).
◆ Monitor and record intake and output and daily weight *to detect fluid volume overload.*
◆ Administer medications as prescribed *to lower blood pressure.*
◆ Make sure the client maintains a low-sodium, low-cholesterol diet *to help minimize hypertension.*
◆ Encourage the client to express feelings about daily stress *to reduce anxiety.*
◆ Maintain a quiet environment *to reduce stress.*

Evaluation

◆ The client maintains reduced blood pressure.
◆ The client expresses understanding of the need for a low-cholesterol, low-calorie, low-sodium diet.
◆ The client has made necessary lifestyle changes.
◆ The client describes the medication regimen.

MYOCARDIAL INFARCTION

With MYOCARDIAL INFARCTION (MI), reduced blood flow in one of the coronary arteries leads to myocardial ischemia, injury, and necrosis. With a Q-wave MI, tissue damage extends through all myocardial layers. With a non-Q-wave MI, usually only the innermost layer is damaged.

Possible causes

◆ Coronary artery occlusion
◆ Coronary artery spasm
◆ Coronary artery stenosis

Risk factors

◆ Aging
◆ Decreased serum HDL levels
◆ Diabetes mellitus
◆ Drug use, specifically use of amphetamines or cocaine
◆ Elevated serum triglyceride, LDL, and cholesterol levels
◆ Excessive intake of saturated fats, carbohydrates, or salt
◆ Family history of CAD
◆ Hypertension
◆ Obesity
◆ Postmenopausal woman
◆ Sedentary lifestyle
◆ Smoking
◆ Stress

Assessment findings

◆ Crushing substernal chest pain that may radiate to the jaw, back, and arms; may wax and wane (because angina is a crescendo pain); is unrelieved by rest or nitroglycerin; or may not be present (in clients with no symptoms or with silent MI.)
◆ Dyspnea
◆ Diaphoresis
◆ Arrhythmias
◆ Tachycardia
◆ Anxiety
◆ Pallor
◆ Hypotension
◆ Nausea and vomiting
◆ Elevated temperature

Diagnostic evaluation

◆ ECG shows a deep, wide Q wave; an elevated or depressed ST segment; and T-wave inversion or cardiac arrhythmias.
◆ Blood chemistry test results show increased creatine kinase (CK), lactate dehydrogenase (LD), lipid, and troponin T levels; increased WBC count; positive CK-MB fraction; and elevated myoglobin levels. Elevated homocysteine and C-reactive protein levels found incidentally in MI, but practical value is unknown.
◆ Coronary angiography visualizes affected vessels.

◆ Echocardiography may show ventricular wall abnormalities.
◆ Nuclear ventriculography identifes acutely damaged muscles as "hot spots."

Nursing diagnoses

◆ Acute pain
◆ Anxiety
◆ Activity intolerance
◆ Decreased cardiac output
◆ Ineffective tissue perfusion (cardiopulmonary)

Treatment

◆ Bed rest with bedside commode
◆ Bleeding precautions (if thrombolytic therapy was administered)
◆ Coronary artery bypass grafting
◆ IABP
◆ Left ventricular assist device
◆ Low-calorie, low-cholesterol, and low-fat diet
◆ Monitoring of vital signs, urine output, ECG results, and hemodynamic status
◆ Ongoing laboratory studies (ABG, CK with isoenzymes, electrolyte, and cardiac troponin levels)
◆ Oxygen therapy
◆ Percutaneous coronary intervention
◆ Possibly a pacemaker for symptomatic bradycardia or heart block
◆ Pulmonary artery catheterization (to detect left- or right-sided heart failure)

Drug therapy options

◆ Analgesic: morphine sulfate
◆ ACE inhibitors: captopril (Capoten), enalapril (Vasotec)
◆ Antiarrhythmics: lidocaine (Xylocaine), procainamide (Pronestyl)
◆ Anticoagulant: heparin I.V. after thrombolytic therapy
◆ Antihypertensive: hydralazine (Apresoline)
◆ Antiplatelet: aspirin
◆ Atropine I.V. for symptomatic bradycardia or heart block
◆ Beta-adrenergic blockers (contraindicated if client also has hypotension or bronchospasm): metoprolol (Lopressor), nadolol (Corgard), propranolol (Inderal)
◆ Calcium channel blockers: diltiazem (Cardizem), nifedipine (Procardia), verapamil (Calan)
◆ Insulin to maintain tight glycemic control
◆ Nitrates: nitroglycerin I.V. (Nitro-Bid, Tridil)
◆ Platelet GP IIb/IIIa receptor antagonists (for non-Q-wave MI): abciximab (Reopro), tirofiban (Aggrastat)
◆ Thrombolytics (for ST-segment elevation or MI): anistreplase (Eminase), streptokinase (Streptase), tissue plasminogen activator (Activase) (given within 6 hours of onset of symptoms but most effective when started within 3 hours)

Planning and goals

◆ The client won't develop preventable complications.
◆ The client will understand the necessary treatment and lifestyle changes.
◆ The client will maintain adequate cardiac output and perfusion.
◆ The client will report decreased pain.

Implementation

◆ Monitor ECG results *to detect ischemia, injury, new or extended infarction, arrhythmias, and conduction defects.*
◆ Monitor and record vital signs and hemodynamic variables *to monitor response to therapy and detect complications.*
◆ Monitor and record intake and output *to assess renal perfusion and possible fluid retention.*
◆ Monitor laboratory values *to detect myocardial damage, abnormal electrolyte levels, drug levels, renal function, and coagulation.*
◆ Assess cardiovascular and respiratory status *to watch for signs of heart failure, such as an S_3 or S_4 gallop, crackles, cough, tachypnea, and edema.*
◆ Make sure the client maintains bed rest *to reduce oxygen demands on the heart.*
◆ Administer oxygen therapy, as prescribed, *to improve oxygen supply to the heart.*
◆ Obtain an ECG reading during acute pain *to detect myocardial ischemia, injury, or infarction.*
◆ Maintain the client's prescribed diet *to reduce fluid retention and cholesterol levels.*
◆ Provide postoperative care, if necessary, *to avoid postoperative complications and help the client achieve a full recovery.*
◆ Allay the client's anxiety *because anxiety increases oxygen demands.*
◆ Administer pain medication to reduce pain.
◆ Monitor glucose levels and administer insulin as prescribed to maintain blood glucose level of 80 to 100 mg/dl *to prevent cardiac complication associated with elevated blood glucose levels.*

Evaluation

◆ The client explains how and when to take medication and states reportable adverse reactions.

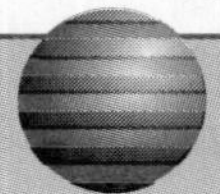

CLINICAL SITUATION

Caring for the client with myocardial infarction

A female client, age 54, is the assistant director of nursing at a large hospital. Married and the mother of three children, she has a history of angina pectoris. Today, her pain is severe and radiates down the left arm. She's also short of breath and diaphoretic. She's admitted to the coronary care unit with a suspected diagnosis of myocardial infarction (MI).

The client reports substernal chest pain. Test results show electrocardiographic changes and an elevated cardiac troponin level.

What should be the focus of nursing care?

A. Improving myocardial oxygenation and reducing cardiac workload
B. Confirming a suspected diagnosis and preventing complications
C. Reducing anxiety and relieving pain
D. Eliminating stressors and providing a nondemanding environment

Answer: A. The client is exhibiting signs and symptoms of MI; therefore, nursing care should focus on improving myocardial oxygenation and reducing cardiac workload. Confirming the diagnosis of MI and preventing complications, reducing anxiety and relieving pain, and providing a nondemanding environment are secondary to improving myocardial oxygenation and reducing workload. Stressors can't be eliminated, only reduced.

The client experiences acute myocardial ischemia. The nurse administers oxygen and sublingual nitroglycerin. When assessing an ECG for evidence that blood flow to the myocardium has improved, the nurse should focus on the:

A. widening of the QRS complex.
B. lengthening of the P-R interval.
C. return of the ST segment to baseline.
D. presence of a significant Q wave.

Answer: C. During episodes of myocardial ischemia, an ECG may show ST-segment elevation or depression. With successful treatment, the ST segment should return to baseline. Other changes – widening QRS complex, presence of a Q wave, and lengthening of the P-R interval – aren't directly indicative of myocardial ischemia.

Questions for further thought

- What types of statements would indicate that the client understands lifestyle changes she needs to make?
- What steps can be taken to decrease the client's anxiety?

- The client describes appropriate lifestyle changes to reduce the risk of a future cardiac event.
- The client experiences no complications. (See *Caring for the client with myocardial infarction.*)
- The client's pain level is relieved.
- The client maintains adequate cardiac output.

MYOCARDITIS

MYOCARDITIS is focal or diffuse inflammation of the cardiac muscle (myocardium). It may be acute or chronic and can occur at any age. Commonly, myocarditis fails to produce specific cardiovascular symptoms or ECG abnormalities, and recovery is usually spontaneous, without residual defects. Occasionally, myocarditis is complicated by heart failure; rarely, it may lead to cardiomyopathy.

Possible causes

- Bacterial infections, such as diphtheria, tuberculosis (TB), typhoid fever, tetanus, and staphylococcal, pneumococcal, and gonococcal infections
- Chemical poisons such as chronic alcoholism
- Helminthic infections such as trichinosis
- Hypersensitive immune reactions, such as acute rheumatic fever and postcardiotomy syndrome
- Parasitic infections, such as toxoplasmosis and, especially, South American trypanosomiasis (Chagas' disease) in infants and immunosuppressed adults
- Radiation therapy including large doses of radiation to the chest in treating lung or breast cancer
- Viral infections (most common cause in the United States and western Europe) such as coxsackievirus A and B strains and, possibly, poliomyelitis, influenza, rubeola, rubella, adenoviruses, and echoviruses

Assessment findings

- Arrhythmias (S_3 and S_4 gallops, faint S_1)
- Dyspnea
- Fatigue
- Fever
- Mild, continuous pressure or soreness in the chest (unlike the recurring, stress-related pain of angina pectoris)

◆ Palpitations
◆ Chronic valvulitis (when myocarditis results from rheumatic fever)
◆ Thromboembolism

Diagnostic evaluation

◆ Blood tests show elevated cardiac enzyme levels (CK, the CK-MB isoenzyme, AST, and LD), increased WBC count and ESR, and elevated antibody titers (such as antistreptolysin-O titer in rheumatic fever).
◆ ECG typically shows diffuse ST-segment and T-wave abnormalities (as in pericarditis), conduction defects (prolonged PR interval), and other supraventricular arrhythmias.
◆ Echocardiography may show weak heart muscle, an enlarged heart, or fluid surrounding the heart.
◆ Endomyocardial biopsy confirms the diagnosis, but a negative biopsy doesn't exclude the diagnosis. A repeat biopsy may be needed.
◆ Stool and throat cultures may identify the causative bacteria.

Nursing diagnoses

◆ Decreased cardiac output
◆ Activity intolerance
◆ Anxiety
◆ Ineffective tissue perfusion (cardiopulmonary)

Treatment

◆ Bed rest
◆ Sodium-restricted diet

Drug therapy options

◆ Antiarrhythmics: quinidine (Quinora), procainamide (Pronestyl), amniodarone (Cordone)
◆ Antibiotic: according to sensitivity of infecting organism
◆ Anticoagulants: warfarin (Coumadin), heparin
◆ Cardiac glycoside: digoxin (Lanoxin) to increase myocardial contractility
◆ Diuretic: furosemide (Lasix)

Planning and goals

◆ The client will maintain hemodynamic stability and adequate cardiac output and will exhibit no arrhythmias.
◆ The client will carry out activities of daily living (ADLs) without weakness or fatigue.
◆ The client will verbalize an understanding of his medical condition and treatment regimen without demonstrating severe signs of anxiety.

Implementation

◆ Assess cardiovascular status frequently to monitor for signs of heart failure, such as dyspnea, hypotension, and tachycardia. Check for changes in cardiac rhythm or conduction. *Rhythm disturbances may indicate early cardiac decompensation.*
◆ Observe for signs of digoxin toxicity (anorexia, nausea, vomiting, blurred vision, cardiac arrhythmias) and for complicating factors that may potentiate toxicity, such as electrolyte imbalances and hypoxia, *to prevent further complications.*
◆ Stress the importance of bed rest. Assist with bathing as necessary; provide a bedside commode, which puts less stress on the heart than using a bedpan. Reassure the client that activity limitations are temporary but necessary *to decrease oxygen demands on the heart.*
◆ Offer diversional activities that are physically undemanding *to decrease anxiety.*

Evaluation

◆ The client has stable vital signs, adequate gas exchange and appropriate urine output.
◆ The client has increased his ADLs without fatigue.
◆ The client complies with therapy and discusses his condition calmly, without evidence of anxiety.

PERICARDITIS

PERICARDITIS is an inflammation of the pericardium, the fibroserous sac that envelops, supports, and protects the heart. It occurs in acute and chronic forms. Acute pericarditis can be fibrinous or effusive with purulent, serous, or hemorrhagic exudate; chronic constrictive pericarditis is characterized by dense fibrous pericardial thickening. The prognosis depends on the underlying cause but is generally good in acute pericarditis unless constriction occurs.

Possible causes

◆ Bacterial, fungal, or viral infection (infectious pericarditis)
◆ Drugs such as procainamide (Pronestyl)
◆ High-dose radiation to the chest
◆ Hypersensitivity or autoimmune disease, such as acute rheumatic fever (most common cause of pericarditis in children), systemic lupus erythematosus, and rheumatoid arthritis
◆ Idiopathic factors (most common in acute pericarditis)
◆ Neoplasms (primary or metastasis from lungs, breasts, or other organs)

◆ Postcardiac injury, such as MI (which later causes an autoimmune reaction [Dressler's syndrome] in the pericardium), trauma, and surgery that leaves the pericardium intact but causes blood to leak into the pericardial cavity
◆ Uremia

Assessment findings

Acute pericarditis

◆ Sharp, sudden pain that usually starts over the sternum and radiates to the neck, shoulders, back, and arms (Unlike the pain of MI, pericardial pain is commonly pleuritic, increasing with deep inspiration and decreasing when the client sits up and leans forward, pulling the heart away from the diaphragmatic pleurae of the lungs.)
◆ Pericardial friction rub (grating sound heard as the heart moves)
◆ Symptoms of cardiac tamponade (pallor, clammy skin, hypotension, pulsus paradoxus, neck vein distention)
◆ Symptoms of heart failure (dyspnea, orthopnea, tachycardia, ill-defined substernal chest pain, feeling of fullness in the chest)

Chronic pericarditis

◆ Pericardial friction rub
◆ Symptoms similar to those of chronic right-sided heart failure (fluid retention, ascites, hepatomegaly)
◆ Gradual increase in systemic venous pressure

Diagnostic evaluation

◆ Blood tests reflect inflammation and may show normal or elevated WBC count, especially in infectious pericarditis; elevated ESR; and slightly elevated cardiac enzyme levels with associated myocarditis.
◆ Culture of pericardial fluid obtained by open surgical drainage or cardiocentesis sometimes identifies a causative organism in bacterial or fungal pericarditis.
◆ Echocardiography confirms the diagnosis when it shows an echo-free space between the ventricular wall and the pericardium (in cases of pleural effusion).
◆ ECG shows the following changes in acute pericarditis: elevation of ST segments in the standard limb leads and most precordial leads without significant changes in QRS morphology that occur with MI, atrial ectopic rhythms such as AF, and diminished QRS voltage in pericardial effusion.

Nursing diagnoses

◆ Acute pain
◆ Decreased cardiac output
◆ Deficient knowledge regarding disorder and treatment
◆ Ineffective tissue perfusion (cardiopulmonary)

Treatment

◆ Bed rest
◆ Pericardiocentesis (in cases of cardiac tamponade), partial pericardectomy (for recurrent pericarditis), total pericardectomy (for constrictive pericarditis)

Drug therapy options

◆ Analgesic: morphine sulfate
◆ Antibiotic: according to sensitivity of infecting organism
◆ Corticosteroid: methylprednisolone (Solu-Medrol)
◆ Nonsteroidal anti-inflammatory drugs (NSAIDs): aspirin, indomethacin (Indocin)

Planning and goals

◆ The client will have relief of pain.
◆ The client will maintain hemodynamic stability.
◆ The client will verbalize an understanding of his current illness and treatment and comply with treatment.

Implementation

◆ Provide complete bed rest *to decrease oxygen demands on the heart.*
◆ Assess pain in relation to respiration and body position *to distinguish pericardial pain from myocardial ischemic pain.*
◆ Place the client in an upright position *to relieve dyspnea and chest pain.*
◆ Provide analgesics and oxygen and reassure the client with acute pericarditis that his condition is temporary and treatable *to promote client comfort and allay anxiety.*
◆ Monitor the client for signs of cardiac compression or cardiac tamponade, possible complications of pericardial effusion. Signs include decreased blood pressure, increased CVP, and pulsus paradoxus. Keep a pericardiocentesis set handy whenever pericardial effusion is suspected *because cardiac tamponade requires immediate treatment.*
◆ Explain tests and treatments to the client. If surgery is necessary, he should learn deep-breathing and coughing exercises beforehand *to alleviate fear and anxiety and promote compliance with the postoperative treatment regimen.* Postoperative care is similar to that given after cardiothoracic surgery.

Evaluation

◆ The client will verbalize relief of pain.
◆ The client states an understanding of his current illness and necessary treatment.
◆ The client has stable vital signs.

PULMONARY EDEMA

PULMONARY EDEMA is a complication of left-sided heart failure. It occurs when pulmonary capillary pressure exceeds intravascular osmotic pressure, resulting in increased pressure in the capillaries of the lungs and acute transudation of fluid. Such increased pressure and fluid accumulation leads to impaired oxygenation and hypoxia.

Possible causes

- Acute respiratory distress syndrome
- Atherosclerosis
- Drug overdose (heroin, barbiturates, morphine sulfate)
- Heart failure
- Hypertension
- MI
- Myocarditis
- Overload of I.V. fluids
- Smoke inhalation
- Valvular disease

Assessment findings

- Agitation, restlessness, intense fear
- Blood-tinged, frothy sputum and paroxysmal cough
- Cold, clammy skin
- Crackles auscultated over lung fields
- Dyspnea, orthopnea, tachypnea
- Jugular vein distention
- Syncope
- Tachycardia, S_3 and S_4 heart sounds, chest pain

Diagnostic evaluation

- ABG levels show respiratory alkalosis or acidosis and hypoxemia.
- ECG reveals tachycardia and ventricular enlargement.
- Hemodynamic monitoring shows increases in PAP, PAWP, and CVP as well as decreased cardiac output.
- Pulse oximetry reveals hypoxia.

Nursing diagnoses

- Impaired gas exchange
- Excess fluid volume
- Anxiety
- Ineffective tissue perfusion (cardiopulmonary)

Treatment

- Bed rest and ROM isometric exercises
- Low-sodium diet and limited intake of oral fluids
- Oxygen therapy with possible intubation and mechanical ventilation
- Hemodialysis or continuous renal replacement therapy

Drug therapy options

- Analgesic: morphine sulfate
- Angiotensin-converting enzyme (ACE) inhibitor: captopril (Capoten), enalapril (Vasotec), lisinopril (Prinivil)
- Beta-adrenergic blockers: carvedilol (Coreg), metoprolol (Lopressor)
- Cardiac glycoside: digoxin (Lanoxin)
- Diuretics: bumetanide (Bumex), furosemide (Lasix), metolazone (Zaroxolyn)
- Human B-type natriuretic peptide: nesiritide (Natrecor)
- Inotropic agents: Inamrinone lactate (Inocor), dobutamine hydrochloride (Dobutrex), milrinone (Primacor)
- Nitrates: isosorbide dinitrate (Isordil), nitroglycerin (Nitro-Bid)
- Vasodilator: nitroprusside (Nitropress)

Planning and goals

- The client will demonstrate adequate gas exchange and fluid volume within normal parameters.
- The client will experience no preventable complications.
- The client will demonstrate improvement in physiologic and psychological comfort.

Implementation

- Assess cardiovascular status, hemodynamic variables, and respiratory status *to detect changes in fluid balance.* Tachycardia, S_3 heart sounds, hypotension, increased respiratory rate, and crackles indicate increased fluid volume.
- Monitor and record intake and output. *Intake greater than output and elevated specific gravity suggest fluid retention.*
- Weigh the client daily *to detect fluid retention. A weight gain of 2 lb (0.9 kg) in 1 day or 5 lb (2.3 kg) in 1 week indicates fluid gain.*
- Track laboratory values. *BUN and creatinine levels indicate renal function; electrolyte and hemoglobin (Hb) levels and hematocrit (HCT) indicate fluid status.*
- Keep the client in high Fowler's position if blood pressure tolerates; if he's hypotensive, keep him in a semi-Fowler's position if tolerated. *Elevating the head of the bed reduces venous return to the heart and promotes chest expansion.*
- Administer oxygen therapy, as prescribed, *to increase alveolar oxygen concentration and enhance arterial blood oxygenation.*
- Administer medications *to improve gas exchange, improve myocardial function, and reduce anxiety.*
- Note the color, amount, and consistency of sputum. *Sputum amount and consistency may indicate hydration*

status. A change in color or foul-smelling sputum may indicate a respiratory tract infection.

◆ Encourage the client to express feelings such as a fear of suffocation *to reduce anxiety and lessen oxygen demands.*

Evaluation

◆ The client demonstrates improved respiratory effort and oxygenation.
◆ The client doesn't develop complications.
◆ The client states anxiety is decreased.

RAYNAUD'S DISEASE

RAYNAUD'S DISEASE is characterized by episodic vasospasm in the small peripheral arteries and arterioles, precipitated by exposure to cold or stress. This condition occurs bilaterally and usually affects the hands or, less commonly, the feet.

Raynaud's disease is most prevalent in women, particularly between puberty and age 40. A benign condition, it requires no specific treatment and has no serious sequelae.

Raynaud's phenomenon, however, a condition commonly associated with several connective tissue disorders — such as scleroderma, systemic lupus erythematosus, and polymyositis — has a progressive course, leading to ischemia, gangrene, and amputation. Differentiating the two disorders is difficult because some clients who experience mild symptoms of Raynaud's disease for several years may later develop overt connective tissue disease — most commonly scleroderma.

Possible causes

◆ Unknown (most probable theory involves sympahtetic response and an antigen antibody immune response)

Assessment findings

◆ Blanching of skin on the fingers, typically, that then becomes cyanotic before changing to red (after exposure to cold or stress)
◆ Numbness and tingling relieved by warmth
◆ Trophic changes, such as sclerodactyly, ulcerations, and chronic paronychia (in longstanding disease)

Diagnostic evaluation

◆ Arteriography reveals vasospasm.
◆ Cold stimulation test reveals skin color changes induced by cold or stress.
◆ Plethysmography reveals intermittent vessel occlusion.

Nursing diagnoses

◆ Ineffective tissue perfusion (peripheral)
◆ Risk for injury
◆ Acute pain

Treatment

◆ Avoidance of cold
◆ Smoking cessation (if appropriate)
◆ Sympathectomy (used in fewer than one-quarter of clients)

Drug therapy options

◆ Calcium channel blockers: diltiazem (Cardizem), nifedipine (Procardia)
◆ Vasodilators: phenoxybenzamine (Dibenzyline), reserpine (Diupres)

Planning and goals

◆ The client will have improved peripheral circulation.
◆ The client won't develop complications from repeated peripheral vasospasm.
◆ The client will have relief from pain.

Implementation

◆ Warn against exposure to the cold. Tell the client to wear mittens or gloves in cold weather or when handling cold items or defrosting the freezer *to prevent vasospasm, which causes an onset of symptoms.*
◆ Advise the client to avoid stressful situations and to stop smoking *to prevent exacerbation of symptoms from vasoconstriction and sympathetic nervous system response.*
◆ Instruct the client to inspect the skin frequently and seek immediate care for signs of skin breakdown or infection *to prevent complications.*
◆ Teach the client about drugs, their use, and their adverse effects *to prevent further complications.*
◆ Provide psychological support and reassurance *to allay the client's fear of amputation and disfigurement.*

Evaluation

◆ The client reports decreased incidents of peripheral vasoconstriction.
◆ The client doesn't develop complications of illness.
◆ The client verbalizes pain relief.

RHEUMATIC FEVER AND RHEUMATIC HEART DISEASE

Commonly recurrent, acute RHEUMATIC FEVER is a systemic inflammatory disease of childhood that follows a group A beta-hemolytic streptococcal infection. RHEUMATIC HEART DISEASE refers to the cardiac manifestations of rheumatic fever and includes pancarditis (myocarditis, pericarditis, and endocarditis) during the early acute phase and chronic valvular disease later. Although rheumatic fever usually affects children age 5 to 15, its ensuing cardiac manifestations can be lifelong.

Long-term antibiotic therapy can minimize recurrence of rheumatic fever, reducing the risk of permanent cardiac damage and eventual valvular deformity. However, severe pancarditis occasionally produces fatal heart failure during the acute phase. Of the clients who survive this complication, about 20% die within 10 years.

This disease strikes most commonly during cool, damp weather in the winter and early spring. In the United States, it's most common in the northern states.

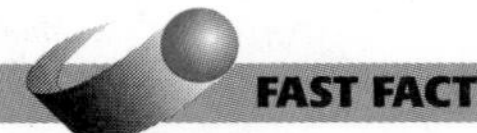

FAST FACT

Rheumatic fever follows a group A beta-hemolytic streptococcal infection. Rheumatic heart disease refers to the cardiac manifestations of rheumatic fever.

Possible causes

- Hypersensitivity reaction to a group A beta-hemolytic streptococcal infection

Assessment findings

Assess the client for the following:

- Carditis
- Temperature of at least 100.4° F (38° C)
- Migratory joint pain or polyarthritis
- Skin lesions such as erythema marginatum (in only 5% of clients)
- Transient chorea (can develop up to 6 months after the original streptococcal infection)

Diagnostic evaluation

- Blood tests show elevated WBC count and ESR and slight anemia during inflammation.
- Cardiac catheterization evaluates valvular damage and left ventricular function in severe cardiac dysfunction.
- Cardiac enzyme levels may be increased in severe carditis.
- Chest X-rays show normal heart size (except with myocarditis, heart failure, or pericardial effusion).
- C-reactive protein is positive (especially during the acute phase).
- Echocardiography helps evaluate valvular damage, chamber size, and ventricular function.
- ECG shows prolonged PR interval in 20% of clients.

Nursing diagnoses

- Decreased cardiac output
- Activity intolerance
- Chronic pain

Treatment

- Strict bed rest for about 5 weeks or until temperature returns to normal without medication, the ESR is normal, and the ECG returns to baseline.
- Corrective valvular surgery (in cases of persistent heart failure)

Drug therapy options

- Antibiotics: erythromycin (Erythrocin), penicillin (Pfizerpen)
- Anti-inflammatories: NSAIDs, aspirin, prednisone (Orasone)

Planning and goals

- The client will maintain hemodynamic stability and adequate cardiac output and will exhibit no arrhythmias.
- The client will increase activity as infection subsides.
- The client will obtain relief from pain.
- The client will verbalize understanding of his current illness and comply with treatment.

Implementation

- Before giving penicillin, ask the client if he has ever had a hypersensitivity reaction to it. Even if the client has never had a reaction to penicillin, warn that such a reaction is possible *to adequately inform the client about possible treatment complications.*
- Tell the client to stop taking the drug and immediately report the development of a rash, fever, chills, or other signs of allergy at any time during penicillin therapy *to prevent anaphylaxis.*
- Instruct the client to watch for and report early signs of heart failure, such as dyspnea and a hacking, nonproductive cough, *to prevent further cardiac decompensation.*
- Stress the need for bed rest during the acute phase and suggest appropriate, physically undemanding diversions. *These measures decrease oxygen demands of the heart.*
- After the acute phase, encourage the client's family and friends to spend as much time as possible with the client *to minimize boredom.*

◆ If the client has severe carditis, help him prepare for permanent changes in his lifestyle *to promote positive coping strategies.*
◆ Warn the client to watch for and immediately report signs of recurrent streptococcal infection — sudden sore throat, diffuse throat redness and oropharyngeal exudate, swollen and tender cervical lymph glands, pain on swallowing, a temperature of 101° to 104° F (38.3° to 40° C), headache, and nausea *to prevent complications associated with delayed treatment such as heart valve damage.* Urge the client to avoid people with respiratory tract infections *to prevent reinfection.*
◆ Make sure the client understands the need to comply with prolonged antibiotic therapy and follow-up care and the need for additional antibiotics before dental surgery *to prevent reinfection.*
◆ Arrange for a visiting nurse to oversee home care if necessary *to promote compliance*

Evaluation
◆ The client reports decreased pain.
◆ The client has stable vital signs.
◆ The client tolerates increased activity.
◆ The client verbalizes an understanding of treatment and complies with regimen.

THROMBOPHLEBITIS
THROMBOPHLEBITIS is marked by inflammation of the venous wall and thrombus formation. It may affect deep veins or superficial veins. The thrombus may occlude a vein or detach and embolize to the lungs.

Possible causes
◆ Hypercoagulability (from cancer, blood dyscrasias, oral contraceptives)
◆ Injury to the venous wall (from I.V. injections, fractures, antibiotics)
◆ Venous stasis (from varicose veins, pregnancy, heart failure, prolonged bed rest)
◆ Major abdminal or pelvic operations

Assessment findings
Deep vein thrombophlebitis
◆ Tenderness to touch in calf or thigh
◆ Positive Homans' sign
◆ Edema
◆ Cramping pain

Superficial vein thrombophlebitis
◆ Induration and redness along a superficial vein
◆ Warmth and tenderness along a superficial vein

Diagnostic evaluation
◆ Hematology reveals increased WBC count.
◆ Phlebography shows filling defects and diverted blood flow.
◆ Plethysmography shows venous-filling defects.
◆ Ultrasonography reveals decreased blood flow.

Nursing diagnoses
◆ Acute pain
◆ Ineffective tissue perfusion (peripheral)
◆ Impaired skin integrity

Treatment
◆ Bed rest and elevation of the affected extremity
◆ Embolectomy and insertion of a vena cava umbrella or filter
◆ Antiembolism stockings
◆ Warm, moist compresses

Drug therapy options
◆ Anticoagulants: heparin, enoxaparin, warfarin (Coumadin) for deep vein thrombophlebitis
◆ Anti-inflammatories: aspirin, NSAIDs

Planning and goals
◆ The client will report pain relief.
◆ The client will exhibit healing of injured site.
◆ The client will demonstrate improved circulation to affected area.

Implementation
◆ Assess pulmonary status. *Crackles, dyspnea, tachypnea, hemoptysis, and chest pain suggest pulmonary embolism.*
◆ Assess cardiovascular status. *Tachycardia and chest pain may indicate pulmonary embolism.*
◆ Check for Homans' sign. *Although it suggests deep vein thrombosis, it may be unreliable because it isn't specific to this condition.*
◆ Assess the client for bleeding *due to anticoagulant therapy.*
◆ Monitor and record vital signs, such as hypotension, tachycardia, tachypnea, and restlessness. Observe the client for bruising, epistaxis, blood in stool, bleeding gums, and painful joints. *Tachypnea and tachycardia may suggest pulmonary embolism or hemorrhage.*

◆ Perform neurovascular checks *to detect nerve or vascular damage.*
◆ Monitor laboratory values. *Partial thromboplastin time (PTT) and platelet count in a client on heparin and prothrombin time (PT) in a client receiving warfarin should be 1½ to 2 times the control. International normalized ratio (INR) value should be between 2 and 3. A decreasing hemoglobin level and hematocrit indicate blood loss.*
◆ Keep the client in bed and elevate the affected extremity *to promote venous return and reduce swelling.*
◆ Administer medications, as prescribed, *to control or dissolve blood clots.*
◆ Apply warm, moist compresses *to improve circulation to the affected area and to relieve pain and inflammation.*
◆ Measure and record the circumference of the client's thighs and calves. Compare the measurement to the unaffected leg *to assess for worsening inflammation.*

Evaluation

◆ The client verbalizes pain relief.
◆ The client exhibits complete healing at the injury site.
◆ The client has improved circulation to the affected area.

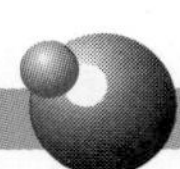

SPOT CHECK

The nurse administers warfarin (Coumadin) to a client with deep vein thrombophlebitis. Which laboratory value indicates that the client has a therapeutic level of warfarin: PTT 1¼ to 2 times the control, PT 1½ to 2 times the control, INR 3 to 4, or hematocrit 32%?

Answer: Warfarin is at a therapeutic level when the PT is 1½ to 2 times the control. Values greater than this increase the risk of bleeding and hemorrhage; lower values increase the risk of blood clot formation. Heparin, not warfarin, prolongs the PTT. The INR may also be used to determine whether warfarin is at a therapeutic level; a therapeutic INR of 2 to 3 is considered therapeutic. Hematocrit doesn't provide information on the effectiveness of warfarin; however, decreasing hematocrit in a client taking warfarin may be a sign of hemorrhage.

VALVULAR HEART DISEASE

With VALVULAR HEART DISEASE, three types of mechanical disruption can occur: stenosis, or narrowing, of the valve opening; incomplete closure of the valve; or prolapse of the valve. These conditions can result from such disorders as endocarditis (most common), congenital defects, and inflammation, and can lead to heart failure.

Valvular heart disease occurs in several forms. The most common include:
◆ AORTIC INSUFFICIENCY or regurgitation, in which blood flows back into the left ventricle during diastole, causing fluid overload in the ventricle, which dilates and hypertrophies (The excess volume causes fluid overload in the left atrium and, finally, the pulmonary system; left-sided heart failure and pulmonary edema eventually result.)
◆ MITRAL INSUFFICIENCY or regurgitation, in which blood from the left ventricle flows back into the left atrium during systole, causing the atrium to enlarge to accommodate the backflow (As a result, the left ventricle also dilates to accommodate the increased volume of blood from the atrium and compensate for diminishing cardiac output.)
◆ MITRAL STENOSIS, in which narrowing of the valve by valvular abnormalities, fibrosis, or calcification obstructs blood flow from the left atrium to the left ventricle (Consequently, left atrial volume and pressure rise and the chamber dilates.)
◆ MITRAL VALVE PROLAPSE (MVP), in which one or both valve leaflets protrude into the left atrium (*MVP syndrome* is the term used when the anatomic prolapse is accompanied by assessment findings unrelated to the valvular abnormality.)
◆ TRICUSPID INSUFFICIENCY or regurgitation, in which blood flows back into the right atrium during systole, decreasing blood flow to the lungs and left side of the heart. (Cardiac output also lessens; fluid overload in the right side of the heart can eventually lead to right-sided heart failure.)

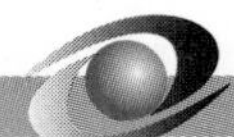

QUICK STUDY

To distinguish the types of mechanical disruption that occur in heart valves, remember the word **SIP**:

Stenosis
Incomplete closure
Prolapse

Possible causes

Aortic insufficiency

◆ Endocarditis
◆ Hypertension
◆ Idiopathic origin
◆ Rheumatic fever
◆ Syphilis

Mitral insufficiency

- Hypertrophic cardiomyopathy
- Left-sided heart failure
- MVP
- Rheumatic fever

Mitral stenosis

- Rheumatic fever

Mitral valve prolapse

- Neuroendocrine and metabolic abnormalities

Tricuspid insufficiency

- Endocarditis
- Rheumatic fever
- Right-sided heart failure
- Trauma

Assessment findings

Aortic insufficiency

- Dyspnea
- Palpitations
- Angina
- Fatigue
- Cough
- Pulmonary vein congestion
- Rapidly rising and collapsing pulses

Mitral insufficiency

- Angina
- Dyspnea
- Fatigue
- Orthopnea
- Peripheral edema

Mitral stenosis

- Dyspnea on exertion
- Palpitations
- Fatigue
- Orthopnea
- Weakness
- Peripheral edema

Mitral valve prolapse

- Possibly asymptomatic
- Dizziness
- Chest pain
- Fatigue
- Palpitations
- Headache

Tricuspid insufficiency

- Dyspnea
- Fatigue
- Peripheral edema

Diagnostic evaluation

Aortic insufficiency

- Cardiac catheterization shows reduction in arterial diastolic pressures.
- Echocardiography shows left ventricular enlargement, alterations in mitral valve movement, and mitral thickening
- ECG shows sinus tachycardia and left ventricular hypertrophy.
- X-ray shows left ventricular enlargement and pulmonary vein congestion.

Mitral insufficiency

- Cardiac catheterization shows mitral regurgitation and elevated atrial pressures and pulmonary artery wedge pressures (PAWP).
- Echocardiography shows abnormal valve leaflet motion and left atrial enlargement.
- ECG may show left atrial and ventricular hypertrophy, sinus tachycardia, and AF.
- X-ray shows left atrial and ventricular enlargement.

Mitral stenosis

- Cardiac catheterization shows diastolic pressure gradient across the valve, elevated left atrial pressures and PAWP, and abnormal contraction of the left ventricle.
- Echocardiography shows thickened mitral valve leaflets.
- ECG shows left atrial hypertrophy, AF, right ventricular hypertrophy, and right axis deviation.
- X-ray shows left atrial and ventricular enlargement and mitral calcifcation.

Mitral valve prolapse

- Color-flow Doppler studies show mitral insufficiency.
- ECG shows ST changes and biphasic or inverted T waves in leads II, III, or AVF.
- Two-dimensional echocardiography shows prolapse of mitral leaf valves into the left atrium.

Tricuspid insufficiency

- Echocardiography shows systolic prolapse of the tricuspid valve and right atrial enlargement.
- ECG shows right atrial or right ventricular hypertrophy and AF.

◆ X-ray shows right atrial dilation and right ventricular enlargement.
◆ Cardiac catheterization shows high atrial pressure, tricuspid regurgitation, and decreased or normal cardiac output.

Nursing diagnoses

◆ Decreased cardiac output
◆ Activity intolerance
◆ Anxiety
◆ Ineffective tissue perfusion (cardiopulmonary)

Treatment

◆ Sodium restrictions (in cases of heart failure)
◆ Open-heart surgery using cardiopulmonary bypass for valve replacement (in severe cases)

Drug therapy options

◆ Anticoagulant: warfarin (Coumadin) to prevent thrombus formation if the client is in atrial fibrillation and after valve replacement surgery
◆ Digoxin (Lanoxin) to treat heart failure
◆ Diuretics to reduce pulmonary and peripheral edema

Planning and goals

◆ The client will remain hemodynamically stable.
◆ The client will demonstrate decreased anxiety over illness after appropriate education.
◆ The client will tolerate increased activity.
◆ The client will verbalize understanding of treatment and comply with therapy.

Implementation

◆ Watch closely for signs of heart failure or pulmonary edema and adverse effects of drug therapy *to prevent cardiac decompensation.*
◆ Place the client in an upright position *to relieve dyspnea.*
◆ Make sure the client maintains bed rest and provide assistance with bathing, if necessary, *to decrease oxygen demands on the heart.*
◆ If the client undergoes surgery, watch for hypotension, arrhythmias, and thrombus formation. Monitor vital signs, ABG levels, intake and output, daily weight, blood chemistry test results, chest X-rays, and pulmonary artery catheter readings *to detect early signs of postoperative complications and ensure early intervention and treatment.*
◆ Allow the client to verbalize concerns over being unable to meet life demands because of activity restrictions *to reduce anxiety.*

Evaluation

◆ The client has stable vital signs and a controlled cardiac rhythm.
◆ The client verbalizes decreased anxiety about the medical condition, discusses treatment, and states an understanding of the illness.
◆ The client demonstrates improved activity tolerance as the medical condition permits, such as taking part in ADLs with no significant change in heart rate or vital signs.
◆ The client complies with treatment.

VENOUS INSUFFICIENCY, CHRONIC

CHRONIC VENOUS INSUFFICIENCY generally results from physiologic changes secondary to deep vein thrombophlebitis. It's a reverse flow of blood in the lower extremities caused by incompetent vessels and resulting in increased pressure in the vessels during ambulation.

Possible causes

◆ Leg trauma
◆ Superficial venous insufficiency secondary to congenital or acquired arteriovenous fistula
◆ Tumor (causing obstruction in the pelvic veins)

Assessment findings

◆ Progressive edema of the leg (particularly the lower leg)
◆ Itching of the skin
◆ Dull discomfort of the lower legs worsened by periods of standing
◆ Pain (if ulceration is present)
◆ Thin, shiny, atrophic and cyanotic skin on legs
◆ Brownish pigmentation of legs
◆ Eczema, with superficial weeping dermatitis

Diagnostic evaluation

◆ Duplex Doppler ultrasonography and impedence plethysmography rule out phlebitis.

Nursing diagnoses

◆ Activity intolerance
◆ Risk for injury
◆ Ineffective tissue perfusion (peripheral)

Planning and goals

◆ The client will demonstrate increased activity tolerance.
◆ The client will maintain skin integrity.
◆ The client will have improved circulation to the lower extremities.

Implementation

◆ Instruct the client to maintain bed rest initially with legs elevated *to diminish chronic edema.*
◆ Suggest intermittent elevation of the legs during the day and elevation of the legs at night (above the level of the heart) *to promote circulation.*
◆ Advise the client to avoid long periods of sitting or standing *to decrease venous stasis.*
◆ Make sure to use properly fitting graduated compression stockings *to avoid venous compression.*
◆ Administer wet compresses to weeping dermatitis four times daily *to facilitate drainage.*
◆ Apply an Unna boot to affected extremity *to promote healing.*

Drug therapy options

◆ Antibiotic (if active infection is present)
◆ Anticoagulant (if recurrent thrombophlebitis): warfarin (Coumadin)

Evaluation

◆ The client has increased activity tolerance.
◆ The client maintains skin integrity.
◆ The client demonstrates improved circulation to the lower extremities.

NEUROLOGIC SYSTEM

The neurologic system serves as the body's communication network. It processes information from the outside world (through the sensory portion) and coordinates and organizes the functions of all other body systems.

NEUROLOGIC SYSTEM STRUCTURE AND FUNCTION

Major parts of the neurologic system include the brain, spinal cord, and peripheral nerves. The complex tissues that make up the neurologic system include billions of neurons (nerve cells).

Neurons

A neuron is a highly specialized conductor cell that receives, integrates, and transmits electrochemical nerve impulses. Delicate, threadlike nerve fibers called *axons* and *dendrites* extend from the neuron cell body and transmit signals. Axons carry impulses away from the cell body; dendrites carry impulses toward the cell body. A covering called a *myelin sheath* protects the entire neuron. Neurotransmitters — including the substances acetylcholine, serotonin, dopamine, endorphins, gamma-aminobutyric acid, and norepinephrine — conduct impulses across a synapse and into the next neuron.

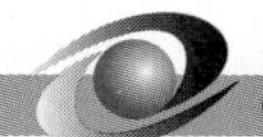

QUICK STUDY

To help you remember the cranial nerves (and their order) think of the mnemonic "**O**n **O**ld **O**lympus's **T**owering **T**ops, **a** **F**inn **a**nd **G**erman **V**iewed **S**ome **H**ops."

Olfactory (CN I)
Optic (CN II)
Oculomotor (CN III)
Trochlear (CN IV)
Trigeminal (CN V)
Abducens (CN VI)
Facial (CN VII)
Acoustic (CN VIII)
Glossopharyngeal (CN IX)
Vagus (CN X)
Spinal accessory (CN XI)
Hypoglossal (CN XII)

Central nervous system

The central nervous system (CNS) includes the brain and spinal cord. These fragile structures are protected by the skull and vertebrae, cerebrospinal fluid (CSF), and three membranes: the dura mater, the pia mater, and the arachnoid membrane.

Brain

The brain is a mass of neural tissue that includes the lobed cerebrum and other related structures.

Cerebrum

The cerebrum, the largest part of the brain, houses the nerve center that controls motor and sensory functions and intelligence. It's divided into hemispheres. Because motor impulses descending from the brain cross in the medulla, the right hemisphere controls the left side of the body and the left hemisphere controls the right side of the body. Several fissures divide the cerebrum into four lobes:
◆ frontal lobe — the site of personality, memory, reasoning, concentration, and motor control of speech
◆ parietal lobe — the site of sensation, integration of sensory information, and spatial relationships
◆ temporal lobe — the site of hearing, speech, memory, and emotion

◆ occipital lobe — the site of vision and involuntary eye movements.

Other structures

Other parts of the brain include the thalamus, hypothalamus, cerebellum, and brain stem:

◆ The thalamus is a structure located deep in the brain that consists of two oval-shaped parts, one located in each hemisphere. The thalamus is referred to as "the relay station of the brain" because it receives input from all of the senses except olfaction (smell), analyzes that input, and then transmits that information to other parts of the brain.

◆ The hypothalamus, located beneath the thalamus, controls sleep and wakefulness, temperature, respiration, blood pressure, sexual arousal, fluid balance, and emotional response.

◆ The cerebellum, at the base of the brain, coordinates muscle movements, regulates muscle tone, maintains balance, and controls posture.

◆ The brain stem provides the connection between the spinal cord and the brain. It contains three sections:

- The *midbrain* mediates pupillary reflexes and eye movements; it's also the reflex center for the third and fourth cranial nerves.
- The *pons* helps regulate respiration; it's also the reflex center for the fifth through eighth cranial nerves and mediates chewing, tasting, saliva secretion, and equilibrium.
- The *medulla oblongata* contains the vomiting, vasomotor, respiratory, and cardiac centers.

Spinal cord

The spinal cord functions as a two-way conductor pathway between the brain stem and the peripheral nervous system. It consists of gray matter and white matter:

◆ The gray matter is made up of cell bodies, dendrites, and axons.

◆ The white matter contains ascending (sensory) and descending (motor) tracts, sending signals up to the brain and motor signals out to the muscles.

Peripheral nervous system

The peripheral nervous system delivers messages from the spinal cord to outlying areas of the body. The main nerves of this system are grouped into:

◆ 31 pairs of spinal nerves, which carry mixed impulses (motor and sensory) to and from the spinal cord

◆ 12 pairs of cranial nerves, including olfactory, optic, oculomotor, trochlear, trigeminal, abducent, facial, acoustic, glossopharyngeal, vagus, spinal accessory, and hypoglossal.

Autonomic nervous system

The autonomic nervous system, a subdivision of the peripheral nervous system, controls involuntary body functions, such as digestion, respiration, and cardiovascular function. It's divided into two cooperating systems to maintain homeostasis, the sympathetic nervous system and the parasympathetic nervous system:

◆ The sympathetic nervous system coordinates activities that handle stress (the fight or flight response).

◆ The parasympathetic nervous system conserves and replenishes energy stores.

NEUROLOGIC DISORDERS

Major neurologic disorders include acute head injury, amyotrophic lateral sclerosis (ALS), Bell's palsy, brain abscess and tumor, cerebral aneurysm, encephalitis, Guillain-Barré syndrome, Huntington's disease, increased intracranial pressure (ICP), meningitis, multiple sclerosis (MS), myasthenia gravis (MG), Parkinson's disease, seizure disorders (epilepsy), spinal cord injury, stroke, and trigeminal neuralgia.

ACUTE HEAD INJURY

ACUTE HEAD INJURY results from a trauma to the head, leading to brain injury or bleeding within the brain. Effects of injury may include edema and hypoxia. Manifestations of the injury can vary greatly from a mild cognitive effect to severe functional deficits.

A head injury is classified by brain injury type: fracture, hemorrhage, or trauma. Fractures can be depressed, comminuted, or linear. Hemorrhages are classified as epidural, subdural, intracerebral, or subarachnoid.

Possible causes

◆ Assault
◆ Motor vehicle accident
◆ Blunt trauma
◆ Fall
◆ Penetrating trauma

Assessment findings

◆ Amnesia
◆ Disorientation to time, place, or person
◆ Unequal pupil size, loss of pupillary reaction (if edema is present) (see *Using the Glasgow Coma Scale,* page 346)
◆ Decreased LOC

Using the Glasgow Coma Scale

To quickly assess a patient's level of consciousness and uncover baseline changes, use the Glasgow Coma Scale. This assessment tool grades consciousness in relation to eye-opening and motor and verbal responses. A decreased reaction score in one or more categories warns of impending neurologic crisis. A patient who scores 7 or less is comatose and probably has severe neurologic damage.

If the patient has an endotracheal tube or a tracheostomy tube and can't respond verbally, use the abbreviation "T" to score this patient. For example, if the patient scores a 5 for best verbal response but he has a tracheostomy tube in place, this score is noted as 5T.

TEST	PATIENT'S REACTION	SCORE
Eye-opening response	Opens spontaneously	4
	Opens to verbal command	3
	Opens to pain	2
	No response	1
Best motor response	Obeys verbal command	6
	Localizes painful stimuli	5
	Flexion-withdrawal	4
	Flexion-abnormal (decorticate rigidity)	3
	Extension (decerebrate rigidity)	2
	No response	1
Best verbal response	Oriented and converses	5
	Disoriented and converses	4
	Inappropriate words	3
	Incomprehensible sounds	2
	No response	1
Total		**3 to 15**

- Paresthesia
- Posturing
- Otorrhea, rhinorrhea, frequent swallowing (if a CSF leak occurs)
- Vomiting

Diagnostic evaluation

- CT scan shows hemorrhage, cerebral edema, or shift of midline structures.
- EEG may reveal seizure activity.
- ICP monitoring shows increased ICP.
- Magnetic resonance imaging (MRI) shows hemorrhage, cerebral edema, or shift of midline structures.
- Skull X-ray may show skull fracture.

Nursing diagnoses

- Ineffective tissue perfusion (cerebral)
- Decreased intracranial adaptive capacity
- Risk for injury

Treatment

- Cervical collar (until neck injury is ruled out)
- Craniotomy: surgical incision into the cranium (may be necessary to evacuate a hematoma or evacuate contents to make room for swelling to prevent herniation)
- Oxygen therapy: intubation and mechanical ventilation (to provide controlled hyperventilation to decrease elevated ICP)
- Restricted oral intake for 24 to 48 hours
- Ventriculostomy: insertion of a drain into the ventricles (to drain CSF in the presence of hydrocephalus, which may occur as a result of head injury; can also be used to monitor ICP)

Drug therapy options

- Analgesic: codeine phosphate
- Anticonvulsant: phenytoin (Dilantin)
- Barbiturate: pentobarbital (Nembutal) if unable to control ICP with diuresis

- CNS depressants: fentanyl (Sublimaze), sufentanil (Sufenta) to lower ICP by reducing metabolic demand or to relieve anxiety and pain
- Diuretics: mannitol (Osmitrol), furosemide (Lasix) to combat cerebral edema
- Glucocorticoid: dexamethasone (Decadron) to reduce cerebral edema
- Histamine-2 (H_2) receptor antagonists: cimetidine (Tagamet), ranitidine (Zantac), famotidine (Pepcid), nizatidine (Axid)
- Mucosal barrier fortifier: sucralfate (Carafate)
- Neuromuscular blocking agent: vecuronium to induce paralysis for ventilation control and reduce metabolic demand
- Posterior pituitary hormone: vasopressin (Pitressin) if client develops diabetes insipidus
- Vasopressors: dopamine (Intropin), phenylephrine (Neo-Synephrine) to maintain cerebral perfusion pressure above 60 mm Hg (if blood pressure is low and ICP is elevated)

Planning and goals

- The client will have improved cerebral perfusion.
- The client will have decreased ICP.
- The client will remain free from injury.

Implementation

- Assess neurologic and respiratory status *to monitor for signs of increased ICP and respiratory distress.*
- Observe for signs of increasing ICP (including ICP greater than 20 mm Hg for more than 10 minutes) *to avoid treatment delay and prevent neurologic compromise.*
- Monitor and record vital signs, intake and output, hemodynamic variables, ICP, cerebral perfusion pressure, specific gravity, laboratory studies, and pulse oximetry *to detect early signs of compromise.*
- Assess for CSF leak as evidenced by otorrhea or rhinorrhea. *CSF leak could leave the client at risk for infection.*
- Assess pain. *Pain may cause anxiety and increase ICP.*
- Check cough and gag reflex *to prevent aspiration.*
- Check for signs of diabetes insipidus (low urine specific gravity, high urine output) *to maintain hydration.*
- Administer I.V. fluids *to maintain hydration.*
- Administer oxygen therapy and maintain position and patency of the endotracheal tube, if present, *to maintain airway and hyperventilate the client to lower ICP.*
- Provide suctioning; if the client is able, assist with turning, coughing, and deep breathing *to prevent pooling of secretions.*
- Maintain position, patency, and low suction of the NG tube *to prevent vomiting.*
- Maintain seizure precautions *to maintain client safety.*
- Administer medications as prescribed *to decrease ICP and pain.*
- Monitor blood glucose levels and administer insulin as prescribed to maintain glucose levels between 80 and 110 mg/dl *to prevent complications of elevated blood glucose levels.*
- Allow a rest period between nursing activities *to avoid an increase in ICP.*
- Encourage the client to express feelings about changes in body image *to allay anxiety.*
- Provide appropriate sensory input and stimuli with frequent reorientation *to foster awareness of the environment.*
- Provide a means of communication, such as a communication board, *to prevent anxiety.*
- Provide eye, skin, and mouth care *to prevent tissue damage.*
- Turn the client every 2 hours or maintain him in a rotating bed if his condition allows *to prevent skin breakdown.*
- Consult various therapies (such as physical, occupational, and speech) *to optimize the client's outcome.*
- Consult social services and home care as appropriate *to help meet the client's ongoing needs.*

Evaluation

- The client's LOC has improved.
- The client doesn't exhibit signs of increased ICP.
- The client remains free from injury.

AMYOTROPHIC LATERAL SCLEROSIS

AMYOTROPHIC LATERAL SCLEROSIS (ALS), commonly known as *Lou Gehrig disease,* is a progressive, degenerative disorder that leads to decreased motor function in the upper and lower motor neuron systems. In ALS, myelin sheaths are destroyed and replaced with scar tissue, resulting in distorted or blocked nerve impulses. Nerve cells die and muscle fibers have atrophic changes resulting in progressive motor dysfunction. The disease affects males three times more commonly than females.

Possible causes

- Autoimmune disorder
- Genetic predisposition
- Nutritional deficiency related to a disturbance in enzyme metabolism
- Physical exhaustion
- Slow-acting virus
- Trauma

Assessment findings

◆ Muscle weakness, especially of limb muscles
◆ Fasciculations
◆ Dysphagia
◆ Awkwardness of fine finger movements
◆ Fatigue
◆ Atrophy
◆ Dyspnea
◆ Nasal quality of speech
◆ Spasticity

Diagnostic evaluation

◆ Creatinine kinase level is elevated.
◆ EMG shows decreased amplitude of evoked potentials.
◆ Muscle biopsy differentiates nerve from muscle disease.

Nursing diagnoses

◆ Ineffective airway clearance
◆ Impaired physical mobility
◆ Ineffective health maintenance

Treatment

◆ Symptomatic relief

Drug therapy options

◆ Anticholinergic: dicyclomine (Bentyl)
◆ Anticonvulsant: gabapentin (Neurontin)
◆ Antispasmodics: baclofen (Lioresal), lorazepam (Ativan)
◆ Interferon therapy
◆ Neuroprotective agent: riluzole (Rilutek)

Planning and goals

◆ The client will maintain a patent airway and adequate ventilation.
◆ The client will maintain joint mobility and range of motion.
◆ The client will maintain care of himself and his environment to the best of his ability.

Implementation

◆ Assess neurologic and respiratory status *to detect decreases in neurologic functioning.*
◆ Assess swallow and gag reflexes *to decrease the risk of aspiration.*
◆ Monitor and record vital signs and intake and output *to determine a baseline and detect changes from the baseline assessment.*
◆ Administer medications as prescribed *to help the client achieve his maximal potential.*
◆ Devise an alternate method of communication, when necessary, *to help the client communicate and decrease his anxiety and frustration.*
◆ Encourage the client to verbalize his feelings and maintain his independence for as long as possible *to decrease anxiety and promote self-esteem.*
◆ Suction the oral pharynx, as necessary, *to stimulate cough and clear airways.*
◆ Maintain the client's diet *to improve nutritional status.*

Evaluation

◆ The client has adequate gas exchange.
◆ The client demonstrates ability to use his muscles and joints effectively.
◆ The client demonstrates ability to perform self-care.

BELL'S PALSY

BELL'S PALSY affects cranial nerve VII (facial) and produces unilateral facial weakness or paralysis. Onset is rapid. While it affects all age-groups, it occurs most commonly in persons younger than age 60. In 80% to 90% of clients, it subsides spontaneously, with complete recovery in 1 to 8 weeks; however, recovery may be delayed in older adults. If recovery is partial, contractures may develop on the paralyzed side of the face. Bell's palsy may recur on the same or opposite side of the face.

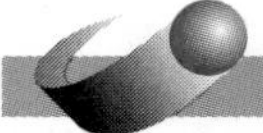

FAST FACT

There are two facial nerves, one on each side. Bell's palsy occurs when one of those nerves becomes swollen and pinched.

Possible causes

◆ Blockage of cranial nerve VII resulting from infection, hemorrhage, tumor, meningitis, or local trauma

Assessment findings

◆ Inability to close eye completely on the affected side, wrinkle forehead, smile, whistle, or grimace
◆ Facial appearance that's masklike and sagging
◆ Pain around the jaw or ear
◆ Unilateral facial weakness
◆ Eye that rolls upward and tears excessively when the client attempts to close it
◆ Ringing in the ears
◆ Taste distortion on the affected anterior portion of the tongue

Diagnostic evaluation

◆ EMG helps predict the level of expected recovery by distinguishing temporary conduction defects from a pathologic interruption of nerve fibers.

Nursing diagnoses

◆ Acute pain
◆ Disturbed sensory perception (gustatory)
◆ Disturbed body image

Treatment

◆ Moist heat
◆ Facial sling
◆ Surgery to decompress facial nerve

Drug therapy options

◆ Corticosteroid: prednisone (Deltasone) to reduce facial nerve edema and improve nerve conduction and blood flow

Planning and goals

◆ The client will experience increased comfort and relief from pain.
◆ The client will report improved sensation and function in the affected area.
◆ The client will state positive feelings about himself.

Implementation

◆ During treatment with prednisone, watch for adverse reactions, especially GI distress and fluid retention. If GI distress is troublesome, a concomitant antacid usually provides relief *to prevent further complications.*
◆ If the client has diabetes, prednisone must be used with caution and necessitates frequent monitoring of serum glucose levels. *Hyperglycemia is an adverse reaction to prednisone therapy.*
◆ Apply moist heat to the affected side of the face, taking care not to burn the skin, *to reduce pain.*
◆ Massage the client's face with a gentle upward motion two to three times daily for 5 to 10 minutes, or have him massage his face himself *to help maintain muscle tone.* When he's ready for active exercises, teach him to exercise by grimacing in front of a mirror.
◆ Arrange for privacy at mealtimes *to reduce embarrassment.*
◆ Instruct the client to always sit up straight when eating, chew on the unaffected side, take small bites, and eat nutritionally balanced meals while refraining from eating foods that are hard to chew *to avoid aspiration and weight loss.*
◆ Apply a facial sling *to improve lip alignment.*
◆ Give the client frequent, complete mouth care, being careful to remove residual food that collects between the cheeks and gums *to prevent breakdown of the oral mucosa.*
◆ Offer psychological support. Give reassurance that recovery is likely within 1 to 8 weeks *to allay the client's anxiety.*

Evaluation

◆ The client reports adequate pain control.
◆ The client has improved sensation and function in the affected area.
◆ The client provides positive statements regarding facial appearance and functional ability.

BRAIN ABSCESS

BRAIN ABSCESS is a free or encapsulated collection of pus that usually occurs in the temporal lobe, cerebellum, or frontal lobes. Brain abscess is rare. Although it can occur at any age, it's most common in people ages 10 to 35 and is rare in older adults.

An untreated brain abscess is usually fatal; with treatment, the prognosis is only fair.

Possible causes

◆ Infection, especially otitis media, sinusitis, dental abscess, and mastoiditis
◆ Subdural empyema
◆ Penetrating head trauma

Assessment findings

◆ Malaise
◆ Headache
◆ Chills
◆ Fever
◆ Confusion
◆ Drowsiness
◆ Lethargy

Temporal lobe abscess

◆ Auditory-receptive dysphasia
◆ Central facial weakness
◆ Hemiparesis

Cerebellar abscess

◆ Dizziness
◆ Coarse nystagmus
◆ Gaze weakness on lesion side
◆ Tremor
◆ Ataxia

Frontal lobe abscess
- Expressive dysphasia
- Hemiparesis with unilateral motor seizure
- Drowsiness
- Inattention
- Mental function impairment
- Seizures

Diagnostic evaluation
- Physical examination shows increased ICP.
- Enhanced CT scanning reveals the abscess site.
- Arteriography highlights the abscess, giving it a halo appearance.
- WBC count and ESR are usually elevated.
- CT-guided stereotactic biopsy may be performed to drain and culture the abscess.
- Culture and sensitivity of drainage identifies the causative organism.

Nursing diagnoses
- Decreased intracranial adaptive capacity
- Disturbed thought processes
- Impaired physical mobility
- Ineffective tissue perfusion (cerebral)

Treatment
- ET intubation and mechanical ventilation
- I.V. therapy
- Surgical aspiration or drainage of the abscess

Drug therapy options
- Diuretics: urea (Ureaphil), mannitol (Osmitrol)
- Corticosteroids: dexamethasone (Decadron)
- Penicillinase-resistant antibiotics: nafcillin, methicillin
- Anticonvulsants: phenytoin (Dilantin), phenobarbital (Luminal)

Planning and goals
- The client will have ICP within normal limits.
- The client will exhibit improved neurologic functioning.
- The client will maintain baseline physical mobility.

Implementation
- Provide intensive care and monitoring to the client with an acute brain abscess *to closely monitor ICP and provide necessary life-support.*
- Frequently assess neurologic status, especially cognition and mentation, speech, and sensorimotor and cranial nerve function (Glasgow Coma Scale) *to detect early signs of increased ICP.*
- Assess and record vital signs at least every hour *to detect trends that may signify increasing ICP,* such as increasing blood pressure and slowing heart rate.
- Monitor fluid intake and output carefully *because fluid overload could contribute to cerebral edema.*
- If surgery is necessary, explain the procedure to the client and answer his questions *to allay anxiety.*
- After surgery, continue frequent neurologic assessment *to detect rises in ICP and deteriorating neurologic status.* Monitor vital signs and intake and output.
- Watch for signs of meningitis (nuchal rigidity, headaches, chills, sweats) *to avoid treatment delay.*
- Change a damp dressing often. Never allow bandages to remain damp. *Damp dressings are a good medium for bacterial growth.*
- Position the client on the operative side *to promote drainage and prevent reaccumulation of the abscess.*
- Measure drainage from Jackson-Pratt or other types of drains as instructed by the surgeon *to assess the effectiveness of the drain and detect signs of hemorrhage if blood should begin to accumulate in the drain.*
- Give meticulous skin care and reposition the client frequently *to prevent pressure ulcers.* Perform ROM exercises *to preserve function and prevent contractures.*
- If the client requires isolation because of postoperative drainage, make sure he and his family understand why *to promote compliance with isolation precautions and to allay anxiety.*
- Ambulate the client as soon as possible *to prevent immobility and encourage independence.*
- Give prophylactic antibiotics as needed after a compound skull fracture or penetrating head wound *to prevent brain abscess.*

Evaluation
- The client doesn't exhibit signs of increased ICP.
- The client demonstrates appropriate thought processes and neurologic functioning.
- The client maintains baseline physical mobility.

BRAIN TUMOR
A BRAIN TUMOR is an abnormal mass found in the brain that results from unregulated cell growth and division. This tumor can infiltrate and destroy surrounding tissue or can be encapsulated and displace brain tissue. The presence of the lesion causes compression of blood vessels, producing ischemia, edema, and increased ICP.

Symptoms and manifestations vary depending on the location of the tumor in the brain. The tumor can be primary (originating in the brain tissue) or secondary (metastasizing from another area of the body). Tumors are classified according to the tissue of origin, such as gliomas (composed of neuroglial cells), meningiomas (originating in the meninges), and astrocytomas (composed of astrocytes).

Possible causes

- ◆ Environmental factors
- ◆ Genetic factors

Assessment findings

Any brain area

- ◆ Deficits in cerebral function
- ◆ Headache

Frontal lobe

- ◆ Aphasia
- ◆ Memory loss
- ◆ Personality changes

Temporal lobe

- ◆ Aphasia
- ◆ Seizures

Parietal lobe

- ◆ Motor seizures
- ◆ Sensory impairment

Occipital lobe

- ◆ Homonymous hemianopsia (defective vision or blindness affecting the right halves or the left halves of the visual field of the two eyes)
- ◆ Visual hallucinations
- ◆ Visual impairment

Cerebellum

- ◆ Impaired coordination
- ◆ Impaired equilibrium

Diagnostic evaluation

- ◆ CT scanning shows the location and size of the tumor.
- ◆ MRI also shows the location and size of the tumor.

Nursing diagnoses

- ◆ Disturbed sensory perception (kinesthetic)
- ◆ Ineffective tissue perfusion (cerebral)
- ◆ Decreased intracranial adaptive capacity
- ◆ Anxiety
- ◆ Risk for injury

Treatment

- ◆ Chemotherapy for malignant tumors
- ◆ Craniotomy
- ◆ High-calorie diet
- ◆ Radiation therapy for malignant tumors
- ◆ Ventriculostomy

Drug therapy options

- ◆ Analgesics: codeine, acetaminophen (for headache)
- ◆ Anticonvulsant: phenytoin (Dilantin)
- ◆ Antineoplastics: vincristine (Oncovin), lomustine (CeeNu), carmustine (BiCNU)
- ◆ Antiemetic: prochlorperazine dimaleate (Compazine) to treat nausea and vomiting
- ◆ Diuretics: mannitol (Osmitrol), furosemide (Lasix) if increased ICP
- ◆ Glucocorticoid: dexamethasone (Decadron)
- ◆ H_2-receptor antagonists: cimetidine (Tagamet), ranitidine (Zantac), famotidine (Pepcid), nizatidine (Axid)
- ◆ Mucosal barrier fortifier: sucralfate (Carafate)
- ◆ Insulin to maintain tight glycemic control

Planning and goals

- ◆ The client will recognize limitations imposed by his illness and express his feelings about these limitations.
- ◆ The client will express feelings about his diminished capacity to perform usual roles.
- ◆ The client will remain free from injury.
- ◆ The client's ICP will remain within normal parameters.

Implementation

- ◆ Assess neurologic and respiratory status *to determine a baseline and deviations from the baseline assessment.*
- ◆ Assess pain. *Continuous assessment correlates the client's subjective complaints and behavior with organic pathology.*
- ◆ Assess for increased ICP *to facilitate early intervention and prevent neurologic complications.*
- ◆ Monitor and record vital signs and intake and output, ICP, and laboratory studies *to determine a baseline and detect early deviations from the baseline assessment.*
- ◆ Monitor for signs and symptoms of SYNDROME OF INAPPROPRIATE ANTIDIURETIC HORMONE (edema, weight gain, positive fluid balance, high urine specific gravity) *to facilitate early intervention and prevent increased ICP* (through fluid restriction and I.V. infusion of normal saline solution).
- ◆ Turn and reposition the client every 2 hours *to maintain skin integrity.*
- ◆ Maintain the client's diet *to promote healing.*

◆ Encourage the client to drink fluids *to maintain hydration.*
◆ Administer I.V. fluids *to maintain hydration if the client can't drink adequate amounts.*
◆ Administer oxygen *to prevent ischemia.*
◆ Administer enteral nutrition or total parenteral nutrition (TPN), as indicated, *to meet nutritional needs.*
◆ Limit environmental noise. *Auditory stimuli can contribute to increased ICP.*
◆ Monitor ABG levels. *Hypercapnia results in vasodilation, increased cerebral blood volume, and increased ICP.*
◆ Maintain normothermia and control shivering. *Shivering causes isometric muscle contraction, which can increase ICP.*
◆ Provide rest periods. *Cerebral blood flow increases during rapid–eye-movement sleep.*
◆ Monitor blood glucose levels and administer insulin as prescribed to maintain blood glucose levels of 80 to 110 mg/dl *to prevent complications of elevated blood glucose levels.*
◆ Maintain seizure precautions and administer anticonvulsants, as ordered. *Seizures increase intrathoracic pressure, decrease cerebral venous outflow, and increase cerebral blood volume, thereby increasing ICP.*
◆ Encourage the client to express feelings about changes in body image and a fear of dying *to decrease anxiety.*
◆ Consult hospice and social servies *to help meet the client's needs in the home.*

Evaluation
◆ The client demonstrates ability to function despite sensory or motor deficits.
◆ The client demonstrates effective coping mechanisms in dealing with the limitations of his illness.
◆ The client remains free from injury.
◆ The client's ICP remains within normal parameters.

CEREBRAL ANEURYSM
A CEREBRAL ANEURYSM is an abnormal outpouching of a cerebral artery that results from weakness of the middle layer of an artery. It usually results from a congenital weakness in the structure of the artery and remains asymptomatic until it ruptures.

Cerebral aneurysms are classified by type: saccular (berry), fusiform, and giant. Saccular aneurysms, the most common, occur at the base of the brain at the juncture where the large arteries bifurcate.

Possible causes
◆ Atherosclerosis
◆ Congenital weakness (structure of artery)
◆ Head trauma

Assessment findings
◆ Asymptomatic until aneurysm ruptures
◆ Headache (commonly described by the client as "the worst ever")
◆ Decreased LOC
◆ Diplopia, ptosis, blurred vision
◆ Fever
◆ Hemiparesis
◆ Nuchal rigidity
◆ Seizure activity

Ruptured cerebral aneurysms are grouped as:
◆ Grade I — minimal bleeding and no defects, slight headache and nuchal rigidity
◆ Grade II — mild bleeding; client alert with mild headache, nuchal rigidity and, possibly, nerve III palsy
◆ Grade III — moderate bleeding; client drowsy or confused, with nuchal rgidity and mild focal deficit
◆ Grade IV — severe bleeding; client stuporous with nuchal rigidity, and mild to severe hemiparesis
◆ Grade V — moribund (fatal); if nonfatal, client decerebrate and in deep coma.

Diagnostic evaluation
◆ Cerebral angiography identifies the aneurysm.
◆ CT scanning shows a shift of intracranial midline structures and blood in the subarachnoid space.
◆ Lumbar puncture (contraindicated with increased ICP) shows increased CSF pressure, protein level, and WBCs and grossly bloody and xanthochromic CSF.
◆ MRI shows shift of intracranial midline structures and blood in the subarachnoid space.

Nursing diagnoses
◆ Ineffective tissue perfusion (cerebral)
◆ Decreased intracranial adaptive capacity
◆ Anxiety

Treatment
◆ Aneurysm and seizure precautions
◆ Aneurysm clipping to isolate the aneurysm without blocking off small arteries nearby
◆ Bed rest
◆ Head of bed elevated 30 degrees
◆ I.V. therapy
◆ Oxygen therapy (intubation and mechanical ventilation with hyperventilation if increased ICP)

Drug therapy options

◆ Analgesic: codeine sulfate
◆ Anticonvulsant: phenytoin (Dilantin)
◆ Antihypertensives: hydralazine (Apresoline), nitroprusside (Nitropress), labetalol (Trandate), metoprolol (Lopressor), esmolol (Brevibloc)
◆ Calcium channel blocker: nimodipine (Nimotop), preferred drug to prevent cerebral vasospasm
◆ Diuretic: furosemide (Lasix) if ICP becomes elevated
◆ Glucocorticoid: dexamethasone (Decadron)
◆ H_2-receptor antagonists: cimetidine (Tagamet), ranitidine (Zantac), famotidine (Pepcid)
◆ Insulin to maintain tight glycemic control
◆ Vasopressors: dopamine (Intropin), phenylephrine (Neo-Synephrine) to maintain systolic blood pressure at 140 to 160 mm Hg
◆ Mucosal barrier fortifier: sucralfate (Carafate)
◆ Stool softener: docusate sodium (Colace)

Planning and goals

◆ The client will maintain adequate ventilation and oxygenation.
◆ The client will have stable cerebral perfusion and neurologic status within normal parameters.
◆ The client will express feelings of calmness.

Implementation

◆ Assess neurologic status *to screen for changes in the client's condition.*
◆ Keep the environment and client quiet using sedatives and pain medication *to reduce increased ICP.*
◆ Administer diuretics *to prevent or treat increased ICP.*
◆ Administer crystalloid solutions after aneurysm clipping *to induce hypervolemia and increase cerebral perfusion, thus decreasing the risk of vasospasm.*
◆ Administer oxygen (may require intubation and mechanical ventilation). *Hypercapnia results in vasodilation, increased cerebral blood volume, and increased ICP.*
◆ Keep the head of the bed elevated to 30 degrees *to reduce increased ICP.*
◆ Monitor for CUSHING'S TRIAD (bradycardia, systolic hypertension, and wide pulse pressure), *which is a sign of impending hemorrhage.*
◆ Monitor blood glucose levels and administer insulin to maintain a blood glucose level of 80 to 110 mg/dl *to prevent complications of elevated blood glucose level.*
◆ Take vital signs every 15 minutes initially, then every 1 to 2 hours as stability increases, then every 4 hours when the client becomes stable *to detect early signs of decreased cerebral perfusion pressure or increased ICP.*
◆ Allow a rest period between nursing activities *to prevent a rise in ICP.*
◆ Maintain seizure precautions and administer anticonvulsants, as ordered. *Seizures increase intrathoracic pressure, decrease cerebral venous outflow, and increase cerebral blood volume, thereby increasing ICP.*
◆ Provide skin care and turn the client every 2 hours *to prevent pressure ulcers.*
◆ Maintain adequate nutrition *to facilitate tissue healing and meet metabolic needs.*
◆ Minimize constipation and straining at defecation *to prevent increased ICP.*
◆ If the client has a potentially compromised airway, use antiemetics or NG suctioning *to prevent nausea and vomiting, which may increase ICP.*
◆ Consult various therapies (such as physical, speech, and occupational) as well as social services *to help meet the needs of the client.*

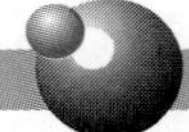

SPOT CHECK

A client undergoes surgical clipping of a cerebral aneurysm. To prevent vasospasm, postsurgical care focuses on maintaining an optimal cerebral perfusion pressure. This goal is best accomplished by administering:

A. diuretics such as furosemide (Lasix).
B. blood products such as cryoprecipitate.
C. the calcium channel blocker nifedipine (Procardia).
D. volume expanders such as crystalloids.

Answer: D. To prevent vasospasm following repair of a cerebral aneurysm, treatment focuses on increasing cerebral perfusion. This goal can be accomplished by giving volume expanders such as crystalloids. Diuretics would decrease cerebral perfusion by reducing volume. Cryoprecipitate isn't used as a volume expander. Nimodipine (Nimotop), not nifedipine (Procardia), is the calcium channel blocker indicated for use in cerebral vasospasm treatment and prevention.

Evaluation

◆ The client has adequate ventilation and oxygenation.
◆ The client is alert and oriented.
◆ The client demonstrates calm behavior.

ENCEPHALITIS

ENCEPHALITIS is a severe inflammation and swelling of the brain, usually caused by a mosquito-borne or, in some areas, a tick-borne virus. Transmission also may occur through ingestion of infected goat's milk and accidental injection or inhalation of the virus. Eastern equine encephalitis may produce permanent neurologic damage and is commonly fatal. The most recent outbreak of mosquito-borne encephalitis was West Nile encephalitis.

In encephalitis, intense lymphocytic infiltration of brain tissues and the leptomeninges causes cerebral edema, degeneration of the brain's ganglion cells, and diffuse nerve cell destruction.

Possible causes

- Exposure to virus

Assessment findings

- Coma (following the acute phase of illness)
- Delirium or confusion
- Headache
- Meningeal irritation (stiff neck and back) and neuronal damage (drowsiness, coma, paralysis, seizures, ataxia, organic psychoses)
- Sensory alterations (seizures, abnormal reflexes)
- Sudden onset of fever
- Vomiting

Diagnostic evaluation

- Blood studies identify the virus and confirm the diagnosis.
- CSF analysis identifies the virus.
- Lumbar puncture shows elevated CSF pressure and, despite inflammation, the fluid is commonly clear. WBC and protein levels in CSF are slightly elevated, but the glucose level remains normal.
- EEG reveals abnormalities such as generalized slowing of waveforms.
- CT scanning may be ordered to rule out cerebral hematoma.

Nursing diagnoses

- Ineffective tissue perfusion (cerebral)
- Decreased intracranial adaptive capacity
- Disturbed thought processes
- Hyperthermia
- Impaired physical mobility

Treatment

- ET intubation and mechanical ventilation
- I.V. fluids
- NG tube feedings or TPN

Drug therapy options

- Anticonvulsants: phenytoin (Dilantin), phenobarbital (Luminal)
- Antiviral: acyclovir (Zovirax) (effective only against herpes encephalitis and only if administered before the onset of coma)
- Analgesics and antipyretics: aspirin, acetaminophen (Tylenol) (relieves headache and reduces fever)
- Diuretics: furosemide (Lasix), mannitol (Osmitrol) (reduces cerebral swelling)
- Corticosteroid: dexamethasone (Decadron) (reduces cerebral inflammation and edema)
- Laxative: bisacodyl (Dulcolax)
- Sedative: lorazepam (Ativan) for restlessness
- Stool softener: docusate (Colace)

Planning and goals

- The client will have appropriate thought processes and neurologic examinations within normal parameters.
- The client will exhibit temperature within normal limits.
- The client will have improved physical mobility.

Implementation

- Assess neurologic function often (every 15 minutes to 1 hour initially, then every 2 to 4 hours as the client stabilizes). Observe the client's mental status and cognitive abilities. *If the tissue within the brain becomes edematous, changes will occur in the client's mental status and cognitive abilities.*
- Maintain adequate fluid intake *to prevent dehydration* but avoid fluid overload, *which may increase cerebral edema.* Measure and record intake and output accurately *to assess fluid status.*
- Give acyclovir by slow I.V. infusion only. The client must be well-hydrated and the infusion given over 1 hour *to avoid kidney damage.* Watch for adverse effects, such as nausea, diarrhea, pruritus, and rash, and adverse effects of other drugs *to prevent complications.* Check the infusion site often *to avoid infiltration and phlebitis.*
- Carefully position the client *to prevent joint stiffness and neck pain,* and turn him often *to prevent skin breakdown.*
- Assist with ROM exercises *to maintain joint mobility.*
- Maintain adequate nutrition *to meet increased metabolic needs and promote healing.* It may be necessary to give the client small, frequent meals or supplement these meals with an NG tube or parenteral feedings.
- Give a stool softener or mild laxative *to prevent constipation and minimize the risk of increased ICP from straining during defecation.*

- Provide good mouth care *to prevent breakdown of oral mucous membranes.*
- Maintain a quiet environment *to promote comfort and decrease stimulation, which can cause ICP to rise.* Darkening the room *may decrease photophobia and headache.*
- If the client naps during the day and is restless at night, plan daytime activities *to minimize napping and promote sleep at night.*
- Provide emotional support and reassurance *because the client is apt to be frightened by the illness and frequent diagnostic tests.*
- Reassure the client and his family that behavioral changes caused by encephalitis usually disappear *to decrease anxiety.*

Evaluation

- The client has appropriate thought processes and neurologic assessments within normal parameters.
- The client has a normal temperature.
- The client has returned to baseline physical mobility.

GUILLAIN-BARRÉ SYNDROME

GUILLAIN-BARRÉ SYNDROME is an acute, rapidly progressive, and potentially fatal form of polyneuritis (inflammation of several peripheral nerves at once) that causes muscle weakness and mild distal sensory loss.

Recovery is spontaneous and complete in about 95% of clients, although mild motor or reflex deficits in the feet and legs may persist. The prognosis is best when symptoms clear between 15 and 20 days after onset.

This disorder is also known as *infectious polyneuritis, Landry-Guillain-Barré syndrome,* and *acute idiopathic polyneuritis.*

Possible causes

- Cell-mediated immune response with an attack on peripheral nerves in response to a virus
- Demyelination of the peripheral nerves
- Respiratory infection

Risk factors

- Surgery
- Rabies or swine influenza vaccination
- Viral illness
- Hodgkin's or another malignant disease
- Systemic lupus erythematosus

Assessment findings

- Muscle weakness without atrophy (ascending from the legs to the arms)
- Dysphagia (difficulty swallowing) or dysarthria (poor speech caused by impaired muscular control)
- Facial diplegia (affecting like parts on both sides of the face; possibly accompanied by ophthalmoplegia [ocular paralysis])
- Hypertonia (excessive muscle tone) and areflexia (absence of reflexes)
- Paresthesia
- Stiffness and pain in the form of a severe "charley horse"
- Weakness of the muscles supplied by cranial nerve XI, the spinal accessory nerve, affecting shoulder movement and head rotation (a less common finding).

Diagnostic evaluation

- History of preceding febrile illness (usually a respiratory tract infection) and typical clinical features suggest Guillain-Barré syndrome.
- CSF protein level begins to rise, peaking in 4 to 6 weeks. The CSF WBC count remains normal but, in severe disease, CSF pressure may rise above normal.
- Blood studies reveal a CBC that shows leukocytosis with the presence of immature forms early in the illness, but blood study results soon return to normal.
- EMG may show repeated firing of the same motor unit, instead of widespread sectional stimulation.
- Nerve conduction velocities are slowed soon after paralysis develops. Diagnosis must rule out similar diseases such as acute poliomyelitis.

Nursing diagnoses

- Ineffective breathing pattern
- Impaired physical mobility
- Anxiety
- Ineffective tissue perfusion (peripheral)

Treatment

- ET intubation or tracheotomy if the client has difficulty clearing secretions; possible mechanical ventilation
- NG tube feedings or parenteral nutrition
- I.V. fluid therapy
- Specialty bed or support surfaces
- Plasmapheresis

Drug therapy options

- Corticosteroid: prednisone (Deltasone)
- Antiarrhythmics: propranolol (Inderal), atropine

◆ Anticoagulants: heparin (Liquaemin), warfarin (Coumadin)
◆ Immunoglobulin to decrease autoimmune response

Planning and goals

◆ The client will maintain adequate ventilation.
◆ The client will return to baseline motor ability.
◆ The client will use available support systems and develop adequate coping mechanisms.

Implementation

◆ Watch for ascending sensory loss, which precedes motor loss. Also, monitor vital signs and LOC *to detect disease progression.*
◆ Assess and treat respiratory dysfunction *to prevent respiratory arrest.* If respiratory muscles are weak, take serial vital capacity recordings. Use a respirometer with a mouthpiece or a facemask for bedside testing *to ensure rapid measurement.*
◆ Obtain ABG measurements. Because neuromuscular disease results in primary hypoventilation with hypoxemia and hypercapnia, watch for a partial pressure of arterial oxygen (Pao_2) below 70 mm Hg, *which signals respiratory failure.*
◆ Be alert for signs of a rising partial pressure of carbon dioxide ($Paco_2$) (confusion, tachypnea) *to detect early signs of hypoventilation and avoid treatment delay.*
◆ Auscultate for breath sounds to detect early changes in respiratory function, and encourage coughing and deep breathing *to mobilize secretions and prevent atelectasis.*
◆ Begin respiratory support at the first sign of dyspnea (in adults, a vital capacity less than 800 ml) or a decreasing Pao_2 *to prevent hypoxemia.*
◆ If respiratory failure becomes imminent, establish an emergency airway with an ET tube *to prevent organ damage from anoxia.*
◆ Provide meticulous skin care *to prevent skin breakdown and contractures.*
◆ Establish a strict turning schedule; inspect the skin (especially the sacrum, heels, and ankles) for breakdown, and reposition the client every 2 hours. *These measures prevent skin breakdown and pressure ulcer development.*
◆ After each position change, stimulate circulation by carefully massaging pressure points. Also, use foam, gel, or alternating-pressure pads at points of contact *to prevent skin breakdown.*
◆ Perform passive ROM exercises within the client's pain limits. Remember that the proximal muscle groups of the thighs, shoulders, and trunk will be the most tender and cause the most pain on passive movement and turning. *Passive ROM exercises maintain joint function.*
◆ When the client's condition stabilizes, change to gentle stretching and active-assistance exercises *to strengthen muscles and maintain joint function.*
◆ Assess the client for signs of dysphagia (coughing, choking, "wet"-sounding voice, increased presence of rhonchi after feeding, drooling, delayed swallowing, regurgitation of food, and weakness in cranial nerves V, VII, IX, X, XI, or XII). *These measures help prevent aspiration.*
◆ Elevate the head of the bed, position the client upright and leaning forward when eating; feed semisolid food, and check the mouth for food pockets *to minimize aspiration risk.*
◆ Encourage the client to eat slowly and remain upright for 15 to 20 minutes after eating *to prevent aspiration.*
◆ If aspiration can't be minimized by diet and position modification, expect to provide NG feeding *to prevent aspiration and ensure that nutritional needs are met.*
◆ As the client regains strength and can tolerate a vertical position, be alert for postural hypotension. Monitor blood pressure and pulse rate during tilting periods and, if necessary, apply toe-to-groin elastic bandages or an abdominal binder *to prevent orthostatic hypotension.*
◆ Inspect the client's legs regularly for orthostatic localized pain, tenderness, erythema, edema, and positive Homans' sign *to detect thrombophlebitis, a common complication of Guillain-Barré syndrome.*
◆ Apply antiembolism stockings and give prophylactic anticoagulants, as needed *to prevent thrombophlebitis.*
◆ If the client has facial paralysis, provide eye and mouth care every 4 hours *to prevent corneal damage and breakdown of the oral mucosa.*
◆ Protect the corneas with isotonic eyedrops and conical eye shields *to prevent corneal injury.*
◆ Encourage adequate fluid intake (2,000 ml/day), unless contraindicated, *to prevent dehydration, constipation, and renal calculi formation.*
◆ Measure and record intake and output every 8 hours, and offer the bedpan every 3 to 4 hours *to monitor for urine retention.*
◆ Begin intermittent catheterization as needed *to relieve urine retention.* The client may need manual pressure on the bladder (Credé's method) before urination *because the abdominal muscles are weak.*
◆ Offer prune juice and a high-bulk diet *to prevent and relieve constipation.* If necessary, give daily or alternate-day suppositories (glycerin or bisacodyl) or Fleet enemas *to relieve constipation.*
◆ Refer the client for physical therapy, occupational therapy, and speech therapy as needed *to promote recovery.*

Evaluation

◆ The client has adequate ventilation as evidenced by a stable pulse oximetry and ABG levels.
◆ The client's joint mobility and ROM are at the same level as before the illness.
◆ The client demonstrates effective coping abilities in dealing with his illness.

HUNTINGTON'S DISEASE

HUNTINGTON'S DISEASE is an autosomal-dominant hereditary disease in which degeneration in the cerebral cortex and basal ganglia causes chronic, progressive chorea (involuntary and irregular movements) and cognitive deterioration, ending in dementia.

Huntington's disease usually strikes people between ages 25 and 55 (average age, 35). Death usually results 10 to 15 years after onset from suicide, heart failure, or pneumonia. The disorder is also called *Huntington's chorea, hereditary chorea, chronic progressive chorea,* and *adult chorea.*

Possible causes

◆ Genetic transmission: autosomal-dominant trait (Either sex can transmit and inherit the disease. Each child of a parent with this disease has a 50% chance of inheriting it; however, a child who doesn't inherit it can't pass it on to his own children.)

Assessment findings

◆ Gradual loss of musculoskeletal control, eventually leading to total dependence
◆ Dementia (can be mild at first but eventually disrupts the client's personality)
◆ Choreic movements that are rapid and usually violent and purposeless, become progressively severe, and may include mild fidgeting, tongue smacking, dysarthria (indistinct speech), athetoid movements (slow, sinuous, writhing movements, especially of the hands), and torticollis (twisting of the neck)
◆ Personality changes, such as obstinacy, carelessness, untidiness, moodiness, apathy, loss of memory and, possibly, paranoia (in later stages of dementia)

Diagnostic evaluation

◆ Positive-emission tomography (PET) scanning detects the disease.
◆ Deoxyribonucleic acid analysis detects the disease.
◆ CT scanning reveals brain atrophy.
◆ MRI reveals brain atrophy.
◆ Molecular genetics testing may detect the gene for Huntington's disease in people at risk while they're still asymptomatic.

Nursing diagnoses

◆ Impaired physical mobility
◆ Ineffective health maintenance
◆ Ineffective tissue perfusion (cerebral)
◆ Risk for injury

Treatment

◆ Because Huntington's disease has no known cure, treatment is supportive, protective, and aimed at relieving symptoms.

Drug therapy options

◆ Antipsychotics: chlorpromazine (Thorazine), haloperidol (Haldol) to help control choreic movements
◆ Antidepressant: imipramine (Tofranil) to help control choreic movements
◆ Antitoxin: botulinum injected directly into the affected muscle for dystonia in selected clients

Planning and goals

◆ The client will maintain functional joint mobility and ROM.
◆ The client will perform ADLs within the confines of the disorder.
◆ The client will remain free from injury.

Implementation

◆ Provide physical support by attending to the client's basic needs, such as hygiene, skin care, bowel and bladder care, and nutrition. Increase this support as mental and physical deterioration make him increasingly immobile. *These measures help prevent complications of immobility.*
◆ Assist in designing a behavioral plan that deals with disruptive and aggressive behavior and impulse control problems. Reinforce positive behaviors, and maintain consistency with all caregiving. *These interventions consistently limit the client's negative behaviors.*
◆ Offer emotional support to the client and his family *to relieve anxiety and enhance coping.* Keep in mind the client's dysarthria, and allow him extra time to express himself, *thereby decreasing frustration.*
◆ Stay alert for possible suicide attempts. Control the client's environment *to protect him from suicide or other self-inflicted injury.* The client may be unable to cope with the devastating nature of the disease.

◆ Pad the side rails of the bed but avoid restraints, *which may cause the client to injure himself with violent, uncontrolled movements.*
◆ If the client has difficulty walking, provide a walker *to help him maintain his balance.*
◆ Consult various therapists (such as speech, physical, and occupatonal) *to help optimize the client's outcome.*
◆ Refer the client and his family to appropriate community organizations *for support and information and for genetic counseling, as appropriate.*

Evaluation

◆ The client has functional mobility and ROM.
◆ The client can care for himself in specific capacities.
◆ The client is free from injury.

INCREASED INTRACRANIAL PRESSURE

INTRACRANIAL PRESSURE (ICP) is the pressure that three different components — brain tissue (84%), CSF (12%), and cerebral blood volume (4%) — exert inside the rigid, unyielding skull. The Monroe-Kellie hypothesis states that, because of the limited space in the skull, an increase in any one component must cause a compensatory change in the volume of the others, by displacing or shifting CSF, increasing the absorption of CSF, or decreasing cerebral blood volume in order to maintain normal ICP of 5 to 15 mm Hg. Typically, these compensatory mechanisms keep the volume and pressure of these three components in a state of equilibrium, resulting in normal ICP.

When a pathologic condition causes these compensatory mechanisms to fail, ICP begins to increase. Increased ICP is characterized by pressure greater than 15 mm Hg and is potentially life threatening. The increasing pressure in the skull diminishes the functioning of various cranial areas and, if unrelieved, affects the vital centers. Aggressive treatment of increased ICP pressure is thought to improve survival and function in clients who have a pathologic condition associated with increased ICP.

Possible causes

Increased brain volume

◆ Abscess
◆ Edema
◆ Neoplasm

Increased blood volume

◆ Decreased venous return
◆ Hemorrhage and hematoma formation
◆ Hypercapnia
◆ Hypoxemia
◆ Increased arterial blood flow
◆ Increased intrathoracic pressure
◆ Pooling of venous blood

Increased CSF flow

◆ Deficient CSF absorption
◆ Increased production of CSF
◆ Obstruction

Assessment findings

◆ Alterations in LOC
◆ Headache
◆ Motor, sensory, or reflex dysfunction
◆ Respiratory dysfunction
◆ Vomiting with or without nausea
◆ Oculomotor dysfunction
◆ Pupillary dysfunction
◆ Papilledema
◆ Posturing (decerebrate, decorticate)
◆ Brain herniation syndromes
◆ Cushing's phenomenon or response

Diagnostic evaluation

◆ CT scanning, MRI, skull X-ray, or cerebral angiography reveal underlying pathology precipitating the signs and symptoms of increased ICP.
◆ PET scanning may reveal decreased cerebral metabolism and blood flow characteristics.
◆ Evoked potential studies are used to locate brain lesions and evaluate brain stem integrity.
◆ Transcranial Doppler ultrasonography may reveal decreased cerebral metabolism and blood flow characteristics.

Nursing diagnoses

◆ Decreased intracranial adaptive capacity
◆ Ineffective tissue perfusion (cerebral)
◆ Ineffective breathing pattern

Treatment

◆ Mechanical ventilation, if needed to maintain oxygenation
◆ Restricted fluid intake
◆ 30- to 45-degree elevation of the head of the bed as well as avoidance of extreme neck flexion or turning, extreme hip flexion, Valsalva's maneuver, and isometric muscle contractions
◆ Maintenance of normothermia

◆ Control of noxious auditory, tactile, and visual environmental stimuli
◆ Avoidance of clustering nursing care
◆ ICP monitoring (for example, with an epidural probe, a subarachnoid screw, or an intraventricular catheter)
◆ Craniotomy

Drug therapy options

◆ Analgesics: acetaminophen (Tylenol), codeine phosphate, codeine sulfate
◆ Antipyretic: acetaminophen (Tylenol)
◆ Antishivering agent: chlorpromazine (Thorazine)
◆ Barbiturates: thiopental sodium (Pentothal), pentobarbital (Nembutal)
◆ Diuretics: ethacrynic acid (Edecrin), furosemide (Lasix), mannitol (Osmitrol)
◆ Glucocorticoid: dexamethasone (Decadron)
◆ H_2 receptor antagonists: cimetidine (Tagamet), famotidine (Pepcid), ranitidine (Zantac)
◆ Hyperosmolar agents: mannitol (Osmitrol) 20%, glycerol 10%
◆ Neuromuscular blocking agent: pancuronium bromide (Pavulon)
◆ Insulin

Planning and goals

◆ The client will have an ICP of 5 to 15 mm Hg.
◆ The client won't have sustained increases in ICP during nursing interventions, monitoring activities, or nursing care activities.
◆ The client will regain his normal LOC, cognition, and sensory-motor function.
◆ The client will avoid preventable complications associated with increased ICP.

Implementation

◆ Maintain a patent airway *to promote oxygenation of cerebral tissues.*
◆ Administer oxygen, as ordered, *to maintain a partial pressure of arterial oxygen ($Pa{O_2}$) between 80 and 100 mm Hg, which promotes oxygenation of cerebral tissues.*
◆ Monitor ABG levels *to help determine if $Pa{O_2}$ is in the desired range and if $Pa{CO_2}$ is between 25 and 30 mm Hg. These ranges are ideal for cerebral vasoconstriction and decreased blood flow, and help to decrease ICP.*
◆ Hyperventilate the client *to maintain hypocapnia with $Pa{CO_2}$ in the desired range.*
◆ Administer medications (such as a hyperosmolar agent, diuretic, and glucocorticoid) *to reduce cerebral edema and increase serum osmolality,* which causes water to move from extracellular brain tissue into the intravascular space. *Excess body water is thus eliminated by pulling it from the brain and depositing it in the cardiovascular system.*
◆ Raise the head of the client's bed 30 to 45 degrees *to reduce edema of cerebral tissues by promoting cerebral venous drainage.*
◆ Assess neurologic status every 15 minutes, and then, as the patient stabilizes, every 1 to 2 hours *to determine a baseline and then to detect changes in neurologic status and signs and symptoms of increased ICP.*
◆ Avoid extreme flexion of the client's head and neck *to reduce edema of cerebral tissues and decrease ICP by promoting cerebral venous drainage.*
◆ Avoid extreme flexion of the client's hips *to prevent trapping of venous blood in the intra-abdominal space, which increases intra-abdominal and intrathoracic pressure, and reduces cerebral venous drainage.*
◆ Administer medications (such as a neuromuscular blocking agent, an analgesic, and an anti-shivering drug) *to control posturing, restlessness, and shivering, and to reduce the metabolic rate and, consequently, the needs of cerebral tissue.*
◆ Control noxious auditory, tactile, and visual stimuli in the client's environment *to prevent increases in ICP.*
◆ Monitor blood glucose levels and administer insulin as prescribed to maintain a blood glucose level of 80 to 110 mg/dl *to prevent complications of elevated blood glucose levels.*

Evaluation

◆ The client has an ICP of 5 to 15 mm Hg.
◆ The client doesn't have sustained increases in ICP during nursing interventions, monitoring activities, or nursing care activities.
◆ The client regains normal LOC, cognition, and motor-sensory function.
◆ The client avoids preventable complications associated with increased ICP.

MENINGITIS

In MENINGITIS, the brain and the spinal cord meninges become inflamed as a result of bacterial, viral, fungal, or protozoal infection. Such inflammation may involve all three meningeal membranes: the dura mater, arachnoid, and pia mater.

The prognosis is good and complications are rare, especially if the disease is recognized early and the infecting organism responds to antibiotics. The prognosis is poorer for infants and elderly people. Mortality is high in untreated meningitis.

Possible causes

- Bacterial infection, which may occur secondary to bacteremia (especially from pneumonia, empyema, osteomyelitis, and endocarditis), sinusitis, otitis media, encephalitis, myelitis, or brain abscess
- Head trauma, which may follow a skull fracture, penetrating head wound, lumbar puncture, or ventricular shunting procedure
- Virus in aseptic viral meningitis, which is usually mild and self-limiting
- Fungal or protozoal infection (less common)

Assessment findings

- Malaise
- Chills
- Fever
- Headache
- Stiff neck and back
- Photophobia
- Positive BRUDZINSKI'S SIGN, in which the client flexes his hips or knees when the nurse places her hands behind his neck and bends it forward (a sign of meningeal inflammation and irritation)
- Positive KERNIG'S SIGN (pain or resistance when the client's leg is flexed at the hip or knee while he's in a supine position)
- Vomiting
- Exaggerated deep tendon reflexes
- Visual alterations (diplopia — two images of a single object)
- Confusion
- Delirium
- Deep stupor
- Coma
- Increased ICP
- Irritability
- Opisthotonos (a spasm in which the back and extremities arch backward so that the body rests on the head and heels)
- Petechial, purpuric, or ecchymotic rash on the lower part of the body (meningococcal meningitis)
- Seizures
- Twitching

Diagnostic evaluation

- Lumbar puncture shows elevated CSF pressure, cloudy or milky-white CSF, high protein level, positive Gram stain and culture that usually identifies the infecting organism (unless it's a virus), and depressed CSF glucose concentration.
- Chest X-rays may reveal pneumonitis or lung abscess, tubercular lesions, or granulomas secondary to fungal infection.
- Sinus and skull films may help identify the presence of cranial osteomyelitis, paranasal sinusitis, or skull fracture.
- WBC count reveals leukocytosis.
- CT scanning can rule out cerebral hematoma, hemorrhage, or tumor.

Nursing diagnoses

- Decreased intracranial adaptive capacity
- Hyperthermia
- Risk for injury

Treatment

- Bed rest
- Hypothermia
- I.V. fluid administration
- Oxygen therapy, possibly with ET intubation and mechanical ventilation

Drug therapy options

- Antibiotics: penicillin G (Pfizerpen), ampicillin (Omnipen); if allergic to penicillin: nafcillin, tetracycline (Achromycin V), chloramphenicol (Chloromycetin)
- Corticosteroid: dexamethasone
- Diuretic: mannitol (Osmitrol)
- Anticonvulsants: phenytoin (Dilantin), phenobarbital (Luminal)
- Analgesics or antipyretics: acetaminophen (Tylenol), aspirin
- Laxative: bisacodyl (Dulcolax)
- Stool softener: docusate (Colace)
- Sedative: midazolam

Planning and goals

- The client will maintain normal ICP.
- The client will exhibit a normal temperature.
- The client will remain free from injury.

Implementation

- Assess neurologic function often *to detect early signs of increased ICP,* such as plucking at the bedcovers, vomiting, seizures, and a change in motor function and vital signs. *Detecting early signs of increased ICP prevents treatment delay.*

◆ Watch for deterioration in the client's condition, *which may signal an impending crisis.*
◆ Monitor fluid balance. Maintain adequate fluid intake *to avoid dehydration without causing fluid overload, which may lead to cerebral edema.*
◆ Measure CVP and intake and output accurately *to determine fluid volume status.*
◆ Suction the client only if necessary. Limit suctioning to 10 to 15 seconds per pass of the catheter. Suctioning stimulates coughing and Valsalva's maneuver; *Valsalva's maneuver increases intrathoracic pressure, decreases cerebral venous drainage, and increases cerebral blood volume, resulting in increased ICP.*
◆ Hyperoxygenate the lungs with 100% oxygen for 1 minute before and after suctioning. Hypercapnia results in cerebral vasodilation, increased blood volume, and increased ICP. *Preoxygenation helps avoid hypoxemia and tissue ischemia.*
◆ Watch for adverse reactions to I.V. antibiotics and other drugs *to prevent complications such as anaphylaxis.*
◆ Institute seizure precautions *to protect the client from injury.*
◆ Position the client carefully *to prevent joint stiffness and neck pain.*
◆ Turn the client often, according to a planned positioning schedule, *to prevent skin breakdown.*
◆ Assist with ROM exercises *to prevent contractures.*
◆ Provide small, frequent meals or supplement meals with NG tube or parenteral feedings (when and if this becomes necessary) *to maintain adequate nutrition and elimination.*
◆ Give the client a mild laxative or stool softener *to prevent constipation and minimize the risk of increased ICP resulting from straining during defecation.*
◆ Ensure the client's comfort *to prevent rises in ICP.*
◆ Provide mouth care regularly *to prevent breakdown of oral mucosa and promote client comfort.*
◆ Maintain a quiet environment. *Auditory stimuli can contribute to increased ICP.*
◆ Darken the room *to decrease photophobia.*
◆ Administer an analgesic as needed *to manage pain;* use narcotics with caution *because they interfere with accurate neurologic assessment.*
◆ Provide reassurance and support. The client may be frightened by his illness and frequent lumbar punctures. *Reassurance and support decrease anxiety; emotional upsets may increase ICP.*
◆ Reassure the family that the delirium and behavior changes caused by meningitis usually disappear *to allay anxiety.*
◆ Follow strict aseptic technique when treating clients with head wounds or skull fractures *to prevent meningitis.*
◆ Institute droplet precautions *to prevent spread of meningococcal infections.*

Evaluation

◆ The client has normal ICP and adequate cerebral perfusion.
◆ The client has a normal temperature.
◆ The client is free from injury.

MULTIPLE SCLEROSIS

MULTIPLE SCLEROSIS (MS) is a progressive, degenerative disease that affects the myelin sheath surrounding the axons in the CNS. It's a leading cause of neurologic disability between ages 20 and 40.

MS is characterized by periods of exacerbation and remission:
◆ During periods of exacerbation, well-circumscribed areas of patchy demyelination, or *plaques,* are scattered along the myelin sheath. Conduction of nerve impulses along affected axons is slowed or inhibited, producing neurologic deficits.
◆ During periods of remission, the myelin sheath affected during exacerbation undergoes myelinization. Conduction of nerve impulses along affected axons returns to normal, and the neurologic deficits that developed during exacerbation are reversed. In most instances, however, recovery from each period of exacerbation is incomplete, causing a stepwise decline in neurologic function.

Possible causes

◆ Autoimmune response
◆ Cell-mediated immune reaction
◆ Emotional stress, overwork, fatigue, pregnancy, and acute respiratory infections possibly preceding onset
◆ Environmental or genetic factors
◆ Infection by a slow, latent virus
◆ Susceptibility gene

Assessment findings

◆ Cerebellar dysfunction (Signs and symptoms include ataxia, dysarthria, incoordination, tremor, and vertigo.)
◆ Cognitive dysfunction (Signs and symptoms include decreased concentration and short-term memory, depression, difficulty finding words and learning new information, euphoria, and short attention span.)

- ◆ Cranial nerve dysfunction (Signs and symptoms include blind spots, blurred central vision, diplopia, dysphagia, facial weakness, faded colors, numbness, and pain.)
- ◆ Motor dysfunction (Signs and symptoms include abnormal gait, paralysis, spasticity, and weakness.)
- ◆ Sensory dysfunction (Signs and symptoms include decreased proprioception and temperature perception, Lhermitte's sign, and paresthesia.)
- ◆ Bowel and bladder dysfunction (Signs and symptoms include constipation; fecal incontinence and urgency; nocturia; urinary frequency, hesitancy, incontinence, and urgency; and urine retention.)
- ◆ Sexual dysfunction (Signs and symptoms include decreased libido, orgasmic ability, and genital sensation [in women]; ejaculatory, erectile, and orgasmic dysfunction and fatigue [in men].)

Diagnostic evaluation

- ◆ CT scanning or MRI may reveal plaques and demyelination in the CNS or an underlying pathology precipitating the signs and symptoms of MS.
- ◆ Evoked potentials may reveal slowing or absence of nerve conduction along the visual, auditory, and somatosensory pathways.
- ◆ PET scanning may reveal altered locations and patterns of cerebral glucose metabolism.
- ◆ EMG may reveal slowing of nerve conduction.

Nursing diagnoses

- ◆ Impaired physical mobility
- ◆ Disturbed body image
- ◆ Self-care deficit: Bathing or hygiene, dressing or grooming, or toileting
- ◆ Interrupted family processes

Treatment

- ◆ High-fiber diet adjusted to the client's ability to chew or swallow
- ◆ Active or passive ROM exercises
- ◆ Dietary consultation
- ◆ Physical therapy
- ◆ Speech therapy
- ◆ Plasmapheresis (for antibody removal)

Drug therapy options

- ◆ Cholinergic: bethanechol (Urecholine)
- ◆ Glucocorticoids: corticotropin, dexamethasone (Decadron), prednisone (Deltasone)
- ◆ Immunosuppressants: cyclophosphamide (Cytoxan), interferon beta-1b (Betaseron), methotrexate (Folex), glatiramer (a combination of four amino acids)
- ◆ Skeletal muscle relaxants: baclofen (Lioresal), dantrolene (Dantrium)
- ◆ Tricyclic antidepressants: phenytoin (Dilantin), carbamazepine (Tegretol) to relieve pain, numbness, burning, and tingling

Planning and goals

- ◆ The client will retain a usual or an improved level of neurologic functioning.
- ◆ The client will develop maximal self-care abilities and physical mobility and an effective means of communication within the limits imposed by MS.
- ◆ The client will experience no preventable complications associated with MS.
- ◆ The client will develop strategies to effectively cope with health problems and body image disturbances associated with MS.
- ◆ The client's family and caregivers will be able to provide needed support.

Implementation

- ◆ Assess neurologic status and vital signs at least every 8 hours *to determine baseline and detect changes.*
- ◆ Encourage the client to eat a high-fiber diet, adjusted to his ability to chew or swallow, *to promote adequate nutritional status, meet metabolic needs, and promote bowel regularity.*
- ◆ Consult a speech therapist *to evaluate and treat communication or swallowing problems.*
- ◆ Assess gag reflex and ability to swallow *to prevent aspiration of food particles.*
- ◆ Monitor weight on a weekly basis *to determine nutritional status.*
- ◆ Encourage fluid intake of $2^1/_2$ qt (2.5 L) every 24 hours, unless contraindicated, *to promote normovolemia and optimal urinary function.*
- ◆ Institute a bowel and bladder program *to promote urinary and fecal continence.*
- ◆ Encourage communication *to promote independence and self-esteem.*
- ◆ Administer prescribed medications on schedule *to maintain therapeutic drug levels and an optimal level of neurologic functioning.*
- ◆ Consult a physical and an occupational therapist *to evaluate which adaptive assistive devices the client may need to independently and safely perform ADLs.*
- ◆ Provide uninterrupted periods of rest *to help conserve energy, reduce the client's oxygen demand, reduce fatigue, and restore the client to an optimal level of neurologic functioning.*

◆ Perform active or passive ROM exercises *to maintain joint mobility and prevent contractures.*
◆ Encourage the client to express feelings about changes in his body image and neurologic functioning *to help him cope with the body changes that MS can cause.*
◆ Refer the client and his family to an MS support group *for additional information and support.*

Evaluation

◆ The client regains his normal level of neurologic functioning.
◆ The client develops maximal self-care abilities and physical mobility and an effective means of communication within the limits imposed by MS.
◆ The client avoids preventable complications associated with MS.
◆ The client develops strategies to effectively cope with health problems and body image disturbances associated with MS.

MYASTHENIA GRAVIS

MYASTHENIA GRAVIS (MG) is a chronic, progressive neuromuscular disorder that affects normal conduction of nerve impulses across the neuromuscular junction. Under normal circumstances, the neurotransmitter acetylcholine (ACh) is released from storage vesicles in the axonal ending. ACh then diffuses across the synaptic cleft between the axonal ending and the muscle fiber, attaches to ACh receptor sites located primarily on the peaks of the junctional folds of the muscle fiber, and stimulates the muscle fiber to contract. The enzyme acetylcholinesterase then destroys the ACh, thus terminating nerve impulse conduction across the neuromuscular junction.

Clients with MG have a normal amount of ACh available at the neuromuscular junction, but the structure of the junction is altered. An autoimmune mechanism is thought to be the cause of this alteration The antibodies in this mechanism change the structure of the neuromuscular junction by accelerating the degeneration of ACh receptor sites. The outcome of this process is a 70% to 80% reduction of the absolute number of functioning ACh receptor sites, development of a decreased number of shallow junctional folds, and a widened synaptic cleft. These structural changes result in the typical symptoms of MG: weakness and abnormal fatigability of skeletal muscles — especially those involved in ocular movements, facial expression, respiration, chewing, and swallowing — that's exacerbated by exercise and relieved by rest.

Possible causes

◆ Autoimmune response
◆ Ineffective ACh release
◆ Inadequate muscle fiber response to acetylcholine

Assessment findings

◆ Muscle weakness and fatigue (Typically, muscles are strongest in the morning but weaken throughout the day, especially after exercise.)
◆ Blurred vision
◆ Difficulty chewing
◆ Diminished vital capacity
◆ Diplopia
◆ Drooling
◆ Dysarthria
◆ Dysphagia
◆ Dyspnea
◆ Facial droop
◆ Flat facial affect
◆ Nasal regurgitation
◆ Nasal, monotone speech
◆ Ptosis
◆ Shallow, slowed respirations
◆ Soft or inaudible voice
◆ Strabismus

Diagnostic evaluation

◆ EMG may reveal a decrease in amplitude of muscle contraction with progressive stimulation.
◆ Chest X-ray or CT scanning may reveal thyoma or hyperplasia of the thymus gland.
◆ I.V. drug challenge with neostigmine (Prostigmin) or edrophonium (Tensilon) may relieve symptoms in clients with MG.
◆ Blood chemistry test results may reveal ACh receptor antibody levels and elevated thyroid function tests.

Nursing diagnoses

◆ Impaired physical mobility
◆ Ineffective breathing pattern
◆ Risk for aspiration
◆ Ineffective coping
◆ Disturbed body image

Treatment

◆ Oxygen therapy
◆ Intermittent positive-pressure breathing (IPPB) and chest physiotherapy
◆ Mechanical ventilation and suctioning
◆ Active or passive ROM exercises

- Small, frequent, high-calorie meals and high-calorie snacks and supplements adjusted for the client's ability to chew or swallow
- Dietary consultation
- Physical therapy
- Speech therapy
- Plasmapheresis (in clients with severe exacerbation) to remove circulating ACh receptor antibodies
- Thymectomy to remove thyoma or thyomic hyperplasia, which is suspected of synthesizing ACh receptor antibodies
- Tracheostomy and vigorous suctioning to remove secretions

Drug therapy options
- Anticholinesterase inhibitors: neostigmine (Prostigmin), pyridostigmine (Mestinon)
- Glucocorticoids: dexamethasone (Decadron), prednisone (Deltasone)
- Immunosuppressants: azathioprine (Imuran), cyclophosphamide (Cytoxan)

Planning and goals
- The client will retain a usual or an improved level of functioning in affected muscles.
- The client will develop maximal self-care abilities and physical mobility and an effective means of communication within the limits imposed by MG.
- The client will avoid preventable complications associated with MG.
- The client will develop strategies to effectively cope with health problems and body image disturbances associated with MG and its treatments (glucocorticoids).

Implementation
- Maintain a patent airway and administer oxygen *to promote oxygenation of tissues.*
- Encourage the client to cough and deep-breathe *to help mobilize secretions in the airway.*
- Provide IPPB and chest physiotherapy, as prescribed, *to mobilize secretions in the airway and expand the lungs.*
- Have emergency intubation equipment readily available. *Respiratory muscle weakness may be severe enough in a myasthenic crisis to require emergency intubation and mechanical ventilation.*
- Assess neurologic status at least once every 8 hours or as indicated *to determine a baseline and detect changes in neurologic status as well as early signs and symptoms of myasthenic or cholinergic crisis.*
- Assess the client for signs and symptoms of a myasthenic or cholinergic crisis. A myasthenic crisis can occur as a result of undermedication and a cholinergic crisis can occur as a result of overmedication.
- Assess respiratory status at least once every 8 hours or as indicated *to determine a baseline and detect changes in respiratory status as well as early signs and symptoms of respiratory distress resulting from respiratory muscle weakness during a myasthenic crisis.*
- Assess the client's gag reflex and ability to swallow *to prevent aspiration and determine the extent of the neurologic deficit.*
- Administer prescribed medications on schedule *to maintain continuous therapeutic drug levels and an optimal level of neurologic functioning.*
- Plan activities early in the day or during energy peaks that follow administration of medications *to ensure that the client is at an optimal level of neurologic functioning during these activities.*
- Encourage the client to eat small, frequent, high-calorie meals and high-calorie snacks and supplements adjusted to his ability to chew or swallow, *to help conserve energy, promote adequate nutritional status, and meet metabolic demands.*
- Consult a speech therapist *to evaluate the client's ability to communicate and swallow and determine an effective regimen for doing both.*
- Monitor weight on a weekly basis *to help determine the client's nutritional status.*
- Consult a physical and an occupational therapist *to evaluate which adaptive assistive devices the client may need to independently and safely perform ADLs.*
- Encourage the client to express feelings about changes in body image *to reduce his tendency to suppress or repress those feelings and to help him cope.*
- Determine the level of support from the client's family and caregivers *to ensure optimal home care and assistance.*

Evaluation
- The client regains his normal level of functioning of affected muscles.
- The client develops maximal self-care abilities and physical mobility and an effective means of communication within the limits imposed by MG.
- The client avoids preventable complications associated with MG.
- The client develops strategies to effectively cope with health problems associated with MG.

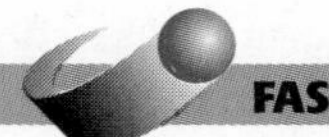

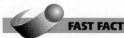

FAST FACT

A client with MG can develop cholinergic crisis due to overmedication. Expect to see these muscarinic or nicotinic effects of cholinergic (anticholinesterase) drugs:
- Abdominal cramping
- Constricted pupils
- Diaphoresis
- Diarrhea
- Fasciculations of eyes and mouth
- Increased salivation.

PARKINSON'S DISEASE

PARKINSON'S DISEASE is a CNS disorder that results in widespread, progressive degeneration of dopamine-producing cells of the substantia nigra in the brain and, consequently, a decrease in the level of the neurotransmitter dopamine.

When dopamine levels are normal, the excitatory cholinergic pathways and the inhibitory dopaminergic pathways are usually balanced, so the client is able to control or limit voluntary motor movement. However, when dopamine levels are decreased, the pathways are unbalanced, so the client is unable to control or limit voluntary motor movement, resulting in the signs and symptoms of Parkinson's disease: tremors, muscular rigidity, bradykinesia, akathisia, dyskinesia, weakness, and fatigue. These signs and symptoms typically occur when 70% of the dopamine-producing cells in the substantia nigra have degenerated.

Possible causes

- Drug therapy (for example, with alpha-methyldopa [Aldomet] or reserpine [Ravdixin])
- Genetic factors (familial forms with autosomal-dominant or autsomal-recessive inheritance)
- Metabolic conditions (for example, Huntington's chorea and Wilson's disease)
- Neurotoxins
- Oxidative stress
- Postencephalitis
- Structural conditions (for example, basal ganglia infarction, hydrocephalus, repeated head trauma, tumors)

Assessment findings

- Akathisia
- Bradykinesia
- Cogwheel, plastic, or lead-pipe rigidity
- Difficulty swallowing, drooling
- Dyskinesia
- Dementia
- Dysphagia
- Fatigue
- Flexed trunk and stooped posture
- Hypophonia, dysarthria
- Masklike facies with wide-open, fixed, staring eyes
- Muscular rigidity
- Restricted chest wall movement
- Shuffling gait
- Small handwriting
- Tremors (pill-rolling, resting)
- Weakness

Diagnostic evaluation

- Diagnosis of Parkinson's disease is made on the basis of a comprehensive history and physical examination; there are no specific diagnostic tests for Parkinson's disease.
- The following tests may be ordered to reveal whether other underlying pathology is precipitating the signs and symptoms of Parkinson's disease:
  - skull X-rays
  - CT scan
  - MRI
  - EEG
  - EMG
  - urinalysis
  - CSF analysis
  - drug screen.

Nursing diagnoses

- Impaired physical mobility
- Risk for injury
- Disturbed body image
- Ineffective coping

Treatment

- Small, frequent, high-calorie meals and high-calorie snacks and supplements adjusted to the client's ability to chew or swallow
- Active or passive ROM exercises
- Deep brain stimlation with electrodes
- Dietary consultation
- Occupational therapy
- Physical therapy
- Speech therapy
- Stereotactic neurosurgery (for example, thalamotomy or pallidotomy)

Drug therapy options

- Anticholinergic: trihexyphenidyl (Artane)
- Antihistamine: diphenhydramine (Benadryl)
- Antiviral: amantadine (Symmetrel)
- Dopaminergics: benztropine (Cogentin), carbidopa-levodopa (Sinemet), levodopa (Larodopa)
- Dopamine agonists: bromocriptine (Parlodel), pergolide (Permax)
- Monoamine oxidase inhibitor: selegiline (Deprenyl)
- Antispasmodic: procyclidine (Kemadrin)
- Antidepressant: amitriptyline (Elavil)

Planning and goals

- The client will retain a usual or an improved level of neurologic functioning.
- The client will develop maximal self-care abilities and physical mobility, and an effective means of communication within the limits imposed by Parkinson's disease.
- The client will avoid preventable complications associated with Parkinson's disease.
- The client will develop strategies to effectively cope with health problems and body image disturbances associated with Parkinson's disease.

Implementation

- Assess neurologic status at least once every 8 hours *to determine a baseline and detect changes in neurologic status.*
- Encourage the client to eat small, frequent, high-calorie meals and high-calorie snacks and supplements adjusted to his ability to chew or swallow *to promote adequate nutritional status and meet his metabolic needs.*
- Consult a speech therapist *to evaluate the client's ability to communicate and swallow and determine an effective regimen for doing both.*
- Assess the client's gag reflex and ability to swallow *to prevent aspiration of food particles.*
- Monitor the client's weight on a weekly basis *to determine nutritional status.*
- Provide ample time for communicating *to decrease the client's frustration and promote independence and self-esteem.*
- Administer prescribed medications on schedule *to maintain continuous therapeutic drug levels and an optimal level of neurologic functioning.*
- Consult a physical and an occupational therapist *to evaluate which adaptive assistive devices the client may need to perform ADLs independently and safely.*
- Provide ample time for the client to perform ADLs and to move around *to decrease the client's frustration and promote safety, independence, and self-esteem.*
- Manipulate the environment (for example, by removing clutter) *to promote client safety and prevent injury.*
- Encourage the client to express his feelings about changes in his body image *to reduce his tendency to suppress or repress those feelings and to help him cope.*

Evaluation

- The client regains his normal level of neurologic functioning.
- The client develops maximal self-care abilities and physical mobility and an effective means of communication within the limits imposed by Parkinson's disease.
- The client avoids preventable complications associated with Parkinson's disease.
- The client develops strategies to effectively cope with health problems and body image disturbances associated with Parkinson's disease.

SEIZURE DISORDERS (EPILEPSY)

A seizure is an uncontrolled discharge of neurons in the cerebral cortex. It interferes with normal CNS function, altering sensation, behavior, movement, perception, or consciousness. This alteration may be as brief as a blank stare, lasting a second, or as long as a TONIC-CLONIC SEIZURE, lasting several minutes, accompanied by loss of consciousness, bowel and bladder incontinence, and respiratory cessation. Signs and symptoms depend on the region of the cerebral cortex in which the seizure originates and the path of spread.

EPILEPSY is defined as recurrent seizures. It isn't a disease but rather a sign of a CNS disorder. Epilepsy can be classified as partial (seizure begins in a local area), generalized (associated with loss of consciousness; convulsive or nonconvulsive, bilateral without focal onset), or unclassified (because of inadequate data). (See *Classifying seizures.*)

Possible causes

Structural factors

- Cerebrovascular disorder (such as embolism, hemorrhage, or ischemia)
- Head trauma
- Infection (such as brain abscess, encephalitis, meningitis, or opportunistic lesions from acquired immune deficiency syndrome)

Classifying seizures

Seizures can take various forms depending on their origin and whether they're localized to one area of the brain (partial seizures) or occur in both hemispheres (generalized seizures). This chart describes each type of seizure and lists common signs and symptoms.

TYPE	DESCRIPTION	SIGNS AND SYMPTOMS
Partial		
Simple partial	Symptoms confined to one hemisphere	May have motor (change in posture), sensory (hallucinations), or autonomic (flushing, tachycardia) symptoms; no loss of consciousness
Complex partial	Begins in one focal area but spreads to both hemispheres (more common in adults)	Loss of consciousness; aura of visual disturbances; postictal symptoms (depression, anxiety, paralysis)
Generalized		
Absence (petit mal)	Sudden onset; lasts 5 to 10 seconds; can have 100 daily; precipitated by stress, hyperventilation, hypoglycemia, fatigue; differentiated from daydreaming	Loss of responsiveness but continued ability to maintain posture control and not fall; twitching eyelids; lip smacking; no postictal symptoms
Myoclonic	Movement disorder (not a true seizure); seen as child awakens or falls asleep; may be precipitated by touch or visual stimuli; focal or generalized; symmetrical or asymmetrical	No loss of consciousness; sudden, brief, shocklike involuntary contraction of one muscle group
Clonic	Opposing muscles contract and relax alternately in rhythmic pattern; may occur in one limb more than others	Mucus production
Tonic	Muscles are maintained in continuous contracted state (rigid posture)	Variable loss of consciousness; pupils dilate; eyes roll up; glottis closes; possible incontinence; may foam at mouth
Tonic-clonic (grand mal, major motor)	Violent, total-body seizure	Aura; tonic first (20 to 40 seconds); clonic next; postictal symptoms
Atonic	Drop and fall attack; needs to wear protective helmet	Loss of posture tone
Akinetic	Sudden, brief loss of muscle tone or posture	Temporary loss of consciousness
Miscellaneous		
Febrile	Seizure threshold lowered by elevated temperature; only one seizure per fever; common in 4% of population younger than age 5; occurs when temperature is rapidly rising; lasts less than 5 minutes	Generalized, transient, and nonprogressive; doesn't generally result in brain damage; EEG is normal after 2 weeks
Status epilepticus	Prolonged or frequent repetition of seizures without interruption; results in anoxia and cardiac and respiratory arrest	Consciousness not regained between seizures; lasts more than 30 minutes

◆ Space-occupying lesions (such as arteriovenous malformation [AVM], neurofibromatosis, primary and metastatic brain tumors, or subdural hematoma)

Metabolic-nutritional factors

◆ Acidosis
◆ Amino acid or fat metabolism disorder
◆ Drug withdrawal (for example, from alcohol, barbiturates, or diazepam [Valium])
◆ Electrolyte or water imbalance (for example, hypocalcemia, hypocapnia, hypoglycemia, or hyponatremia)
◆ Hypoxia
◆ Pyridoxine deficiency
◆ Toxins and toxic factors (such as heavy metals, "street" drugs, systemic disorders [such as toxemia and uremia], and toxic levels of any drug)

Genetic factors

◆ Chromosomal abnormalities

Assessment findings

◆ Aura just before the seizure's onset (client reports unusual tastes, feelings, or odors)
◆ Eyes deviating to a particular side or blinking
◆ Irregular breathing with spasms
◆ Usually unresponsive during tonic-clonic muscular contractions; may experience incontinence
◆ Possibly disoriented to time and place, drowsy, and uncoordinated immediately after a seizure

Diagnostic evaluation

◆ EEG may reveal abnormal patterns of electrical activity.
◆ CT scanning or MRI may reveal that an underlying pathology precipitated the seizures.
◆ ABG levels may reveal acidosis, hypocapnia, or hypoxia.
◆ CSF analysis may point to increased ICP or infection (for example, meningitis) as the underlying pathology that precipitated the seizures.
◆ Blood chemistry test results may reveal acidosis, elevated prescription drug levels, hypoglycemia, hyponatremia, toxic conditions (such as uremia), or toxic substances (such as cocaine or heavy metals).

Nursing diagnoses

◆ Risk for injury
◆ Ineffective airway clearance
◆ Risk for aspiration
◆ Disturbed body image

Treatment

◆ Correction of underlying condition precipitaing the seizure
◆ Supportive oxygen therapy and suctioning, as needed (maintaining airway and preventing injury), until seizure ends
◆ Cortical resection of epileptic focus
◆ Corpus callosotomy
◆ Anterior temporal lobe resection
◆ Vagal nerve stimulator implant (focal seizures)
◆ Transcranial magnetic stimulators

Drug therapy options

◆ Barbiturate: phenobarbital (Luminol)
◆ Benzodiazepine: diazepam (Valium)
◆ Deoxybarbiturate: primidone (Mysoline)
◆ Hydantoin: phenytoin (Dilantin)
◆ Iminostilbene: carbamazepine (Tegretol)
◆ Miscellaneous drugs: felbamate (Felbatol), gabapentin (Neurotonin), lamotrigine (Lamictal), valproic acid (Depakene)
◆ Oxazolidinedione: trimethadione (Tridione)
◆ Succinimide: ethosuximide

Planning and goals

◆ The client will maintain a patent airway.
◆ The client will regain his normal LOC, cognition, and motor-sensory function after and between seizures.
◆ The client will avoid preventable complications and injuries associated with seizures.
◆ The client will develop strategies to effectively cope with health problems and body image disturbances associated with seizures.

Implementation

Before seizure

◆ If the client has a seizure disorder, pad the side rails of the bed *to prevent him from injuring himself during a seizure.*

During seizure

◆ Note the date, time of onset, and duration of the seizure as well as what the client was doing when the seizure started *to help diagnose the type of seizure and develop a therapeutic treatment plan.*
◆ Provide privacy, asking nonessential people to leave the room, *to preserve the client's dignity and self-esteem during the seizure.*
◆ If client is standing, lower him to a flat surface *so that he doesn't injure himself.*

◆ Maintain a patent airway and administer oxygen *to promote oxygenation of the client's tissues.*
◆ Suction as needed *to clear secretions from the client's airway.*
◆ Turn the client's head to one side *to allow secretions to drain from his mouth.*
◆ Guide, if necessary, but don't restrain the movement of the client's limbs *to prevent injury to the client.*
◆ Note the seizure activity (including the body parts involved, sequence, character of movements, head and eye deviation, and behavior) *to help diagnose the type of seizure and develop a therapeutic treatment plan.*
◆ Administer prescribed medications on schedule *to maintain continuous therapeutic drug levels and an optimal level of neurologic functioning.*
◆ If the client is to continue medication for seizures after discharge, discuss the importance of the regimen and the need for compliance *to prevent further seizure activity.*

After seizure

◆ Assess the client's vital signs and neurologic status *to detect changes from baseline.*
◆ Encourage the client to express his feelings about changes in his body image *to help him cope with changes that a seizure disorder can cause.*

Evaluation

◆ The client maintains a patent airway.
◆ The client regains his normal level of LOC, cognition, and motor-sensory function after seizures.
◆ The client avoids preventable complications and injuries associated with seizures.
◆ The client develops strategies to effectively cope with health problems and body image disturbances associated with seizures.

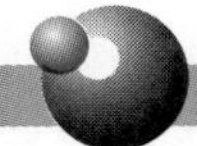

SPOT CHECK

Would you expect all clients with epilepsy to have abnormal EEGs?

Answer: No. A normal EEG doesn't always exclude a diagnosis of epilepsy; conversely, an abnormal EEG doesn't always confirm the diagnosis. During a seizure, EEG abnormalities are present; between seizures, a client with epilepsy may show no abnormalities or abnormalities that aren't characteristic of a seizure disorder.

SPINAL CORD INJURY

SPINAL CORD INJURY usually results from a traumatic force to the vertebral column. This injury typically has lifelong consequences, not only for the client but also for family members and society.

Spinal cord injuries are classified by type, level, degree, mechanism, and force of injury:
◆ Types of injury are classified as concussion, contusion, laceration, transection, or hemorrhage.
◆ Levels of injury are classified as cervical, thoracic, or lumbar. An injury to the spinal cord at the cervical level may result in paralysis of all four extremities (quadriplegia). An injury to the spinal cord at the thoracic or lumbar level may result in paralysis of the lower extremities (paraplegia).
◆ Degrees of injury are classified as complete or incomplete:
– A complete injury initially results in flaccid paralysis and total loss of motor, sensory, reflex, and bowel and bladder function below the level of injury.
– An incomplete injury is a mixed pattern of motor, sensory, reflex, and bowel and bladder function below the level of injury because some spinal cord tracts remain intact.
◆ The major mechanisms of injury are acceleration, deceleration, deformation, axial loading or vertical compression, and penetration.
◆ The four forces of injury are flexion, extension, rotation, and compression.

After a spinal cord injury, necrosis and scar tissue form in the area of the traumatized spinal cord, resulting in varying, and commonly catastrophic, degrees of permanent neurologic deficits, depending on the specific nerve tracts damaged.

Possible causes

◆ Congenital anomalies
◆ Diving into shallow water
◆ Falling
◆ Gunshot wounds
◆ Infections
◆ Sports injuries
◆ Stab wounds
◆ Tumors
◆ Vehicular accidents

Assessment findings

◆ Complete or incomplete loss of the following functions below the level of the injury:
– Voluntary motor movement

- Pain, light touch, temperature, and pressure sensation, and proprioception
- Reflex activity
- Autonomic activity
- Localized pain or tenderness over the site of injury
- Bowel and bladder function
- Respiratory function

Diagnostic evaluation

◆ CT scanning or MRI may reveal changes in the spinal cord, vertebrae, and soft tissue surrounding the spine.
◆ Myelography may reveal blockage or disruption of the spinal canal.
◆ Spinal X-rays may reveal fracture, deformity, or displacement of vertebrae as well as soft-tissue masses such as hematomas.

Nursing diagnoses

◆ Disturbed sensory perception (kinestetic, tactile)
◆ Impaired physical mobility
◆ Impaired gas exchange
◆ Powerlessness
◆ Disturbed body image

Treatment

◆ Immobilization, reduction, and alignment of injured area of spinal column (for example, tongs with cervical traction, halo external fixation device)
◆ Cervical traction
◆ Pin care
◆ Bed rest on a firm surface (for example, on a kinetic or rotating frame) with a hard-cervical collar and log-rolling until the client is stable and allowed to ambulate
◆ Oxygen therapy
◆ IPPB and chest physiotherapy
◆ Mechanical ventilation and suctioning
◆ Enteral nutrition through an enteral feeding tube (for example, a gastrostomy tube, percutaneous gastrostomy [PEG], or percutaneous jejunostomy [PEJ]) or TPN, as prescribed
◆ High-protein, high-fiber diet
◆ Consultation with a dietitian
◆ Physical therapy
◆ Occupational therapy
◆ Antiembolism hose or sequential compression stockings
◆ Bowel and bladder program
◆ Surgery to stabilize the injured spine (for example, insertion of Harrington rods)

Drug therapy options

◆ Analgesics: acetaminophen (Tylenol), codeine
◆ Anticoagulant: heparin
◆ Anxiolytic: lorazepam (Ativan)
◆ Glucocorticoid: methylprednisolone (Solu-Medrol)
◆ H_2 receptor antagonists: cimetidine (Tagamet), famotidine (Pepcid), ranitidine (Zantac)
◆ Laxative: bisacodyl (Dulcolax)
◆ Muscle relaxants: dantrolene (Dantrium), lioresal (Baclofen)

Planning and goals

◆ The client will retain a usual or an improved level of neurologic functioning.
◆ The client will develop maximal self-care abilities and physical mobility within the limitations imposed by spinal cord injury.
◆ The client will avoid preventable complications associated with spinal cord injury.
◆ The client will develop strategies to effectively cope with health problems and body image disturbances associated with spinal cord injury.
◆ The client will make use of forms of therapy aimed at maintaining or improving his level of independence to the extent possible within the confines of his injury.

Implementation

◆ Maintain immoblization of the spine and log-roll the client *to prevent further injury to the spine.*
◆ Immobilize, reduce, and align the injured area of the spinal column, using tongs with cervical traction, a halo external fixation device, or another device *to prevent further trauma to the spinal cord, and extension of the spinal cord injury.*
◆ If the client is in cervical traction, assess and clean the pin sites as prescribed *to detect signs and symptoms of infection.* Make sure the weights are free-hanging and not lying on the floor or headboard *to ensure they're easily accessible.*
◆ If the client is in halo fixation, assess and clean the pin sites as prescribed; assess pins, bolts, and vest structure for looseness; keep a torque screwdriver readily available and in a secure place so that tension on bars can be adjusted; and keep an open-end wrench readily available and in a secure place so that bolts can be released and the vest temporarily removed in the case of cardiac arrest *to detect signs and symptoms of infection, ensure that traction is being applied to the spinal column, and allow access to the client's chest if cardiopulmonary resuscitation is required.*

◆ Provide bed rest on a firm-surface rotating bed *to keep the spinal column aligned while allowing you to move and turn the client.*
◆ Maintain a patent airway and administer oxygen *to promote oxygenation of tissues.*
◆ Assist the client with coughing and deep breathing *to mobilize secretions in the airway and expand the lungs.*
◆ Assess the client's neurologic status and vital signs every 1 to 2 hours initially, then every 4 hours when the client's condition becomes stable *to determine a baseline, detect changes in neurologic status and early signs and symptoms of spinal shock, and determine a possible need for changes in the treatment plan.*
◆ Encourage the client to eat a high-protein, high-fiber diet or, if necessary, administer enteral nutrition through an enteral feeding tube (for example, a gastrostomy, PEG, or a PEJ tube) or TPN *to promote adequate nutritional status, facilitate tissue healing, and meet metabolic demands.*
◆ Monitor the client's weight weekly *to determine nutritional status.*
◆ Provide urinary catheterization during the acute phase *to provide bladder decompression when spinal shock is likely.*
◆ Institute a bowel and bladder program *to promote urinary and fecal continence and avoid stimuli that could trigger autonomic dysreflexia (AD).* (AD is an exaggerated sympathetic response to a noxious stimulus that occurs in clients with a spinal cord injury above T_7. Signs and symptoms include extreme hypertension, pounding headache, flushing, diaphoresis, blurred vision, and bradycardia. Treatment consists of removing the noxious stimulus.)
◆ Assess the client for signs and symptoms of AD *to prevent complications such as severely elevated blood pressure.*
◆ Consult a physical and an occupational therapist *to evaluate which adaptive assistive devices the client may need to independently and safely perform ADLs.*
◆ Perform active or passive ROM exercises *to help maintain joint mobility and prevent contractures.*
◆ Apply antiembolism hose or sequential compression stockings, as prescribed, *to promote venous return and prevent deep vein thrombosis of the lower extremities.*
◆ Assess the client for signs and symptoms of depression *to detect the need for possible intervention.*
◆ Encourage the client to express his feelings about changes in his body image *to reduce his tendency to suppress or repress those feelings and to help him cope.*
◆ Provide sexual counseling *to encourage the client to ask questions and avoid misunderstandings.*
◆ Assist with discharge planning to help meet the client's continuing needs.

Evaluation

◆ The client regains his normal level of neurologic functioning.
◆ The client develops maximal self-care abilities and physical mobility within the limitations imposed by spinal cord injury.
◆ The client avoids preventable complications associated with spinal cord injury.
◆ The client develops strategies to effectively cope with health problems and body image disturbances associated with spinal cord injury.

STROKE

STROKE, previously known as a *cerebrovascular accident* (CVA), is a sudden disruption in normal cerebral circulation from occlusion of an intracranial or extracranial blood vessel or hemorrhage in the brain from rupture of an intracranial blood vessel. No matter what the cause of a stoke, the extent of the cerebral ischemia, neuronal death, and subsequent neurologic impairment depends on numerous factors.

When a stroke results from occlusion of an intracranial or extracranial blood vessel (ischemic stroke), the location, size, and degree of occlusion as well as the adequacy of collateral circulation to the area of the brain supplied by the affected blood vessel have a significant impact on the client's recovery from the event. When a stroke results from hemorrhage in the brain caused by rupture of an intracranial blood vessel, the location, size, and mass of the hematoma as well as the adequacy of collateral circulation to the area of the brain affected by the hematoma have a significant impact on the client's recovery from the event.

Possible causes

◆ Thrombosis, embolism, and hemorrhage are the most common causes of stroke. (See *Causes of stroke,* page 372.)

Thrombosis

◆ Atherosclerosis
◆ Diabetes mellitus
◆ Hyperlipidemia
◆ Hypertension
◆ Hypovolemia
◆ Obesity
◆ Polycythemia
◆ Sedentary lifestyle

Causes of stroke

Thrombosis, the most common cause of stroke among middle-aged and elderly clients, typically occurs when an extracerebral vessel becomes occluded. Embolism, the second-leading cause of stroke, can happen at any age. It occurs when a fragmented clot, tumor, fat, bacteria, or air lodges in the cerebral circulation. Hemorrhage, the third most common cause of stroke, can occur in any vessel. It results in diminished blood supply to the cerebral area.

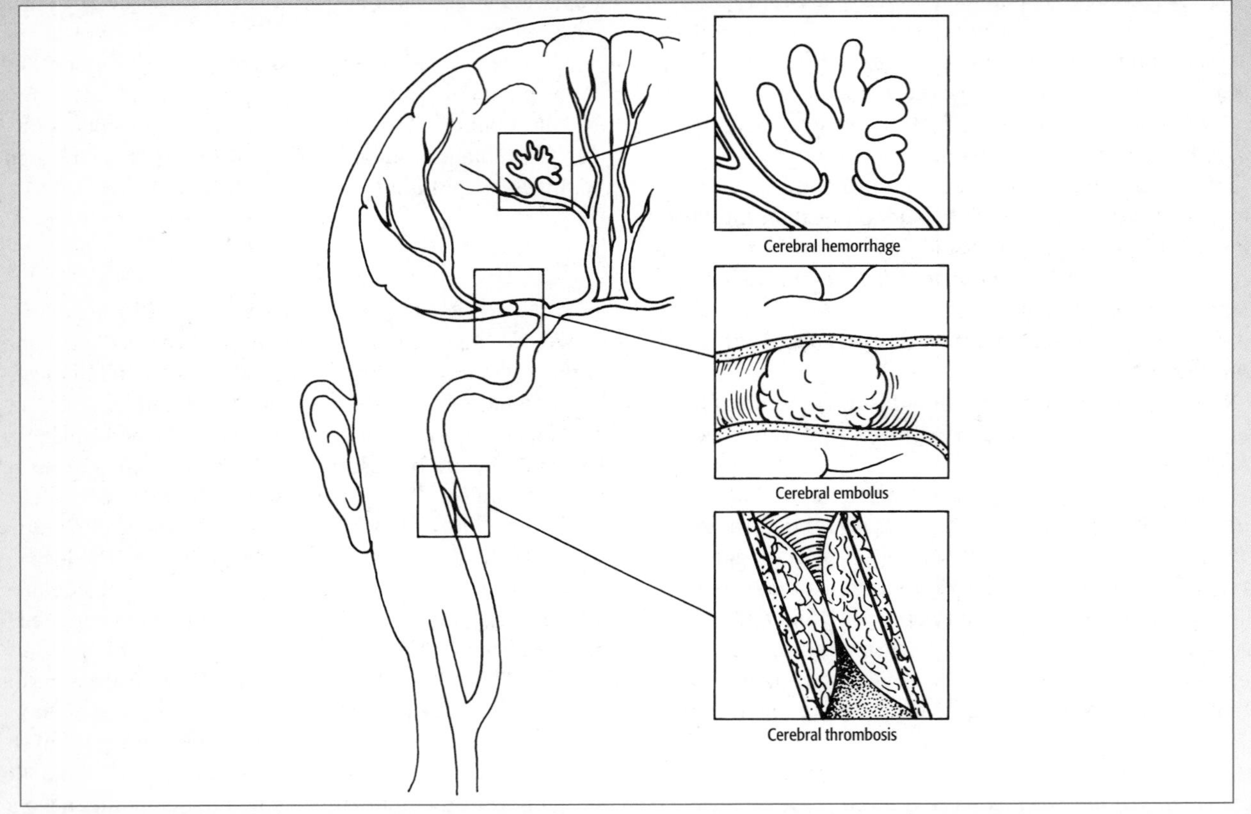

- Sickle cell anemia
- Smoking
- Stress
- Transient ischemic attack

Embolism
- Air or fat emboli
- Atrial fibrillation
- Cardiac arrhythmias
- Heart valve replacement
- Oral contraceptives

Hemorrhage
- Aneurysm rupture
- Anticoagulants
- Aplastic anemia
- AVM rupture
- Hemophilia
- Hypertension
- Liver disease
- Metastatic brain tumor rupture
- Substance abuse (for example, cocaine)
- Vasopressors

Assessment findings
- Neurologic deficits (progressive or abrupt in onset)
- Altered LOC (wakefulness to coma)
- Headache

◆ Fever
◆ Nuchal rigidity
◆ Seizures (See *Stroke sites.*)

Diagnostic evaluation

◆ CT scanning or MRI may reveal the site of infarction, hematoma, and shift of brain structures.
◆ Cerebral angiography is used to identify collateral blood circulation and may reveal the site of rupture or occlusion.
◆ PET scanning may reveal information on cerebral metabolism and blood flow characteristics.
◆ EEG may reveal abnormal electrical activity, such as focal slowing, which helps locate the lesion or assess the client's amount of brain wave activity.
◆ ECG may reveal atrial fibrillation as the source of emboli.
◆ Echocardiography may reveal thrombus on valvular heart structures and mural thrombi on the myocardial walls as the possible sources of emboli.
◆ Oculoplethysmography may reveal decreased intraocular systolic pressure and, thus, carotid blood flow.
◆ Transcranial Doppler ultrasonography may reveal decreased cerebral metabolism and characteristics of blood flow.
◆ Blood chemistry studies may reveal decreased hemoglobin level, hematocrit, and RBC count; increased PT, PTT, and liver function test results, and elevated cholesterol, triglycerides, and glucose levels; and positive sickle cell trait.
◆ CSF analysis, which isn't routinely done, may reveal bloody CSF with hemorrhagic CVA.
◆ Lumbar puncture, which isn't routinely done, may reveal increased CSF pressure.

Nursing diagnoses

◆ Decreased intracranial adaptive capacity
◆ Disturbed body image
◆ Disturbed sensory perception (visual, auditory, kinesthetic, gustatory, tactile, or olfactory, depending on the area of the brain affected and extent of cerebral tissue affected)
◆ Disturbed thought processes
◆ Ineffective tissue perfusion (cerebral)
◆ Interrupted family processes (See *Caring for the client with stroke,* page 374.)

Treatment

◆ Oxygen (may require mechanical ventilation)
◆ IPPB and chest physiotherapy
◆ I.V. fluids

Stroke sites

Clinical features of stroke vary with the artery affected (and, consequently, the portion of the brain the artery supplies), the severity of damage, and the extent of collateral circulation that develops to help the brain compensate for decreased blood supply.

Typical arteries affected and their associated signs and symptoms are described below.

Middle cerebral artery

Injury to this artery causes aphasia, dysphasia, visual field cuts, and hemiparesis on the affected side (more severe in the face and arm than in the leg).

Carotid artery

If the carotid artery is affected, the client may develop weakness, paralysis, numbness, sensory changes, and visual disturbances on the affected side; altered level of consciousness, bruits, headaches, aphasia, and ptosis may also occur.

Vertebrobasilar artery

A stroke affecting this artery may lead to weakness on the affected side, numbness around the lips and mouth, visual field cuts, diplopia, poor coordination, dysphagia, slurred speech, dizziness, amnesia, and ataxia.

Anterior cerebral artery

If this artery is affected, the client may develop confusion, and weakness and numbness (especially in the leg) on the affected side; incontinence, loss of coordination, impaired motor and sensory functions, and personality changes may also occur.

Posterior cerebral arteries

If posterior cerebral arteries are affected, the patient may develop visual fields cuts, sensory impairment, dyslexia, coma, and cortical blindness.

◆ Bed rest during the acute stage (until the client's condition stabilizes) with head of bed elevated 30 to 45 degrees, or as prescribed
◆ Active and passive ROM exercises
◆ Enteral nutrition through an enteral feeding tube (for example, a gastrostomy, PEG, or PEJ tube) or TPN
◆ Low-sodium, low-cholesterol, low-fat diet adjusted for the client's ability to chew and swallow
◆ Dietary consultation
◆ Physical and occupational therapy

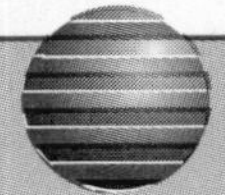

CLINICAL SITUATION

Caring for the client with stroke

A 68-year-old African-American male had a stroke due to a right cerebral thrombosis 1 week ago that resulted in left hemiplegia. He's a history instructor at the local community college. His hobby is woodcarving, and he spends hours each week working in his garden. The client is also an active member of his church. For the past 2 years, he has been taking medication for hypertension, but his wife reports that he often forgets to take it and that his blood pressure was high at his last physical examination. She tells the nursing staff that she has never had to worry about her husband's health before and that she wants to learn everything she can to care for him at home. However, she says that her husband was always the one to make the decisions and pay the bills. She adds that all the children, grandchildren, neighbors, and family pastor want to see her husband back at home as soon as possible.

What are three appropriate nursing diagnoses for this situation?

◆ Ineffective tissue perfusion (cerebral) (related to disruption of blood flow)
◆ Interrupted family processes (related to the change in the client's function and needs secondary to stroke)
◆ Disturbed body image (related to residual deficits caused by stroke)

Questions for further thought

◆ Would you expect the client to have difficulty with his speech? If so, why?
◆ What considerations must be included when planning for the client's discharge to the home and community?
◆ What would you reply if, after you've completed passive range-of-motion exercises on the client's left arm, he states, "I just ignore that part of my body; it doesn't work anyway."

◆ Speech therapy
◆ Antiembolism hose or sequential compression stockings, as prescribed
◆ Bowel and bladder program
◆ Carotid endarterectomy, embolization of AVM, clipping of aneurysm, evacuation of hematoma

Drug therapy options

◆ Antipyretic analgesic: acetaminophen (Tylenol)
◆ Analgesics: codeine phosphate, codeine sulfate
◆ Anticoagulants: heparin, ticlopidine (Ticlid), warfarin (Coumadin)
◆ Antiplatelet aggregation drugs: aspirin, dipyridamole (Persantine)
◆ Anticonvulsant: phenytoin (Dilantin)
◆ Antihypertensive: nifedipine (Procardia)
◆ Diuretic: furosemide (Lasix)
◆ Glucocorticoid: dexamethasone (Decadron)
◆ H_2-receptor antagonists: cimetidine (Tagamet), famotidine (Pepcid), ranitidine (Zantac)
◆ Insulin to maintain tight glycemic control
◆ Thrombolytic enzyme: tissue plasminogen activator for embolic or thrombotic stroke

Planning and goals

◆ The client will regain his normal LOC, cognition, and motor-sensory function.
◆ The client will develop maximal self-care abilities and physical mobility and an effective means of communication within the limitations imposed by the stroke.
◆ The client will experience no preventable complications associated with a stroke.
◆ The client will develop strategies to effectively cope with health problems and body image disturbances associated with a stroke.

Implementation

◆ Maintain a patent airway and administer oxygen, as prescribed, *to help promote oxygenation of cerebral tissues.*
◆ Encourage the client to cough and deep-breathe *to help mobilize secretions in the airway and expand the lungs.*
◆ Monitor pulse oximetry and ABG levels, as prescribed, *to evaluate the effectiveness of gas exchange and ventilatory effort.*
◆ Make sure the client maintains bed rest during the acute phase *to conserve energy, reducing the oxygen demands of cerebral tissues and the body, and restoring the client to an optimal level of neurologic functioning.*
◆ Assess neurologic status using the Glasgow Coma scale at least every 2 hours initially, then every 2 to 4 hours when the client's condition becomes stable *to detect changes in neurologic status.*
◆ Maintain nothing-by-mouth status and possible NG decompression during the acute phase *to help prevent gastric distention, nausea, and vomiting.*
◆ Encourage the client to eat a low-sodium, low cholesterol and, if needed, low-fat diet. The diet should be adjusted for his ability to chew and swallow, and determined in collaboration with the registered dietitian *to promote*

nutritional status, facilitate tissue healing, and meet metabolic demands.

◆ If necessary, administer enteral nutrition through an enteral feeding tube (for example, a gastrostomy tube, PEG, or PEJ) or TPN, as prescribed, *until oral intake is sufficient to meet metabolic demands.*

◆ Consult a speech therapist *to evaluate the client's ability to communicate and swallow.*

◆ Assess gag reflex and ability to swallow *to prevent aspiration of food particles.*

◆ Institute a bowel and bladder program *to help promote urinary and fecal continence.*

◆ Administer I.V. fluids, as prescribed, *to help promote normovolemia and electrolyte balance.*

◆ Monitor blood glucose levels and administer insulin as prescribed to maintain a blood glucose level of 80 to 110 mg/dl *to prevent complications of elevated blood glucose levels.*

◆ Monitor intake and output *to help detect the need for early intervention for fluid volume overload or deficit.*

◆ Administer prescribed medications *to help the client maintain continuous therapeutic drug levels and an optimal level of neurologic functioning.*

◆ Consult a physical and an occupational therapist *to evaluate which adaptive assistive devices the client may need to perform ADLs independently and safely.*

◆ Perform active or passive ROM exercises *to help the client maintain joint mobility and prevent contractures.*

◆ Apply antiembolism hose or sequential compression stockings, as prescribed, *to promote venous return and prevent deep vein thrombosis of lower extremities.*

◆ Institute seizure precautions *to prevent the client from injuring himself during a seizure.*

◆ Encourage the client to express feelings about changes in body image *to reduce the tendency to suppress or repress those feelings and to help him cope.*

◆ Consult with social services *to help meet the needs of the client at home or after discharge.*

Evaluation

◆ The client regains his normal LOC, cognition, and motor-sensory function.

◆ The client develops maximal self-care abilities and physical mobility and an effective means of communication within the limitations imposed by the stroke.

◆ The client avoids preventable complications associated with the stroke.

◆ The client develops strategies to effectively cope with health problems and body image disturbances associated with the stroke.

TRIGEMINAL NEURALGIA

TRIGEMINAL NEURALGIA is a painful disorder of one or more branches of the fifth cranial (trigeminal) nerve that produces paroxysmal attacks of excruciating facial pain. Attacks are precipitated by stimulation of a trigger zone, a hypersensitive area of the face.

It occurs mostly in people older than age 40, in women more commonly than men, and on the right side of the face more commonly than the left. Trigeminal neuralgia can subside spontaneously, with remissions lasting from several months to years. The disorder is also called *tic douloureux.*

Possible causes

Although the cause remains undetermined, trigeminal neuralgia may:

◆ reflect an afferent reflex phenomenon located centrally in the brain stem or more peripherally in the sensory root of the trigeminal nerve

◆ be related to compression of the nerve root by posterior fossa tumors, middle fossa tumors, or vascular lesions (subclinical aneurysm), although such lesions usually produce simultaneous loss of sensation

◆ occasionally be a manifestation of multiple sclerosis or herpes zoster.

Assessment findings

◆ Searing pain in the facial area

Triggers

◆ Light touch to a sensitive area of the face (trigger zone)

◆ Exposure to hot or cold temperatures

◆ Eating, smiling, or talking

◆ Drinking hot or cold beverages

Diagnostic evaluation

◆ Observation during the examination shows the client favoring (splinting) the affected area. To ward off a painful attack, the client commonly holds her face immobile when talking. She may also leave the affected side of her face unwashed and, in men, unshaven.

◆ Skull X-rays, MRI, and CT scanning rule out sinus or tooth infections, tumors, or aneurysm.

Nursing diagnoses

◆ Acute pain

◆ Powerlessness

◆ Anxiety

Treatment

◆ Percutaneous radio frequency procedure, which causes partial root destruction and relieves pain
◆ Microsurgery for vascular decompression
◆ Percutaneous electrocoagulation of nerve rootlets, under local anesthesia

Drug therapy options

◆ Anticonvulsants: carbamazepine (Tegretol), phenytoin (Dilantin) to temporarily relieve or prevent pain

Planning and goals

◆ The client will experience increased comfort and relief from pain.
◆ The client will identify triggers that intensify the disorder and develop methods to control them.
◆ The client will use available support systems to cope with the effects of the disorder.

Implementation

◆ Observe and record the characteristics of each attack, including the client's protective mechanisms *to gain information for developing the treatment plan.*
◆ Provide adequate nutrition in small, frequent meals at room temperature *to ensure nutritional needs are met. Temperature extremes may cause an attack.*
◆ If the client is receiving carbamazepine, watch for cutaneous and hematologic reactions (erythematous and pruritic rashes, urticaria, photosensitivity, exfoliative dermatitis, leukopenia, agranulocytosis, eosinophilia, aplastic anemia, thrombocytopenia) and, possibly, urine retention and transient drowsiness. *Identifying adverse reactions early helps limit complications.*
◆ For the first 3 months of carbamazepine therapy, complete blood count and liver function should be monitored weekly, then monthly thereafter. Warn the client to report fever, sore throat, mouth ulcers, easy bruising, or petechial or purpuric hemorrhage immediately. *Hematologic toxicity is rare but serious.*
◆ If the client is receiving phenytoin, watch for adverse effects, including ataxia, skin eruptions, gingival hyperplasia, and nystagmus. *Early detection and treatment of adverse reactions limits complications.*
◆ After resection of the first division of the trigeminal nerve, tell the client to avoid rubbing her eyes and using aerosol spray. Advise her to wear glasses or goggles outdoors and to blink often *to prevent injury.*
◆ After surgery to sever the second or third division, tell the client to avoid hot foods and drinks, which could burn her mouth, and to chew carefully *to avoid biting her mouth.*
◆ Advise the client to place food in the unaffected side of her mouth when chewing, to brush her teeth often, and to see a dentist twice per year to detect cavities. *Cavities in the area of the severed nerve won't cause pain.*
◆ After surgical decompression of the root or partial nerve dissection, check neurologic and vital signs often *to detect early signs of postoperative complications.*
◆ Reinforce natural avoidance of stimulation (air, heat, cold) of trigger zones (lips, cheeks, gums) *to prevent further episodes.*

Evaluation

◆ The client reports adequate pain control.
◆ The client demonstrates appropriate measures to limit exacerbation of her disorder.
◆ The client displays appropriate coping mechanisms.

RESPIRATORY SYSTEM

The respiratory system is made up of the lungs and other structures that conduct air to and from the lungs and are involved in related functions. The major function of the respiratory system is gas exchange.

RESPIRATORY STRUCTURE AND FUNCTION

During gas exchange, air is taken into the body by inhalation and travels through respiratory passages to the lungs. In the lungs, oxygen (O_2) diffuses into the blood, and carbon dioxide (CO_2) is removed by exhalation.

Lungs and related structures

As a unit, the lungs are composed of three lobes on the right side and two lobes on the left side. The respiratory process involves the lungs and related structures, such as the nose and mouth, trachea, bronchi, and alveoli.
◆ The nose and mouth allow airflow into and out of the body. They also humidify inhaled air, which reduces irritation of the mucous membranes. Within the nose, the nares (nostrils) contain olfactory receptor sites, providing the body's sense of smell.
◆ The paranasal sinuses are air-filled, cilia-lined cavities within the nose. Their function is to trap particles of for-

eign matter that might interfere with the workings of the respiratory system.

◆ The pharynx serves as a passageway to the digestive and respiratory tracts. The pharynx maintains air pressure in the middle ear and also contains a mucosal lining. This lining humidifies and warms inhaled air and traps foreign particles.

◆ The larynx, known as the voice box, connects the upper and lower airways. It contains vocal cords that produce sounds. The larynx also initiates the cough reflex, which is part of the respiratory system's defense mechanisms.

◆ The trachea contains C-shaped cartilaginous rings composed of smooth muscle. It connects the larynx to the bronchi.

◆ The trachea branches into the right and left bronchi, the large air passages that lead to the right and left lungs. The right main bronchus is slightly larger and more vertical than the left.

◆ As they pass into the lungs, the bronchi form smaller branches called bronchioles, which branch into terminal bronchioles and alveoli.

◆ Alveoli are clustered microscopic sacs enveloped by capillaries. The lungs contain millions of alveoli, and it's there that gas exchange occurs. The lungs regulate air exchange by a concentration gradient in the alveoli as gases diffuse across the alveolar-capillary membrane. The alveoli also contain a coating of surfactant, which reduces surface tension and keeps them from collapsing.

◆ In the alveoli, gases move from an area of high concentration to an area of low concentration. Because the concentration of CO_2 is greater in the venous blood, it diffuses across the alveolar-capillary membrane into the alveoli and is exhaled. O_2 diffuses across the alveolar-capillary membrane and into the blood, to be carried to the rest of the body.

◆ Pleura is a mebraneous sac that covers the lungs and lines the thoracic cavity. The visceral pleura covers the lungs; the parietal pleura covers the thoracic cavity. Pleural fluid inside the pleural sac provides lubrication to reduce friction during respiration.

RESPIRATORY DISORDERS

Major respiratory disorders include acute respiratory distress syndrome (ARDS), acute respiratory failure, asbestosis, asphyxia, asthma, atelectasis, bronchiectasis, chronic bronchitis, chronic obstructive pulmonary disease (COPD), cor pulmonale, emphysema, Legionnaires' disease, lung cancer, pleural effusion and empyema, pleurisy, *Pneumocystis carinii* pneumonia, pneumonia, pneumothorax and hemothorax, pulmonary embolism, respiratory acidosis, respiratory alkalosis, sarcoidosis, and TB.

ACUTE RESPIRATORY DISTRESS SYNDROME

ACUTE RESPIRATORY DISTRESS SYNDROME (ARDS), is a form of pulmonary edema that causes acute respiratory failure. It results from increased permeability of the alveolocapillary membrane. Fluid accumulates in the lung interstitium, alveolar spaces, and small airways, causing the lung to stiffen. Effective ventilation is thus impaired. When severe, the syndrome can cause an unmanageable and ultimately fatal lack of oxygen. However, people who recover may have little or no permanent lung damage.

Possible causes

◆ Aspiration
◆ Blood transfusion
◆ Cardiopulmonary bypass
◆ Decreased surfactant production
◆ Drug overdose (barbiturates, glutethimide, opioids)
◆ Fluid overload
◆ Hypertransfusion
◆ Microemboli (fat, air emboli or disseminated intravascular coagulation [DIC])
◆ Near-drowning
◆ Neurologic injuries
◆ Oxygen toxicity
◆ Pancreatitis
◆ Respiratory tract infection
◆ Sepsis
◆ Severe acute respiratory syndrome (SARS)
◆ Shock
◆ Smoke or chemical inhalation (nitrous oxide, chlorine, ammonia)
◆ Trauma
◆ Viral, bacteria, or fungal pneumonia

Assessment findings

◆ Crackles, decreased breath sounds, rhonchi
◆ Dyspnea, tachypnea
◆ Cyanosis
◆ Cough
◆ Anxiety, restlessness

Diagnostic evaluation

◆ ABG analysis on room air initially shows a decreased PaO_2 (less than 60 mm Hg) and a decreased $PaCO_2$ (less than 35 mm Hg). The resulting pH reflects respiratory alkalosis. As ARDS becomes more severe, ABG levels show respiratory acidosis, metabolic acidosis, and hypoxemia that doesn't respond to increased fraction of inspired oxygen (FIO_2).
◆ Blood culture reveals the infectious organism.
◆ Chest X-ray shows bilateral infiltrates (in early stages) and lung fields with a ground-glass appearance and, with irreversible hypoxemia, massive consolidation ("white-outs") of both lung fields (in later stages).
◆ Sputum study reveals the infectious organism.

Nursing diagnoses

◆ Anxiety
◆ Impaired gas exchange
◆ Ineffective breathing pattern
◆ Ineffective tissue perfusion (cardiopulmonary)

Treatment

◆ Bed rest with prone positioning, if possible, and passive ROM exercises
◆ Rotating bed therapy
◆ Chest physiotherapy, postural drainage, and suction
◆ Restricted fluid intake or, if intubated, nothing by mouth
◆ Extracorporeal membrane oxygenation, if available
◆ Intubation and mechanical ventilation using PEEP or pressure-controlled inverse ratio ventilation
◆ Oxygen therapy
◆ Transfusion therapy: platelets, packed RBCs

Drug therapy options

◆ Analgesic: morphine sulfate
◆ Antacid: aluminum hydroxide gel (AlternaGEL)
◆ Antibiotics: according to susceptibility of infecting organism
◆ Anticoagulant: heparin
◆ Diuretics: ethacrynic acid (Edecrin), furosemide (Lasix)
◆ Exogenous surfactant: beractant (Survanta)
◆ Histamine-2 blockers: cimetidine (Tagamet), ranitidine (Zantac), famotidine (Pepcid)
◆ Mucosal barrier fortifier: sucralfate (Carafate)
◆ Neuromuscular blockers: pancuronium bromide (Pavulon), vecuronium bromide (Norcuron)
◆ Proton pump inhibitor: Pantoprazole (Protonix)
◆ Steroids: hydrocortisone (Solu-Cortef), methylprednisolone sodium succinate (Solu-Medrol)

Planning and goals

◆ The client will demonstrate improved oxygenation.
◆ The client will demonstrate adequate breathing pattern.
◆ The client wll exhibit decreased anxiety.

Implementation

◆ Assess respiratory, cardiovascular, and neurologic status *to detect evidence of hypoxemia, such as tachycardia, tachypnea, and irritability.*
◆ Monitor pulse oximetry continuously *to determine the effectiveness of therapy.*
◆ Monitor blood chemistry test results. *A decrease in hemoglobin levels and hematocrit affects oxygen-carrying capacity of the blood. An increase in WBC count suggests an infection such as pneumonia.* Monitor platelet count, fibrinogen level, PT, and PTT *to detect DIC, a complication of ARDS.*
◆ Monitor and record intake and output and central venous pressure *to determine fluid status and hemodynamic variables.*
◆ Monitor mechanical ventilation (high PEEP increases the risk for pneumothorax) *to increase PaO_2 without raising FIO_2, thereby reducing the risk of oxygen toxicity,* and provide suction, as necessary, *to aid removal of secretions.*
◆ Make sure the client maintains bed rest with prone positioning, if possible, *to promote oxygenation.*
◆ Maintain fluid restrictions *to reduce fluid volume overload.*
◆ Suction the patient and provide turning, chest physiotherapy, and postural drainage *to promote drainage and keep airways clear.*
◆ Position client *to promote oxygenation and ventilation.*
◆ Administer total parenteral nutrition or enteral feedings, as appropriate, *to prevent respiratory muscle impairment and maintain nutritional status.*
◆ Administer medications, as prescribed, *to optimize respiratory and hemodynamic status.*
◆ Organize nursing care to allow rest periods *to conserve energy, and avoid overexertion and fatigue.*
◆ Weigh the client daily *to detect fluid retention.*
◆ Encourage the client to express feelings about fear of suffocation *to reduce anxiety and, therefore, oxygen demands.*

Evaluation

◆ The client has adequate oxygenation.
◆ The client is breathing without difficulty.
◆ The client has decreased anxiety.

ACUTE RESPIRATORY FAILURE

With ACUTE RESPIRATORY FAILURE, the respiratory system can't adequately supply the body with the oxygen it needs or adequately remove carbon dioxide. Respiratory failure occurs when PaO_2 is 50 mm Hg or less or $PaCO_2$ is 50 mm Hg or greater.

Acute respiratory failure can be classified as ventilatory failure or oxygenation failure:

- Ventilatory failure is characterized by alveolar hypoventilation.
- Oxygenation failure is characterized by ventilation-perfusion mismatching (blood flow to areas of the lung with reduced ventilation, or ventilation to lung tissue that's experiencing reduced blood flow) or physiologic shunting (blood moving from the right side of the heart to the left without being oxygenated).

Possible causes

- Abdominal or thoracic surgery
- Anesthesia
- ARDS
- Atelectasis
- Brain tumors
- Chronic obstructive pulmonary disease (COPD)
- Drug overdose
- Encephalitis
- Flail chest
- Guillain-Barré syndrome
- Head trauma
- Hemothorax
- Meningitis
- Multiple sclerosis
- Muscular dystrophy
- Myasthenia gravis
- Pleural effusion
- Pneumonia
- Pneumothorax
- Poliomyelitis
- Polyneuritis
- Pulmonary edema
- Pulmonary embolism
- Stroke

Assessment findings

- Adventitious breath sounds, including crackles, pleural friction rub, rhonchi, and wheezing
- Difficulty breathing, shortness of breath, dyspnea, tachypnea, orthopnea
- Cough, sputum production, hemoptysis
- Decreased respiratory excursion, accessory muscle use, retractions
- Tachycardia
- Chest pain
- Change in mentation, anxiety, restlessness
- Nasal flaring
- Fatigue
- Cyanosis, diaphoresis

Diagnostic evaluation

- ABG levels show hypoxemia, acidosis, alkalosis, and hypercapnia.
- Chest X-ray shows pulmonary infiltrates, interstitial edema, and atelectasis.
- Hematology reveals increased WBC count and erythrocyte sedimentation rate (ESR).
- Lung scan shows ventilation-perfusion ratio mismatches.
- Sputum study identifies causative organism.

Nursing diagnoses

- Ineffective breathing pattern
- Ineffective airway clearance
- Ineffective tissue perfusion (cardiopulmonary)
- Anxiety

Treatment

- Chest physiotherapy, coughing, deep-breathing exercises, postural drainage (positioning the client in a prone or supine position, with the foot of the bed elevated higher than the head), and incentive spirometry
- Chest tube insertion if pneumothorax develops from high positive end-expiratory pressure (PEEP) administration
- High-calorie, high-protein diet and decreased or increased intake of fluids, depending on cause of disorder
- Oxygen therapy, intubation, and mechanical ventilation (possibly with PEEP)

Drug therapy options

- Analgesic: morphine sulfate
- Antibiotics: according to susceptibility of infecting organism
- Anticoagulants: heparin, enoxaparin (Lovenox), warfarin (Coumadin)
- Anxiolytic: lorazepam (Ativan)
- Bronchodilators: aminophylline (Aminophyllin), terbutaline (Brethine), theophylline (Theo-Dur); via nebulizer: albuterol (Proventil), ipratropium bromide (Atrovent), metaproterenol sulfate (Alupent)
- Diuretic: furosemide (Lasix)
- Expectorant: guaifenesin (Robitussin, Mucinex)

◆ Histamine-2 blockers: cimetidine (Tagamet), famotidine (Pepcid), ranitidine (Zantac), nizatidine (Axid)
◆ Neuromuscular blockers: atracurium besylate (Tracrium), pancuronium bromide (Pavulon), vecuronium bromide (Norcuron)
◆ Proton pump inhibitor: pantoprazole sodium (Protonix)
◆ Steroids: hydrocortisone sodium succinate (Solu-Cortef), methylprednisolone sodium succinate (Solu-Medrol)

Planning and goals

◆ The client will maintain a patent airway.
◆ The client will exhibit normal breathing pattern.
◆ The client will verbalize fears and concerns related to breathing difficulties.
◆ The client will demonstrate adequate oxygenation.

Implementation

◆ Assess respiratory status *to detect early signs of compromise and hypoxemia.*
◆ Monitor and record intake and output *to detect fluid volume excess,* which may lead to pulmonary edema.
◆ Track laboratory test results and report deteriorating ABG values, such as a decrease in $Pa{O_2}$ levels and an increase in $Pa{CO_2}$ levels. *Low hemoglobin levels and hematocrit reduce oxygen-carrying capacity of the blood. Electrolyte abnormalities may result from use of a diuretic.*
◆ Monitor pulse oximetry *to detect a drop in arterial oxygen saturation ($Sa{O_2}$).*
◆ Monitor and record vital signs. *Tachycardia and tachypnea may indicate hypoxemia.*
◆ Monitor and record color, consistency, and amount of sputum *to determine hydration status, effectiveness of therapy, and presence of infection.*
◆ Administer oxygen *to reduce hypoxemia and relieve respiratory distress.*
◆ Monitor mechanical ventilation *to prevent complications and optimize $Pa{O_2}$.*
◆ Provide suctioning; assist with turning, coughing, and deep breathing; and perform chest physiotherapy and postural drainage *to facilitate removal of secretions.*
◆ Make sure the client maintains bed rest *to reduce the amount of oxygen required.*
◆ Keep the client in semi- or high-Fowler's position *to promote chest expansion and ventilation.*
◆ Maintain diet restrictions. *Fluid restrictions and a low-sodium diet may be necessary to avoid fluid overload.*
◆ Administer medications, as prescribed, *to treat infection, dilate airways, and reduce inflammation.*
◆ Monitor the chest tube system *to assess for lung reexpansion.*

Evaluation

◆ The client demonstrates decreased anxiety with improved ventilation.
◆ The client maintains a patent airway and exhibits normal breathing patterns.
◆ The client demonstrates adequate oxygenation.

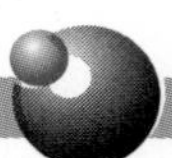

SPOT CHECK

A client experiencing acute respiratory failure is most likely to demonstrate:
A. hypocapnia, hypoventilation, hyperoxemia.
B. hypocapnia, hyperventilation, hyperoxemia.
C. hypercapnia, hyperventilation, hypoxemia.
D. hypercapnia, hypoventilation, hypoxemia.
Answer: D. Acute respiratory failure is marked by hypercapnia (elevated arterial carbon dioxide), hypoventilation, and hypoxemia (subnormal oxygen).

ASBESTOSIS

ASBESTOSIS is characterized by widespread filling and inflammation of lung spaces with asbestos fibers. In asbestosis, asbestos fibers assume a longitudinal orientation in the airway. These fibers move in the direction of airflow and penetrate respiratory bronchioles and alveolar walls, causing diffuse interstitial fibrosis (tissue filled with fibers).

Asbestosis can develop as long as 15 to 20 years after regular exposure to asbestos has ended. It increases the risk of lung cancer in cigarette smokers.

Possible causes

◆ Inhalation of asbestos fibers

Assessment findings

◆ Dyspnea on exertion (usually first symptom)
◆ Dyspnea at rest (in advanced disease)
◆ Pleuritic chest pain
◆ Dry crackles at lung bases
◆ Dry cough
◆ Recurrent respiratory infections
◆ Tachypnea
◆ Finger clubbing
◆ Pulmonary hypertension
◆ Cor pulmonale
◆ Right ventricular hypertrophy

Diagnostic evaluation

◆ ABG analysis may be within normal limits or, if client is having respiratory distress, it reveals decreased PaO_2 and low $PaCO_2$.
◆ Chest X-rays show fine, irregular, and linear diffuse infiltrates; extensive fibrosis results in a "honeycomb" or "ground-glass" appearance. X-rays may also show pleural thickening and pleural calcification, with bilateral obliteration of costophrenic angles and, in later stages, an enlarged heart with a classic "shaggy" heart border.
◆ Pulmonary function tests show decreased vital capacity, forced vital capacity, and total lung capacity and reduced diffusing capacity of the lungs.

Nursing diagnoses

◆ Impaired gas exchange
◆ Imbalance nutrition: Less than body requirements
◆ Ineffective tissue perfusion (cardiopulmonary)
◆ Fatigue

Treatment

◆ Chest physiotherapy
◆ Fluid intake of at least 3 L/day
◆ Oxygen therapy or mechanical ventilation (in advanced cases)

Drug therapy options

◆ Antibiotic: according to susceptibility of infecting organism (for treatment of respiratory tract infections)
◆ Cardiac glycoside: digoxin (Lanoxin)
◆ Diuretic: furosemide (Lasix)
◆ Mucolytic inhalation therapy: acetylcysteine (Mucomyst)

Planning and goals

◆ The client will demonstrate adequate ventilation and oxygenation.
◆ The client will maintain calorie intake specific to meet needs.
◆ The client will identify measures to prevent or reduce fatigue.

Implementation

◆ Perform chest physiotherapy *to promote mobilization of secretions.*
◆ Administer diuretics and cardiac glycoside preparations for clients with cor pulmonale *to treat dyspnea, tachycardia, and dependent edema.*
◆ Monior intake and output *to evaluate fluid balance.*
◆ Administer oxygen by cannula or mask (1 to 2 L/minute), or by mechanical ventilation if PaO_2 can't be maintained above 40 mm Hg *to prevent complications of hypoxemia.*
◆ Administer antibiotics, as ordered, for respiratory infections *to prevent complications such as sepsis.*
◆ Consult a registered dietitian *to help meet the client's nutritional needs.*

Evaluation

◆ The client maintains adequate gas exchange as evidenced by stable or improved pulse oximetry.
◆ The client maintains his present weight.
◆ The client reports feeling less fatigued.

ASPHYXIA

In ASPHYXIA, interference with respiration leads to insufficient oxygen and accumulating carbon dioxide in the blood and tissues. Asphyxia leads to cardiopulmonary arrest and is fatal without prompt treatment.

Possible causes

◆ Extrapulmonary obstruction, such as tracheal compression from a tumor, strangulation, trauma, or suffocation
◆ Hypoventilation as a result of opioid overdose, medullary disease, hemorrhage, pneumothorax, respiratory muscle paralysis, or cardiopulmonary arrest
◆ Inhalation of toxic agents, such as carbon monoxide and smoke, and excessive oxygen inhalation
◆ Intrapulmonary obstruction, such as airway obstruction, severe asthma, foreign body aspiration, pulmonary edema, pneumonia, and near-drowning

Assessment findings

◆ Agitation, restlessness
◆ Central and peripheral cyanosis (cherry-red mucous membranes in late-stage carbon monoxide poisoning)
◆ Dyspnea
◆ Altered respiratory rate (apnea, bradypnea, occasional tachypnea)
◆ Decreased breath sounds
◆ Anxiety
◆ Confusion leading to coma
◆ Fast, slow, or absent pulse
◆ Seizures

Diagnostic evaluation

◆ ABG measurement indicates decreased PaO_2 (less than 60 mm Hg) and increased $PaCO_2$ (greater than 50 mm Hg).
◆ Chest X-rays may show a foreign body, pulmonary edema, or atelectasis.

◆ Pulmonary function tests may indicate respiratory muscle weakness.
◆ Pulse oximetry reveals decreased hemoglobin (Hb) saturation of oxygen.
◆ Toxicology tests may show drugs, chemicals, or abnormal Hb.

Nursing diagnoses

◆ Anxiety
◆ Impaired gas exchange
◆ Impaired spontaneous ventilation
◆ Ineffective breathing pattern
◆ Risk for suffocation

Treatment

◆ Bronchoscopy (for extraction of a foreign body)
◆ Cardiopulmonary resuscitation
◆ Gastric lavage (for poisoning)
◆ Oxygen therapy, which may include ET intubation and mechanical ventilation

Drug therapy options

◆ Opioid antagonist: Naloxone (for opioid overdose)

Planning and goals

◆ The client will demonstrate decreased anxiety.
◆ The client will maintain adequate ventilation and oxygenation.
◆ The client will maintain an adequate breathing pattern.
◆ The client will remain safe from injury caused by suffocation.

Implementation

◆ Assess cardiac and respiratory status *to detect early signs of compromise.*
◆ Position the client upright, if his condition tolerates, *to promote lung expansion and improve oxygenation.*
◆ Reassure the client during treatment *to ease anxiety associated with respiratory distress.*
◆ Give prescribed medications *to promote ventilation and oxygenation.*
◆ Suction carefully, as needed, and encourage deep breathing *to mobilize secretions and maintain a patent airway.*
◆ Closely monitor vital signs and laboratory test results *to guide the treatment plan.*

Evaluation

◆ The client demonstrates decreased anxiety.
◆ The client has adequate gas exchange as evidenced by stable pulse oximetry and arterial blood gases.
◆ The client's breathing pattern remains within normal parameters.
◆ The client has a safe environment and is free from injury related to suffocation.

ASTHMA

ASTHMA is a form of chronic obstructive airway disease in which the bronchial linings overreact to various stimuli, causing episodic spasms and inflammation that can severely restrict the airways. Symptoms range from mild wheezing and labored breathing to life-threatening respiratory failure.

Asthma can be result from a number of causes.

Possible causes

◆ Allergens (pollen, dander, dust, sulfite food additives)
◆ Drugs, chemicals
◆ Exercise
◆ Endocrine changes
◆ Noxious fumes
◆ Respiratory infection
◆ Stress
◆ Temperature and humidity

Assessment findings

◆ Anxiety, fear
◆ Chest tightness
◆ Dyspnea
◆ Wheezing, primarily on expiration but also sometimes on inspiration
◆ Absent or diminished breath sounds during severe obstruction
◆ Tachypnea, tachycardia
◆ Cough
◆ Prolonged expiration
◆ Use of accessory muscles
◆ Usually asymptomatic between attacks

Diagnostic evaluation

◆ ABG analysis in acute severe asthma shows decreased Pa_{O_2} and decreased, normal, or increased Pa_{CO_2}.
◆ Blood tests: Serum immunoglobulin E may increase from an allergic reaction; CBC may reveal an increased eosinophil count.
◆ Chest X-ray shows hyperinflated lungs with air trapping during an attack.

◆ Pulmonary function tests during attacks show decreased forced expiratory volumes that improve with therapy, and increased residual volume and total lung capacity.
◆ Skin tests may identify allergens.

Nursing diagnoses

◆ Ineffective airway clearance
◆ Ineffective breathing pattern
◆ Ineffective tissue perfusion (cardiopulmonary)
◆ Impaired gas exchange
◆ Ineffective therapeutic regimen management

Treatment

◆ Desensitization to allergens
◆ Intubation and mechanical ventilation if respiratory status worsens
◆ Oxygen therapy at 2 L/minute
◆ Fluids up to 3,000 ml/day, as tolerated
◆ Relaxation exercises (yoga)

Drug therapy options

◆ Antibiotics: according to susceptibility of infecting organism
◆ Beta-adrenergic drugs: epinephrine hydrochloride (Adrenalin), salmeterol (Serevent)
◆ Bronchodilators: terbutaline (Brethine), aminophylline (Aminophyllin), theophylline (Theo-Dur); via nebulizer: albuterol (Proventil), ipratropium bromide (Atrovent), metaproterenol sulfate (Alupent)
◆ Leukotriene modifier: zileuton (Zyflo)
◆ Leukotriene receptor antagonists: montelukast (Singulair), zafirlukast (Accolate)
◆ Mast cell stabilizer therapy: cromolyn sodium (Intal)
◆ Steroids: hydrocortisone (Solu-Cortef), methylprednisolone sodium succinate (Solu-Medrol); via nebulizer: beclomethasone (Vanceril), triamcinolone (Azmacort)

Planning and goals

◆ The client will maintain a patent airway.
◆ The client will exhibit a normal breathing pattern.
◆ The client will maintain adequate oxygenation.
◆ The client will maintain adequate ventilation.
◆ The client and his family will indicate verbally or through demonstration that they learned what was taught.

Implementation

◆ Administer low-flow humidified oxygen *to reduce inflammation of the airways, ease breathing, and increase* Sao_2.
◆ Administer medications, as prescribed, *to reduce inflammation and obstruction of airways.* Auscultate lungs for improved breath sounds. Observe for complications of drug therapy.
◆ Encourage the client to express feelings about fear of suffocation *to reduce anxiety.* As breathlessness and hypoxemia are relieved, anxiety should be reduced.
◆ Allow activity, as tolerated, with rest periods *to reduce work of breathing and reduce oxygen demands.*
◆ Assess respiratory status *to determine effectiveness of therapy,* such as clear breath sounds and improved airflow, pulmonary function tests, Sao_2, and ease of breathing. Louder wheezing may be heard as airways respond to therapy and open up. As the client's condition improves and airflow increases, wheezing should diminish and breath sounds improve.
◆ Assist with turning, coughing, deep breathing, and breathing retraining *to mobilize and clear secretions. Pursed-lip and diaphragmatic breathing promote more effective ventilation.*
◆ Keep the client in high-Fowler's position *to improve ventilation.*
◆ Maintain the client's diet and administer small, frequent feedings *to reduce pressure on the diaphragm and increase caloric intake.*
◆ Encourage fluids *to treat dehydration and liquefy secretions to facilitate their removal.*
◆ Monitor and record the color, amount, and consistency of sputum. *Changes in sputum characteristics may signal a respiratory infection.*
◆ Monitor and record vital signs *to assess overall condition. Tachycardia may indicate worsening asthma or drug toxicity. Hypertension may indicate hypoxemia. Fever may signal infection.*
◆ Monitor laboratory studies *to identify potential problems. An increase in WBC count may signal infection. Eosinophilia may indicate an allergic response. Drug levels may reveal toxicity.*
◆ Provide chest physiotherapy, postural drainage, incentive spirometry, and suction *to aid in the removal of secretions.*

Evaluation

◆ The client maintains improved ventilation and oxygenation.
◆ The client has adequate gas exchange as evidenced by stable pulse oximetry and ABG levels.
◆ The client exhibits appropriate knowledge of the therapeutic regimen.

ATELECTASIS

ATELECTASIS is marked by incomplete expansion of lobules (clusters of alveoli) or lung segments, which may result in partial or complete lung collapse. The collapsed areas are unavailable for gas exchange; blood that lacks oxygen passes through unchanged, thereby producing hypoxia.

Atelectasis may be chronic or acute. It occurs to some degree in many clients undergoing upper abdominal or thoracic surgery. The prognosis depends on prompt removal of an airway obstruction, relief of hypoxia, and reexpansion of the collapsed lung.

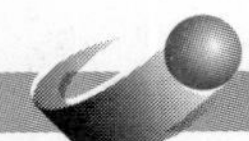

FAST FACT

Atelectasis can cause hypoxemia and acute respiratory failure. Additionally, static secretions from atelectasis may lead to pneumonia.

Possible causes

- Bronchial occlusion by mucus plugs, as in clients with COPD, bronchiectasis, or cystic fibrosis, or those who smoke heavily
- CNS depression
- External compression, such as from upper abdominal surgical incisions, rib fractures, pleuritic chest pain, tight dressings around the chest, or obesity
- Occlusion by foreign bodies, bronchogenic carcinoma, and inflammatory lung disease
- Prolonged immobility

Assessment findings

- Diminished breath sounds or crackles
- Dyspnea

In severe cases

- Severe dyspnea
- Cyanosis
- Diaphoresis
- Anxiety
- Substernal or intercostal retraction
- Tachycardia
- Hyperinflation of unaffected areas of the lung
- Peripheral circulatory collapse

Diagnostic evaluation

- Chest X-ray shows characteristic horizontal lines in the lower lung zones and, with segmental or lobar collapse, characteristic dense shadows commonly associated with hyperinflation of neighboring lung zones (in widespread atelectasis).
- Bronchoscopy rules out neoplasm or obstruction.

Nursing diagnoses

- Impaired gas exchange
- Ineffective airway clearance
- Ineffective breathing pattern
- Risk for infection

Treatment

- Bronchoscopy
- Chest physiotherapy and postural drainage
- Deep breathing and coughing exercises
- Surgery or radiation therapy to remove an obstructing neoplasm

Drug therapy options

- Analgesic: morphine
- Bronchodilator: albuterol (Proventil)
- Mucolytic inhalation therapy: acetylcysteine (Mucomyst)

Planning and goals

- The client will maintain a patent airway.
- The client will maintain adequate ventilation.
- The client will have a temperature and a WBC count within normal limits.

Implementation

- Encourage postoperative and other high-risk clients to cough and deep-breathe every 1 to 2 hours *to prevent atelectasis.*
- In postoperative clients, hold a pillow tightly over the incision; teach the client this technique as well *to minimize pain during coughing exercises.* Gently reposition these clients often and help them walk as soon as possible *to prevent atelectasis.*
- Administer analgesics to control pain and prior to deep breathing and coughing exercises. *Pain may prevent the client from taking deep breaths, which leads to atelectasis.*
- During mechanical ventilation, maintain tidal volume at 10 to 15 ml/kg of the client's body weight *to ensure adequate lung expansion.* Use the sigh mechanism on the ventilator, if appropriate, to intermittently increase tidal volume at the rate of 10 to 15 sighs/hour.
- Use an incentive spirometer *to encourage deep inspiration through positive reinforcement.* Teach the client how to use the spirometer and encourage him to use it every 1 to 2 hours.
- Humidify inspired air and encourage adequate fluid intake *to mobilize secretions.* Use postural drainage and

chest percussion *to promote loosening and clearance of secretions.*

◆ If the client is intubated or uncooperative, provide suctioning as needed *to maintain a clear airway.* Use sedatives with discretion *because they depress respirations and the cough reflex and suppress sighing.*

◆ Assess breath sounds and ventilatory status frequently and be alert for changes *to prevent respiratory compromise.*

◆ Encourage the client to stop smoking, lose weight, or both, as needed. Refer him to appropriate support groups *for help to modify risk factors.*

◆ Provide reassurance and emotional support *because the client may be frightened by his limited breathing capacity.*

Evaluation

◆ The client maintains a patent airway.

◆ The client has adequate ventilation and oxygenation.

◆ The client doesn't exhibit any signs of infection.

BRONCHIECTASIS

BRONCHIECTASIS is marked by chronic, abnormal dilation of bronchi (large air passages of the lungs) and destruction of bronchial walls.

Bronchiectasis has three forms: cylindrical (fusiform), varicose, and saccular (cystic). It can occur throughout the tracheobronchial tree or can be confined to one segment or lobe. However, it's usually bilateral and involves the basilar segments of the lower lobes.

The disorder affects people of both sexes and all ages and, once established, is irreversible. Because of the availability of antibiotics to treat acute respiratory tract infections, the incidence of bronchiectasis has dramatically decreased in the past 20 years.

Possible causes

◆ Congenital abnormalities, such as bronchomalacia, congenital bronchiectasis, immotile cilia syndrome, and Kartagener's syndrome.

◆ Inhalation of corrosive gas or repeated aspiration of gastric juices into the lungs

◆ Immunologic disorders such as agammaglobulinemia

◆ Mucoviscidosis (in cases of cystic fibrosis)

◆ Obstruction (by a foreign body, tumor, or stenosis) in association with recurrent infection

◆ Recurrent, inadequately treated bacterial respiratory tract infections, such as TB, and complications of measles, pneumonia, pertussis, or influenza

Assessment findings

◆ Dyspnea

◆ Chronic cough that produces copious, foul-smelling, mucopurulent secretions, possibly totaling several cupfuls daily

◆ Clubbing of the fingers

◆ Coarse crackles during inspiration over involved lobes or segments

◆ Malaise

◆ Weight loss

◆ Occasional wheezes

◆ Recurrent fever, chills, and other signs and symptoms of infection

◆ Sinusitis

Diagnostic evaluation

◆ Bronchoscopy helps identify the source of secretions or the bleeding site in hemoptysis.

◆ Chest X-rays show peribronchial thickening, areas of atelectasis, and scattered cystic changes.

◆ CBC detects anemia and leukocytosis.

◆ CT scanning shows characteristic changes.

◆ Pulmonary function tests detect decreased vital capacity, expiratory flow, and hypoxemia.

◆ Sputum culture and Gram stain identify predominant organisms.

Nursing diagnoses

◆ Ineffective airway clearance

◆ Impaired gas exchange

◆ Imbalanced nutrition: Less than body requirements

Treatment

◆ Bronchoscopy (to mobilize secretions)

◆ Chest physiotherapy

◆ Oxygen therapy

Drug therapy options

◆ Antibiotics: according to susceptibility of infecting organism

◆ Bronchodilator: albuterol (Proventil)

Planning and goals

◆ The client will maintain a patent airway.

◆ The client will maintain adequate oxygenation.

◆ The client will consume a specific number of calories daily.

Bronchiectasis care

Review the following home-care points with the client and his family regarding bronchiectasis:

- Ensure that the client can perform coughing and deep-breathing exercises prior to discharge.
- The client should be encouraged to rest as much as possible.
- The client should be encouraged to eat a balanced, high-protein diet and drink plenty of fluids to promote healing and expectoration of secretions.
- Postural drainage, percussion, and mouth care should be taught to the family to promote bronchial hygiene and prevention of infection.
- Proper disposal of secretions should be discussed.
- Review the need to avoid infection and smoking (including second-hand smoke) to promote health and well-being.

Implementation

- Assess respiratory status *to detect early signs of decompensation.*
- Provide supportive care and help the client adjust to the permanent changes in lifestyle that irreversible lung damage necessitates *to facilitate positive coping.* (See *Bronchiectasis care.*)
- Administer antibiotics as needed *to eradicate infection.*
- Explain all diagnostic tests to the client *to decrease anxiety.*
- Perform chest physiotherapy, including postural drainage and chest percussion designed for involved lobes, several times per day. The best times to do this are early morning and just before bedtime. Instruct the client to maintain each position for 10 minutes; then perform percussion and tell him to cough. *These measures mobilize secretions.*

Evaluation

- The client maintains a patent airway.
- The client has adequate ventilation and oxygenation.
- The client has maintained or improved weight.

CHRONIC BRONCHITIS

CHRONIC BRONCHITIS, a form of COPD, results from irritants and infections that increase mucus production, impair airway clearance, and cause irreversible narrowing of the small airways. These changes cause a severe ventilation-perfusion imbalance, leading to hypoxemia and CO_2 retention.

Possible causes

- Airborne irritants and pollutants
- Chronic respiratory infections
- Smoking

Assessment findings

- Dyspnea
- Increased sputum production
- Productive cough
- Prolonged expiration
- Rhonchi, wheezes
- Tachypnea
- Use of accessory muscles
- Weight gain, edema, jugular vein distention
- Wheezing
- Finger clubbing, later in the disease

Diagnostic evaluation

- ABG analysis shows decreased Pao_2 and normal or increased $Paco_2$.
- Chest X-ray shows hyperinflation.
- ECG shows atrial arrhythmias, peaked P waves in leads II, III, and aV_F and, occasionally, right ventricular hypertrophy.
- Pulmonary function tests may reveal increased residual volume, decreased vital capacity and forced expiratory volumes, and normal static compliance and diffusion capacity.
- Sputum culture may reveal many microorganisms and neutrophils.

Nursing diagnoses

- Deficient knowledge related to the disease process and treatment
- Ineffective airway clearance
- Ineffective breathing pattern
- Activity intolerance
- Risk for infection

Treatment

- Avoidance of smoking and air pollutants
- Chest physiotherapy, postural drainage, and incentive spirometry
- Dietary changes, including establishing a diet high in protein and vitamin C
- Fluid intake up to 3,000 ml/day, if not contraindicated
- Intubation and mechanical ventilation if respiratory status deteriorates
- Low-flow oxygen therapy at 2 to 3 L/minute
- Ultrasonic or mechanical nebulizer treatments

Drug therapy options

◆ Antibiotics: according to susceptibility of infecting organism
◆ Bronchodilators: terbutaline (Brethine), aminophylline (Aminophyllin), theophylline (Theo-Dur); via nebulizer: albuterol (Proventil), ipratropium bromide (Atrovent), metaproterenol sulfate (Alupent)
◆ Diuretic: furosemide (Lasix) for edema
◆ Expectorant: guaifenesin (Robitussin, Mucinex)
◆ Influenza and Pneumovax vaccines
◆ Steroids: hydrocortisone (Solu-Cortef), methylprednisolone sodium succinate (Solu-Medrol) (via nebulizer): beclomethasone (Vanceril), triamcinolone (Azmacort)

Planning and goals

◆ The client will maintain adequate ventilation.
◆ The client will identify measures to prevent or reduce fatigue.
◆ The client will verbalize understanding of the disease process and comply with the therapy regimen.
◆ The client won't exhibit signs of infection.

Implementation

◆ Administer low-flow oxygen. Because clients with chronic bronchitis have chronic hypercapnia, they have a hypoxic respiratory drive. Higher flow rates may eliminate this hypoxic respiratory drive. *Low flow rates may not eliminate this drive.*
◆ Administer medications, as prescribed, *to relieve symptoms and prevent complications.*
◆ Allow activity, as tolerated, *to avoid fatigue and reduce oxygen demands.*
◆ Assess respiratory status, ABG levels, and pulse oximetry *to detect respiratory compromise, severe hypoxemia, and hypercapnia.*
◆ Assist with turning, coughing, and deep breathing *to mobilize secretions and facilitate removal.*
◆ Assist with diaphragmatic and pursed-lip breathing *to strengthen respiratory muscles.*
◆ Keep the client in high-Fowler's position *to improve ventilation.*
◆ Maintain the client's diet and administer small, frequent feedings *to avoid fatigue when eating and reduce pressure on the diaphragm from a full stomach.*
◆ Monitor and record the color, amount, and consistency of sputum. *Changes in sputum characteristics may signal a respiratory infection.*
◆ Monitor and record cardiovascular status and vital signs *to assess for complications.* Edema, jugular vein distention, tachycardia, and an elevated CVP suggest right-sided heart failure. An irregular pulse may indicate an arrhythmia caused by altered ABG levels. Tachycardia and tachypnea may indicate hypoxemia.
◆ Monitor laboratory studies *to identify potential problems.* Follow drug levels for evidence of toxicity. Electrolyte imbalances may occur with the use of diuretics. Reduced Hb level and hematocrit (HCT) affect the oxygen-carrying capacity of the blood.
◆ Monitor intake and output and daily weights *to detect fluid overload associated with right-sided heart failure. Dehydration impairs the removal of secretions.*
◆ Provide chest physiotherapy, postural drainage, incentive spirometry, and suction *to aid in removal of secretions.*
◆ Weigh the client daily *to detect edema caused by right-sided heart failure.*

Evaluation

◆ The client has adequate ventilation, as exhibited by stable ABG levels.
◆ The client reports less incidence of fatigue.
◆ The client verbalizes an understanding of the disease process and complies with treatment.
◆ The client remains free from infection.

CHRONIC OBSTRUCTIVE PULMONARY DISEASE

CHRONIC OBSTRUCTIVE PULMONARY DISEASE (COPD), also known as *chronic airflow limitation,* is a group of conditions that obstruct pulmonary air outflow, resulting in air being trapped in the alveoli.

Chronic obstructive bronchitis, a productive cough persisting for 3 months of the year for at least 2 consecutive years, causes inflamed airways that lead to increased mucus production and bronchospasms. Mucus plugs entrap air and result in alveolar hyperinflation. Clients with severe chronic bronchitis usually have severe hypoxemia and polycythemia, with HCT values from 50% to 55%.

Emphysema, characterized by enlargement of the alveoli distal to the terminal bronchioles, leads to alveolar wall destruction, obstructed expiratory airflow, and irreversible loss of lung elasticity. Emphysema causes less hypoxemia than chronic bronchitis does, and HCT values are commonly normal.

Asthma, marked by a widespread airway narrowing in response to various stimuli, is considered COPD only if airway obstruction becomes irreversible.

Possible causes

◆ Airborne irritants and pollutants

- ◆ Allergens
- ◆ $Alpha_1$-antitrypsin deficiency
- ◆ Chronic respiratory tract infection
- ◆ Smoking

Assessment findings

- ◆ Anatomic changes (such as barrel chest and clubbing of fingers) in late disease
- ◆ Cor pulmonale (right-sided heart failure)
- ◆ Cough (evaluate character, frequency, and time of day)
- ◆ Decreased breath sounds, hyperresonant breath sounds on percussion, wheezing
- ◆ Dyspnea
- ◆ Jugular vein distention
- ◆ Peripheral edema
- ◆ Posturing (leaning forward)
- ◆ Prolonged expiration
- ◆ Pursed-lip breathing
- ◆ Sputum (evaluate amount, color, and consistency)
- ◆ Use of accessory muscles

Diagnostic evaluation

- ◆ Pulmonary function tests, especially spirometry, reveal diminished lung function.
- ◆ Chest X-ray provides baseline norms; in late disease, the client's diaphragm appears flat; with cardiac involvement, cardiomegaly is present.
- ◆ ABG levels show hypercapnia and hypoxemia. Bicarbonate levels may increase to compensate for chronic hypercapnia and the resultant respiratory acidosis.
- ◆ CBC shows elevated hemoglobin and hematocrit.
- ◆ Pulse oximetry may show a decrease in arterial oxygen saturation, which indicates hypoxia.
- ◆ ECG shows signs of right ventricular hypertrophy in late disease.

Nursing diagnoses

- ◆ Ineffective airway clearance
- ◆ Ineffective breathing pattern
- ◆ Imbalanced nutrition: Less than body requirements
- ◆ Impaired gas exchange
- ◆ Fatigue
- ◆ Deficient knowledge related to disease process and treatment

Treatment

- ◆ Chest physiotherapy, postural drainage, and incentive spirometry
- ◆ Fluid intake up to 3,000 ml per day if not contraindicated by heart failure
- ◆ Oxygen therapy as ordered and transtracheal therapy for home oxygen therapy
- ◆ Diet high in protein, vitamin C, and nitrogen. Clients with advanced disease may require a diet that's low in carbohydrates and higher in fats.

Drug therapy options

- ◆ $Alpha_1$-antitrypsin
- ◆ Antibiotics: according to susceptibility of the infecting organism
- ◆ Bronchodilators: aminophylline (Aminophyllin), terbutaline (Brethine), theophylline (Theo-Dur); via nebulizer: albuterol (Proventil), ipratropium bromide (Atrovent), metaproterenol sulfate (Alupent)
- ◆ Diuretic: furosemide (Lasix)
- ◆ Expectorant: guaifenesin (Robitussin)
- ◆ Histamine-2 blockers: cimetidine (Tagamet), ranitidine (Zantac), famotidine (Pepcid)
- ◆ Proton pump inhibitor: pantoprazole (Protonix)
- ◆ Steroids: hydrocortisone (Solu-Cortef), methylprednisolone sodium succinate (Solu-Medrol); via nebulizer: beclomethasone (Vanceril), triamcinolone (Azmacort)
- ◆ Influenza and Pneumovax vaccines

Planning and goals

- ◆ The client will maintain a patent airway.
- ◆ The client will maintain adequate gas exchange.
- ◆ The client will establish an effective breathing pattern.
- ◆ The client will verbalize understanding of disease process and comply with treatment.
- ◆ The client will maintain weight within normal parameters.

Implementation

- ◆ Assess respiratory status and ABG and pulse oximetry studies *to evaluate oxygenation.* Administer low-flow oxygen, if indicated, usually 1 to 2 L per minute in 24% to 28% concentrations.

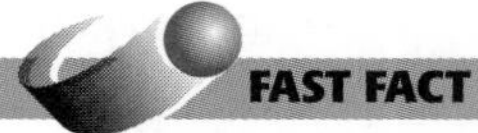

FAST FACT

Some clients with emphysema respond only to low oxygen tension. Giving this client too much oxygen reduces the drive to breathe and contributes to respiratory failure.

- ◆ Monitor cardiovascular status *to detect arrhythmias related to hypoxia or adverse response to medications.*

- Encourage the client to drink plenty of fluids, and weigh him daily *to monitor for fluid overload and right-sided heart failure.*
- Monitor and record color, amount, and consistency of sputum; *change may indicate infection.*
- Monitor electrolyte levels, blood counts, and drug levels *for indications of a possible toxic reaction.*
- Administer medications as prescribed *to relieve symptoms and prevent complications.*
- Encourage the client to pace his activity as tolerated *to prevent fatigue.*
- Instruct the client about breathing exercises, and proper deep breathing and coughing *to maintain a patent airway.*
- Provide chest physiotherapy, as needed, including postural drainage, postural drainage and percussion, incentive spirometry, and suction *to aid in removal of secretions.*
- Consult a registered dietitian *to help meet the client's nutritional needs.*
- Instruct the client about the disease process and treatment *to aid compliance.*

Evaluation

- The client maintains a patent airway and improved gas exchange.
- The client exhibits less fatigue.
- The client maintains proper weight.
- The client complies with treatment.

COR PULMONALE

A chronic heart condition, COR PULMONALE is hypertrophy (enlargement) of the heart's right ventricle that results from diseases affecting the function or the structure of the lungs. To compensate for the extra work needed to force blood through the lungs, the right ventricle dilates and enlarges. Right-sided heart failure may progress to biventricular heart failure.

Invariably, cor pulmonale follows some disorder of the lungs, pulmonary vessels, chest wall, or respiratory control center. For instance, COPD produces pulmonary hypertension, which leads to right ventricular hypertrophy and right-sided heart failure. Because cor pulmonale generally occurs late during the course of COPD and other irreversible diseases, the prognosis is generally poor.

Possible causes

- COPD (about 25% of clients with COPD eventually develop cor pulmonale)
- Living at high altitudes (chronic mountain sickness)
- Loss of lung tissue after extensive lung surgery
- Obesity-hypoventilation syndrome (pickwickian syndrome) and upper airway obstruction
- Obstructive lung diseases, such as bronchiectasis and cystic fibrosis
- Pulmonary vascular diseases, such as recurrent thromboembolism, primary pulmonary hypertension, schistosomiasis, and pulmonary vasculitis
- Respiratory insufficiency without pulmonary disease, as seen in chest wall disorders, such as kyphoscoliosis, neuromuscular incompetence resulting from muscular dystrophy and amyotrophic lateral sclerosis, polymyositis, and spinal cord lesions above C6
- Restrictive lung diseases, such as pneumoconiosis, interstitial pneumonitis, scleroderma, and sarcoidosis

Assessment findings

- Dyspnea on exertion
- Edema
- Orthopnea
- Tachypnea
- Fatigue
- Weakness
- Wheezing respirations
- Chronic productive cough

Diagnostic evaluation

- ABG analysis shows decreased PaO_2 (less than 70 mm Hg).
- Blood tests may show HCT greater than 50%.
- Chest X-ray shows large central pulmonary arteries and suggests right ventricular enlargement by rightward enlargement of cardiac silhouette on an anterior chest film.
- Echocardiography or angiography indicates right ventricular enlargement; echocardiography can estimate pulmonary artery pressure (PAP).
- ECG commonly shows arrhythmias, such as premature atrial and ventricular contractions and atrial fibrillation, during severe hypoxia. It may also show right bundle-branch block, right axis deviation, prominent P waves and an inverted T wave in right precordial leads, and right ventricular hypertrophy.
- PAP measurements show increased right ventricular pressure as a result of increased pulmonary vascular resistance.
- Pulmonary function tests show results consistent with the underlying pulmonary disease.

Nursing diagnoses

- Impaired gas exchange
- Ineffective tissue perfusion (cardiopulmonary)

- Excess fluid volume
- Activity intolerance

Treatment

- Low-salt diet, with restricted fluid intake
- Lung transplantation
- Tracheostomy for upper airway obstruction
- Oxygen therapy by mask or cannula in concentrations ranging from 24% to 40%, depending on Pa_{O_2}, as necessary; in acute cases, mechanical ventilation

Drug therapy options

- Angiotensin-converting enzyme inhibitor: captopril (Capoten)
- Angiotensin II receptor blocker: losartan potassium (Cozaar)
- Antibiotic: when respiratory infection is present
- Anticoagulant: heparin
- Beta-adrenergic blockers: atenolol (Tenormin), metoprolol (Lopressor)
- Cardiac glycoside: digoxin (Lanoxin)
- Diuretic (to reduce edema): furosemide (Lasix)
- Vasodilators: diazoxide (Proglycem), hydralazine (Apresoline), nitroprusside (Nipride), prostaglandins (in primary pulmonary hypertension)

Planning and goals

- The client will maintain a patent airway and adequate ventilation.
- The client will identify the need to control fluid intake and follow a therapeutic regimen to decrease fluid overload.
- The client will demonstrate skill in conserving energy while carrying out activities according to his tolerance level.

Implementation

- Consult the dietary staff, and provide small, frequent feedings rather than three heavy meals *because the client may lack energy and tire easily when eating.*
- Limit the client's fluid intake to 1,000 to 2,000 ml/day, and provide a low-sodium diet *to prevent fluid retention.*
- Monitor the client's serum potassium levels closely if the client is receiving diuretics. *Low serum potassium levels can potentiate the risk of arrhythmias associated with cardiac glycosides.*
- Monitor the client's digoxin level *to prevent symptoms of digoxin toxicity,* such as anorexia, nausea, vomiting, and yellow halos around visual images.
- Teach the client to check his radial pulse before taking digoxin or any cardiac glycoside and to report changes in his pulse rate *to avoid complications of digoxin therapy.*
- Reposition bedridden clients often *to prevent atelectasis.*
- Provide respiratory care, including oxygen therapy and, for COPD clients, pursed-lip breathing exercises, *to improve oxygenation.*
- Periodically measure ABG levels and watch for signs of respiratory failure, such as a change in pulse rate; deep, labored respirations; and increased fatigue produced by exertion. *Monitoring these parameters helps detect early signs of worsening respiratory status.*
- Consult social services *to help obtain necessary equipment the client may need at home.*

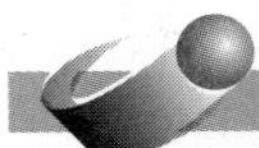

FAST FACT

Cor pulmonale clients with underlying COPD shouldn't receive high doses of oxygen. It could lead to subsequent respiratory depression.

Evaluation

- The client maintains a patent airway with adequate oxygenation as evidenced by stable ABG levels.
- The client maintains fluid balance.
- The client demonstrates energy conservation measures while performing ADLs.

EMPHYSEMA

EMPHYSEMA is a form of COPD in which recurrent pulmonary inflammation damages and eventually destroys the alveolar walls, creating large air spaces. This breakdown leaves the alveoli unable to recoil normally after expanding and, upon expiration, results in bronchiolar collapse. This collapse traps air in the lungs, leading to overdistention and reduced gas exchange.

Possible causes

- Deficiency of alpha$_1$-antitrypsin
- Smoking

Assessment findings

- Dyspnea
- Pursed-lip breathing
- Decreased breath sounds
- Prolonged expiration
- Use of accessory muscles for breathing
- Anorexia, weight loss

- Barrel chest
- Finger clubbing (late in the disease)
- Chronic cough

Diagnostic evaluation

- ABG analysis shows reduced PaO_2, with normal $PaCO_2$ until late in the disease.
- Pulmonary function tests show increased residual volume, total lung capacity, and compliance as well as decreased vital capacity, diffusing capacity, and expiratory volumes.
- Chest X-ray in advanced disease reveals a flattened diaphragm, reduced vascular markings in the lung periphery, enlarged anteroposterior chest diameter, and a vertical heart.
- CBC shows increased Hb level late in the disease when client has severe persistent hypoxia.
- ECG shows tall, symmetrical P waves in leads II, III, and aV_F, vertical QRS axis, and signs of right ventricular hypertrophy.

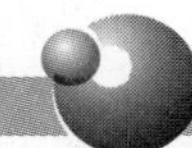

SPOT CHECK

In a client with emphysema, the initiative to breathe is triggered by:

A. high CO_2 levels.
B. low CO_2 levels.
C. high O_2 levels.
D. low O_2 levels.

Answer: D. Because of long-standing hypercapnia, breathing in a client with emphysema is triggered by low O_2 levels. In a client with a normal respiratory drive, the initiative to breathe is triggered by increased CO_2 levels.

Nursing diagnoses

- Impaired gas exchange
- Ineffective tissue perfusion (cardiopulmonary)
- Fatigue
- Imbalanced nutrition: Less than body requirements

Treatment

- Chest physiotherapy, postural drainage, and incentive spirometry
- Dietary changes, including establishing a diet high in protein, vitamin C, calories, and nitrogen
- Fluid intake up to 3,000 ml/day if not contraindicated by heart failure
- Intubation and mechanical ventilation if respiratory status deteriorates
- Oxygen therapy as ordered; transtracheal therapy for home oxygen therapy
- Ultrasonic or mechanical nebulizer treatments
- Lung volume reduction surgery

Drug therapy options

- $Alpha_1$-antitrypsin therapy
- Antibiotic: according to susceptibility of infective organism
- Bronchodilators: terbutaline (Brethine), aminophylline (Aminophyllin), theophylline (Theo-Dur); via nebulizer: albuterol (Proventil), ipratropium bromide (Atrovent), metaproterenol sulfate (Alupent)
- Diuretic (to reduce edema): furosemide (Lasix)
- Expectorant: guaifenesin (Robitussin, Mucinex)
- Histamine-2 blockers: cimetidine (Tagamet), ranitidine (Zantac), famotidine (Pepcid)
- Influenza and Pneumovax vaccines
- Proton pump inhibitor: pantoprazole (Protonix)
- Steroids: hydrocortisone (Solu-Cortef), methylprednisolone sodium succinate (Solu-Medrol) (via nebulizer): beclomethasone (Vanceril), triamcinolone (Azmacort)

Planning and goals

- The client will maintain a patent airway and adequate ventilation.
- The client will identify measures to prevent or reduce fatigue.
- The client will consume adequate daily calories, as required.

Implementation

- Administer low-flow oxygen *because emphysema clients have chronic hypercapnia, and, therefore, a hypoxic respiratory drive resulting in further increases in CO_2 and the need for respiratory therapy. Higher flow rates may eliminate this hypoxic respiratory drive.*
- Administer medications, as prescribed, *to relieve symptoms and prevent complications.*
- Allow activity, as tolerated, *to avoid fatigue and reduce oxygen demands.*
- Assess respiratory status, ABG levels, and pulse oximetry *to detect respiratory compromise, severe hypoxemia, and hypercapnia.*
- Monitor and record cardiovascular status and vital signs *to assess for complications.* An irregular pulse may indicate an arrhythmia caused by altered ABG levels. Tachycardia and tachypnea may indicate hypoxemia. Late in the disease, pulmonary hypertension may lead to right ventricular hypertrophy and right-sided heart failure. Jugular

vein distention, edema, hypotension, tachycardia, S_3 heart sound, a loud pulmonic component of S_2, heart murmurs, and hepatojugular reflux may be present.

- Assist with turning, coughing, and deep breathing *to mobilize secretions and facilitate their removal.*
- Assist with diaphragmatic and pursed-lip breathing *to improve ventilation and reduce air trapping.*
- Keep the client in high-Fowler's position *to improve ventilation.*
- Maintain the client's diet and administer small, frequent feedings *to avoid fatigue when eating. Small meals relieve pressure on the diaphragm and allow fuller lung movement.*
- Consult a registered dietitian *to meet the client's nutritional needs.*
- Monitor and record the color, amount, and consistency of sputum. *Changes in sputum may signal a respiratory infection.*
- Monitor laboratory studies *to identify potential problems.* Track drug levels for evidence of toxicity. *Electrolyte imbalances may occur with the use of diuretics. Reduced Hb level and HCT affect the oxygen-carrying capacity of the blood.*
- Monitor intake and output and daily weights *to detect fluid overload and edema associated with right-sided heart failure. Dehydration may impair the removal of secretions.*
- Encourage fluids, unless contraindicated, *to liquefy secretions.*
- Provide chest physiotherapy, postural drainage, incentive spirometry, and suction *to aid removal of secretions.*

Evaluation

- The client has adequate gas exchange as exhibited by stable ABG levels.
- The client reports increased energy and tolerance of activities of daily living.
- The client has maintained stable weight.

LEGIONNAIRES' DISEASE

LEGIONNAIRES' DISEASE is an acute type of bronchopneumonia, an inflammation of the lungs that begins in the terminal bronchioles. It's produced by a fastidious, gram-negative bacillus (rod-shaped bacterium).

This disease may occur epidemically or sporadically, usually in late summer or early fall. Its severity ranges from a mild illness, with or without pneumonitis, to multilobar pneumonia, with a mortality as high as 15%. A milder, self-limiting form (Pontiac syndrome) subsides within a few days but leaves the client fatigued for several weeks; this form mimics Legionnaires' disease but produces few or no respiratory symptoms, no pneumonia, and no fatalities.

Possible causes

- *Legionella pneumophila*

Assessment findings

- Cough that's initially nonproductive but that can eventually produce grayish, nonpurulent, blood-streaked sputum
- Dyspnea
- Pleuritic chest pain
- Fine crackles
- Delirium
- Heart failure
- Renal failure
- Shock
- Fever
- Recurrent chills
- Malaise
- Generalized weakness
- Bradycardia
- Headache
- Diffuse myalgias
- Anorexia
- Diarrhea
- Mental sluggishness
- Amnesia (mild, temporary)

Diagnostic evaluation

- Blood tests show leukocytosis, increased ESR, increased liver enzyme levels (alanine aminotransferase, aspartate aminotransferase, alkaline phosphatase), and hyponatremia.
- Chest X-ray shows patchy, localized infiltration, which progresses to multilobar consolidation (usually involving the lower lobes), pleural effusion and, in fulminant disease, opacification of the entire lung.
- Direct immunofluorescence of *L. pneumophila* and indirect fluorescent serum antibody testing compare findings from initial blood studies with findings from those done at least 3 weeks later. A convalescent serum sample showing a fourfold or greater rise in antibody titer for *L. pneumophila* confirms the diagnosis.
- Sputum test eliminates other organisms.

Nursing diagnoses

- Impaired gas exchange
- Ineffective tissue perfusion (cardiopulmonary)
- Hyperthermia

Treatment
◆ Oxygen therapy, which may require intubation and mechanical ventilation

Drug therapy options
◆ Antibiotics: erythromycin (Erythrocin), rifampin (Rifadin)
◆ Antipyretics: acetaminophen (Tylenol), aspirin
◆ Inotropic agent: dopamine (Intropin)

Planning and goals
◆ The client will have adequate gas exchange.
◆ The client will maintain adequate ventilation.
◆ The client will remain normothermic.

Implementation
◆ Closely monitor the client's respiratory status. Evaluate chest wall expansion, depth and pattern of respirations, cough, and chest pain *to detect respiratory decompensation.*
◆ Continually monitor the client's vital signs, pulse oximetry or ABG values, LOC, and dryness and color of the lips and mucous membranes. Watch for signs of shock (decreased blood pressure, thready pulse, diaphoresis, clammy skin) *to avoid crisis.*
◆ Keep the client comfortable; avoid chills and exposure to drafts, *which increase metabolic demands.* Provide mouth care frequently. If necessary, apply soothing cream to the nostrils *to promote comfort and prevent skin breakdown.*
◆ Replace fluid and electrolytes as needed *to maintain homeostasis.* The client with renal failure may require dialysis.
◆ Provide mechanical ventilation and other respiratory therapy as needed *to promote oxygenation.*
◆ Give antibiotics as necessary to eradicate infection, and observe carefully for adverse effects *to prevent complications.*

Evaluation
◆ The client has adequate gas exchange as evidenced by stable pulse oximetry and ABG levels.
◆ The client has maintained a normal temperature.

LUNG CANCER
In lung cancer, unregulated cell growth and uncontrolled cell division result in the development of a neoplasm. Cancer may also reach the lungs due to metastasis from other organs, mainly the liver, brain, bone, kidneys, and adrenal glands.

Four histologic types of lung cancer include:
◆ squamous cell (epidermoid), a slow-growing cancer that originates from bronchial epithelium. It metastasizes late to the surrounding area, but may cause bronchial obstruction.
◆ adenocarcinoma, a moderately growing cancer located in peripheral areas of the lung. It metastasizes through the bloodstream to other organs.
◆ large-cell anaplastic, a very fast-growing cancer associated with early and extensive metastasis. It's more common in peripheral lung tissue.
◆ small-cell (oat cell cancer), a very fast-growing cancer that metastasizes very early through lymph vessels and the bloodstream to other organs.

Possible causes
◆ Cigarette smoking
◆ Exposure to environmental pollutants, including second-hand smoke
◆ Exposure to occupational pollutants
◆ Familial susceptibility

Assessment findings
◆ Cough, hemoptysis
◆ Weight loss, anorexia
◆ Chest pain
◆ Chills, fever
◆ Dyspnea, wheezing
◆ Weakness, fatigue
◆ Gynecomastia
◆ Cushing's and carcinoid syndrome
◆ Bronchial obstruction
◆ Hoarseness, vocal cord paralysis

Diagnostic evaluation
◆ Bronchoscopy reveals a positive biopsy.
◆ CT scanning of the chest delineates tumor size and relationship.
◆ PET, bone marrow biopsy, or CT scanning of the brain or abdomen detects metastasis.
◆ Chest X-ray shows a lesion or mass.
◆ Lung scan shows a mass.
◆ Lung biopsy reveals a positive biopsy.
◆ Sputum study reveals positive cytology for cancer cells.

Nursing diagnoses
◆ Impaired gas exchange
◆ Activity intolerance
◆ Acute pain
◆ Imbalanced nutrition: Less than body requirements
◆ Risk for infection

Disposable drainage systems

Commercially prepared disposable drainage systems combine drainage collection, water seal, and suction control in one unit (as shown here). These systems ensure client safety with positive- and negative-pressure relief valves and have a prominent air-leak indicator. Some systems produce no bubbling sound.

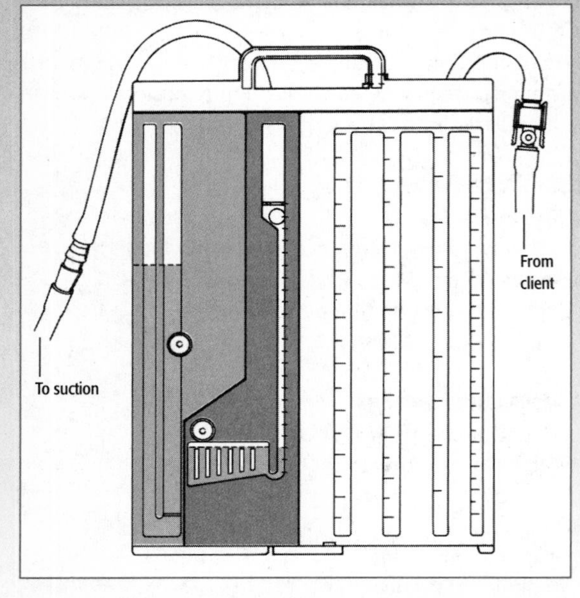

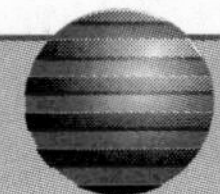

CLINICAL SITUATION

Caring for the client with lung cancer

A 55-year-old male client is diagnosed with lung cancer and is to receive radiation and chemotherapy. He expresses extreme anxiety over his diagnosis and treatment.

How can you reduce some of this client's anxiety?
Urge the client to express his concerns. Answer all questions honestly. Include family members or significant others in the discussion. Explain all procedures that the client will experience. Reassure the client that adverse effects will be treated and that the client's comfort is of utmost importance. Suggest that the client and family contact the American Cancer Society for information on local support groups.

Questions for future thought
- What measures could be done to decrease anxiety concerning future surgery for lung cancer?
- How would decreasing anxiety improve the client's recovery?

Treatment

- Dietary changes, including establishing a high-protein, high-calorie diet and providing small, frequent meals
- Incentive spirometry
- Laser therapy through a bronchoscope to destroy local tumor
- Oxygen therapy, intubation and, if the condition deteriorates, mechanical ventilation
- Radiation therapy
- Resection of the affected lobe (lobectomy) or lung (pneumonectomy) followed by chest drainage to maintain lung expansion (See *Disposable drainage systems*.)

Drug therapy options

- Analgesics: morphine sulfate, fentanyl (Sublimaze), oxycodone (OxyContin)
- Antiemetics: prochlorperazine (Compazine), ondansetron hydrochloride (Zofran)
- Antineoplastics: cyclophosphamide (Cytoxan), doxorubicin hydrochloride (Adriamycin), cisplatin (Platinol), vincristine (Oncovin)
- Diuretics: furosemide (Lasix), ethacrynic acid (Edecrin)

Planning and goals

- The client will maintain adequate ventilation.
- The client will carry out ADLs without weakness or fatigue.
- The client will express feelings of comfort and decreased pain and anxiety. (See *Caring for the client with lung cancer.*)
- The client will maintain adequate nutritional balance.
- The client won't exhibit signs of infection.

Implementation

- Assess respiratory status *to detect respiratory complications.* Cyanosis may suggest respiratory failure while an increase in sputum production may suggest an infection.
- Assess the client's pain and administer analgesics, as prescribed, *to control pain.* Assessment allows for care plan modification, as needed.

- Monitor and record vital signs *to assess for complications.* Tachycardia and tachypnea may indicate hypoxemia. An elevated temperature suggests an infection.
- Monitor and record intake and output *to assess fluid status.*
- Track laboratory values *to identify potential problems.* Monitor for bleeding, infection, and electrolyte imbalance due to effects of chemotherapy. *A low WBC count increases the risk of infection. Low platelets increase the risk of bleeding.* Electrolyte abnormalities, especially hypercalcemia, may also occur.
- Monitor pulse oximetry values and report a drop in oxygen saturation *to avoid hypoxemia.*
- Administer oxygen therapy *to maintain tissue oxygenation.*
- Encourage fluids and administer I.V. fluids *to provide hydration and liquefy secretions to facilitate removal. Drinking moistens mucous membranes.*
- Provide suctioning, and assist with turning, coughing, and deep breathing *to facilitate removal of secretions.*
- Keep the client in semi-Fowler's position *to maximize ventilation.*
- Administer TPN or enteral feeding, as indicated, *to optimize nutrition and bolster the immune system.*
- Administer medications, as prescribed, *to treat the cancer and provide pain relief.*
- Encourage the client to express feelings about changes in body image and a fear of dying *to reduce anxiety.*
- Maintain the chest drainage system if resection of the affected lobe or lung was performed *to maintain lung expansion.*
- Provide mouth care *to improve comfort and reduce the risk of stomatitis (with chemotherapy).* Provide skin care *to minimize adverse effects of radiation therapy.*
- Provide rest periods *to enhance tissue oxygenation.*
- Consult a registered dietitian *to help meet the client's nutritional needs.*
- Consult social services home care and hospice *to help meet the client's needs.*

Evaluation

- The client has adequate gas exchange as evidenced by stable pulse oximetry and ABG gas results.
- The client reports ability to perform ADLs without fatigue.
- The client maintains normal weight.
- The client remains free from infection.
- The client reports adequate pain control.

PLEURAL EFFUSION AND EMPYEMA

PLEURAL EFFUSION is an excess of fluid in the pleural space (the thin space between the lung tissue and the membranous sac that protects it). Normally, the pleural space contains a small amount of extracellular fluid that lubricates the pleural surfaces. Increased production or inadequate removal of this fluid results in pleural effusion.

There are two types of pleural effusion:

- TRANSUDATIVE PLEURAL EFFUSION, an ultrafiltrate of plasma containing low concentrations of protein, results when excessive hydrostatic pressure or decreased osmotic pressure causes excessive amounts of fluid to pass across intact capillaries.
- EXUDATIVE PLEURAL EFFUSION results when capillaries exhibit increased permeability with or without changes in hydrostatic and colloid osmotic pressures, allowing protein-rich fluid to leak into the pleural space.

EMPYEMA is the accumulation of pus and necrotic tissue in the pleural space. Blood (hemothorax) and chyle (chylothorax) may also collect in this space.

Possible causes

Transudative pleural effusion

- Disorders resulting in overexpanded intravascular volume
- Heart failure
- Hepatic disease with ascites
- Hypoalbuminemia
- Peritoneal dialysis

Exudative pleural effusion

- Bacterial or fungal pneumonitis or empyema
- Chest trauma
- Collagen disease (lupus erythematosus and rheumatoid arthritis)
- Malignancy
- Myxedema
- Pancreatitis
- Pulmonary embolism (with or without infarction)
- Subphrenic abscess
- Tuberculosis

Empyema

- Carcinoma
- Esophageal rupture
- Idiopathic disease
- Perforation
- Pneumonitis

Assessment findings

- Pleuritic chest pain
- Dyspnea
- Decreased breath sounds
- Fever
- Malaise

Diagnostic evaluation

- Chest X-ray shows radiopaque fluid in dependent regions.
- Thoracentesis shows lactate dehydrogenase (LD) levels less than 200 International units and protein levels less than 3 g/dl (in transudative effusions); ratio of protein in pleural fluid to serum greater than or equal to 0.5, LD in pleural fluid greater than or equal to 200 International units, and ratio of LD in pleural fluid to LD in serum greater than 0.6 (in exudative effusions); and acute inflammatory WBCs and microorganisms (in empyema).
- Tuberculin skin test rules out TB as the cause.

Nursing diagnoses

- Acute pain
- Impaired gas exchange
- Hyperthermia
- Risk for infection

Treatment

- Heimlich valve with chest tube
- Thoracentesis (to remove fluid)
- Thoracotomy if thoracentesis isn't effective

Drug therapy options

- Analgesic: morphine
- Antibiotic for empyema: according to infecting organism

Planning and goals

- The client will state that pain is decreased.
- The client will maintain adequate ventilation.
- The client will remain free from signs and symptoms of infection.
- The client will remain normothermic.

Implementation

- Explain thoracentesis to the client. Before the procedure, tell the client to expect a stinging sensation from the local anesthetic and a feeling of pressure when the needle is inserted *to allay the client's anxiety.*
- Instruct the client to tell you immediately if he feels uncomfortable or has trouble breathing during the procedure. *Difficulty breathing may indicate pneumothorax, which requires immediate chest tube insertion.*
- Reassure the client during thoracentesis *to allay anxiety.*
- Remind the client to breathe normally and to avoid sudden movements, such as coughing and sighing, *to prevent improper placement of the needle.*
- Monitor vital signs and watch for syncope *to prevent injury.*
- Watch for respiratory distress or pneumothorax (sudden onset of dyspnea, cyanosis) after thoracentesis *to detect complications of thoracentesis.*
- Administer oxygen *to improve oxygenation.*
- Administer antibiotics *to treat empyema.*
- Administer pain medication prior to deep-breathing and coughing exercises and ambulating or turning the client *to promote comfort.*
- Encourage the client to do deep-breathing exercises *to promote lung expansion.* Also encourage the use of an incentive spirometer *to promote deep breathing.*
- Provide meticulous chest tube care and use aseptic technique for changing dressings around the tube insertion site in empyema *to prevent infection at the insertion site.*
- Ensure chest tube patency by watching for bubbles in the underwater seal chamber *to prevent respiratory distress resulting from chest tube malfunction.*
- Record the amount, color, and consistency of tube drainage *to monitor the effectiveness of treatment.*
- Arrange visiting nurse referrals for clients who will be discharged with the tube in place *to evaluate the healing process.*

Evaluation

- The client is free from pain.
- The client has adequate gas exchange as evidenced by a stable pulse oximetry and ABG levels.
- The client has no complications caused by infection.
- The client has a normal temperature.

PLEURISY

Also known as *pleuritis,* PLEURISY is inflammation of the visceral and parietal pleurae, the serous membranes that line the inside of the thoracic cage and envelop the lungs.

Possible causes

- Cancer
- Chest trauma
- Dressler's syndrome
- Pneumonia

◆ Pulmonary infarction
◆ Rheumatoid arthritis
◆ Systemic lupus erythematosus
◆ TB
◆ Uremia
◆ Viruses

Assessment findings

◆ Sharp, stabbing pain that increases with respiration
◆ Pleural friction rub (a coarse, creaky sound heard during late inspiration and early expiration)
◆ Dyspnea
◆ Possible vibration felt with palpation over affected area

Diagnostic evaluation

Although diagnosis generally rests on the client's history and the nurse's respiratory assessment, diagnostic tests help rule out other causes and pinpoint the underlying disorder.

◆ ECG rules out CAD as the source of the client's pain.
◆ Chest X-rays and ultrasound can aid the diagnosis.

Nursing diagnoses

◆ Ineffective breathing pattern
◆ Acute pain
◆ Activity intolerance

Treatment

◆ Bed rest
◆ Thoracentesis (for pleurisy with pleural effusion)

Drug therapy options

◆ Analgesic: acetaminophen with oxycodone (Percocet)
◆ Anti-inflammatory: indomethacin (Indocin)
◆ Interstitial nerve block with local anesthetic: novacaine

Planning and goals

◆ The client will maintain adequate gas exchange.
◆ The client will express feelings of comfort and relief of pain.
◆ The client will demonstrate skill in conserving energy while carrying out ADLs to tolerance level.

Implementation

◆ Stress the importance of bed rest and plan your care *to allow the client as much uninterrupted rest as possible.*
◆ Administer pain medication as necessary *to relieve pain.*
– If the pain requires an opioid analgesic, warn the client about to be discharged to avoid overuse *because such medication depresses coughing and respiration.*
◆ Encourage the client to deep-breathe and cough while applying firm pressure at the pain site (splinting) during coughing exercises *to minimize pain.*

Evaluation

◆ The client has adequate gas exchange as evidenced by stable pulse oximetry and ABG levels.
◆ The client reports adequate pain control.
◆ The client reports increased activity level.

PNEUMOCYSTIS CARINII PNEUMONIA

The microorganism *Pneumocystis carinii* is part of the normal flora in most healthy people. However, in the immunocompromised client, *P. carinii* becomes an aggressive pathogen. *PNEUMOCYSTIS CARINII* PNEUMONIA (PCP) is an opportunistic infection strongly associated with HIV infection.

PCP occurs in up to 90% of HIV-infected clients in the United States at some point during their lifetime. It's the leading cause of death in these clients. Disseminated infection doesn't occur.

PCP is also associated with other conditions involving immunocompromise, including organ transplantation, leukemia, and lymphoma.

Possible causes

◆ *P. carinii*

Assessment findings

◆ Generalized fatigue
◆ Low-grade, intermittent fever
◆ Nonproductive cough
◆ Shortness of breath
◆ Dyspnea
◆ Tachypnea
◆ Anorexia
◆ Weight loss
◆ Crackles
◆ Decreased breath sounds
◆ Cyanosis
◆ Accessory muscle use

Diagnostic evaluation

◆ ABG analysis detects hypoxia and an increased alveolar-arterial gradient.
◆ Chest X-ray may show slowly progressing, fluffy infiltrates and, occasionally, nodular lesions or a spontaneous

pneumothorax, but these findings must be differentiated from findings in other types of pneumonia or ARDS.

◆ Fiber-optic bronchoscopy confirms PCP.

◆ Gallium scan may show increased uptake over the lungs, even when the chest X-ray appears relatively normal.

◆ Histologic studies confirm *P. carinii.* In clients with HIV infection, initial examination of a first-morning sputum specimen (induced by inhaling an ultrasonically dispersed saline mist) may be sufficient; however, this technique is usually ineffective in clients without HIV infection.

Nursing diagnoses

◆ Ineffective breathing pattern

◆ Impaired gas exchange

◆ Imbalanced nutrition: Less than body requirements

◆ Risk for infection

◆ Deficient knowledge regarding disease process and treatment

Treatment

◆ Dietary therapy to maintain adequate nutrition

◆ Oxygen therapy, which may include ET intubation and mechanical ventilation

Drug therapy options

◆ Antibiotics: co-trimoxazole (Bactrim), pentamidine (NebuPent)

Planning and goals

◆ The client will maintain adequate oxygenation and ventilation.

◆ The client will have adequate daily calorie intake.

◆ The client will remain free from infection.

◆ The client will verbalize understanding of the disorder and treatment.

Implementation

◆ Frequently assess the client's respiratory status and monitor ABG levels every 4 hours *to detect early signs of hypoxemia.*

◆ Administer oxygen therapy as necessary. Encourage the client to ambulate and to perform deep-breathing exercises and incentive spirometry *to facilitate effective gas exchange.*

◆ Administer antipyretics, as required, *to relieve fever.*

◆ Monitor intake and output and daily weight *to evaluate fluid balance.* Replace fluids as necessary *to correct fluid volume deficit.*

◆ Give antimicrobial drugs as required. Never give pentamidine I.M. *because it can cause pain and sterile abscesses.* Administer the I.V. drug form slowly over 60 minutes *to reduce the risk of hypotension.*

◆ Monitor the client for adverse reactions to antimicrobial drugs. If he's receiving co-trimoxazole, watch for nausea, vomiting, rash, bone marrow suppression, thrush, fever, hepatotoxicity, and anaphylaxis. If he's receiving pentamidine, watch for cardiac arrhythmias, hypotension, dizziness, azotemia, hypocalcemia, hyperkalemia, hyperglycemia, hypoglycemia, bronchospasm, and hepatic disturbances. *These measures detect problems early to avoid crisis.*

◆ Provide diversional activities and coordinate health care activities *to allow adequate rest periods between procedures.*

◆ Supply nutritional supplements as needed. Encourage the client to eat a high-calorie, protein-rich diet. Offer small, frequent meals if the client can't tolerate large amounts of food. Consult a registered dietitian regarding the client's diet. *These measures ensure that the client's nutritional intake meets metabolic needs.*

◆ Provide a relaxing environment, eliminate excessive environmental stimuli, and allow ample time for meals *to reduce anxiety.*

◆ Give emotional support and help the client identify and use meaningful support systems *to promote emotional well-being.*

◆ Provide education regarding the disease process and treatment *to ensure compliance with the treatment regimen.*

Evaluation

◆ The client has adequate gas exchange as evidenced by stable pulse oximetry and ABG levels.

◆ The client has maintained an appropriate weight.

◆ The client is free from infection.

◆ The client complies with the treatment regimen.

PNEUMONIA

PNEUMONIA is a bacterial, viral, parasitic, or fungal infection that causes inflammation of the alveolar spaces. In pneumonia, microorganisms enter alveolar spaces through droplet inhalation, resulting in inflammation and an increase in alveolar fluid. Ventilation decreases as secretions thicken.

Possible causes

◆ Aspiration

- Chemical irritants
- Organisms, such as *Escherichia coli, Haemophilus influenzae, Staphylococcus aureus, Pneumocystis carinii, Streptococcus pneumoniae,* and *Pseudomonas*

Assessment findings

- Shortness of breath, dyspnea, tachypnea, accessory muscle use
- Sputum production that's rusty, green, or bloody with pneumococcal pneumonia and yellow-green with bronchopneumonia
- Chills, fever
- Crackles, rhonchi, pleural friction rub on auscultation
- Cough
- Malaise
- Pleuritic pain
- Restlessness, confusion

Diagnostic evaluation

- ABG levels show hypoxemia and respiratory alkalosis.
- Chest X-ray shows pulmonary infiltrates.
- Hematology study shows increased WBCs and ESR.
- Sputum study identifies the causative organism.

(See *Caring for the client with pneumonia.*)

Nursing diagnoses

- Impaired gas exchange
- Ineffective airway clearance
- Imbalanced nutrition: Less than body requirements
- Hyperthermia

Treatment

- Chest physiotherapy, postural drainage, and incentive spirometry
- Dietary changes, including establishing a high-calorie, high-protein diet and forcing fluids
- Intubation and mechanical ventilation if condition deteriorates
- Nutritional support, including enteral nutrition if client requires intubation

Drug therapy options

- Antibiotics: according to susceptibility of infecting organism
- Antipyretics: aspirin, acetaminophen (Tylenol)
- Antitussive with codeine
- Bronchodilators: metaproterenol sulfate (Alupent), isoetharine (Bronkosol), albuterol (Proventil)
- Expectorants: guaifenisin (Robitussin, Mucinex)

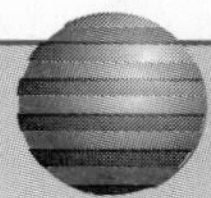

CLINICAL SITUATION

Caring for the client with pneumonia

A 60-year-old female client arrives at the clinic complaining of malaise, productive cough, fever with chills, and pleuritic chest pain.

Which diagnostic measures should be taken to confirm a diagnosis of pneumonia?

A. Chest X-ray, urinalysis, bronchoscopy
B. Chest X-ray, sputum and blood culture, complete blood count (CBC)
C. Throat culture, CBC, arterial blood gas (ABG) analysis
D. Throat culture, urinalysis, chest X-ray

Answer: B. Chest X-ray discloses infiltrates, confirming the diagnosis. Sputum specimen for Gram stain and culture and sensitivity shows acute inflammatory cells, and can direct antibiotic therapy. Blood cultures reflect bacteremia and help to determine the causative organism.

ABG analysis results help evaluate oxygenation but don't help diagnose pneumonia. A throat culture helps diagnose the causative agent of a sore throat; it doesn't diagnose pneumonia. Urinalysis helps diagnose a urinary tract infection.

White blood cell count indicates leukocytosis in bacterial pneumonia and a normal or low count in viral or mycoplasmal pneumonia. Bronchoscopy isn't necessary to diagnose pneumonia; however it may be necessary to remove secretions to isolate the causative organism if a sputum specimen can't be obtained.

Which nursing diagnoses would be appropriate when caring for a client with pneumonia?

A. Imbalanced nutrition: Less than body requirements
B. Impaired gas exchange
C. Ineffective airway clearance
D. Acute pain
E. Risk for deficient fluid volume
F. Risk for infection

Answer: All of these nursing diagnoses would apply to caring for a client with pneumonia.

Questions for further thought

- What measures would decrease the incidence of pneumonia in an elderly, pediatric, or immunosuppressed client?
- What teaching should be done to maximize oxygenation in a client with pneumonia?

Planning and goals

◆ The client will maintain adequate ventilation and oxygenation.
◆ The client will maintain appropriate weight.
◆ The client with be normothermic.

Implementation

◆ Monitor and record intake and output. *Insensible water loss secondary to fever may cause dehydration.*
◆ Monitor laboratory studies. *An elevated WBC count suggests infection. Blood and sputum cultures may identify the causative agent.*
◆ Monitor pulse oximetry *to detect respiratory compromise.*
◆ Assess respiratory status *to detect early signs of compromise.*
◆ Monitor and record vital signs. *An elevated temperature increases oxygen demands. Hypotension and tachycardia may suggest hypovolemic shock.*
◆ Monitor and record color, consistency, and amount of sputum. *Sputum amount and consistency may indicate hydration status and effectiveness of therapy. Foul-smelling sputum suggests respiratory infection.*
◆ Administer oxygen *to help relieve respiratory distress.*
◆ Consult a registered dietitian *to help meet the client's metabolic needs.*
◆ Force fluids to 3,000 ml/day and administer I.V. fluids *to help liquefy secretions and aid in their removal.*
◆ Provide suction and chest physiotherapy and assist with turning, coughing, and deep breathing *to promote mobilization and removal of secretions.*
◆ Administer medications, as prescribed, *to treat infection and improve ventilation.*
◆ Encourage the client to express feelings about fear of suffocation *to reduce anxiety.*
◆ Provide tissues and a bag for hygienic sputum disposal *to prevent spread of infection.*
◆ Provide oral hygiene *to promote comfort and improve nutrition.*

Evaluation

◆ The client has adequate oxygenation as evidenced by stable pulse oximetry and ABG levels.
◆ The client has maintained appropriate weight.
◆ The client is normothermic.

PNEUMOTHORAX AND HEMOTHORAX

In PNEUMOTHORAX, loss of negative intrapleural pressure results in the collapse of the lung. Pneumothorax may be described as spontaneous, open, or tension:
◆ Spontaneous pneumothorax results from the rupture of a bleb.
◆ Open pneumothorax occurs when an opening through the chest wall allows air to flow between the pleural space and the outside of the body.
◆ Tension pneumothorax results from a buildup of air in the pleural space that can't escape.

In all cases, the surface area for gas exchange is reduced, resulting in hypoxia and hypercapnia.

In HEMOTHORAX, blood accumulates in the pleural space when a rib lacerates lung tissue or an intercostal artery. This laceration compresses the lung and limits respiratory capacity. Hemothorax can also result from rupture of large or small pulmonary vessels.

Possible causes

◆ Blunt chest trauma
◆ Central venous catheter insertion
◆ Penetrating chest injuries
◆ Rupture of a bleb
◆ Thoracentesis
◆ Thoracic surgeries

Assessment findings

◆ Dyspnea, tachypnea, subcutaneous emphysema, cough
◆ Diminished or absent breath sounds unilaterally
◆ Sharp pain that increases with exertion
◆ Dullness on chest percussion (in the case of hemothorax and tension pneumothorax)
◆ Tracheal shift, decreased chest expansion unilaterally
◆ Paradoxical chest movement
◆ Anxiety
◆ Diaphoresis, pallor
◆ Hypotension (with hemothorax)
◆ Tachycardia

Diagnostic evaluation

◆ ABG levels show respiratory acidosis and hypoxemia.
◆ Chest X-ray reveals pneumothorax or hemothorax.
◆ Ventilation-perfusion scintigraphy is decreased.
◆ Lung scan shows ventilation-perfusion ratio mismatches.

Nursing diagnoses

◆ Impaired gas exchange

◆ Ineffective breathing pattern
◆ Acute pain
◆ Anxiety

Treatment
◆ Active ROM exercises to affected arm
◆ Blood transfusions for hemothorax, as indicated
◆ Chest tube to water-seal drainage
◆ Incentive spirometry
◆ Occlusive dressing (for open pneumothorax)
◆ Oxygen therapy
◆ Surgical repair

Drug therapy options
◆ Analgesic: morphine sulfate

Planning and goals
◆ The client will maintain adequate ventilation.
◆ The client will achieve a normal breathing pattern.
◆ The client will express feelings of comfort and a decrease in pain and anxiety.

Implementation
◆ Monitor and record vital signs. *Hypotension, tachycardia, and tachypnea suggest tension pneumothorax.*
◆ Check the chest drainage system for air leaks *that can impair lung expansion.*
◆ Monitor chest tube drainage *to ensure proper placement. An increase in the amount of bloody drainage suggests new bleeding or an increase in bleeding.* Check tubing for blockage or kinks if there's a sudden reduction in drainage.
◆ Assess respiratory status *to identify possible complications. Dyspnea, tachypnea, diminished breath sounds, subcutaneous emphysema, and use of accessory muscles suggest accumulation of air in the pleural space.*
◆ Assess cardiovascular status *to identify possible complications. Tachycardia, hypotension, and jugular vein distention suggest tension pneumothorax.*
◆ Assess the client's pain and administer medications, as prescribed, *to control pain.*
◆ Administer oxygen *to relieve respiratory distress caused by hypoxemia.*
◆ Assist with turning, coughing, deep breathing, and incentive spirometry *to enhance mobilization of secretions and prevent atelectasis.*
◆ Maintain chest tube to water-seal drainage *to prevent air from entering the chest tube when the client inhales.*
◆ Keep the client in high-Fowler's position, if tolerated and not contraindicated, *to enhance chest expansion.*

Evaluation
◆ The client has adequate gas exchange as evidenced by stable pulse oximetry and ABG levels.
◆ The client has a normal breathing pattern.
◆ The client reports adequate pain control and decreased anxiety.

PULMONARY EMBOLISM
PULMONARY EMBOLISM results from an undissolved substance (such as fat, air, or thrombus) in the pulmonary vessels that obstructs blood flow. The embolus travels from the venous circulation to the right side of the heart and pulmonary artery, obstructing blood flow and resulting in pulmonary hypertension and possible infarction.

Possible causes
◆ Abdominal, pelvic, or thoracic surgery
◆ Central venous catheter insertion
◆ Flat, long bone fractures
◆ Heart failure
◆ Hypercoagulability
◆ Malignant tumors
◆ Obesity
◆ Hormonal contraceptives
◆ Polycythemia vera
◆ Pregnancy
◆ Prolonged bed rest
◆ Sickle cell anemia
◆ Thrombophlebitis
◆ Venous stasis

Assessment findings
◆ Sudden onset of dyspnea, tachypnea, crackles
◆ Chest pain
◆ Tachycardia, arrhythmias
◆ Hypotension
◆ Anxiety
◆ Cough, hemoptysis
◆ Fever

Diagnostic evaluation
◆ ABG levels show respiratory alkalosis and hypoxemia.
◆ Blood chemistry tests reveal an increased LD level.
◆ Chest X-ray shows dilated pulmonary arteries, pneumoconstriction, and diaphragm elevation on the affected side.
◆ ECG shows tachycardia, nonspecific ST-segment changes, and right axis deviation.
◆ Pulmonary angiography shows the location of the embolism and the filling defect of pulmonary artery.

◆ Lung scan shows ventilation-perfusion mismatch.
◆ Spinal CT scanning may identify a thrombus in the pulmonary vasculature.

Nursing diagnoses

◆ Impaired gas exchange
◆ Ineffective tissue perfusion (cardiopulmonary)
◆ Anxiety
◆ Deficient knowledge related to disease condition and therapy

Treatment

◆ Bed rest with active and passive ROM and isometric exercises
◆ Vena cava filter insertion, or other surgery (vena cava ligation or plication)
◆ Oxygen therapy, intubation, and mechanical ventilation, if necessary

Drug therapy options

◆ Analgesic: morphine sulfate
◆ Anticoagulant: heparin followed by warfarin (Coumadin)
◆ Diuretic: furosemide (Lasix) if right ventricular failure develops
◆ Fibrinolytic: streptokinase (Streptase)

Planning and goals

◆ The client will have adequate gas exchange.
◆ The client will have improved tissue perfusion.
◆ The client will use support systems to assist with coping.
◆ The client will verbalize understanding of the disease and treatment regimen.

Implementation

◆ Assess respiratory status *to detect respiratory distress.*
◆ Assess cardiovascular status *to identify complications.* An irregular pulse may signal arrhythmia caused by hypoxemia. If pulmonary embolism is caused by thrombophlebitis, temperature may be elevated.
◆ Monitor laboratory studies *to identify possible problems.* Maintain PTT at 1½ to 2 times control in clients receiving heparin. Maintain PT at 1½ to 2 times control or INR at 2 to 3 for the client receiving warfarin. Monitor ABGs for evidence of pulmonary compromise.
◆ Monitor and record CVP. *CVP may rise if right-sided heart failure develops.*
◆ Monitor and record intake and output *to detect fluid volume overload and renal perfusion.*
◆ Assess for positive Homans' sign *to detect thromboembolism as a cause of pulmonary embolus.*
◆ Administer oxygen *to enhance arterial oxygenation.*
◆ Assist with turning, coughing, and deep breathing *to mobilize secretions and clear the airways.*
◆ Keep the client in high-Fowler's position *to enhance ventilation.*
◆ Provide suctioning and monitor and record color, consistency, and amount of sputum *to assess for complications.* A productive cough and blood-tinged sputum may be present with pulmonary embolism.
◆ Administer I.V. fluids, as ordered, *to maintain hydration.*
◆ Administer medications, as prescribed, *to enhance tissue oxygenation.*
◆ Assess for bleeding and prevent trauma to the client *to decrease the incidence of bleeding while on anticoagulant therapy.*
◆ Provide client teaching *to decrease the incidence of thrombophlebitis and embolism.*

Evaluation

◆ The client has adequate gas exchange and cardiac perfusion as evidenced by stable vital signs.
◆ The client demonstrates calm behavior and appropriate coping skills.
◆ The client verbalizes understanding of the underlying disease, causative factors, prevention, and treatment.

SARCOIDOSIS

SARCOIDOSIS is a multisystemic, granulomatous disorder (meaning it affects many body systems and produces nodules of chronically inflamed tissue). Sarcoidosis may lead to lymphadenopathy (disease of the lymph nodes), pulmonary infiltration, and skeletal, liver, eye, or skin lesions.

Sarcoidosis occurs most commonly in young adults (ages 20 to 40). In the United States, sarcoidosis occurs predominantly among blacks and affects twice as many women as men.

Acute sarcoidosis usually resolves within 2 years. Chronic, progressive sarcoidosis, which is uncommon, is associated with pulmonary fibrosis and progressive pulmonary disability.

Possible causes

Although the cause of sarcoidosis is unknown, the following explanations are possible:
◆ Hypersensitivity response (possibly from a T-cell imbalance) to such agents as mycobacteria, fungi, and pine pollen

◆ Genetic predisposition (suggested by a slightly higher incidence of sarcoidosis within the same family)
◆ Chemicals, such as zirconium or beryllium, which can lead to illnesses resembling sarcoidosis.

Assessment findings

Initial signs

◆ Arthralgia (in the wrists, ankles, and elbows)
◆ Fatigue
◆ Malaise
◆ Weight loss

Respiratory

◆ Substernal pain
◆ Breathlessness
◆ Cor pulmonale (in advanced pulmonary disease)
◆ Cough (usually nonproductive)
◆ Pulmonary hypertension (in advanced pulmonary disease)

Cutaneous

◆ Erythema nodosum
◆ Subcutaneous skin nodules with maculopapular eruptions
◆ Extensive nasal mucosal lesions

Ophthalmic

◆ Anterior uveitis (common)
◆ Glaucoma and blindness (rare)

Lymphatic

◆ Lymphadenopathy
◆ Splenomegaly (enlarged spleen)

Musculoskeletal

◆ Muscle weakness
◆ Pain
◆ Polyarthralgia (pain affecting many joints)
◆ Punched-out lesions on phalanges

Hepatic

◆ Granulomatous hepatitis (usually asymptomatic)

Genitourinary

◆ Hypercalciuria (excessive calcium in the urine)

Cardiovascular

◆ Arrhythmias (premature beats, bundle-branch block, or complete heart block)
◆ Cardiomyopathy (rare)

CNS

◆ Cranial or peripheral nerve palsies
◆ Basilar meningitis (inflammation of the meninges at the base of the brain)
◆ Seizures
◆ Pituitary and hypothalamic lesions producing diabetes insipidus

Diagnostic evaluation

◆ ABG analysis shows decreased PaO_2.
◆ Chest X-ray shows bilateral hilar and right paratracheal adenopathy with or without diffuse interstitial infiltrates; occasionally, large nodular lesions are present in lung parenchyma.
◆ Lymph node, skin, or lung biopsy reveals noncaseating granulomas with negative cultures for mycobacteria and fungi.
◆ Negative tuberculin skin test, fungal serologies, and sputum cultures for mycobacteria and fungi as well as negative biopsy cultures help rule out infection.
◆ Other laboratory data sometimes reveal increased serum calcium, mild anemia, leukocytosis, or hyperglobulinemia.
◆ Pulmonary function tests show decreased total lung capacity and compliance and decreased diffusing capacity.

Nursing diagnoses

◆ Impaired gas exchange
◆ Ineffective tissue perfusion (cardiopulmonary)
◆ Imbalanced nutrition: Less than body requirements
◆ Activity intolerance

Treatment

◆ Low-calcium diet and avoidance of direct exposure to sunlight (in clients with hypercalcemia)
◆ Oxygen therapy
◆ No treatment (for asymptomatic sarcoidosis)

Drug therapy options

◆ Systemic or topical steroid, if sarcoidosis causes ocular, respiratory, CNS, cardiac, or systemic symptoms (such as fever and weight loss), hypercalcemia, or destructive skin lesions

Planning and goals

◆ The client will maintain adequate ventilation and oxygenation.
◆ The client will maintain weight within normal parameters.
◆ The client will perform ADLs without fatigue.

Implementation

◆ Monitor laboratory results *to identify possible problems.* Be aware of abnormal laboratory results (anemia, for example) *that could alter client care.*

◆ For the client with arthralgia, administer analgesics as needed *to promote client comfort.* Record signs of progressive muscle weakness *to detect deterioration in the client's condition.*

◆ Provide a nutritious, high-calorie diet and plenty of fluids *to ensure that nutritional intake meets the client's metabolic needs.* If the client has hypercalcemia, suggest a low-calcium diet *to prevent complications of hypercalcemia, such as muscle weakness, heart block, hypertension, and cardiac arrest.* Weigh the client regularly *to detect weight loss.*

◆ Monitor respiratory function. Check chest X-rays for the extent of lung involvement; note and record bloody sputum or increase in sputum. If the client has pulmonary hypertension or end-stage cor pulmonale, check ABG values, watch for arrhythmias, and administer oxygen as needed. *These measures promptly detect deterioration in the client's condition.*

◆ Perform fingerstick glucose tests at least every 12 hours at the beginning of steroid therapy *because steroids may induce or worsen diabetes mellitus.*

◆ Assess for fluid retention, electrolyte imbalance (especially hypokalemia), moon face, hypertension, and personality changes, *which are adverse effects of steroids.*

◆ Instruct the patient to pace activity *to avoid fatigue.*

Evaluation

◆ The client has adequate gas exchange as evidenced by stable pulse oximetry and ABG levels.

◆ The client maintains adequate body weight.

◆ The client is able to perform ADLs without fatigue.

TUBERCULOSIS

TUBERCULOSIS (TB) is an airborne, infectious, communicable disease that can occur acutely or chronically. It occurs most commonly in lower socioeconomic groups and immigrants, and is associated with overwork, poor nutrition, and overcrowding combined with poor ventilation. Individuals with immunosuppression (for example, cancer or HIV) are at increased risk.

Inhaled mycobacteria, carried by droplet nuclei, usually settle in alveolar lung tissue, where they begin an inflammatory process. Cell-mediated immunity to the mycobacteria develops within 3 to 6 weeks and arrests the disease. If the infection reactivates, the inflammatory process can lead to necrosis in the center of the inflamed area, causing caseation (a process that changes dead tissue into a cheeselike substance). The caseum may localize, undergo fibrosis, or excavate and form cavities, the walls of which are studded with multiplying mycobacteria. If this occurs, infected caseous debris may spread by the tracheobronchial tree to other areas throughout the lungs.

Possible causes

◆ *Mycobacterium tuberculosis*

Assessment findings

◆ Cough, hemoptysis, or mucoid sputum

◆ Dyspnea

◆ Crackles

◆ Low-grade fever

◆ Night sweats, crackles

◆ Fatigue, malaise

◆ Anorexia

◆ Weight loss

◆ Pleuritic chest pain

Diagnostic evaluation

◆ Chest X-ray shows active or calcified lesions.

◆ Hematology shows increased WBC count and ESR.

◆ Sputum smear is positive for acid bacilli.

◆ Culture is positive for *M. tuberculosis.*

◆ Mantoux skin test result is positive. Induration is localized. The amount of induration considered positive ranges from 5 to 15 mm, depending on the risk category. Old infections may no longer be positive. A two-step method may be used to boost response.

Nursing diagnoses

◆ Ineffective airway clearance

◆ Ineffective tissue perfusion (cardiopulmonary)

◆ Ineffective health maintenance

◆ Imbalanced nutrition: Less than body requirements

◆ Deficient knowledge related to disease process and treatment

Treatment

◆ Standard airborne precautions (As long as the client is contagious, everyone entering the client's room must wear a respirator with high-efficiency particulate air filter.)

◆ Diet high in carbohydrates, protein, vitamins B_6 and C, and calories

◆ Chest physiotherapy, postural drainage, and incentive spirometry

Medications for clients with tuberculosis

These medications are commonly used to treat or to prevent tuberculosis (TB) in those who have been exposed. They are used in different combinations according to the client's age and condition.

Streptomycin
- Streptomycin is an aminoglycoside antibiotic and is used in combination with other antituberculotic drugs. It's administered only by deep I.M. injection.
- Central nervous system depression syndrome has been reported in infants on high doses.
- Avoid direct contact with the drug because sensitization may occur.
- Monitor the client for ototoxicity and nephrotoxicity.

Isoniazid (INH)
- Isoniazid is used to treat those with active TB and to prevent the disorder in high-risk clients.
- The oral form is best administered on an empty stomach.
- A client taking the drug should avoid tyramine- and histamine-containing foods.
- If the solution crystallizes, warm it to room temperature to dissolve the crystals.
- Monitor the client for visual changes.
- This drug causes vitamin B_6 deficiency. Monitor the client for paresthesia of the hands and feet, and administer pyridoxine as ordered.
- Monitor blood pressure for orthostatic hypotension.
- Monitor liver enzyme levels.
- Monitor weight.

Ethambutol (Myambutol)
- Ethambutol is an antituberculotic drug and is given with at least one other drug.
- Protect this drug from light, moisture, and heat.
- Monitor vision.
- Monitor hepatic and renal function.
- Monitor blood counts and serum uric acid levels.

Rifampin (Rifadin, Rimactane, Rofact)
- Rifampin is an antituberculotic drug and is given in combination with other antituberculotic drugs.
- Administer oral medication on an empty stomach.
- Monitor hepatic function.
- Monitor prothrombin time if the client is also taking an anticoagulant.
- Urine, feces, sputum, and sweat may be stained red-orange.
- Rifampin can decrease the effectiveness of hormonal contraceptives.

Pyrazinamide (Pyrazinamide, Tebrazid)
- Pyrazinamide may affect glycemic control in diabetics.
- Monitor hepatic function and uric acid levels.
- Encourage the client to drink plenty of fluids.

Drug therapy options
- Directly observed combination therapy with isoniazid (INH), rifampin (Rifadin), pyrazinamide (Pyrazinamide), and ethambutol (Myambutol). (Clients with atypical mycobacterial disease or drug-resistant TB require treatment with second-line drugs, such as streptomycin, capreomycin, para-aminosalicylic acid, cycloserine, amikain or quinolone.) (See *Medications for clients with tuberculosis.*)

Planning and goals
- The client will maintain a patent airway with adequate ventilation and oxygenation.
- The client will maintain adequate body weight.
- The client will verbalize understanding of the disease process and transmission and will comply with therapy.

Implementation
- Provide a negative-pressure room *to prevent the spread of infection.* (See *Guidelines for respiratory isolation,* page 406.)
- Monitor respiratory status, vital signs, and laboratory test results *to detect signs of respiratory compromise and adverse reactions to drug therapy.*
- If ordered, perform chest physiotherapy *to help mobilize secretions.*
- Encourage frequent oral hygiene *to promote comfort and appetite.*
- Encourage the client to eat foods rich in protein, calcium, and vitamins C, D, and B complex *to improve nutritional status.*
- Encourage the client to drink plenty of fluids *to liquefy sputum.*

> **Guidelines for respiratory isolation**
>
> Here are the guidelines to follow when providing care to a client in respiratory isolation:
> - ◆ Provide a private, negative-pressure room for the client, and keep the door closed.
> - ◆ Wash your hands before entering and leaving the client's room.
> - ◆ Use special handling procedures for sputum and secretions.
> - ◆ Have the client wear a mask when being transported outside the room.
> - ◆ Instruct everyone entering the client's room to wear a respirator with a high-efficiency particulate filter while the client is contagious.

◆ Administer medications as prescribed *to avoid development of drug-resistant organisms.*
◆ Teach the client the importance of following a prescribed regimen *to promote compliance.*
◆ Advise the client to cover his mouth when coughing, sneezing, or raising sputum *to reduce droplet transmission.*

Evaluation
◆ The client demonstrates adequate oxygenation through improvement in pulse oximetry and ABG levels.
◆ The client verbalizes understanding of the disease process, transmission, and treatment, and follows the medication regimen.
◆ The client maintains a normal weight.

MUSCULOSKELETAL SYSTEM

The musculoskeletal system has two main functions: to provide support and to produce movement. In addition, the musculoskeletal system protects internal tissues and organs, produces RBCs in the bone marrow, and stores mineral salts such as calcium.

MUSCULOSKELETAL STRUCTURE AND FUNCTION
The musculoskeletal system is made up of the skeleton, skeletal muscles, and associated structures, such as tendons and ligaments.

Bones, muscles, and other structures
◆ The skeleton consists of 206 bones that work with the muscles to support and protect internal organs. The bones store calcium, magnesium, and phosphorus. Bone marrow produces RBCs.
◆ Skeletal muscles are attached to the bones by tendons and provide body movement and posture by tightening and shortening. They begin contracting when stimulated by a motor neuron, and derive energy for muscle contraction from hydrolysis of adenosine triphosphate to adenosine diphosphate and phosphate. The skeletal muscles relax with the breakdown of acetylcholine by cholinesterase. Even then, they retain some contraction to maintain muscle tone.
◆ Ligaments and tendons are tough bands of collagen fibers. Ligaments connect bones to bones and encircle joints to add strength and stability. Tendons connect muscles to bones.
◆ Joints are formed by the articulation of two bone surfaces. Joints provide stabilization and permit locomotion. The degree of joint movement is called *range of motion (ROM).*
◆ The synovium is a membrane that lines a joint's inner surfaces. In conjunction with cartilage, the synovium reduces friction in joints through its production of synovial fluid.
◆ Cartilage is a specialized tissue that serves as a smooth surface for articulating bones. It absorbs shock to joints and serves as padding to reduce friction. Cartilage atrophies with limited ROM or in the absence of weight-bearing bursae (small sacs of synovial fluid).

MUSCULOSKELETAL DISORDERS

Disorders of the musculoskeletal system may be acute or chronic. Disorders include arm and leg fractures, carpal tunnel syndrome, compartment syndrome, gout, herniated disk, hip fracture, osteoarthritis, osteomyelitis, and osteoporosis.

ARM AND LEG FRACTURES
Fractures of the arms and legs usually result from trauma and commonly cause substantial muscle, nerve, and other soft-tissue damage. The prognosis varies with the extent of disability or deformity, the amount of tissue and vascular damage, the adequacy of reduction and immobilization, and the client's age, health, and nutritional status.

Children's bones usually heal rapidly and without deformity. Bones of adults in poor health and with impaired circulation may never heal properly. Severe open fractures, especially of the femoral shaft, may cause substantial blood loss and life-threatening hypovolemic shock.

Possible causes

- Bone tumors
- Trauma
- Osteoporosis

Assessment findings

- Discoloration
- Decreased sensory and motor function
- Pain
- Swelling
- Deformity
- Crepitus
- Diminished or absent distal pulses

Diagnostic evaluation

- Anteroposterior and lateral radiographs of the suspected fracture as well as radiographs of the joints above and below it confirm the diagnosis.
- CT scanning or MRI visualizes fracture and surrounding area.

Nursing diagnoses

- Impaired physical mobility
- Acute pain
- Deficient fluid volume
- Anxiety
- Deficient knowledge related to injury and treatment process.

Treatment

Emergency care

- Splinting the limb above and below the suspected fracture
- Cold-pack application and elevation of the extremity to reduce edema and pain
- Direct pressure to control bleeding in severe fractures that cause blood loss
- If blood loss occurs, fluid replacement as soon as possible to prevent hypovolemic shock

After confirming diagnosis

- Closed reduction (restoring displaced bone segments to their normal position), which is usually followed by splinting or casting
- Open reduction during surgery to reduce and immobilize the fracture using rods, plates, and screws when closed reduction is impossible
- Immobilization with a splint, cast, or traction
- Skin or skeletal traction (if splint or cast fails to maintain the reduction, or in elderly clients if surgery for hip fracture is delayed)

Open fractures

- Surgery to repair soft-tissue damage
- Thorough debridement of the wound

Drug therapy options

- Analgesics: codeine, morphine sulfate, acetaminophen, and oxycodone (Percocet)
- NSAID: ibuprofen (Motrin, Advil)
- Prophylactic antibiotics: cefazolin (Ancef), vancomycin (Vancocin)
- Tetanus prophylaxis: tetanus toxoid

Planning and goals

- The client's fracture will heal without complications.
- The client will have increased mobility.
- The client's fluid and electrolyte balance will be within normal parameters.
- The client will demonstrate decreased anxiety and verbalize relief from pain.
- The client will verbalize understanding of the treatment process and signs of complications to report.

Implementation

- Observe the client for signs of shock, such as rapid pulse, decreased blood pressure, pallor, and cool, clammy skin. *Severe open fracture of a large bone such as the femur can cause increased blood loss, leading to hypovolemic shock.*
- Assess the affected limb *for color, motion, sensation, temperature, and signs of compartment syndrome.* (See "Compartment syndrome," page 409.)
- Administer I.V. fluids as needed *to replace fluid loss.*
- Offer reassurance. *With any fracture, the client is likely to be frightened and in pain.*
- Ease pain with analgesics as needed *to promote comfort.*
- Reassure and help the client set realistic goals for recovery *to prevent frustration with the recovery process.*
- If the fracture requires long-term immobilization with traction, reposition the client often *to increase comfort and prevent pressure ulcers.* Assist with active ROM exercises *to prevent muscle atrophy.* Encourage deep breathing and coughing *to avoid hypostatic pneumonia.*

Cast care

Care of a client with a new cast should include these steps:

- Support and elevate a plaster cast with pillows while it's drying (up to 72 hours, depending on cast size) to maintain proper shape. Keep the cast dry at all times.
- Mark on the cast the time and date of any drainage sites. Observe for increases in these sites, which may indicate bleeding or infection beneath the cast.
- Demonstrate to the client proper body mechanics for movement with larger casts.
- Perform regular neurovascular checks.
- Tell the client to report extreme pain or pressure beneath the cast. Note any drainage or fever, which may indicate infection under the cast.
- Check the skin along the edges of the cast and protect it as necessary.
- Allow family or friends to sign the cast; however, discourage covering large areas of the cast with markings because this may obscure drainage sites.

- Make sure that the immobilized client receives adequate fluid *to prevent urinary stasis and constipation.* Watch for signs of renal calculi, such as flank pain, nausea, and vomiting, *to ensure early recognition and treatment.*
- Provide good cast care *to avoid skin breakdown.* (See *Cast care.*)
- Encourage the client to start moving around as soon as possible *to prevent complications of immobility.* Help him walk. (Remember that the client who has been bedridden for some time may be dizzy at first.)
- Demonstrate how to use crutches properly *to prevent injury.*
- After cast removal, refer the client for physical therapy *to restore limb mobility.*

Evaluation

- The client's fluid volume remains within normal parameters and circulation remains adequate to the distal extremity.
- The client learns safe mobility techniques such as crutch walking.
- The client verbalizes that pain is relieved or decreased.
- The client complies with required treatment of the injury.

CARPAL TUNNEL SYNDROME

CARPAL TUNNEL SYNDROME results from compression of the median nerve at the wrist, within the carpal tunnel. This nerve, along with blood vessels and flexor tendons, passes through to the fingers and thumb. Compression neuropathy causes sensory and motor changes in the median distribution of the hand. Carpal tunnel is the most common of the nerve entrapment syndromes.

Carpal tunnel syndrome usually occurs in women ages 30 to 60 and poses a serious occupational health problem. Assembly-line workers and packers, typists, and persons who repeatedly use poorly designed tools are most likely to develop this disorder. Any strenuous use of the hands — sustained grasping, twisting, or flexing — aggravates this condition.

Possible causes

- Flexor tenosynovitis (commonly associated with rheumatic disease)
- Nerve compression
- Physical trauma
- Pregnancy (due to hormonally induced swelling)
- Rheumatoid arthritis

Assessment findings

- Numbness, burning, or tingling
- Pain
- Weakness
- Atrophic nails

Diagnostic evaluation

- Physical examination reveals decreased sensation to light touch or pinpricks in the affected fingers. Thenar muscle atrophy occurs in about half of all cases of carpal tunnel syndrome. The client exhibits a positive TINEL'S SIGN (tingling over the median nerve on light percussion). He also responds positively to PHALEN'S WRIST-FLEXION TEST, in which holding the forearms vertically and allowing both hands to drop into complete flexion at the wrists for 1 minute reproduces symptoms of carpal tunnel syndrome.
- A blood pressure cuff inflated above systolic pressure on the forearm for 1 to 2 minutes provokes pain and paresthesia along the distribution of the median nerve.
- EMG detects a median nerve motor conduction delay of more than 5 msec.

Nursing diagnoses

- Chronic pain
- Impaired physical mobility
- Disturbed sensory perception (kinesthetic, tactile)

Treatment

◆ Resting the hands by splinting the wrist in neutral extension for 1 to 2 weeks (If a definite link has been established between the client's occupation and the development of carpal tunnel syndrome, he may have to seek other work.)
◆ Modifications in the work area, work duties, or recreation activities may be needed
◆ Correction of an underlying disorder
◆ Surgical decompression of the nerve by resecting the entire transverse carpal tunnel ligament or by using endoscopic surgical techniques (Neurolysis [releasing of nerve fibers] may also be necessary.)

Drug therapy options

◆ NSAIDs: indomethacin (Indocin), ibuprofen (Motrin), naproxen (Naprosyn)
◆ Corticosteroid (injections): betamethasone (Celestone), hydrocortisone (Hydrocortone)

Planning and goals

◆ The client will express feelings of comfort and pain relief.
◆ The client will maintain joint mobility and ROM.
◆ The client will maintain tactile and kinesthetic sensation.

Implementation

◆ Administer NSAIDs as needed *to reduce inflammation and pain.*
◆ Encourage the client to use his hands as much as possible *to maintain ROM.*
◆ If the client's dominant hand has been impaired, assist with eating and bathing as needed. *Mobility may be limited with carpal tunnel syndrome.*
◆ Regularly assess the client's degree of physical immobility *to evaluate the effectiveness of the current treatment plan.*
◆ After surgery, monitor vital signs and regularly check the color, sensation, and motion of the affected hand *to detect signs of compromised circulation.*
◆ Advise the client who's about to be discharged to occasionally exercise his hands. If the arm is in a sling, tell him to remove the sling several times per day and perform elbow and shoulder exercises *to maintain ROM.*

Evaluation

◆ The client reports adequate pain control.
◆ The client demonstrates functional joint mobility and ROM.
◆ The client reports decreased numbness and tingling and improved sensation.

COMPARTMENT SYNDROME

COMPARTMENT SYNDROME occurs when the pressure within a muscle and its surrounding structures increases. If the pressure becomes greater than diastolic blood pressure, circulation can be impaired or interrupted completely. Tissue damage occurs after 30 minutes; after 4 hours, irreversible damage may occur.

Possible causes

◆ Application of a dressing or cast that's too tight
◆ Burns
◆ Closed fracture injury
◆ Crushing injuries
◆ Muscle swelling after exercise

Assessment findings

◆ Severe or increased pain in the affected area with stretching or muscle elevation that's unrelieved by narcotics
◆ Tense, swollen muscle
◆ Decreased movement, strength, and sensation
◆ Increased pain with muscle stretching
◆ Loss of distal pulse
◆ Numbness and tingling distal to the involved muscle
◆ Paralysis

Diagnostic evaluation

◆ Intracompartment pressure is elevated, as indicated by a compartment measuring device.

Nursing diagnoses

◆ Acute pain
◆ Impaired physical mobility
◆ Risk for peripheral neurovascular dysfunction

Treatment

◆ Fasciotomy
◆ Positioning affected extremity lower than the heart
◆ Removal of dressings or constrictive coverings of the area

Drug therapy options

◆ Analgesic: morphine sulfate
◆ NSAID: ibuprofen (Motrin)

Planning and goals

◆ The client will express feelings of comfort and pain relief.
◆ The client will maintain muscle strength and ROM.
◆ The client will maintain peripheral circulation.

Implementation

◆ Monitor vital signs *to detect early changes and prevent complications.*
◆ Monitor the affected extremity and perform neurovascular checks *to detect signs of impaired circulation.*
◆ Maintain the extremity in a position lower than the heart *to ensure adequate circulation and to reduce pressure.*
◆ Assess the client for pain and anxiety *because stress may lead to vasoconstriction.*
◆ Administer medications as ordered *to maintain or improve the client's condition.*
◆ Perform dressing changes after the fasciotomy and reinforce dressings frequently *to facilitate monitoring of the extremity.* (A large amount of bloody drainage should be expected.)

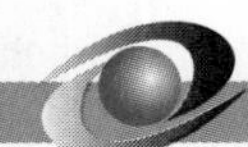

QUICK STUDY

Numbers to remember for compartment syndrome: 30 to 4. Tissue damage after 30 minutes; permanent damage after 4 hours.

Evaluation

◆ The client reports adequate pain control.
◆ The client has appropriate muscle strength and ROM.
◆ The client has adequate peripheral circulation.

GOUT

GOUT is a metabolic disease marked by urate deposits in the joints, which cause painfully arthritic joints. It can strike any joint but favors those in the feet and legs, most notably the joints of the great toes and ankles. Primary gout usually occurs in men older than age 30 and in postmenopausal women. Secondary gout occurs in older people.

Gout follows an intermittent course and commonly leaves clients free from symptoms for years between attacks. Gout can lead to chronic disability or incapacitation and, rarely, severe hypertension and progressive renal disease. The prognosis is good with treatment.

Possible causes

◆ Certain drugs, especially hydrochlorothiazide (Diuril), which interfere with urate excretion.
◆ Obesity, diabetes mellitus, hypertension, sickle cell anemia, and renal disease
◆ Genetic predisposition
◆ Increased uric acid

Assessment findings

◆ Inflamed, painful joints
◆ Hypertension
◆ Back pain

Diagnostic evaluation

◆ Arthrocentesis reveals the presence of monosodium urate monohydrate crystals or needlelike intracellular crystals of sodium urate in synovial fluid taken from an inflamed joint or a tophus.
◆ Blood studies show serum uric acid levels above normal. The urine uric acid level is usually higher in secondary gout than in primary gout.
◆ X-ray examination results are initially normal. X-rays show damage of the articular cartilage and subchondral bone in chronic gout and outward displacement of the overhanging margin from the bone contour.

Nursing diagnoses

◆ Chronic pain
◆ Impaired physical mobility
◆ Risk for injury

Treatment

◆ Ambulation without bearing weight
◆ Immobilization and protection of the inflamed joints
◆ Local application of heat and cold
◆ Diet changes (with the goal of weight loss)

Drug therapy options

◆ Analgesic: acetaminophen
◆ Antigout drugs: colchicine, allopurinol (Zyloprim)
◆ Uricosuric drugs: probenecid (Benemid), sulfinpyrazone (Anturane)
◆ Alkalinizing drug: sodium bicarbonate
◆ Corticosteroids: betamethasone (Celestone), hydrocortisone (Hydrocortone)

Planning and goals

◆ The client will express feelings of comfort and pain relief.
◆ The client will maintain joint mobility and ROM.
◆ The client will remain free from injury.

Implementation

◆ Allow the client to be out of bed with the affected extremity elevated; use a bed cradle *to keep bedcovers off extremely sensitive, inflamed joints.*
◆ Give pain medication as needed, especially during acute attacks, *to promote comfort.*

◆ Apply hot or cold packs to inflamed joints *to promote comfort.*
◆ Administer anti-inflammatory medication and other drugs *to decrease inflammation and increase excretion of uric acid.*
◆ Be alert for GI disturbances with colchicine administration *to prevent complications.*
◆ Urge the client to drink plenty of fluids (up to 2 L per day) *to prevent formation of renal calculi.*
◆ When forcing fluids, record intake and output accurately *to detect fluid volume excess.*
◆ Be sure to monitor serum uric acid levels regularly *to evaluate the effectiveness of the treatment plan.*
◆ Alkalinize urine with sodium bicarbonate or another agent, as needed, *to prevent formation of renal calculi.*
◆ Make sure the client understands the importance of having serum uric acid levels checked periodically *to help ensure compliance.*
◆ Advise the client receiving allopurinol, probenecid, and other drugs to immediately report adverse effects, such as drowsiness, dizziness, nausea, vomiting, urinary frequency, and dermatitis, *to prevent complications.*
◆ Warn the client taking probenecid or sulfinpyrazone to avoid aspirin and other salicylates. *Their combined effect causes urate retention.*
◆ Inform the client that long-term colchicine therapy is essential during the first 3 to 6 months of treatment with uricosuric drugs or allopurinol *to prevent further acute attacks.*

Evaluation

◆ The client reports adequate pain control.
◆ The client demonstrates adequate joint mobility and ROM.
◆ The client hasn't experienced injury.

HERNIATED DISK

With a HERNIATED DISK (herniated nucleus pulposus), the intervertebral disk ruptures, causing a protrusion of the nucleus pulposus (the soft, central portion of a spinal disk) into the spinal canal. (See *What happens when a disk herniates.*) This protrusion causes compression of the spinal cord or nerve roots, resulting in pain, numbness, and loss of motor function. The neurologic deficits experienced vary in relation to the level of the spinal cord involved, with lumbosacral levels L4, L5, and S1 and cervical levels C5, C6, and C7 being the most common levels involved. Herniation typically occurs on only one side due to vertical support provided by the longitudinal ligament. Subsequently, pain and neurologic deficits are usually experienced on only one side of the body.

What happens when a disk herniates

The spinal column is made up of vertebrae that are separated by cartilage called *disks*. Within each disk is a soft, gelatinous center (nucleus pulposus) that acts as a cushion during vertebral movement. When there's severe trauma or strain or intervertebral joint degeneration, the outer ring of the disk or anulus fibrosus can weaken or tear, and the nucleus pulposus is forced through this opening. The extruded disk can impinge on the spinal nerve root or the spinal cord.

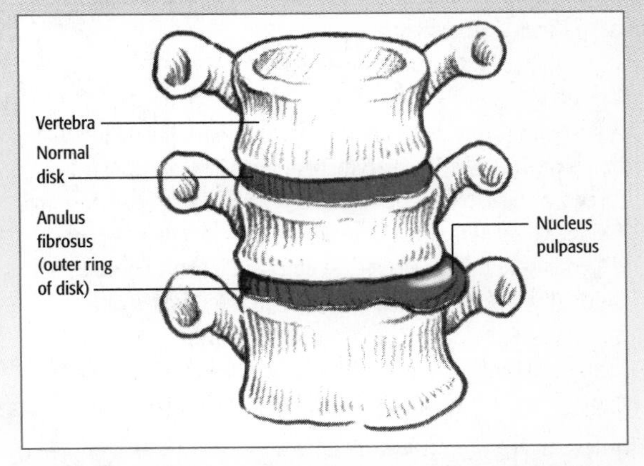

Possible causes

◆ Accidents, trauma
◆ Congenital or developmental bone deformity
◆ Degeneration of disk

Assessment findings

Cervical area

◆ Neck pain that radiates down the arm to the hand
◆ Neck stiffness
◆ Weakness of affected upper extremities with numbness and tingling of the hand
◆ Atrophy of biceps and triceps

Lumbosacral area

◆ Acute pain in the lower back radiating across the buttock and down the leg
◆ Pain on ambulation
◆ Weakness, numbness, and tingling of the foot and leg

Surgeries for ruptured disk

Laminectomy or hemilaminectomy

A laminectomy or hemilaminectomy consists of removing the vertebral lamina (wing) to gain access to the disk area. The disk pieces are then removed from the annulus, the cartilage ring between the vertebrae. After a laminectomy, the client can get up (on the same day, if able) and move with minimal restrictions. Recovery proceeds fairly steadily after the ruptured disk pieces are removed, relieving nerve pressure and pain. The client should be taught proper lifting techniques to prevent additional trauma, and exercises to strengthen back and abdominal muscles after discharge.

Spinal fusion

A spinal fusion involves laminectomy to remove the ruptured disk pieces followed by placement of bone inserts (grafts), screws, or pins to fuse the vertebral segments solidly. After spinal fusion, the client may require bed rest for 1 to 3 days or more, depending on the fusion type. At times, a client may need a brace, which helps stabilize the fused parts for the lengthy healing time required (9 to 12 months for solid fusion). Postoperatively, the client must be positioned with the logrolling maneuver and will have limited ability to bend when the fusion heals.

Chemonucleolysis

Chemonucleolysis is the dissolution of ruptured disk pieces by injecting chymopapain, an enzyme from the papaya plant, into the affected disk. The enzyme dissolves the disk, which is replaced with scar tissue. Chymopapain can elicit severe anaphylactic responses and may result in death. Preoperative preparation includes obtaining a thorough allergy history and administering I.V. preoperative corticosteroids, antihistamines, and cimetidine to block histamine release.

Postoperatively, the client may have back muscle spasms of varying intensity and duration. Pain relief may be temporary, with pain returning 6 or more months later, possibly from scar tissue formation. The safety and effectiveness of this procedure is controversial. Although initial enthusiasm for chemonucleolysis appears to be waning, the procedure is still being performed. For some clients, results have been good; other clients have resorted to laminectomy.

Microdiskectomy

Microdiskectomy is similar to laminectomy but requires an incision measuring 1″ to 3″ (2.5 to 7.5 cm); only the disk fragments are removed, and recovery is faster. Sometimes, multiple operations are required because of retained disk fragments.

- Straightening of normal lumbar curve with scoliosis away from the affected side

Diagnostic evaluation

- Deep-tendon reflexes are depressed or absent in the affected extremity.
- EMG shows spinal nerve involvement.
- Lasègue's sign is positive.
- MRI depicts disk bulges and protrusions.
- Myelography and contrast-enhanced CT show compression of the spinal cord.
- Radiography shows a narrowing of disk space.

Nursing diagnoses

- Acute pain
- Activity intolerance
- Impaired physical mobility

Treatment

- Bed rest with knees slightly bent and active and passive ROM and isometric exercises
- Diet that includes increased fiber and fluids
- Heating pad and moist, hot compresses
- Orthopedic devices, including back brace and cervical collar
- Transcutaneous electrical nerve stimulation (TENS)
- Laminectomy, spinal fusion, chemonucleolysis, or microdiskectomy (see *Surgeries for ruptured disk*)

Drug therapy options

- Corticosteroid: cortisone (Cortone)
- Fecal softeners or fiber stimulants: docusate sodium (Colace), psyllium (Metamucil)
- Muscle relaxants: cyclobenzaprine (Flexeril), diazepam (Valium), metaxalone (Skelaxin)
- Analgesics: codeine, morphine sulfate, oxycodone (OxyContin)
- NSAIDs: ibuprofen (Motrin), indomethacin (Indocin), ketorolac tromethamine (Toradol), naproxen (Naprosyn), piroxicam (Feldene)

Planning and goals

- The client will tolerate increased activity.
- The client will regain musculoskeletal and neurologic tissue function without complications.
- The client will verbalize understanding of the implications of a spinal injury and will participate in rehabilitation.

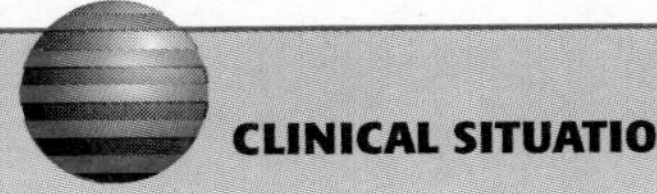

CLINICAL SITUATION

Caring for a client with a compression fracture

A 40-year-old male construction worker is hospitalized after falling from a scaffold. He complains of bilateral numbness of his fourth and fifth toes and pain that radiates down his buttocks and the back of his thighs. Radiographic studies indicate that the client has a compression fracture of the fourth lumbar vertebra (L4). He's admitted to the orthopedic unit for further evaluation and treatment.

Describe the appropriate conservative treatment for a client with a compression fracture.

Conservative treatment includes bed rest with active and passive range-of-motion and isometric exercises; heating pad and moist, hot compresses; orthopedic devices; and transcutaneous electrical nerve stimulation.

Name potential surgical interventions for a client with a compression fracture.

Surgical intervention may include laminectomy, spinal fusion, chemonucleolysis, or microdiskectomy.

Questions for further thought

- Why does the nurse need to continue to assess *all* body systems?
- What are some key assessments when checking the client's neurovascular status? What findings could indicate progression of symptoms?
- What should be included in client teaching if the client is placed in a body cast?

Implementation

- Assess neurovascular status *to determine a baseline and detect early changes.*
- Monitor and record vital signs, intake and output, and results of laboratory studies *to detect changes in the client's condition.*
- Maintain the client's diet; increase fluid intake *to maintain hydration.*
- Keep the client in semi-Fowler's position with moderate hip and knee flexion *to promote comfort.*
- Administer medications, as prescribed, *to maintain or improve the client's condition.*
- Encourage the client to express feelings about changes in his body image and fears of disability *to help him resolve feelings.*
- Provide skin and back care *to promote comfort and prevent skin breakdown.*
- Turn the client every 2 hours using the logrolling technique *to prevent injury.*
- Continue bed rest and body alignment *to maintain joint function and prevent neuromuscular deformity.*
- Maintain traction, braces, and cervical collar *to prevent further injury and promote healing.*
- Promote independence in ADLs *to maintain self-esteem.*

Evaluation

- The client is regaining full motor and sensory functions in the limb as healing continues.
- The client has regained limited mobility initially, working up to full rehabilitation. (See *Caring for a client with a compression fracture.*)

HIP FRACTURE

A fracture occurs when too much stress is placed on the bone in relation to its stress tolerance. As a result, the bone breaks and local tissue becomes injured, causing muscle spasm, edema, hemorrhage, compressed nerves, and ecchymosis.

Sites of hip fractures include intracapsular (within the capsule of the femur), extracapsular (outside the capsule of the femur), intertrochanteric (within the trochanter), and subtrochanteric (below the trochanter).

Possible causes

- Aging
- Bone tumors
- Cushing's syndrome
- Immobility
- Malnutrition
- Multiple myeloma
- Osteomyelitis
- Osteoporosis
- Steroid therapy
- Trauma (especially falls)

Assessment findings

◆ Shorter appearance and outward rotation of affected leg resulting in limited or abnormal ROM
◆ Edema and discoloration of surrounding tissue
◆ Pain in the affected hip and leg, exacerbated by any movement
◆ History of a fall or other trauma to the bones

Diagnostic evaluation

◆ CT (for complicated fractures) scanning pinpoints abnormalities.
◆ Hematologic studies show decreased hemoglobin level and hematocrit.
◆ Radiography reveals a break in the continuity of the bone.

Nursing diagnoses

◆ Acute pain
◆ Deficient fluid volume
◆ Impaired physical mobility

Treatment

◆ Abductor splint or trochanter roll between legs to maintain alignment
◆ Skin traction, such as Buck's or Russell's until surgically corrected (see *Types of skin traction*)
◆ Surgical immobilization or joint replacement

Drug therapy options

◆ Analgesics: codeine, meperidine (Demerol), morphine sulfate
◆ NSAIDs: ibuprofen (Motrin), naproxen (Naprosyn)

Planning and goals

◆ The client will avoid complications from injury or treatment.
◆ The client will increase physical mobility through use of a walker.
◆ The client will use appropriate supportive services, such as physical therapy and home health care.

Implementation

◆ Assess neurovascular and respiratory status. Most important, check for compromised circulation, hemorrhage, and neurologic impairment in the affected extremity and pneumonia in the bedridden client *to detect changes and prevent complications.*
◆ Monitor and record vital signs, intake and output, and results of laboratory studies *to detect early changes in the client's condition.*
◆ Maintain the client's diet; increase fluid intake *to maintain hydration.*
◆ Keep the client in a flat position with the foot of the bed elevated 25 degrees when in traction *to prevent further injury.*
◆ Keep the legs abducted and avoid hip flexion greater than 90 degrees *to prevent dislocation of the hip joint.*
◆ Administer medications, as prescribed, *to improve or maintain the client's condition.*
◆ Provide skin care, and logroll the client every 2 hours *to maintain skin integrity and prevent pressure ulcers.*
◆ Assist with coughing, deep breathing, and incentive spirometry *to maintain a patent airway.*
◆ Keep the hip extended *to prevent further injury and maintain circulation.*
◆ Promote independence in ADLs *to promote self-esteem.*
◆ Provide active and passive ROM and isometric exercises for unaffected limbs *to maintain joint mobility.*
◆ Provide an over-the-bed trapeze *to promote independence in self-care.*
◆ Maintain traction at all times *to ensure proper body alignment and promote healing.*
◆ Keep side rails up *to prevent injury.*
◆ Provide appropriate sensory stimulation with frequent reorientation *to reduce anxiety.*
◆ Encourage increased fiber, fluids, and activity, as allowed, as well as medication, as needed, *to prevent constipation.*
◆ Provide diversional activities *to reduce boredom.*
◆ Apply antiembolism stockings or a sequential compression device *to promote venous circulation.*

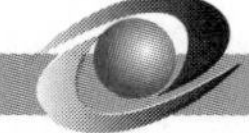

QUICK STUDY

Remember, don't **CFR** a **THR.** That means don't:

Cross
Flex
Rotate
a
Total
Hip
Replacement.

Types of skin traction

This chart lists types of skin traction, along with the site, appropriate weight, and care factors for each. Although each traction type has unique application and care factors, all types require neurovascular assessments of the client to ensure that circulation remains adequate.

TRACTION TYPE	APPLICATION SITE	WEIGHT	CARE FACTORS
Buck's extension	Arm or leg (one or both)	5 to 7 lb per extremity	◆ Clean and dry the skin. Be sure the client has no open cuts or wounds. ◆ Make sure equipment (tape, bandages, traction straps, or boot) is new (when appropriate) and functioning properly. ◆ Remove the traction apparatus to care for and observe tissues. ◆ Keep the client recumbent to obtain the most effective traction. ◆ Teach the client how to use traction at home.
Russell's extension	Leg only (one or both)	5 to 10 lb per leg	◆ Arrange pulleys and ropes, and determine the weight by applying the principle "for every force in one direction, there's an equal force in the opposite direction." ◆ Loosen the knee sling for care and observation. ◆ Keep the client recumbent. ◆ Remove the traction to care for the client. (Always check with the physician before removing it.)
Pelvic belt	Around abdomen and pelvis, like a girdle	20 to 35 lb	◆ Use for conservative low-back pain and possible ruptured disk. ◆ Use traction intermittently and never at night. ◆ Keep the client recumbent, with knees and hips flexed at 45-degree angles. ◆ Teach the client how to use traction at home.
Pelvic sling	Under the pelvis, like a hammock	20 to 35 lb	◆ Use for stable pelvic bone fractures. ◆ Advise the client to stay in the sling except when it's removed for care. ◆ Wean the client from the sling to prevent dependency. ◆ Keep the sling clean and dry to prevent pressure areas. ◆ Position the client's buttocks slightly off the bed to ensure correct use of the sling. ◆ One person can remove the client from the sling, but two are needed to reapply it to center the client properly.
Head halter	Under the chin and around the skull base	5 to 15 lb (8 to 10 lb most common)	◆ Use for neck muscle disorders, degenerative cervical conditions, and (rarely) cervical vertebral fractures. ◆ Explain that the pull comes mostly from the occipital area of the halter, not from the chin. ◆ Tell the client that pressure exerted on the chin reverts to the temporomandibular joint, causing pain and soreness when chewing.

(continued)

Types of skin traction *(continued)*

TRACTION TYPE	APPLICATION SITE	WEIGHT	CARE FACTORS
Head halter *(continued)*			◆ Remove the client from the traction for care before inserting skull tongs. (If the client has a fractured cervical vertebra, only the physician removes the traction.) ◆ Show the client (especially one with arthritis) how to use traction at home. ◆ Avoid pressure exerted over the facial nerve by a halter that's too small or incorrectly applied.
90-90 (ninety-ninety)	Lower legs and thighs	5 to 15 lb	◆ Relieves lumbosacral muscle spasms by applying the principle of 90-degree angle of knees and hips. ◆ Keep the client flat in bed while in this traction. ◆ Use traction intermittently, and usually not at night.
Dunlop's	Humerus	8 to 15 lb	◆ Use for humeral fractures to decrease muscle spasms and align bone fragments. ◆ Hold the client's forearm in Buck's extension vertically, with the elbow at a 90-degree angle to the arm for the most effective traction. ◆ Keep the client recumbent for effective traction.
Cotrel's	Head halter to the head and a pelvic belt to the pelvis	8 to 15 lb for head halter; 15 to 30 lb for pelvic belt	◆ Use to assist straightening scoliotic curvature (commonly used before brace application or surgical correction). ◆ Maintain the client flat in bed so that the spine is pulled lengthwise in opposite directions by the head halter and pelvic belt. ◆ Use intermittently but not at night unless curvature and muscle spasms are severe.

Evaluation

- The client avoids complications from the injury or treatment.
- The client uses a walker effectively to increase mobility.
- The client uses supportive services appropriately.

OSTEOARTHRITIS

OSTEOARTHRITIS, also known as *degenerative joint disease,* is characterized by degeneration of cartilage in weight-bearing joints, such as the spine, knees, and hips. It occurs when cartilage softens with age, narrowing the joint space. This softening allows bones to rub together, causing pain and limiting joint movement. Osteoarthritis also occurs in the small joints of the hands and feet. Heberden's nodules usually occur in distal joints of the hands.

Osteoarthritis can be primary or secondary. Primary osteoarthritis, a normal part of aging, results from metabolic, genetic, chemical, and mechanical factors. Secondary osteoarthritis usually follows an identifiable cause, such as obesity and congenital deformity, and leads to degenerative changes. A client suffering from rheumatoid arthritis who's receiving long-term corticosteroid therapy is also at risk for osteoarthritis. (See *Comparing rheumatoid arthritis to osteoarthritis.*)

Possible causes

- Aging
- Chemical causes
- Congenital abnormalities
- Joint trauma
- Metabolic changes
- Obesity

Comparing rheumatoid arthritis to osteoarthritis

This chart lists characteristics of rheumatoid arthritis and osteoarthritis.

RHEUMATOID ARTHRITIS	OSTEOARTHRITIS
◆ Systemic disease: affects multiple body systems	◆ Local disease of joints only
◆ Affects synovial membranes initially, then other joint structures	◆ Affects cartilage initially, then other joint structures
◆ Affects symmetrical joints bilaterally; affects proximal joints and smaller joints most commonly	◆ Asymmetrical joint involvement; distal joints and larger weight-bearing joints most likely to be involved
◆ Multiple subcutaneous nodules under skin surfaces, not in joints	◆ Bony enlargements of distal joints common (Heberden's nodes)
◆ Dislocations, subluxations (partial dislocations), and deformities common (swan-neck and boutonnière deformities of joints such as the hands)	◆ Dislocation and subluxation uncommon; deformity from bony outgrowths
◆ Signs of inflammation: heat, fever, swelling, malaise, elevated erythrocyte sedimentation rate	◆ No systemic signs of inflammation; joints may be swollen but rarely hot
◆ Three times more common in women than in men; affects those ages 30 to 55	◆ Not gender-specific; affects those age 45 and older

Assessment findings
- Crepitation
- Enlarged, edematous joints
- Heberden's nodes
- Increased pain in damp, cold weather and late in day
- Joint stiffness in the morning and after exercise
- Limited ROM
- Pain relieved by resting joints
- Smooth, taut, shiny skin

Diagnostic evaluation
- Arthroscopy reveals bone spurs and narrowing of joint space.
- Radiography shows joint deformity, narrowing of joint space, and bone spurs.

Nursing diagnoses
- Impaired physical mobility
- Activity intolerance
- Chronic pain

Treatment
- Joint-protective exercises, such as walking, swimming, and water aerobics
- Canes or walkers or other supportive devices
- Cold therapy
- Heat therapy
- Low-calorie diet if the client is over optimal weight
- Isometric exercises
- Paraffin dips for hands
- Surgical treatment: arthroplasty, arthrodesis, osteoplasty, osteotomy

Drug therapy options
- Analgesic: aspirin
- Artificial joint fluids: Synvisc, Hyalgan
- Glucosamine
- Chondroitin sulfate
- Corticosteroids: intra-articular injections
- NSAIDs: diclofenac (Voltaren), diflunisal (Dolobid), flurbiprofen (Ansaid), ibuprofen (Motrin), indomethacin (Indocin), naproxen (Naprosyn), piroxicam (Feldene), sulindac (Clinoril)

Planning and goals
- The client's joint mobility will improve.
- The client will have an increased ability to perform ADLs.
- The client will state that pain is decreased.

Implementation
- Assess musculoskeletal status *to determine a baseline and detect changes.*
- Assess pain. *Correlating the client's pain with the time of day and visits may be useful in modifying tasks.*
- Keep joints extended *to prevent contractures and maintain joint mobility.*
- Administer medications as prescribed *to relieve pain and encourage mobility.*

◆ Assess for increased bleeding or bruising tendency *to facilitate early intervention for drug adverse effects.*
◆ Urge the client to express feelings about changes in body image *to promote effective communication about changes.*
◆ Provide rest periods *to conserve energy.*
◆ Maintain a calorie count *to promote nutrition and healing and keep weight within normal limits.*
◆ Provide moist compresses and paraffin baths (heat therapy) as prescribed *to promote comfort.*
◆ Teach proper body mechanics *to prevent injury.*
◆ Provide passive ROM exercises *to maintain joint mobility.*

Evaluation
◆ The client demonstrates improved mobility of joints.
◆ The client is able to perform ADLs.
◆ The client expresses a decreased amount of pain.

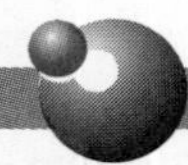

SPOT CHECK

When assessing a client with osteoarthritis of the knees, when are you most likely to detect crepitation?

Answer: Crepitus is a grating sensation associated with degenerative joint disease and it can be felt or heard. You're most likely to detect it during palpation of the affected joint.

OSTEOMYELITIS

OSTEOMYELITIS is a pyogenic (pus-producing) bone infection. It may be chronic or acute and commonly results from a combination of local trauma — usually quite trivial but resulting in hematoma formation — and an acute infection originating elsewhere in the body. Although osteomyelitis commonly remains localized, it can spread through the bone to the marrow, cortex, and periosteum (the membrane that covers the bone).

Acute osteomyelitis is usually a blood-borne disease that most commonly affects rapidly growing children. Chronic osteomyelitis (rare) is characterized by multiple draining sinus tracts and metastatic lesions.

Osteomyelitis occurs more commonly in children than adults — and particularly in boys — usually as a complication of an acute, localized infection. The most common sites in children are the lower end of the femur and the upper ends of the tibia, humerus, and radius. In adults, the most common sites are the pelvis and vertebrae, generally the result of contamination associated with surgery or trauma.

Possible causes
◆ Exposure to disease-causing organisms

Assessment findings
◆ Pain
◆ Tenderness
◆ Swelling

Diagnostic evaluation
◆ Blood and wound cultures identify the causative organism.
◆ ESR is elevated.
◆ WBC count shows leukocytosis.
◆ Bone scan shows the infection site.
◆ CT scanning and MRI delineate the extent of infection.

Nursing diagnoses
◆ Activity intolerance
◆ Acute pain
◆ Impaired physical mobility

Treatment
◆ Early surgical excision and drainage to relieve pressure buildup and sequestrum (dead bone that has separated from sound bone) formation
◆ High-protein diet with extra vitamin C
◆ Immobilization of the affected bone by plaster cast, traction, or bed rest
◆ I.V. fluids

Drug therapy options
◆ Antibiotics: broad-spectrum antibiotics after cultures are taken
◆ Analgesics: ibuprofen (Motrin), acetaminophen and oxycodone (Percocet)

Planning and goals
◆ The client will perform ADLs within the confines of the disease.
◆ The client will express feelings of comfort and pain relief.
◆ The client will maintain joint mobility and ROM.

Implementation
◆ Use strict aseptic technique when changing dressings and irrigating wounds *to prevent infection.*
◆ If the client is in skeletal traction for compound fractures, cover insertion points of pin tracks with small, dry dressings, and tell him not to touch the skin around the pins and wires *to prevent infection.*

◆ Administer I.V. fluids *to maintain adequate hydration as necessary.*
◆ Provide a diet high in protein and vitamin C *to promote healing.*
◆ Assess vital signs and wound appearance daily and monitor daily for new pain, *which may indicate secondary infection.*
◆ Support the affected limb with firm pillows. Keep the limb level with the body (don't let it sag) *to prevent injury.*
◆ Provide good skin care. Turn the client gently every 2 hours *to prevent skin breakdown,* and watch for signs of developing pressure ulcers *to ensure early intervention and treatment.*
◆ Provide good cast care. Support the cast with firm pillows and "petal" the edges with pieces of adhesive tape or moleskin to smooth rough edges *to prevent skin breakdown, which may lead to infection.*
◆ Check circulation and drainage. If a wet spot appears on the cast, circle it with a marking pen and note the time of appearance (on the cast). Be aware of how much drainage is expected. Check the circled spot at least every 4 hours. Watch for enlargement. *These measures help detect early signs of hemorrhage.*
◆ Protect the client from mishaps, such as jerky movements and falls, which may threaten bone integrity *to prevent injury.*
◆ Be alert for sudden pain, crepitus, or deformity. Watch for sudden malposition of the limb *to detect fracture.*
◆ Provide emotional support and appropriate diversions *to reduce anxiety.*

Evaluation

◆ The client reports the ability to adequately perform ADLs.
◆ The client reports adequate pain control.
◆ The client demonstrates adequate joint mobility and ROM.

OSTEOPOROSIS

In OSTEOPOROSIS, a metabolic bone disorder, the rate of bone resorption accelerates while the rate of bone formation slows down, causing a progressive loss of bone mass. Bones affected by this disease lose calcium and phosphate salts, and thus become porous, brittle, and abnormally vulnerable to fracture.

Osteoporosis may be primary or secondary to an underlying disease. Primary osteoporosis is typically called *senile* or *postmenopausal osteoporosis* because it most commonly develops in elderly, postmenopausal women. Secondary osteoporosis results from an underlying condition, such as hyperparathyroidism or long-term corticosteroid therapy.

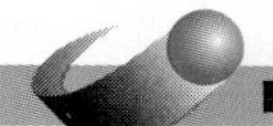

FAST FACT

In osteoporosis, bone deteriorates faster than the body can restore it.

Possible causes

◆ Lactose intolerance
◆ Osteogenesis imperfecta
◆ Hyperthyroidism
◆ Alcoholism
◆ Malnutrition
◆ Malabsorption
◆ Scurvy
◆ Total immobilization or disuse of bone, such as in hemiplegia
◆ Decreased hormonal function (drops in estrogen at time of menopause; drop in testosterone in men)
◆ Long-term corticosteroid therapy
◆ Negative calcium balance
◆ Sedentary lifestyle

Assessment findings

◆ Compression fractures of spine, Colles' fracture of wrist, hip fracture (usually first indication)
◆ Height loss
◆ Kyphosis
◆ Pain

Diagnostic evaluation

◆ Bone-mineral density (BMD) testing shows demineralization.
◆ Bone biopsy specimen shows thin and porous, but otherwise normal-looking bone.
◆ Dual or single photon absorptiometry, which aids assessment of the extremities, hips, heels, and spine, reveals decreased bone mass.
◆ Serum calcium, phosphorus, and alkaline phosphatase levels are within reference limits, but parathyroid hormone level may be increased.
◆ Radiographs show degeneration in the lower thoracic and lumbar vertebrae; the vertebral bodies appear flattened and may look more dense than normal.

Nursing diagnoses
- ◆ Risk for injury
- ◆ Impaired physical mobility
- ◆ Chronic pain

Treatment
- ◆ Physical therapy with gentle exercise and activity
- ◆ Supportive devices for weakened vertebrae
- ◆ Balanced diet high in vitamin D, calcium, and protein

Drug therapy options
- ◆ Analgesics: aspirin, indomethacin (Indocin)
- ◆ Antihypercalcemic drugs: etidronate (Didronel), alendronate (Fosamax)
- ◆ Hormonal agent: calcitonin (Calcimar), estrogen, started 3 years after menopause; testosterone in men without prostate cancer
- ◆ Vitamin D supplements, calcium supplements
- ◆ Sodium fluoride therapy

Planning and goals
- ◆ The client will remain free from injury.
- ◆ The client will have improved mobility.
- ◆ The client will state pain is decreased.

Implementation
- ◆ Focus on the client's fragility, stressing careful positioning, ambulation, and prescribed exercises *to prevent injury.*
- ◆ Provide a balanced diet high in such nutrients as vitamin D, calcium, and protein *to support skeletal metabolism.*
- ◆ Administer analgesics and heat *to relieve pain.*
- ◆ Advise the client to sleep on a firm mattress *to promote comfort* and avoid excessive bed rest *to slow disease progression.*
- ◆ Make sure the client knows how to wear a back brace *to prevent back injury.*
- ◆ Encourage appropriate exercises *to help slow disease progression.*
- ◆ Assess the client's risk of falling *to prevent injury and maintain client safety.*

Evaluation
- ◆ The client avoids injury.
- ◆ The client exhibits improved mobility.
- ◆ The client states that her pain is decreased.

INTEGUMENTARY SYSTEM

The integumentary system protects the body's inner organs. It also helps regulate body temperature through function of the sweat glands.

INTEGUMENTARY STRUCTURE AND FUNCTION

Skin, hair, nails, and certain glands make up the integumentary system:

- ◆ The skin provides the first line of defense against microorganisms and is composed of three layers:
  - – epidermis (outer layer), which contains keratinocytes and melanocytes
  - – dermis (middle layer), a collagen layer that supports the epidermis contains nerves, elastic fibers, and blood vessels; and is the origin of hair, nails, sebaceous glands, eccrine sweat glands, and apocrine sweat glands
  - – hypodermis (third layer), which is composed of loose connective tissue filled with fatty cells and provides heat, insulation, shock absorption, and a reserve of calories (also known as *subcutaneous tissue*)
- ◆ Hair also provides protection and coverage for most of the body, with the exception of the palms, lips, soles of the feet, nipples, penis, and labia.
- ◆ The nails, protecting the tips of the fingers and toes, are composed of dead cells filled with keratin.

The integumentary system contains three types of glands:

- ◆ sebaceous (oil) glands, which lubricate hair and the epidermis and are stimulated by sex hormones
- ◆ eccrine sweat glands, which excrete waste products through the pores and regulate body temperature through water secretion
- ◆ apocrine sweat glands, which are located in the axilla, nipple, anal, and pubic areas and secrete odorless fluid (decomposition of this fluid by bacteria causes odor).

INTEGUMENTARY DISORDERS

Major integumentary disorders include atopic dermatitis, burns, herpes zoster, pressure ulcers, psoriasis, and skin cancer.

ATOPIC DERMATITIS

ATOPIC DERMATITIS is a chronic skin disorder characterized by superficial skin inflammation and intense itching. It may also be called *atopic eczema* or *infantile eczema.*

Atopic dermatitis may be associated with other atopic diseases, such as bronchial asthma and allergic rhinitis. It usually develops in infants and toddlers between ages 1 month and 1 year, usually in those with strong family histories of atopic disease. These children commonly acquire other atopic disorders as they grow older.

Typically, this form of dermatitis flares and subsides repeatedly before finally resolving during adolescence. However, it can persist into adulthood.

Possible causes

◆ Chemical irritants
◆ Food allergies
◆ Genetic predisposition
◆ Immune dysfunction (possibly linked to elevated serum immunoglobulin E [IgE] levels or defective T-cell function)
◆ Infections (with *Staphylococcus aureus*)

Assessment findings

◆ Characteristic location of lesions in areas of flexion and extension, such as the neck, antecubital fossa (behind the elbow), popliteal folds (posterior surface of the knee), and behind the ears
◆ Erythematous lesions that eventually become scaly and lichenified
◆ Excessive dry skin
◆ Hyperpigmentation
◆ Pruritus
◆ Skin eruptions

Diagnostic evaluation

◆ Serum IgE levels are commonly elevated, but this finding isn't diagnostic.

Nursing diagnoses

◆ Impaired skin integrity
◆ Body image disturbance
◆ Anxiety
◆ Risk for infection

Treatment

◆ Washing lesions with water and a little soap and keeping skin mildly lubricated
◆ Environmental control of offending allergens
◆ Phototherapy

Drug therapy options

◆ Antibiotics for secondary infection
◆ Antihistamines: methdilazine (Phenergan), diphenhydramine (Benadryl)
◆ Corticosteroid ointments: fluocinolone acetonide (Tri-Luma), flurandrenolide (Cordran)

Planning and goals

◆ The client will exhibit improved or healed lesions or wounds.
◆ The client will express feelings about his changed body image.
◆ The client will use support systems to assist with coping mechanisms.
◆ The client won't develop symptoms of infection

Implementation

◆ *To prevent injury,* warn that using antihistamines that relieve daytime itching may cause drowsiness.
◆ If nocturnal itching interferes with sleep, suggest methods for inducing natural sleep, such as drinking a glass of warm milk, *to prevent overuse of sedatives.*
◆ Explain that antihistamines may also be useful at bedtime *because antihistamines relieve itching and cause drowsiness.*
◆ Help the client set up an individual schedule and plan for daily skin care *to help the client cope with the chronic condition and promote compliance.*
◆ Instruct the client to bathe in plain water. (He may have to limit bathing, depending on the severity of the lesions.) Tell him to bathe with a special nonfatty soap and tepid water (96° F [35.6° C]), to avoid using soap when lesions are acutely inflamed, and to limit baths or showers to 5 to 7 minutes. *These measures prevent worsening of the condition.*
◆ For scalp involvement, advise the client to shampoo frequently and to apply a corticosteroid solution to the scalp afterward *to improve skin integrity.*
◆ Keep fingernails short *to limit excoriation and secondary infections caused by scratching.*
◆ Lubricate the skin after a shower or bath *to prevent excessive dryness.*
◆ Instruct the client to apply cortiosteroid cream after bathing *for optimal penetration.*
◆ Apply occlusive dressings (such as plastic film) over a corticosteroid cream intermittently as necessary *to help clear lichenified skin.*
◆ Be careful not to show anxiety or revulsion when touching the lesions during treatment. Help the client accept his altered body image, and encourage him to verbal-

ize his feelings. *Coping with disfigurement is extremely difficult, especially for children and adolescents.*

Evaluation

- The client displays healing lesions.
- The client demonstrates a positive attitude regarding his self-image.
- The client demonstrates appropriate coping abilities.
- The client doesn't develop a secondary infection.

BURNS

A burn is a destruction of skin that causes loss of intracellular fluid and electrolytes. A burn is characterized as first, second, third, or fourth degree, depending on the extent (area) and degree (depth) of the burn (most burns include a combination of degrees):

- A first-degree (superficial partial-thickness) burn involves the epidermal layer.
- A second-degree (dermal partial-thickness) burn involves the epidermal and dermal layers.
- A third-degree (full-thickness) burn involves epidermal, dermal, and subcutaneous layers and nerve endings.
- A fourth-degree burn involves deeply charred subcutaneous tissue, down to muscle and bone.

The RULE OF NINES is a method used to estimate the size of a burned area. In this method, a person's skin area is divided into several sections, each representing 9% (or multiples of 9%) of the total body area. By observing the size and location of a burn and assigning the appropriate body percentage, the nurse can roughly determine what percentage of a client's body has been burned. (See *Emergency burn care.*)

The LUND AND BROWDER CHART is another method of estimating body surface area that has been burned. This method accounts for changes in body proportion that occur with age. Its greater accuracy can be used to help determine a client's exact fluid replacement requirements after a burn injury.

Possible causes

- Chemicals (acids, alkalies, vesicants)
- Electrical (lightning, electrical wires)
- Mechanical (friction)
- Radiation (X-rays, sun, nuclear)
- Thermal (flame, frostbite, scald)

Assessment findings

First-degree burn

- Erythema
- Edema
- Pain
- Blanching on pressure

Second-degree burn

- Pain
- Oozing, fluid-filled vesicles
- Erythema
- Shiny, wet subcutaneous layer after vesicles rupture
- Mild to moderate edema

Third-degree burn

- Eschar
- Edema
- Little or no pain

Fourth-degree burn

- Deeply charred subcutaneous tissue, muscle, and bone

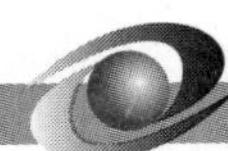

QUICK STUDY

When assessing a burn victim, obtain an **AMPLE** history, including:

Allergies
Medications
Past medical history
Last meal
Events surrounding the injury.

Diagnostic evaluation

- Urinalysis of a 24-hour collection specimen shows decreased creatinine clearance and negative nitrogen balance.
- ABG analysis shows metabolic acidosis.
- Blood studies show increased potassium, Hb, and HCT levels, and decreased sodium, albumin, complement fixation, fibrinogen, platelets, WBC and immunoglobulin levels.
- Decreased fibrinogen, platelets and WBC count.
- Urine chemistry results show hematuria and myoglobinuria.
- Visual examination is used to estimate the extent of the burn (determined by Rule of Nines and Lund and Browder chart).

Nursing diagnoses

- Acute pain
- Risk for infection
- Deficient fluid volume
- Impaired gas exchange

Emergency burn care

Nursing interventions

1. Stop the burning process.
– *Chemical burn* – Remove clothes if splattered; flush burned areas with cool, clean water for 10 to 15 minutes. Wear double gloves.
– *Thermal burn* – Remove objects that retain heat (such as rings and medals). Remove the client's clothes, if dirty, and cover the client with clean cloths or dressings, moistening them for easy removal.
– *Electrical burn* – Monitor vital functions of the brain, heart, and lungs. The human body is electrolytic. (It conducts electricity.) Make sure the current is off.
2. Prevent infection.
3. Determine the extent and degree of tissue burned.

Nursing rationales

◆ Flushing the area dilutes the chemicals and washes them away. Wearing double gloves aids in avoiding contact with the chemical.
◆ Electricity that passes through the body (with an entrance and exit site) affects all body systems.
◆ Because skin is the body's first line of defense against infecting organisms, its disruption by burning predisposes the client to infection, which is the major cause of death among burn victims. When caring for a burned client, always use aseptic technique and equipment. Cover the burn area to keep it soil-free, prevent heat loss, and protect exposed nerve endings, thereby decreasing pain.
◆ The Rule of Nines is a formula used to estimate body surface area burned. The body is visually divided into percentages: 9% to the head and each arm, 18% to each leg and to the posterior and anterior trunk, and 1% to the perineum. The percentages of burned areas are added to estimate the percent of total body surface area burned. When used for children, the age and size are considered, but this isn't done for adults, making it a valid guideline only in an emergency.

Depth of burns

◆ *Partial thickness* – superficial; epidermis only (example: sunburn-marked reddening from dilated dermal blood vessels)
◆ *Deep* – between dermis and epidermis; plasma leaking from dilated vessels and formation of blisters of plasma fluid between the skin layers
◆ *Full thickness* – complete damage of epidermis, dermis, and skin appendages (sweat glands, sebaceous glands, and hair follicles); black, brownish, and leathery burned areas that fail to heal (reepithelialize) without grafting

RULE OF NINES

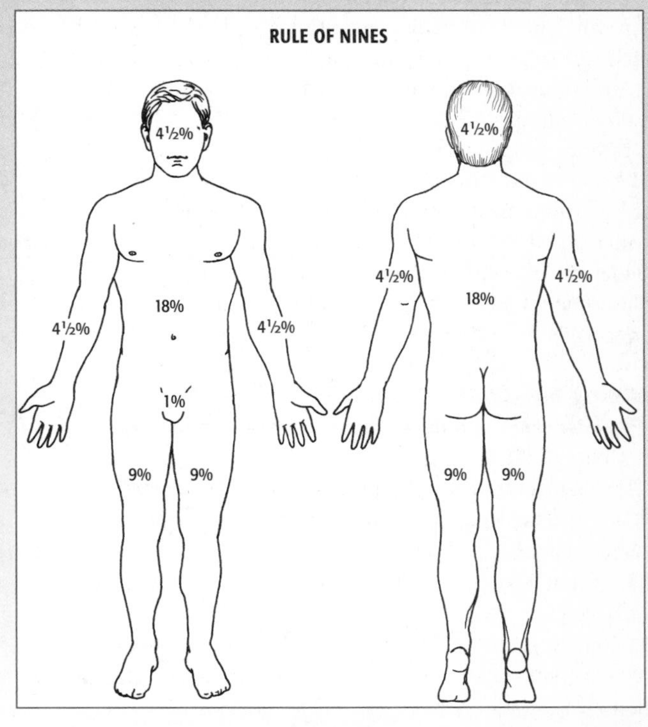

◆ Disturbed body image
◆ Anxiety
◆ Imbalanced nutrition: Less than body requirements

Treatment

◆ Oxygen therapy to maintain airway patency and oxygenate tissue; mechanical ventilation, if needed
◆ Biological dressings
◆ Diet high in protein, fat, calories, and carbohydrates, with small, frequent feedings; TPN or parenteral nutrition as needed
◆ Early excisional therapy
◆ Escharotomy (surgical excision of burned tissue)
◆ I.V. therapy, including hydration and electrolyte replacement (I.V. administration is gauged according to the amount of fluid it takes to maintain a urine output of 30 to 50 ml/hour). Usually, the Parkland formula is used as a general guideline for fluid replacement: Administer

4 ml/kg of crystalloid × % total burn surface area; give half of the solution over the first 8 hours, calculated from the time of injury, and the balance over the next 16 hours.)

- Protective isolation to protect the client from infection
- Skin grafts
- Splints to maintain proper joint position and prevent contractures
- Transfusion therapy of fresh frozen plasma, platelets, packed RBCs, and plasma

Drug therapy options

- Analgesic: morphine
- Antianxiety agent: lorazepam (Ativan)
- Antibiotic: gentamicin (Garamycin)
- Anti-infectives: mafenide (Sulfamylon), povidone-iodine (Betadine), silver sulfadiazine (Silvadene), silver nitrate
- Antitetanus agent: tetanus toxoid
- Colloid: albumin 5% (Albuminar-5)
- Diuretic: mannitol (Osmitrol)
- Histamine antagonists: cimetidine (Tagamet), famotidine (Pepcid), nizatidine (Axid), ranitidine (Zantac)
- Mucosal barrier fortifier: sucralfate (Carafate)
- Sedative: oxazepam (Serax)
- Vitamins: phytonadione (AquaMEPHYTON), cyanocobalamin (vitamin B_{12})

Planning and goals

- The client will exhibit signs of comfort and pain relief and anxiety will decrease.
- The client will heal without infection or complications.
- The client will maintain an adequate airway and adequate oxygenation.
- The client's fluid, electrolyte, and cellular balances will be restored.
- The client will maintain adequate nutritional needs.
- The client's self-concept will be restored without lasting deficits.

Implementation

- Assess respiratory status. Secure the client's airway, and provide oxygenation and ventilation. *Upper airway injury is common with burns to the face, neck, and chest. Edema may narrow airways initially, and again as fluid shifts back into the circulation.*
- Assess fluid and electrolyte status and maintain fluid requirements as ordered. *Hypovolemia is indicated by a decreasing LOC, urine output less than 30 ml/hour, blood pressure less than 90/60 mm Hg, heart rate greater than 100 beats/minute, dry mucous membranes, and delayed capillary refill. Topical burn therapy treatments will be altered systemically and may alter the electrolyte values.*
- Assess the client for hypervolemia and pulmonary edema as fluid shifts back into the circulation *to prevent life-threatening complications.*
- Assess for concurrent injuries if the client was traumatized. Maintain cervical spine immobilization *to prevent further injury until injury to the client's vertebral column is ruled out.*
- If the client underwent skin grafting, keep pressure off the donor side *to maintain blood flow to the site and promote wound healing.*
- Monitor for signs of infection *to determine if the treatment plan must be altered.*
- Assess the effectiveness of pain medication *to promote comfort.*
- Monitor and record vital signs, fluid intake and output, laboratory studies, hemodynamic variables, stool for occult blood, specific gravity, calorie count, daily weight, neurovascular checks, and pulse *to detect complications.*
- Assess bowel sounds *to determine motility of the GI tract.*
- Administer I.V. fluids *to maintain hydration and replace fluid loss.*
- Administer oxygen *to meet cellular demands.*
- Provide suctioning; assist with turning, coughing, and deep breathing, and perform chest physiotherapy and postural drainage *to maintain the client's airway.*
- Maintain the position, patency, and low suction of the NG tube *to prevent vomiting.*
- Consult a registered dietitian *to help meet the client's nutritional needs.* Administer TPN or enteral feedings *to meet the client's increased metabolic demands.*
- Administer medications, as prescribed, *to maintain or improve the client's condition.*
- Encourage the client to express feelings about disfigurement, immobility from scarring, and a fear of dying *to encourage coping mechanisms.*
- Provide treatments, such as ROM exercises, immersion tank, skin treatments and dressing changes, bed cradle, splints, and Jobst clothing *to maintain ROM and prevent complications.*
- Elevate the affected extremities *to promote venous drainage and decrease edema.*
- Maintain a warm environment during the acute period *because the client is unable to regulate body temperature.*
- Maintain protective precautions *to prevent the transmission of infection to the client.*
- Provide skin and mouth care *to promote comfort.*

◆ Consult with physical therapy and occupational therapy *to help optimize the client's outcome and meet his needs.*

Evaluation

◆ The client reports decreased pain and anxiety.
◆ The client regains skin integrity and is free from infection.
◆ The client maintains fluid and nutritional status.
◆ The client maintains optimal oxygenation.
◆ The client resumes social roles and accepts his altered body image.

HERPES ZOSTER

HERPES ZOSTER, also known as *shingles,* is an acute viral infection of nerve structures caused by varicella zoster. Affected areas include the spinal and cranial sensory ganglia and posterior gray matter of the spinal cord. Herpes zoster produces localized vesicular skin lesions confined to a dermatome and severe neurologic pain in peripheral areas innervated by nerves arising in the inflamed root ganglia.

Possible causes

◆ Cytotoxic drug-induced immunosuppression
◆ Chronic or debilitating disease
◆ Exposure to varicella zoster

Assessment findings

◆ Usually unilaterally clustered skin vesicles along peripheral sensory nerves on the trunk, thorax, or face
◆ Erythema
◆ Pruritus
◆ Malaise
◆ Neuralgia
◆ Severe, deep pain
◆ Fever
◆ Anorexia
◆ Edematous skin
◆ Headache
◆ Paresthesia

Diagnostic evaluation

◆ Skin study identifies the organism.
◆ Visual examination shows vesicles along the peripheral sensory nerves.

Nursing diagnoses

◆ Impaired skin integrity
◆ Acute pain
◆ Risk for infection

Treatment

◆ No specific treatment. (The primary goal is to relieve itching and pain.)

Drug therapy options

◆ Analgesic: acetaminophen (Tylenol) with codeine
◆ Antianxiety agents: lorazepam (Ativan), hydroxyzine (Vistaril)
◆ Antipruritic: diphenhydramine (Benadryl)
◆ Antiviral agents: acyclovir (Zovirax), famciclovir (Famvir), valacyclovir (Valtrex)
◆ Miscellaneous: gabapentin (Neurontin) for neuropathic pain

Planning and goals

◆ The client will exhibit improved or healed lesions or wounds.
◆ The client will express feelings of comfort and pain relief.
◆ The client will remain free from signs and symptoms of infection.

Implementation

◆ Assess the client's neurologic status *to determine a baseline and detect changes.*
◆ Assess pain and note the effectiveness of analgesics *to promote comfort and evaluate the need for a change in the current treatment plan.*
◆ Monitor and record vital signs, laboratory results, and cranial nerve function *to assess the baseline and detect changes.*
◆ Administer medications, as directed, *to maintain or improve the client's condition.*
◆ Encourage the client to express feelings about changes in his physical appearance and the recurrent nature of the illness *to help him adapt to his illness.*
◆ Instruct the client to avoid scratching and rubbing affected areas *to prevent infection.*
◆ Provide diversional activities *to help the client take his mind off pain and pruritus.*

Evaluation

◆ The client displays healing lesions.
◆ The client reports adequate pain control.
◆ The client remains free from infection.

PRESSURE ULCERS

Pressure ulcers are localized areas of cellular necrosis that occur most commonly in skin and subcutaneous tissue over bony prominences. These ulcers may be superficial, caused by local skin irritation with subsequent surface maceration, or deep, originating in underlying tissue. Deep lesions commonly go undetected until they penetrate the skin but, by then, subcutaneous damage has occurred.

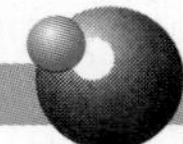

SPOT CHECK

What are the characteristics of a stage 3 pressure ulcer?

- Deep crater with or without undermining of adjacent tissue
- Full-thickness skin loss involving damage or necrosis of subcutaneous tissue that may extend down to, but not through, underlying fasciae

Possible causes

- ◆ Pressure, particularly over bony prominences
- ◆ Prolonged immobility
- ◆ Inadequate nutrition
- ◆ Breakdown of skin or subcutaneous tissue

Assessment findings

Signs and symptoms of pressure ulcers occur in four stages.

Stage 1

- ◆ Nonblanchable erythema of intact skin
- ◆ Skin discoloration
- ◆ Warmth or coolness
- ◆ Pain or pruritus

Stage 2

- ◆ Abrasion
- ◆ Blister
- ◆ Partial-thickness skin loss involving the epidermis and dermis
- ◆ Shallow crater

Stage 3

- ◆ Deep crater with or without undermining of adjacent tissue
- ◆ Full-thickness skin loss involving damage or necrosis of subcutaneous tissue that may extend down to, but not through, underlying fasciae

Stage 4

- ◆ Damage to muscle, bone, tendon, or joint
- ◆ Full-thickness skin loss with extensive destruction
- ◆ Tissue necrosis
- ◆ Possible presence of sinus tracts

Diagnostic evaluation

- ◆ Visual inspection reveals the pressure ulcer.
- ◆ Wound culture and sensitivity tests identify the infecting organism.

Nursing diagnoses

- ◆ Impaired skin integrity
- ◆ Impaired tissue integrity
- ◆ Imbalanced nutrition: Less than body requirements
- ◆ Impaired physical mobility
- ◆ Risk for infection

Treatment

- ◆ High-protein, high-calorie diet in small, frequent feedings; parenteral or enteral feedings if the client is unable or unwilling to take adequate nutrients orally
- ◆ Topical wound care according to the facility's protocol
- ◆ Wound debridement; tissue flap
- ◆ Vaccum-assisted wound closure

Planning and goals

- ◆ The client will have improved nutritional status.
- ◆ The client will have evidence of pressure ulcer healing and improved skin integrity.
- ◆ The client will increase his physical mobility.
- ◆ The client won't show evidence of infection.

Implementation

- ◆ Assess skin integrity and watch for signs of infection *to detect complications.*
- ◆ Check the bedridden client for possible changes in skin color, turgor, temperature, and sensation *to prevent further skin breakdown.*
- ◆ Reposition the client every 2 hours *to prevent pressure ulcers.*
- ◆ Use a special mattress, bed cradle, or other device *to avoid skin breakdown.*
- ◆ Provide meticulous skin care and check bony prominences *to reduce the chance of pressure ulcer development.*
- ◆ Provide wound care, as ordered, *to promote healing.*
- ◆ Maintain the client's diet and encourage oral fluid intake *to promote wound healing.* Consult a registered dietitian *to help meet the client's nutritional needs.*
- ◆ Provide ROM exercises *to promote joint mobility.*

◆ Consult a wound care specialist or an enterstomal therapist *to optimize wound care treatment.*

Evaluation

◆ The client maintains skin integrity.
◆ The client has improved physical mobility.
◆ The client has adequate nutritional intake.
◆ The client doesn't demonstrate signs of infection

PSORIASIS

PSORIASIS is a chronic, recurrent disease marked by epidermal proliferation. Lesions appear as erythematous papules and plaques covered with silver scales; they vary widely in severity and distribution.

Although this disorder most commonly affects young adults, it may strike at any age, including infancy. Psoriasis is characterized by recurring partial remissions and exacerbations.

Possible causes

◆ Genetic predisposition
◆ Trauma (develops at site of injury)
◆ Infection (especially beta-hemolytic streptococci)
◆ Pregnancy
◆ Endocrine changes
◆ Climate
◆ Emotional stress

Assessment findings

◆ Itching
◆ Lesions (red, and usually forming well-defined patches) characteristically located on the scalp, chest, elbows, knees, back, and buttocks or at site of trauma
◆ Pustules
◆ Pain
◆ Patches, consisting of silver scales that flake off or thicken and cover the lesions
◆ Arthritic symptoms

Diagnostic evaluation

◆ Skin biopsy is positive for the disorder.
◆ Blood studies reveal elevated serum uric acid level in severe cases, due to accelerated nucleic acid degradation; however, indications of gout are absent.

Nursing diagnoses

◆ Impaired skin integrity
◆ Risk for infection
◆ Disturbed body image
◆ Chronic pain

Treatment

◆ Emollients, tar, wet dressings, or oatmeal baths
◆ Ultraviolet light to retard cell production (may be used in the form of ultraviolet B or may be used in conjunction with psoralen-ultraviolet-light [PUVA] therapy)

Drug therapy options

◆ Antihistamine: diphenhydramine (Benedryl)
◆ Corticosteroid ointment: hydrocortisone (Dermacort)
◆ Corticosteroid: intralesional steroid injections
◆ Antipsoriatic agents: calcipotriene (Dovonex), anthralin (Anthraderm)
◆ Immunomodulators: alefacept (Amevive), methotrexate (Trexall)

Planning and goals

◆ The client will exhibit improved or healed lesions or wounds.
◆ The client will remain free from signs and symptoms of infection.
◆ The client will express feelings about his changed body image.
◆ The client will express feelings of comfort.

Implementation

◆ Make sure the client understands his prescribed therapy; provide written instructions *to promote compliance and avoid confusion.*
◆ Apply fluorinated steroid cream after bathing *to facilitate absorption.* Occlusive dressings or a vinyl exercise suit may be necessary *to promote absorption.*
◆ Apply petroleum jelly around the affected skin before applying anthralin *to prevent seepage to adjacent tissues.*
◆ Watch for adverse reactions, especially allergic reactions to anthralin, atrophy and acne from steroids, and burning, itching, nausea, and squamous cell epitheliomas from PUVA *to prevent complications.*
◆ Caution the client receiving PUVA therapy to stay out of the sun on the day of treatment and to protect his eyes with sunglasses for 24 hours after treatment. Tell him to wear goggles during exposure to this light. *These measures protect the client from injury caused by excessive UVA exposure.*
◆ Be aware that psoriasis can cause psychological problems. Assure the client that psoriasis isn't contagious and, although exacerbations and remissions occur, they're con-

trollable with treatment. However, make sure he understands there's no cure. *Appropriate teaching helps the client develop healthy coping strategies.*

◆ Help the client learn to cope with stressful situations and employ relaxation techniques *because stressful situations tend to exacerbate psoriasis.*

Evaluation

◆ The client displays healing lesions.

◆ The client remains free from signs and symptoms of infection.

◆ The client demonstrates a positive attitude regarding his self-image.

◆ The client expresses decreased pain and increased comfort.

SKIN CANCER

Skin cancer is a malignant primary tumor of the skin. There are three types:

◆ BASAL CELL EPITHELIOMA is a tumor commonly caused by prolonged exposure to the sun.

◆ MELANOMA is a neoplasm that arises from melanocytes. Melanoma spreads through the lymph and vascular systems and metastasizes to the lymph nodes, skin, liver, lungs, and CNS.

◆ SQUAMOUS CELL CARCINOMA is a slow-growing cancer that causes airway obstruction, cough, and sputum production.

Possible causes

◆ Chemical irritants (squamous cell)

◆ Arsenic ingestion (squamous cell)

◆ Friction or chronic irritation (squamous cell)

◆ Heredity (squamous cell)

◆ Immunosuppression

◆ Prolonged sun exposure (most commonly basal cell)

◆ Vaccination

◆ Precancerous lesions, such as leukoplakia, nevi, and senile keratoses

◆ Radiation

Assessment findings

◆ Change in color, size, or shape of preexisting lesion

◆ Circular, irregular, bordered lesion with hues of tan, black, or blue (melanoma)

◆ Local soreness

◆ Oozing, bleeding, crusting lesion

◆ Pruritus

◆ Small, red, nodular lesion that begins as an erythematous macule or plaque with indistinct margins (squamous cell carcinoma)

◆ Waxy nodule with telangiectasis (basal cell epithelioma)

Diagnostic evaluation

◆ Skin biopsy specimen shows cancer cells.

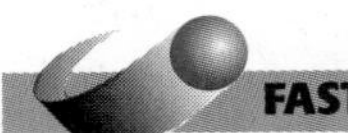

FAST FACT

Remember, a change in color, size, or shape of a skin lesion may indicate a cancerous growth.

Nursing diagnoses

◆ Risk for infection

◆ Anxiety

◆ Disturbed body image

◆ Deficient knowledge related to disease process and treatment

Treatment

◆ Chemosurgery with zinc chloride

◆ Cryosurgery with liquid nitrogen

◆ Curettage and electrodesiccation

◆ Radiation therapy

Drug therapy options

◆ Alkylating agents: carmustine (BiCNU), dacarbazine (DTIC-Dome)

◆ Antiemetics: prochlorperazine (Compazine), ondansetron (Zofran)

◆ Antimetabolite: fluorouracil (Adrucil)

◆ Antineoplastics: hydroxyurea (Hydrea), vincristine sulfate (Oncovin)

◆ Immunotherapy for melanoma: Bacillus Calmette-Guérin (BCG) vaccine

Planning and goals

◆ The client will remain free from infection.

◆ The client will have decreased anxiety regarding the treatment and outcome of lesion removal.

◆ The client will develop a positive self-image.

◆ The client will verbalize an understanding of the disease process and treatment. (See *Caring for the client with a cancerous lesion.*)

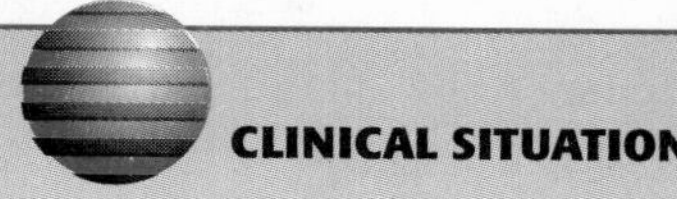

CLINICAL SITUATION

Caring for the client with a cancerous lesion

A 62-year-old female client recently had a cancerous lesion diagnosed by results of a circular skin punch procedure.

Immediately after the procedure, the nurse should observe for which significant finding?

A. Infection
B. Dehiscence
C. Hemorrhage
D. Swelling

Answer: C. The nurse's main concern after a circular skin punch procedure is to monitor for bleeding. Infection is a later possible consequence of a skin punch. Dehiscence is more likely in larger wounds, such as surgical wounds of the abdomen or thorax. Swelling is a normal reaction associated with any event that traumatizes the skin.

What teaching should the nurse include regarding skin care?

The client should be taught to:

- avoid contact with chemical irritants
- use sunblock and layered clothing when outdoors
- self-monitor for lesions and moles that don't heal or that change characteristics
- have moles removed if they're subject to chronic irritation.

Questions for further thought

- What are appropriate outcomes for this client after the procedure?
- What types of statements indicate that the client understands necessary precautions?

Implementation

- Monitor a skin punch biopsy site *to detect bleeding.*
- Assess lesions. *Regular assessment prevents recurrence.*
- Monitor and record vital signs *to determine a baseline and detect changes.*
- Administer medications, as prescribed, *to maintain and improve the client's condition.*
- Encourage the client to express feelings about changes in his body image and a fear of dying *to help him accept changes in body image.*
- Provide postchemotherapy and postradiation nursing care *to promote healing.*
- Tell the client about the disease process and treatment *to promote compliance with the treatment plan and reduce anxiety.*
- Consult additional assistance as required *to meet the client's needs (such as home care, hospice, wound care specialists, and counselors).*

Evaluation

- The client remains free from infection.
- The client has decreased anxiety.
- The client develops a positive self-image.
- The client verbalizes an understanding of the disease process and complies with treatment.

EYE, EAR, NOSE, AND THROAT

The senses of sight, hearing, smell, and taste allow us to communicate with others, connect with the world around us, and take pleasure in life.

SENSORY STRUCTURE AND FUNCTION

The structures discussed below include the sensory organs (the eyes, ears, and nose) and the throat.

Eye

About 70% of all sensory information reaches the brain through the eyes. The eyes are composed of external and internal structures. External structures include the eyelid, conjunctiva (a thin, transparent mucous membrane that lines the lid), lacrimal apparatus (which lubricates and protects the cornea and conjunctiva by producing and absorbing tears), six extraocular muscles (which hold the eyes parallel to create binocular vision), and the eyeball itself.

The eye also contains numerous internal structures. Some of the most important include the:

- IRIS — thin, circular pigmented muscular structure in the eye that gives color to the eye, divides the space between the cornea and lens into anterior and posterior chambers, and controls the amount of light admitted to the retina

- CORNEA — transparent, dome-shaped structure covering the front of the eye that consists of five layers of cells and proteins and refracts light
- PUPIL — circular aperture in the iris that changes size as the iris adapts to the amount of light entering the eye
- LENS — biconvex, avascular, colorless, transparent structure that's suspended behind the iris by the ciliary zonulae and focuses light
- VITREOUS BODY — clear, transparent, avascular, gelatinous fluid that fills the space in the posterior portion of the eye and maintains the transparency and form of the eye
- RETINA — thin, semitransparent layer of nerve tissue that lines the back of the eye
- RETINAL CONES — visual cell segments responsible for visual acuity and color discrimination
- RETINAL RODS — visual cell segments responsible for peripheral vision under decreased light conditions
- OPTIC NERVE — nerve located at the posterior portion of the eye that transmits visual impulses from the retina to the brain.

Ear

The ears are composed of three sections: external, middle, and inner. The external ear includes the pinna (auricle) and external auditory canal. It's separated from the middle ear by the tympanic membrane.

The middle ear, known as the *tympanum,* is a tiny, air-filled cavity in the temporal bone. It contains three small bones (malleus, incus, and stapes).

The inner ear, known as the *bony labyrinth,* is the portion of the ear that consists of the cochlea, vestibule, and semicircular canals.

Nose

The nose is more than the sensory organ of smell. It also plays a key role in the respiratory system by filtering, warming, and humidifying inhaled air.

The lower two-thirds of the external nose consists of flexible cartilage, and the upper one-third is rigid bone.

Posteriorly, the internal nose merges with the pharynx. Anteriorly, it merges with the external nose.

The internal and external nose are divided vertically by the nasal septum, which is straight at birth and in early life but becomes slightly deviated or deformed in almost every adult. Only the posterior end, which separates the posterior nares, remains constantly in the midline. Kiesselbach's plexus, the most common site of nosebleeds, is located in the anterior portion of the septum.

Air entering the nose passes through the vestibule, which is lined with coarse hair that helps filter dust. Olfactory receptors lie above the vestibule in the roof of the nasal cavity and the upper one-third of the septum. Known as the *olfactory region,* this area is rich in capillaries and mucus-producing goblet cells that help warm, moisten, and clean inhaled air. Because of its rich blood supply, the nasal mucosa is redder than the oral mucosa.

Farther along the nasal passage are the superior, middle, and inferior turbinates. The curved, bony turbinates and their mucosal covering ease breathing by warming, filtering, and humidifying inhaled air.

The sinuses lighten the weight of the cranium, serve as resonators for sound production, and provide mucus. Four pairs of paranasal sinuses open into the internal nose, including the:

- maxillary sinuses, located on the cheeks below the eyes
- frontal sinuses, located above the eyebrows
- ethmoidal and sphenoidal sinuses, located behind the eyes and nose.

Throat

The throat is composed of various structures:

- The nasopharynx is continuous with the nasal passage and is located behind and above the soft palate. The adenoids and eustachian tube opening are located here.
- The oropharynx extends from the soft palate to just above the hyoid bone.
- The laryngopharynx is located above the larynx and is the lower part of the pharynx.
- Located within the throat are the hard and soft palates, the uvula, and the tonsils.
- The mucous membrane lining the throat is usually smooth and bright pink to light red.

EYE, EAR, NOSE, AND THROAT DISORDERS

Major eye, ear, nose, and throat disorders include cataracts, conjunctivitis, corneal abrasion, deviated septum, glaucoma, laryngeal cancer, Ménière's disease, otosclerosis, and retinal detachment.

CATARACT

A CATARACT occurs when the normally clear, transparent crystalline lens becomes opaque. With age, lens fibers become more densely packed, making the lens less transparent and giving the lens a yellowish hue. These changes result in vision loss.

A cataract usually develops first in one eye but, in many cases, is followed by the development of a cataract in the other eye. Cataracts are removed surgically by intracapsular or extracapsular extraction followed by artificial intraocular lens implantation.

Possible causes

- Aging
- Anterior uveitis
- Atopic dermatitis
- Blunt or penetrating trauma
- Chemical toxicity (certain drugs)
- Congenital factors
- Diabetes mellitus
- Glaucoma
- Hypoparathyroidism
- Infrared rays
- Long-term steroid treatment
- Radiation exposure
- UV light exposure

Assessment findings

- Disabling glare
- Distorted images
- Gradual dimmed or blurred vision
- Poor vision at night and in bright sunlight
- Red reflex lost as cataract matures
- Yellow, gray, or white pupil

Diagnostic evaluation

- Ophthalmoscopy or slit-lamp examination is used to confirm the diagnosis by revealing a dark area in the normally homogeneous red reflex.

Nursing diagnoses

- Disturbed sensory perception (visual)
- Impaired physical mobility
- Risk for infection
- Risk for injury

Treatment

- Intracapsular or extracapsular cataract extraction with intraocular lens implantation

Drug therapy options

- Opthalmic antibiotics: gentamycin (Garamycin) postoperatively
- Opthalmic antibiotic with corticosteroid ointment: neomycin and polymixin B sulfate, hydrocortisone opthalmic suspension

Planning and goals

- The client will demonstrate improved vision.
- The client will demonstrate improved mobility.
- The client will take steps to prevent infection and reduce intraocular pressure.
- The client won't injure himself.

Implementation

- Provide a safe environment for the client. Orient the client to his surroundings *to reduce the risk of injury.*
- Modify the environment to help the client meet self-care needs by placing items on the unaffected side *to discourage movement or positions that would apply pressure to the operative site or cause increased intraocular pressure (IOP).*
- Caution the client not to rub the eyes *to decrease the risk of infection and damage to the surgical site.*
- Enforce postoperative care teaching, including no bending, straining at stool, coughing, sneezing, or squeezing eyes shut, *to prevent increased IOP.*
- Provide sensory stimulation (such as large print or audiotapes) *to help compensate for vision loss.*
- Instruct the client on proper application of eyedrops and ointments if prescribed *to prevent infection from improper application.*

Evaluation

- The client has improved vision.
- The client demonstrates adequate mobility.
- The client remains free from infection.
- The client remains free from injury.

CONJUNCTIVITIS

CONJUNCTIVITIS is characterized by inflammation of the conjunctiva, the delicate membrane that lines the eyelids and covers the exposed surface of the eyeball. It may result from infection, allergy, radiation, or chemical reactions.

Conjunctivitis is common. Bacterial and viral conjunctivitis are highly contagious but are also self-limiting after a couple weeks' duration. Chronic conjunctivitis may result in degenerative changes to the eyelids.

Possible causes

- Bacterial — *Staphylococcus aureus, Streptococcus pneumoniae, Neisseria gonorrhoeae, Neisseria meningitidis, Haemophilis influenzae*
- Chlamydial — *Chlamydia trachomatis* (inclusion conjunctivitis)
- Viral — adenovirus types 3 and 7; type 1 herpes simplex virus; enteroviruses

Other possible causes

- Allergic reactions to pollen, grass, topical medications, air pollutants, and smoke
- Fungal infections (rare)
- Occupational irritants (acids and alkalies)
- Parasitic diseases caused by *Phthirus pubis* or *Schistosoma haematobium*
- Rickettsial diseases (Rocky Mountain spotted fever, petechial conjunctivitis)

Assessment findings

- Itching, burning
- Excessive tearing
- Mucopurulent discharge
- Hyperemia (engorgement) of the conjunctiva, sometimes accompanied by discharge and tearing

Diagnostic evaluation

- Culture and sensitivity tests identify the causative bacterial organism and indicate appropriate antibiotic therapy.

Nursing diagnoses

- Disturbed sensory perception (visual)
- Risk for infection
- Disturbed body image

Treatment

- Cold compresses to relieve itching for allergic conjunctivitis
- Warm compresses to treat bacterial or viral conjunctivitis

Drug therapy options

- Antiviral agent: vidarabine ointment (Vira-A); oral acyclovir (Zovirax) if herpes simplex is the cause
- Corticosteroids: dexamethasone (Maxidex), fluorometholone (Fluor-Op Ophthalmic)
- Mast cell stabilizer: cromolyn (Opticrom) for allergic conjunctivitis
- Topical antibiotic according to susceptibility of infecting organism, if caused by bacteria

Planning and goals

- The client will have improved visual ability.
- The client will prevent the spread of infection to other individuals.
- The client will have a positive body image.

Implementation

- Teach proper hand-washing technique *because certain forms of conjunctivitis are highly contagious.*
- Stress the risk of spreading infection to family members by sharing washcloths, towels, and pillows. Warn against rubbing the infected eye, which can spread the infection to the other eye and to other persons. *These measures prevent the spread of infection.*
- Apply warm compresses and therapeutic ointment or drops. *Don't irrigate the eye because doing so will spread infection.*
- Have the client wash his hands before he uses the medication, and use clean washcloths or towels frequently *so he doesn't infect his other eye.*
- Teach the client to instill eyedrops and ointments correctly — without touching the bottle tip to his eye or lashes — and to avoid sharing medications with others *to prevent the spread of infection.*
- Stress the importance of safety glasses for the client who works near chemical irritants *to prevent further episodes of conjunctivitis.*
- Notify public health authorities if cultures show *N. gonorrhoeae. Public health authorities track sexually transmitted diseases.*

Evaluation

- The client has returned to baseline visual acuity.
- The client demonstrates safe practices to avoid transmission of infection.
- The client has a positive body image.

CORNEAL ABRASION

A CORNEAL ABRASION is a scratch on the surface epithelium of the cornea, the dome-shaped transparent structure in front of the eye. This type of eye injury is commonly caused by a foreign body, such as a cinder or piece of dirt, or by improper use of a contact lens.

Possible causes

- Improper use of contact lenses
- Trauma caused by a foreign body (such as a cinder or a piece of dust, dirt, or grit)

Assessment findings

- Burning
- Edema of eyelid
- Redness
- Increased tearing
- Sensation of "something in the eye"
- Sensitivity to light
- Pain disproportionate to the size of the injury
- Change in visual acuity (depending on the size and location of the injury)

Diagnostic evaluation

- Staining the cornea with fluorescein stain confirms the diagnosis — the injured area appears green when examined with a Woods lamp or black light.
- Slit-lamp examination discloses the depth of the abrasion.

Nursing diagnoses

- Acute pain
- Risk for infection
- Disturbed sensory perception (visual)

Treatment

- Irrigation with saline solution
- Pressure patch (a tightly applied eye patch)
- Removal of a deeply embedded foreign body with a foreign body spud, using a topical anesthetic

Drug therapy options

- Antibiotic: sulfisoxazole (Gantrisin)
- Cycloplegic agent: tropicamide (Paremyd)

Planning and goals

- The client will express feelings of comfort and pain relief.
- The client will remain free from signs and symptoms of infection.
- The client will regain visual function.

Implementation

- Assist with examination of the eye. Check visual acuity before beginning treatment *to assess visual loss from injury.*
- If the foreign body is visible, carefully irrigate the eye with normal saline solution *to wash away the foreign body without damaging the eye.*
- Tell the client with an eye patch to leave the patch in place for 6 to 8 hours *to protect the eye from further corneal irritation when the client blinks.*
- Warn the client with an eye patch that wearing a patch alters depth perception; advise caution in everyday activities, such as climbing stairs, stepping off a curb, and driving a car, *to prevent injury.*
- Reassure the client that the corneal epithelium usually heals in 24 to 48 hours *to allay anxiety.*
- Stress the importance of instilling prescribed antibiotic eyedrops *because an untreated corneal infection can lead to ulceration and permanent loss of vision.*
- Emphasize the importance of safety glasses *to protect the eyes from flying fragments.*

Evaluation

- The client reports adequate pain control.
- The client doesn't display signs or symptoms of infection.
- The client has regained baseline visual acuity.

DEVIATED SEPTUM

Deviated septum is a shift of the nasal septum from the midline, which is common in adults, and may be severe enough to obstruct the passage of air through the nostrils. With surgery, the prognosis is good.

Possible causes

- Nasal trauma
- Shift of the septum from one side to the other during growth

Assessment findings

- Difficulty breathing through the nostrils
- Dry, cracked, or crusted nasal mucosa
- Ecchymosis from trauma
- Edema in the nasal mucosa
- Feeling of fullness in the face
- Noisy breathing during sleep
- Recurring epistaxis, infection, sinusitis, and headache
- Shortness of breath

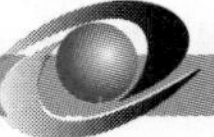

QUICK STUDY

Remember that a "deviated" septum may cause a "deviation" from normal breathing.

Diagnostic evaluation

- X-ray reveals nasal fracture and a deviated septum.
- Skull X-rays are used to rule out skull fracture.

Nursing diagnoses

- Ineffective airway clearance
- Acute pain
- Risk for infection
- Anxiety

Treatment

- Reconstruction of the nasal septum, rhinoplasty, or septoplasty to relieve nasal obstruction
- Vasoconstrictors, nasal packing, or cauterization to control hemorrhage

Drug therapy options

- Analgesics: acetaminophen (Tylenol), ibuprofen (Motrin)
- Decongestant: pseudoephedrine (Sudafed)

Planning and goals

- The client will exhibit a patent airway and adequate breathing patterns.
- The client will verbalize that pain and anxiety are decreased.
- The client won't develop signs of infection.

Implementation

- Encourage verbalization of concerns and answer questions *to allay anxiety.*
- *To relieve nasal congestion,* instill normal saline solution and provide a humidifier.
- If the client experiences epistaxis, elevate the head of the bed, compress the outer nose, and apply ice packs *to alleviate bleeding.*
- Postoperatively, place a small ice bag over the eyes and nose intermittently *to reduce facial edema and pain.*
- Provide good mouth care *because the postoperative client will be breathing through the mouth.*
- Warn the client not to blow the nose for 48 hours after the packing is removed *to decrease the risk of bleeding.*
- Limit physical activity for 2 to 3 days postoperatively *to reduce the risk for injury.*
- Allow verbalization of feelings regarding changes in appearance *to decrease anxiety.*

Evaluation

- The client maintains a patent airway.
- The client exhibits decreased anxiety and is pain-free.
- The client is free from infection.

Normal flow of aqueous humor

Aqueous humor, a plasmalike fluid produced by the ciliary epithelium of the ciliary body, flows from the posterior chamber to the anterior chamber through the pupil. Here it flows peripherally and filters through the trabecular meshwork to the canal of Schlemm, through which the fluid ultimately enters venous circulation.

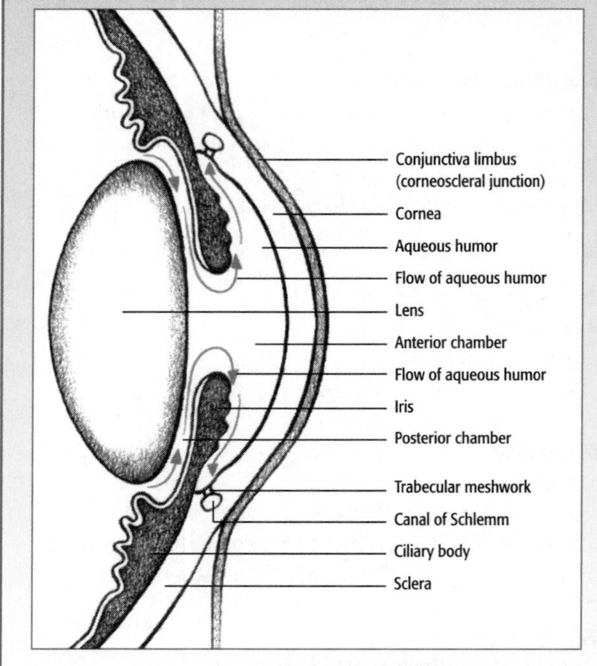

Glaucoma

In GLAUCOMA, the client experiences visual field loss due to damage to the optic nerve resulting from increased IOP caused by impaired flow of aqueous humor (a fluid in the front of the eye). If left untreated, glaucoma can lead to blindness.

Glaucoma is classified as either open-angle or angle-closure, depending on where the flow and resorption of aqueous humor is compromised. In open-angle glaucoma, increased IOP is caused by overproduction of or obstructed outflow of aqueous humor. Primary open-angle glaucoma is characterized by an abnormal increase in IOP caused by an abnormality of the trabecular meshwork, which controls the flow of aqueous humor. In angle-closure glaucoma, the anterior chamber is smaller than average. (See *Normal flow of aqueous humor.*)

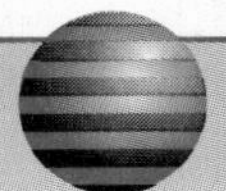

CLINICAL SITUATION

Caring for the client with primary open-angle glaucoma

A 55-year-old female client sees halos around lights and has had mild pain in both eyes for several weeks. She works as a bookkeeper and lives alone. Primary open-angle glaucoma was previously diagnosed. She arrives at the ambulatory surgical unit on the morning she's scheduled for a laser trabeculoplasty. She'll be discharged the same day.

What postoperative measures should be stressed to the client before she goes home?

- Wear an eye shield or eyeglasses to protect the affected eye.
- Adjust the home environment to avoid injury.
- Report eye pain that's unrelieved by analgesics and accompanied by nausea or decreased vision.
- Adhere to instructions for the proper administration of eye medications.
- Keep follow-up appointments with the health care provider.

Questions for further thought

- Based on the client's medical condition, what assessment findings would the nurse anticipate?
- Why should the nurse caution the client to avoid bending, sneezing, straining, and coughing after the procedure?

Possible causes

- Age over 45
- Diabetes mellitus
- Family history of glaucoma
- Long-term steroid treatment
- Myopia
- Previous eye trauma or surgery
- Race (blacks have a higher incidence)
- Uveitis

Assessment findings

Chronic open-angle glaucoma

- Initially asymptomatic
- Atrophy and cupping of optic nerve head
- Increased IOP
- Narrowed field of vision
- Possible asymmetric involvement

Acute angle-closure glaucoma

- Acute ocular pain
- Blurred vision
- Dilated pupil
- Halo vision
- Increased IOP
- Nausea and vomiting

Diagnostic evaluation

- Gonioscopy reveals if the angle is open or closed.
- Ophthalmoscopy shows atrophy and cupping of the optic nerve head.
- Perimetry shows a decreased field of vision.
- Tonometry shows increased IOP.

Nursing diagnoses

- Acute pain
- Anxiety
- Disturbed sensory perception (visual)
- Powerlessness
- Risk for injury

Treatment

Chronic open-angle glaucoma

- Reduction of IOP by decreasing aqueous humor production with medication
- Argon laser trabeculoplasty (for those who don't respond to drug therapy) to create an opening for outflowing aqueous humor (See *Caring for the client with primary open-angle glaucoma.*)

Acute angle-closure glaucoma

- Ocular emergency that requires immediate treatment to decrease IOP
- Laser iridectomy or surgical iridectomy if IOP doesn't decrease with drug therapy

Drug therapy options

Chronic open-angle glaucoma

- Alpha-adrenergic agonist: brimonidine (Alphagan) to reduce aqueous humor production and increase outflow

◆ Beta-adrenergic antagonist: timolol (Timoptic) to decrease the rate fluid flows into the eye

Acute angle-closure glaucoma

◆ Cholinergic: pilocarpine to reduce pressure by increasing flow rate out of the eye.

Planning and goals

◆ The client's anxiety and pain will decrease.

◆ The client's vision will increase and he'll be more independent.

◆ The client won't develop an injury.

Implementation

◆ Explain the disease process or surgical procedure *to reduce the client's anxiety.*

◆ Assess eye pain and administer medication as prescribed. *Medication reduces pain and may control disease progression.*

◆ Provide a safe environment. *Orienting the client to the surroundings reduces the risk of injury.*

◆ Modify the environment *to meet the client's self-care needs.*

◆ During an acute episode, limit activities that increase IOP *to reduce the risk of complications.*

◆ Advise the client to wear an eye shield or eye glasses *to protect the affected eye.*

◆ Tell the client to report eye pain that's unrelieved by analgesics and accompanied by nausea or decreased vision *to prevent complications.*

◆ Make sure the client understands the discharge instructions and proper administration of eye medications *to ensure proper self-care.*

◆ Encourage the client to express feelings about changes in his body image *to aid acceptance of vision loss.*

Evaluation

◆ The client has relief of pain and anxiety.

◆ The client's vision is improved.

◆ The client plans to modify his lifestyle as necessary to cope effectively with glaucoma and prevent injury.

LARYNGEAL CANCER

Laryngeal cancer occurs in several forms: An intrinsic cancerous tumor that's on the true vocal cords tends not to spread because underlying connective tissues lack lymph nodes. An extrinsic tumor is on some other part of the larynx and tends to spread easily. Squamous cell carcinomas constitute about 95% of laryngeal tumors. Laryngeal cancer is more common in men than in women, and among blacks; most victims are between ages 50 and 65.

Possible causes

◆ Unknown

Risk factors

◆ Smoking

◆ Alcoholism

◆ Chronic inhalation of noxious fumes

◆ Familial disposition

Assessment findings

◆ Local throat irritation

◆ Hoarseness

◆ Pain or burning in the throat when drinking citrus juice or hot liquid

◆ Pain radiating to the ear

◆ Dysphagia

◆ Dyspnea

◆ Enlarged cervical lymph nodes

◆ Cough

Diagnostic evaluation

◆ Laryngoscopy allows visualization of the tumor.

◆ Chest X-ray reveals metastasis.

◆ Laryngeal CT scanning shows lymph node metastasis.

◆ Biopsy results reveal the type of cancer.

◆ Laryngography is used to define the tumor and its borders.

Nursing diagnoses

◆ Impaired verbal communication

◆ Acute pain

◆ Impaired gas exchange

◆ Imbalanced nutrition: Less than body requirements

◆ Anxiety

Treatment

◆ Early lesions: laser surgery or radiation therapy

◆ Advanced lesions: laser surgery, radiation therapy, and chemotherapy

Drug therapy options

◆ Analgesic: morphine sulfate

◆ Chemotherapy: cisplatin (Platinol), 5-fluorouracil (5-FU)

Planning and goals

◆ The client will be able to communicate his needs.

- The client will have adequate pain control.
- The client will have an unobstructed airway.
- The client's nutrition will be adequate to meet his needs.
- The client's anxiety will be decreased.

Implementation

- Instruct the client about the procedure and postoperative care *to allay his anxiety.*
- Encourage the client to express concerns and choose an alternative method of communication *to decrease anxiety.*

After total laryngectomy

- Position the client on his side and elevate the head of the bed 30 to 45 degrees *to relieve pressure on the operative site.*
- Provide adequate humidification *to prevent crusting on the stoma and skin breakdown.*
- Monitor vital signs, especially temperature, which may indicate infection if elevated, *to assess for complications.*
- Give analgesics *to relieve discomfort.*
- Monitor for bleeding, adequate oxygenation, and fluid balance *to prevent complications.*
- Consult a registered dietitian *to meet nutritional needs.*
- Consult with home care and hospice *to help meet the client's needs.*
- Encourage the client to cough and deep-breathe every 1 to 2 hours *to prevent pneumonia.*
- If the client requires mechanical ventilation, suction the client as needed *to maintain a patent airway.*
- Turn and reposition the client every 2 hours *to prevent complications of immobility such as skin breakdown.*

Evaluation

- The client communicates effectively.
- The client is pain-free.
- The client maintains a patent airway.
- The client maintains adequate nutrition.
- The client expresses that his anxiety is decreased.

MÉNIÈRE'S DISEASE

MÉNIÈRE'S DISEASE is a dysfunction in the labyrinth (the part of the ear that produces balance) that causes severe vertigo, sensorineural hearing loss, and tinnitus. It usually affects adults between ages 30 and 60, men slightly more commonly than women. After multiple attacks over several years, this disorder leads to residual tinnitus and hearing loss. This disorder is also called *endolymphatic hydrops.*

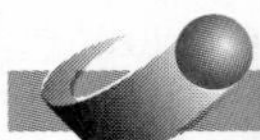

FAST FACT

In Ménière's disease, an increase in the amount of fluid in the labyrinth increases pressure in the inner ear and leads to a disruption of the client's sense of balance.

Possible causes

- Autonomic nervous system dysfunction that produces a temporary constriction of blood vessels supplying the inner ear
- Overproduction or decreased absorption of endolymph, which causes endolymphatic hydrops or endolymphatic hypertension, with consequent degeneration of the vestibular and cochlear hair cells

Assessment findings

- Severe vertigo
- Tinnitus
- Feeling of fullness or blockage in the ear
- Severe nausea
- Vomiting
- Sweating
- Giddiness
- Nystagmus
- Sensorineural hearing loss

Diagnostic evaluation

- Electronystagmography, electrocochleography, CT scanning, MRI, and X-rays of the internal meatus may be necessary for a differential diagnosis.
- Audiometric studies indicate a sensorineural hearing loss and loss of discrimination and recruitment.

Nursing diagnoses

- Disturbed sensory perception (auditory)
- Powerlessness
- Risk for injury

Treatment

- Restriction of sodium intake to less than 2 g per day.
- Surgery to destroy the affected labyrinth (If medical treatment fails, destruction of the labyrinth permanently relieves symptoms but results in irreversible hearing loss.)

Drug therapy options

- Anticholinergic: atropine (may stop an attack in 20 to 30 minutes)
- Cardiac stimulant: epinephrine (Adrenalin)

◆ Diuretic: furosemide (Lasix) to prevent excess fluid in the labyrinth (long-term management)
◆ Antihistamines: diphenhydramine (Benadryl) (may be necessary in a severe attack)
◆ Antihistamines: meclizine (Antivert), dimenhydrinate (Dramamine) (for milder attacks; may also be administered as part of prophylactic therapy)
◆ Sedatives: phenobarbital (Luminal), diazepam (Valium) as part of prophylactic therapy

Planning and goals

◆ The client will regain hearing or develop alternate means of communication.
◆ The client will use available support systems to develop coping abilities for dealing with the disorder.
◆ The client will remain free from injury.

Implementation

◆ Advise the client against reading and exposure to glaring lights *to reduce dizziness.*
◆ Keep the side rails of the client's bed up *to prevent falls.* Tell him not to get out of bed or walk without assistance *to prevent injury.*
◆ Instruct the client to avoid sudden position changes and tasks that vertigo makes hazardous *because an attack can begin quite rapidly.*

Before surgery

◆ If the client is vomiting, record fluid intake and output and characteristics of vomitus *to prevent dehydration.* Administer antiemetics as necessary, and give small amounts of fluid frequently *to prevent vomiting.*

After surgery

◆ Record intake and output carefully *to monitor fluid status and direct the treatment plan.*
◆ Tell the client to expect dizziness and nausea for 1 or 2 days after surgery *to relieve anxiety.*
◆ Give prophylactic antibiotics and antiemetics as required *to decrease the chance of infection and combat nausea.*

Evaluation

◆ The client has appropriate communication abilities.
◆ The client demonstrates appropriate coping behaviors.
◆ The client hasn't experienced injury.

OTOSCLEROSIS

OTOSCLEROSIS is characterized by abnormal overgrowth of the ear's spongy bone around the oval window and stapes footplate. This overgrowth curtails movement of the stapes in the oval window, preventing sound from being transmitted to the cochlea and resulting in conductive hearing loss. Sensorineural hearing loss can also occur along with conductive hearing loss.

Possible causes

◆ Familial tendency
◆ Pregnancy

Assessment findings

◆ Progressive hearing loss
◆ Tinnitus

Diagnostic evaluation

◆ Audiometric testing confirms hearing loss.
◆ Weber's test detects sound lateralizing to the more affected ear.

Nursing diagnoses

◆ Disturbed sensory perception (auditory)
◆ Impaired verbal communication
◆ Risk for infection
◆ Anxiety

Treatment

◆ Hearing aid (air conduction aid with molded ear insert receiver)
◆ Stapedectomy and insertion of a prosthesis to restore partial or total hearing

Drug therapy options

◆ Oral fluoride, calcium, Vitamin D to help minimize hearing loss.

Planning and goals

◆ The client will communicate effectively with others.
◆ The client won't develop an infection.
◆ The client will state his anxiety is decreased.

Implementation

◆ Don't shout, particularly if the client uses a hearing aid *because hearing aids increase sensitivity to loud noises.*
◆ Monitor vital signs and check the dressing postoperatively for signs of bleeding *to detect complications.*
◆ Develop alternative means of communication *to decrease anxiety and communicate effectively with the client.*

◆ If the client has speech limitations or can't understand you, use gestures, allow time for responses, repeat words if necessary, remain calm, and avoid distractions *to communicate effectively with the client.*
◆ Tell the client that hearing may not be immediately restored postoperatively due to edema and packing *to decrease anxiety.*

Evaluation
◆ The client maintains effective communication.
◆ The client accurately describes measures to prevent infection.
◆ The client states anxiety is decreased.

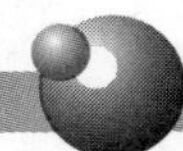

SPOT CHECK

Why doesn't hearing improve immediately after a stapedectomy?
Answer: Immediately after stapedectomy, the client experiences some postoperative edema. Also, packing must remain in place for a short time after surgery.

RETINAL DETACHMENT
Retinal detachment is the separation of the retina from the choroid (the middle vascular coat of the eye between the retina and the sclera). It occurs when the retina develops a hole or tear and the vitreous seeps between the retina and choroid. If left untreated, retinal detachment can lead to vision loss.

Possible causes
◆ Aging
◆ Cataract surgery
◆ Diabetic neovascularization
◆ Familial tendency
◆ Hemorrhage
◆ Inflammatory process
◆ Myopia
◆ Prematurity
◆ Systemic diseases
◆ Trauma
◆ Tumor
◆ Uveitis

Assessment findings
◆ Blurred vision, worsening as the detachment increases
◆ Painless change in vision (floaters caused by blood cells in the vitreous humor and flashes of light as the vitreous humor pulls on the retina)
◆ Photopsia (recurrent flashes of light)
◆ With progression of detachment, painless vision loss that may be described as a veil, curtain, or cobweb that eliminates part of the visual field

Diagnostic evaluation
◆ Indirect ophthalmoscopy shows retinal tear or detachment.
◆ Slit-lamp examination reveals retinal tear or detachment.
◆ Ultrasonography shows a retinal tear or detachment in the presence of a cataract.

Nursing diagnoses
◆ Disturbed sensory perception (visual)
◆ Risk for injury
◆ Anxiety

Treatment
◆ Complete bed rest and restriction of eye movement to prevent further detachment
◆ Cryopexy, if there's a hole in the peripheral retina
◆ Laser therapy, if there's a hole in the posterior portion of the retina
◆ Scleral buckling to reattach the retina

Planning and goals
◆ The client's vision will improve.
◆ The client won't develop an injury.
◆ The client will express anxiety is decreased.

Implementation
◆ Assess the client's visual status and functional vision in the unaffected eye *to determine his self-care needs.*
◆ Prepare the client for surgery by explaining possible surgical interventions and techniques *to alleviate the client's anxiety.*
◆ Postoperatively, instruct the client to lie on his back or on his unoperated side *to reduce IOP on the affected side.*
◆ Discourage straining during defecation, bending down, and hard coughing, sneezing, or vomiting *to prevent increased IOP.*
◆ Provide assistance with ADLs *to minimize frustration and strain.*
◆ Assist with ambulation, as needed, *to help the client remain independent.*

◆ Approach the client from the unaffected side *to avoid startling him.*
◆ Orient the client to his environment *to reduce the risk of injury.*

Evaluation

◆ The client's vision doesn't deteriorate.
◆ The client remains free from injury.
◆ The client states that his anxiety is decreased.

ENDOCRINE SYSTEM

The endocrine system is a complex network of hormone-secreting structures that regulate metabolism and other body processes.

ENDOCRINE STRUCTURE AND FUNCTION

The endocrine system consists of glands, which are made up of specialized cell clusters, and hormones, which are released by the glands and act as chemical transmitters throughout the body.

Glands and hormones

The primary structures of the endocrine system include the hypothalamus, pituitary gland, thyroid gland, parathyroid glands, adrenal gland, and pancreas.

Hypothalamus

The hypothalamus controls temperature, respiration, and blood pressure. Its functions affect emotional states. The hypothalamus also produces hypothalamic-stimulating hormones, which affect the inhibition and release of pituitary hormones.

Pituitary gland

The pituitary gland is composed of anterior and posterior lobes. Each lobe produces a variety of hormones that affect the body.

Anterior lobe

The anterior lobe of the pituitary gland secretes:
◆ follicle-stimulating hormone, which stimulates graafian follicle growth and estrogen secretion in women
◆ luteinizing hormone, which induces ovulation and development of the corpus luteum in women and stimulates testosterone secretion in men
◆ corticotropin, also called *adrenocorticotropic hormone,* which stimulates the secretion of hormones from the adrenal cortex
◆ thyroid-stimulating hormone (TSH), which regulates the secretory activity of the thyroid gland
◆ growth hormone, which is an insulin antagonist that stimulates the growth of cells, bones, muscle, and soft tissue.

Posterior lobe

The posterior lobe of the pituitary gland secretes:
◆ vasopressin (antidiuretic hormone), which helps the body retain water
◆ oxytocin, which stimulates uterine contractions during labor and milk secretion in lactating women.

Thyroid gland

The thyroid gland accelerates growth and cellular reactions, including basal metabolic rate. TSH controls hormones released by the thyroid gland. The thyroid gland produces thyrocalcitonin, triiodothyronine (T_3), and thyroxine (T_4), which are necessary for growth and development.

Parathyroid gland

The parathyroid gland secretes parathyroid hormone (parathormone), which regulates calcium and phosphorus levels and promotes the resorption of calcium from bones.

Adrenal glands

The adrenal glands include the adrenal cortex and the adrenal medulla.

Adrenal cortex

The adrenal cortex secretes three major types of hormone:
◆ glucocorticoids (cortisol, cortisone, and corticosterone), which mediate the stress response, promote sodium and water retention and potassium secretion, and suppress corticotropin secretion
◆ mineralocorticoids (aldosterone and deoxycorticosterone), which promote sodium and water retention and potassium secretion
◆ sex hormones (androgens, estrogens, and progesterone), which develop and maintain secondary sex characteristics and libido.

Adrenal medulla

The adrenal medulla secretes two hormones:

◆ norepinephrine, which regulates generalized vasoconstriction

◆ epinephrine, which regulates instantaneous stress reaction and increases metabolism, blood glucose levels, and cardiac output.

Pancreas

The pancreas is an accessory gland of digestion. It has exocrine and endocrine functions:

◆ In its exocrine function, it secretes digestive enzymes (amylase, lipase, and trypsin). Amylase breaks down starches into smaller carbohydrate molecules. Lipase breaks down fats into fatty acids and glycerol. Trypsin breaks down proteins. Note that exocrine glands discharge secretions through a duct; the pancreas secretes enzymes into the duodenum through the pancreatic duct.

◆ In its endocrine function, the pancreas secretes hormones (insulin, glucagon, and somatostatin) from the islets of Langerhans into the blood or lymph. Insulin regulates fat, protein, and carbohydrate metabolism and decreases blood glucose levels by promoting glucose transport into cells. Glucagon increases blood glucose levels by promoting hepatic glyconeogenesis. Somatostatin inhibits the release of insulin, glucagon, and somatotropin.

ENDOCRINE DISORDERS

Major endocrine disorders include acromegaly and gigantism, Addison's disease, Cushing's syndrome, diabetes insipidus, diabetes mellitus, hyperthyroidism, hypothyroidism, pancreatic cancer, thyroid cancer, and thyroiditis.

ACROMEGALY AND GIGANTISM

ACROMEGALY and GIGANTISM are marked by hormonal dysfunction and startling skeletal overgrowth. Both are chronic, progressive diseases that occur when the pituitary gland produces too much growth hormone, causing excessive growth. Acromegaly develops slowly; gigantism develops abruptly.

Acromegaly occurs after epiphyseal closure, causing bone thickening and transverse growth and visceromegaly (enlargement of the viscera). In other words, acromegaly may occur any time after adolescence, when the arms and legs have stopped growing. The signs of this disorder are swelling and enlargement of the arms, legs, and face.

Gigantism begins before epiphyseal closure and causes proportional overgrowth of all body tissues. In other words, gigantism begins in childhood or adolescence when the arms and legs are still growing. That's why clients with gigantism may attain giant proportions.

Possible causes

◆ Genetic predisposition

◆ Oversecretion of human growth hormone (HGH)

◆ Tumors of the anterior pituitary gland (which lead to oversecretion of HGH)

Assessment findings

Acromegaly

◆ Enlarged supraorbital ridge

◆ Thickened ears and nose

◆ Paranasal sinus enlargement

◆ Thickening of the tongue

◆ Marked prognathism (projection of the jaw) that may interfere with chewing

◆ Laryngeal hypertrophy

◆ Oily skin

◆ Diaphoresis

◆ Severe headache

◆ Bitemporal hemianopia

◆ Loss of visual acuity

◆ Blindness

Gigantism

◆ Excessive growth in all parts of the body (Gigantism causes remarkable height increases, as much as 6″ (15.2 cm) per year; infants and children may grow to three times the normal height for their age; adults may reach heights above 80″ [203.2 cm].)

Diagnostic evaluation

◆ Glucose normally suppresses HGH secretion; therefore, a glucose infusion that doesn't suppress the hormone level to below the accepted normal value of 2 ng/ml, when combined with characteristic clinical features, strongly suggests hyperpituitarism.

◆ Plasma HGH levels measured by radioimmunoassay are typically elevated. However, because HGH secretion is pulsatile, the results of random sampling may be misleading. Insulin-like growth factor I levels offer a better screening alternative.

◆ Skull X-rays, a CT scan, arteriography, and MRI determine the presence and extent of the pituitary lesion.

Nursing diagnoses

- Disturbed body image
- Risk for disproportionate growth
- Impaired physical mobility

Treatment

- Surgery to remove affecting tumor (transsphenoidal hypophysectomy)
- Pituitary radiation therapy

Drug therapy options

- Thyroid hormone replacement therapy: levothyroxine (Synthroid) after surgery
- Corticosteroid: cortisone (Cortone)
- Inhibitor of growth hormone release: bromocriptine (Parlodel)
- Somatotropic hormone: octreotide (Sandostatin)

Planning and goals

- The client will express positive feelings about himself.
- The client will demonstrate age-appropriate skills and behaviors to the extent possible.
- The client will maintain joint mobility and ROM.

Implementation

- Provide the client with emotional support *to help him cope with his body image. Grotesque body changes characteristic of this disorder can cause severe psychological stress.*
- Examine the client for skeletal manifestations, such as arthritis of the hands and osteoarthritis of the spine, *to detect complications.*
- Administer prescribed medications *to improve the client's condition.*
- Perform or assist with ROM exercises *to promote maximum joint mobility.*
- Evaluate muscular weakness, especially in the client with late-stage acromegaly. Check the strength of his handclasp *to monitor for disease progression.* If it's very weak, help with tasks such as cutting food.
- Keep the skin dry. Avoid using an oily lotion *because the skin is already oily.*
- Test blood glucose to detect early signs of hyperglycemia. Check for signs of hyperglycemia (fatigue, polyuria, polydipsia) *to avoid treatment delay.*
- Be aware that the client's tumor may cause visual problems. If the client has hemianopia, stand where he can see you *to reduce anxiety.*
- Keep in mind that this disease can also cause inexplicable mood changes. Reassure the family that these mood changes result from the disease and can be modified with treatment *to help the family cope with the client's condition.*
- Before surgery, reinforce what the surgeon has told the client, and provide a clear and honest explanation of the scheduled operation *to allay the client's fears and anxiety.*
- If the client is a child, explain to his parents that such surgery prevents permanent soft-tissue deformities but won't correct bone changes that have already taken place. Arrange for counseling, if necessary, *to help the child and parents cope with permanent defects.*
- After surgery, diligently monitor vital signs and neurologic status. Be alert for alterations in LOC, pupil equality, or visual acuity as well as vomiting, falling pulse rate, and rising blood pressure. *These changes may signal an increase in intracranial pressure due to intracranial bleeding or cerebral edema.*
- Check blood glucose level often *because HGH levels usually fall rapidly after surgery, eliminating an insulin antagonist effect in many clients and, possibly, precipitating hypoglycemia.*
- Measure intake and output hourly, watching for large increases. *Transient diabetes insipidus, which sometimes occurs after surgery for hyperpituitarism, can cause such increases in urine output.*
- If the transsphenoidal approach is used, a large nasal pack is kept in place for several days. Because the client must breathe through his mouth, give good mouth care *to prevent breakdown of the oral mucosa.*
- The surgical site is packed with a piece of tissue generally taken from a midthigh donor site. Watch for CSF leaks from the packed site. Look for increased external nasal drainage or drainage into the nasopharynx. CSF leaks may necessitate additional surgery to repair the leak. *These measures detect complications quickly and avoid treatment delays.*
- Encourage the client to ambulate on the 1st or 2nd day after surgery *to prevent complications of immobility.*
- If client is a child, instruct the parents to follow up closely with the pediatrician *to ensure continuation of care and an optimal outcome for the child.*

Evaluation

- The client demonstrates positive self-esteem and body image.
- The client demonstrates age-appropriate behavior.
- The client demonstrates functional joint mobility and ROM.

ADDISON'S DISEASE

ADDISON'S DISEASE, also known as *primary adrenal hypofunction,* occurs when the adrenal gland fails to secrete sufficient mineralocorticoids, glucocorticoids, and androgens. Secondary adrenal hypofunction is due to impaired pituitary secretion of corticotropin and is characterized by decreased glucorticoid secretions. Secretion of aldosterone, the major mineral corticord, is commonly unaffected.

ADDISONIAN CRISIS (adrenal crisis) is a critical deficiency of mineralocorticoids and glucocorticoids. It generally occurs in clients who have chronic adrenal insufficiency, and follows acute stress, sepsis, trauma, surgery, or omission of steroid therapy. It's a medical emergency that necessitates immediate, vigorous treatment.

Possible causes

- Autoimmune process
- Bilateral adrenalectomy
- Family history (rare)
- Hemorrhage into the adrenal gland
- Infections
- Neoplasms
- Tuberculosis

Assessment findings

- Hypoglycemia
- Weakness and lethargy
- Bronzed skin pigmentation of nipples, scars, and buccal mucosa
- Depression and personality changes
- Anorexia, diarrhea, and nausea
- Orthostatic hypotension
- Weight loss
- Dehydration and thirst
- Decreased pubic and axillary hair

Diagnostic evaluation

- Corticotropin-stimulation test indicates secondary adrenal insufficiency if cortisol levels are less than 18 mcg/dl and aldosterone levels measured on the same blood samples are normal (greater than or equal to 5 ng/dl).

Nursing diagnoses

- Ineffective tissue perfusion: Renal
- Imbalanced nutrition: Less than body requirements
- Risk for infection
- Decreased cardiac output

Treatment

- High-carbohydrate, high-protein, high-sodium, low-potassium diet in small, frequent feedings before steroid therapy; high-potassium and low-sodium diet while on steroid therapy
- In adrenal crisis, I.V. hydrocortisone (Solu-Cortif) administered promptly along with 3 to 5 L of normal saline solution

Drug therapy options

- Glucocorticoids: cortisone (Cortone), hydrocortisone (Solu-Cortef)
- Mineralocorticoid: fludrocortisone (Florinef)
- Vasopressor: phenylephrine (Neo-Synephrine)

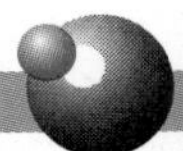

SPOT CHECK

Clients receiving long-term therapy with corticosteroids must not abruptly stop taking the drug but must have the dosage gradually reduced. What's the rationale for this?

Answer: An abrupt withdrawal of corticosteroids may trigger addisonian crisis. Gradual withdrawal of the medication will prevent this situation because the body will produce some corticosteroids.

Planning and goals

- The client will maintain adequate urine output.
- The client will maintain an adequate nutritional level for age and weight.
- The client won't show signs of infection.
- The client will remain hemodynamically stable.

Implementation

- Be prepared to administer I.V. hydrocortisone and saline solution promptly if the client is in adrenal crisis *to reverse shock and hyponatremia.*
- Assess fluid balance (and tell the client to increase fluid intake in hot weather) *to prevent addisonian crisis,* which may be precipitated by salt or fluid loss in hot weather and during exercise.
- Monitor and record vital signs, intake and output, urine specific gravity, and laboratory studies *to assess for deficient fluid volume.*
- Maintain the client's diet *to promote nutritional balance.*
- Administer I.V. fluids *to maintain hydration and prevent addisonian crisis.*
- Weigh the client daily *to determine nutritional status and detect fluid loss.*
- Administer medications, as prescribed, *to maintain or improve the client's condition.*
- Don't allow the client to sit up or stand quickly *to avoid orthostatic hypotension.*

◆ Assist with ADLs and maintain a quiet environment *to conserve energy and decrease metabolic demands.*

Evaluation

◆ The client has normal urine output and hemodynamic states.
◆ The client maintains an adequate nutritional level.
◆ The client doesn't demonstrate signs and symptoms of infection.

CUSHING'S SYNDROME

Cushing's syndrome, also known as *hypercortisolism,* is hyperactivity of the adrenal cortex. It results in excessive secretion of glucocorticoids, particularly cortisol. There may be an increase in mineralocorticoids and sex hormones.

Possible causes

◆ Cortisol-secreting adrenal tumor
◆ Adrenal adenoma or carcinoma
◆ Excessive or prolonged administration of glucocorticoids
◆ Corticotropin-producing tumor in another organ (particularly a bronchogenic or pancreatic carcinoma)
◆ Hyperplasia of the adrenal glands
◆ Pituitary hyperactivity

Assessment findings

◆ Weight gain, especially truncal obesity, buffalo hump, and moonface
◆ Hypertension
◆ Muscle wasting
◆ Fragile skin
◆ Amenorrhea
◆ Mood swings
◆ Acne
◆ Decreased libido
◆ Ecchymosis
◆ Edema
◆ Enlarged clitoris
◆ Gynecomastia
◆ Hirsutism
◆ Pain in joints
◆ Poor wound healing
◆ Purple striae on abdomen
◆ Recurrent infections
◆ Weakness and fatigue

QUICK STUDY

Remember, the signs of Cushing's syndrome are *cushioning* of the face, neck, and trunk from fat.

Diagnostic evaluation

◆ Blood chemistry studies show increased cortisol, aldosterone, sodium, corticotropin, and glucose levels and a decreased potassium level.
◆ CT scanning, MRI, ultrasonography, or angiography shows location of tumors.
◆ Dexamethasone suppression test shows no decrease in 17-hydroxycorticosteroids.
◆ Glucose tolerance test results show hyperglycemia.
◆ Hematology shows increased WBC and RBC counts and decreased eosinophils.
◆ Urine chemistry shows increased 17-hydroxycorticosteroids and 17-ketosteroids, decreased urine specific gravity, and glycosuria.

Nursing diagnoses

◆ Disturbed body image
◆ Excessive fluid volume
◆ Risk for infection

Treatment

◆ Hypophysectomy or bilateral adrenalectomy
◆ Diet low in sodium, carbohydrates, calories and high in protein and potassium
◆ Radiation therapy

Drug therapy options

◆ Adrenal suppressants: aminoglutethimide (Cytadren), metyrapone (Metopirone)
◆ Antidiabetic agent: insulin or oral antidiabetic agents (sulfonylurea [Diabenese, Glucotrol, Micronase]) if hyperglycemic
◆ Diuretics: ethacrynic acid (Edecrin), furosemide (Lasix)

Planning and goals

◆ The client will maintain a positive self-image.
◆ The client wil exhibit hemodynamic stability.
◆ The client won't show evidence of infection.

Implementation

◆ Perform postoperative care *to prevent complications.*
◆ Assess fluid balance and edema *to detect fluid deficit or overload.*
◆ Monitor and record vital signs, intake and output, urine specific gravity, fingersticks, urine glucose and ketones,

and laboratory studies. *Altered parameters may indicate altered fluid or electrolyte status.*
- Apply antiembolism stockings or sequential compression devices if the client is bedridden *to promote venous return and prevent thromboembolism formation.*
- Maintain the client's diet *to ensure nutritional status.*
- Maintain standard precautions *to protect the client from infection.*
- Provide meticulous skin care and reposition the client every 2 hours if he's unable to ambulate *to prevent skin breakdown.*
- Limit water intake *to prevent fluid volume excess.*
- Weigh the client daily *to detect fluid retention.*
- Administer medications, as prescribed, *to maintain or improve the client's condition.*
- Encourage the client to express feelings about changes in his body image and sexual function *to help the client cope effectively.*
- Provide rest periods *to prevent fatigue.*
- Provide postradiation nursing care *to prevent complications.*

Evaluation
- The client is coping with an altered body image.
- The client is hemodynamically stable.
- The client remains free from infection and trauma.

DIABETES INSIPIDUS

DIABETES INSIPIDUS stems from a deficiency of antidiuretic hormone (ADH), also called *vasopressin,* which is secreted by the posterior lobe of the pituitary gland. Decreased ADH reduces the ability of distal and collecting renal tubules in the kidneys to concentrate urine, resulting in excessive urination, excessive thirst, and excessive fluid intake.

Possible causes
- Brain surgery
- Head injury or trauma
- Idiopathy
- Infection
- Granulomatous disease
- Vascular lesions
- Tumor of the posterior lobe of the pituitary gland

Assessment findings
- Polyuria (greater than 5 L/day)
- Polydipsia (excessive thirst)
- Dehydration
- Fatigue
- Headache
- Muscle weakness and pain
- Tachycardia
- Weight loss

Diagnostic evaluation
- Blood chemistry shows decreased ADH by radioimmunoassay and increased potassium, sodium, and osmolality levels.
- Urine chemistry shows urine specific gravity less than 1.005, osmolality of 50 to 200 mOsm/kg, decreased urine pH, and decreased sodium and potassium levels.

Nursing diagnoses
- Deficient fluid volume
- Ineffective tissue perfusion: Cardiopulmonary, renal
- Deficient knowledge related to disease process and treatment

Treatment
- I.V. therapy, including electrolyte replacement and hydration (when first diagnosed, intake and output must be matched milliliter to milliliter to prevent dehydration.)
- Regular diet with restriction of foods that exert a diuretic effect

Drug therapy options
- ADH replacements: vasopressin (Pitressin), desmopressin acetate

Planning and goals
- The client's fluid volume will remain within normal limits.
- The client will remain hemodynamically stable.
- The client will verbalize an understanding of his illness and comply with treatment.

Implementation
- Assess fluid balance *to avoid dehydration.*
- Monitor and record vital signs, intake and output (urine output every hour when first diagnosed), urine specific gravity (every 1 to 2 hours when first diagnosed), and laboratory studies *to assess for fluid volume deficit.*
- Maintain the client's diet *to maintain nutritional balance.*
- Force fluids *to keep intake equal to output and prevent dehydration.*
- Administer I.V. fluids *to replace fluid and electrolyte loss.*
- Maintain patency of the indwelling urinary catheter *to allow accurate measuring of urine output.*

◆ Administer medications, as prescribed, *to enable concentration of urine and prevent dehydration.*
◆ Weigh the client daily *to detect fluid loss.*
◆ Teach the client about stress reduction or techniques *to prevent complications.*
◆ Explain signs of fluid overload to report to the physician (weight gain, tight clothes, edema) *to prevent complications.*

Evaluation

◆ The client has adequate intake and output values.
◆ The client is hemodynamically stable.
◆ The client relates appropriate knowledge of his illness.

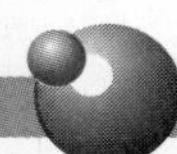

SPOT CHECK

Which nursing diagnosis is most applicable for a client with an acute episode of diabetes insipidus?

A. Imbalanced nutrition: Less than body requirements
B. Deficient fluid volume
C. Impaired gas exchange
D. Ineffective tissue perfusion: Cerebral

Answer: B. Diabetes insipidus causes a pronounced loss of intravascular volume. The most prominent risk to the client is deficient fluid volume. Nutrition, gas exchange, and tissue perfusion are at risk as a result of the deficient fluid volume caused by diabetes insipidus.

DIABETES MELLITUS

DIABETES MELLITUS is a chronic disorder resulting from a disturbance in the production, action, and rate of insulin utilization. There are several types of diabetes mellitus:

◆ Type 1 (insulin-dependent diabetes mellitus) usually develops in childhood.
◆ Type 2 (non-insulin–dependent diabetes mellitus) usually develops after age 30.
◆ Gestational diabetes mellitus occurs with pregnancy.
◆ Secondary diabetes mellitus is induced by trauma, surgery, pancreatic disease, or medications and can be treated as type 1 or type 2.

Factors that increase blood glucose include glucocorticoids, epinephrine, glucagon, somatotropin, emotional stress, pregnancy with multiple births, surgery or trauma, and obesity (overeating). Factors that decrease blood glucose include insulin, exercise, and decreased food intake. (See *Major complications of diabetes mellitus.*)

Possible causes

◆ Autoimmune disease
◆ Blockage of insulin supply
◆ Cushing's syndrome
◆ Exposure to chemicals
◆ Failure of the body to produce insulin
◆ Genetics
◆ Hyperpituitarism
◆ Hyperthyroidism
◆ Infection
◆ Medications
◆ Pregnancy
◆ Receptor defect in normally insulin-responsive cells
◆ Stress
◆ Surgery
◆ Trauma

Assessment findings

◆ Polyuria
◆ Polydipsia
◆ Polyphagia
◆ Weight loss
◆ Dehydration
◆ Acetone breath
◆ Anorexia
◆ Atrophic muscles
◆ Blurred vision
◆ Fatigue
◆ Flushed, warm, smooth, shiny skin
◆ Kussmaul's respirations
◆ Mottled extremities
◆ Multiple infections and boils
◆ Pain
◆ Paresthesia
◆ Peripheral and visceral neuropathies
◆ Poor wound healing
◆ Retinopathy
◆ Sexual dysfunction
◆ Weakness

Diagnostic evaluation

◆ Blood chemistry shows increased glucose, potassium, chloride, ketone, cholesterol, and triglyceride levels; decreased carbon dioxide level; and pH less than 7.4.
◆ Fasting blood glucose level is increased (126 mg/dl or greater).
◆ Glycosylated hemoglobin assay (Hb A_{1c}) is increased.
◆ Glucose tolerance test results show hyperglycemia.
◆ Two-hour postprandial blood glucose level shows hyperglycemia (greater than 200 mg/dl).

Major complications of diabetes mellitus

Major complications of diabetes mellitus include arteriosclerosis, metabolic acidosis, hyperosmolar hyperglycemic nonketotic syndrome (HHNS), and hypoglycemia.

Arteriosclerosis

To check for arteriosclerosis, assess for ulcers on the legs, lack of sensation in the legs and feet, angina pectoris, pyelonephritis and reduced renal function, and retinopathy (observe for visual impairment). Note that the client should undergo an annual vision examination by an ophthalmologist. The diabetic client is susceptible to peripheral vascular disease, neuropathy, and early coronary artery disease. Glomerulosclerosis is a common complication. Retinopathy is the major cause of acquired blindness in diabetic adults. With severely impaired vision, the client may require modifications in self-care management.

Metabolic acidosis

Diabetic ketoacidosis, a type of metabolic acidosis that occurs in diabetes, is more common in type 1 diabetes, and has a slow onset. It results from acute insulin deficiency, causing acidosis from metabolism of fats (ketone bodies). Assess for dehydration caused by polyuria and hypovolemia as well as acid-base imbalance and electrolyte changes caused by acidosis and ketone excretion. Determine the client's blood glucose level and assess the client's history for recent infection, severe stress, and noncompliance with insulin therapy. Depending on the severity of the acidosis, the client may need I.V. insulin, plasma expanders to prevent shock, and electrolyte replacement. Monitor the client's blood glucose level frequently to assess progress. Teach the client how to avoid recurrence by adhering to the planned diet, exercise, and medication program.

HHNS

The client with type 2 diabetes is at risk for HHNS, a life-threatening complication that occurs when an elevated blood glucose level leads to severe dehydration and electrolyte imbalance. Treatment resembles that for ketoacidosis; however, correcting dehydration is even more important.

Hypoglycemia (insulin reaction)

To check for hypoglycemia, assess the client for hunger, anxiety, blurred vision, sweating, and tremors. Unconsciousness can occur if the blood glucose level falls below 50 mg/dl, or below the normal level for the client. Provide a source of rapidly absorbed carbohydrate (for example, 4 oz of orange juice, regular soda pop, or five LifeSavers). If the client can't swallow, administer 25 ml of 50% glucose by I.V. bolus, as ordered. (Glucagon, which converts glycogen stored in the liver to glucose, can also be administered to a client who can't swallow; for example, a family member can administer glucagon I.M. to an unconscious client. When the client regains consciousness, the family member should provide small, frequent meals.) Monitor the blood glucose level to prevent relapse. Teach the client to avoid hypoglycemia by regulating diet, exercise, and insulin or oral hypoglycemic drugs.

- Urine chemistry shows increased glucose and ketone levels.

Nursing diagnoses

- Risk for deficient fluid volume
- Risk for impaired skin integrity
- Risk for infection
- Deficient knowledge regarding disease process and treatment
- Imbalanced nutrition: More than body requirements

Treatment

- Dietary restrictions
- Exercise
- Pancreas transplant

Drug therapy options

- Insulin or oral antidiabetic agent
- Vitamin and mineral supplement (see *Treating clients with diabetes,* page 448)

Planning and goals

- The client will remain hemodynamically stable.
- The client will maintain intact skin.
- The client won't exhibit evidence of infection.
- The client will verbalize an understanding of his treatment and disease process.
- The client's blood glucose level, HbA_{1c} level, and body weight will approach acceptable levels.

Implementation

- Assess acid-base and fluid balance *to monitor for signs of hyperglycemia.*

Treating clients with diabetes

Effective treatment for clients with diabetes optimizes blood glucose levels and decreases complications. In type 1 diabetes, treatment includes insulin replacement, meal planning, and exercise. Current forms of insulin replacement include single-dose, mixed-dose, split-mixed-dose, and multiple-dose regimens. The multiple-dose regimen may use an insulin pump.

Insulin action

Insulin may be rapid-acting (Humalog), fast-acting (Regular), intermediate-acting (NPH and Lente), long-acting (Ultralente), or a premixed combination of fast-acting and intermediate-acting. Insulin may be derived from beef, pork, or human sources. Purified human insulin is commonly used today.

Personalized meal plan

Treatment for clients with either type of diabetes also requires a meal plan to meet nutritional needs, control blood glucose levels, and help the client reach and maintain his ideal body weight. In type 1 diabetes, the calorie allotment may be high, depending on the client's growth stage and activity level. Weight reduction is a goal for the obese client with type 2 diabetes.

Other treatments

Exercise is also useful in managing type 2 diabetes because it increases insulin sensitivity, improves glucose tolerance, and promotes weight loss. In addition, clients with type 2 diabetes may need oral antidiabetic drugs to stimulate endogenous insulin production and increase insulin sensitivity at the cellular level.

Thinking long-term

Treatment for clients with long-term complications may include dialysis or kidney transplantation for renal failure, photocoagulation for retinopathy, and vascular surgery for large-vessel disease. Pancreas transplantation is also an option.

- Monitor for signs of hypoglycemia (vagueness, slow cerebration, dizziness, weakness, pallor, tachycardia, diaphoresis, seizures, and coma), ketoacidosis (acetone breath, dehydration, weak or rapid pulse, Kussmaul's respirations), and hyperosmolar coma (polyuria, thirst, neurologic abnormalities, stupor) *to ensure early intervention and prevent complications.*
- Be prepared to treat hypoglycemia; immediately give carbohydrates in the form of fruit juice, hard candy, or honey. If the client is unconscious, administer glucagon or dextrose I.V. *to prevent neurologic complications.*
- Be prepared to administer I.V. fluids, insulin and, usually, potassium replacement for ketoacidosis or hyperosmolar coma *to reduce the risk of potentially life-threatening complications.*
- Monitor and record vital signs, intake and output, fingersticks for blood glucose, and laboratory studies *to assess fluid and electrolyte balance.*
- Monitor wound healing *to assess for infection.*
- Maintain the client's diet *to prevent complications of diabetes,* such as hyperglycemia and hypoglycemia.
- Consult a registered dietitian and a diabetic educator *to help meet the client needs.*
- Force fluids *to keep the client hydrated.*
- Administer medications, as prescribed. *Diabetic control requires a dynamic balance between diet, the prescribed antidiabetic agent, and exercise.*
- Encourage the client to express feelings about diet, medication regimen, and body image changes *to facilitate coping mechanisms.*
- Encourage exercise, as tolerated, *to prevent long-term complications of diabetes.*
- Weigh the client weekly *to determine nutritional status.*
- Provide meticulous skin and foot care. *Clients with diabetes are at increased risk for infection from impaired leukocyte activity. These practices minimize the risk of infection and promote early detection of health problems.*
- Maintain a warm, quiet environment *to provide rest and reduce metabolic demands.*
- Foster independence *to promote self-esteem.*
- Determine the client's compliance with diet, exercise, and medication regimens *to help develop appropriate interventions.*

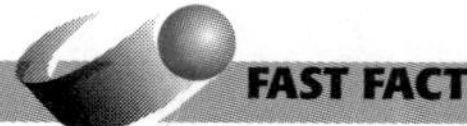

FAST FACT

Signs of hypoglycemia include vagueness, slow cerebration, dizziness, weakness, pallor, tachycardia, diaphoresis, seizures, and coma.

Evaluation

- The client is hemodynamically stable.
- The client demonstrates intact skin.
- The client remains free from infection.
- The client verbalizes knowledge of his medication regimen, diet, and potential complications of the disease.
- The client's blood studies are within acceptable limits and his weight is well controlled.

GOITER

A GOITER is an enlargement of the thyroid gland that isn't caused by inflammation or a neoplasm. This condition is typically referred to as *nontoxic* or *simple goiter.*

A goiter is commonly classified as endemic or sporadic. With appropriate treatment, the prognosis is good for either type.

Endemic goiter usually results from inadequate dietary intake of iodine associated with such factors as iodine-depleted soil and malnutrition. Endemic goiter affects females more than males, especially during adolescence and pregnancy, when the demand on the body for thyroid hormone increases.

Sporadic goiter follows ingestion of certain drugs or foods. It doesn't affect any specific population more than others.

Possible causes

- Insufficient thyroid gland production
- Depletion of glandular iodine
- Ingestion of goitrogenic foods (rutabagas, cabbage, soybeans, peanuts, peaches, peas, strawberries, spinach, and radishes)
- Use of goitrogenic drugs (propylthiouracil, methimazole, iodides, and lithium)

Assessment findings

- Single or multinodular, firm, irregular enlargement of the thyroid gland
- Dizziness or syncope when the client raises his arms above his head (Pemberton's sign)
- Dysphagia
- Respiratory distress

Diagnostic evaluation

- Testing for Graves' disease, Hashimoto's thyroiditis, and thyroid carcinoma rules out these conditions as causes of the goiter.
- Laboratory tests reveal high or normal TSH, low serum T_4 concentrations, and increased radioactive iodine (^{131}I) uptake.

Nursing diagnoses

- Imbalanced nutrition: Less than body requirements
- Disturbed body image
- Deficient knowledge of disease and treatment

Treatment

- Subtotal thyroidectomy

Drug therapy options

- Thyroid hormone replacement: levothyroxine (Synthroid)
- Iodine: small doses (Lugol's iodine or potassium iodide solution)

Planning and goals

- The client will consume a specific number of calories daily.
- The client will express positive feelings about himself.
- The client will relate knowledge regarding his illness.

Implementation

- Measure the client's neck circumference *to check for progressive thyroid gland enlargement.* Also check for the development of hard nodules in the gland, *which may indicate carcinoma.*
- Provide preoperative teaching and postoperative care if subtotal thyroidectomy is indicated. *These measures allay the client's anxiety and prevent postoperative complications.*
- Teach the client about iodized salt, medications, and symptoms of thyrotoxicosis to ensure compliance with treatment and prevent complications.

Evaluation

- The client has maintained an appropriate weight.
- The client makes positive comments regarding his self-image.
- The client relates appropriate knowledge regarding his illness.

HYPERTHYROIDISM

HYPERTHYROIDISM is the increased synthesis of thyroid hormone. It can result from overactivity (Graves' disease) or a change in the thyroid gland (toxic nodular goiter).

Possible causes

- Autoimmune disease
- Genetic factors
- Infection
- Pituitary tumors
- Psychological or physiologic stress
- Thyroid adenomas

Assessment findings

- Anxiety and mood swings
- Atrial fibrillation
- Bruit or thrill over thyroid

- Diaphoresis
- Diarrhea
- Dyspnea
- Exophthalmos
- Fine hand tremors
- Flushed, smooth skin
- Heat intolerance
- Hyperhidrosis
- Increased hunger
- Increased systolic blood pressure
- Palpitations
- Tachycardia
- Tachypnea
- Weakness
- Weight loss

Diagnostic evaluation

- Blood chemistry shows increased T_3, T_4, and free T_4 levels, and decreased TSH and cholesterol levels.
- ^{131}I uptake is increased.
- Thyroid scan shows nodules.

Nursing diagnoses

- Activity intolerance
- Risk for imbalanced body temperature
- Deficient knowledge regarding disease process and treatment

Treatment

- High-protein, high-carbohydrate, high-calorie diet; restriction of stimulants, such as coffee and caffeine
- Radiation therapy
- Thyroidectomy (see *Nursing care after thyroidectomy*)

Drug therapy options

- Adrenergic-blocking agents: guanethidine (Ismelin), propranolol (Inderal), reserpine (Serpasil)
- Antithyroid agents: methimazole (Tapazole), propylthiouracil
- Cardiac glycoside: digoxin (Lanoxin)
- Glucocorticoids: cortisone (Cortone), hydrocortisone (Solu-Cortef)
- Iodine preparations: potassium iodide (SSKI), ^{131}I
- Sedative: oxazepam (Serax)
- Vitamins: ascorbic acid (vitamin C), thiamine (vitamin B_1)

Planning and goals

- The client will be able to perform ADLs.
- The client will have normal temperature.
- The client will verbalize an understanding of the disease process and recommended treatment.

Implementation

- Assess cardiovascular status for signs of hyperthyroidism, such as tachycardia, increased blood pressure, palpitations, and atrial arrhythmias. *Presence of these signs may require a change in the treatment regimen.*
- Assess fluid balance *for signs of fluid volume deficit.*
- Monitor and record vital signs, intake and output, and laboratory studies *to detect early changes and guide treatment.*
- Maintain the client's diet *to promote adequate nutrition.*
- Avoid stimulants, such as drugs and foods that contain caffeine, *to reduce or eliminate arrhythmias.*
- Administer I.V. fluids *to promote hydration.*
- Administer medications, as prescribed, *to maintain or improve the client's condition.*
- Weigh the client daily *to ensure consistent readings.*
- Provide postoperative nursing care *to promote healing and prevent complications.*

Nursing care after thyroidectomy

Keep these crucial points in mind when caring for the client who has undergone thyroidectomy:

- Keep the client in Fowler's position to promote venous return from the head and neck and to decrease oozing into the incision.
- Watch for signs of respiratory distress (tracheal collapse, tracheal mucus accumulation, and laryngeal edema).
- Note that vocal cord paralysis can cause respiratory obstruction with sudden stridor and restlessness.
- Keep a tracheotomy tray at the client's bedside for 24 hours after surgery and be prepared to assist with emergency tracheotomy if necessary.
- Assess for signs of hemorrhage.
- Assess for hypocalcemia (tingling and numbness of the extremities, muscle twitching, cramps, laryngeal spasm, cramps, and positive Chvostek's and Trousseau's signs), which may occur when parathyroid glands are damaged.
- Keep calcium gluconate available for emergency I.V. administration.
- Be alert for signs of thyroid storm (tachycardia, hyperkinesis, fever, vomiting, and hypertension).

- Provide rest periods and a quiet, cool environment *to reduce metabolic demands and promote comfort.*
- Provide skin and eye care *to prevent complications.*
- Encourage the client to express feelings about changes in his body image *to reduce anxiety and facilitate coping mechanisms.*
- Provide postradiation nursing care *to prevent complications associated with treatment.*

Evaluation

- The client tolerates increased activity.
- The client exhibits normothermia.
- The client verbalizes an understanding of the disease and follows the recommended treatment.

HYPOTHYROIDISM

HYPOTHYROIDISM, which affects women more commonly than men, occurs when the thyroid gland fails to produce sufficient thyroid hormone. This deficiency causes an overall decrease in metabolism.

Possible causes

- Hashimoto's thyroiditis
- Malfunction of pituitary gland
- Overuse of antithyroid drugs
- Thyroidectomy
- Use of ^{131}I

Assessment findings

- Fatigue
- Hypothermia
- Constipation
- Menstrual disorders
- Weight gain and anorexia
- Mental sluggishness
- Dry, flaky skin and thinning nails
- Coarse hair and alopecia
- Cold intolerance
- Decreased diaphoresis
- Edema
- Hypersensitivity to narcotics, barbiturates, and anesthetics
- Thick tongue and swollen lips

Diagnostic evaluation

- Blood chemistry shows decreased T_3, T_4, and sodium levels, and increased TSH and cholesterol levels.
- ^{131}I uptake is decreased.

Nursing diagnoses

- Activity intolerance
- Decreased cardiac output
- Ineffective coping
- Deficient knowledge related to disease process and treatment

Treatment

- High-fiber, high-protein, low-calorie diet

Drug therapy options

- Stool softener: docusate sodium (Colace)
- Thyroid hormone replacement: levothyroxine (Synthroid), liothyronine (Cytomel), thyroglobulin (Proloid)

Planning and goals

- The client will resume a normal activity level.
- The client will remain hemodynamically stable.
- The client will exhibit adequate coping skills.
- The client verbalizes an understanding of the disease process and treatment.

Implementation

- Avoid sedation. Administer one-half to one-third the normal dose of sedatives or opioids *to prevent complications.* (See *Caring for the client with hypothyroidism,* page 452.)
- Monitor for drug interactions and adverse effects *to avoid complications.*
- Assess fluid balance *to determine fluid volume deficit or excess.*
- Check for constipation and edema *to detect early changes.*
- Monitor and record vital signs, intake and output, and laboratory studies *to determine fluid status.*
- Maintain the client's diet *to facilitate nutritional balance.*
- Force fluids *to maintain hydration.*
- Administer medications, as prescribed, *to maintain or improve the client's condition.*
- Encourage the client to express feelings of depression *to promote coping mechanisms.*
- Encourage physical activity and mental stimulation *to enhance self-esteem.*
- Provide a warm environment *to promote comfort because the client with hypothyroidism may be sensitive to cold.*
- Turn the client every 2 hours while on bed rest and provide skin care *to prevent skin breakdown.*
- Provide frequent rest periods *because clients diagnosed with hypothyroidism are commonly fatigued.*

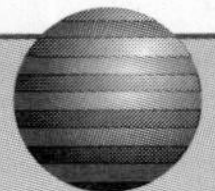

CLINICAL SITUATION

Caring for the client with hypothyroidism

A 65-year-old male client recently retired after 50 years as a butcher. He has gradually become lethargic and usually sits all day. His physician has diagnosed his condition as hypothyroidism.

How would the client's condition be confirmed?
Laboratory tests could confirm hypothyroidism. The thyroid-stimulating hormone level would be increased and T_3 and T_4 levels would be decreased.

Why should the nurse instruct the client to monitor his pulse rate?
A rapid pulse rate may indicate signs of drug toxicity. Other adverse reactions include palpitations, nervousness, increased blood pressure, weight loss, heat intolerance, and insomnia.

How should sedatives be prescribed for this client?
A client with hypothyroidism should be given sedatives at one-half to one-third the normal dose to prevent complications.

Questions for further thought

- What are appropriate nursing diagnoses for this client?
- What effects does thyroid hormone replacement have on a client's metabolism? Why would such treatment put a client who's susceptible to cardiac problems (such as angina) at risk?

Evaluation

- The client resumes his previous activity level.
- The client has stable vital signs.
- The client develops adequate coping skills.
- The client verbalizes an understanding of the chronic illness and required treatment.

PANCREATIC CANCER

Pancreatic cancer progresses rapidly and is deadly. Treatment is rarely successful because the disease has usually widely metastasized by the time it's diagnosed. Therapeutic care focuses on helping the client and family come to terms with the end of life.

Pancreatic tumors are almost always adenocarcinomas and most arise in the head of the pancreas. Tumors of the body and tail of the pancreas and of the islet cells are less common. The two main tissue types are cylinder cell and large, fatty, granular cell.

Possible causes

- Foods high in fat and protein
- Food additives
- Industrial chemicals, such as naphthalene, benzidine, and urea
- Smoking

Assessment findings

- Dull, intermittent epigastric pain (early in disease)
- Continuous pain that radiates to the right upper quadrant or dorsolumbar area (may be colicky, dull, or vague and unrelated to activity or posture)
- Anorexia
- Nausea
- Vomiting
- Diarrhea
- Jaundice
- Pruritus
- Clay-colored stools
- Splenomegaly
- Hepatomegaly
- Steatorrhea
- Rapid, profound weight loss
- Palpable mass in the subumbilical or left hypochondrial region

Diagnostic evaluation

- Percutaneous fine-needle aspiration biopsy of the pancreas may detect tumor cells.
- Laparotomy with a biopsy allows definitive diagnosis.
- Ultrasonography and CT scanning can identify a mass but not its histology.
- Angiography can reveal the vascular supply of a tumor.

◆ MRI shows tumor size and location in great detail.
◆ Blood studies reveal increased serum bilirubin, increased serum amylase and lipase, prolonged PT, elevated alkaline phosphatase (with biliary obstruction), and elevated aspartate aminotransferase and alanine aminotransferase (when liver cell necrosis is present).
◆ Fasting blood glucose may indicate hyperglycemia or hypoglycemia.
◆ Plasma insulin immunoassay shows measurable serum insulin in the presence of islet cell tumors.
◆ Stool studies may show occult blood if ulceration in the GI tract or ampulla of Vater has occurred.
◆ Tumor markers for pancreatic cancer, including carcinoembryonic antigen, alpha-fetoprotein, and serum immunoreactive elastase I, are elevated.

Nursing diagnoses

◆ Disturbed sensory perception: Tactile
◆ Acute pain
◆ Imbalanced nutrition: Less than body requirements
◆ Powerlessness

Treatment

◆ Blood transfusion
◆ I.V. fluid therapy
◆ Total pancreatectomy (surgical removal of the pancreas)
◆ Cholecystojejunostomy (surgical anastomosis of the gallbladder and the jejunum)
◆ Choledochoduodenostomy (surgical anastomosis of the common bile duct and the duodenum)
◆ Choledochojejunostomy (surgical anastomosis of the common bile duct and the jejunum)
◆ Whipple's operation or pancreatoduodenectomy (excision of the head of the pancreas along with the encircling loop of the duodenum)
◆ Gastrojejunostomy (surgical creation of an anastomosis between the stomach and the jejunum)
◆ Radiation therapy
◆ Chemotherapy

Drug therapy options

◆ Antineoplastic combination: fluorouracil (Adrucil), streptozocin (Zanosar), ifosfamide (IFEX), doxorubicin (Adriamycin)
◆ Antibiotic: cefmetazole (Zefazone) to prevent infection and relieve symptoms
◆ Anticholinergic: propantheline (Pro-Banthine) to decrease GI tract spasm and motility and reduce pain and secretions
◆ Histamine-2 receptor antagonists: cimetidine (Tagamet), ranitidine (Zantac), famotidine (Pepcid), nizatidine (Axid)
◆ Diuretic: furosemide (Lasix) to mobilize extracellular fluid from ascites
◆ Insulin to provide an adequate exogenous insulin supply after pancreatic resection
◆ Narcotic analgesics: morphine, meperidine (Demerol), codeine (can lead to biliary tract spasm and increased common bile duct pressure; used when other methods fail)
◆ Pancreatic enzyme: pancrelipase (Pancrease)
◆ Vitamin K: phytonadione (AquaMEPHYTON)

Planning and goals

◆ The client will express feelings of comfort and pain relief.
◆ The client will demonstrate improved nutritional status.
◆ The client will demonstrate adequate coping mechanisms.

Implementation

Before surgery

◆ Ensure that the client is medically stable, particularly regarding nutrition (which may take 4 to 5 days). If the client can't tolerate oral feedings, provide TPN and I.V. fat emulsions *to correct deficiencies and maintain a positive nitrogen balance.*
◆ Give blood transfusions *to combat anemia,* vitamin K *to overcome prothrombin deficiency,* antibiotics *to prevent postoperative infection,* and gastric lavage *to maintain gastric decompression, as necessary.*
◆ Tell the client about expected postoperative procedures and expected adverse effects of radiation and chemotherapy *to allay anxiety.*

After surgery

◆ Watch for and report complications, such as fistula, pancreatitis, fluid and electrolyte imbalance, infection, hemorrhage, skin breakdown, nutritional deficiency, hepatic failure, renal insufficiency, and diabetes *to ensure early detection and treatment of complications.*
◆ If the client is receiving chemotherapy, treat adverse effects symptomatically *to promote client comfort and prevent complications.*

Throughout illness

◆ Monitor fluid balance, abdominal girth, metabolic state, and weight daily *to determine fluid volume status.* Replace nutrients I.V., orally, or by NG tube *to combat weight loss.*

Impose dietary restrictions, such as a low-sodium or low-fluid retention diet as required, *to combat weight gain (due to ascites)*. Maintain a 2,500-calorie diet for the client *to meet increased nutritional needs.*

- Administer an oral pancreatic enzyme at mealtimes, if needed, *to aid digestion.*
- Consult a registered dietitian *to help meet the clients nutritional needs.* Serve small, frequent, nutritious meals *to help the client meet increased metabolic demands.*
- Position the client properly at mealtime and help him walk when he can *to increase GI motility.*
- Administer pain medication *to promote comfort;* antibiotics *to combat infection;* and antipyretics *to reduce fever,* as necessary.
- Watch for signs of hypoglycemia or hyperglycemia; administer glucose or an antidiabetic agent as necessary *to prevent complications of hypoglycemia or hyperglycemia.* Monitor blood glucose levels *to detect early signs of hypoglycemia or hyperglycemia*
- Provide meticulous skin care *to avoid pruritus and necrosis.*
- Watch for signs of upper GI bleeding; test stools and vomitus for occult blood and keep a flow sheet of Hb and HCT values *to prevent hemorrhage.*
- Promote gastric vasoconstriction with prescribed medication *to control active bleeding.* Replace any fluid loss *to prevent hypovolemia.*
- Ease discomfort from pyloric obstruction with an NG tube *to provide gastric decompression.*
- Apply antiembolism stockings and assist in ROM exercises while on bed rest *to prevent thrombosis.* If thrombosis occurs, elevate the client's legs *to promote venous return* and give an anticoagulant or aspirin as required *to decrease blood viscosity and prevent further thrombosis.*

Evaluation

- The client reports comfort and adequate pain control.
- The client's nutritional status has improved, as evidenced by laboratory values.
- The client employs adequate coping skills.

THYROID CANCER

Thyroid cancer is a malignant, primary tumor of the thyroid. It doesn't affect thyroid hormone secretion. (See *Anaplastic thyroid cancer.*)

Possible causes

- Chronic overstimulation of the pituitary gland
- Chronic overstimulation of the thymus gland
- Familiar disposition
- Radiation exposure

Assessment findings

- Enlarged thyroid gland
- Painless, firm, irregular, enlarged thyroid nodule or mass
- Hoarseness
- Dysphagia
- Dyspnea
- Palpable cervical lymph nodes

Diagnostic evaluation

- Blood chemistry shows increased calcitonin, serotonin, and prostaglandin levels.
- ^{131}I uptake shows a "cold," or nonfunctioning, nodule.
- Thyroid biopsy shows cytology positive for cancer cells.
- Thyroid function test is normal.

Nursing diagnoses

- Anxiety
- Impaired swallowing
- Acute pain

Treatment

- High-protein, high-carbohydrate, high-calorie diet with supplemental feedings
- Radiation therapy
- Thyroidectomy (total or subtotal); total thyroidectomy and radical neck excision

Drug therapy options

- Antiemetics: prochlorperazine (Compazine), ondansetron (Zofran)
- Chemotherapy: chlorambucil (Leukeran), doxorubicin (Adriamycin), vincristine (Oncovin)
- Thyroid hormone replacement: levothyroxine (Synthroid), liothyronine (Cytomel), thyroglobulin (Proloid)

Planning and goals

- The client will use available support systems to help with coping mechanisms.
- The client won't aspirate.
- The client will express feelings of comfort and pain relief.

Anaplastic thyroid cancer

The most disfiguring, destructive, and deadly form of thyroid cancer, anaplastic carcinoma, has the poorest prognosis. Although this tumor rarely metastasizes to distant organs, its rapid growth and size produce severe anatomic distortion of nearby structures. Treatment usually consists of total thyroidectomy, which is seldom successful.

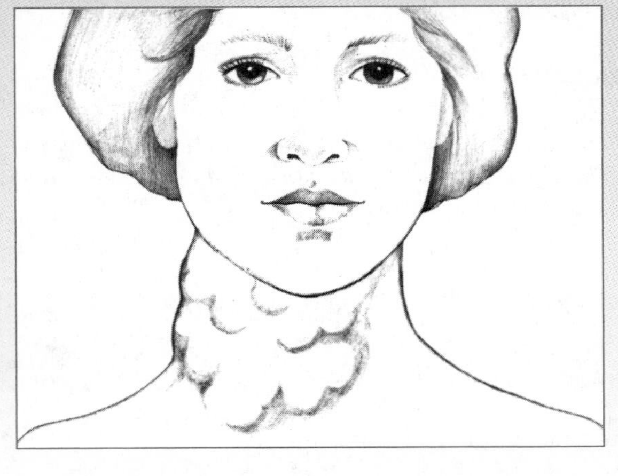

Implementation

◆ Assess respiratory status for signs of airway obstruction. A tracheotomy set should be kept at the bedside *because swelling may cause airway obstruction.*

◆ Assess the client's ability to swallow *to maintain a patent airway.*

◆ Provide postoperative thyroidectomy care *to promote healing and prevent postoperative complications.*

◆ Monitor and record vital signs, intake and output, and laboratory studies *to determine a baseline and detect early changes that may occur with hemorrhage, airway obstruction, or hypocalcemia.*

◆ Administer medications, as prescribed, *to maintain or improve the client's condition.*

◆ Maintain the client's diet *to improve nutritional status.*

◆ Encourage the client to express his feelings *to facilitate coping mechanisms.*

◆ Provide postchemotherapy and postradiation nursing care *to prevent and treat complications associated with therapy.*

◆ Consult home care and hospice services *to help meet the client's needs.*

Evaluation

◆ The client demonstrates appropriate coping mechanisms in dealing with his illness.

◆ The client doesn't display signs or symptoms of aspiration.

◆ The client reports adequate pain control.

THYROIDITIS

THYROIDITIS is inflammation of the thyroid gland. It may occur in various forms: autoimmune thyroiditis or Hashimoto's thyroiditis (long-term inflammatory disease); subacute granulomatous thyroiditis or DeQuervain's thyroiditis (self-limiting inflammation); silent thyroiditis (postpartum thyroiditis occurring within 1 year after delivery); and miscellaneous thyroiditis (acute suppurative, chronic infective, and chronic noninfective types).

Possible causes

◆ Antibodies to thyroid antigens

◆ Bacterial invasion

◆ Mumps, influenza, coxsackievirus, or adenovirus infection

◆ Recent pregnancy

◆ Sarcoidisis and amyloidasis

◆ Tuberculosis, syphilis, actinomycosis or other infectious agents in chronic infective form.

Assessment findings

◆ Thyroid enlargement

◆ Fever

◆ Pain

◆ Tenderness and reddened skin over the thyroid gland

Diagnostic evaluation

Autoimmune thyroiditis

◆ Blood studies show high titers of thyroglobulin and microsomal antibodies present in serum.

Subacute granulomatous thyroiditis

◆ Laboratory tests show an ESR, increased thyroid hormone levels, decreased thyroidal ^{131}I uptake.

Acute suppurative, chronic infective, and noninfective thyroiditis

◆ Laboratory studies show varied findings, depending on underlying infection or other disease.

Nursing diagnoses

- Risk for infection
- Acute pain
- Disturbed body image

Treatment

- Partial thyroidectomy to relieve tracheal or esophageal compression in Riedel's thyroiditis (rare, chronic type of thyroiditis)

Drug therapy options

- Thyroid hormone replacement: levothyroxine (Synthroid) for accompanying hypothyroidism
- Analgesic and anti-inflammatory agent: indomethacin (Indocin) for mild subacute granulomatous thyroiditis
- Beta-adrenergic blocker: propranolol (Inderal) for transient thyrotoxicosis

Planning and goals

- The client won't have signs or symptoms of infection.
- The client will express feelings of comfort and pain relief.
- The client will express a positive image of himself.

Implementation

Before thyroidectomy

- Obtain a client history *to identify underlying diseases that may cause thyroiditis, such as tuberculosis and a recent viral infection.*
- Check vital signs and examine the client's neck for unusual swelling, enlargement, or redness *to detect disease progression and signs of airway occlusion.*
- Consult a registered dietitian *to help meet the client's nutritional needs.*
- If the neck is swollen, measure and record the circumference daily *to monitor progressive enlargement.*
- Check for signs of thyrotoxicosis (nervousness, tremor, weakness), which commonly occur in subacute thyroiditis. *Checking for early signs prevents treatment delay.*
- Instruct the client to watch for and report signs of hypothyroidism (lethargy, restlessness, sensitivity to cold, forgetfulness, dry skin) *to prevent complications.*

After thyroidectomy

- Check vital signs every 15 to 30 minutes until the client's condition stabilizes. Stay alert for signs of tetany secondary to accidental parathyroid injury during surgery. Keep 10% calcium gluconate available for I.V. use if needed. *These measures help prevent serious postoperative complications.*
- Assess dressings frequently for excessive bleeding *to detect signs of hemorrhage.*
- Watch for signs of airway obstruction, such as difficulty talking and increased swallowing; keep tracheotomy equipment handy. *The airway may become obstructed because of postoperative edema; tracheotomy equipment should be handy to avoid treatment delay if the airway becomes obstructed.*

Evaluation

- The client doesn't exhibit signs of infection.
- The client reports adequate pain control.
- The client demonstrates a positive body image and attitude toward himself.

HEMATOLOGIC AND IMMUNE SYSTEMS

The hematologic and immune systems are closely related. The immune system consists of specialized cells and structures that defend the body against invasion by harmful organisms or chemical toxins. The hematologic system also functions as an important part of the body's defenses. Blood transports the components of the immune system throughout the body. In addition, blood delivers oxygen and nutrients to all tissues and removes wastes. Immune system cells and blood cells originate in the bone marrow. Blood components play a vital role in transporting electrolytes and regulating acid-base balance.

HEMATOLOGIC AND IMMUNE STRUCTURE AND FUNCTION

The key structures of the immune system are the:

- lymph nodes
- thymus
- spleen
- tonsils.

The key structures of the hematologic system are the:

- blood
- bone marrow.

Lymphatic vessels and nodes

Lymphatic vessels include capillaries that are permeable to large molecules. Lymphatic vessels prevent edema by

moving fluid and proteins from interstitial spaces to venous circulation. Lymph nodes are patches of lymphatic tissue regionally dispersed throughout the body in clusters. They filter lymph fluid as it flows through the lymphatic vessels. These clusters include:
- cervical nodes — drain the head and neck
- axillary nodes — drain the upper extremities and chest
- inguinal nodes — drain the lower extremities and genitals.

Lymph is a clear fluid resembling plasma. Lymph is composed of water, the end product of cell metabolism, protein, and electrolytes.

Thymus
The thymus gland is located in the neck. This structure forms thymosin, which is involved in the development of lymphocytes and T cells.

Spleen
The spleen is a collection of lymph tissue. Here are some major characteristics of the spleen:
- It's the largest lymphoid organ.
- It destroys bacteria entering by the splenic artery.
- It filters blood rather than lymph.
- It serves as a blood reservoir.
- Lymphocytes and monocytes are located in the spleen.
- The spleen traps formed particles, which are destroyed in the spleen by leukocytes.

Tonsils
Tonsils are a large collection of lymph nodes in the oropharynx that filter pathogens entering the mouth or nose. There are three sets of tonsils, including the palatine, pharyngeal, and lingual tonsils.

Blood
Blood is composed of several components, including erythrocytes, thrombocytes, leukocytes, and plasma.

Erythrocytes
ERYTHROCYTES, also called *red blood cells* (RBCs), are formed in the bone marrow and contain Hb. Oxygen binds with Hb to form oxyhemoglobin, which is transported throughout the body.

Thrombocytes
THROMBOCYTES, also called *platelets,* are formed in the bone marrow and function in the coagulation of blood. They are produced from fragments of megakaryocytes.

Leukocytes
LEUKOCYTES, also called *white blood cells* (WBCs) are formed in the bone marrow and lymphatic tissue and include nuclei. They're white because they lack Hb. WBCs provide protection from infection by phagocytosis (engulfing, digesting, and destroying microorganisms).

Plasma
Plasma is the liquid portion of the blood and is composed of water, proteins (albumin and globulin), glucose, and electrolytes.

Blood type
A person's BLOOD TYPE is determined by a system of antigens located on the surface of RBCs. The four blood types are:
- A antigen
- B antigen
- AB (both A and B) antigens
- O (no antigens).

Because group O lacks certain antigens, it can be transfused in limited amounts in an emergency to individuals of other blood types. People with that blood type are called *universal donors.* A person with AB negative lacks certain antigens and can receive blood from people of other blood types. This person is sometimes called a *universal recipient.*

The antigen Rh factor is found on the RBCs of approximately 85% of people. A person with the Rh factor is said to have Rh-positive blood. A person without the factor is Rh-negative. A person may receive blood only from a person with the same Rh factor.

Bone marrow
Bone marrow is involved in blood cell production. Hematopoiesis is carried out by red marrow and produces erythrocytes, leukocytes, and thrombocytes. Red bone marrow is a source of stem cells that differentiate into the three previously mentioned cells.
- Some stem cells evolve into lymphocytes; lymphocytes may become B cells or T cells.
- Other stem cells evolve into monocytes or megakaryocytes, also called *thrombocytes* or *platelets.*

Immune system
In cell-mediated immunity, T cells respond directly to antigens (foreign substances such as bacteria or toxins that induce antibody formation). This response involves destruction of target cells — such as virus-infected cells and

cancer cells — through secretion of lymphokines (lymph proteins). Examples of cell-mediated immunity are rejection of transplanted organs and delayed immune responses that fight disease.

T cells

T CELLS can be killers, helpers, or suppressors:
- Killer T cells bind to the surface of the invading cell, disrupt the membrane, and destroy it by altering its internal environment.
- Helper T cells stimulate other T cells and B cells to mature, enhancing the immune response.
- Suppressor T cells reduce the humoral response when the antigen is destroyed.

B cells

B CELLS act differently from T cells to recognize and destroy antigens. B cells are responsible for humoral, or immunoglobulin-mediated, immunity. B cells originate in the bone marrow and mature into plasma cells that produce antibodies (immunoglobulin molecules that interact with a specific antigen).

Immunoglobulins

There are five major classes of IMMUNOGLOBULIN:
- Immunoglobulin G (IgG) is found in the circulation and tissue spaces. It activates complement proteins.
- Immunoglobulin M (IgM) is the first immunoglobulin produced during an immune response. It's too large to easily cross membrane barriers and is usually present only in the vascular system. It activates complement proteins.
- Immunoglobulin A (IgA) is found mainly in body secretions, such as saliva, sweat, tears, mucus, bile, and colostrum. It defends against pathogens on body surfaces, especially those that enter the respiratory and GI tracts.
- Immunoglobulin D (IgD) is found on the cell membrane of the surface of B cells. Its exact function is unknown; it may be active in antigen recognition.
- Immunoglobulin E (IgE) is the antibody involved in immediate hypersensitivity reactions, or allergic reactions that develop within minutes of exposure to an antigen. IgE stimulates the release of mast cell granules, which contain histamine and heparin.

HEMATOLOGIC AND IMMUNE DISORDERS

Major immune disorders include acquired immunodeficiency syndrome (AIDS), anemia (aplastic, iron deficiency, pernicious, and sickle cell), ankylosing spondylitis, disseminated intravascular coagulation (DIC), hemophilia, Kaposi's sarcoma, leukemia, lymphoma, multiple myeloma, polycythemia vera, rheumatoid arthritis, scleroderma, systemic lupus erythematosus, and vasculitis.

ACQUIRED IMMUNODEFICIENCY SYNDROME

AIDS is a defect in T cell–mediated immunity caused by HIV. AIDS places a client at significant risk for the development of potentially fatal opportunistic infections. A diagnosis of AIDS is based on laboratory evidence of HIV infection coexisting with one or more indicator diseases, such as herpes simplex virus, cytomegalovirus, mycobacteria, candidal infection, *Pneumocystis carinii* pneumonia, Kaposi's sarcoma, wasting syndrome, or dementia.

Possible causes

- Exposure to blood containing HIV (transfusions, contaminated needles, handling of blood, in utero)
- Exposure to semen and vaginal secretions containing HIV (sexual intercourse, handling of semen and vaginal secretions)

Assessment findings

- Anorexia, weight loss, recurrent diarrhea
- Disorientation, confusion, dementia
- Fatigue and weakness
- Fever
- Lymphadenopathy
- Malnutrition
- Night sweats
- Opportunistic infections
- Pallor

Diagnostic evaluation

- Blood chemistry shows increased transaminase, alkaline phosphatase, and gamma globulin levels and a decreased albumin level.
- $CD4^+$ T-cell level is less than 200 cells/µl.
- Enzyme-linked immunosorbent assay shows positive HIV antibody titer.

◆ Hematologic studies show decreased WBCs, RBCs, and platelets.
◆ Western blot test result is positive.

Nursing diagnoses

◆ Ineffective protection
◆ Hopelessness
◆ Social isolation

Treatment

◆ Activity, including active and passive ROM exercises, as tolerated
◆ High-calorie, high-protein diet and small, frequent feedings (see *Nutrition and AIDS*)
◆ Nutritional support, including TPN and enteral feedings, if necessary
◆ Plasmapheresis
◆ Respiratory treatments, including chest physiotherapy, postural drainage, and incentive spirometry
◆ Specialized air therapy bed
◆ Standard precautions
◆ Transfusion therapy, including fresh frozen plasma, platelets, and packed RBCs

Drug therapy options

◆ Antibiotic: co-trimoxazole (Bactrim)
◆ Antiemetic: prochlorperazine (Compazine)
◆ Antifungals: amphotericin B (Fungizone), fluconazole (Diflucan)
◆ Antivirals: acyclovir (Zovirax), aerosolized pentamidine (Nebupent), dapsone, didanosine (Videx), ganciclovir (Cytovene), pentamidine (Pentam 300), zidovudine (Retrovir, AZT)
◆ Interferon α-2a, recombinant (Roferon-A)

Medications used in combination to fight HIV

◆ Nonnucleoside reverse transcriptase inhibitors: delavirdine (Rescriptor), nevirapine (Viramune) to block conversion of RNA to DNA, preventing incorporation into the nucleus of the infected cell
◆ Nucleoside reverse transcriptase inhibitors: lamivudine (Epivir), zalcitabine (Dideoxycytidine, ddC), zidovudine (Retrovir, AZT) to interrupt viral DNA synthesis by substituting a "look-alike" compound resembling one of the normal nucleisides the virus uses to construct DNA from RNA
◆ Protease inhibitors: indinavir (Crixivan), nelfinavir (Viracept), ritonavir (Norvir), saquinavir (Invirase) to block protease enzymes needed to cut the viral protein into short segments around viral RNA

Nutrition and AIDS

Clinical manifestations of altered nutritional status in a patient with acquired immunodeficiency syndrome (AIDS) include:
◆ Weight loss that is:
– progressive and unexplained loss (wasting syndrome)
– Massive loss (20 to 40 lb [9 to 18 kg]) with severe diarrhea.
◆ Reduced appetite secondary to malaise, depression, or drug therapy
◆ Early satiety related to massive hepatomegaly or splenomegaly
◆ Diarrhea (can be severe)
◆ Other GI symptoms, including:
– dysphagia
– steatorrhea
– lactose intolerance
– nausea and vomiting
– abdominal pain
– taste alterations
– malabsorption
– alterations in metabolism of nutrients.

Nutritional support

◆ For outpatient clients to supplement calories and protein:
– whole milk and cream
– liberal use of butter, margarine, and mayonnaise
– sauces and gravies
– toppings (nuts, whipped cream, sour cream, frostings)
– nonfat dry milk added to home-baked goods, hot cereals, soups, and desserts.
◆ For inpatient clients who have good appetite, minimal malabsorption, moderate diarrhea, and semisolid stool:
– high calories
– high protein
– low fat (about 3% of total calorie intake)
– lactose-free dairy foods
– oral food supplement.
◆ For inpatient clients with severe diarrhea:
– short-term use of the BRAT diet (Bananas, Rice, Apples, and Tea and Toast)
– oral food supplement.

Planning and goals

◆ The client will remain free from infection and complications as long as possible.

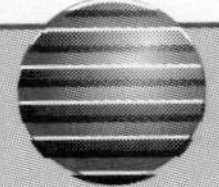

CLINICAL SITUATION

Caring for the client with HIV infection

A 30-year-old male client has a history of I.V. drug abuse. He arrives at the medical clinic complaining of shortness of breath, hacking cough, and loss of appetite. He has lost 20 lb (9.1 kg) during the past several months. Diagnostic testing reveals that he has Pneumocystis carinii *pneumonia and human immunodeficiency virus (HIV) infection. His CD4+ lymphocyte count has decreased from 220 cells/µl to 160/µl.*

Can you identify at least four appropriate nursing diagnoses?

There are a number of appropriate nursing diagnoses for this client, including:

- Impaired gas exchange related to respiratory infection
- Imbalanced nutrition: Less than body requirements related to anorexia, weight loss, and possible GI manifestations
- Risk for infection related to impaired immunocompetence
- Diarrhea related to GI infection
- Activity intolerance related to weakness and air hunger
- Disturbed body image related to weight loss
- Impaired home maintenance management related to debilitation
- Social isolation related to possible rejection by peers
- Fear related to the disease's life-threatening consequences
- Disturbed sensory perception (visual) related to neurologic complications.

What steps could be taken to relieve respiratory distress?

Respiratory distress warrants immediate relief. Appropriate interventions include:

- administering oxygen to relieve hypoxemia present with extensive *Pneumocystis* infection
- instituting chest physiotherapy to mobilize secretions from the chest and help maintain a patent airway
- teaching the client diaphragmatic and pursed-lip breathing (because breathing exercises enhance respirations)
- instructing the client to avoid smoking (because smoking and other forms of smoke should be avoided to prevent further lung damage)
- administering antibiotics, such as co-trimoxazole and pentamidine (an antiprotozoal agent), as ordered, and monitoring the client for adverse effects. (Preventive treatment is recommended for a client whose CD4+ lymphocyte count drops below 200/µl.)

Questions for further thought

- Why is it so important to monitor for signs of immunosuppression?
- What should be included in instructions regarding sexual practices?

- The client will identify a support system, be able to verbalize feelings, and learn lifestyle adjustments needed to cope with AIDS.
- The client will experience decreased feelings of isolation.

Implementation

- Assess respiratory and neurologic systems *to detect AIDS-related dementia.* Other factors, such as anemia, fever, hypoxemia, and fluid balance, can affect neurologic status.
- Monitor and record vital signs *to detect evidence of compromise.*
- Monitor for opportunistic infections *because early treatment may limit complications.*
- Administer oxygen *to enhance oxygenation.*
- Provide incentive spirometry and assist with turning, coughing, and deep breathing *to mobilize and remove secretions.*
- Encourage fluids or administer I.V. fluids *to prevent dehydration.*
- Maintain the client's diet *to fight opportunistic infection and maintain weight.*
- Consult a registered dietitian *to optimize nutritional status.* Administer TPN and enteral feedings if necessary *to bolster nutritional reserves and immune system.*
- Administer medications, as prescribed, *to reduce the risk of complications and halt the reproduction of HIV.*
- Maintain activity, as tolerated, *to encourage independence.*
- Provide rest periods *to reduce oxygen demands and prevent fatigue.* (See *Caring for the client with HIV infection.*)
- Provide mouth care *to prevent infection, provide comfort, and enhance the taste of meals.*

◆ Maintain standard precautions *to avoid exposure to blood, body fluids, and secretions.*
◆ Provide pain medication as prescribed *to relieve pain and decrease anxiety.*
◆ Encourage the client to express feelings about changes in his body image, a fear of dying, and social isolation *to help him cope with chronic illness and reduce his anxiety.*
◆ Make referrals to community agencies for support *to enhance quality of life and independence.*
◆ Monitor intake and output, daily weight, and urine specific gravity *for early recognition and treatment of dehydration.*
◆ Assess respiratory status *to detect complications, such as pneumonia and malignancies.*
◆ Monitor laboratory values *for early detection of complications. Thrombocytopenia requires precautions to prevent bleeding. Leukopenia requires precautions to prevent infection.*
◆ Review key teaching topics with the client *to ensure adequate knowledge about the condition and treatment,* including:
– refraining from donating blood
– avoiding use of alcohol and recreational drugs
– using condoms during sexual intercourse
– avoiding anal sex
– getting laboratory testing performed every 3 months or as ordered
– adhering to the medication regimen
– speaking with a health care professional about vaccine status
– cleaning drug paraphernalia with bleach (if using I.V. drugs).

Evaluation

◆ The client remains afebrile and exhibits no sign of infections, including wound, respiratory, skin, and oral infections.
◆ The client expresses feelings, learns coping skills, and is able to identify personal and community support systems.
◆ The client participates in care and unit activities as much as possible and maintains prior social relationships.

ANEMIA, APLASTIC

APLASTIC ANEMIA, also known as *normocytic anemia* is an immune-medicated illness that results from suppression, damage, or infiltration of the bone marrow. This damage to the bone marrow causes an inability to produce adequate amounts of erythrocytes, leukocytes, and platelets. Aplastic anemia may be congenital or acquired.

Possible causes

◆ Chemotherapy agents
◆ Drug-use (some anti-inflammatory, antibiotic, or anticonvulsant agents)
◆ Exposure to toxic chemicals
◆ Autoimmune diseases
◆ Radiation
◆ Viral and bacterial infections

Assessment findings

◆ Fatigue, weakness
◆ Purpura, petechiae, ecchymosis, pallor
◆ Dyspnea, tachypnea
◆ Bleeding (epistaxis, hematuria, melena)
◆ Anorexia
◆ Gingivitis
◆ Headache
◆ Multiple infections, fever
◆ Palpitations, tachycardia

Diagnostic evaluation

◆ Bone marrow biopsy specimen shows fatty marrow with reduction of stem cells.
◆ Fecal occult blood test result is positive.
◆ Hematologic studies show decreased granulocytes, thrombocytes, and RBCs.
◆ Peripheral blood smear shows pancytopenia.
◆ Urine chemistry reveals hematuria.

Nursing diagnoses

◆ Risk for infection
◆ Risk for deficient fluid volume
◆ Activity intolerance

Treatment

◆ Bone marrow transplantation
◆ Dietary changes, including establishing a high-protein, high-calorie, high-vitamin diet
◆ Supportive care to prevent or treat infections and hemorrhage
◆ Transfusion of platelets and packed RBCs

Drug therapy options

◆ Analgesics: ibuprofen (Motrin), acetaminophen (Tylenol)
◆ Androgens: fluoxymesterone (Halotestin), oxymetholone (Anadrol-50)
◆ Antibiotic, according to the susceptibility of the infecting organism

◆ Immunosupressants: antithymocyte globulin (ATG) and cyclosporine
◆ Hematopoietic growth factor: epoetin alfa (Epogen)
◆ Human granulocyte colony-stimulating factor: filgastim (Neupogen)

Planning and goals

◆ The client will maintain an adequate fluid balance.
◆ The client will remain free from infection.
◆ The client will be free from complications caused by decreased activity.

Implementation

◆ Assess respiratory status *to detect hypoxemia caused by low Hb levels.*
◆ Assess vital signs *for signs of hemorrhage, infection, and activity intolerance.*
◆ Assess cardiovascular status *to detect arrhythmias or myocardial ischemia.*
◆ Monitor and record intake and output and urine specific gravity *to determine fluid balance.*
◆ Monitor laboratory values *to determine the effectiveness of therapy.*
◆ Assess stool, urine, and emesis *for occult blood loss caused by reduced platelet levels.*
◆ Monitor for infection, bleeding, and bruising *caused by reduced levels of WBCs and platelets.*
◆ Encourage fluids and administer I.V. fluids *to replace fluids lost by fever and bleeding.*
◆ Administer oxygen to improve tissue oxygenation *because low Hb levels reduce the oxygen-carrying capacity of the blood.*
◆ Assist with turning, coughing, and deep breathing *to mobilize and remove secretions.*
◆ Administer transfusion therapy, as prescribed, *to replace low blood components.*
◆ Administer medications, as prescribed, *to treat the disorder and prevent complications.*
◆ Maintain the client's diet *to promote RBC production and fight infection.*
◆ Encourage verbalization of concerns and fears *to allay the client's anxiety.*
◆ Alternate rest periods with activity *to conserve energy and reduce weakness caused by anemia.*
◆ Provide cooling blankets and tepid sponge baths for fever *to promote comfort and reduce metabolic demands.*
◆ Maintain protective precautions *to prevent infection and hemorrhage.*
◆ Provide mouth care before and after meals *to enhance the taste of meals.*
◆ Provide skin care *to prevent skin breakdown due to bed rest, dehydration, and fever.*
◆ Protect the client from falls *to reduce the risk of hemorrhage.*
◆ Avoid giving the client I.M. injections *to reduce the risk of hemorrhage.*
◆ Avoid using hard toothbrushes and straight razors on the client *to reduce the risk of hemorrhage.*
◆ Provide genetic counseling resources for the client for futher information *so the client can make informed decisions.*
◆ Review key teaching topics with the client *to ensure adequate knowledge about his condition and treatment,* including:
– recognizing the early signs and symptoms of bleeding and infection
– avoiding contact sports
– wearing a medical identification bracelet
– refraining from using over-the-counter medications
– monitoring stool for occult blood
– using an electric razor to avoid bleeding
– refraining from taking aspirin.

Evaluation

◆ The client is afebrile and free from signs of infection, including respiratory infections and skin breakdown.
◆ The client has a balanced intake and output and normal vital signs.
◆ The client displays no complications from inactivity.

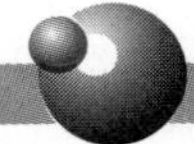

SPOT CHECK

What are three possible causes of aplastic anemia?
Answer: Three possible causes of aplastic anemia are chemotherapy, radiation, and viral hepatitis.

ANEMIA, IRON DEFICIENCY

IRON DEFICIENCY ANEMIA is a chronic, slowly progressing disease involving circulating RBCs. Iron deficiency results when an individual absorbs inadequate amounts of iron or loses excessive amounts (such as through chronic bleeding). This decreased iron affects the formation of Hb and RBCs which, in turn, decreases the capacity of the blood to transport oxygen.

Possible causes

- Acute and chronic bleeding
- Alcohol abuse
- Chronic renal failure
- Dialysis treatment
- Drugs
- Surgery involving bypass of the duodenum
- Inadequate intake of iron-rich foods
- Malabsorption syndrome
- Menstruation
- Pregnancy
- Vitamin B_6 deficiency

Assessment findings

- Pallor (most common symptom)
- Glossitis
- Headache
- Irritability
- Impaired thought processes
- Depression
- Paresthesias
- Weakness and fatigue
- Sensitivity to cold
- Dizziness
- Dyspnea
- Palpitations
- Cheilosis (scalp and fissures of the lips)
- Koilonychia (spoon-shaped nails)
- Pale, dry mucous membranes
- Stomatitis

Diagnostic evaluation

- Hematology shows decreased Hb level, HCT, iron, ferritin, reticulocytes, red cell indices, transferrin, and saturation; absent hemosiderin; and increased iron-binding capacity.
- Peripheral blood smear reveals microcytic and hypochromic RBCs.

Nursing diagnoses

- Activity intolerance
- Imbalanced nutrition: Less than body requirements
- Impaired gas exchange

Treatment

- Diet high in iron, roughage, and protein with increased fluids and avoidance of teas and coffee, which reduce iron absorption
- Transfusion therapy with packed RBCs, if necessary

Drug therapy options

- Antianemics: ferrous sulfate (Feosol), iron dextran (Dexferrum)
- Vitamins: pyridoxine hydrochloride (vitamin B_6), ascorbic acid (vitamin C), cyanocobalamin (Vitamin B_{12})

Planning and goals

- The client will express feelings of increased energy.
- The client will maintain weight without further loss.
- The client will maintain adequate ventilation.

Implementation

- Monitor intake and output *to detect fluid imbalances.*
- Monitor laboratory studies *to determine the effectiveness of therapy.*
- Assess cardiovascular and respiratory status *to detect decreased activity intolerance and dyspnea on exertion.*
- Monitor and record vital signs *to determine activity intolerance.*
- Monitor stool, urine, and emesis for occult blood *to identify the cause of anemia.*
- Administer oxygen, as necessary, *to treat hypoxemia caused by reduced Hb levels.*
- Provide a diet high in iron *to replace iron stores in the body.*
- Administer medications, as prescribed, *to replace iron stores in the body.* Administer an iron injection deep into muscle using the Z-track technique *to avoid subcutaneous irritation and discoloration from a leaking drug.*
- Monitor for constipation; administer stool softeners and increase fiber in the diet *to prevent constipation, which may occur from iron administration.*
- Encourage fluids *to avoid dehydration.*
- Provide rest periods *to avoid fatigue and reduce oxygen demands.*
- Provide mouth, skin, and foot care *because the tongue and lips may be dry or inflamed and nails may be brittle.*
- Protect the client from falls caused by weakness and fatigue. *Falls may result in bleeding and bruising.*
- Keep the client warm *to enhance comfort.*

Evaluation

- The client reports increased energy and decreased periods of fatigue.
- The client maintains a stable weight.
- The client has adequate ventilation as evidenced by normal respirations.

ANEMIA, PERNICIOUS

PERNICIOUS ANEMIA, also called *amegaloblastic anemia* or *Addison's anemia,* is a chronic, progressive, macrocytic anemia caused by a deficiency of intrinsic factor, a substance normally secreted by the stomach. Without intrinsic factor, dietary vitamin B_{12} can't be absorbed by the ileum, inhibiting normal deoxyribonucleic acid synthesis and resulting in defective maturation of RBCs. The resulting vitamin B_{12} deficiency causes serious neurologic, gastric, and intestinal abnormalities. Untreated, pernicious anemia may lead to permanent neurologic disability and death.

Possible causes

- Autoimmune disease
- Bacterial or parasitic infections
- Deficiency of intrinsic factor
- Gastric mucosal atrophy
- Genetics
- Lack of administration of vitamin B_{12} after small-bowel resection or total gastrectomy
- Malabsorption
- Prolonged iron deficiency

Assessment findings

- Weakness, fatigue
- Glossitis, sore mouth
- Tingling and paresthesia of hands and feet
- Constipation or diarrhea
- Depression, delirium
- Dyspnea
- Mild jaundice of sclera
- Pallor
- Paralysis, gait disturbances
- Positive Babinski's and Romberg's signs
- Loss of bowel and bladder control
- Impotence (males)
- Altered vision (diplopia, blurred vision), taste, and hearing (tinnitus)
- Tachycardia, palpitations
- Weight loss, anorexia, dyspepsia

Diagnostic evaluation

- Blood chemistry test results reveal increased bilirubin and lactate dehydrogenase levels.
- Bone marrow aspiration specimen shows increased megaloblasts, few maturing erythrocytes, and defective leukocyte maturation.
- Gastric analysis shows hypochlorhydria.
- Hematology shows decreased HCT and Hb levels.
- Peripheral blood smear reveals oval, macrocytic, hyperchromic erythrocytes.
- Romberg test and/or Schilling test are positive.
- Upper GI series shows atrophy of gastric mucosa.

Nursing diagnoses

- Imbalanced nutrition: Less than body requirements
- Impaired gas exchange
- Risk for injury

Treatment

- Establishing a diet high in iron and protein and restricting highly seasoned, coarse, or extremely hot foods
- Transfusion therapy with packed RBCs

Drug therapy options

- Antianemics: ferrous sulfate (Feosol), iron dextran (Dexferrum)
- Vitamins: pyridoxine hydrochloride (vitamin B_6), ascorbic acid (vitamin C), cyanocobalamin (vitamin B_{12}), folic acid (vitamin B_9)

Planning and goals

- The client will maintain diet as prescribed.
- The client will demonstrate signs of adequate gas exchange.
- The client will identify precautions to prevent injury.

Implementation

- Assess cardiovascular status to detect signs of compromise because the heart works harder *to compensate for the reduced oxygen-carrying capacity of the blood.*
- Monitor and record vital signs *to enable early detection of compromise.*
- Monitor and record amount, consistency, and color of stools *to enable early detection and treatment of diarrhea and constipation.*
- Consult a registered dietitian *to ensure proper nutrition.* Maintain the client's diet *to ensure adequate intake of vitamins, iron, and protein.*
- Administer medications as prescribed. *Vitamin B_{12} injections are given monthly and are lifelong.*

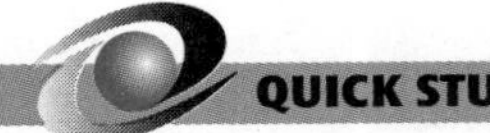

QUICK STUDY

Remember that pernicious anemia results from a lack of vitamin B_{12} absorption, so it's easy to recall that vitamins are an important part of treating clients with this disorder.

- Maintain activity, as tolerated, *to avoid fatigue.*
- Provide mouth care before and after meals *for comfort and to reduce the risk of oral mucous membrane breakdown.*
- Use soft toothbrushes *to avoid injuring mucous membranes.*
- Maintain a warm environment *for client comfort.*
- Provide foot and skin care *because sensation in the feet may be reduced.*
- Prevent the client from falling *due to reduced coordination, paresthesia of the feet, and reduced thought processes.*
- Assess neurologic status *because poor memory and confusion increase the risk of injury.*
- Monitor laboratory studies *to determine the effectiveness of therapy.*
- Review key teaching topics with the *client to ensure adequate knowledge about his condition and treatment,* including:
  - recognizing the signs and symptoms of skin breakdown
  - altering ADLs to compensate for paresthesia
  - complying with lifelong, monthly injections of vitamin B_{12}
  - avoiding the use of heating pads and electric blankets.

Evaluation

- The client verbalizes the importance of maintaining a diet high in iron and protein and of taking vitamins and supplements as prescribed.
- The client has normal vital signs and exhibits no signs of respiratory distress.
- The client verbalizes the appropriate injury-preventing precautions, such as performing mouth care, protecting the extremities, and avoiding falls.

ANEMIA, SICKLE CELL

SICKLE CELL ANEMIA is a congenital hematologic disease that causes impaired circulation, chronic ill health, and premature death. Although it's most common in tropical Africa and in people of African descent, it also occurs in people from Puerto Rico, Turkey, India, the Middle East, and the Mediterranean.

In clients with sickle cell anemia, a change in the gene that encodes the beta chain of Hb results in a defect. This abnormal Hb is called *HbS.* When hypoxia (oxygen deficiency) occurs, the HbS in the RBCs becomes insoluble. The cells become rigid and rough, forming an elongated sickle shape and impairing circulation. Infection, stress, dehydration, and conditions that provoke hypoxia (strenuous exercise, high altitude, unpressurized aircraft, cold, and vasoconstrictive drugs) may provoke periodic crisis. Crises can occur in different forms, including painful crisis, aplastic crisis, and acute sequestration crisis.

Possible causes

- Genetic homozygous inheritance of an autosomal recessive gene that produces a defective Hb molecule (HbS). Heterozygous inheritance results in sickle cell trait. (People with this trait are carriers who can then pass the gene to their offspring.)

Assessment findings

- Aching bones
- Chronic fatigue
- Family history of the disease
- Frequent infections
- Tachycardia
- Unexplained dyspnea or dyspnea on exertion
- Jaundice, pallor
- Joint swelling
- Leg ulcers (especially on ankles)
- Severe localized and generalized pain
- Unexplained, painful erections (priapism)

Sickle cell crisis (general symptoms)

- Hematuria
- Irritability
- Lethargy
- Pale lips, tongue, palms, and nail beds
- Severe pain

Painful crisis (vaso-occlusive crisis, which appears periodically after age 5)

- Dark urine
- Low-grade fever
- Severe abdominal, thoracic, muscle, or bone pain
- Tissue anoxia and necrosis caused by blood vessel obstruction from tangled sickle cells
- Worsening of jaundice

Aplastic crisis (generally associated with viral infection)

- Dyspnea
- Lethargy, sleepiness
- Markedly decreased bone marrow activity
- Pallor
- Possible coma
- RBC hemolysis (destruction)

Acute sequestration crisis (rare; occuring in infants ages 8 months to 2 years)

- Hypovolemic shock caused by entrapment of RBCs in spleen and liver
- Lethargy
- Liver congestion and enlargement
- Pallor
- Worsened chronic jaundice

Diagnostic evaluation

- Blood tests show low RBC counts, elevated WBC and platelet counts, decreased ESR, increased serum iron levels, decreased RBC survival, and reticulocytosis.
- Hb electrophoresis shows HbS.
- Hb levels may be low or normal.
- Stained blood smear shows sickle cells.

Nursing diagnoses

- Impaired gas exchange
- Acute pain
- Ineffective tissue perfusion (peripheral, renal)

Treatment

- Application of warm compresses for pain relief
- Blood transfusion therapy to treat crisis or partial exchange transfusion
- Bone marrow transplantation
- Iron and folic acid supplements to prevent anemia
- I.V. fluid therapy to prevent dehydration and vessel occlusion

Drug therapy options

- Analgesics: meperidine (Demerol), morphine to relieve pain from vaso-occlusive crises
- Antisickling agents: hydroxyurea (Droxia); Erythropoietin if unresponsive to hydroxyurea

Planning and goals

- The client will maintain adequate ventilation.
- The client will express feelings of comfort and pain relief.
- The client will have improved circulation.

Implementation

- Provide emotional support *to allay the client's anxiety.*
- Refer the client for genetic counseling *to decrease his anxiety and help him understand the chances of passing the disease to his offspring.*
- Refer the client and his family to community support groups *to help them cope with the illness.*

During a crisis

- Apply warm compresses to painful areas and cover the client with a blanket. *Cold compresses and temperature can aggravate his condition.*
- Administer an analgesic-antipyretic such as aspirin or acetaminophen *for pain relief.* (Additional pain relief may be necessary during an acute crisis.)
- Maintain bed rest *to reduce the heart's workload and reduce pain.*
- Administer blood components (packed RBCs), as ordered, *for aplastic crisis caused by bone marrow suppression.*
- Administer oxygen *to enhance oxygenation and reduce sickling.*
- Encourage fluid intake *to prevent dehydration, which can precipitate a crisis.*
- Administer prescribed I.V. fluids *to ensure fluid balance and renal perfusion.*
- Give antibiotics as ordered *to treat infections and avoid precipitating a crisis.*

Evaluation

- The client has adequate ventilation as evidenced by normal respiratory rate and effort.
- The client reports adequate pain control.
- The client doesn't display signs of diminished circulatory perfusion.

ANKYLOSING SPONDYLITIS

ANKYLOSING SPONDYLITIS is a chronic, usually progressive inflammatory disease that primarily affects the spine and adjacent soft tissue. Generally, the disease begins in the sacroiliac joints (between the sacrum and the ileum) and gradually progresses to the lumbar, thoracic, and cervical regions of the spine. Deterioration of bone and cartilage can lead to fibrous tissue formation and eventual fusion of the spine or peripheral joints.

Ankylosing spondylitis affects five times as many males as females. Progressive disease is well recognized in men, but the diagnosis is commonly overlooked in women, who tend to have more peripheral joint involvement.

Possible causes

- Familial tendency (strongly suggested)
- Possible link to underlying infection
- Presence of histocompatibility antigen (HLA-B27) and circulating immune complexes (suggests immunologic activity)

◆ Secondary ankylosing spondylitis possibly associated with reactive arthritis (Reiter's syndrome), psoriatic arthritis, or inflammatory bowel disease

Assessment findings

◆ Intermittent lower back pain (the first indication), usually most severe in morning or after a period of inactivity
◆ Mild fatigue, fever, anorexia, or weight loss
◆ Unilateral acute anterior uveitis
◆ Aortic insufficiency and cardiomegaly
◆ Upper lobe pulmonary fibrosis (mimics tuberculosis)
◆ Stiffness and limited motion of the lumbar spine
◆ Symptoms that progress unpredictably (disease can go into remission, exacerbation, or arrest at any stage)
◆ Pain and limited expansion of the chest due to involvement of the costovertebral joints
◆ Pain or tenderness at tendon insertion sites (enthesitis), especially at the Achilles or patellar tendon
◆ Tenderness over the site of inflammation
◆ Peripheral arthritis involving the shoulders, hips, and knees
◆ Severe neurologic complications, such as cauda equina syndrome or paralysis, secondary to fracture of a rigid cervical spine or C1-C2 subluxation
◆ Kyphosis in advanced stages, caused by chronic stooping to relieve symptoms, and hip deformity and associated limited ROM

Diagnostic evaluation

◆ Characteristic X-ray findings confirm the diagnosis (blurring of the bony margins of joints in the early stage, bilateral sacroiliac involvement, patchy sclerosis with superficial bony erosions, eventual squaring of vertebral bodies, and "bamboo spine" with complete ankylosis).
◆ Blood studies show slight elevation in ESR, alkaline phosphatase, and creatine kinase levels. A negative rheumatoid factor helps rule out rheumatoid arthritis, which produces similar symptoms.
◆ Typical symptoms, a family history, and the presence of HLA-B27 strongly suggest ankylosing spondylitis.

Nursing diagnoses

◆ Chronic pain
◆ Impaired physical mobility
◆ Activity intolerance

Treatment

◆ Good posture, stretching, and deep-breathing exercises and, in some clients, braces and lightweight supports to delay further deformity (because ankylosing spondylitis progression can't be stopped)
◆ Long-term daily exercise program (essential to delay loss of function)
◆ Spinal wedge osteotomy to separate and reposition the vertebrae in case of severe spinal involvement (performed only on selected clients because of the risk of spinal cord damage and long convalescence)
◆ Surgical hip replacement in cases of severe hip involvement

Drug therapy options

◆ Anti-inflammatory agents: aspirin, indomethacin (Indocin), sulfasalazine (Azulfidine) to control pain and inflammation

Planning and goals

◆ The client will express feelings of comfort and pain relief.
◆ The client will maintain joint mobility and ROM.
◆ The client will perform ADLs within the confines of the disease.

Implementation

◆ Offer support and reassurance *because ankylosing spondylitis can be an extremely painful and crippling disease.* The caregiver's main responsibility is to promote the client's comfort while preserving as much mobility as possible. Keep in mind that the client's limited ROM makes simple tasks difficult.
◆ Administer medications as needed *to decrease inflammation and pain.*
◆ Apply local heat and massage the affected area *to relieve pain.* Assess mobility and degree of discomfort frequently *to monitor disease progression.*
◆ Teach and assist with daily exercises as needed *to maintain strength and function.* Stress the importance of maintaining good posture *to prevent kyphosis.*
◆ If treatment includes surgery, provide good postoperative care *to prevent postoperative complications, such as wound infection, thrombophlebitis, and pneumonia.*
◆ Ensure that the client receives comprehensive treatment, including counseling from a social worker, visiting nurse, and dietitian *because ankylosing spondylitis is a chronic, progressively crippling condition.*

Evaluation

◆ The client reports adequate pain control.
◆ The client demonstrates adequate mobility.
◆ The client verbalizes the ability to perform ADLs.

DISSEMINATED INTRAVASCULAR COAGULATION

DISSEMINATED INTRAVASCULAR COAGULATION (DIC), also called *consumption coagulopathy and defibrination syndrome,* occurs as a complication of diseases and conditions that accelerate clotting. This accelerated clotting process causes small blood vessel occlusion, organ necrosis, depletion of circulating clotting factors and platelets, and activation of the fibrinolytic system, which in turn can lead to severe hemorrhage.

Clotting in the microcirculation usually affects the kidneys and extremities but may occur in the brain, lungs, pituitary and adrenal glands, and GI mucosa. Other conditions, such as vitamin K deficiency, hepatic disease, and anticoagulant therapy, may cause a similar hemorrhage.

DIC is generally an acute condition but may be chronic in clients with cancer. The prognosis depends on early detection and treatment, the severity of the hemorrhage, and treatment of the underlying disease or condition.

Possible causes

- Disorders that produce necrosis, such as extensive burns and trauma, brain tissue destruction, transplant rejection, and hepatic necrosis
- Infection (the most common cause), including gram-negative or gram-positive septicemia; viral, fungal, or rickettsial infection; and protozoal infection (falciparum malaria)
- Neoplastic disease, including acute leukemia and metastatic carcinoma
- Obstetric complications, such as abruptio placentae, amniotic fluid embolism, and retained dead fetus
- Other causes including heatstroke, shock, poisonous snakebite, cirrhosis, fat embolism, incompatible blood transfusion, cardiac arrest, surgery necessitating cardiopulmonary bypass, giant hemangioma, severe venous thrombosis, and purpura fulminans

Assessment findings

- Abnormal bleeding without an accompanying history of a serious hemorrhagic disorder (petechiae, hematomas, ecchymosis, cutaneous oozing)
- Oliguria
- Shock
- Dyspnea
- Nausea
- Vomiting
- Severe muscle, back, and abdominal pain
- Seizures
- Coma

Diagnostic evaluation

- Blood tests show prolonged PT greater than 15 seconds; prolonged PTT greater than 60 to 80 seconds; fibrinogen levels less than 150 mg/dl; platelets less than 100,000/µl; fibrin degradation products commonly greater than 100 µg/ml; positive D-dimer test specific for DIC; positive fibrin monomers; diminished levels of factors V and VIII; fragmentation of RBCs; and decreased hemoglobin (less than 10 g/dl).

Nursing diagnoses

- Ineffective tissue perfusion (peripheral)
- Fatigue
- Risk for deficient fluid volume

Treatment

- Prompt recognition and treatment of the underlying disorder
- Bed rest
- Transfusion therapy, including fresh frozen plasma, platelets, and packed RBCs

Drug therapy options

- Anticoagulants: heparin I.V. (controversial)
- Antithrombin III agent: gabexate mesylate to inhibit clotting cascade (investigational drug)

Planning and goals

- The client will exhibit signs of adequate tissue perfusion and no signs of hemorrhage.
- The client will exhibit less fatigue.
- The client will maintain an adequate fluid balance.

Implementation

- Don't scrub bleeding areas *to prevent clots from dislodging and causing fresh bleeding.* Use pressure, cold compresses, and topical hemostatic agents *to control bleeding.*
- Enforce complete bed rest during bleeding episodes. If the client is very agitated, pad the side rails *to protect from injury.*
- Check all I.V. and venipuncture sites frequently for bleeding. Apply pressure to the injection sites for at least 10 minutes. Alert other personnel to the client's tendency to hemorrhage. *These measures prevent hemorrhage.*

◆ Monitor intake and output hourly in acute DIC, especially when administering blood products, *to monitor the effectiveness of fluid volume replacement.*
◆ Watch for transfusion reactions and signs of fluid overload. Weigh dressings and linen and record drainage *to measure the amount of blood lost.* Weigh the client daily, particularly in renal involvement, *to monitor for fluid volume excess.*
◆ Watch for bleeding from the GI and genitourinary tracts *to detect early signs of hemorrhage.* Measure the client's abdominal girth at least once every 4 hours, and monitor closely for signs of shock *to detect intra-abdominal bleeding.*
◆ Monitor the results of serial blood studies (particularly HCT, Hb, and coagulation times) *to guide the treatment plan.*
◆ Inform family members of the client's progress. Prepare them for his appearance (I.V. lines, nasogastric tubes, bruises, dried blood). Provide emotional support to the client and his family. Enlist the aid of a social worker, chaplain, and other members of the health care team as needed. *Providing support in a crisis situation reduces family members' anxiety.*
◆ Review key teaching topics with the client and family members *to ensure adequate knowledge about the condition and treatment,* including:
- understanding the disorder and treatment options
- preventing bleeding.

Evaluation

◆ The client displays normal or maintained peripheral pulses, adequate color, and capillary refill.
◆ The client verbalizes decreased fatigue, energy-saving measures, and the need for rest.
◆ The client has a balanced intake and output and normal vital signs.

HEMOPHILIA

HEMOPHILIA is a hereditary bleeding disorder that affects only males and produces mild to severe abnormal bleeding. After a platelet plug develops at a bleeding site, the lack of clotting factor prevents the formation of a stable fibrin clot. Although hemorrhaging doesn't usually happen immediately, delayed bleeding is common. The severity of hemophilia and the client's prognosis vary with the degree of deficiency and the site of bleeding.

There are two types of hemophilia:
◆ hemophilia A, or *classic hemophilia* (deficiency or nonfunction of factor VIII)
◆ hemophilia B, or *Christmas disease* (deficiency or nonfunction of factor IX).

Possible causes

◆ Genetic inheritance (both types of hemophilia are inherited as X-linked recessive traits)

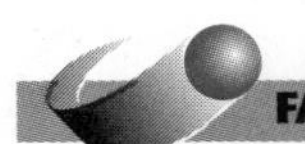

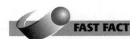

FAST FACT

Hemophilia is an inherited X-linked recessive trait. A female carrier has a 50% chance of transmitting the trait to her daughter (making her daughter a carrier), and a 50% chance of transmitting it to her son.

Assessment findings

Severe hemophilia

◆ Excessive bleeding after circumcision (in many cases, this is the first sign of the disease)
◆ Large subcutaneous and deep intramuscular hematomas
◆ Spontaneous or severe bleeding after minor trauma

Moderate hemophilia

◆ Occasional spontaneous bleeding
◆ Subcutaneous and intramuscular hematomas

Mild hemophilia

◆ No spontaneous bleeding
◆ Prolonged bleeding after major trauma or surgery (Blood may ooze slowly or intermittently for up to 8 days after surgery.)

All degrees of severity

◆ Hematemesis (bloody vomit)
◆ Hematomas on the extremities or torso
◆ Hematuria (bloody urine)
◆ History of prolonged bleeding after surgery, dental extractions, or trauma
◆ Joint tenderness
◆ Limited ROM
◆ Pain and swelling in a weight-bearing joint (such as the hip, knee, or ankle)
◆ Signs of decreased tissue perfusion, such as chest pain; confusion; cool, clammy skin; decreased urine output; hypotension; pallor; restlessness; anxiety; and tachycardia
◆ Signs of internal bleeding, such as abdominal, chest, or flank pain
◆ Tarry stools

Diagnostic evaluation

Hemophilia A

◆ Activated PTT is prolonged.

◆ Factor VIII assay reveals 0% to 25% of normal factor VIII.

◆ Platelet count and function, bleeding time, and PT are normal.

Hemophilia B

◆ Baseline coagulation result is similar to that of hemophilia A, with normal factor VIII.

◆ Factor IX assay shows deficiency.

Nursing diagnoses

◆ Risk for imbalanced fluid volume

◆ Ineffective tissue perfusion (cardiopulmonary)

◆ Impaired physical mobility

Treatment

Hemophilia A

◆ Administration of cryoprecipitate antihemophilic factor (AHF) and lyophilized (dehydrated) AHF to encourage normal hemostasis (arrest of bleeding)

◆ Immediate notification of physician following injury, especially to the head, neck, or abdomen

Hemophilia B

◆ Administration of recombinant factor VIII and purified factor IX to promote hemostasis

◆ Immediate notification of doctor following injury, especially to the head, neck, or abdomen

Drug therapy options

◆ Analgesics (morphine) to control joint pain

Planning and goals

◆ The client will maintain adequate urine output and heart rate.

◆ The client will demonstrate adequate tissue perfusion.

◆ The client will maintain joint mobility.

Implementation

◆ Provide emotional support *because hemophilia is a chronic disorder.*

◆ Refer new clients to a hemophilia treatment center *for education, evaluation, and development of a treatment plan.*

◆ Refer clients and carriers for genetic counseling *to determine the risk of passing the disease to their offspring.*

During bleeding episodes

◆ Apply pressure to cuts and during epistaxis *to stop bleeding. Pressure is commonly the only treatment needed for surface cuts.*

◆ Apply cold compresses or ice bags and elevate the injured part *to control bleeding.*

◆ Give sufficient clotting factor or plasma, as ordered, *to promote hemostasis.* The body uses AHF in 48 to 72 hours, so repeat infusions may be necessary.

◆ Administer analgesics *to control pain.* Avoid I.M. injections *because they may cause hematomas at the injection site.* Remember that aspirin and aspirin-containing medications are contraindicated *because they decrease platelet adherence and may increase bleeding.*

Bleeding into joint

◆ Immediately elevate the joint *to control bleeding.*

◆ Begin ROM exercises, if ordered, at least 48 hours after the bleeding has been controlled *to restore joint mobility.*

◆ Don't allow the client to bear weight on the affected joint until bleeding stops and swelling subsides *to prevent deformities due to hemarthrosis.*

After bleeding episodes and surgery

◆ Watch for signs of further bleeding *to detect and control bleeding as soon as possible.*

◆ Closely monitor PTT. *Prolonged times increase the risk of bleeding.*

◆ Review key teaching topics with the client and his family *to ensure adequate knowledge about the condition and treatment,* including:

– recognizing signs of severe internal bleeding

– knowing when to notify the primary care provider; for example, after even a minor injury

– wearing a medical identification bracelet

– protecting a child from injury

– understanding the importance of medical follow-up

– understanding the risk of infection such as hepatitis from blood component administration

– caring for injuries

– administering blood factor components at home, as appropriate.

Evaluation

◆ The client maintains adequate fluid volume as evidenced by vital signs within normal parameters and adequate urine output.

◆ The client maintains tissue perfusion.

◆ The client maintains joint mobility.

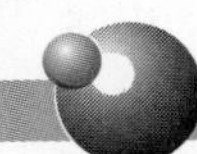

SPOT CHECK

If a client with hemophilia has an increased PTT, are bleeding tendencies decreased or increased?

Answer: Increased PTT indicates increased bleeding tendencies.

KAPOSI'S SARCOMA

Previously considered a rare type of cancer that primarily affected elderly Italian and Jewish men, KAPOSI'S SARCOMA (cancer of the lymphatic cell wall) is now the most common AIDS-related cancer, its incidence rising dramatically along with the incidence of AIDS. Kaposi's sarcoma causes structural and functional damage. When associated with AIDS, it progresses aggressively, involving the lymph nodes, the viscera and, possibly, GI structures.

Possible causes

- Immunosuppression (mechanism unclear)
- Human herpes virus 8 (HHV 8) (has been strongly associated with Kaposi's sarcoma)

Assessment findings

- One or more obvious lesions in various shapes, sizes, and colors (ranging from red-brown to dark purple) appearing most commonly on the skin, buccal mucosa, hard and soft palates, lips, gums, tongue, tonsils, conjunctiva, and sclera
- Pain (if the sarcoma advances beyond the early stages or if a lesion breaks down or impinges on nerves or organs)
- Dyspnea (in cases of pulmonary involvement), wheezing, hypoventilation, and respiratory distress from bronchial blockage
- Edema from lymphatic obstruction

Diagnostic evaluation

- CT scanning detects and evaluates possible metastasis.
- Tissue biopsy identifies the lesion's type and stage.

Nursing diagnoses

- Risk for infection
- Imbalanced nutrition: Less than body requirements
- Disturbed body image

Treatment

- High-calorie, high-protein diet
- Radiation therapy
- I.V. fluid therapy

Drug therapy options

- Chemotherapy agents: doxorubicin (Adriamycin), etoposide (VePesid), vinblastine (Velban), vincristine (Oncovin)
- Biological response modifier: interferon alfa-2b (ineffective in advanced disease)
- Antiemetic: trimethobenzamide (Tigan)
- Vitamin A: 9-cis retinoic acid applied directly to skin lesions.
- Anti-HIV drugs used in combination of three or more

Planning and goals

- The client will remain free from signs and symptoms of infection.
- The client will maintain weight within an acceptable range.
- The client will express positive feelings about himself.

Implementation

- Provide a referral for psychological counseling *to assist the client who's coping poorly.* Family members may also need help coping with the client's disease and associated demands that the disorder places on them.
- As appropriate, allow the client to participate in self-care decisions whenever possible and encourage him to participate in self-care measures as much as he can. *Involving the client in the treatment plan helps him gain some sense of control over his situation.*
- Inspect the client's skin every shift. Look for new lesions and skin breakdown. If the client has painful lesions, help him into a more comfortable position *to alleviate pain and promote client comfort.*
- Administer pain medications. Suggest distractions, and help the client with relaxation techniques *to divert him from his pain and promote comfort.*
- Urge the client to share his feelings, and provide encouragement *to help him adjust to changes in his appearance.*
- Monitor the client's weight daily *to evaluate if nutritional needs are being met.*
- Consult a registered dietitian to meet the client's nutritional needs. Supply the client with high-calorie, high-protein meals. If he can't tolerate regular meals, provide frequent smaller meals. Plan meals around the client's treatment. *Adverse reactions to medications and the disease itself may make it difficult for the client's nutritional intake to meet his metabolic needs.*
- If the client can't take food by mouth, administer I.V. fluids *to maintain hydration.* Also, provide antiemetics *to combat nausea and encourage nutritional intake.*

- Be alert for adverse reactions to radiation therapy or chemotherapy (such as anorexia, nausea, vomiting, and diarrhea) and take steps to prevent or alleviate them. *Adverse reactions are common and can further compromise the client's condition.*
- Reinforce the explanation of treatments. Make sure the client understands which adverse reactions to expect and how to manage them *to ensure prompt intervention and treatment.* For example, during radiation therapy, instruct the client to keep irradiated skin dry *to avoid possible breakdown and subsequent infection.*
- Explain all prescribed medications, including possible adverse effects and drug interactions, *to promote compliance with the medication regimen.*
- Explain infection prevention techniques and, if necessary, demonstrate basic hygiene measures *to prevent infection.* Advise the client not to share his toothbrush, razor, or other items that may be contaminated with blood. *These measures are especially important if the client also has AIDS, as they prevent the spread of infection to others.*
- Encourage the client to set priorities, accept the help of others, and delegate nonessential tasks. Help the client plan daily periods of alternating activity and rest *to help him cope with fatigue.*
- Explain the proper use of assistive devices, when appropriate, *to ease ambulation and promote independence.*
- As appropriate, refer the client to support groups offered by the social services department *to promote emotional well-being.*
- If the client's prognosis is poor (less than 6 months to live), suggest immediate hospice care. *Hospice care provides much needed support to caregivers and helps the client through the dying process.*

Evaluation
- The client has no signs or symptoms of infection.
- The client maintains an acceptable weight.
- The client expresses a positive self-image.

LEUKEMIA
LEUKEMIA is characterized by an uncontrolled proliferation of WBC precursors that fail to mature. Leukemia occurs when normal hematopoietic cells are replaced by leukemic cells in bone marrow. Immature forms of WBCs circulate in the blood, infiltrating the liver, spleen, and lymph nodes. Types of leukemia include:
- acute lymphocytic (lymphoblastic)
- acute myelogenous (myeloblastic)
- chronic lymphocytic
- chronic granulocytic (myelogenous or myelocytic).

Possible causes
- Altered immune system
- Exposure to chemicals
- Genetics
- Radiation
- Virus

Assessment findings
- Enlarged lymph nodes, spleen, and liver
- Frequent infections
- Weakness and fatigue
- Epistaxis
- Fever
- Generalized pain
- Gingivitis and stomatitis
- Hematemesis
- Hypotension
- Jaundice
- Joint, abdominal, and bone pain
- Melena
- Night sweats
- Petechiae and ecchymoses
- Prolonged menses
- Tachycardia

Diagnostic evaluation
- Bone marrow biopsy reveals a large number of immature leukocytes.
- Hematology shows decreased HCT, Hb, RBCs, and platelets and increased ESR, immature WBCs, and prolonged bleeding time. (See *Caring for the client with leukemia.*)

Nursing diagnoses
- Imbalanced nutrition: Less than body requirements
- Chronic pain
- Risk for infection

Treatment
- High-protein, high-vitamin and high-mineral diet, involving soft, bland foods in small, frequent feedings
- Stem cell transplant
- Transfusion of platelets, packed RBCs, and whole blood

Drug therapy options
- Alkylating agents: busulfan (Myleran), chlorambucil (Leukeran), cyclophosphamide (Cytoxan)
- Antitumor antibiotics: doxorubicin (Adriamycin), plicamycin (Mithracin), daunorubicin (Cerubidine), mitoxantrone (Novantrone), idarubicin (Idamycin)

◆ Antimetabolites: fluorouracil (Adrucil), methotrexate (Folex), cytarabine (Cyrasar, Ara-C), 6-mercaptopurine (Purinethol), 6-thioguanine (6-TG), fludarabine (Fludara)
◆ Antineoplastic (mitotic inhibitors): vinblastine (Velban), vincristine sulfate (Oncovin)
◆ Corticosteroid: prednisone
◆ Hematopoietic growth factor: epoetin alfa (Epogen)
◆ Monoclonal antibodies: rituximab (Riruxan), alemtuzumab (Campath)
◆ Nitrosourea: Carmustine (BiCNU)
◆ Miscellaneous drugs: L-asparaginase (Elspar), hydroxyurea (Hydrea), etoposide (Vepsid), retinoic acid (Tretinoin), arsenic trioxide (Trisenox), imatinib mesylate (Gleevic)

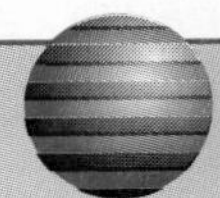

CLINICAL SITUATION

Caring for the client with leukemia

A 25-year-old male client is seeing his health care provider because of his recent history of extreme fatigue and swollen glands in his neck. He has also had some spontaneous nosebleeds. The health care provider orders a complete blood count that reveals immature white blood cells. Then the health care provider orders a bone marrow biopsy.

What finding would most strongly support a diagnosis of acute leukemia?

A. Large number of immature lymphocytes
B. Large number of immature thrombocytes
C. Large number of immature reticulocytes
D. Large number of immature leukocytes

Answer: D. Leukemia is manifested by an abnormal overproduction of immature leukocytes in the bone marrow.

Questions for future thought

◆ What would you tell the client regarding bleeding tendencies?
◆ What symptoms would you warn the client about regarding infection?

Planning and goals

◆ The client will maintain weight within an acceptable range.
◆ The client will express feelings of comfort and pain relief.
◆ The client will remain free from signs and symptoms of infection.

Implementation

◆ Monitor and record vital signs *to promptly detect deterioration in the client's condition.*
◆ Monitor intake, output, and daily weight *because body weight may decrease as a result of fluid loss.*
◆ Monitor laboratory studies *to help establish blood replacement needs, assess fluid status, and detect possible infection.*
◆ Monitor for bleeding. *Regular assessment may help anticipate or alleviate problems.*
◆ Place the client with epistaxis in an upright position, leaning slightly forward, *to reduce vascular pressure and prevent aspiration.*
◆ Monitor for infection. *Damage to bone marrow may suppress WBC formation.* Promptly report fever over 101° F (38.3° C) and decreased WBC counts *so that antibiotic therapy may be initiated.*
◆ Monitor oxygen therapy. *Oxygen therapy increases alveolar oxygen concentration and enhances arterial blood oxygenation.*
◆ Force fluids *to maintain adequate hydration.*
◆ Administer I.V. fluids *to replace fluid loss.*
◆ Encourage turning every 2 hours *to prevent venous stasis and skin breakdown.*
◆ Encourage coughing and deep breathing *to help remove secretions and prevent pulmonary complications.*
◆ Keep the client in semi-Fowler's position when in bed *to promote chest expansion and ventilation of basilar lung fields.*
◆ Maintain the client's diet *to provide necessary nutrition.*
◆ Administer TPN, if needed, *to provide the client with electrolytes, amino acids, and other nutrients tailored to his needs.*
◆ Administer transfusion therapy as prescribed and monitor for adverse reactions. *Transfusion reactions may occur during blood administration and may further compromise the client's condition.*
◆ Administer medications as prescribed *to combat disease and promote wellness.*
◆ Provide gentle mouth and skin care *to prevent oral mucous membrane or skin breakdown.*
◆ Encourage the client to express his feelings about changes in his body image and his fear of dying *to reduce anxiety.*
◆ Avoid giving the client I.M. injections and enemas and taking rectal temperature *to prevent bleeding.*

◆ Consult home care and hospice services *to help meet the client's needs.*

Evaluation
◆ The client maintains adequate weight.
◆ The client reports adequate pain control.
◆ The client has no signs or symptoms of infection.

LYMPHOMA
LYMPHOMA can be classified as Hodgkin's disease or malignant lymphoma (also called *non-Hodgkin's lymphoma*).

In HODGKIN'S DISEASE, Reed-Sternberg cells proliferate in a single lymph node and travel contiguously through the lymphatic system to other lymphatic nodes and organs. (See *Progression of Hodgkin's disease.*)

In malignant lymphoma, tumors occur throughout lymph nodes and lymphatic organs in unpredictable patterns. Malignant lymphoma may be categorized as:
◆ lymphocytic
◆ histiocytic
◆ mixed cell types.

Progression of Hodgkin's disease

Hodgkin's disease occurs in four stages.

Stage 1
Disease occurs in a single lymph node region or single extralymphatic organ.

Stage 2
Disease occurs in two or more lymph nodes on the same side of the diaphragm or in an extralymphatic organ.

Stage 3
Disease spreads to both sides of the diaphragm and perhaps to an extralymphatic organ, the spleen, or both.

Stage 4
Disease disseminates.

Possible causes
◆ Environmental factors (Hodgkin's disease)
◆ Genetic factors (Hodgkin's disease)
◆ Immunologic factors
◆ Viruses

Assessment findings
Hodgkin's disease
◆ Bone pain
◆ Dysphagia
◆ Dyspnea
◆ Edema and cyanosis of face and neck
◆ Enlarged, nontender, firm, movable lymph nodes in lower cervical regions
◆ Predictable pattern of spread

Malignant lymphoma
◆ Less predictable pattern of spread
◆ Prominent, painless, generalized lymphadenopathy

Both lymphomas
◆ Anorexia and weight loss
◆ Cough
◆ Hepatomegaly
◆ Malaise and lethargy
◆ Night sweats
◆ Recurrent infection
◆ Recurrent, intermittent fever
◆ Severe pruritus
◆ Splenomegaly

Diagnostic evaluation
◆ Bone marrow aspiration and biopsy specimens reveal small, diffuse lymphocytic or large, follicular-type cells (malignant lymphoma).
◆ Blood chemistry shows increased alkaline phosphatase levels (Hodgkin's disease).
◆ Chest X-ray reveals lymphadenopathy.
◆ Hematology shows decreased Hb level, HCT, and platelets and increased ESR, immature leukocytes, and gamma globulin (Hodgkin's disease).
◆ Lymph node biopsy specimen is positive for Reed-Sternberg cells (Hodgkin's disease).
◆ Lymphangiogram shows positive lymph node involvement (Hodgkin's disease).
◆ Lactate dehydrogenase is increased (Hodgkin's disease).

Nursing diagnoses
◆ Ineffective protection
◆ Impaired tissue integrity
◆ Risk for infection

Treatment
◆ Diet high in protein, calories, vitamins, minerals, iron, and calcium that consists of bland, soft foods

- Radiation therapy
- Transfusion of packed RBCs
- Bone marrow and stem cell transplantation

Drug therapy options

- Chemotherapy: most effective with multiple combinations of antineoplastic agents

Planning and goals

- The client will be free from complications.
- The client will exhibit no signs of skin breakdown.
- The client will be free from infection.

Implementation

- Monitor and record vital signs *to allow for early detection of complications.*
- Monitor intake and output and urine specific gravity. *Low urine output and high specific gravity indicate hypovolemia.*
- Monitor laboratory studies. *Electrolyte level, Hb levels, and HCT help indicate fluid status; WBC measurement may indicate bone marrow suppression.*
- Monitor for bleeding, infection, jaundice, and electrolyte imbalance *to detect complications associated with lymphoma.*
- Keep the client in semi-Fowler's position when in bed *to promote chest expansion and ventilation of basilar lung fields.*
- Administer oxygen. *Supplemental oxygen helps reduce hypoxemia.*
- Encourage turning every 2 hours *to prevent skin breakdown,* and encourage coughing and deep breathing *to help remove secretions and prevent pulmonary complications.*
- Provide mouth and skin care *to prevent the breakdown of the oral mucous membranes and skin.*
- Help the client maintain his diet *to ensure nutritional requirements are met.*
- Encourage fluids *to prevent dehydration and complications associated with chemotherapeutic drugs.*
- Administer I.V. fluids as prescribed *to replace fluid loss.*
- Administer medications as prescribed, and monitor for adverse effects *to prevent further complications.*
- Administer transfusion therapy as prescribed, and monitor for adverse reactions. *Transfusion reactions during blood administration may further compromise the client's condition.*
- Provide rest periods *to enhance immune function and decrease weakness caused by anemia.*
- Encourage the client to express his feelings about changes in his body image and a fear of dying (indolent type of lymphoma isn't curable) *to allay the client's anxiety.*
- Consult home care and hospice services *to help meet the client's needs.*
- Review key teaching topics with the client *to ensure adequate knowledge about his condition and treatment,* including:
  - recognizing early signs and symptoms of motor and sensory deficits
  - increasing fluid intake
  - using only an electric razor
  - refraining from using over-the-counter medications (unless cleared by the physician)
  - contacting the American Cancer Society.

Evaluation

- The client displays no signs of complications, such as bleeding, dehydration, jaundice, or hypoxemia.
- The client's skin remains intact.
- The client remains afebrile and exhibits no sign of infections, including wound, respiratory, skin, and oral infections.

MULTIPLE MYELOMA

MULTIPLE MYELOMA involves the abnormal proliferation of plasma cells. These plasma cells are immature and malignant and invade the bone marrow, lymph nodes, liver, spleen, and kidneys, triggering osteoblastic activity and leading to bone destruction throughout the body.

Possible causes

- Environmental factors
- Genetic factors

Assessment findings

- Anemia, thrombocytopenia, hemorrhage
- Constant, severe bone pain
- Fever
- Headaches
- Hepatomegaly
- Malaise
- Multiple infections
- Pathologic fractures, skeletal deformities of the sternum and ribs, loss of height
- Pneumonia
- Pyelonephritis
- Renal calculi

- Splenomegaly
- Vascular insufficiency
- Weight loss

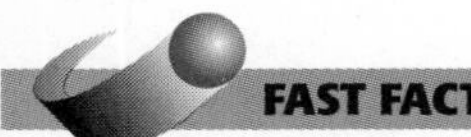

FAST FACT

A client with multiple myeloma may have bone demineralization and may lose large amounts of calcium into the urine and blood, resulting in renal calculi, nephrocalcinosis and, eventually, renal failure due to hypocalcemia.

Diagnostic evaluation

- Bence Jones protein is present in the urine.
- Blood chemistry tests show increased calcium, uric acid, blood urea nitrogen, and creatinine levels.
- Bone marrow biopsy specimen shows an increased number of immature plasma cells.
- Bone scan reveals increased uptake.
- Hematology shows decreased HCT, WBCs, and platelets and increased ESR.
- Immunoelectrophoresis shows monoclonal spike.
- Urine chemistry shows increased calcium and uric acid.
- X-rays show diffuse, round, punched-out bone lesions; osteoporosis; osteolytic lesions of the skull; and widespread demineralization.

Nursing diagnoses

- Acute pain
- Chronic pain
- Impaired physical mobility
- Risk for infection

Treatment

- Allogenic bone marrow transplantation
- Diet that's high in protein, carbohydrates, vitamins, and minerals given in small, frequent feedings
- Orthopedic devices, such as braces, splints, and casts
- Peritoneal dialysis and hemodialysis
- Radiation therapy
- Surgery (aminectomy for spinal cord compression)
- Transfusion therapy, including packed RBCs

Drug therapy options

- Alkylating agents: melphalan (Alkeran), cyclophosphamide (Cytoxan), carmustine (BiCNU)
- Analgesic: morphine sulfate
- Androgen: fluoxymesterone (Halotestin)
- Antibiotics: doxorubicin (Adriamycin), plicamycin (Mithracin)
- Antiemetic: prochlorperazine (Compazine)
- Antigout: allopurinol (Zyloprim)
- Antineoplastics: vinblastine (Velban), vincristine sulfate (Oncovin)
- Diuretic: furosemide (Lasix)
- Glucocorticoid: prednisone (Deltasone)

Planning and goals

- The client will verbalize pain relief.
- The client will demonstrate maintained or improved mobility.
- The client will be free from signs of infection.

Implementation

- Assess renal status *to detect renal calculi and renal failure secondary to hypercalcemia.*
- Monitor and record vital signs *to enable early detection of complications.*
- Monitor intake and output, urine specific gravity, and daily weight *to identify fluid volume excess or deficit.*
- Monitor laboratory studies. *RBCs, WBCs, Hb, HCT, and platelets may be affected by chemotherapy.*
- Assess cardiovascular and respiratory status *to detect signs of compromise.*
- Assess bone pain *to determine the client's response to analgesics.*
- Monitor for infection and bruising *to detect complications.*
- Encourage the client to maintain a balanced diet *to ensure nutritional requirements are met.*
- Encourage fluids *to prevent dehydration and dilute calcium.*
- Administer I.V. fluids *to replace fluid loss, dilute calcium, and prevent renal protein precipitation.*
- Assist with turning, coughing, and deep breathing *to mobilize and remove secretions.*
- Administer transfusion therapy as prescribed *to replace blood components.*
- Administer medications, as prescribed, and monitor for adverse effects *to prevent complications.*
- Maintain seizure precautions *to prevent injury.*
- Provide skin and mouth care *to prevent the breakdown of the oral mucous membranes and skin.*
- Alternate rest periods with activity *to prevent fatigue.*
- Prevent the client from falling *because he's vulnerable to fractures.*
- Move the client gently, keeping his body in alignment, *to prevent injury.*
- Apply and maintain braces, splints, and casts *to prevent injury and reduce pain.*

◆ Consult home care and hospice services *to meet the client's needs.*
◆ Review key teaching topics with the client *to ensure adequate knowledge about his condition and treatment,* including:
- exercising regularly, with particular attention to muscle-strengthening exercises
- recognizing signs and symptoms of renal calculi, fractures, and seizures
- avoiding lifting, constipation, and over-the-counter medications
- monitoring stool for occult blood
- using braces, splints, and casts
- contacting the American Cancer Society.

Evaluation

◆ The client verbalizes that he experiences adequate pain relief with treatment.
◆ The client remains free from complications caused by immobility, maintains or improves mobility, and verbalizes the appropriate use of splints or braces and appropriate activities to maintain and improve muscle strength.
◆ The client is afebrile and free from signs of infection, including respiratory infections and skin breakdown.

POLYCYTHEMIA VERA

POLYCYTHEMIA VERA is a chronic myeloproliferative disorder characterized by increased RBC mass, leukocytosis, thrombocytosis, and increased Hb concentration with normal or increased plasma volume. It usually occurs in clients ages 40 to 60 and is most common among males of Jewish ancestry; it rarely affects children or blacks and doesn't appear to be familial. It may also be known as *primary polycythemia, erythremia, polycythemia rubra vera, splenomegalic polycythemia,* or *Vaquez-Osler disease.*

The prognosis depends on the client's age at diagnosis, the treatment used, and complications. Mortality is high if polycythemia isn't treated or is associated with leukemia or myeloid metaplasia.

Possible causes

◆ Unknown (possibly due to a multipotential stem cell defect)

Assessment findings

◆ Congestion of the conjunctiva, retina, and retinal veins
◆ Dizziness (vertigo)
◆ Dyspnea
◆ Ecchymosis
◆ Feeling of fullness in the head
◆ Headache
◆ Hemorrhage
◆ Hepatosplenomegaly
◆ Hypertension
◆ Pruritus
◆ Ruddy cyanosis of the nose
◆ Thrombosis of smaller vessels
◆ Tinnitus
◆ Visual disturbances (blurring, diplopia, engorged veins of fundus and retina)
◆ Weight loss

Diagnostic evaluation

◆ Blood test results show increased RBC mass and normal arterial oxygen saturation in association with splenomegaly or two of the following:
- thrombocytosis
- leukocytosis
- elevated leukocyte alkaline phosphatase level
- elevated serum vitamin B_{12} or unbound B_{12} binding capacity.

◆ WBC count is increased to 10,000 to 20,000 units/L.
◆ Platelets are increased to 1,000,000 units/L.
◆ HCT is increased to greater than 60% above normal.
◆ Serum uric acid levels show increased uric acid production, leading to hyperuricemia and hyperuricuria.
◆ Serum iron levels show decreased concentration.
◆ Erythropoietin levels are inappropriately elevated.
◆ Bone marrow biopsy reveals panmyelosis.

Nursing diagnoses

◆ Ineffective tissue perfusion (cardiovascular)
◆ Deficient knowledge of disease process and treatment

Treatment

◆ Phlebotomy (typically, 350 to 500 ml of blood removed at variable intervals, depending on the client, until the client's HCT is reduced to the low-normal range)
◆ Pheresis to permit return of plasma to the client, diluting the blood and reducing hypovolemic symptoms
◆ Hydration therapy to reduce blood viscosity.

Drug therapy options

◆ Chemotherapy agents: busulfan (Myleran), chlorambucil (Leukeran), melphalan (Alkeran)
◆ Myelosuppressives: hydroxyurea (Hydrea), radioactive phosphorus (^{32}P)
◆ Antiplatelet agents: aspirin, dipyridamole (Persantine)

Planning and goals

◆ The client will maintain adequate tissue perfusion.
◆ The client will verbalize an understanding of the disease, treatment course, and complications.

Implementation

◆ Check blood pressure, pulse rate, and respiratory rate prior to and during phlebotomy *to monitor the client's tolerance of the procedure.*
◆ During phlebotomy, make sure the client is lying down comfortably *to prevent vertigo and syncope.*
◆ Stay alert for tachycardia, clamminess, or complaints of vertigo. If these effects occur, the procedure should be stopped. *These signs and symptoms indicate hypovolemia.*
◆ Immediately after phlebotomy, check the client's blood pressure and pulse rate. Have him sit up for about 5 minutes before allowing him to walk *to prevent vasovagal attack or orthostatic hypotension.* Also, administer 24 oz (720 ml) of juice or water *to replace fluid volume lost during the procedure.*
◆ Tell the client to watch for and report signs or symptoms of iron deficiency (pallor, weight loss, weakness, glossitis). *After repeated phlebotomies, iron deficiency will develop, which stabilizes RBC production and reduces the need for phlebotomy.*
◆ Keep the client active and ambulatory to prevent thrombosis. If bed rest is absolutely necessary, prescribe a daily program of active and passive ROM exercises *to prevent thrombosis and maintain joint mobility.*
◆ Watch for complications, such as hypervolemia, thrombocytosis, and signs of an impending stroke (decreased sensation, numbness, transitory paralysis, fleeting blindness, headache, and epistaxis) *to ensure early treatment.*
◆ Regularly examine the client closely for bleeding. Advise him about common bleeding sites (such as the nose, gingiva, and skin) so he can check for bleeding. Advise the client to report abnormal bleeding promptly. *These measures decrease the risk of hemorrhage.*
◆ Give additional fluids, as ordered, and alkalinize the urine *to compensate for increased uric acid production and prevent uric acid calculi.*
◆ If the client has symptomatic splenomegaly, suggest or provide small, frequent meals followed by a rest period *to prevent nausea and vomiting.*
◆ Report acute abdominal pain immediately *to avoid treatment delay.* Acute pain may signal splenic infarction, renal calculi, or abdominal organ thrombosis.

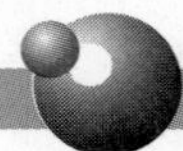

SPOT CHECK

What can acute abdominal pain signify in a client with polycythemia vera?

Answer: Acute pain may signal splenic infarction, renal calculi, or abdominal organ thrombosis.

During myelosuppressive treatment

◆ Monitor CBC and platelet counts before and during therapy. Warn an outpatient who develops leukopenia that resistance to infection is low; advise the client to avoid crowds and watch for symptoms of infection. *These measures protect the client from life-threatening infection.*
◆ If leukopenia develops in a hospitalized client who needs reverse isolation, follow facility guidelines. If thrombocytopenia develops, tell the client to watch for signs of bleeding (blood in urine, nosebleeds, black stools) *to prevent hemorrhage.*
◆ Tell the client about possible adverse effects of alkylating agents (nausea, vomiting, and the risk of infection) of alkylating agents *to allay anxiety and ensure early treatment.*
◆ Watch for adverse reactions. If nausea and vomiting occur, begin antiemetic therapy and adjust the client's diet *to promote comfort.*
◆ Take a blood sample for CBC and platelet count before beginning treatment with ^{32}P. Use of ^{32}P requires radiation precautions *to prevent contamination.*
◆ Have the client lie down during I.V. administration *to facilitate the procedure and prevent extravasation* and for 15 to 20 minutes afterward *to monitor the client's tolerance of the procedure.*
◆ Review key teaching topics with the client *to ensure adequate knowledge about the condition and treatment,* including:
– understanding the disease process and treatment options
– understanding the importance of remaining as active as possible
– avoiding infection
– keeping the environment free from hazards that could cause falls
– using a safety razor to prevent bleeding
– preventing adverse reactions to treatment, such as using antiemetics to prevent nausea and vomiting
– using community resources
– understanding warnings against fingerstick blood tests because of compromised circulation.

Evaluation

- The client has a heart rate and blood pressure within normal range; warm, dry skin; and decreased dyspnea.
- The client demonstrates knowledge about the disease, treatment, and signs and symptoms that should be reported.

RHEUMATOID ARTHRITIS

Believed to be an autoimmune disorder, RHEUMATOID ARTHRITIS is a systemic inflammatory disease that affects the synovial lining of the joints. Antibodies first attack the synovium of the joint, causing it to become inflamed and swollen. Eventually, the articular cartilage and surrounding tendons and ligaments are affected.

Inflammation of the synovial membranes is followed by formation of pannus (granulation tissue) and destruction of cartilage, bone, and ligaments. Pannus is replaced by fibrotic tissue and calcification, which causes subluxation of the joint. The joint becomes ankylosed — or fused — leaving a very painful joint and limited ROM.

Possible causes

- Autoimmune disease
- Genetic transmission

Assessment findings

- Symmetrical joint swelling (mirror image of affected joints)
- Painful, swollen joints; crepitus; and morning stiffness
- Fatigue
- Malaise
- Anorexia and weight loss
- Dry eyes and mucous membranes
- Enlarged lymph nodes
- Fever
- Leukopenia and anemia
- Limited ROM
- Paresthesia of the hands and feet
- Pericarditis
- Raynaud's phenomenon
- Splenomegaly
- Subcutaneous nodules

Diagnostic evaluation

- B-lymphocyte alloantigen (HLA-DR4) is positive in 60% to 80% of clients.
- Antinuclear antibody (ANA) test is positive.
- Hematology shows increased ESR, C-reactive protein, WBC, platelets, and anemia.
- Rheumatoid factor test is positive.
- Serum protein electrophoresis shows elevated serum globulins.
- Synovial fluid analysis shows increased WBCs, increased volume and turbidity, and decreased viscosity and complement (C_3 and C_4 levels).
- X-rays reveal bone demineralization and soft-tissue swelling in early stages; in later stages, X-rays reveal loss of cartilage, narrowing of joint spaces, cartilage and bone destruction, and erosion, subluxations, and deformity.

Nursing diagnoses

- Chronic pain
- Activity intolerance
- Disturbed body image

Treatment

- Cold therapy during acute episodes
- Heat therapy to relax muscles and relieve pain for chronic disease
- Physical therapy (to forestall loss of joint function), passive ROM exercises, and observance of rest periods
- Surgery to relieve deformity, improve function, and decrease pain
- Weight control because obesity adds stress to joints
- Well-balanced diet

Drug therapy options

- Analgesic: aspirin
- Antimetabolite: methotrexate (Rheumatrex)
- Antirheumatic: hydroxychloroquine (Plaquenil)
- Glucocorticoids: prednisone (Deltasone) and hydrocortisone (Hydrocortone)
- Gold therapy: gold sodium thiomalate (Myochrysine)
- Nonsteroidal anti-inflammatory drugs (NSAIDs): indomethacin (Indocin), ibuprofen (Advil, Motrin), sulindac (Clinoril), piroxicam (Feldene), flurbiprofen (Ansaid), diclofenac sodium (Voltaren), naproxen (Naprosyn), diflunisal (Dolobid)

Planning and goals

- The client will express feelings of comfort and pain relief.
- The client will attain the highest level of mobility possible within the confines of his disease.
- The client will express a positive self-image.

Implementation

- Monitor vital signs *to allow for early detection of complications.*

- Monitor neuromuscular status *to determine the client's capabilities.*
- Check joints for swelling, pain, and redness *to determine the extent of the disease and the effectiveness of treatment.*
- Monitor laboratory studies *to detect remissions and exacerbations.*
- Administer medications as prescribed *to enhance the treatment regimen.*
- Provide passive ROM exercises *to prevent joint contractures and muscle atrophy.*
- Consult a physical therapist and occupational therapist *to maximize the client's mobility and function.*
- Splint inflamed joints *to maintain joints in a functional position and prevent musculoskeletal deformities.*
- Provide warm or cold therapy as prescribed *to help alleviate pain.*
- Provide skin care *to prevent skin breakdown.*
- Minimize environmental stress and plan rest periods *to help the client cope with the disease.*
- Encourage the client to express his feelings about changes in his body image *to help him express doubts and resolve concerns.*

Evaluation

- The client reports adequate pain control.
- The client demonstrates maximum mobility.
- The client displays a positive attitude regarding his self-image.

SCLERODERMA

SCLERODERMA is a diffuse connective tissue disease characterized by inflammatory and then degenerative and fibrotic changes in skin, blood vessels, synovial membranes, skeletal muscles, and internal organs (especially the esophagus, intestinal tract, thyroid, heart, lungs, and kidneys). The disease, also known as *progressive systemic sclerosis,* affects more women than men, especially between ages 30 and 50.

Possible causes

- Unknown

Assessment findings

- Signs and symptoms of Raynaud's phenomenon, such as blanching, cyanosis, and erythema of the fingers and toes in response to stress or exposure to cold
- Pain
- Stiffness
- Swelling of fingers and joints
- Taut, shiny skin over the entire hand and forearm
- Tight and inelastic facial skin, causing a masklike appearance and "pinching" of the mouth
- Slowly healing ulcerations on the tips of the fingers or toes that may lead to gangrene
- Cardiac and pulmonary fibrosis (in advanced disease)
- Renal involvement accompanied by malignant hypertension (the main cause of death)

Diagnostic evaluation

- Blood studies show slightly elevated ESR, positive rheumatoid factor in 25% to 35% of clients, and positive antinuclear antibody test.
- Chest X-rays show bilateral basilar pulmonary fibrosis.
- Electrocardiogram reveals possible nonspecific abnormalities related to myocardial fibrosis.
- GI X-rays show distal esophageal hypomotility and stricture, duodenal loop dilation, small-bowel malabsorption pattern, and large diverticula.
- Hand X-rays show terminal phalangeal tuft resorption, subcutaneous calcification, and joint space narrowing and erosion.
- Pulmonary function studies show decreased diffusion and vital capacity.
- Skin biopsy may show changes consistent with the progress of the disease, such as marked thickening of the dermis and occlusive vessel changes.
- Urinalysis reveals proteinuria, microscopic hematuria, and casts (with renal involvement).

Nursing diagnoses

- Chronic pain
- Impaired physical mobility
- Impaired skin integrity

Treatment

- Palliative measures, including drug therapy and physical therapy to maintain function and promote muscle strength (currently, no cure exists for scleroderma)

Drug therapy options

- Immunosuppressants: cyclosporine (Sandimmune), chlorambucil (Leukeran)
- Antineoplastics: interferon-alpha, interferon-gamma
- Antineoplastics: methotrexate, interferon-alpha, interferon-gamma

Planning and goals

◆ The client will express feelings of comfort and pain relief.
◆ The client will maintain maximum functional mobility within the confines of the disease.
◆ The client will maintain skin integrity.

Implementation

◆ Assess motion restrictions, pain, vital signs, intake and output, respiratory function, and daily weight *to monitor disease progression and guide the treatment plan.*
◆ Teach the client to monitor blood pressure at home and report increases above baseline. *Malignant hypertension is the main cause of death in clients diagnosed with scleroderma.*
◆ Warn against fingerstick blood tests *because of compromised circulation.*
◆ Help the client and her family adjust to the client's new body image and to the limitations and dependence that these changes cause. *Clients and their families need time to adjust to the overwhelming effects of illness.*
◆ Help the client and her family accept the fact that this condition is incurable. Encourage them to express their feelings, and help them cope with their fears and frustrations by offering information about the disease, its treatment, and relevant diagnostic tests. *Such information helps to alleviate anxiety and provides the client with the knowledge that's necessary for informed decision making.*
◆ Whenever possible, let the client participate in treatment by measuring her intake and output, planning her diet, assisting in dialysis, giving herself heat therapy, and doing prescribed exercises *to help her gain a sense of control over her condition.*
◆ Involve the client's family in treatment *to help them overcome feelings of helplessness.*
◆ Encourage the client to contact local scleroderma support *to obtain support and current information on treatments and therapies.*

Evaluation

◆ The client reports adequate pain control.
◆ The client demonstrates functional mobility.
◆ The client maintains skin integrity.

SYSTEMIC LUPUS ERYTHEMATOSUS

SYSTEMIC LUPUS ERYTHEMATOSUS (SLE) is an autoimmune disorder that involves most organ systems. It's chronic in nature and characterized by periods of exacerbation and remission.

In SLE, there's a depression of T-cell activity and an increase in the production of antibodies, specifically antibodies to deoxyribonucleic acid and ribonucleic acid and antierythrocyte, antinuclear, and antiplatelet antibodies. The immune response results in an inflammatory process involving the veins and arteries (vasculitis), which causes pain, swelling, and tissue damage in any area of the body.

Possible causes

◆ Autoimmune factors
◆ Effects of drugs, such as procainamide (Pronestyl), hydralazine (Apresoline), and phenytoin (Dilantin)
◆ Environmental factors
◆ Exposure to sunlight or UV-light
◆ Hormonal factors
◆ Physical or mental stress
◆ Genetics
◆ Viral

Assessment findings

◆ Fatigue
◆ Butterfly rash on face (may vary in severity from malar erythema to discoid lesions)
◆ Low-grade fever
◆ Migratory pain, stiffness, and joint swelling
◆ Photosensitivity
◆ Anorexia and weight loss
◆ Anemia, leukopenia, and thrombocytopenia
◆ Erythema on palms
◆ Oral and nasopharyngeal ulcerations
◆ Alopecia
◆ Raynaud's phenomenon
◆ Lymphadenopathy, splenomegaly, and hepatomegaly
◆ Glomerulonephritis and renal dysfunction and failure (renal involvement)
◆ Impaired cognitive function, psychosis, depression, seizures, peripheral neuropathies, strokes, and organic brain syndrome (central nervous system involvement)
◆ Pleurisy, pericarditis, myocarditis, noninfectious endocarditis, and hypertension (cardiac involvement)

Diagnostic evaluation

◆ ANA test is positive.
◆ Anti-double stranded deoxyribonucleic acid (ds DNA) test is positive.
◆ Blood chemistry shows decreased complement fixation.
◆ Hematology shows decreased Hb, HCT, WBC, and platelets and an increased ESR.
◆ Lupus erythematosus cell preparation is positive.
◆ Rheumatoid factor is positive.
◆ Urine chemistry shows proteinuria and hematuria.

Nursing diagnoses

◆ Ineffective tissue perfusion (peripheral, cardiopulmonary)
◆ Risk for infection
◆ Impaired mobility

Treatment

◆ Diet high in iron, protein, and vitamins (especially vitamin C)
◆ Hemodialysis or kidney transplant if renal failure occurs
◆ Limited exertion and maintenance of adequate rest
◆ Plasmapheresis
◆ Hematopoietic stem cell transplantation

Drug therapy options

◆ Analgesic: aspirin
◆ Antianemics: ferrous sulfate (Feosol), ferrous gluconate (Fergon)
◆ Antirheumatic: hydroxychloroquine (Plaquenil)
◆ Antineoplastic drug: methotrexate (Rheumatrex) (may delay or prevent deteriorating renal status)
◆ Glucocorticoid: prednisone (Deltasone)
◆ Immunosuppressants: azathioprine (Imuran), cyclophosphamide (Cytoxan) (Some biologic agents and immunosuppressants under investigation include dehydroepiandrosterone, LJP 394, B-lymphocyte stimulators, LJP 1082, bromocriptine, and thalidamide.)
◆ NSAIDs: indomethacin (Indocin), ibuprofen (Motrin), sulindac (Clinoril), piroxicam (Feldene), flurbiprofen (Ansaid), diclofenac sodium (Voltaren), naproxen (Naprosyn), diflunisal (Dolobid)

Planning and goals

◆ The client will maintain adequate tissue perfusion.
◆ The client will remain free from signs and symptoms of infection.
◆ The client will maintain joint mobility and ROM.

Implementation

◆ Assess musculoskeletal status *to determine the client's baseline functional abilities.*
◆ Monitor renal status. *Decreased urine output without lowered fluid intake may indicate decreased renal perfusion, a possible indication of decreased cardiac output.*
◆ Monitor vital signs *to determine promptly if the client's condition is deteriorating and evaluate the effectiveness of treatment.* Fever can signal an exacerbation.
◆ Provide prophylactic skin, mouth, and perineal care *to prevent skin and oral mucous membrane breakdown.*
◆ Administer medications as prescribed *to enhance the treatment regimen.*
◆ Maintain seizure precautions *to prevent client injury.*
◆ Monitor dietary intake *to help ensure adequate nutritional intake.*
◆ Teach the client relaxation techniques, minimize environmental stress, and provide rest periods *to avoid fatigue and help the client cope with illness.*
◆ Promote independence in ADLs *to help the client develop self-esteem.*
◆ Administer antiemetics *to alleviate nausea and vomiting.*
◆ Administer antidiarrheals as prescribed *to alleviate diarrhea.*
◆ Encourage the client to avoid triggers, such as exposure to sunlight, and to take preventive measures, such as using sunscreen and hats, *to reduce the risk of relapse.*
◆ Encourage the client to discuss feelings about changes in his body image and the chronic nature of the disease *to help him express doubts and resolve concerns.*
◆ Encourage the client to contact local support group for lupus erythomatosis *to provide ongoing information and support.*

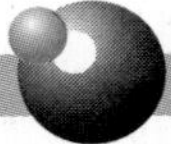

SPOT CHECK

The nurse is preparing a client with SLE for discharge. Which instructions should she include in the teaching plan?

A. Exposure to sunlight will help control skin rashes.
B. There are no activity limitations between flare-ups.
C. Monitoring body temperature is important to treatment.
D. Corticosteroids may be stopped when symptoms are relieved.

Answer: C. The client should monitor his temperature because fever can signal an exacerbation and should be reported to the physician. Sunlight and other sources of ultraviolet light may precipitate severe skin reactions and exacerbate the disease. Fatigue can cause an SLE flare-up, and clients should be encouraged to pace activities and plan for rest periods. Corticosteroids must be gradually tapered because they can suppress the function of the adrenal gland. Abruptly stopping corticosteroids can cause adrenal insufficiency, a potentially life-threatening situation.

Evaluation

◆ The client has adequate tissue perfusion as evidenced by stable vital signs and adequate urine output.
◆ The client doesn't show signs or symptoms of infection.
◆ The client demonstrates functional mobility.

VASCULITIS

VASCULITIS is a broad spectrum of disorders characterized by inflammation and necrosis of blood vessels. Its clinical effects depend on the vessels involved and reflect tissue ischemia caused by blood flow obstruction.

Prognosis is also variable. For example, hypersensitivity vasculitis is usually a benign disorder limited to the skin, but more extensive polyarteritis nodosa can be rapidly fatal.

Vasculitis can occur at any age, except for mucocutaneous lymph node syndrome, which occurs only during childhood. Vasculitis may be a primary disorder or secondary to other disorders, such as rheumatoid arthritis or SLE. Some types of vasculitis include Wegener's granulomatosis, giant cell arteritis, and Takayasu's arteritis.

Possible causes

- Excessive levels of antigen
- High-dose antibiotic therapy
- Immune response
- Serious infectious disease, such as hepatitis B or bacterial endocarditis

Assessment findings

Wegener's granulomatosis

- Cough
- Fever
- Malaise
- Mild to severe hematuria
- Pulmonary congestion
- Anorexia
- Weight loss

Giant cell arteritis

- Fever
- Headache (associated with polymyalgia rheumatica syndrome)
- Jaw claudication
- Myalgia
- Visual changes

Takayasu's arteritis

- Malaise
- Arthralgias
- Pain or paresthesia distal to the affected area
- Bruits
- Syncope
- Stroke (with disease progression)
- Diplopia and transient blindness, if carotid artery is involved
- Heart failure (with disease progression)
- Loss of distal pulses
- Anorexia
- Nausea
- Night sweats
- Pallor
- Weight loss

Diagnostic evaluation

Wegener's granulomatosis

- Tissue biopsy shows necrotizing vasculitis with granulomatous inflammation.
- Blood studies show leukocytosis; elevated ESR, IgA, and IgG; low titer rheumatoid factor; and circulating immune complexes (antineutrophil cytoplasmic antibody in more than 90% of clients)
- Renal biopsy shows focal segmental glomerulonephritis.

Giant cell arteritis

- Blood studies show decreased Hb level and elevated ESR.
- Tissue biopsy shows panarteritis with infiltration of mononuclear cells, giant cells within the vessel wall (seen in 50% of cases), fragmentation of the internal elastic lamina, and proliferation of the intima.

Takayasu's arteritis

- Blood studies show decreased Hb level, leukocytosis, positive lupus erythematosus cell preparation, and elevated ESR.
- Arteriography shows calcification and obstruction of affected vessels.
- Tissue biopsy shows inflammation of the adventitia and intima of vessels and thickening of vessel walls.

Nursing diagnoses

- Ineffective tissue perfusion (systemic)
- Acute pain
- Disturbed sensory perception (tactile)

Treatment

- Removal of identified environmental antigen
- Elimination of antigenic food, if identifiable
- Treatment of underlying disorder

Drug therapy options

- Corticosteroid: prednisone (Deltasone)
- Antineoplastic: cyclophosphamide (Cytoxan)
- Antiinflammatory: ibuprofen

Planning and goals

- The client will have improved tissue perfusion.

◆ The client will express feelings of comfort and pain relief.
◆ The client will have an improved sense of touch.

Implementation

◆ Assess for dry nasal mucosa in clients with Wegener's granulomatosis. Instill nose drops *to lubricate the mucosa and help diminish crusting.* Alternatively, irrigate the nasal passages with warm normal saline solution *to combat drying.*
◆ Regulate environmental temperature *to prevent additional vasoconstriction caused by cold.*
◆ Monitor vital signs. Use a Doppler ultrasonic flowmeter, if available, *to auscultate blood pressure in clients with Takayasu's arteritis, whose peripheral pulses are commonly difficult to palpate.*
◆ Monitor intake and output. Check daily for edema. Keep the client well-hydrated (3 L daily) *to reduce the risk of hemorrhagic cystitis associated with cyclophosphamide therapy.*
◆ Provide emotional support *to help the client and his family cope with an altered body image — the result of the disorder or its therapy.* (For example, Wegener's granulomatosis may be associated with saddle nose, steroids may cause weight gain, and cyclophosphamide may cause alopecia.)
◆ Monitor the client's WBC count during cyclophosphamide therapy *to prevent severe leukopenia.*

Evaluation

◆ The client displays improved systemic circulation and tissue perfusion.
◆ The client reports adequate pain control.
◆ The client has improved tactile perception.

GASTROINTESTINAL SYSTEM

The GI system is the body's food processing complex. This section provides a brief review of the structures of the GI system and some of the major disorders that affect the GI system.

GI STRUCTURE AND FUNCTION

The GI system includes the GI tract and related structures, such as the tongue, as well as the liver and other accessory organs.

GI tract

The GI tract is basically a hollow, muscular tube through which food passes as it's digested. Accessory organs, such as the liver and pancreas, contribute substances that are vital to digestion.

Mouth and esophagus

The digestive process begins in the mouth, where a mechanical (tongue and teeth) and chemical (saliva) combination begins to break down food.

The esophagus transfers food from the oropharynx (behind the palate) to the stomach. The esophagus contains two structures, the epiglottis and the cardiac sphincter, that direct food into the stomach. The epiglottis closes to prevent food from entering the trachea; the cardiac sphincter closes to prevent reflux of gastric contents.

Stomach

The stomach is a hollow muscular pouch that secretes pepsin, mucus, and hydrochloric acid for digestion. In the stomach, food mixes with gastric juices to become chyme, which the stomach stores before parceling it into the small intestine. The stomach also secretes the intrinsic factor necessary for absorption of vitamin B_{12}.

Small intestine

The small intestine consists of the duodenum, jejunum, and ileum. Nearly all digestion and absorption of nutrients takes place in the small intestine, which contains digestive agents, such as bile and pancreatic secretions. The small intestine is also lined with villi, which contain capillaries and lymphatics that transport nutrients from the small intestine to other parts of the body.

Large intestine

The large intestine consists of the ascending colon, transverse colon, descending colon, sigmoid colon, and rectum. It absorbs fluids and electrolytes, synthesizes vitamin K, and stores fecal material.

Liver and accessory organs

The liver is one of the largest organs of the body. Its many functions include:
◆ producing and conveying bile
◆ metabolizing carbohydrates, fats, and proteins
◆ synthesizing coagulation factors VII, IX, and X and prothrombin
◆ storing copper, iron, and vitamins A, D, E, K, and B_{12}

- detoxifying chemicals, excreting bilirubin, and producing and storing glycogen
- promoting erythropoiesis when bone marrow production is insufficient.

Gallbladder

The gallbladder is a hollow, pear-shaped organ that stores bile and then delivers it through the cystic duct to the common bile duct.

Pancreas

The pancreas secretes three digestive enzymes: amylase, lipase, and trypsin. It also secretes the hormones insulin, glucagon, and somatostatin from the islets of Langerhans into the blood. In addition, the pancreas secretes large amounts of sodium bicarbonate, which neutralizes the acid in chyme.

GI DISORDERS

The major GI disorders include appendicitis, cholecystitis, cirrhosis, colorectal cancer, Crohn's disease, diverticular disease, esophageal cancer, gastric cancer, gastritis, gastroenteritis, gastroesophageal reflux disease, hepatitis, hiatal hernia, intestinal obstruction, irritable bowel syndrome, pancreatitis, peptic ulcer, peritonitis, and ulcerative colitis.

APPENDICITIS

APPENDICITIS is an inflammation of the appendix. Although the appendix has no known function, it regularly fills with and empties itself of food. Appendicitis occurs when the appendix becomes inflamed from ulceration of the mucosa or from obstruction of the lumen.

Possible causes

- Barium ingestion
- Fecal mass
- Stricture
- Viral infection

Assessment findings

- Abdominal rigidity
- Anorexia
- Client lying in knee-bent position
- Constipation
- Fever
- Generalized abdominal pain that becomes localized in the right lower abdomen (McBurney's point)
- Malaise
- Nausea and vomiting
- Rebound abdominal tenderness
- Sudden cessation of pain (indicates rupture)

Diagnostic evaluation

- Hematology shows a moderately elevated WBC count.

Nursing diagnoses

- Acute pain
- Imbalanced nutrition: Less than body requirements
- Risk for infection

Treatment

- Appendectomy
- I.V. fluids to prevent dehydration
- Nothing by mouth

Drug therapy options

- Analgesics: meperidine (Demerol), morphine sulfate (administered only when diagnosis is confirmed)
- Antibiotic therapy specific to infecting organism if peritonitis develops

Planning and goals

- The client will express pain relief.
- The client will maintain optimum nutritional status.
- The client will remain free from infection.

Implementation

- Assess GI status and pain. *Sudden cessation of pain preoperatively may indicate appendix rupture.*
- Monitor and record vital signs and intake and output *to determine fluid volume.*
- Administer I.V. fluids *to prevent dehydration.*
- Place the client in semi-Fowler's position *to reduce pain and tension on the incision postoperatively.*
- Maintain nothing-by-mouth status until bowel sounds return postoperatively; then advance the diet as tolerated *to promote healing and meet metabolic needs.*
- Assist the client with incentive spirometry, turning, coughing, and deep breathing *to mobilize secretions and promote lung expansion.*
- Monitor dressings for drainage and incision for infection postoperatively *to detect early signs of infection and prevent complications.*

◆ Review key teaching topics with the client and family members *to ensure adequate knowledge about the condition and treatment,* including:
- completing follow-up medical care
- caring for the incision
- following activity restrictions
- recognizing the signs and symptoms of infection.

Evaluation

◆ The client expresses pain relief.
◆ Adequate fluid and caloric intake has been maintained.
◆ Skin is intact without signs of infection.

CHOLECYSTITIS

CHOLECYSTITIS is an acute or chronic inflammation of the gallbladder most commonly associated with cholelithiasis (presence of gallstones). It occurs when an obstruction, such as calculi or edema, prevents the gallbladder from contracting when fatty foods enter the duodenum.

Based on the results of diagnostic studies, a client may undergo surgical removal of the stones in the bile duct and removal of the inflamed gallbladder by traditional cholecystectomy. (Some clients don't undergo surgical removal of gallstones.) (See *Alternative treatments for gallstones.*)

Clients who require gallbladder removal increasingly are undergoing laparoscopic cholecystectomy. In this ambulatory surgery, the surgeon makes four small incisions into the abdomen. Pain is minimal; the client is discharged the same day or on the first postoperative day and can resume activities after a few days. In contrast, the client undergoing traditional cholecystectomy is typically discharged in about 5 days. Postoperatively, the client may have a T tube in place. (See *T tube placement.*)

Possible causes

◆ Cholelithiasis
◆ Estrogen therapy
◆ Infection of the gallbladder with *Escherichia coli*
◆ Obesity

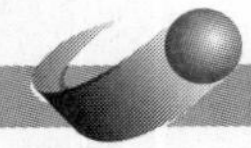

FAST FACT

Incidence of gallstone formation increases with the use of oral contraceptives, estrogens, and clofibrate because these drugs increase biliary cholesterol.

Alternative treatments for gallstones

Extracorporeal shock wave lithotripsy

Extracorporeal shock wave lithotripsy is designed for a client with a small number of stones and mild to moderate symptoms. The client sits in a tank of water or holds a water-filled cushion against the appropriate place on the abdomen. Shock waves are sent through the water until the stones disintegrate (1 to 2 hours). The client is on a cardiac monitor throughout the procedure because shock waves must be coordinated with cardiac rhythm to prevent arrhythmias. After the procedure, observe the client for hematuria, hematoma, nausea, and biliary colic.

Endoscopic sphincterotomy

Endoscopic sphincterotomy uses an endoscope to remove stones from the common bile duct. After the procedure, monitor the client for bleeding, pain, and fever. Promote bed rest for 6 to 8 hours, and give the client nothing by mouth until the gag reflex returns.

Cholesterol dissolvent

Moctanin is administered through a nasal biliary catheter to dissolve stones left in the bile duct after cholecystectomy. Dissolution may take 1 to 3 weeks. Observe the client for anorexia, nausea, vomiting, and abdominal pain.

Oral bile acids

Chenodiol (Chenix) and ursodiol (Actigall) are administered to dissolve small stones. Adverse effects include diarrhea (especially with chenodiol), elevation of hepatic enzymes, gastritis, and gastric ulcers. Dissolution takes between 6 months and 2 years, and the success rate is only about 30%.

Assessment findings

◆ Belching
◆ Clay-colored stools
◆ Dark amber urine
◆ Ecchymosis
◆ Episodic colicky pain in the epigastric area, which radiates to the back and shoulder
◆ Fever
◆ Flatulence
◆ Indigestion or chest pain after eating fatty or fried foods
◆ Jaundice
◆ Nausea and vomiting

T tube placement

A biliary tube, or T tube, is a flexible catheter that's placed within the common bile duct to facilitate bile drainage.

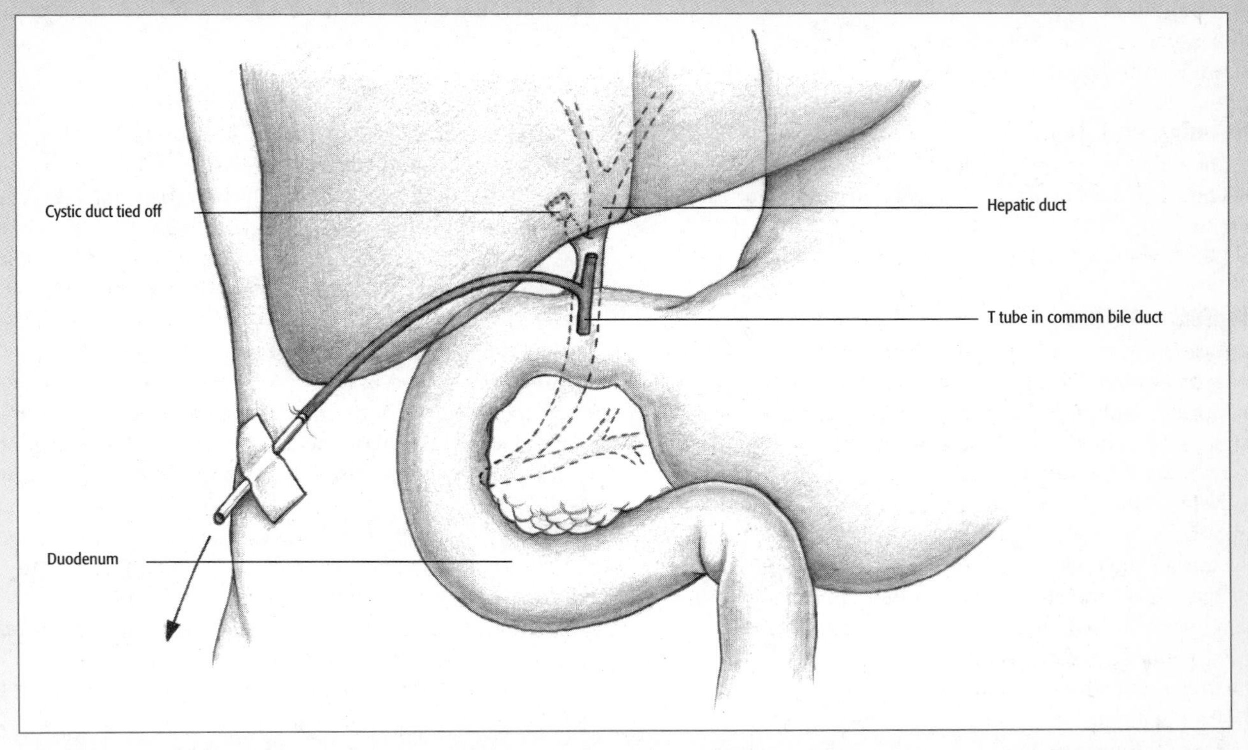

- ◆ Pruritus
- ◆ Steatorrhea

Diagnostic evaluation

◆ Blood studies, such as CBC, serum bilirubin levels, aspartate aminotransferase (AST), alanine aminotransferase (ALT), alkaline phosphatase, and serum amylase, reveal elevated enzyme levels if the liver has stasis or cell destruction. Elevated bilirubin levels (as well as alkaline phosphatase) indicate obstructed bile flow through the common bile duct, and elevated serum amylase levels may indicate concurrent pancreatitis. WBC count may also be elevated.

◆ Radiologic studies include GI series, ultrasound, chest X-ray, cholecystogram (rare), and endoscopic retrograde cholangiopancreatography, which show any abnormalities, the extent of the disease, and the client's ability to tolerate the proposed surgery.

◆ Urinalysis show darkened urine (cola-colored) and stool examination shows clay-colored stools if there's an obstruction.

Nursing diagnoses

- ◆ Acute pain
- ◆ Imbalanced nutrition: Less than body requirements
- ◆ Risk for infection

Treatment

- ◆ Small, frequent meals of a low-fat, low-calorie diet high in carbohydrates, protein, and fiber with restricted intake of gas-forming foods or no foods or fluids, as directed
- ◆ Extracorporeal shock wave lithotripsy
- ◆ Incentive spirometry
- ◆ Laparoscopic cholecystectomy or open cholecystectomy

Drug therapy options

◆ Analgesic: meperidine (Demerol)
◆ Antibiotic: cephalothin (Keflin)
◆ Anticholinergics: dicyclomine (Bentyl), propantheline (Pro-Banthine)
◆ Antiemetic: prochlorperazine (Compazine)
◆ Antipruritic: diphenhydramine (Benadryl)

Planning and goals

◆ The client will express pain relief.
◆ The client will maintain or regain adequate nutritional intake.
◆ The client won't develop an infection.

Implementation

◆ Assess abdominal status and pain *to determine baselines and detect changes in the client's condition.*
◆ Monitor and record vital signs and intake and output, laboratory studies, and urine specific gravity *to assess fluid and electrolyte balance.*
◆ Weigh the client daily *to detect signs of decreased food intake.*
◆ Monitor the client's appetite, food intake, and food tolerance; assess the client for pain after eating, abdominal distention, nausea, and vomiting *to help determine the client's nutritional status and detect passage of stones from the duct or increasing obstruction.*
◆ Use the guaiac test *to detect occult blood in stools.* Guaiac testing detects occult bleeding caused by decreased prothrombin synthesis if the liver is inflamed.
◆ Administer I.V. fluids *to provide needed fluids and electrolytes.*

For diagnostic testing

◆ Prepare the client for upper GI studies, including explaining procedures and rationales, administering a laxative if ordered, and instituting any dietary restrictions required by testing, such as clear liquids the evening before, *to decrease client anxiety and help reduce contents in the GI tract.*
◆ If necessary, prepare the client for ultrasonography or cholecystogram, *as directed by facility guidelines.*
◆ Administer enemas, as ordered. One or two enemas may be needed *to clean the colon.*
◆ Provide only clear liquids or nothing by mouth after midnight, if ordered, *to keep the colon free from contents.*
◆ After the client returns from the examination, resume the client's diet and fluids, as ordered *to promote return to a normal bowel pattern.*

Preoperative care (traditional surgery)

◆ Perform usual preoperative preparations, including an explanation of the T tube the client may have after surgery. If the surgery involves exploration of the common bile duct, the client will have a T tube placed in the common duct *to promote drainage.*

Postoperative care

◆ Perform routine postoperative care. Check the client's vital signs, fluid and electrolyte levels, Hb level, WBC count, and partial pressure of arterial carbon dioxide level *to help determine his postoperative status.*
◆ Check the client's skin for relief from jaundice and edema. *Jaundice should gradually fade. Edema shouldn't be present postoperatively.*
◆ Have the client turn, deep-breathe, cough, and use a respiratory aid every 2 hours; increase walking as tolerated *to help prevent complications such as atelectasis after surgery;* administer pain medications as needed *to relieve pain with breathing caused by the right upper quadrant incision.*
◆ Observe drainage in the T tube bile collection container, and keep the container below the incisional level; maintain the client on I.V. fluids only, as ordered. *The T tube uses gravity. I.V. fluids nourish the client until GI functions return; then food intake provides nourishment.*
◆ Clamp the T tube, when ordered, *to aid fat digestion.* If the client experiences no pain, nausea, or vomiting after eating, the physician removes the T tube. (A cholangiogram may be performed to confirm the absence of stones before the T tube is removed.) If the client is discharged with a T tube in place, provide instructions for home care *to ensure adequate care.* Maintain gravity drainage until the surgeon decides healing has occurred and bile is draining into the duodenum. The tube will then be clamped. Instruct the client to take a daily shower *to keep the insertion site clean.*
◆ Check the wound site every 4 hours for 24 to 48 hours *to observe for signs of bleeding and infection.* Change the dressing as needed and perform wound care, using aseptic technique.
◆ Measure the client's abdominal girth, check stool color, and monitor for flatus. Begin a clear liquid diet, when ordered, after bowel sounds return and the client can pass flatus; advance to a regular diet as tolerated. (The GI tract begins to regain function after the second postoperative day. *Passage of flatus represents significant progress.* The client's appetite slowly increases. *Abdominal girth measurement will detect the development of ileus.)*
◆ Prepare the client for discharge by reviewing home-care instructions and activity restrictions *to ensure appropriate*

Pathophysiologic changes caused by cirrhosis

This table outlines and defines the pathophysiologic changes as they occur in the client with cirrhosis.

CHANGES	DEFINITION
Portal vein hypertension	The portal vein empties into the liver. Scarring or obstruction in the liver causes backup in the portal vein, producing portal vein hypertension.
Hypoalbuminemia	The contents of the portal vein and blood serum contain albumin and globulin, two serum proteins. Albumin leaks out of the portal vein into the peritoneal cavity because the portal vein is distended by portal vein hypertension. Hypoalbuminemia is a loss of albumin from the blood serum.
Esophageal varices	Portal vein hypertension leads to increased pressures in veins, causing esophageal varices and hemorrhoids.
Ascites	Albumin draws fluids with it into the abdominal cavity, causing a fluid accumulation called *ascites.*
Hyperaldosteronism	Only the liver metabolizes aldosterone. A cirrhotic liver can't perform its normal functions. Therefore, aldosterone builds up (hyperaldosteronism), leading to fluid retention and edema.
Portal-systemic (hepatic) encephalopathy	Build-up of nitrogenous and biliary products in the blood causes a pathologic brain cell condition (encephalopathy). The wastes accumulate because the dysfunctional liver can't metabolize and excrete them.

care. Wound care includes washing the area while the client is bathing, noting untoward signs (drainage, warmth, tenderness), and keeping the area free from dressings and pressure from clothing. The client may not lift or carry heavy items for 6 weeks but can perform light household activities and cooking, as desired. The client should return to the physician if pain or food intolerance recurs.

Evaluation

- ◆ The client states pain is relieved.
- ◆ The client maintains nutritional intake to restore nutritional balance.
- ◆ The client remains free from signs or symptoms of infection.

CIRRHOSIS

CIRRHOSIS of the liver is a severe, life-threatening condition. Fibrotic, scarred tissues and fatty deposits gradually replace functioning liver cells. About 50% of cirrhosis results from alcoholism. Other causes include hepatitis, chemical destruction (from drugs, such as vinyl chloride), and bacterial liver infections. The cirrhotic liver shows patchy areas of regenerated cells that give the liver capsule a hobnailed, irregular appearance.

The pathophysiologic changes of cirrhosis arise from portal vein hypertension, leading to hypoalbuminemia and excessive venous pressures and causing esophageal varices and hemorrhoids, ascites, hyperaldosteronism, and hepatic encephalopathy. (See *Pathophysiologic changes caused by cirrhosis.*)

Possible causes

- ◆ Alcoholism and resulting malnutrition
- ◆ Autoimmune disease, such as sarcoidosis and chronic inflammatory bowel disease
- ◆ Cholestatic diseases
- ◆ Exposure to hepatitis (types A, B, C, and D viral hepatitis) or toxic substances

Assessment findings

- ◆ Weakness
- ◆ Nausea
- ◆ Vomiting
- ◆ Fatigue
- ◆ Diarrhea
- ◆ Edema

- Bleeding tendencies
- Constipation
- Anorexia
- Indigestion
- Gynecomastia
- Muscle cramps
- Petechiae
- Jaundice
- Asterixis
- Ascites
- Abdominal pain (possibly because of an enlarged liver)
- Decreased mental function and fine motor skills

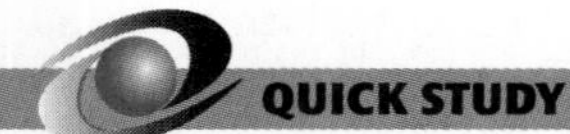

QUICK STUDY

To remember the signs of impending hepatic encephalopathy, know your **ABC**s.

Asterixis: Ask the client to hold his arms straight in front and look for hand tremors.

Behavioral changes: Assess the client for personality changes.

Clarity: Assess the client for mental status changes.

Diagnostic evaluation

- Esophagogastroduodenoscopy reveals bleeding esophageal varices, stomach irritation or ulceration, or duodenal bleeding and irritation.
- Chest X-ray determines pulmonary condition.
- Liver biopsy confirms the diagnosis.
- EEG determines cerebral functioning.
- Blood studies reveal decreased platelet count; decreased levels of Hb and HCT, albumin, serum electrolytes (sodium, potassium, chloride, magnesium), and folate; elevated levels of globulin, ammonia, total bilirubin, alkaline phosphatase, AST, ALT, and LD; and increased thymol turbidity.
- Urine studies show increased levels of bilirubin and urobilinogen.
- Stool studies reveal decreasing urobilinogen levels.

Nursing diagnoses

- Imbalanced nutrition: Less than body requirements
- Ineffective breathing pattern
- Risk for impaired skin integrity
- Risk for injury

Treatment

- Blood transfusions for bleeding
- Fluid restriction (usually to 1,500 ml/day)
- Gastric intubation and esophageal balloon tamponade for bleeding esophageal varices (Sengstaken-Blakemore method and Minnesota tube method)
- High-calorie, sodium-restricted, moderate- to high-protein diet (Protein is restricted in encephalopathy.)
- I.V. therapy using colloid volume expanders or crystalloids
- Oxygen therapy (may require endotracheal intubation and mechanical ventilation)
- Paracentesis to reduce abdominal pressure from ascites
- Portal-systemic shunting for a client with bleeding esophageal varices and portal hypertension
- Sclerotherapy (if the client continues to experience repeated hemorrhagic episodes despite conservative treatment)

Drug therapy options

- Antibiotic: Neomycin
- Antiemetic: trimethobenzamide (Tigan)
- Beta-adrenergic blocker: propranolol (Inderal)
- Diuretics: furosemide (Lasix), spironolactone (Aldactone)
- Hemostatic: vasopressin (Pitressin) for esophageal varices
- Laxative or ammonia detoxicant: lactulose
- Vitamin K: phytonadione (AquaMEPHYTON) for bleeding tendencies

Planning and goals

- The client will maintain optimum nutritional level.
- The client will maintain a patent airway and normal breathing patterns.
- The client's skin will remain intact.
- The client will not incur an injury.

Implementation

- Assess respiratory status frequently *because abdominal distention may interfere with lung expansion.* Position the client to facilitate breathing.
- Check skin, gums, stool, and emesis regularly for bleeding *to recognize early signs of bleeding and prevent hemorrhage.*
- Apply pressure to injection sites *to prevent bleeding.*
- Warn the client against taking aspirin, straining during defecation, and blowing his nose or sneezing too vigorously *to avoid bleeding.* Also, suggest using an electric razor and soft toothbrush.
- Observe the client closely for signs of behavioral or personality changes — especially increased stupor, lethargy,

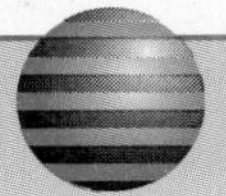

CLINICAL SITUATION

Caring for the client with cirrhosis

A 54-year-old male client, a manufacturer of plastic ornaments, enters the hospital with a tentative medical diagnosis of cirrhosis of the liver. The client has been ill at home for the past 6 weeks after developing viral hepatitis B. For 25 years, he has worked in a plastics factory, handling liquid materials. The client appears pale, weak, and fatigued. He's scheduled for a liver biopsy.

What nursing measures can help prevent hemorrhage after the liver biopsy?

◆ Apply a snug dressing over the biopsy site and have the client lie on his right side to assist in splinting the site for 1 to 4 hours, as ordered.

◆ Check vital signs frequently to ensure the client's safety. For example, check vital signs every 15 minutes for 1 hour, then every 30 minutes for 1 hour, and then every hour for the first 8 to 12 hours. After 8 to 12 hours, begin ambulation, if ordered.

The nurse is monitoring the client for nausea and vomiting. If vomitus contains blood, the nurse should prepare for treatment of esophageal varices. What treatment would be anticipated?

Treatment can vary as follows:

◆ Minor bleeding may warrant nasogastric tube insertion and antacid administration.

◆ Major bleeding may require I.V. administration of vasopressin to cause splanchnic vasoconstriction.

◆ Uncontrolled bleeding may necessitate a Sengstaken-Blakemore (S-B) tube. The S-B tube has a triple lumen to the esophageal balloon, gastric balloon, and gastric suction. Periodically, the esophageal balloon must be deflated and reinflated to prevent compression trauma to the esophageal venous circulation. The physician may order ice-water saline lavages to decrease the client's bleeding. The nurse must deflate and reinflate the esophageal balloon, as ordered.

Questions for further thought

◆ Why would vitamin K be ordered for a client with bleeding?

◆ What are key assessments after the removal of a S-B tube?

hallucinations, and neuromuscular dysfunction — *that may indicate increased ammonia levels.*

◆ Wake the client periodically *to determine LOC.*

◆ Watch for asterixis, *a sign of developing hepatic encephalopathy.*

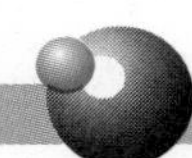

SPOT CHECK

What's the underlying cause of hepatic encephalopathy?

Answer: Elevated blood ammonia levels

◆ Monitor ammonia levels *to determine the effectiveness of lactulose therapy.*

◆ Weigh the client and measure abdominal girth daily, inspect the ankles and sacrum for dependent edema, and accurately record intake and output *to assess fluid retention.*

◆ Carefully evaluate the client before, during, and after paracentesis *because drastic loss of fluid may induce shock.*

◆ Avoid using soap when bathing the client; instead, use lubricating lotion or moisturizing agents *to prevent skin breakdown associated with edema and pruritus.*

◆ Handle the client gently, and turn and reposition him often *to keep the skin intact.*

◆ Encourage rest and good nutrition *to help the client conserve energy and decrease metabolic demands on the liver.*

◆ Instruct the client to avoid ingesting substances that are toxic to the liver, including alcohol, acetaminohen, and other over-the-counter or illicit drugs, *to prevent further deterioration of the liver.*

◆ Review dietary instructions *to ensure nutritional needs are met,* including following a diet of modified protein (70 to 100 g daily), carbohydrate intake to spare protein, and modified fat as desired; total intake should range from 2,000 to 3,000 calories daily. *Dietary needs result from the liver's inability to use nutrients properly.*

Evaluation

◆ The client verbalizes an understanding of dietary restrictions, the medication regimen, and the need to avoid exposure to infections and abstain from alcohol. (See *Caring for the client with cirrhosis.*)

- The client exhibits no evidence of respiratory distress.
- The client's skin exhibits no evidence of redness, breakdown, or infection.
- The client doesn't experience an injury during hospitalization.

COLORECTAL CANCER

Colorectal cancer is a malignant tumor of the colon or rectum. It may be primary or metastatic. It begins when unregulated cell growth and uncontrolled cell division develop into a neoplasm. Adenocarcinomas then infiltrate and cause obstruction, ulcerations, and hemorrhage.

Possible causes

- Aging
- Chronic constipation
- Chronic ulcerative colitis
- Diverticulosis
- Familial polyposis
- Family history of colon cancer or inflammatory bowel disease
- Low-fiber, high-carbohydrate diet
- Diet high in animal fat

Assessment findings

- Abdominal cramping
- Abdominal distention
- Anorexia
- Change in bowel habits and shape of stools
- Diarrhea and constipation
- Fecal oozing
- Melena
- Pallor
- Palpable mass
- Passage of blood in stools
- Vomiting
- Weakness
- Weight loss

Diagnostic evaluation

- Barium enema is used to locate a mass.
- Biopsy is positive for cancer cells.
- Carcinoembryonic antigen (CEA) is positive.
- Colonoscopy or sigmoidoscopy is used to identify and locate a mass.
- Digital rectal examination is used to detect a mass.
- Fecal occult blood test is positive.
- Lower GI series shows location of a mass.
- Hematology shows decreased Hb level and HCT.

Nursing diagnoses

- Anxiety
- Risk for deficient fluid volume
- Imbalanced nutrition: Less than body requirements

Treatment

- Radiation therapy
- Surgery, depending on tumor location

Drug therapy options

- Antiemetics: prochlorperazine (Compazine), ondansetron (Zofran)
- Antineoplastics: doxorubicin (Adriamycin), 5-fluorouracil (Adrucil)
- Folic acid derivative: leucovorin (citrovorum factor)

Planning and goals

- The client will verbalize decreased anxiety.
- The client will maintain adequate fluid balance.
- The client will maintain adequate nutritional intake.

Implementation

- Assess GI status *to determine a baseline and detect changes in the client's condition.*
- Monitor and record vital signs and intake and output, laboratory studies, and daily weight *to assess fluid and electrolyte status.*
- Monitor and record the color, consistency, amount, and frequency of stools *to detect early changes and bleeding.*
- Monitor for bleeding, infection, and electrolyte imbalance *to detect early changes and prevent complications.*
- Maintain the client's diet *to meet metabolic needs and promote healing.*
- Keep the client in semi-Fowler's position *to promote emptying of the GI tract.*
- Consult a registered dietitian *to help meet the client's nutritional needs.*
- Administer TPN *to improve nutritional status when the client can't consume adequate calories through the GI tract.*
- Administer postoperative care if indicated (including monitoring vital signs and intake and output; making sure the NG tube is kept patent; monitoring the dressing for drainage; assessing the wound for infection; assisting with turning, coughing, deep breathing, and incentive spirometry; administering pain medication as necessary or guiding

the client in use of patient-controlled analgesia) *to prevent complications and promote healing.*

◆ Encourage the client to express feelings about changes in his body image and a fear of dying, and support coping mechanisms *to increase the potential for further adaptive behavior.*

◆ Provide skin and mouth care *to maintain tissue integrity.*

◆ Provide rest periods *to promote healing and conserve energy.*

◆ Provide postchemotherapeutic and postradiation nursing care *to promote healing and prevent complications.*

◆ Administer antiemetics and antidiarrheals, as prescribed, *to prevent further fluid loss.*

◆ Consult home care and hospice services *to assist in meeting the client's needs.*

◆ Review key teaching topics with the client *to ensure adequate knowledge about his condition and treatment,* including:

– performing ostomy self-care if indicated
– monitoring changes in bowel elimination
– self-monitoring for infection
– alternating rest periods with activity
– contacting the United Ostomy Association and the American Cancer Society.

Evaluation

◆ The client verbalizes knowledge about the disease and treatment, expresses feelings of anxiety, and describes coping skills to help manage increased anxiety.

◆ The client has a balanced intake and output and normal vital signs.

◆ The client maintains adequate nutritional intake through diet or TPN and understands dietary instructions for discharge.

CROHN'S DISEASE

CROHN'S DISEASE is a chronic inflammatory disease of the small intestine, usually affecting the terminal ileum. It also sometimes affects the large intestine, usually in the ascending colon. It's slowly progressive with exacerbations and remissions.

Possible causes

◆ Allergies
◆ Emotional upset
◆ Immune disorder
◆ Genetic transmission

Assessment findings

◆ Abdominal cramps and spasms after meals
◆ Chronic diarrhea with blood
◆ Fever
◆ Flatulence
◆ Nausea
◆ Pain in lower right quadrant
◆ Weight loss

Diagnostic evaluation

◆ Abdominal X-ray shows congested, thickened, fibrosed, narrowed intestinal wall.

◆ Barium enema shows lesions in the terminal ileum.

◆ Fecal occult blood test is positive.

◆ Flexible sigmoidoscopy and colonscopy show ulceration, inflammation, strictures, and granulomes.

◆ Upper GI series shows a classic string sign: segments of stricture separated by normal bowel.

◆ CBC usually shows a decreased Hb level and HCT; WBC may be elevated.

◆ Low albumin and protein levels reflect poor absorption of protein.

◆ ESR is elevated due to inflammation.

Nursing diagnoses

◆ Anxiety
◆ Diarrhea
◆ Imbalanced nutrition: Less than body requirements

Treatment

◆ Colectomy with ileostomy in clients with extensive disease of the large intestine and rectum

◆ Small, frequent meals of a diet high in protein, calories, and carbohydrates and low in fat, fiber, and residue with bland foods, elimination of dairy products (if lactose intolerate) and gas-forming foods, or no food or fluids

◆ TPN to rest the bowel

Drug therapy options

◆ Analgesics: meperidine (Demerol), morphine sulfate

◆ Antianemics: ferrous sulfate (Feosol), ferrous gluconate (Fergon)

◆ Antibiotics: sulfasalazine (Azulfidine), metronidazole (Flagyl)

◆ Anticholinergics: propantheline (Pro-Banthine), dicyclomine (Bentyl)

◆ Antidiarrheal: diphenoxylate (Lomotil)

◆ Antiemetic: prochlorperazine (Compazine)

◆ Anti-inflammatory: olsalazine (Dipentum)

◆ Corticosteroid: prednisone (Deltasone)
◆ Immunosuppressants: mercaptopurine (Purinethol), azathioprine (Imuran)
◆ Potassium supplements: potassium chloride (K-Lor) administered with food, potassium gluconate (Kaon)

Planning and goals

◆ The client will verbalize decreased anxiety.
◆ The client will regain normal bowel function.
◆ The client will maintain adequate nutritional intake.

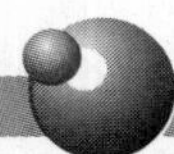

SPOT CHECK

Why is TPN commonly administered to a client with Crohn's disease?

Answer: To allow the bowel to rest and to treat the client for malnutrition

Implementation

◆ Assess GI status (noting excessive abdominal distention) and fluid balance *to determine baseline and detect changes in the client's condition.*
◆ Monitor and record vital signs and intake and output, laboratory studies, daily weight, urine specific gravity, and fecal occult blood *to detect bleeding and dehydration.*
◆ Monitor the number, amount, and character of stools *to detect deterioration in GI status.*
◆ Administer TPN *to rest the bowel and promote nutritional status.*
◆ Administer medications, as prescribed, *to maintain or improve the client's condition.*
◆ Maintain the client's diet; withhold food and fluids as necessary *to minimize GI discomfort.*
◆ Minimize stress and encourage verbalization of feelings *to allay the client's anxiety.*
◆ Provide skin and perianal care *to prevent skin breakdown.*
◆ If surgery is necessary, provide postoperative care (including monitoring vital signs, dressings for drainage, and ileostomy drainage, performing ileostomy care as needed; assessing incision for signs of infection; assisting with turning, coughing, and deep breathing; assisting with use of an incentive spirometer; and getting the client out of bed on the first postoperative day if stable) *to promote healing and prevent complications.*
◆ Review key teaching topics with the client *to ensure adequate knowledge about his condition and treatment,* including:
– performing ileostomy self-care
– avoiding laxatives and aspirin
– performing perianal care daily
– reducing stress
– recognizing the signs and symptoms of rectal hemorrhage and intestinal obstruction.

Evaluation

◆ The client verbalizes knowledge about the disease and treatment, expresses feelings of anxiety, and relates coping skills to help manage increased anxiety.
◆ The client is free from diarrhea and abdominal cramps.
◆ The client maintains adequate nutritional intake and verbalizes an understanding of dietary instructions for discharge.

DIVERTICULAR DISEASE

Diverticular disease has two clinical forms: diverticulosis and diverticulitis. DIVERTICULOSIS occurs when the intestinal mucosa protrudes through the muscular wall. The common sites for diverticula are in the descending and sigmoid colon, but they may develop anywhere from the proximal end of the pharynx to the anus.

DIVERTICULITIS is an inflammation of the diverticula that may lead to infection, hemorrhage, or obstruction.

Possible causes

◆ Age (most common in people older than age 40)
◆ Chronic constipation
◆ Congenital weakening of the intestinal wall
◆ Low intake of roughage and fiber
◆ Straining during defecation
◆ Stress

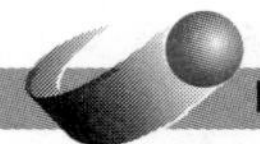

FAST FACT

The incidence of diverticular disease increases with age, secondary to structural changes in the muscle layers of the colon. Symptoms may be less pronounced and blood in the stool may go undetected due to poor vision of an elderly client.

Assessment findings

◆ Anorexia
◆ Bloody stools
◆ Change in bowel habits
◆ Constipation and diarrhea
◆ Fever
◆ Flatulence

◆ Left lower quadrant pain or midabdominal pain that radiates to the back
◆ Nausea, vomiting
◆ Rectal bleeding
◆ Signs of shock (high fever, chills, hypotension) if peritonitis develops

Diagnostic evaluation

◆ Barium enema (contraindicated in clients with acute diverticulitis) shows inflammation, narrow lumen of the bowel, and diverticula.
◆ Biopsy confirms cancer (colonoscopic biopsy contraindicated during acute diverticular disease because of risk of perforation)
◆ Blood studies show increased WBC count and ESR.
◆ Sigmoidoscopy (contraindicated in clients with acute diverticulitis) shows a thickened wall in the diverticula.
◆ CT scanning shows abscesses or thickening of the bowel.
◆ Upper GI series confirms diverticulosis of the esophagus and small bowel.

Nursing diagnoses

◆ Acute pain
◆ Chronic pain
◆ Constipation
◆ Diarrhea
◆ Imbalanced nutrition: Less than body requirements

Treatment

◆ Generally no treatment for asymptomatic diverticulosis
◆ Colon resection (for diverticulitis refractory to medical treatment)
◆ Liquid or low-residue diet, stool softeners, and occasional doses of mineral oil for diverticulitis or diverticulosis that's accompanied by pain, mild GI distress, or difficult defecation
◆ Low-residue diet, bulk-forming medication (psyllium), and increased water consumption for diverticulosis or diverticulitis after pain subsides
◆ Temporary colostomy possible for perforation, peritonitis, obstruction, or fistula that accompanies diverticulitis

Drug therapy options

◆ Analgesic: meperidine (Demerol)
◆ Antibiotics: metronidazole, (Flagyl), ciprofloxacin (Cipro), co-triamoxazole (Bactrim)
◆ Anticholinergic: propantheline (Pro-Banthine)
◆ Stool softener: docusate sodium (Colace) (for diverticulosis or mild diverticulitis)
◆ Bulk laxative

Planning and goals

◆ The client will verbalize pain relief.
◆ The client's diarrhea or constipation will be controlled.
◆ The client will maintain or regain adequate nutrition.

Implementation

◆ Assess abdominal distention and bowel sounds *to determine a baseline and detect changes in the client's condition.*
◆ Monitor and record vital signs, intake and output, and laboratory studies *to assess fluid status.*
◆ Monitor stools for occult blood *to detect bleeding.*
◆ Maintain the client's diet *to improve nutritional status and promote healing.*
◆ Maintain position, patency, and low suction of NG tube *to prevent nausea and vomiting.* (See *GI tubes,* page 496.)
◆ Keep the client in semi-Fowler's position *to promote comfort and GI emptying.*
◆ Prepare the client for surgery (administering cleansing enemas, osmotic purgative, and oral and parenteral antibiotics), if necessary, *to avoid wound contamination from bowel contents during surgery.*
◆ Provide postoperative care (watching for signs of infection; performing meticulous wound care; watching for signs of postoperative bleeding; assisting with turning, coughing, and deep breathing; and teaching ostomy self-care) *to promote healing and prevent complications.*
◆ Consult a registered dietitian *to help meet the client's nutritional needs.* Administer TPN *to improve nutritional status when the client can't receive nutrition through the GI tract.*
◆ Administer medications as prescribed *to maintain or improve the client's condition.*
◆ Review key teaching topics with the client *to ensure adequate knowledge about his condition and treatment,* including:
– decreasing constipation
– following dietary recommendations and restrictions
– avoiding corn, nuts, and fruits and vegetables with seeds
– monitoring stools for bleeding.

Evaluation

◆ The client verbalizes adequate pain relief or pain control and can demonstrate pain-relief measures.
◆ The client exhibits improved stool consistency and decreased incidence of constipation or diarrhea.
◆ The client maintains adequate nutrition.

GI tubes

The chart below lists types of GI tubes, along with their site, purpose, and appropriate nursing interventions.

TYPE	SITE AND PURPOSE	NURSING CONSIDERATIONS
Salem sump	Nasogastric (NG) Suctioning or feeding	◆ Make sure that blue tubing is free from secretions. ◆ Clamp tube for ambulation and note its tolerance. ◆ Irrigate tube with 20 to 30 ml of normal saline solution.
Levin tube	NG Suctioning or feeding	◆ Make sure to connect tube to low intermittent suction to prevent gastric irritation. ◆ Irrigate tube with 20 to 30 ml of normal saline solution.
Nutriflex	NG Feeding	◆ Use 50-ml syringe with 20 ml of water to irrigate. (Small syringe may cause tube to rupture from excessive pressure.) ◆ Use infusion pump, which can exert only up to 40 psi. (Tube bursting pressure is 80 psi).
Gastrostomy	Stomach Suctioning or feeding	◆ Know that tube uses gravity drainage. ◆ As required, clamp tube and open for residuals.
Sengstaken-Blakemore	Esophagus and stomach Compressing esophageal varices	◆ Inflate (never irrigate) esophageal balloon with air and irrigate stomach tube with 20 to 30 ml normal saline solution as required.
Jejunostomy	Jejunum Feeding	◆ Know that feedings may be intermittent or continuous with an infusion pump.
Dobhoff	Jejunum Feeding	◆ Know that tube has mercury tip for X-ray visualization and assists in passage. ◆ Know that tube has same cautions as Nutriflex tube.
Cantor	Small to large intestine Suctioning	◆ Know that mercury is inserted into balloon before insertion to aid passage. ◆ Connect tube to suction. ◆ Irrigate tube with 20 to 30 ml of normal saline solution.
Miller-Abbott	Small to large intestine Suctioning	◆ Know that mercury is instilled into properly marked opening after tube reaches stomach to aid passage. ◆ Irrigate tube with 20 to 30 ml normal saline solution.

ESOPHAGEAL CANCER

Esophageal cancer attacks the esophagus, the muscular tube that runs from the back of the throat to the stomach. Cells in the lining of the esophagus start to multiply rapidly and form a tumor that may spread to other parts of the body.

Nearly always fatal, esophageal cancer usually develops in men older than age 50. This disease occurs worldwide, but incidence varies geographically. It's most common in Japan, China, the Middle East, and parts of South Africa.

Possible causes

- ◆ Excessive use of alcohol
- ◆ Nutritional deficiency
- ◆ Smoking

Assessment findings

- ◆ Dysphagia
- ◆ Weight loss
- ◆ Pain
- ◆ Hoarseness
- ◆ Coughing

Diagnostic evaluation

◆ Endoscopic examination of the esophagus, punch and brush biopsies, and an exfoliative cytologic test confirm esophageal tumors.

◆ X-rays of the esophagus with barium swallow and motility studies reveal structural and filling defects and reduced peristalsis.

Nursing diagnoses

- ◆ Impaired swallowing
- ◆ Imbalanced nutrition: Less than body requirements
- ◆ Risk for aspiration

Treatment

◆ Endoscopic laser treatment and bipolar electrocoagulation to help restore swallowing by vaporizing cancerous tissue

◆ Esophageal dilation

◆ Gastrostomy or jejunostomy to help provide adequate nutrition

◆ Radiation therapy

◆ Radical surgery to excise the tumor and resect the esophagus or the stomach and the esophagus

Drug therapy options

◆ Analgesics: morphine (MS Contin), fentanyl (Duragesic)

◆ Antineoplastic: porfimer (Photofrin)

Planning and goals

◆ The client will have improved swallowing abilities related to diet modification.

◆ The client will maintain weight within an acceptable range.

◆ The client won't aspirate.

Implementation

◆ Before surgery, answer the client's questions and let him know what to expect after surgery (gastrostomy tubes, closed chest drainage, NG suctioning) *to allay anxiety.*

◆ After surgery, monitor vital signs and watch for unexpected changes *to detect early signs of complications and avoid treatment delay.* If surgery included an esophageal anastomosis, keep the client flat on his back *to avoid tension on the suture line.*

◆ Promote adequate nutrition, and assess the client's nutritional and hydration status *to determine the need for supplementary parenteral feedings.*

◆ Place the client in Fowler's position for meals and allow plenty of time to eat *to avoid aspiration of food.*

◆ Provide high-calorie, high-protein, pureed food as needed *to meet increased metabolic demands and to prevent aspiration.*

◆ If the client has a gastrostomy tube, give food slowly, using gravity to adjust the flow rate *to prevent abdominal discomfort.* The prescribed amount usually ranges from 200 to 500 ml. Offer something to chew before each feeding *to promote gastric secretions and a semblance of normal eating.*

◆ Instruct the family in gastrostomy tube care (checking tube patency before each feeding, providing skin care around the tube, and keeping the client upright during and after feedings) *to avoid complications.*

◆ Provide emotional support to the client and his family *to help them cope with the terminal illness.*

◆ Consult home care and hospice services to help meet the client's needs.

Evaluation

◆ The client reports improved swallowing abilities.

◆ The client maintains an adequate weight.

◆ The client doesn't display signs or symptoms of aspiration.

GASTRIC CANCER

Gastric cancer involves a malignant stomach tumor. It may be primary or metastatic. Its precise cause is unknown, but it's commonly associated with gastritis, gastric atrophy, and other conditions. About one-half of gastric cancers occur in the pyloric area of the stomach. It metastasizes rapidly to the regional lymph nodes, omentum, liver, and lungs.

Possible causes

◆ Chronic gastritis, ulceration, *Helicobacter pylori*

◆ Dietary factors: type of food preparation, physical properties of some foods, and certain methods of food preservation (especially smoking, pickling, and salting)

◆ Environmental factors (smoking, high alcohol intake)

◆ Familial history of gastric cancer

◆ Genetic factors

◆ Peptic ulcer

Assessment findings

- ◆ Indigestion
- ◆ Pain after eating that isn't relieved by antacids
- ◆ Fatigue
- ◆ Malaise
- ◆ Anorexia
- ◆ Nausea and vomiting
- ◆ Epigastric fullness and pain
- ◆ Weakness
- ◆ Hematemesis
- ◆ Melena
- ◆ Weight loss

Diagnostic evaluation

◆ Blood studies show increased levels of AST, LD, and amylase.

◆ CEA test is positive.

◆ Fecal occult blood test is positive.

◆ Gastroscopy or endoscopy for biopsy is positive for cancer cells.

◆ Barium X-ray of GI tract with fluorscopy reveals a tumor or abnormal gastric mucosal outline.

◆ Hematology shows decreased Hb level and HCT.

◆ Liver, CT, and bone scans and liver biopsy may show metastasis.

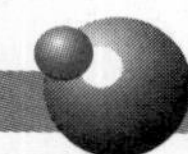

SPOT CHECK

The nurse is reviewing the diagnostic data of a client suspected of having gastric cancer. What laboratory finding is the nurse most likely to find?

A. Elevated Hb level and HCT

B. Negative fecal occult blood test

C. Subnormal gastric hydrochloric acid level

D. Negative CEA test

Answer: C. One manifestation of gastric cancer is achlorhydria, an absence of free hydrochloric acid in the stomach. In gastric cancer, subnormal Hb level and HCT is most likely; fecal occult blood test is most likely to be positive. The CEA test would most likely be positive in gastric cancer.

Nursing diagnoses

- ◆ Acute pain
- ◆ Anxiety
- ◆ Risk for deficient fluid volume
- ◆ Imbalanced nutrition: Less than body requirement

Treatment

◆ Gastric surgery: gastroduodenostomy, gastrojejunostomy, partial gastric resection, total gastrectomy

◆ TPN

◆ High-calorie diet

◆ Radiation therapy

Drug therapy options

◆ Analgesics: meperidine (Demerol), morphine

◆ Antiemetic: prochlorperazine (Compazine)

◆ Antineoplastics: carmustine (BiCNU), 5-fluorouracil (Adrucil), doxorubicin (Adriamycin), cisplatin (Platinol-AQ), methotrexate (Rheumatrex), mitomycin (Mutamycin)

◆ Vitamin supplements: folic acid (Folvite), cyanocobalamin (vitamin B_{12}) for clients who have undergone total gastrectomy

Planning and goals

- ◆ The client will express feelings of increased comfort.
- ◆ The client will verbalize feelings of decreased anxiety.
- ◆ The client will maintain adequate fluid status.
- ◆ The client will maintain adequate nutritional balance.

Implementation

◆ Assess GI status postoperatively *to monitor the client for dumping syndrome (weakness, nausea, flatulence, and palpitations 30 minutes after a meal).*

◆ Monitor and record vital signs, intake and output, laboratory studies, and daily weight *to determine a baseline and early changes in condition.*

◆ Monitor the consistency, amount, and frequency of stools *to detect GI compromise.*

◆ Monitor the color of stools *to detect bleeding and to prevent hemorrhage.*

◆ Maintain the client's diet *to promote nutritional balance.*

◆ Maintain position, patency, and low suction of NG tube (without irrigating or repositioning the NG tube because it may put pressure on the suture line) *to prevent complications, nausea, and vomiting.*

◆ Consult a registered dietitian *to help meet the client's nutritional needs.* Administer TPN for 1 week or longer if gastric surgery is extensive *to meet metabolic needs and promote wound healing.*

◆ Administer medications, as prescribed, *to maintain or improve the client's condition.*

◆ Support client coping mechanisms *to increase the potential for adaptive behavior.*

◆ Provide skin and mouth care *to prevent skin breakdown and damage to the oral mucosa and improve nutritional intake.*

◆ Provide rest periods *to conserve energy.*

◆ Consult home care and hospice services *to help meet the client's needs.*

Evaluation

◆ The client reports adequate pain control and decreased anxiety.
◆ The client doesn't display signs of dehydration.
◆ The client maintains adequate nutritional balance.

GASTRITIS

GASTRITIS is an inflammation of the gastric mucosa (stomach lining). It may be acute or chronic. Acute gastritis produces mucosal reddening, edema, hemorrhage, and erosion. Chronic gastritis is common among elderly people and those with pernicious anemia. In chronic atrophic gastritis, all stomach mucosal layers are inflamed.

Possible causes

Acute gastritis

◆ Ingestion of irritating foods, spicy foods, or alcohol
◆ Drugs, such as aspirin and other NSAIDs, cytotoxic agents, caffeine, and corticosteroids
◆ Infecton, such as *H. pylori* or other acute infectious organisms
◆ Ingestion of poisons or corrosive substances

Chronic gastritis

◆ Alcohol ingestion
◆ Autoimmune factor
◆ Cigarette smoke
◆ *H. pylori* infection
◆ Peptic ulcer disease
◆ Pernicious anemia

Assessment findings

◆ Abdominal cramping
◆ Anorexia
◆ Epigastric discomfort
◆ Hematemesis
◆ Indigestion
◆ Nausea and vomiting

Diagnostic evaluation

◆ Fecal occult blood test can detect occult blood in vomitus and stools if the client has gastric bleeding.
◆ Blood studies show low Hb level and HCT when significant bleeding has occurred.
◆ Upper GI endoscopy with biopsy confirms the diagnosis when performed within 24 hours of bleeding (contraindicated after ingestion of a corrosive agent).
◆ Upper GI series may be performed to exclude serious lesions.

Nursing diagnoses

◆ Risk for deficient fluid volume
◆ Imbalanced nutrition: Less than body requirements
◆ Acute pain

Treatment

◆ Angiography with vasopressin infused in normal saline solution (when gastritis causes massive bleeding)
◆ Blood transfusion
◆ I.V. fluid therapy
◆ NG lavage to control bleeding
◆ Oxygen therapy, if necessary
◆ Partial or total gastrectomy (rare)
◆ Vagotomy and pyloroplasty (limited success when conservative treatments have failed)

Drug therapy options

◆ Antacids used as buffers (if pH of stomach is less than 4.0)
◆ Analgesics for pain relief
◆ Antibiotics: according to susceptibility of the infecting organism (if the cause is bacterial)
◆ Antidote: according to the ingested poison (if the cause is poisoning)
◆ H_2-receptor antagonists: cimetidine (Tagamet), ranitidine (Zantac), famotidine (Pepcid), nizatidine (Axid) to block gastric secretions
◆ Vitamin B_{12} if pernicious anemia is the cause

Planning and goals

◆ The client will maintain normal fluid volume.
◆ The client will maintain weight.
◆ The client will express feelings of increased comfort and pain relief.

Implementation

◆ If the client is vomiting, give antiemetics and I.V. fluids *to prevent dehydration and electrolyte imbalance.*
◆ Monitor fluid intake and output and electrolyte levels *to detect early signs of dehydration and electrolyte loss.*
◆ Consult a registered dietitian *to meet the client's nutritional needs.* Monitor the client for recurrent symptoms as food is reintroduced.
◆ Offer smaller, more frequent meals *to reduce irritating gastric secretions.* Eliminate foods that cause gastric upset *to prevent gastric irritation.*
◆ If surgery is necessary, prepare the client preoperatively and provide appropriate postoperative care *to decrease preoperative anxiety and prevent intraoperative and postoperative complications.*

◆ Administer antacids and other prescribed medications *to promote gastric healing.*
◆ Urge the client to seek immediate attention for recurring symptoms, such as hematemesis, nausea, and vomiting, *to prevent complications such as GI hemorrhage.*
◆ Urge the client to take prophylactic medications as prescribed *to prevent recurring symptoms.*
◆ Provide emotional support to the client *to help him manage his symptoms.*

Evaluation

◆ The client doesn't display signs of dehydration.
◆ The client has maintained his weight.
◆ The client reports adequate pain control.

GASTROENTERITIS

GASTROENTERITIS is irritation and inflammation of the digestive tract characterized by diarrhea, nausea, vomiting, and abdominal cramping. It occurs in all age-groups and is usually self-limiting in adults.

In the United States, gastroenteritis ranks second to the common cold as a cause of lost work time and fifth as the cause of death among young children. It also can be life-threatening in elderly and debilitated persons. It's a major cause of morbidity and mortality in developing nations.

This disorder is also called *intestinal flu, traveler's diarrhea, viral enteritis,* and *food poisoning.*

Possible causes

◆ Amoebae, especially *Entamoeba histolytica*
◆ Bacteria (responsible for acute food poisoning), such as *Staphylococcus aureus,* salmonella, shigella, *Clostridium botulinum, Escherichia coli,* and *Clostridium perfringens*
◆ Drug reactions (especially antibiotics)
◆ Enzyme deficiencies
◆ Food allergens
◆ Ingestion of toxins, such as plants and toadstools (mushrooms)
◆ Parasites, such as ascaris, enterobius, *Trichinella spiralis*
◆ Viruses (may be responsible for traveler's diarrhea), such as adenovirus, echovirus, and coxsackievirus

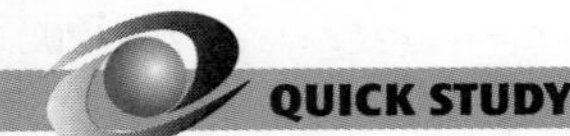

QUICK STUDY

Fight the WAR against gastroenteritis by remembering these tips:

Wash your hands before handling all foods.
Always cook food thoroughly and keep hot foods hot.
Refrigerate perishable foods promptly and keep cold foods cold.

Assessment findings

◆ Abdominal discomfort
◆ Diarrhea
◆ Nausea and vomiting

Diagnostic evaluation

◆ Stool culture identifies the causative bacterium, parasite, or amoeba.
◆ Blood culture identifies causative organism.

Nursing diagnoses

◆ Diarrhea
◆ Risk for deficient fluid volume
◆ Acute pain

Treatment

◆ Increased fluid intake
◆ I.V. fluid and electrolyte replacement
◆ Nutritional support

Drug therapy options

◆ Antibiotic: according to the susceptibility/infecting of the organism
◆ Antidiarrheals: camphorated opium tincture (Paregoric), diphenoxylate with atropine (Lomotil), loperamide (Imodium)
◆ Antiemetics: prochlorperazine (Compazine), trimethobenzamide (Tigan) (should be avoided in clients with viral or bacterial gastroenteritis)

Planning and goals

◆ The client's stools will return to normal.
◆ The client will maintain adequate fluid volume.
◆ The client will express feeling of comfort and pain relief.

Implementation

◆ Administer medications and correlate dosages, routes, and times appropriately with the client's meals and activities; for example, give antiemetics 30 to 60 minutes before meals *to prevent onset of symptoms.*
◆ If the client is unable to tolerate food, replace lost fluids and electrolytes with clear liquids and sport drinks *to prevent dehydration.*
◆ Vary the client's diet *to make eating more enjoyable and allow some choice of foods.*
◆ Instruct the client to avoid milk and milk products, *which may exacerbate the condition.*
◆ Record strict intake and output. Watch for signs of dehydration, such as dry skin and mucous membranes, fever, and sunken eyes, *to prevent complications of dehydration.*

◆ Wash your hands thoroughly after giving care *to avoid the spread of infection.*
◆ Instruct the client to perform warm sitz baths three times per day *to relieve anal irritation.*
◆ Educate the client regarding proper food handling and hygiene *to prevent recurrence.* Report cases of food poisoning to public health authorities *to aid in community surveillance of outbreaks.*

Evaluation

◆ The client has normal bowel movements.
◆ The client doesn't display signs of dehydration.
◆ The client reports adequate pain control.

GASTROESOPHAGEAL REFLUX DISEASE

GASTROESOPHAGEAL REFLUX DISEASE (GERD) refers to the backflow, or reflux, of gastric and duodenal contents past the lower esophageal sphincter and into the esophagus. Reflux may cause symptoms or pathologic changes. Persistent reflux may cause reflux esophagitis (inflammation of the esophageal mucosa). The prognosis varies with the underlying cause.

Possible causes

◆ Any action that decreases lower esophageal sphincter (LES) pressure, such as smoking cigarettes and ingesting certain food (fats, whole milk, orange juice, tomatoes chocolate), alcohol, anticholinergics (atropine, belladonna, propantheline), and other drugs (morphine, diazepam, meperidine)
◆ Any condition or position that increases intra-abdominal pressure
◆ Hiatal hernia (especially in children)
◆ Long-term NG intubation (more than 5 days)
◆ Pressure within the stomach that exceeds LES pressure
◆ Pyloric surgery (alteration or removal of the pylorus), which allows reflux of bile or pancreatic juice

Assessment findings

◆ Heartburn (burning sensation in the upper abdomen)
◆ Dysphagia
◆ Pain radiating to the neck, jaws, and arms
◆ Odynophagia followed by a dull, stomachache
◆ Nocturnal regurgitation

Diagnostic evaluation

◆ Barium swallow fluoroscopy indicates reflux.
◆ Esophageal pH probe reveals reflux.
◆ Esophagoscopy shows reflux.
◆ Acid perfusion (Bernstein) test shows that reflux is the cause of symptoms.
◆ Endoscopy allows visualization and confirmation of pathologic changes in the mucosa.
◆ Biopsy allows visualization and confirmation of pathologic changes in the mucosa.

Nursing diagnoses

◆ Risk for aspiration
◆ Chronic pain
◆ Deficient knowledge regarding disease process and treatment

Treatment

◆ Positional therapy to help relieve symptoms by decreasing intra-abdominal pressure
◆ Dietary modifications (see *Dietary factors affecting LES pressure,* page 502)
◆ Surgery, which reduces reflux by creating an artificial closure at the gastroesophageal junction (in severe and unresponsive cases, hemorrhage, pulmonary aspiration, severe pain, perforation, incompetent LES, and associated hiatal hernia)

Drug therapy options

◆ Antacid: aluminum hydroxide (AlternaGEL) administered 1 hour and 3 hours after meals and at bedtime
◆ H_2-receptor antagonists: cimetidine (Tagamet), ranitidine (Zantac), famotidine (Pepcid), nizatidine (Axid)
◆ Proton pump inhibitors: omeprazole (Prilosec), lansoprazole (Prevacid), pantoprazole (Protonix) or rabeprazole (Aciphex)

Planning and goals

◆ The client won't show signs of aspiration.
◆ The client will express feelings of comfort and pain relief.
◆ The client will verbalize knowledge regarding dietary guidelines and treatment for GERD.

Implementation

◆ Consult a registered dietitian *to help meet the client's nutritional needs.* Develop a diet that takes food preferences into account while helping to minimize reflux symptoms *to ensure compliance.*
◆ Have the client sleep in reverse Trendelenburg's position (with the head of the bed elevated 6″ to 12″ [15 to 30 cm]) or raise the head of the bed at home by placing it on cinderblocks *to reduce intra-abdominal pressure.*

Dietary factors affecting LES pressure

Various dietary and lifestyle elements can increase or decrease lower esophageal sphincter (LES) pressure. Take these into account as you plan the patient's treatment program.

Increase LES pressure
- Protein
- Carbohydrate
- Nonfat milk
- Low-dose ethanol

Decrease LES pressure
- Fat
- Whole milk
- Orange juice
- Carbonated beverages
- Tomatoes
- Chocolate
- Antiflatulent (simethicone)
- High-dose ethanol
- Cigarette smoking
- Lying on right or left side
- Sitting

After surgery using a thoracic approach
- Carefully watch and record chest tube drainage and respiratory status *to detect early signs of respiratory distress.*
- If needed, give chest physiotherapy and oxygen *to mobilize secretions and prevent hypoxemia.*
- Place the client with an NG tube in semi-Fowler's position *to help prevent reflux.*
- Offer reassurance and emotional support *to help the client cope with pain and discomfort.*

Evaluation
- The client doesn't display signs of aspiration.
- The client reports adequate pain control.
- The client relates appropriate treatment guidelines.

HEPATITIS
HEPATITIS is an inflammation of liver tissue that causes hypertrophy and proliferation of Kupffer's cells and bile stasis. Hepatitis is typically caused by one of six viruses: hepatitis A, B, C, D, E, or G. Hepatitis may also be nonviral, such as drug- or toxin-induced or secondary to infection.

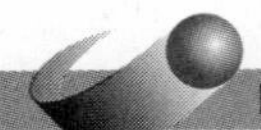

FAST FACT

All health care workers and others at risk should be vaccinated with hepatitis B vaccine. Boosters are given 1 month and 6 months after the initial dose. Antibody response can be checked 1 to 3 months after completing the course of vaccination.

Possible causes
Hepatitis A
- Contaminated food, milk, or water
- Contact with infected feces

Hepatitis B
- Parenteral exposure (needle sticks)
- Contact with infected blood
- Contact with infected secretions or body fluids (sexual contact)
- Perinatal transmission (from mother to infant)

Hepatitis C
- Contact with infected blood or serum (blood transfusions)
- Contact with infected secretions or body fluids (sexual contact)
- Tattooing

Hepatitis D
- Contact with infected blood and blood products (occurs with frequent exposure, as in hemophilia or I.V. drug abuse)
- Contact with infected secretions or body fluids (sexual contact)

Hepatitis E
- Fecal-oral transmission

Hepatitis G
- Blood-borne transmission (blood transfusions)

Nonviral hepatitis
- Autoimmune and metabolic diseases (Wilson's disease, autoimmune hepatitis)
- Infectious agents (systemic viruses, such as Epstein-Barr virus, cytomegalovirus, measles, varicella zoster, herpes simplex, HIV, and coxsackie virus) or spirochetes (syphilis, leptospirosis)

◆ Hepatotoxins, such as alcohol, medications, and industrial toxins

Assessment findings

Assessment findings are consistent for the different types of hepatitis, but signs and symptoms progress over several stages: the preicteric phase (usually 1 to 5 days), the icteric phase (usually 1 to 2 weeks), and the posticteric, or recovery, phase (usually 2 to 12 weeks but sometimes longer in clients with hepatitis B, C, or E). (See *Recognizing fulminant hepatitis.*)

Preicteric phase

◆ Anorexia
◆ Constipation and diarrhea
◆ Fatigue
◆ Fever
◆ Headache
◆ Hepatomegaly
◆ Malaise
◆ Nasal discharge
◆ Nausea and vomiting
◆ Pharyngitis
◆ Pruritus
◆ Right upper quadrant pain
◆ Splenomegaly
◆ Weight loss

Icteric phase

◆ Clay-colored stools
◆ Dark urine
◆ Fatigue
◆ Hepatomegaly
◆ Jaundice
◆ Pruritus
◆ Splenomegaly
◆ Weight loss

Posticteric phase

◆ Decreased hepatomegaly
◆ Decreased jaundice
◆ Fatigue
◆ Improved appetite

Recognizing fulminant hepatitis

Fulminant hepatitis is a rare but severe form of hepatitis that rapidly causes massive liver necrosis. It usually occurs in clients with hepatitis B, D, or E. Mortality is extremely high (more than 80% of clients lapse into deep coma), but those who survive may recover completely.

Assessment

In a client with viral hepatitis, suspect fulminant hepatitis if you detect:

◆ confusion
◆ somnolence
◆ ascites
◆ edema
◆ rapidly rising bilirubin level
◆ markedly prolonged prothrombin time.

As the disease progresses quickly to the terminal phase, the client may experience cerebral edema, brain stem compression, GI bleeding, sepsis, respiratory failure, cardiovascular collapse, and renal failure.

Emergency actions

If you suspect fulminant hepatitis, you should:

◆ notify the physician immediately
◆ provide supportive care, such as maintaining fluid volume, supporting ventilation through mechanical means, controlling bleeding, and correcting hypoglycemia
◆ restrict protein intake
◆ expect to administer oral lactulose or neomycin and, possibly, massive doses of glucocorticoids
◆ prepare the client for a liver transplant if necessary and if the client meets the criteria.

Diagnostic evaluation

◆ Blood studies show increased ALT, AST, alkaline phosphatase, lactate dehydrogenase, bilirubin, and ESR; positive antibody to hepatitis A; positive immunoglobulin anti-delta antigens (in type D); positive hepatitis B surface antigen; and positive hepatitis E antigen, and hepatitis G surface antigen; and increased prothrombin time and fibrin-split products.
◆ Stool specimen reveals hepatitis A virus (in hepatitis A cases).
◆ Urine chemistry shows increased urobilinogen.

Nursing diagnoses

◆ Fatigue
◆ Imbalanced nutrition: Less than body requirements
◆ Risk for deficient fluid volume
◆ Deficient knowledge regarding disease process and treatment

Treatment

- High-calorie, moderate-protein, high-carbohydrate, low-fat diet given in small, frequent meals
- Rest

Drug therapy options

- Antiemetic: prochlorperazine (Compazine)
- Vitamins and minerals: vitamin K (AquaMEPHYTON), ascorbic acid (vitamin C), vitamin B-complex (Mega-B)
- Alpha-interferon and ribavirin (Rebetron): may be given for hepatitis B and C; has demonstrated efficacy in the treatment of hepatitis C

Planning and goals

- The client will exhibit a decreased level of fatigue.
- The client will regain adequate nutritional and fluid intake.
- The client will verbalize an understanding about the disease and how to prevent infection and transmission.

Implementation

- Assess GI status and watch for bleeding and fulminant hepatitis *to detect early complications.*
- Consult a registered dietitian *to establish the client's nutritional and metabolic needs.* Encourage small, frequent meals *to improve his nutrition.*
- Monitor and record vital signs, intake and output, and laboratory studies *to detect early signs of deficient fluid volume.*
- Administer medications, as prescribed, *to maintain or improve the client's condition.*
- Maintain standard precautions. *Hand washing prevents the spread of pathogens to others.*
- Provide rest periods *to conserve the client's energy and reduce his metabolic demands.*
- Change the client's position every 2 hours *to reduce the risk of skin breakdown.*
- Monitor for signs of bleeding *to prevent hemorrhage.*
- Review key teaching topics with the client *to ensure adequate knowledge about his condition and treatment,* including:
  - avoiding exposure to people with infections
  - avoiding alcohol
  - maintaining good personal hygiene
  - refraining from donating blood
  - increasing fluid intake to 3,000 ml/day (approximately 12 8-oz glasses)
  - abstaining from sexual intercourse until serum liver studies are within normal limits
  - avoiding over-the-counter medications, such as acetaminophen, until discussing their use with a health care professional.

Evaluation

- The client verbalizes decreased fatigue, use of energy-saving measures, and the need for rest.
- The client exhibits balanced intake and output, adequate nutritional intake, and normal vital signs.
- The client demonstrates an understanding about the disease process, the need for follow-up care, the necessity for good personal hygiene, and practices to avoid disease infection and transmission.

HIATAL HERNIA

A HIATAL HERNIA, also known as an *esophageal hernia,* is a protrusion of the stomach through the diaphragm into the thoracic cavity. Hiatal hernia is the most common problem of the diaphragm affecting the alimentary canal. Incidence of hiatal hernia is higher in women than men and increases with age.

Possible causes

- Aging
- Congenital weakness
- Increased abdominal pressure
- Obesity
- Pregnancy
- Trauma

Assessment findings

- Cough
- Dysphagia
- Dyspnea
- Feeling of fullness
- Pyrosis
- Regurgitation
- Sternal pain after eating
- Tachycardia
- Vomiting

Diagnostic evaluation

- Barium swallow reveals protrusion of the hernia.
- Chest X-ray shows protrusion of abdominal organs into the thorax.
- Esophageal motility studies assess the presence of esophageal motor abnormality before surgical repair of the hernia.
- Esophagoscopy shows incompetent cardiac sphincter.
- Gastric analysis reveals increased pH.

Nursing diagnoses

- ◆ Acute pain
- ◆ Anxiety
- ◆ Chronic pain
- ◆ Imbalanced nutrition: Less than body requirements

Treatment

◆ Antireflux surgical repair, if complications develop

◆ Bland diet with decreased intake of caffeine and spicy foods, and small frequent meals

◆ Weight loss, if necessary, and restrictions on activity that increases intra-abdominal pressure such as bending, lifting, coughing, and straining

◆ Putting head of bed on blocks to elevate

Drug therapy options

◆ Antacids: (Mylanta)

◆ H_2-receptor antagonists: cimetidine (Tagamet), famotidine (Pepcid), ranitidine (Zantac)

Planning and goals

◆ The client will experience pain relief.

◆ The client will have a decreased level of anxiety.

◆ The client will have improved nutritional status.

Implementation

◆ Assess respiratory status *to detect early signs of respiratory distress.*

◆ Monitor and record vital signs, intake and output, and daily weight *to determine baselines and detect early signs of nutritional deficit.*

◆ Administer oxygen *to help relieve respiratory distress.*

◆ Avoid flexion at the waist in positioning the client *to promote comfort.*

◆ Consult a registered dietitian *to help establish the client's nutritional needs.* Maintain the client's diet *to ensure nutritional status.*

◆ Maintain position, patency, and low suction of the NG tube *to prevent nausea and vomiting.*

◆ Keep the client in semi-Fowler's position *to promote comfort.*

◆ Administer medications, as prescribed, *to improve GI function.*

◆ Review key teaching topics with the client *to ensure adequate knowledge about his condition and treatment,* including:

- eating small, frequent meals
- avoiding hot, spicy foods, carbonated beverages, and alcohol
- remaining upright for 2 hours after eating
- avoiding constrictive clothing
- avoiding lifting, bending, straining, and coughing
- sleeping with upper body elevated to reduce gastric reflux.

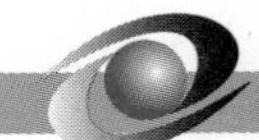

QUICK STUDY

When teaching your client with a hiatal hernia what to avoid, just keep the word **HIATAL** in mind.

Hot and spicy foods
Ingestion of large meals
Apparel that's constrictive
Twisting, bending, and lifting
Alcohol
Limit carbonated beverages

Evaluation

◆ The client acknowledges changes in his eating habits and interventions that can help promote comfort before, during, and after eating.

◆ The client expresses feelings, verbalizes decreased anxiety, and discusses coping skills to handle anxiety.

◆ The client regains and maintains adequate nutritional intake.

INTESTINAL OBSTRUCTION

An INTESTINAL OBSTRUCTION occurs when the intestinal lumen becomes blocked, causing gas, fluid, and digested substances to accumulate near the obstruction and increasing peristalsis in the area of the obstruction. Water and electrolytes are then secreted into the blocked bowel, causing inflammation and inhibiting absorption. Signs and symptoms depend on the location and extent of the obstruction.

Possible causes

- ◆ Adhesions
- ◆ Diverticulitis
- ◆ Fecal impaction
- ◆ Hernias
- ◆ Inflammation (Crohn's disease)
- ◆ Mesenteric thrombosis
- ◆ Paralytic ileus
- ◆ Tumors
- ◆ Volvulus

Assessment findings

- ◆ Nausea
- ◆ Cramping pain
- ◆ Abdominal distention

- ◆ Diminished or absent bowel sounds
- ◆ Constipation
- ◆ Fever
- ◆ Vomiting fecal material
- ◆ Weight loss

Diagnostic evaluation

◆ Abdominal X-ray shows an increased amount of gas in the bowel.

◆ Barium enema stops at obstruction.

◆ Blood studies show decreased sodium and potassium levels and increased WBC count.

Nursing diagnoses

- ◆ Ineffective tissue perfusion (GI)
- ◆ Acute pain
- ◆ Imbalanced nutrition: Less than body requirements

Treatment

◆ Bowel resection with or without anastomosis, if other treatment fails

◆ GI decompression using an NG tube, a Miller-Abbott tube, or Cantor tube

◆ Withholding food and fluids

◆ Correcting fluid and electrolyte imbalances with I.V. therapy and replacements

Drug therapy options

- ◆ Analgesic: meperidine (Demerol)
- ◆ Antibiotic: gentamicin (Garamycin)

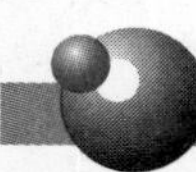

SPOT CHECK

A physician orders gastric decompression for a client with small-bowel obstruction. The nurse should plan for the suction to be:

A. low pressure and intermittent.

B. low pressure and continuous.

C. high pressure and intermittent.

D. high pressure and continuous.

Answer: A. Gastric decompression is typically low pressure and intermittent. High pressure and continuous gastric suctioning predisposes the gastric mucosa to injury and ulceration.

Planning and goals

◆ The client will have adequate perfusion of the GI system as exhibited by normal bowel sounds and movements.

◆ The client will express feelings of comfort and pain relief.

◆ The client will maintain adequate caloric intake.

Implementation

◆ Assess GI status. Assess and record bowel sounds once per shift *to determine GI status.*

◆ Monitor and record vital signs, intake and output, and laboratory studies *to detect early signs of fluid volume deficit.*

◆ Withhold food and fluids *to prevent nausea and vomiting.*

◆ Monitor and record the frequency, color, and amount of stools *to assess and determine nutritional status.*

◆ Measure and record the client's abdominal girth *to determine the presence of distention.*

◆ Administer I.V. fluids *to maintain hydration.*

◆ Maintain position, patency, and low intermittent suction of the NG tube and Miller-Abbott tube *to prevent nausea and vomiting and to resolve the obstruction, if possible.*

◆ Consult with a registered dietitian *to help meet the client's nutritional needs.* (TPN may be required.)

◆ Keep the client in semi-Fowler's position *to promote comfort.*

◆ Administer postoperative care if indicated (monitoring vital signs and intake and output; making sure the NG tube is kept patent; monitoring the dressing for drainage; assessing the wound for infection; assisting with turning, coughing, and deep breathing; medicating for pain as necessary or guiding the client with use of postoperative client-controlled analgesia) *to promote healing and detect early postoperative complications.*

◆ Administer medications as prescribed *to maintain or improve the client's condition.*

Evaluation

- ◆ The client doesn't display signs of ischemic bowel.
- ◆ The client reports adequate pain control.
- ◆ The client maintains an adequate weight.

IRRITABLE BOWEL SYNDROME

IRRITABLE BOWEL SYNDROME is marked by chronic symptoms of abdominal pain, alternating constipation and diarrhea, and abdominal distention. This disorder is extremely common (about 20% more common in women than men); a substantial portion of clients, however, never seek medical attention.

This disorder may also be referred to as *spastic colon* or *spastic colitis.*

Possible causes

- Diverticular disease
- Irritants (caffeine, alcohol)
- Stress
- Lactose intolerance
- Abuse of laxatives
- Food poisoning
- Colon cancer

Assessment findings

- Abdominal bloating
- Constipation, diarrhea, or both
- Dyspepsia
- Faintness
- Heartburn
- Lower abdominal pain that intensifies with stress or 1 to 2 hours after eating
- Passage of mucus with stools
- Pasty, pencil-like stools
- Weakness

Diagnostic evaluation

- Barium enema may reveal colonic spasm and tubular appearance of the descending colon. It also rules out certain other disorders, such as diverticula, tumors, and polyps.
- Sigmoidoscopy and colonoscopy may disclose spastic contractions.
- Stool examination for occult blood, parasites, and pathogenic bacteria is negative.

Nursing diagnoses

- Chronic pain
- Diarrhea
- Constipation

Treatment

- Elimination diet to determine if symptoms result from food intolerance (In this type of diet, certain foods, such as citrus fruits, coffee, corn, dairy products, tea, and wheat, are sequentially eliminated; then each food is gradually reintroduced to identify which foods, if any, trigger the client's symptoms)
- Diet containing 15 to 20 g/day of bulky foods, such as wheat bran, oatmeal, oat bran, rye cereals, prunes, dried apricots, and figs (if the client has constipation and abdominal pain)
- Increasing fluid intake to at least eight 8-oz glasses per day
- Stress management
- Heat application

Drug therapy options

- Sedative: diazepam (Valium)
- Antiflatulent: simethicone (Mylicon)
- Antispasmodic: propantheline (Pro-Banthine)
- Antidiarrheal: diphenoxylate with atropine (Lomotil)
- Sertonin 4 receptor agonist: tegaserod (Zelnorm)

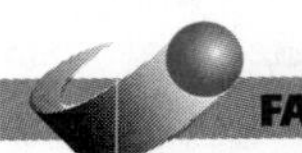

FAST FACT

The client with irritable bowel syndrome needs to ingest 15 to 20 g of bulk per day.

Planning and goals

- The client will express feelings of comfort and pain relief.
- The client's bowel function will return to normal.

Implementation

- Help the client deal with stress, and warn against dependence on sedatives or antispasmodics *because stress may be the underlying cause of irritable bowel syndrome.*
- Encourage regular checkups. For clients over age 40, emphasize the need for a yearly flexible sigmoidoscopy and rectal examination. *Irritable bowel syndrome is associated with a higher-than-normal incidence of diverticulitis and colon cancer.*
- Consult a registered dietitian to help meet the client's nutritional needs.

Evaluation

- The client reports adequate pain control.
- The client reports a decreased incidence of diarrhea and constipation.

PANCREATITIS

PANCREATITIS is the inflammation of the pancreas. In acute pancreatitis, pancreatic enzymes are activated in the pancreas rather than the duodenum, resulting in tissue damage and autodigestion of the pancreas.

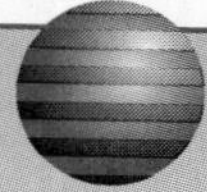

CLINICAL SITUATION

Caring for the client with pancreatitis

The client is a 34-year-old male with a history of alcohol abuse. He complains of severe abdominal pain that radiates to his back. He has also had several incidents of nausea and vomiting.

Which diagnostic tests should be ordered to confirm a diagnosis of pancreatitis?

A. Amylase, lipase, chest X-ray
B. Amylase, lipase, abdominal X-ray
C. Amylase, lipase, computed tomography (CT) scan
D. Complete blood count, urinalysis, electrolytes, electrocardiogram

Answer: C. Elevated serum amylase and lipase are the diagnostic hallmarks that confirm acute pancreatitis. Characteristically, serum amylase reaches peak levels 24 hours after the onset of pancreatitis and then returns to normal within 48 to 72 hours, despite continued symptoms. Serum lipase levels remain elevated longer than amylase levels.

A CT scan reveals an increased pancreatic diameter. Abdominal and chest X-rays rule out other diseases that cause similar symptoms and detect pleural effusions.

True or false?

During acute pancreatitis, the client should be placed on a clear liquid diet.

Answer: False. In acute pancreatitis, the client can't eat or drink. Nasogastric suctioning is usually required to decrease gastric distention and suppress pancreatic secretions.

Questions for further thought

- Which nursing diagnoses would be appropriate for the client with pancreatitis?
- What complications of pancreatitis can occur?

In chronic pancreatitis, chronic inflammation results in fibrosis and calcification of the pancreas, obstruction of the ducts, and destruction of the secreting acinar cells.

Possible causes

- Alcoholism
- Bacterial or viral infection
- Biliary tract disease
- Blunt trauma to the pancreas or abdomen
- Drugs, such as steroids, thiazide diuretics, and oral contraceptives
- Duodenal ulcer
- Hyperlipidemia
- Hyperparathyroidism

Assessment findings

- Abrupt onset of pain in the epigastric area that radiates to the shoulder, substernal area, back, and flank
- Abdominal tenderness and distention
- Aching, burning, stabbing, pressing pain
- Knee-chest position, fetal position, or leaning forward for comfort
- Decreased or absent bowel sounds
- Nausea and vomiting
- Tachycardia
- Dyspnea
- Fever
- Hypotension
- Jaundice
- Steatorrhea
- Weight loss

Diagnostic evaluation

- Arteriography reveals fibrous tissue and calcification of the pancreas.
- Blood studies show increased amylase, lipase, LD, glucose, AST, and lipid levels; decreased calcium and potassium levels; increased WBC count; and decreased Hb and HCT. (See *Caring for the client with pancreatitis.*)
- CT scanning shows an enlarged pancreas.
- Cullen's sign is positive.
- Endoscopic retrograde cholangiopancreatography (ERCP) reveals biliary obstruction.
- Fecal fat test is positive.
- Glucose tolerance test shows decreased tolerance.
- Grey-Turner's sign is positive.
- Ultrasonography reveals cysts, bile duct inflammation, and dilation.
- Urine chemistry shows increased amylase.

Nursing diagnoses

- ◆ Acute pain
- ◆ Ineffective breathing pattern
- ◆ Deficient fluid volume

Treatment

- ◆ Bland, low-fat, high-protein diet of small, frequent meals with restricted intake of caffeine, alcohol, and gas-forming foods (nothing by mouth as the disease progresses)
- ◆ Bed rest
- ◆ I.V. fluids (vigorous replacement of fluids and electrolytes)
- ◆ Dialysis
- ◆ Sequential compression device to prevent blood clot formation
- ◆ Surgical intervention to treat the underlying cause, if appropriate
- ◆ Transfusion therapy with packed RBCs

Drug therapy options

- ◆ Analgesics: meperidine (Demerol) (Morphine is contraindicated.)
- ◆ Anticholinergics: propantheline (Pro-Banthine), dicyclomine (Bentyl)
- ◆ Antidiabetic: insulin (possible infusion to stabilize blood glucose levels)
- ◆ Antiemetic: prochlorperazine (Compazine)
- ◆ Calcium supplement: calcium gluconate (Kalcinate)
- ◆ Corticosteroid: hydrocortisone (Solu-Cortef)
- ◆ Digestant: pancrelipase (Pancrease)
- ◆ H_2-receptor antagonists: cimetidine (Tagamet), ranitidine (Zantac), famotidine (Pepcid), nizatidine (Axid)
- ◆ Mucosal barrier fortifier: sucralfate (Carafate)
- ◆ Potassium supplement: I.V. potassium chloride
- ◆ Tranquilizers: lorazepam (Ativan), alprazolam (Xanax)

Planning and goals

- ◆ The client will express feelings of comfort and pain relief.
- ◆ The client will maintain adequate ventilation.
- ◆ The client will maintain a normal fluid volume.

Implementation

- ◆ Assess abdominal, cardiac, and respiratory status and, as the disease progresses, watch for respiratory failure, tachycardia, and worsening GI status *to determine baselines and detect early changes and signs of complications.*
- ◆ Assess fluid balance *to detect fluid volume deficit or excess.*
- ◆ Monitor and record vital signs, intake and output, laboratory studies, CVP, daily weight, and urine specific gravity *to detect signs of fluid volume deficit.*
- ◆ Monitor urine and stool for color, character, and amount *to detect bleeding.*
- ◆ Maintain the client's diet and withhold food and fluids as necessary *to rest the pancreas and prevent nausea and vomiting.*
- ◆ Perform bedside glucose monitoring *to assess for hyperglycemia.*
- ◆ Administer oxygen and maintain endotracheal tube and mechanical ventilation if necessary *to improve oxygenation* and provide suctioning as needed *to stabilize secretions.*
- ◆ Administer I.V. fluids *to treat or prevent hypovolemic shock and restore electrolyte balance.*
- ◆ Maintain position, patency, and low suction of the NG tube *to prevent nausea and vomiting.*
- ◆ Keep the client in semi-Fowler's position (if his blood pressure allows) *to promote comfort and lung expansion.*
- ◆ Administer TPN. In severe cases, reintroduction of food may be associated with pancreatic abscess. *TPN is necessary to meet the client's metabolic needs.*
- ◆ Keep the client in bed and turn him every 2 hours, or utilize a specialty rotation bed *to prevent pressure ulcers.*
- ◆ Administer medications as prescribed *to improve or maintain the client's condition.*
- ◆ Provide skin, nares, and mouth care *to prevent tissue damage.*
- ◆ Provide a quiet, restful environment *to conserve energy and decrease metabolic demands.*

Evaluation

- ◆ The client reports adequate pain relief.
- ◆ The client's breathing pattern remains normal and unlabored.
- ◆ The client doesn't display signs of dehydration.

PEPTIC ULCER

PEPTIC ULCERS are breaks in the continuity of the esophageal, gastric, or duodenal mucosa. They can occur in any part of the GI tract that comes in contact with gastric substances, hydrochloric acid, and pepsin. The ulcers may be found in the esophagus, stomach, duodenum, or (after gastroenterostomy) jejunum.

Possible causes

◆ Alcohol abuse
◆ Drug-use, such as salicylates, steroids, NSAIDs, and rauwolfia alkaloids (Reserpine)
◆ Gastritis
◆ *Helicobacter pylori* infection
◆ Smoking
◆ Stress
◆ Zollinger-Ellison syndrome

Assessment findings

◆ Anorexia
◆ Diarrhea or constipation (secondary to antacid use)
◆ Dizziness, fainting
◆ Hematemesis
◆ Left epigastric pain 1 to 2 hours after eating
◆ Melena
◆ Nausea and vomiting
◆ Relief from pain after administration of antacids
◆ Weight loss

Diagnostic evaluation

◆ Acid-base studies may indicate metabolic alkalosis caused by overuse of antacids.
◆ Barium swallow shows ulceration of the gastric mucosa.
◆ Fecal occult blood test is positive.
◆ Gastric analysis is normal.
◆ Gastric sampling may be positive for *H. pylori.*
◆ Blood studies show decreased Hb level and HCT (if bleeding is present) and normal or increased serum gastrin level.
◆ Upper GI endoscopy shows location of the ulcer.

Nursing diagnoses

◆ Acute pain
◆ Anxiety
◆ Chronic pain
◆ Risk for deficient fluid volume

Treatment

◆ Endoscopic laser to control bleeding
◆ Gastric surgery (if GI hemorrhage) that may include gastroduodenostomy, gastrojejunostomy, partial gastric resection, and total gastrectomy
◆ Low-fiber diet in small, frequent meals
◆ Photocoagulation to control bleeding
◆ Transfusion therapy with packed RBCs (if bleeding is present and Hb level and HCT are low)

Drug therapy options

◆ Antacids: magnesium and aluminum hydroxide (Maalox), aluminum hydroxide gel (AlternaGEL)
◆ Antibiotic, if *H. pylori* is present
◆ Anticholinergics: propantheline (Pro-Banthine), dicyclomine (Bentyl)
◆ H_2-receptor antagonists: cimetidine (Tagamet), famotidine (Pepcid), nizatidine (Axid), ranitidine (Zantac)
◆ Mucosal barrier fortifier: sucralfate (Carafate)
◆ Pituitary hormone: vasopressin (Pitressin) to manage bleeding
◆ Prostaglandin: misoprostol (Cytotec) to protect the stomach lining
◆ Proton pump inhibitors: lansoprazole (Prevacid), omeprazole (Prilosec)

Planning and goals

◆ The client will experience pain relief through healing.
◆ The client will display decreased anxiety.
◆ The client will regain and maintain adequate fluid balance and nutritional intake.

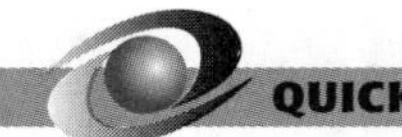

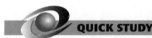

QUICK STUDY

To remember the most common complications of peptic ulcer disease, think **HOP.**

Hemorrhage
Obstruction (pyloric)
Perforation

Implementation

◆ Assess GI status *to monitor for signs of bleeding.*
◆ Assess cardiovascular status *to detect early signs of GI hemorrhage.*
◆ Monitor and record vital signs, intake and output, laboratory studies, fecal occult blood, and gastric pH *to detect signs of bleeding.*
◆ Monitor the consistency, color, amount, and frequency of stools *to detect early signs of GI bleeding.*
◆ Maintain the client's diet with small, frequent feedings *to meet metabolic needs and promote healing.*
◆ Maintain position, patency, and low suction of the NG tube if gastric decompression is ordered *to prevent nausea and vomiting.*
◆ Administer medications, as prescribed, *to maintain or improve the client's condition.*
◆ Provide nose and mouth care *to maintain tissue integrity.*
◆ Provide postoperative care if necessary (avoiding repositioning the NG tube, irrigating the tube gently if ordered,

medicating for pain as needed and ordered, monitoring the dressings for drainage, assessing bowel sounds, and getting the client out of bed as tolerated) *to detect early complications and promote healing.*

◆ Review key teaching topics with the client *to ensure adequate knowledge about his condition and treatment,* including:
- reducing stress
- relaxation techniques
- following dietary recommendations and restrictions such as avoiding caffeine, alcohol, and spicy or fried foods
- following postoperative care and restrictions.

Evaluation

◆ The client remains free from pain.

◆ The client verbalizes decreased anxiety and is able to describe positive outlets for stress and learn stress management techniques.

◆ The client has a balanced intake and output and normal vital signs.

PERITONITIS

PERITONITIS results from a localized or generalized inflammation of the peritoneal cavity. It occurs when irritants in the peritoneal area cause inflammatory edema, vascular congestion, and hypermotility of the bowel.

Possible causes

◆ Bacterial invasion (as in appendicitis, diverticulitis, peptic ulcer, ulcerative colitis, volvulus, strangulated obstruction perforated or ruptured gallbladder, abdominal neoplasm, and a penetrating wound)

◆ Chemical invasion (as in ruptured fallopian tube or bladder, perforated gastric ulcer, and release of pancreatic enzymes)

Assessment findings

◆ Abdominal resonance and tympany on percussion
◆ Abdominal rigidity and distention
◆ Anorexia
◆ Constant, diffuse, intense abdominal pain
◆ Decreased or absent bowel sounds
◆ Decreased peristalsis
◆ Decreased urine output
◆ Fever
◆ Malaise
◆ Nausea
◆ Rebound tenderness
◆ Shallow respirations
◆ Weak, rapid pulse

Diagnostic evaluation

◆ Abdominal CT scan or X-ray shows free air in the abdomen under the diaphragm.

◆ Blood studies show increased WBC count and HCT.

◆ Peritoneal aspiration is positive for blood, pus, bile, bacteria, or amylase.

◆ Laparotomy identifies underlying cause.

Nursing diagnoses

◆ Decreased cardiac output
◆ Acute pain
◆ Deficient fluid volume

Treatment

◆ Withholding food or fluid

◆ Surgical intervention when the client's condition is stabilized (chosen to treat the cause — for example, an appendectomy for a perforated appendix with drains placed for drainage of infected material)

Drug therapy options

◆ Analgesic: meperidine (Demerol)

◆ Antibiotics: gentamicin (Garamycin), clindamycin (Cleocin), cephalothin (Keflex), ampicillin and sulbactam (Unasyn)

Planning and goals

◆ The client will remain hemodynamically stable.

◆ The client will express feelings of comfort and pain relief.

◆ The client will maintain normal fluid volume.

Implementation

◆ Assess abdominal and respiratory status and fluid balance *to detect and assess signs of fluid volume deficit.*

◆ Monitor and record vital signs, intake and output, laboratory studies, CVP, daily weight, and urine specific gravity *to detect signs of fluid volume deficit.*

◆ Measure and record the client's abdominal girth *to assess for abdominal distention.*

◆ Withhold food and fluids *to prevent nausea and vomiting.*

◆ Administer I.V. fluids *to maintain hydration and electrolyte balance.*

◆ Provide routine postoperative care (monitoring vital signs and intake and output, including drainage from drains; assist with turning, incentive spirometry, cough-

Comparing ulcerative colitis and Crohn's disease

Use this table to compare ulcerative colitis and Crohn's disease. Clinical symptoms usually don't aid differentiation.

	ULCERATIVE COLITIS	CROHN'S DISEASE
Site of inflammation	Usually begins in the rectal area and may extend through the entire bowel.	Small intestine (primarily terminal ileum), although the disease may occur in any part of the small or large intestine
Type of lesion	Continuous ulcerated lesions involving mucosal and submucosal layers (may create abscesses)	Skip lesions (inflamed areas skip around in the tract); lesions involve all intestinal layers (mucosa, submucosa, muscle, and serous layers); may abscess or perforate, scar, or form fistulas
Common patterns	Frequent diarrhea (30 to 40 bowel movements per day), that's profuse, mucus-filled, watery, bloody, and debilitating; dehydration and weight loss; electrolyte imbalances (common); fever (common in acute attacks)	Watery, mucus-filled diarrhea that's less bloody than in ulcerative colitis; cramping; distention; and low-grade fever
Treatments	*Medical:* Diet high in protein, calories, and vitamins; anticholinergic drugs and anti-inflammatory, antibacterial, or antibiotic drugs; emotional support *Surgical:* Ileostomy with colectomy and removal of the rectum	*Medical:* Same as for ulcerative colitis *Surgical:* Bowel resection (possibly repeated resections)

ing, and deep breathing; and getting the client out of bed on the first postoperative day if his condition allows) *to promote healing and to prevent and detect early complications.*

◆ Maintain the position, patency, and low suction of the NG tube *to prevent nausea and vomiting.*

◆ Keep the client in semi-Fowler's position *to promote comfort and prevent pulmonary complications.*

◆ Consult a registered dietitian *to help meet the client's nutritional needs.* Administer TPN *to meet the client's metabolic needs.*

◆ Administer medications, as prescribed, *to treat infection and control pain.*

Evaluation

◆ The client has stable vital signs.

◆ The client reports adequate pain control.

◆ The client doesn't display signs of dehydration.

ULCERATIVE COLITIS

ULCERATIVE COLITIS is a major health problem and a potentially debilitating disease. It's a type of inflammatory bowel disease that produces lesions primarily confined to the large bowel, with ulcerations of the large bowel's mucosa and submucosa. Healing of lesions causes scarring and strictures, leading to bowel obstruction, and ulcers may perforate, causing hemorrhage and peritonitis. Ulcerative colitis usually develops in people between ages 15 and 30 with peak occurrence in the 50- to 70-year-old age-group. It occurs more commonly in women than in men. (See *Comparing ulcerative colitis and Crohn's disease.*)

Possible causes

◆ Genetic factors

◆ Idiopathic cause

◆ Allergies

◆ Autoimmune disease

◆ Emotional stress

◆ Viral and bacterial infections

Assessment findings

- ◆ Abdominal cramping, distention, and tenderness
- ◆ Anorexia
- ◆ Bloody, purulent, mucoid, watery stools (15 to 20 per day)
- ◆ Dehydration
- ◆ Fever
- ◆ Hyperactive bowel sounds
- ◆ Nausea and vomiting
- ◆ Weakness
- ◆ Weight loss

Diagnostic evaluation

- ◆ Barium enema shows ulcerations.
- ◆ Blood studies show decreased potassium level, increased osmolality, and decreased Hb level and HCT.
- ◆ Intestinal biopsy helps differentiate between ulcerative colitis and Crohn's disease.
- ◆ Sigmoidoscopy and colonoscopy show ulceration and hyperemia. (Colonoscopy shouldn't be performed during an acute episode because of the risk of perforation.)
- ◆ Stool specimen is positive for blood and mucus.
- ◆ Urine chemistry displays increased urine specific gravity.

Nursing diagnoses

- ◆ Deficient knowledge regarding disease process and treatment
- ◆ Diarrhea
- ◆ Imbalanced nutrition: Less than body requirements
- ◆ Risk for deficient fluid volume

Treatment

- ◆ Surgical treatment, if necessary, for toxic megacolon or clients who fail to respond to drugs and supportive measures; colectomy; or pouch ileostomy
- ◆ High-protein, high-calorie, low-residue diet, with bland foods in small, frequent meals and restricted intake of milk and gas-forming foods; or no food or fluids
- ◆ TPN if necessary to rest the GI tract (see *Total parenteral nutrition*)
- ◆ Transfusion therapy with packed RBCs

Drug therapy options

- ◆ Analgesic: meperidine (Demerol)
- ◆ Antianemics: ferrous gluconate (Fergon), ferrous sulfate (Feosol)
- ◆ Antibiotic: sulfasalazine (Azulfidine)
- ◆ Anticholinergics: dicyclomine (Bentyl), propantheline (Pro-Banthine)
- ◆ Antidiarrheals: diphenoxylate (Lomotil), loperamide (Imodium)
- ◆ Antiemetic: prochlorperazine (Compazine)
- ◆ Anti-inflammatory: olsalazine (Dipentum)
- ◆ Corticosteroid: hydrocortisone (Solu-Cortef)
- ◆ Immunosuppressants: azathioprine (Imuran), cyclophosphamide (Cytoxan)
- ◆ Potassium supplements: potassium chloride (K-Lor), potassium gluconate (Kaon)
- ◆ Sedative: lorazepam (Ativan)

Total parenteral nutrition

Total parenteral nutrition (TPN) is administered to meet a client's total nutritional needs when oral feedings, tube feedings, and standard I.V. feedings are contraindicated. It's used for clients with various GI problems or other conditions that necessitate nutritional support such as some oncology clients.

Key facts

- ◆ In most cases, administer TPN through a central vein such as the subclavian. The fluid is highly concentrated to provide rapid dilution and thus decrease the risks of peripheral inflammation and thrombosis.
- ◆ Administer TPN at a constant rate, using an infusion pump.
- ◆ The infusion should never be stopped abruptly. Administer dextrose 10% in water if you must stop the infusion. During TPN administration, the pancreas secretes increased insulin; abrupt cessation can lead to hypoglycemia. Taper the infusion rate when discontinuing.
- ◆ Maintain strict asepsis. Use an occlusive dressing and change the dressing, tubing, and filter every 48 hours.
- ◆ Monitor blood glucose levels or check urine for glucose every 6 hours. Note that the client might need insulin.
- ◆ Observe the client for headache, nausea, vomiting, and fever. These signs and symptoms indicate an allergy to the protein.
- ◆ Closely monitor intake and output.
- ◆ Weigh the client daily. Expect a weight gain of ¼ lb per day.
- ◆ Never use a filter with fat emulsions. Monitor for nausea and fever, which are common adverse reactions.

Planning and goals

- ◆ The client will verbalize an understanding of the disease process and possible complications of ulcerative colitis.
- ◆ The client will exhibit normal bowel patterns.
- ◆ The client will maintain adequate fluid balance and nutritional intake.

Low-residue diet

A low-residue diet is prescribed to avoid irritation of the mucosal lining. A regular diet containing normal amounts of protein and gradually incorporating fiber should be instituted when the client can tolerate it.

FOODS	ALLOWED	NOT ALLOWED
Breads and cereals	Refined breads without seeds	High-fiber cereals (All Bran, Grape Nuts); whole-grain breads
Fruit	Canned fruits without skins or seeds; ripe banana; strained fruit juice	Raw fruits
Fats	All	None
Meats, fish, poultry	Roasted, baked, or broiled	Fried or highly spiced
Dairy	Milk, eggs, cheese	Fried eggs
Soups	Bouillon, broth, strained cream soups	All others
Vegetables	Canned or cooked strained vegetables; tomato juice	Raw or whole cooked vegetables
Miscellaneous	Salt, gravy, jelly, syrups, chocolate, puddings, and plain cakes	Nuts, olives, pickles, jam, alcohol, rich pastries

Implementation

◆ Assess GI status and fluid balance *to determine deficient fluid volume.*

◆ Monitor and record vital signs, intake and output, laboratory studies, daily weight, urine specific gravity, calorie count, and fecal occult blood *to determine deficient fluid volume.*

◆ Monitor the number, amount, and character of stools *to determine status of nutrient absorption.*

◆ Consult a registered dietitian to meet the client's nutritional needs. Maintain the client's diet; withhold food and fluids as necessary *to prevent nausea and vomiting.*

◆ Administer I.V. fluids and TPN *to maintain hydration and improve nutritional status.*

◆ Maintain position, patency, and low suction of the NG tube *to prevent nausea and vomiting.*

◆ Keep the client in semi-Fowler's position *to promote comfort.*

◆ Administer medications, as prescribed, *to maintain or improve the client's condition.*

◆ Provide skin, mouth, nares, and perianal care *to promote comfort and prevent skin breakdown.*

◆ Review key teaching topics with the client *to ensure adequate knowledge about her condition and treatment,* including:

- monitoring weight
- reducing stress and performing relaxation techniques
- recognizing the early signs and symptoms of rectal hemorrhage and intestinal obstruction
- following a low-residue, high-protein diet during an acute exacerbation (see *Low-residue diet*)
- contacting the United Ostomy Association and the National Foundation of Ileitis and Colitis.

Evaluation

◆ The client can explain the treatment regimen and possible complications.

◆ The client maintains normal bowel movements.

◆ The client has a balanced intake and output and normal vital signs.

◆ The client maintains adequate nutritional intake to restore nutritional balance.

GENITOURINARY SYSTEM

The genitourinary (GU) system serves as the body's water treatment plant, filtering waste products from the body and expelling them as urine through the kidneys and other parts of the urinary system. The major functions of the urinary system include regulating volume, osmolarity, electrolytes, and acid-base balance.

The GU system also encompasses the female and male reproductive systems, including external and internal genitalia.

GENITOURINARY STRUCTURE AND FUNCTION

The key structures of the urinary system include the kidneys, ureter, bladder, urethra, and prostate gland. The urinary system processes and filters waste products by continuously exchanging water and solutes, such as hydrogen, potassium, chloride, bicarbonate, sulfate, and phosphate, across cell membranes.

Kidneys

The kidneys are two bean-shaped organs situated on either side of the vertebral column that produce urine and maintain fluid and acid-base balance. To help maintain acid-base balance, the kidneys secrete hydrogen ions, reabsorb sodium and bicarbonates, acidify phosphate salts, and produce ammonia.

The kidneys have four main components:

- ◆ cortex, which makes up the outer layer of the kidney and contains the glomeruli, the proximal tubules of the nephron, and the distal tubules of the nephron
- ◆ medulla, which makes up the inner layer of the kidney and contains the loops of Henle and the collecting tubules
- ◆ renal pelvis, a reservoir that collects urine from the calices
- ◆ nephron, which makes up the functional unit of the kidney and contains Bowman's capsule and the glomerulus as well as the renal tubule (which consists of the proximal convoluted tubule and collecting segments).

Ureter

The ureter, which transports urine from the kidney to the bladder, is a tubule that extends from the renal pelvis to the bladder floor.

Bladder

The bladder, a muscular, distensible sac, can contain up to 1 L of urine.

Urethra

The urethra, extending from the bladder to the urinary meatus, transports urine from the bladder to the exterior of the body.

Prostate gland

The prostate gland surrounds the male urethra. It contains ducts that secrete the alkaline portion of seminal fluid.

Urine

Urine is produced through a complex process in the kidneys:

- ◆ Blood from the renal artery is filtered across the glomerular capillary membrane in Bowman's capsule. Filtration requires adequate intravascular volume and adequate cardiac output.
- ◆ ADH and aldosterone control the reabsorption of water and electrolytes. The composition of the filtrate is similar to blood plasma without proteins.
- ◆ Formed filtrate moves through the tubules of the nephron, which reabsorb and secrete electrolytes, water, glucose, amino acids, ammonia, and bicarbonate.
- ◆ What remains in the filtrate is excreted as urine.

Blood pressure control

The kidneys are involved in regulating blood pressure by regulating sodium and removing water from the body in the form of urine. The renin-angiotensin system is activated by decreased blood pressure and can be altered by renal disease.

FEMALE EXTERNAL GENITALIA

The external female genitalia include the mons pubis, labia majora, labia minora, clitoris, vestibule, urethral meatus, paraurethral glands, and breasts.

Mons pubis

The mons pubis:

- ◆ provides an adipose cushion over the anterior symphysis pubis
- ◆ protects the pelvic bones and contributes to the rounded contour of the female body.

Labia majora

The labia majora are two folds that converge at the mons pubis and extend to the posterior commissure. The labia majora:
- consist of connective tissue, elastic fibers, veins, and sebaceous glands
- protect components of the vulval cleft.

Labia minora

The labia minora are located within the labia majora. The labia minora:
- consist of connective tissue, sebaceous and sweat glands, nonstriated muscle fibers, nerve endings, and blood vessels
- unite to form the fourchette and vaginal vestibule
- serve to lubricate the vulva, which adds to sexual enjoyment and fights bacteria.

Clitoris

The clitoris — located in the anterior portion of the vulva above the urethral opening — is made up of erectile tissue, nerves, and blood vessels and, homologous to the penis, provides sexual pleasure. The clitoris consists of:
- glans
- body
- two crura.

Vestibule

The vaginal vestibule extends from the clitoris to the posterior fourchette and consists of:
- vaginal orifice
- hymen — a thin, vascularized mucous membrane at the vaginal orifice
- fossa navicularis — a depressed area between the hymen and fourchette
- Bartholin's glands — two bean-shaped glands on either side of the vagina that secrete mucus during sexual stimulation
- perineal body — the area between the vagina and the anus that's the site of episiotomy during childbirth.

Urethral meatus

The urethral meatus is located 1/4″ to 1″ (0.5 to 2.5 cm) below the clitoris.

Paraurethral glands

The paraurethral glands, also called *Skene's glands,* are located immediately inside the urethral meatus.

Breasts

The breasts consist of glandular, fibrous, and adipose tissue. The breasts:
- are stimulated by secretions from the hypothalamus, anterior pituitary, and ovaries
- provide nourishment to the infant and transfer maternal antibodies during breast-feeding
- enhance sexual pleasure.

FEMALE INTERNAL GENITALIA

The internal female genitalia include the vagina, uterus, fallopian tubes, and ovaries.

Vagina

The vagina is a vascularized musculomembranous tube that extends from the external genitals to the uterus.

Uterus

The uterus is a hollow, pear-shaped, muscular organ that's divided by a slight constriction (isthmus) into an upper portion (body or corpus) and a lower portion (cervix). The uterus:
- consists of a body or corpus with three layers (perimetrium, myometrium, and endometrium)
- receives support from broad, round, uterosacral ligaments
- provides an environment for fetal growth and development.

Fallopian tubes

The fallopian tubes are about 4 1/4″ (11 cm) long and consist of four layers (peritoneal, subserous, muscular, mucous) divided into four portions (interstitial, isthmus, ampulla, fimbria). The fallopian tubes:
- transport ovum from the ovary to the uterus
- provide a nourishing environment for zygotes
- serve as the site of fertilization.

Ovaries

The ovaries are two almond-shaped glandular structures that rest below and behind the fallopian tubes on either side of the uterus. The ovaries:
- produce sex hormones (estrogen, progesterone, androgen)
- serve as the site of ovulation.

MALE EXTERNAL GENITALIA

The male external genitalia include the penis and scrotum.

Penis

The penis consists of the body (shaft) and glans and has three layers of erectile tissue — two corpora cavernosa and one corpus spongiosum. The penis deposits spermatozoa in the female reproductive tract and provides sexual pleasure.

Scrotum

The scrotum is a pouchlike structure composed of skin, fascial connective tissue, and smooth muscle fibers. It houses the testes and protects spermatozoa from high body temperature.

MALE INTERNAL GENITALIA

The internal male genitalia produce and transport semen and seminal fluid. They include the testes, epididymides, vas deferens, urethra, seminal vesicles, prostate gland, and bulbourethral glands.

Testes

The testes are two oval-shaped glandular organs inside the scrotum that produce spermatozoa and testosterone.

Epididymides

The epididymides serve as the initial section of the testes' excretory duct system that store spermatozoa as they mature and become motile.

Vas deferens

The vas deferens connect the epididymal lumen and the prostatic urethra and serve as conduits for spermatozoa. The vas deferens:

- consist of ejaculatory ducts
- are located between the seminal vesicles and the urethra
- serve as passageways for semen and seminal fluid.

Urethra

The urethra extends from the bladder through the penis to the external urethral opening, and serves as the excretory duct for urine and semen.

Seminal vesicles

The seminal vesicles are two pouchlike structures between the bladder and the rectum that secrete a viscous fluid that aids in spermatozoa motility and metabolism.

Prostate gland

The prostate gland is located just below the bladder and is considered homologous to Skene's glands in females. The prostate gland:

- produces an alkaline fluid that enhances spermatozoa motility
- lubricates the urethra during sexual activity.

Bulbourethral glands

The bulbourethral glands, also called *Cowper's glands,* are two pea-sized glands opening into the posterior portion of the urethra. They secrete a thick, alkaline fluid that neutralizes acidic secretions in the female reproductive tract, thus prolonging spermatozoa survival.

GENITOURINARY DISORDERS

The major disorders that affect the GU system include acute poststreptococcal glomerulonephritis, acute renal failure, benign prostatic hyperplasia, bladder cancer, breast cancer, cervical cancer, chlamydia, chronic renal failure, cystitis, gonorrhea, herpes simplex virus, neurogenic bladder, ovarian cancer, prostate cancer, renal calculi, syphilis, and testicular cancer.

ACUTE POSTSTREPTOCOCCAL GLOMERULONEPHRITIS

Also called *acute glomerulonephritis,* ACUTE POSTSTREPTOCOCCAL GLOMERULONEPHRITIS (APSGN) is a relatively common bilateral inflammation of the glomeruli, the kidney's blood vessels. It follows a streptococcal infection of the respiratory tract or, less commonly, a skin infection such as impetigo.

Possible causes

- Trapped antigen-antibody complexes (produced as an immunologic mechanism in response to streptococci) in the glomerular capillary membranes, inducing inflammatory damage and impeding glomerular function
- Untreated pharyngitis (inflammation of the pharynx)

Assessment findings

- Oliguria
- Hematuria
- Fatigue
- Azotemia
- Edema

- Proteinuria
- Mild to severe hypertension
- Heart failure
- Pulmonary edema

Diagnostic evaluation

- Blood studies show elevated serum creatinine levels.
- Urinalysis of a 24-hour urine sample shows low creatinine clearance and impaired glomerular filtration.
- Elevated antistreptolysin-O titers (in 80% of clients), elevated streptozyme and anti-DNase B titers, and low serum complement levels verify recent streptococcal infection.
- Renal biopsy may confirm the diagnosis in a client with APSGN or may be used to assess renal tissue status.
- Renal ultrasonography may show a normal or slightly enlarged kidney.
- Throat culture may also show group A beta-hemolytic streptococci.
- Urinalysis typically reveals proteinuria and hematuria. RBCs, WBCs, and mixed cell casts are common findings in urinary sediment.
- Kidney-ureter-bladder X-rays show bilateral kidney enlargement.

Nursing diagnoses

- Impaired urinary elimination
- Excess fluid volume
- Fatigue

Treatment

- Bed rest
- Fluid restriction
- High-calorie, low-sodium, low-potassium, low-protein diet
- Dialysis (occasionally necessary)

Drug therapy options

- Diuretics: metolazone (Zaroxolyn) and furosemide (Lasix) to reduce extracellular fluid overload
- Antihypertensive: hydralazine (Apresoline)

Planning and goals

- The client will maintain urine specific gravity within the designated limits.
- The client will maintain fluid balance.
- The client's energy level will increase.

Implementation

- Check vital signs and electrolyte values. Monitor fluid intake and output and daily weight. Assess renal function daily through serum creatinine and BUN levels and urine creatinine clearance. Watch for signs of acute renal failure (oliguria, azotemia, acidosis). *These measures detect early signs of complications and guide the treatment plan.*
- Consult the dietitian *to provide education regarding a diet high in calories and low in protein, sodium, potassium, and fluids.*
- Provide adequate nutrition, use good hygienic technique, and prevent contact with infected people *to protect the debilitated client against secondary infection.*
- Bed rest is necessary during the acute phase. Encourage the client to gradually resume normal activities as symptoms subside *to prevent fatigue.*
- Provide emotional support for the client and family. If the client is on dialysis, explain the procedure fully. *These measures may help ease his anxiety.*

Evaluation

- The client has normal urine specific gravity.
- The client doesn't display signs of fluid overload.
- The client reports increased energy.

ACUTE RENAL FAILURE

ACUTE RENAL FAILURE is a sudden interruption of renal function resulting from obstruction, poor circulation, or kidney disease. With treatment, this condition is usually reversible; if untreated, it may progress to end-stage renal disease or death.

Acute renal failure is classified as:

- prerenal — results from conditions that diminish blood flow to the kidneys
- intrarenal — results from damage to the kidneys, usually from acute tubular necrosis
- postrenal — results from bilateral obstruction of urine flow.

Acute renal failure has four phases: onset, oliguric-anuric, diuretic, and convalescent. The convalescent period can last up to 12 months.

Possible causes

- Acute glomerulonephritis
- Acute tubular necrosis
- Anaphylaxis
- Benign prostatic hyperplasia
- Blood transfusion reaction
- Burns
- Ischemia
- Cardiogenic shock
- Cardiopulmonary bypass
- Collagen diseases

- ◆ Congenital deformity
- ◆ Dehydration
- ◆ Diabetes mellitus
- ◆ Heart failure
- ◆ Cardiogenic shock
- ◆ Endocarditis
- ◆ Malignant hypertension
- ◆ Obstetric complications (placental abruptio or previa)
- ◆ Hemorrhage
- ◆ Infections, such as pyelonephritis and septicemia
- ◆ Nephrotoxins, such as antibiotics, X-ray dyes, pesticides, and anesthetics
- ◆ Thrombi or emboli

Assessment findings

- ◆ Anorexia
- ◆ Nausea
- ◆ Vomiting
- ◆ Costovertebral pain
- ◆ Headache
- ◆ Diarrhea or constipation
- ◆ Irritability
- ◆ Restlessness
- ◆ Lethargy
- ◆ Drowsiness
- ◆ Stupor
- ◆ Coma
- ◆ Pallor
- ◆ Ecchymosis
- ◆ Stomatitis
- ◆ Thick tenacious sputum
- ◆ Urine output less than 400 ml/day for 1 to 2 weeks, followed by diuresis (3 to 5 L/day) for 2 to 3 weeks
- ◆ Weight gain

Diagnostic evaluation

- ◆ ABG analysis shows metabolic acidosis.
- ◆ Blood studies show increased potassium, phosphorus, magnesium, BUN, creatinine, and uric acid levels; decreased calcium, carbon dioxide, and sodium levels; decreased Hb level, HCT, and erythrocytes; and increased PT and PTT.
- ◆ Creatinine clearance is low.
- ◆ Excretory urography shows decreased renal perfusion and function.
- ◆ Glomerular filtration rate (GFR) is 20 to 40 ml/minute (renal insufficiency); 10 to 20 ml/minute (renal failure); or less than 10 ml/minute (end-stage renal disease).
- ◆ Urine chemistry shows albuminuria; proteinuria; increased sodium levels; casts, RBCs, and WBCs; and urine specific gravity greater than 1.025 and then fixed at less than 1.010.

Nursing diagnoses

- ◆ Excess fluid volume
- ◆ Risk for infection
- ◆ Risk for deficient fluid volume

Treatment

- ◆ Detection and treatment of underlying causes
- ◆ Continuous arteriovenous hemofiltration
- ◆ Low-protein, increased-carbohydrate, moderate-fat, moderate-calorie diet with potassium, sodium, and phosphorus intake regulated according to serum levels
- ◆ Peritoneal dialysis or hemodialysis (see *Types of dialysis*, page 520)
- ◆ Fluid intake restricted to the amount needed to replace fluid loss
- ◆ Transfusion therapy with packed RBCs administered over 1 to 3 hours as tolerated

Drug therapy options

- ◆ Alkalinizing agent: sodium bicarbonate
- ◆ Antacid: aluminum hydroxide (AlternaGEL)
- ◆ Beta-adrenergic blocker: dopamine (Intropin), initially to improve renal perfusion
- ◆ Cation exchange resin: sodium polystyrene sulfonate (Kayexalate)
- ◆ Diuretics: furosemide (Lasix), metolazone (Zaroxolyn)

Planning and goals

- ◆ The client will have normal fluid and electrolyte levels.
- ◆ The client will show no evidence of infection.

Implementation

Oliguric-anuric phase

During the oliguric-anuric phase, the client's urine output falls below 400 ml/day, with resultant electrolyte imbalance, metabolic acidosis, and retention of nitrogenous wastes from nonfunctioning nephrons. This phase may last up to 14 days. The nurse should follow these steps:

- ◆ Maintain the client on complete bed rest; organize care to provide long rest periods. *Activity increases the rate of metabolism, which increases production of nitrogenous waste products.*
- ◆ Implement interventions to prevent infection and the complications of immobility. *Because of bed rest, the client becomes susceptible to the hazards of immobility. Infection is a serious risk and the leading cause of death in clients with acute renal failure.*

Types of dialysis

Dialysis is the process of diffusion, osmosis, and ultrafiltration used to reestablish fluid and electrolyte balance and remove toxic substances and metabolic wastes:

- *Diffusion* is the passage of ions from an area of high concentration across a semipermeable membrane to an area of lower concentration.
- *Osmosis* is the passage of water molecules across a semipermeable membrane from a less concentrated solution to a more concentrated one.
- *Ultrafiltration* uses positive pressure to cause fluid to pass across a semipermeable membrane from an area of lesser concentration to one of greater concentration. It's faster than osmosis.

Peritoneal dialysis

In peritoneal dialysis, a commercially prepared sterile dialysate (an electrolyte solution) flows by gravity through a catheter inserted through the abdominal wall into the peritoneal cavity. The peritoneum acts as a semipermeable membrane for osmosis and diffusion. After the solution has remained in the peritoneal cavity for the prescribed time, the dialysate is removed. The physician will order this process repeated until the client's fluid and electrolyte levels fall within acceptable limits.

Hemodialysis

In hemodialysis, the client's blood is passed through a dialyzer where, through the processes of diffusion and ultrafiltration, body fluids and electrolytes are exchanged with the dialysate. In this way, excess fluid, electrolytes, and nitrogenous wastes are removed from the body. Access to the client's bloodstream is essential in hemodialysis. Access is achieved by external arteriovenous shunt (for acute situations), subclavian or femoral catheters (for acute situations), or internal arteriovenous fistula or graft (for chronic dialysis).

Continuous ambulatory peritoneal dialysis

Continuous ambulatory peritoneal dialysis (CAPD) is a recent variation of peritoneal dialysis. CAPD involves infusing 500 to 1,000 ml of a personalized dialysate through a peritoneal catheter, clamping the catheter with the empty bag still attached, rolling the bag up, and placing it in a waistband, with the client then going about his usual activities. Every 4 hours the client drains the fluid from his peritoneal cavity into the empty bag, removes the bag and drainage from the catheter, aseptically attaches a new bag of dialysate, and repeats the infusion. CAPD proves much less confining to those who can assume the responsibility of maintaining the proper techniques. Major complications of CAPD include peritonitis, fluid and electrolyte imbalances, dehydration, catheter sepsis, abdominal pain and tenderness, organ trauma, and hemorrhage.

Continuous cyclic peritoneal dialysis uses a machine to deliver and drain the peritoneal fluid. Cycling time lasts from 6 to 8 hours, so the client can usually be dialyzed while sleeping at night. The machine has an alarm to protect the client from malfunction.

- Observe the client for metabolic acidosis *to identify complications of renal failure.*
- Observe fluid and electrolyte balance hourly. Insert an indwelling urinary catheter, and measure output and specific gravity hourly. *These actions allow the nurse to monitor the kidneys, which have the major role in regulating fluid and electrolyte balance. High potassium levels can occur.*
- Provide only enough fluid intake to replace urine output *to avoid edema caused by excessive fluid intake.*
- Monitor the client's diet *to provide high carbohydrates, adequate fats, and low protein.* (Protein should be of high biologic value, or complete protein, such as from beef, eggs, milk, and chicken.) Offer carbohydrate supplements (hard candy, jelly beans, Kool-Aid, tapioca, honey, and jelly). *If the client receives adequate calories from fat and carbohydrate metabolism, the body doesn't break down protein for energy. Protein is thus available for growth and repair. There's an accompanying decrease in nonprotein waste products, which result from protein metabolism.*
- Reduce the client's potassium intake *to help prevent elevated potassium levels. Protein catabolism causes potassium release from cells into the serum.*
- Observe for arrhythmias and cardiac arrest *to identify complications of high serum potassium.*
- Provide frequent oral hygiene *to avoid tissue irritation and, sometimes, ulcer formation caused by urea and other acid waste products excreted through the skin and mucous membranes.*
- Provide the client with hard candy and chewing gum *to stimulate saliva flow and decrease thirst.*
- Maintain skin care with cool water *to relieve pruritus and remove uremic frost (white crystals formed on the skin from excretion of urea).*
- Administer stool softeners *to prevent colon irritation from high levels of urea and organic acids.*

◆ Provide emotional reassurance to the client and family members *to help decrease anxiety levels caused by the fact that the client has an acute illness with an unknown prognosis.*
◆ Explain treatments and progress to the client *to help reduce anxiety.*
◆ Provide hemodialysis or peritoneal dialysis, as ordered, *to reduce nonprotein nitrogen waste levels in the blood and improve fluid and electrolyte balance until the kidneys regain function.* (See *Key nursing measures during dialysis.*)

Early diuretic phase

During the early diuretic phase, which lasts about 10 days, the client excretes a large volume (usually over 3,000 ml/day) of very dilute urine. The glomeruli are beginning to function effectively, but the tubules aren't, and the client still experiences electrolyte imbalance, retention of nitrogenous waste products, and metabolic acidosis. The nurse should follow these steps:
◆ Assess fluid and electrolyte balance *to identify any continued imbalance when the renal tubules aren't functioning.*
◆ Assess the emotional status of the client and family members *to provide support because the prognosis is still uncertain.*
◆ Continue interventions used during the oliguric phase, except for:
– increasing fluid intake dramatically to keep up with output *to prevent dehydration that may be experienced during the polyuric phase*
– administering potassium or other electrolyte replacements, if needed, *to prevent imbalances caused by loss of electrolytes and fluid.*

Late diuretic phase

In the late diuretic phase, the client is still excreting more fluid than normal; urine specific gravity is increasing because the tubules are beginning to function effectively; and fluid, electrolyte, and acid-base balances are returning to normal. The nurse should follow these steps:
◆ Continue implementations of the early diuretic phase. Allow the client to engage in nonstrenuous activity for brief periods, and increase the activity level gradually; don't let her become fatigued, *which may increase the rate of metabolism and overwork the kidneys.*
◆ Teach the client to prevent infection and to avoid the factors that caused renal failure *to help prevent a recurrence.*

Key nursing measures during dialysis

Before dialysis

◆ Explain the procedure to the client.
◆ Weigh the client, and measure his vital signs.

Peritoneal dialysis

◆ Ask the client to urinate before you insert the catheter into the peritoneum, to prevent bladder puncture.
◆ Warm the bottles of dialysate in warm water.
◆ Permit 2 L of dialysate to flow unrestricted into the peritoneal cavity (which should take about 10 minutes).
◆ Allow fluid to remain in the cavity for the time ordered by the physician (about 20 to 30 minutes).
◆ Reverse the bottles; allow fluid to drain from the peritoneal cavity unrestricted (about 20 to 30 minutes). Facilitate drainage by changing the client's position or massaging the abdomen.
◆ Keep accurate intake and output records related to the amount of dialysis fluid entering the peritoneal cavity and the amount in the drainage. *Important:* Remove all the dialysis fluid.

Hemodialysis

◆ Observe carefully for breaks or kinks in membranes to prevent hemorrhage.
◆ Monitor the chemical composition of the dialysate solution, the fluid rate and pressure, and blood clotting time (anticoagulants are administered throughout hemodialysis).
◆ Provide shunt care:
– Keep the area clean, dry, and sterile.
– Observe the internal fistula for patency. If it's working, you can feel a thrill on palpation or hear a bruit with a stethoscope; if the shunt is discolored, patency is questionable.
– Immediately report clotting to the physician.
– Avoid trauma to the extremity with the shunt (no blood pressure measurement, intramuscular or intravenous medications, or blood drawn).
– Have clamps available to prevent exsanguination if the external shunt disconnects.
◆ Provide comfort measures for the client.

After dialysis

◆ Monitor the client's pulse rate and blood pressure every 15 minutes until the client becomes stable and then every 4 hours.
◆ Monitor the client's weight daily.
◆ Monitor the client's temperature every 4 hours.

Evaluation

- The client regains fluid and electrolyte balance.
- The client remains infection-free.

BENIGN PROSTATIC HYPERPLASIA

BENIGN PROSTATIC HYPERPLASIA (BPH) affects about one-half of all men older than age 50. In BPH, the prostate gland enlarges, causing compression of the urethra and urinary obstruction. If hyperplasia becomes severe and causes obstruction, infection, or impaired renal function, surgical intervention becomes necessary. Surgeons most commonly use transurethral resection to treat BPH.

Possible causes

- Hormonal alterations
- Neoplasm
- Arteriosclerosis
- Inflammation
- Metabolic or nutritional disturbances

Assessment findings

- Decreased force and amount of urination
- Dribbling
- Hesitancy
- Nocturia
- Urgency, frequency, and burning on urination

Diagnostic evaluation

- BUN level (normally 8 to 20 mg/dl) is elevated, indicating dehydration or renal damage.
- Creatinine level (normally 0.8 to 1.5 mg/dl) is elevated, indicating renal damage.
- Excretory urography, an X-ray of the kidney and pelvis using a contrast material injected I.V., shows urethral obstruction and hydronephrosis. A check for hypersensitivity to the dye may be necessary.
- Cystoscopy, which permits visualization of the bladder and urethra through a lighted tube, shows an enlarged prostate gland, obstructed urine flow, and urinary stasis. (See *Nursing interventions for cystoscopy.*)
- Rectal examination discloses an enlarged prostate gland.
- Urinary flow rate determination shows a small volume, prolonged flow pattern, and low peak flow.
- Urine chemistry shows bacteria, hematuria, alkaline pH, and increased urine specific gravity.

Nursing diagnoses

- Acute pain
- Urinary retention
- Impaired urinary elimination
- Sexual dysfunction

Treatment

- Encourage fluids
- Transurethral resection of the prostate or prostatectomy
- Sitz bath

Drug therapy options

- Alpha-adrenergic blockers: tamsulosin (Flomax), terazosin (Haptrin), prazosin (Minipress) to improve urine flow and relieve bladder outlet obstruction by preventing contractions of prostatic capsule and bladder neck
- Analgesic: oxycodone hydrochloride (Tylox)
- Antianxiety agent: oxazepam (Serax)
- Antibiotic: co-trimoxazole (Bactrim)
- Urinary antiseptic: phenazopyridine (Pyridium)

Planning and goals

- The client will demonstrate normal urine output and unobstructed flow.
- The client will verbalize decreased pain.
- The client will discuss concerns related to temporary sexual dysfunction.

Implementation

Preoperative care

- Gradually drain urine through a urethral catheter *to relieve the obstruction.* With severe obstruction, the bladder may contain more than 1,000 ml of urine; *gradual decompression is necessary to prevent shock and hemorrhage.*
- Prepare the client for the transurethral resection. Tell him to expect a catheter in the bladder. Explain that he'll feel like voiding and that urine will drain through the tube *to ensure that the client doesn't attempt to void around the tube, which would strain the bladder and contribute to spasms.*
- Reassure the client that he'll probably be able to resume sexual activity after he has healed *to help alleviate the client's fears about sexual dysfunction.* Impotence rarely occurs except after a radical prostatectomy for prostate cancer.

Postoperative care

- Inspect the client's urine, and observe him for signs of shock *to monitor response to surgery and identify signs of complications.* Dark red blood in the urine is normal for the first few days after surgery; bright red blood and clots indicate an active hemorrhage. Tissue sloughing and straining can cause delayed hemorrhaging 6 to 10 days postoperatively.

◆ Maintain catheter patency. Keep accurate intake and output records, and account for irrigating fluid *to monitor the client's status.* Assess him for water intoxication *to identify signs of complications.* The client is likely to have a three-way indwelling urinary catheter in place with continuous irrigation for the first 24 hours. The catheter maintains flow and prevents and eliminates clots. The venous sinusoids of the bladder may absorb the irrigating fluid.

◆ Force fluids *to keep urine diluted.*

◆ Remind the client not to void around the catheter, and irrigate as needed *to decrease strain and reduce the discomfort of bladder spasms. Irrigation removes clots. The catheter has a 30-ml balloon, and applied traction prevents bleeding. Both the large balloon and traction contribute to spasms, which usually decrease within 24 to 48 hours.*

◆ Administer anticholinergic drugs (for example, belladonna and opium suppositories) as ordered *to decrease bladder spasms.*

◆ Remove the catheter 2 to 3 days after surgery, as ordered, and periodically check for voiding *to assess urinary status and check for occasional dribbling.* The catheter is typically removed by the time the client is discharged, usually 3 days after surgery.

◆ Teach perineal (Kegel) exercises, with the client tightly squeezing the perineal muscles 5 to 10 times each hour. *Perineal exercises increase sphincter tone. Full bladder capacity may not return for 2 months.*

◆ Help the client walk *to prevent a thromboembolism and reduce bladder spasms.*

◆ Before discharge, provide the following instructions *to protect the client from injury and hemorrhage, which can occur if he sustains trauma before healing is complete:*

- Don't strain at stool.
- Use a stool softener.
- Don't drive a car for 3 weeks.
- Do no heavy lifting for 6 weeks.
- Resume sexual activity when healing is complete.

Without complications, the client is usually discharged on day 4 after the cystoscopy.

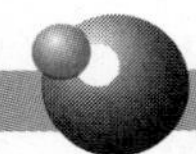

SPOT CHECK

When is surgical intervention necessary for a client with BPH?

Answer: Surgical intervention is performed if prostatic enlargement causes obstruction, infection, or impaired renal function.

Nursing interventions for cystoscopy

Before cystoscopy

◆ Encourage fluids for several hours to maintain a constant flow of urine and prevent bacterial stasis.

◆ Provide sedation 1 hour before the cystoscopy with either diazepam (Valium) or meperidine (Demerol), as ordered, to reduce stress and anxiety in the client.

After cystoscopy

◆ Check the client's voiding to evaluate following the procedure. Urine may be pink-tinged from the trauma of cystoscopy.

◆ Check for complaints of pain, spasms, and urinary frequency. Warm sitz baths, analgesics, or antispasmodics may be needed to promote comfort.

◆ Force fluids to keep the urinary tract flushed and provide internal irrigation.

◆ Observe the client for complications, such as an elevated temperature, chills, flushing, and hypotension, which may signal hemorrhage or infection.

Evaluation

◆ The client has an unobstructed urine flow.

◆ The client verbalizes pain relief.

◆ Follow-up care reveals that the client isn't experiencing sexual dysfunction.

BLADDER CANCER

Bladder cancer is a malignant tumor that invades the mucosal lining of the bladder. It may metastasize to the ureters, prostate gland, vagina, rectum, and periaortic lymph nodes.

Possible causes

◆ Chronic bladder irritation or infection

◆ Environmental carcinogens (2-naphthylamine, benzidine, tobacco, nitrates)

Assessment findings

◆ Urinary frequency

◆ Bladder irritability

◆ Nocturia

◆ Painless hematuria

◆ Dribbling

◆ Pain after voiding

Diagnostic evaluation

- ◆ Cystoscopy reveals a mass.
- ◆ Cytologic examination is positive for malignant cells.
- ◆ Excretory urography shows a mass or an obstruction.
- ◆ Blood studies show decreased RBC count, Hb level, and HCT.
- ◆ Kidney-ureter-bladder X-ray shows mass or obstruction.
- ◆ Urine chemistry shows hematuria.

Nursing diagnoses

- ◆ Impaired urinary elimination
- ◆ Acute pain
- ◆ Anxiety

Treatment

- ◆ Transfusion therapy with packed RBCs
- ◆ Surgery, depending on the location and progress of the tumor
- ◆ Radiation

Drug therapy options

- ◆ Analgesics: meperidine (Demerol), morphine sulfate
- ◆ Antispasmodic: phenazopyridine (Pyridium)
- ◆ Sedative: oxazepam (Serax)
- ◆ Antineoplastics (intravesicular to bladder): doxorubicin (Doxil), mitomycin (Mutamycin), Bacillus Calmette-Guérin (BCG)
- ◆ Immunotherapy: immunoglobulin
- ◆ Biologic response modifier: interferon (Roferon)
- ◆ Chemotherapy drugs: cyclophosphamide (Cytoxan), doxorubicin (Doxil), cisplatin (Platinol-AQ)

Planning and goals

- ◆ The client will maintain adequate intake and output.
- ◆ The client will express feelings of comfort and pain relief.
- ◆ The client will exhibit adequate coping mechanisms.

Implementation

- ◆ Assess renal status *to determine a baseline and detect early changes.*
- ◆ Monitor and record vital signs and intake and output. *Accurate intake and output are essential for correct fluid replacement therapy.*
- ◆ Provide postoperative care *to promote healing and prevent complications.* (Closely monitor urine output. Observe for hematuria [reddish tint to gross bloodiness] or infection [cloudy, foul smelling, with sediment]. Maintain continuous bladder irrigation, if indicated. Assist with turning, coughing and deep breathing.)
- ◆ Consult a registered dietitian *to help meet the client's nutritional needs.* Maintain the client's diet *to improve nutrition and to meet metabolic demands.*
- ◆ Force fluids *to prevent dehydration.*
- ◆ Administer I.V. fluids *to maintain hydration.*
- ◆ Administer medications, as prescribed, *to maintain or improve the client's condition.*
- ◆ Encourage the client to express his fears *to encourage adequate coping mechanisms.*
- ◆ Provide postchemotherapeutic care (watch for myelosuppression, chemical cystitis, and skin rash) and postradiation nursing care *to prevent complications associated with treatment.*

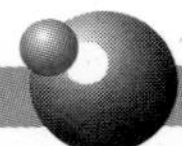

SPOT CHECK

Following a diagnosis of bladder cancer, a client receives local radiation therapy and experiences a dry skin reaction. In recommending care of the skin, the nurse should instruct the client to avoid:

A. lubrication.
B. cleansers.
C. cold packs.
D. cotton garments.

Answer: C. Cold packs over the area of a dry reaction to radiation therapy are contraindicated because they reduce capillary circulation to the site and hamper healing. Lubrication, cleansers, and cotton garments aren't unconditionally contraindicated.

Evaluation

- ◆ The client has an appropriate fluid balance.
- ◆ The client reports adequate pain control.
- ◆ The client demonstrates appropriate coping mechanisms.

BREAST CANCER

Breast cancer is the most common cancer in women in the United States; however, since 1986, breast cancer has been second to lung cancer as the leading cause of death due to cancer in women. Current statistical data indicate that one in every eight American women develops breast cancer in her lifetime. While breast cancer can also develop in men, its incidence is very low.

Most primary breast cancers are adenocarcinomas and occur in the upper outer quadrant of the breast. The most common sites of metastasis from breast cancer are the:

- ◆ liver

- bone
- lungs.

Possible causes

High risk factors

- Female gender
- Personal or family history of breast cancer
- History of endometrial or ovarian cancer
- Early menarche (before age 12)
- Nulliparity or parity (first, full-term pregnancy) after age 35
- Late menopause (after age 55)
- Exposure to ionizing radiation, especially during young adulthood

Other potential risk factors

- Antihypertensives
- Estrogen therapy
- Diet high in fat
- Fibrocystic disease of the breasts

Assessment findings

- Asymmetry of breasts
- Dimpling or puckering of the skin
- Enlargement of axillary or supraclavicular lymph nodes
- Lump or thickening in the breast
- Nipple retraction or inversion
- Peau d'orange skin changes
- Redness, ulceration, edema, or dilated veins in the breast
- Scaly skin around the nipple
- Spontaneous nipple discharge

Diagnostic evaluation

- Sonography or ultrasonography differentiates between a solid or cystic lesion.
- MRI or magnetic resonance mammography (MRM) of the breast can be used to distinguish between a benign or malignant lesion.
- Fine-needle aspiration (FNA) is used when a known lesion is solid or to determine if a lump is cystic. If cystic, a lump should resolve after the FNA is completed.
- Biopsy, such as stereotactic needle-guided biopsy, wire-localized biopsy, or excisional biopsy, reveals a malignant lesion.
- Estrogen-progesterone receptor analysis (biomarker) identifies hormone-dependent tumors that may respond to hormonal therapy. Receptor-positive tumors occur more commonly in postmenopausal women and generally confer an improved overall prognosis.
- Radiographic scans of the bone, brain, liver, and other organs can reveal distant metastases.

Nursing diagnoses

- Disturbed body image
- Fear
- Deficient knowledge regarding disease process and treatment

Treatment

Treatment varies depending on the extent of the disease, and may include:

- surgery, such as lumpectomy, skin-sparing mastectomy, partial mastectomy, total mastectomy, or modified radical mastectomy
- radiation therapy
- peripheral stem cell therapy.

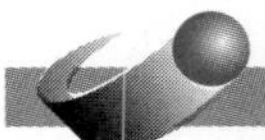

FAST FACT

Breast reconstruction surgery can be performed immediately after mastectomy, or it may be delayed if adjuvant chemotherapy or radiation therapy is necessary.

Drug therapy options

- Analgesics: fentanyl (Actiq), morphine, NSAIDs (Motrin)
- Antiemetics: granisetron hydrochloride (Kytril), ondansetron (Zofran), prochlorperazine (Compazine), trimethobenzamide (Tigan)
- Antineoplastics: cyclophosphamide (Cytoxan), doxorubicin (Adriamycin), methotrexate (Folex, Mexate), vincristine (Oncovin), paclitaxel (Taxol)
- Hormonal therapy: tamoxifen (Nolvadex), letrozole (Femara), toremifene (Fareston)

Planning and goals

- The client will maintain a positive body image and positive self-concept.
- The client will demonstrate a decreased level of fear.
- The client will verbalize an understanding of disease process and treatment.

Implementation

- Assess the client's feelings about her illness, and determine what she knows about breast cancer and her expectations *to identify her needs and aid in developing a care plan.*

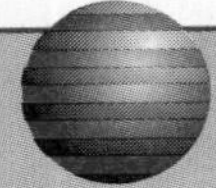

CLINICAL SITUATION

Caring for the client with breast cancer

A 62-year-old female arrives at the ambulatory surgery unit at 6 a.m. on the morning of her scheduled right modified radical mastectomy. One week ago she had a biopsy that showed a 1" (2.5 cm) adenocarcinoma in the upper outer quadrant of her right breast. Since that time, she has had a full workup to check for metastasis. All tests have been negative. Her husband, who seems attentive and concerned about her condition, accompanies her to the hospital. The client had her preoperative teaching 3 days ago at the preadmission testing unit. She'll stay 3 to 4 days if she remains free from complications.

After surgery, what are appropriate nursing actions?

◆ Observe the client's vital signs *to establish her condition.*

◆ Inspect the dressing for bleeding and report any bleeding to the physician immediately. Be sure to check under the client. *Gravity may cause the blood to flow beneath the client, thereby obscuring it.*

◆ Ensure proper functioning of the Hemovac unit, *which removes excess fluid.* Show the client how to empty the drain *because the drain may remain in place after discharge.*

◆ Identify the type and severity of the client's pain. *Initially, the operation causes trauma pain. Later, pain may result from nerve irritation and muscle spasm. The client may also feel a phantom breast if the breast was removed and immediate reconstruction was unable to be performed.*

◆ Elevate the affected arm in an abducted position; observe for edema. Transient or long-term edema can occur after removal of the lymph nodes. *Arm elevation in the abducted position facilitates drainage, increases venous return, and prevents lymphedema and shoulder contracture.*

◆ Encourage ambulation. Have the client deep-breathe every 2 hours. Provide analgesics *to relieve pain.*

◆ Spend time with the client, encourage her to express feelings and concerns, and provide generous emotional support. *The nurse's presence can be a source of comfort during this difficult time.*

Questions for further thought

◆ How can the husband help the nurse to reassure the client of continued love and nurturing?

◆ What actions by the client indicate she's beginning to accept the change to her body?

◆ Provide routine postoperative care *to prevent complications.*

◆ Perform comfort measures *to promote relaxation and relieve anxiety.*

◆ Administer analgesics, as ordered, and monitor their effectiveness *to promote the client's comfort.*

◆ Watch for treatment-related complications, such as nausea, vomiting, anorexia, leukopenia, thrombocytopenia, GI ulceration, and bleeding, *to ensure that measures are taken to prevent further complications.*

◆ Monitor the client's weight and nutritional intake *to detect evidence of malnutrition.* Consult a registered dietitian *to help meet the client's nutritional needs.* Encourage a high-protein diet. Dietary supplements may be necessary to meet increased metabolic demands.

◆ Assess the client's and family member's ability to cope, especially if the cancer is terminal. Counseling may be necessary *to help them cope with the fear of death and dying.*

◆ In the immediate postoperative phase, teach arm exercises, as ordered, *to facilitate drainage, prevent contractures, and relieve muscle spasms.* Such factors as wound healing, grafts, temperature elevation, and increased drainage may delay exercises. Consult the surgeon to determine when to undertake a full regimen.

◆ Before discharge, encourage the client to view her incision *to help her adjust to an altered body image.* Explain that, after healing has occurred, the incision can be massaged with cocoa butter or cold cream to soften it. (See *Caring for the client with breast cancer.*)

◆ Take precautions to prevent lymphedema and infection *to prevent long-term problems.* Permit no invasive procedures on the affected arm, and give the client these instructions:

- Don't permit blood pressure checks on the affected arm.
- Wear gloves when gardening.
- Avoid all burns, including sunburn.
- Wear a thimble when sewing.
- Immediately provide care for even minor cuts and scratches.
- Whenever possible, keep the arm elevated.
- Don't wear constrictive clothing.
- Avoid undue pressure such as from a shoulder purse.

◆ Before discharge, review key teaching topics with the client and her family *to ensure adequate knowledge about her condition and treatment,* including:
- treatment options
- management of adverse reactions to treatment
- importance of immediately reporting signs of infection to the physician
- breast self-examination
- availability of community support services
- contacting the American Cancer Society.

Evaluation

◆ The client expresses her feelings about body image changes and expresses positive feelings about herself.
◆ The client verbalizes a decreased level of fear and can discuss her feelings, the diagnosis, and treatment options.
◆ The client discusses self-care activities to promote full recovery.

CERVICAL CANCER

Cervical cancer is the third most common cause of the female reproductive tract. Preinvasive cancers range from minimal cervical dysplasia, in which the lower third of the epithelium contains abnormal cells, to carcinoma in situ, in which the full thickness of the epithelium contains abnormally proliferating cells.

Most cervical cancers are squamous; only 5% are adenocarcinomas. Invasive carcinoma usually occurs in clients between ages 30 and 50, though in rare cases it can occur in those younger than age 20.

Causes

◆ Multiple sexual partners
◆ Early age at first sexual intercourse, particularly before age 16
◆ Human papillomavirus (HPV)
◆ History of herpes simplex virus II (HSV-2) and other bacterial or viral venereal infections

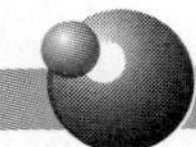

SPOT CHECK

Name two STDs that put a client at risk for cervical cancer.
Answer: Two STDs that put a client at risk for cervical cancer are HPV and HSV-2.

Assessment findings

◆ Abnormal bleeding (amount may vary from scant spotting to frank bleeding)
◆ Prolonged menstrual period or intermittent bleeding
◆ Bleeding following sexual intercourse
◆ Difficulty voiding, urinary urgency, hematuria, rectal tenesmus, or rectal bleeding (direct invasion of the bladder or rectum)
◆ Lower extremity edema (lymphatic involvement)
◆ Odor or pain in the lower back, leg, or groin (extensive tumor involvement)
◆ Serosanguineous discharge (uncommon)

Diagnostic evaluation

◆ Pap test is used for screening purposes.
◆ Colposcopy determines the source of abnormal cells found through the Pap test.
◆ Cone biopsy is performed if endocervical curettage is positive.
◆ Reflex HPV typing distinguishes between cells or lesions requiring aggressive treatment (intermediate or high-risk HPV), such as colposcopy, and those that can be managed conservatively (negative or low-risk HPV) through repeated Pap tests in 3 to 6 months.
◆ Chest X-ray, I.V. pyelogram or CT scan, cystoscopy, proctosigmoidoscopy, and HIV testing — especially for younger at-risk women — for initial workup, clinical staging, and in invasive cervical cancer evaluation of metastasis.
◆ CT scanning reveals enlarged lymph nodes, which can then be assessed histologically and cytologically with surgical excision or FNA.
◆ MRI detects early parametrial and nodal disease.
◆ Barium enema, bone scans, cystography, and lymphangiography detect metastasis.

Nursing diagnoses

◆ Acute pain
◆ Fear
◆ Risk for infection

Treatment

◆ Treatment varies depending on the stage and extent of the cancer

Preinvasive

◆ Laser therapy, cryosurgery, cervical conization
◆ Total excisional biopsy
◆ Hysterectomy (rare)

Invasive

◆ Radiation therapy (internal, external, or both)
◆ Radical hysterectomy
◆ Pelvic exoneration (rare)

Planning and goals

◆ The client will receive adequate pain relief.
◆ The client will have a decreased level of fear.
◆ The client will be free from signs of infection.

Implementation

◆ Encourage the client to use relaxation techniques *to promote comfort during diagnostic procedures.*
◆ When assisting with a biopsy, drape and prepare the client as for a routine pelvic examination. Have a container of formaldehyde ready *to preserve the specimen during transfer to the pathology laboratory.* Assist the physician as needed and provide support for the client throughout the procedure *to allay the client's anxiety.*
◆ If assisting with laser therapy, drape and prepare the client as for a routine pelvic examination. Assist the physician as needed and provide support to the client *to alleviate the client's anxiety.*
◆ Watch for complications related to therapy *to ensure that measures can be instituted to prevent or alleviate complications.*
◆ Administer pain medication, as needed, and note its effectiveness *to relieve pain.* If pain relief isn't achieved, an alternative dose or medication may be required.
◆ Review key teaching topics with the client and family members *to ensure adequate knowledge about her condition and treatment,* including:
– treatment options
– postexcisional biopsy care (expecting discharge or spotting for about 1 week; avoiding douching, using tampons, or engaging in sexual intercourse during this time; reporting signs of infection)
– follow-up Pap tests and pelvic examinations.

Postoperative care

After abdominal hysterectomy:
◆ Check abdominal and perineal dressings for excessive bleeding every 15 minutes for 2 hours, then every 4 hours for at least 8 hours. A moderate amount of sanguineous drainage on the perineal pad is normal. *The risk of hemorrhage after an abdominal hysterectomy is greatest during the first 24 hours because of the abundant blood supply to the pelvis.*
◆ Encourage the client to void or insert an indwelling urinary catheter *to maintain urine output.*
◆ Allow no food or fluids for 24 to 48 hours, as ordered, until peristalsis returns and bowel sounds are normal. When the client is able to eat, allow no gas-forming foods *because flatus causes intense discomfort.*
◆ Encourage ambulation *to promote peristalsis.*
◆ Encourage ambulation and exercises *to promote circulation.* Have the client walk the day after surgery, if ordered. Avoid high Fowler's position, which may result in pelvic congestion. Don't use the knee gatch (resulting in flexed knees) on the bed. Use antiembolism stockings and pneumatic compression stockings as appropriate *to promote venous return.*
◆ Review key teaching topics with the client and family members *to ensure adequate knowledge about the condition and treatment,* including:
– avoiding sexual intercourse and douching until instructed otherwise by the physician
– avoiding heavy lifting and other strenuous activities for about 2 months, as instructed by the physician
– notifying the physician of bleeding or abnormal vaginal discharge
– understanding the importance of continued follow-up care at frequent intervals, which allows for an assessment of the client's psychological adjustment. (While most clients successfully resolve their feelings of loss and fear associated with hysterectomy and a diagnosis of cancer, some will have unusual difficulty coping and may need referral for psychological counseling.)

Evaluation

◆ The client verbalizes relief from pain.
◆ The client verbalizes a decreased level of fear and can discuss her feelings, the diagnosis, and treatment options.
◆ The client has normal vital signs, an incision site without signs of redness or drainage, and exhibits no signs of complication from surgery.

CHLAMYDIA

CHLAMYDIA refers to a group of infections linked to one organism: *Chlamydia trachomatis.* Chlamydia infection causes urethritis in men and urethritis and cervicitis in women. Untreated, chlamydial infections can lead to such complications as acute epididymitis, salpingitis, pelvic inflammatory disease and, eventually, sterility.

Chlamydial infections are the most common sexually transmitted diseases in the United States.

Possible causes

- Exposure to *C. trachomatis* through vaginal or rectal intercourse, or oral-genital contact with an infected person
- Passage through the birth canal (in infants)

Assessment findings

In women

- Pelvic pain
- Dyspareunia
- Mucopurulent discharge
- Cervical erosion

In men

- Urinary frequency
- Dysuria
- Pruritus
- Erythema
- Tenderness of the meatus
- Urethral discharge

Diagnostic evaluation

- Swab from the site of infection (urethra, cervix, or rectum) establishes a diagnosis of urethritis, cervicitis, salpingitis, endometritis, or proctitis.
- Culture of aspirated material establishes a diagnosis of epididymitis.
- Antigen detection methods, including the enzyme-linked immunosorbent assay and the direct fluorescent antibody test, are the diagnostic tests of choice for identifying chlamydial infection, although tissue cell cultures are more sensitive and specific.
- Nucleic acid probes using polymerase chain reactions (newer, commercially available test) detects chlamydia

Nursing diagnoses

- Deficient knowledge regarding disorder and treatment
- Acute pain
- Ineffective sexuality patterns

Treatment

- The only treatment available for chlamydial infection is drug therapy.

Drug therapy options

- Antibiotics: doxycycline (Vibramycin); azithromycin (Zithromax) for pregnant women with chlamydial infections or as alternative treatment

Planning and goals

- The client will relate appropriate information concerning disease transmission and treatment.
- The client will express feelings of comfort and pain relief.
- The client will voice feelings about changes in sexual practice.

Implementation

- Practice standard precautions when caring for a client with a chlamydial infection *to prevent the spread of infection.*
- Make sure that the client fully understands the dosage requirements of all prescribed medications for this infection *to ensure compliance with the treatment regimen.*
- If required in your state, report all cases of chlamydial infection to the appropriate local public health authorities, who will then conduct follow-up notification of the client's sexual contacts. *These measures help ensure that an infected sexual contact will receive medical care to treat the infection.*
- Suggest that the client and sexual partners receive testing for HIV. *The unsafe sex practices that lead to chlamydial infection also place the client at risk for contracting HIV.*
- Check newborns of infected mothers for signs of chlamydial infection *to ensure prompt recognition and treatment of infection.* Obtain appropriate specimens for diagnostic testing *to confirm the diagnosis of chlamydial infection.*

Evaluation

- The client relates appropriate knowledge regarding the disease.
- The client reports adequate pain control.
- The client reports responsible sexual behavior.

CHRONIC GLOMERULONEPHRITIS

A slowly progressive disease, CHRONIC GLOMERULONEPHRITIS is characterized by inflammation of the glomeruli, which results in sclerosis, scarring and, eventually, renal failure. By the time it produces symptoms, chronic glomerulonephritis is usually irreversible.

Possible causes

- Renal disorders
- Systemic disorders (lupus erythematosus, Goodpasture's syndrome, diabetes mellitus)

Assessment findings

- Hematuria
- Edema

- Hypertension
- Uremic symptoms (in the late stages of the disease)
- Heart failure

Diagnostic evaluation

- Kidney biopsy identifies the underlying disease and provides the data needed to guide therapy.
- Blood studies reveal rising blood urea nitrogen and serum creatinine levels, which indicate advanced renal insufficiency.
- Urinalysis reveals proteinuria, hematuria, cylindruria, and RBC casts.
- X-ray or ultrasonography shows smaller kidneys.

Nursing diagnoses

- Impaired urinary elimination
- Excess fluid volume
- Fatigue

Treatment

- Dialysis
- Low-sodium, high-calorie with adequate protein diet
- Kidney transplant

Drug therapy options

- Antibiotics: according to affecting organism for symptomatic urinary tract infections
- Antihypertensive: metoprolol (Lopressor)
- Diuretic: furosemide (Lasix)

Planning and goals

- The client will maintain fluid balance.
- The client will verbalize feelings of increased energy and decreased fatigue.

Implementation

- Understand that client care is primarily supportive, focusing on continual observation and sound client teaching. *Supportive measures encourage the client to cope with chronic disease.*
- Accurately monitor vital signs, intake and output, and daily weight *to evaluate fluid retention.*
- Observe for signs of fluid, electrolyte, and acid-base imbalances *to ensure early treatment and prevent complications.*
- Consult a registered dietitian *to plan low-sodium, high-calorie meals with adequate protein.*
- Administer medications and provide good skin care *to combat pruritus and edema.*
- Provide good oral hygiene *to prevent breakdown of the oral mucosa.*

Evaluation

- The client doesn't display signs of fluid overload.
- The client reports increased energy.

CHRONIC RENAL FAILURE

CHRONIC RENAL FAILURE is progressive, irreversible destruction of the kidneys, leading to loss of renal function. It may result from a rapidly progressing disease of sudden onset that destroys the nephrons and causes irreversible kidney damage.

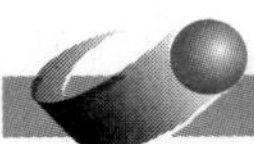

FAST FACT

End-stage renal disease (ESRD) is more common among African-Americans and Native Americans. Incidence is higher in African-Americans when ERSD results from hypertension. Incidence in Native Americans is higher when ERSD results from diabetes.

Possible causes

- Congenital abnormalities
- Dehydration
- Diabetes mellitus
- Exacerbations of nephritis
- Hypertension
- Nephrotoxins
- Recurrent urinary tract infection
- Systemic lupus erythematosus
- Urinary tract obstructions

Assessment findings

- Amenorrhea
- Anemia
- Anorexia, nausea, vomiting
- Apathy
- Arrhythmias
- Azotemia
- Bone pain
- Brittle nails and hair
- Cardiomyopathy
- Coma (late metabolic acidosis)
- Confusion
- Decreased urine output
- Drowsiness
- Dyspnea

- Ecchymosis
- Edema
- Fatigue
- Gastritis, gastric ulceration
- Heart failure
- Hypertension
- Impotence
- Irritability (early metabolic acidosis)
- Lethargy
- Muscle cramping and twitching
- Pain
- Paresthesia
- Pericardial effusion
- Peripheral neuropathy
- Pruritus
- Pulmonary edema
- Restless leg syndrome
- Seizures
- Stomatitis
- Susceptibility to infection
- Uremia
- Weakness
- Weight gain

Diagnostic evaluation

- ABG analysis shows metabolic acidosis.
- Blood studies show increased BUN, creatinine, phosphorus, and lipid levels; decreased calcium, carbon dioxide, and albumin levels; and decreased Hb, HCT, and platelet count.
- Urine chemistry shows proteinuria, increased WBC count and sodium level, and decreased and then fixed urine specific gravity.

Nursing diagnoses

- Excess fluid volume
- Ineffective tissue perfusion (renal)
- Powerlessness

Treatment

- Maintaining fluid balance
- Low-protein, low-sodium, low-potassium, low-phosphorus, high-calorie, high-carbohydrate diet
- Peritoneal dialysis and hemodialysis (For more information on dialysis, see *Types of dialysis,* page 520, and *Key nursing measures during dialysis,* page 521.)
- Transfusion therapy with packed RBCs and platelets

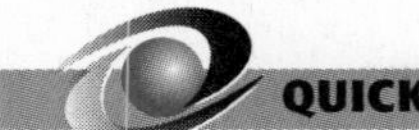

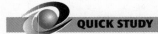

QUICK STUDY

To remember contraindications for peritoneal dialysis, think **SHE:**

Severe obstructive pulmonary diseases
History of multiple abdominal surgical procedures
Excessive obesity, large abdominal wall, and fat deposits

Drug therapy options

- Alkalinizing agent: sodium bicarbonate
- Antacid: aluminum hydroxide gel (AlternaGEL)
- Antianemics: epoetin alfa (recombinant human erythropoietin, Epogen), ferrous sulfate (Feosol), iron dextran (InFed)
- Antiarrhythmic: procainamide (Pronestyl)
- Antibiotic: cefazolin (Ancef)
- Antiemetic: prochlorperazine (Compazine)
- Antipyretic: acetaminophen (Tylenol)
- Beta-adrenergic blocker: dopamine (Intropin)
- Calcium supplement: calcium carbonate (Os-Cal)
- Cation exchange resin: sodium polystyrene sulfonate (Kayexalate)
- Cardiac glycoside: digoxin (Lanoxin)
- Diuretic: furosemide (Lasix)
- Stool softener: docusate sodium (Colace)
- Vitamins: ascorbic acid (vitamin C), pyridoxine hydrochloride (vitamin B_6)

Planning and goals

- The client will demonstrate normal vital signs and fluid balance.
- The client's laboratory values will return to normal limit.
- The client and family members will be able to cope with the prognosis and the need for lifelong dialysis.

Implementation

- Assess renal, respiratory, and cardiovascular status and fluid balance. *An increase in hemodynamic status and vital signs may indicate fluid overload caused by lack of kidney function.*
- Assess the dialysis access site for bruits and thrills *to ensure patency and detect complications.*
- Monitor and record vital signs, intake and output, ECG values, daily weight, laboratory studies, and stools for occult blood *to assess baseline and detect early changes in the client's condition.*

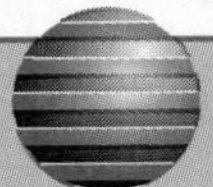

CLINICAL SITUATION

Caring for the client with chronic renal failure

A 57-year-old steelworker has had several urinary tract infections. Recently, he has been experiencing muscle weakness, and he tires more easily than usual, being exhausted at the end of a workday. After a thorough physical examination and diagnostic testing, the client receives a medical diagnosis of chronic renal failure.

The nurse formulates the following nursing diagnoses:

- *Excess fluid volume related to impaired excretory function*
- *Impaired physical mobility related to fatigue and anemia*
- *Powerlessness related to dependence on dialysis.*

The nurse formulates a fourth nursing diagnosis: *Risk for situational low self-esteem.*

Provide at least three reasons why the last nursing diagnosis is appropriate for this medical condition.

Possible reasons that the client's self-esteem may be affected by this medical condition include:

- lifestyle changes
- dependency on dialysis
- chronic fatigue
- body image changes
- role maintenance
- occupational problems.

Questions for further thought

- What medications excreted by the kidney need to be avoided?
- What type of diet is appropriate for the client with chronic renal failure and why?
- When should the nurse instruct the client to take his diuretics and why?

- Monitor for ecchymosis and GI bleeding *because the blood clotting mechanism may be affected.*
- Maintain standard precautions *to prevent the spread of infection.*
- Maintain the client's diet *to promote nutritional status.*
- Allow the client to select foods from the diet prescribed *to encourage him to eat.* (See *Caring for the client with chronic renal failure.*)
- Restrict fluids *to prevent fluid overload.*
- Administer medications, as prescribed, and observe for adverse effects of medications *to improve or maintain the client's condition and monitor his increased sensitivity to medications.*
- Encourage the client to express his feelings about the chronicity of his illness *to encourage the use of coping mechanisms.*
- Provide tepid baths *to promote comfort and reduce skin irritation.*
- Maintain a cool, quiet environment *to reduce metabolic demands.*
- Provide mouth care using plain water *to promote comfort and enhance the ability to eat.* The client's breath will have an ammonia odor, resembling that of urine, which may limit the ability to eat. His gums may bleed and stomatitis or ulcers may form.
- Avoid giving the client I.M. injections *to prevent bleeding from the injection site.*
- The client and family members may become depressed by the problems of continuing therapy and the poor prognosis. Encourage them to express their feelings and provide emotional support *to aid communication, provide an outlet for their feelings, and to identify the need for further support measures.*
- Review key teaching topics with the client and family members *to ensure adequate knowledge about the condition and treatment,* including:
  - required care techniques and what symptoms to report to the physician
  - importance of getting sufficient rest
  - importance of completing skin and mouth care daily
  - ways to avoid infection.

Evaluation

- The client maintains fluid balance within normal parameters.
- The client demonstrates normal laboratory values.
- The client and family members are learning to cope with their situation.

CYSTITIS

CYSTITIS, an inflammation of the urinary bladder, usually results from pathologic microorganisms. Most commonly, it's related to a superficial infection that doesn't extend to the bladder mucosa.

Possible causes

- Diabetes mellitus
- Incorrect aseptic technique during catheterization
- Incorrect perineal care
- Kidney infection

◆ Obstruction of the urethra
◆ Pregnancy
◆ Radiation
◆ Sexual intercourse
◆ Stagnation of urine in the bladder

Assessment findings

◆ Low-grade fever
◆ Urinary burning, frequency, and urgency
◆ Suprapubic or flank tenderness
◆ Pus or blood in the urine (present with advanced infection)
◆ Presence of predisposing factors or disease

Diagnostic evaluation

◆ Cystoscopy shows obstruction or deformity.
◆ Urine chemistry shows hematuria, pyuria, and increased protein, leukocytes, and urine specific gravity.
◆ Urine culture and sensitivity positively identifies organisms (*Escherichia coli, Proteus vulgaris,* or *Streptococcus faecalis*).

Nursing diagnoses

◆ Acute pain
◆ Impaired urinary elimination
◆ Risk for infection

Treatment

◆ Increased intake of fluids and vitamin C

Drug therapy options

◆ Antibiotic: co-trimoxazole (Bactrim)
◆ Antipyretic: acetaminophen (Tylenol)
◆ Urinary antiseptic: phenazopyridine (Pyridium)

Planning and goals

◆ The client will express increased comfort.
◆ The client will demonstrate normal voiding patterns.
◆ The client will verbalize knowledge of how to prevent cystitis.

Implementation

◆ Assess renal status *to determine a baseline and detect changes.*
◆ Monitor and record vital signs, intake and output, and laboratory studies *to assess the client's status and to detect early complications.*
◆ Maintain the client's diet *to promote nutrition.*
◆ Force fluids (cranberry or orange juice) up to 3 qt (3 L)/day *because dilute urine lessens irritation of the bladder mucosa and lowering urine pH with orange juice and cranberry juice consumption helps diminish bacterial growth.*
◆ Administer medications, as prescribed, *to maintain or improve the client's condition.*
◆ Perform sitz baths and perineal care *to relieve perineal or suprapubic discomfort.*
◆ Encourage voiding every 2 to 3 hours *to decrease bladder irritation and prevent urine stasis.*
◆ Review key teaching topics with the client *to ensure adequate knowledge about his condition and treatment,* including:
- avoiding coffee, tea, alcohol, and cola
- increasing fluid intake to 3 L/day using orange juice and cranberry juice
- voiding every 2 to 3 hours and after intercourse
- performing perineal care correctly; wiping the perineal area from front to back after voiding and defecation
- avoiding bubble baths, vaginal deodorants, and tub baths
- recognizing that urine may be orange while taking phenazopyridine
- seeking early treatment if cystitis symptoms are noticed.

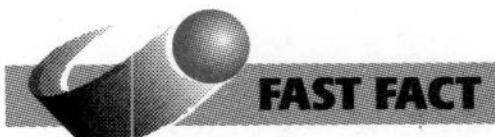

FAST FACT

Encourage the client to void every 2 to 3 hours to empty the bladder completely. Frequent voiding enhances bacteria removal and reduces urinary stasis.

Evaluation

◆ The client reports no pain or bladder spasms.
◆ The client has normal voiding patterns.
◆ The client can explain how to prevent recurrence and avoid infection.

GONORRHEA

A common sexually transmitted disease, GONORRHEA is an infection of the genitourinary tract (especially the urethra and cervix) and, occasionally, the rectum, pharynx, and eyes. Untreated gonorrhea can spread through the blood to the joints, tendons, meninges, and endocardium; in females, it can also lead to chronic pelvic inflammatory disease (PID) and sterility.

After adequate treatment, the prognosis in males and females is excellent, although reinfection is common. Gonorrhea is especially prevalent among young people and people with multiple partners, particularly those between ages 19 and 25.

Possible causes

◆ Exposure to *Neisseria gonorrhoeae* through sexual contact
◆ Maternal-infant transmission (gonococcal ophthalmia neonatorum, which occurs during passage through birth canal)
◆ Touching eyes with contaminated hands

Assessment findings

◆ Dysuria
◆ Purulent urethral or cervical discharge
◆ Unilateral conjunitival redness and swelling
◆ Itching, burning, and pain

Diagnostic evaluation

◆ Culture from the site of infection (urethra, cervix, rectum, or pharynx) grown on a Thayer-Martin or Transgrow medium usually establishes the diagnosis by isolating the organism.
◆ Gram stain showing gram-negative diplococci supports the diagnosis and may be sufficient to confirm gonorrhea in males.

Nursing diagnoses

◆ Risk for infection
◆ Acute pain
◆ Ineffective sexuality patterns

Treatment

◆ Moist heat to affected joints if gonococcal arthritis is present

Drug therapy options

◆ Antibiotics: ceftriaxone (Rocephin), doxycycline (Vibramycin), erythromycin (E-Mycin)
◆ Prophylactic antibiotic: 1% silver nitrate or erythromycin (EryPed) eye drops to prevent infection in neonates

Planning and goals

◆ The client will remain free from signs and symptoms of infection.
◆ The client will express feelings of comfort and pain relief.
◆ The client will voice concerns over alterations in sexual practice.

Implementation

◆ Before treatment, establish whether the client has any drug sensitivities. Watch closely for adverse effects during therapy *to prevent severe adverse reactions.*
◆ Warn the client that, until cultures prove negative, he's still infectious and can transmit gonococcal infection *to prevent the spread of infection to others.*
◆ Practice standard precautions *to prevent the spread of infection.*
◆ In the client with gonococcal arthritis, apply moist heat *to ease pain in affected joints.*
◆ Urge the client to inform his sexual contacts of his *infection so that they can seek treatment, even if cultures are negative.* Advise him to avoid sexual intercourse until treatment is complete *to prevent the spread of infection.*
◆ Routinely instill two drops of 1% silver nitrate or erythromycin in the eyes of all neonates immediately after birth. Check newborn infants of infected mothers for signs of infection. Take specimens for culture from the infant's eyes, pharynx, and rectum. *These measures ensure prompt recognition and treatment of infection in the newborn.*
◆ Report all cases of gonorrhea in children to child abuse authorities.

Evaluation

◆ The client doesn't display signs of infection.
◆ The client reports adequate pain control.
◆ The client reports safe sexual practices.

HERPES SIMPLEX VIRUS

A recurrent viral infection, HERPES SIMPLEX VIRUS is caused by two types of *Herpesvirus hominis* (HVH), a widespread infectious agent.

Type 1 herpes, which is transmitted by oral and respiratory secretions, affects the skin and mucous membranes and commonly produces cold sores and fever blisters.

Type 2 herpes primarily affects the genital area and is transmitted by sexual contact. Cross-infection may result from orogenital sex.

Possible causes

◆ Contact with type 1 herpes through oral or respiratory secretions
◆ Exposure to type 2 herpes through sexual contact

Assessment findings

Neonatal infection

◆ Disseminated infection (liver, lungs, brain): seizures, mental retardation, blindness, deafness, microcephaly, diabetes insipidus, spasticity

Generalized infection

- Blisters on any part of the mouth accompanied by erythema and edema
- Fever
- Swelling of the lymph nodes under the jaw
- Appetite loss
- Increased salivation
- Conjunctivitis (herpetic keratoconjunctivitis, or herpes of the eye)

Localized infection

- Fluid-filled blisters on the genitalia
- Painful urination
- Fever
- Swollen lymph nodes
- Keratoconjunctivitis (unilateral conjunctivitis, excess lacrimation, photophobia, purulent discharge)
- Herpetic whitlow (finger tingling; swollen, painful vesicles)

Diagnostic evaluation

- Isolation of the virus from local lesions and a histologic biopsy confirm the diagnosis.
- Blood studies reveal a rise in antibodies and moderate leukocytosis.

Nursing diagnoses

- Acute pain
- Impaired oral mucous membrane
- Impaired social interaction

Treatment

- Treatment is symptomatic and supportive.

Drug therapy options

- Analgesic-antipyretic: acetaminophen (Tylenol) to reduce fever and relieve pain
- Drying agent: calamine lotion (Calamox) to relieve pain of genital lesions
- Antivirals: famciclovir (Famvir), valacyclovir (Valtrex), trifluridine (Viroptic), vidarabine (Vira-A), 5% acyclovir (Zovirax) ointment (possible relief to clients with genital herpes or to immunosuppressed clients with HVH skin infections; I.V. acyclovir to treat more severe infections)

Planning and goals

- The client will express feelings of comfort and pain relief.
- The client will exhibit improved or healed lesions or wounds.
- The client will resume effective communication patterns.

Implementation

- Observe standard precautions. For clients with extensive cutaneous, oral, or genital lesions, institute contact precautions *to prevent the spread of infection.*
- Administer pain medications and prescribed antiviral agents as ordered *to relieve pain and treat infection.*
- Provide supportive care, as indicated, such as oral hygiene, nutritional supplementation, and antipyretics for fever. *These measures enhance the client's well-being.*
- Abstain from direct client care if you have herpetic whitlow (an HVH finger infection which commonly affects health care workers) *to prevent the spread of infection.*
- Explain the disorder, modes of transmission, treatment, and prevention of recurrence to the client *to optimize his health.*

Evaluation

- The client reports adequate pain control.
- The client displays healing lesions.
- The client reports improved social interaction.

NEUROGENIC BLADDER

NEUROGENIC BLADDER refers to all types of bladder dysfunction caused by an interruption of normal bladder innervation. Subsequent complications include incontinence, residual urine retention, urinary infection, stone formation, and renal failure. A neurogenic bladder may be described as spastic (resulting from an upper motor neuron lesion) or flaccid (resulting from a lower motor neuron lesion).

This disorder is also known as *neuromuscular dysfunction of the lower urinary tract, neurologic bladder dysfunction,* and *neuropathic bladder.*

Possible causes

- Acute infectious diseases such as Guillain-Barré syndrome
- Cerebral disorder (stroke, brain tumor [meningioma and glioma], Parkinson's disease, multiple sclerosis, dementia)
- Chronic alcoholism
- Collagen diseases such as systemic lupus erythematosus
- Disorders of peripheral innervation
- Distant effects of cancer such as primary oat cell carcinoma of the lung
- Heavy metal toxicity
- Herpes zoster

- Metabolic disturbances (hypothyroidism, porphyria, or uremia)
- Sacral agenesis
- Spinal cord disease or trauma
- Vascular diseases such as atherosclerosis

Assessment findings

- Altered micturition
- Flaccid neurogenic bladder (overflow incontinence, diminished anal sphincter tone, greatly distended bladder with an accompanying feeling of bladder fullness)
- Hydroureteronephrosis (distention of the ureter and the renal pelvis and calices)
- Incontinence
- Spastic neurogenic bladder (involuntary or frequent scanty urination without a feeling of bladder fullness, possible spontaneous spasms of the arms and legs, increased anal sphincter tone)
- Vesicoureteral reflux (passage of urine from the bladder back into a ureter)

Diagnostic evaluation

- Voiding cystourethrography evaluates bladder neck function, vesicoureteral reflux, and continence.
- Urodynamic studies help evaluate how urine is stored in the bladder, how well the bladder empties, and the rate of movement of urine out of the bladder during voiding.
- Retrograde urethrography reveals the presence of strictures and diverticula.

Nursing diagnoses

- Impaired urinary elimination
- Disturbed body image
- Impaired skin integrity

Treatment

- Credé's maneuver (application of manual pressure over the lower abdomen) to evacuate the bladder
- Valsalva's maneuver to promote complete emptying of the bladder
- Indwelling urinary catheter insertion, including teaching the client self-catheterization techniques
- Surgical repair if the client has structural impairment
- Surgical insertion of an artificial urinary sphincter

Drug therapy options

- Urinary tract stimulant: bethanechol (Urecholine)
- Antimuscarinics: propantheline (Pro-Banthine), flavoxate (Urispas)

Planning and goals

- The client will demonstrate skill in managing urinary elimination problem.
- The client will maintain a positive self-image.
- The client will maintain skin integrity.

Implementation

- Use strict aseptic technique during insertion of an indwelling urinary catheter (a temporary measure to drain the incontinent client's bladder). Don't interrupt the closed drainage system for any reason *to prevent infection.*
- Obtain urine specimens with a syringe and small-bore needle inserted through the aspirating port of the catheter itself (below the junction of the balloon instillation site). Irrigate in the same manner, if necessary, *to prevent infection.*
- Clean the catheter insertion site with soap and water at least twice per day *to prevent infection.*
- Don't allow the catheter to become encrusted *because crusting is a medium for bacteria growth.*
- Use a sterile applicator to apply antibiotic ointment around the meatus after catheter care, if prescribed. Keep the drainage bag below the tubing, and don't raise the bag above the level of the bladder *to prevent urine reflux and infection.*
- Clamp the tubing or empty the catheter bag before transferring the client to a wheelchair or stretcher *to prevent accidental urine reflux.*
- Watch for signs of infection (fever, cloudy or foul-smelling urine) *to ensure early treatment intervention and prevent complications.*
- Try to keep the client as mobile as possible. Perform passive ROM exercises, if necessary. *These measures prevent complications of immobility.*
- If a urinary diversion procedure is to be performed, arrange for consultation with an enterostomal therapist and coordinate the care *to help the client cope with his change in body image.*

Evaluation

- The client demonstrates the ability to control his urinary problem.
- The client demonstrates a positive self-image.
- The client's skin remains intact.

OVARIAN CANCER

Ovarian cancer attacks the ovaries, which are the organs in women that produce the hormones estrogen and progesterone. After cancers of the lung, breast, and colon, primary ovarian cancer ranks as the most common cause of cancer death among American women. In women with previously treated breast cancer, metastatic ovarian cancer is more common than cancer at any other site.

The prognosis varies with the histologic type and stage of the disease but is generally poor because ovarian tumors produce few early signs and are usually advanced at diagnosis. About 40% of women with ovarian cancer survive for 5 years.

Possible causes

- Age at menopause
- Celibacy
- Exposure to asbestos, talc, and industrial pollutants
- Familial tendency and history of breast or uterine cancer
- High-fat diet
- Infertility
- Upper socioeconomic levels and age between 20 and 54 (highest incidence)

Assessment findings

- Abdominal discomfort, dyspepsia, and other mild GI disturbances
- Pelvic discomfort
- Abdominal distention
- Constipation
- Urinary frequency
- Weight loss

Diagnostic evaluation

Diagnosis requires clinical evaluation, a complete client history, surgical exploration, and histologic studies. Preoperative evaluation includes a complete physical examination, including pelvic examination with a Papanicolaou (Pap) test (positive in only a small number of women with ovarian cancer) and the following special tests:

- Abdominal ultrasonography, CT scanning, or X-ray may delineate tumor size.
- Chest X-ray may reveal distant metastasis and pleural effusions.
- Barium enema (especially in clients with GI symptoms) may reveal obstruction and size of tumor.
- Lymphangiography may show lymph node involvement.
- Mammography may rule out primary breast cancer.
- Liver scanning in clients with ascites may rule out liver metastasis.
- Blood tests such as ovarian carcinoma antigen, carcinoembryonic antigen, and human chorionic gonadotropin reveal the presence of cancer.

Despite extensive testing, accurate diagnosis and staging are impossible without exploratory laparotomy, including lymph node evaluation and tumor resection.

Nursing diagnoses

- Acute pain
- Fear
- Imbalanced nutrition: Less than body requirements

Treatment

Conservative treatment (for girls or young women with a unilateral encapsulated tumor who wish to maintain fertility)

- Resection of the involved ovary
- Biopsies of the omentum and the uninvolved ovary
- Peritoneal washings for cytologic examination of pelvic fluid
- Careful follow-up, including periodic chest X-rays to rule out lung metastasis

Aggressive treatment (for ovarian cancer)

- Total abdominal hysterectomy and bilateral salpingo-oophorectomy with tumor resection, omentectomy, and appendectomy
- Lymph node biopsies with lymphadenectomy, tissue biopsies, and peritoneal washings

Drug therapy options

- Antineoplastics: cisplatin (Platinol), paclitaxel (Taxol), topotecan (Hycamtin)
- Analgesics: morphine, fentanyl (Duragesic)
- Antipyretics: aspirin, acetaminophen (Tylenol)
- Immunotherapy: Bacillus Calmette-Guérin vaccine

Planning and goals

- The client will express feelings of comfort and pain relief.
- The client will express feelings about her illness.
- The client will maintain an appropriate weight.

Implementation

Before surgery

- Thoroughly explain all preoperative tests, the expected course of treatment, and surgical and postoperative procedures *to allay the client's anxiety.*
- For a client who's premenopausal, explain that bilateral oophorectomy artificially induces early menopause, so she

may experience hot flashes, headaches, palpitations, insomnia, depression, and excessive perspiration. *Explaining this will help her cope with changes in her body image that occur as a result of surgery.*

After surgery

- Monitor vital signs frequently *to detect early signs of postoperative complications such as fluid volume deficit.*
- Monitor fluid intake and output *to detect fluid volume excess or deficit,* while maintaining good catheter care *to prevent infection.*
- Check the dressing regularly for excessive drainage or bleeding, and watch for signs of infection. *These measures detect early signs of complications and prevent treatment delay.*
- Provide abdominal support *to promote comfort,* and watch for abdominal distention, *which may indicate the presence of ascites.*
- Encourage coughing and deep breathing *to mobilize secretions and prevent postoperative pneumonia.*
- Reposition the client often *to prevent skin breakdown,* and encourage her to walk shortly after surgery *to prevent complications of immobility.*
- Monitor and treat adverse effects of radiation and chemotherapy *to prevent complications.*
- Enlist the help of a social worker, chaplain, and other members of the health care team *to provide additional supportive care.*

Evaluation

- The client reports adequate pain control.
- The client demonstrates appropriate coping mechanisms.
- The client has an appropriate weight.

PROSTATE CANCER

Prostate cancer is a malignant tumor of the prostate gland, which can obstruct urine flow when encroaching on the bladder neck. It commonly metastasizes to bone, lymph nodes, brain, and lungs. Next to skin cancer, prostate cancer is the most common type of cancer in American men.

Possible causes

- Family history
- Age
- Race
- Vasectomy
- Increased dietary fat

Assessment findings

- Decreased size and force of urine stream
- Difficulty and frequency of urination
- Hematuria
- Urine retention

Diagnostic evaluation

- Digital rectal examination reveals a palpable, firm nodule in the gland or diffuse induration in the posterior lobe.
- Serum acid phosphatase level is increased.
- Radioimmunoassay for acid phosphatase is increased.
- Prostatic-specific antigen is increased.
- Transurethral ultrasound studies show mass or obstruction.
- Prostate biopsy has cytology positive for cancer cells.
- Excretory urogram shows mass or obstruction.

Nursing diagnoses

- Acute pain
- Impaired urinary elimination
- Sexual dysfunction

Treatment

- High-protein diet with restrictions on caffeine and spicy foods
- Radiation implant
- Radical prostatectomy (for localized tumors without metastasis), cryosurgery, or transurethral resection of the prostate (to relieve obstruction in metastatic disease)

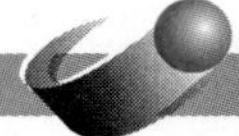

FAST FACT

Because many prostate cancers grow slowly, many elderly men never need treatment. Active treatment can be started later if the cancer begins to grow more quickly or causes other problems.

Drug therapy options

- Analgesics: meperidine (Demerol), morphine sulfate, oxycodone (Tylox)
- Antiemetics: granisetron (Kytril), ondansetron (Zofran)
- Antineoplastics: cisplatin (Platinol), doxorubicin (Adriamycin), cyclophosphamide (Cytoxan), fluorouracil (Adrucil)
- Corticosteroid: prednisone (Deltasone)
- Immunosuppressants: cyclophosphamide (Cytoxan)
- Luteinizing hormone-releasing hormone analogs: goserelin acetate (Zoladex), leuprolide acetate (Lupron)
- NSAIDs: ibuprofen (Motrin), indomethacin (Indocin), sulindac (Clinoril)

◆ Oral flutamide (Eulexin) to block circulating testosterone
◆ Stool softener: docusate sodium (Colace)

Planning and goals

◆ The client will verbalize adequate pain relief.
◆ The client will have normal urine output and unobstructed flow.
◆ The client will discuss concerns related to sexual dysfunction.

Implementation

◆ Assess renal and fluid status *to determine a baseline and detect early changes.*
◆ Monitor and record vital signs, fluid intake and output, and laboratory studies. *Accurate intake and output are essential for correct fluid replacement therapy.*
◆ Monitor for signs of infection *to assess for complications.*
◆ Assess pain and note the effectiveness of analgesia *to promote comfort.*
◆ Administer medications, as prescribed, *to maintain or improve the client's condition.*
◆ Maintain the client's diet *to ensure adequate nutrition and meet increased metabolic demands.*
◆ Maintain patency of the urinary catheter and note drainage *to ensure effective urine drainage.*
◆ Encourage the client to express his feelings about the changes in his body image and fear of sexual dysfunction *to encourage coping and adaptation.*
◆ Encourage ambulation *to prevent complications of immobility.*
◆ Provide postoperative, postchemotherapeutic, and postradiation nursing care *to prevent complications.*
◆ Review key teaching topics with the client and family members *to ensure adequate knowledge about the condition and treatment,* including:
– managing changes in sexual activity
– avoiding prolonged sitting, standing, and walking
– avoiding the strain of exercise and lifting
– urinating frequently
– avoiding coffee and cola beverages
– decreasing fluid intake during evening hours
– performing perineal exercises
– completing catheter care, as directed
– self-monitoring for bloody urine, pain, burning, frequency, decreased urine output, and loss of bladder control
– contacting the American Cancer Society and other community agencies and resources for additional information or support.

Evaluation

◆ The client verbalizes pain relief and has normal vital signs.
◆ The client's urine flow isn't obstructed.
◆ The client indicates he isn't experiencing sexual dysfunction when seen for follow-up care.

RENAL CALCULI

RENAL CALCULI, also known as *kidney stones,* result from the precipitation of substances in the urine including calcium oxalate, calcium phosphate, magnesium ammonium phosphate, urate, and cystine. Under normal circumstances, calculi are dissolved and excreted in the urine. However, larger calculi can cause great pain and may become lodged in the ureter resulting in obstruction and hydronephrosis.

Possible causes

◆ Chemotherapy
◆ Dehydration
◆ Diet high in calcium, vitamin D, milk, protein, oxalate, and alkali
◆ Genetics
◆ Gout
◆ Hypercalcemia
◆ Hyperparathyroidism
◆ Idiopathic origin
◆ Immobility
◆ Infection
◆ Leukemia
◆ Metabolic factors
◆ Polycythemia vera
◆ Urinary stasis
◆ Urinary tract infection
◆ Urinary tract obstruction

Assessment findings

◆ Costovertebral tenderness
◆ Fever, chills
◆ Hematuria
◆ Nausea and vomiting
◆ Pallor, diaphoresis
◆ Renal colic (classic pain)
◆ Urinary frequency and urgency

Diagnostic evaluation

◆ Urinalysis of 24-hour urine collection shows increased uric acid, oxalate, calcium, phosphorus, and creatinine levels.

Diet considerations for the client with renal calculi

Use this table as a guide for what foods to consider and avoid when planning a diet for the client with renal calculi.

FOODS THAT ACIDIFY URINE	FOODS THAT ALKALINIZE URINE	FOODS TO AVOID WITH CALCIUM CALCULI	FOODS TO AVOID WITH OXALATE CALCULI
Fish (halibut)	Dried apricots	Cheddar cheese	Rhubarb
Bacon	Dried figs	Cheese food	Asparagus
Veal	Molasses	Cheese spread	Dandelion greens
Lamb	Beet greens	Whole milk	Spinach
Chicken	Green olives	Evaporated milk	Cranberries
Roast beef	Dandelion greens	Skim milk	Beets and beet greens
Pork	Navy beans	Powdered dry skim milk	Cashew nuts
Cranberries	Milk		Chocolate
Prunes	Milk products		Cocoa
Plums	Citrus fruit and juice		Okra
			Potatoes
			Tomatoes
			Corn
			Swiss chard

- Blood studies show increased calcium, phosphorus, creatinine, BUN, uric acid, protein, and alkaline phosphatase levels.
- Cystoscopy allows visualization of stones.
- Excretory urography reveals stones.
- Kidney-ureter-bladder X-ray reveals stones.
- Ultrasonography reveals obstruction and hydronephosis.
- Urine chemistry shows pyuria, proteinuria, hematuria, presence of WBCs, and increased urine specific gravity.

Nursing diagnoses

- Acute pain
- Impaired urinary elimination
- Risk for infection

Treatment

- Specific diet if type of kidney stone is identified (see *Diet considerations for the client with renal calculi*)
- Extracorporeal shock wave lithotripsy to shatter calculi
- Increased fluid intake to 3 qt (3 L)/day
- Moist heat to flank; hot baths
- Percutaneous nephrostolithotomy
- Surgery if other measures to remove the stone aren't effective (type of surgery depends on the location of the stone)

Drug therapy options

- Acidifiers: ammonium chloride, methenamine mandelate (Mandelamine)
- Alkalinizing agents: potassium acetate, sodium bicarbonate
- Analgesics: meperidine (Demerol), morphine sulfate
- Antibiotics: cefazolin (Ancef), cefoxitin (Mefoxin)
- Antiemetic: prochlorperazine (Compazine)
- Antigout agent: sulfinpyrazone (Anturane)

Planning and goals

- The client will express pain relief.
- The client will exhibit normal voiding patterns.
- The client won't develop symptoms of infection.

Implementation

- Assess the client's renal status *to determine a baseline and detect complications.*
- Assess pain and the effectiveness of analgesia *to enable modification of the care plan as needed.*
- Monitor and record vital signs, intake and output, daily weight, urine specific gravity, laboratory studies, and urine pH *to assess renal status.*
- Monitor the client's urine for evidence of renal calculi. Strain all urine and save all solid material for analysis *to facilitate spontaneous passage of calculi.*

◆ Encourage fluids to 3,000 ml/day *to moisten mucous membranes and dilute chemicals within the body.*

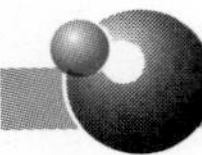

SPOT CHECK

When providing care for a client with renal calculi, the nurse carefully records urine output. What other nursing action must be conducted each time the client voids?

Answer: The urine should be strained for calculi each time the client voids.

◆ Consult a registered dietitian *to meet the client's nutritional needs.* Maintain the client's diet *to promote adequate nutrition.*

◆ Administer medications, as prescribed, *to maintain and improve the client's condition.*

◆ Apply warm soaks to the client's flank *to promote comfort.*

◆ If surgery was performed, check dressings regularly for bloody drainage and report excessive amounts of bloody drainage to the physician; use sterile technique to change the dressing; maintain nephrostomy tube or indwelling urinary catheter if indicated; and monitor incision for signs of infection *to promote healing and detect complications.*

◆ Review key teaching topics with the client *to ensure adequate knowledge about his condition and treatment,* including:

- increasing fluid intake, especially during hot weather, illness, and exercise
- voiding whenever the urge is felt
- testing urine pH
- increasing fluids at night and voiding frequently.

Evaluation

◆ The client verbalizes pain relief.

◆ The client demonstrates normal voiding patterns.

◆ The client is free from infection.

SYPHILIS

SYPHILIS is a chronic, infectious, sexually transmitted disease that begins in the mucous membranes and quickly becomes systemic, spreading to nearby lymph nodes and the bloodstream. This disease, when untreated, is characterized by progressive stages: primary, secondary, latent, and late (formerly called *tertiary*).

In the United States, incidence of syphilis is highest among urban populations, especially in persons ages 15 to 39, drug users, and those infected with HIV. It also is transmitted prenatally to the fetus (congenital syphilis), resulting in 50% mortality rate of the fetus.

Possible causes

◆ Exposure to the spirochete *Treponema pallidum* through sexual contact

◆ Transmission from an infected mother to her fetus

Assessment findings

Primary syphilis

◆ Chancres on the genitalia, anus, fingers, lips, tongue, nipples, tonsils, or eyelids

Secondary syphilis

◆ Symmetrical mucocutaneous lesions

◆ General lymphadenopathy

◆ Headache

◆ Malaise

◆ Anorexia

◆ Weight loss

◆ Nausea

◆ Vomiting

◆ Sore throat

◆ Slight fever

Late syphilis

◆ Gumma-chronic, superficial nodule on long bones

◆ Epigastric pain

◆ Perforated septum on palate

◆ Bone or organ destruction

◆ Aortic fibrosis

◆ Aortic aneurysm

◆ Meningitis

◆ CNS symptoms (paresis, personality changes, weakness)

Diagnostic evaluation

◆ Dark-field examination identifies *T. pallidum* from a lesion. This method is most effective when moist lesions are present, as in primary, secondary, and prenatal syphilis.

◆ Fluorescent treponemal antibody-absorption test identifies antigens of *T. pallidum* in tissue, ocular fluid, CSF, tracheobronchial secretions, and exudates from lesions. This is the most sensitive test available for detecting syphilis at all stages. When reactive, it remains so permanently.

◆ Venereal Disease Research Laboratory (VDRL) slide test and rapid plasma reagin test detect nonspecific antibodies. Both tests, if positive, become reactive within 1 to 2 weeks after the primary lesion appears or 4 to 5 weeks after the infection begins.

◆ CSF examination identifies neurosyphilis when the total protein level is above 40 mg/100 ml, VDRL slide test is reactive, and CSF cell count exceeds five mononuclear cells per microliter.

Nursing diagnoses

◆ Ineffective sexuality patterns
◆ Impaired skin integrity
◆ Deficient knowledge regarding disorder and treatment

Treatment

Antibiotic therapy is the only treatment for syphilis.

Drug therapy options

◆ Antibiotics: penicillin G benzathine (Permapen); if allergic to penicillin, doxycycline (Vibramycin)

Planning and goals

◆ The client will verbalize problems related to sexuality.
◆ The client will exhibit healing lesions or wounds.
◆ The client will relate appropriate information regarding his illness and safe sexual practice.

Implementation

◆ Follow standard precautions when assessing the client, collecting specimens, and treating lesions *to prevent the spread of infection.*

◆ Check for a history of drug sensitivity before administering the first dose of penicillin *to prevent anaphylaxis.*

◆ In secondary syphilis, keep the lesions clean and dry. If they're draining, dispose of contaminated materials properly *to prevent the spread of infection.*

◆ In late syphilis, provide supportive care *to relieve the client's symptoms during prolonged treatment.*

◆ In cardiovascular syphilis, check for signs of decreased cardiac output (decreased urine output, hypoxia, and decreased sensorium) and pulmonary congestion *to prevent shock and respiratory distress.*

◆ In neurosyphilis, regularly check level of consciousness, mood, and coherence. Watch for signs of ataxia. *These measures detect neurologic complications early and prevent treatment delay.*

◆ Urge clients to seek VDRL testing after 3, 6, 12, and 24 months *to detect possible relapse.* Clients treated for latent or late syphilis should receive blood tests at 6-month intervals for 2 years *to detect possible relapse.*

◆ Be sure to report all cases of syphilis to local public health authorities. Urge the client to inform his sexual partners of his infection *so that they can also receive treatment.*

◆ Refer the client and his sexual partners for HIV testing. *High-risk behaviors that caused the client to contract syphilis also place the client at risk for HIV.*

Evaluation

◆ The client expresses feelings regarding sexual practices and alterations.

◆ The client doesn't have any futher lesions; skin is clean, dry, and intact.

◆ The client relates appropriate information regarding his illness and safe sexual practice.

TESTICULAR CANCER

Testicular cancer affects the testes or testicles, the two oval-shaped glandular organs inside the scrotum that produce spermatozoa and testosterone. Malignant testicular tumors primarily affect young to middle-aged men. Testicular tumors in children are rare.

Most testicular tumors originate in gonadal cells. About 40% are seminomas (uniform, undifferentiated cells resembling primitive gonadal cells). The rest are nonseminomas (tumor cells showing various degrees of differentiation).

The prognosis varies with the cell type and disease stage. When treated with surgery and radiation, almost all clients with localized disease survive beyond 5 years.

Possible causes

Contributing factors include:

◆ age (incidence peaks between ages 20 and 40)

◆ higher incidence in men with cryptorchidism and those whose mothers used diethylstilbestrol during pregnancy.

Assessment findings

◆ Firm, painless, smooth testicular mass, varying in size and sometimes producing a sense of testicular heaviness

Advanced stages

◆ Abdominal mass
◆ Cough
◆ Fatigue
◆ Hemoptysis
◆ Lethargy
◆ Pallor

- Shortness of breath
- Ureteral obstruction
- Weight loss

Diagnostic evaluation

- Regular self-examinations and testicular palpation during a routine physical examination may disclose testicular tumors.
- Transillumination can be used to distinguish between a tumor (which doesn't transilluminate) and a hydrocele or spermatocele (which does transilluminate).
- CT scanning can be used to detect metastasis.
- Scrotal ultrasonography can be used to differentiate between a cyst and a solid mass.
- Chest X-ray may show pulmonary metastasis.
- Excretory urography may reveal ureteral deviation resulting from para-aortic node involvement.
- Serum alpha-fetoprotein and beta-human chorionic gonadotropin levels — indicators of testicular tumor activity — provide a baseline for measuring the client's response to therapy and determining the prognosis.
- Surgical excision and biopsy of the tumor and testis permits histologic verification of the tumor cell type.
- Inguinal exploration (examination of the groin) is used to determine the extent of nodal involvement.

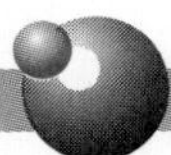

SPOT CHECK

True or False? The incidence of testicular cancer peaks between ages 50 and 75.

Answer: False. Incidence peaks between ages 20 and 40.

Nursing diagnoses

- Disturbed body image
- Fear
- Sexual dysfunction

Treatment

- Radiation therapy
- Orchiectomy: (Most surgeons remove the testicle but not the scrotum to allow for a prosthetic implant.)
- Retroperitoneal lymph node dissection (dissection of lymph nodes posterior to the peritoneum)
- Bone marrow transplantation (follows chemotherapy and radiation therapy in clients with unresponsive tumors)
- High-calorie diet provided in small, frequent feedings
- I.V. fluid therapy

Drug therapy options

- Antineoplastics: bleomycin (Blenoxane), carboplatin (Paraplatin), cisplatin (Platinol), dactinomycin (Cosmegen), etoposide (VePesid), ifosfamide (IFEX), plicamycin (Mithracin), vinblastine (Velban)
- Analgesics: fentanyl (Duragesic), morphine sulfate
- Antiemetics: granisetron hydrochloride (Kytril), ondansetron (Zofran)
- Hormone replacement therapy (after bilateral orchiectomy)

Planning and goals

- The client will maintain a positive body image and positive self-concept.
- The client will demonstrate a decreased level of fear.
- The client will discuss concerns related to sexual dysfunction.

Implementation

- Develop a treatment plan that addresses the client's psychological and physical needs *to enhance his sense of well-being.*

Before orchiectomy

- Reassure the client that sterility and impotence need not follow unilateral orchiectomy, that synthetic hormones can restore hormonal balance, and that most surgeons don't remove the scrotum. In many cases, a testicular prosthesis can correct anatomic disfigurement. *These interventions can help allay the client's anxiety.*
- If bilateral orchiectomy is planned, facilitate the proper referral or discussions about sperm-banking options, as appropriate, *to promote client and family understanding of the available options.*

After orchiectomy

- For the first day after surgery, apply an ice pack to the scrotum *to reduce swelling* and provide analgesics *to promote comfort.*
- Check for excessive bleeding, swelling, and signs of infection *to detect early signs of complications and to prevent treatment delay.*
- Provide a scrotal athletic supporter *to minimize pain during ambulation.*

During chemotherapy

- Give antiemetics, as needed, *to treat or prevent nausea and vomiting.*

◆ Encourage small, frequent meals *to maintain oral intake despite anorexia.*
◆ Establish a mouth care regimen to prevent breakdown of the oral mucosa and check for stomatitis *to detect early signs and avoid treatment delay.*
◆ Watch for signs of myelosuppression so precautions can be taken *to avoid infection.*
◆ Encourage increased fluid intake and provide I.V. fluids, a potassium supplement, and diuretics *to prevent renal damage.*
◆ Review key teaching topics with the client and family members *to ensure adequate knowledge about the condition and treatment,* including:
– understanding the disease process and treatment options
– preventing and reporting infection
– managing adverse reactions to chemotherapy and radiation.

Evaluation

◆ The client verbalizes feelings about his body image change and expresses positive feelings about himself.
◆ The client verbalizes a decreased level of fear and can discuss his feelings, the diagnosis, and treatment options.
◆ The client indicates he isn't experiencing sexual dysfunction when seen for follow-up care.

Appendices

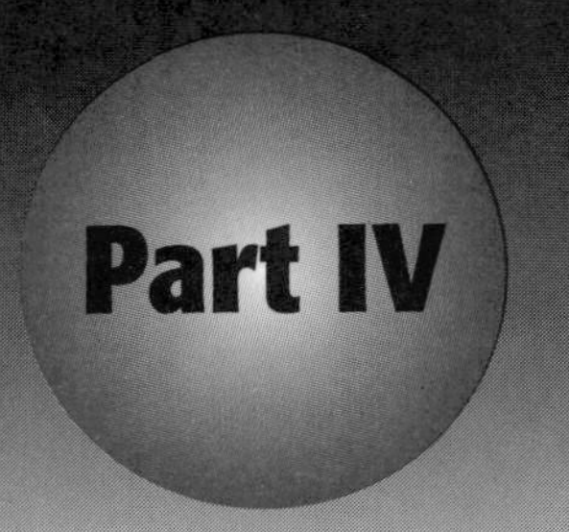

State Boards of Nursing

The following list includes boards of nursing for all U.S. states and territories.

Alabama
Alabama Board of Nursing
770 Washington Avenue
RSA Plaza, Suite 250
Montgomery, AL 36130-3900
Phone: (334) 242-4060
Fax: (334) 242-4360
Web site: http://www.abn.state.al.us/

Alaska
Alaska Board of Nursing
550 West Seventh Avenue, Suite 1500
Anchorage, AK 99501-3567
Phone: (907) 269-8161
Fax: (907) 269-8196
Web site: http://www.dced.state.ak.us/occ/pnur.htm

American Samoa
American Samoa Health Services Regulatory Board
LBJ Tropical Medical Center
Pago, Pago, AS 96799
Phone: (684) 633-1222
Fax: (684) 633-1869

Arizona
Arizona State Board of Nursing
1651 E. Morten Avenue, Suite 210
Phoenix, AZ 85020
Phone: (602) 889-5150
Fax: (602) 889-5115
Web site: http://www.azboardofnursing.org/

Arkansas
Arkansas State Board of Nursing
University Tower Building
1123 S. University, Suite 800
Little Rock, AR 72204-1619
Phone: (501) 686-2700
Fax: (501) 686-2714
Web site: http://www.state.ar.us/nurse

California
California Board of Registered Nursing
400 R St., Suite 4030
Sacramento, CA 95814-6239
Phone: (916) 322-3350
Fax: (916) 327-4402
Web site: http://www.rn.ca.gov/

Colorado
Colorado Board of Nursing
1560 Broadway, Suite 880
Denver, CO 80202
Phone: (303) 894-2430
Fax: (303) 894-2821
Web site: http://www.dora.state.co.us/nursing/

Connecticut
Connecticut Board of Examiners for Nursing
Dept. of Public Health
410 Capitol Ave., #13PHO
P.O. Box 340308
Hartford, CT 06314-0308
Phone: (860) 509-7624
Fax: (860) 509-7553
Web site: http://www.state.ct.us/dph/

Delaware
Delaware Board of Nursing
861 Silver Lake Blvd.
Cannon Building, Suite 203
Dover, DE 19904
Phone: (302) 739-4522
Fax: (302) 739-2711
Web site: http://www.professionallicensing.state.de.us/boards/nursing/index.shtml

District of Columbia
District of Columbia Board of Nursing
Department of Health
717 14th Street, NW
Suite 600
Washington, DC 20005
Phone: (202) 724-4900
Fax: (202) 727-8241
Web site: http://www.dchealth.dc.gov/

Florida
Florida Board of Nursing
4052 Bald Cypress Way BIN CO2
Tallahassee, FL 32399-3252
Phone: (850) 245-4125
Fax: (850) 245-4172
Web site: http://www.doh.state.fl.us/mqa/

Georgia
Georgia Board of Nursing
237 Coliseum Drive
Macon, GA 31217-3858
Phone: (478) 207-1640
Fax: (478)207-1660
Web site: http://www.sos.state.ga.us/plb/rn

Guam
Guam Board of Nurse Examiners
P.O. Box 2816
Hagatna, GU 96932
Phone: (671) 735-7406 or (671) 725-7411
Fax: (671) 735-7413

Hawaii
Hawaii Board of Nursing
King Kalakaua Building
335 Merchant Street, 3rd Floor
Honolulu, HI 96813
Phone: (808) 586-3000
Fax: (808) 586-2689
Web site: http://www.hawaii.gov/dcca/pvl/areas/boards/nursing/

Idaho
Idaho Board of Nursing
280 N. 8th Street, Suite 210
P.O. Box 83720
Boise, ID 83720-0061
Phone: (208) 334-3110
Fax: (208) 334-3262
Web site: http://www2.state.id.us/ibn

Illinois
Illinois Department of Professional Regulation
James R. Thompson Center
100 West Randolph, Suite 9-300
Chicago, IL 60601
Phone: (312) 814-2715
Fax: (312) 814-3145
Web site: http://www.dpr.state.il.us/

Indiana
Indiana State Board of Nursing
Health Professions Bureau
402 W. Washington Street, Room W066
Indianapolis, IN 46204
Phone: (317) 234-2043
Fax: (317) 233-4236
Web site: http://www.state.in.us/hpb/boards/isbn/

Iowa
Iowa Board of Nursing
RiverPoint Business Park
400 S.W. 8th Street, Suite B
Des Moines, IA 50309-4685
Phone: (515) 281-3255
Fax: (515) 281-4825
Web site: http://www.state.ia.us/government/nursing/

Kansas
Kansas State Board of Nursing
Landon State Office Building
900 S.W. Jackson, Suite 1051
Topeka, KS 66612
Phone: (785) 296-4929
Fax: (785) 296-3929
Web site: http://www.ksbn.org

Kentucky
Kentucky Board of Nursing
312 Whittington Parkway, Suite 300
Louisville, KY 40222
Phone: (502) 429-3300
Fax: (502) 429-3311
Web site: http://www.kbn.ky.gov/

Louisiana
Louisiana State Board of Nursing
3510 N. Causeway Blvd., Suite 601
Metairie, LA 70002
Phone: (504) 838-5332
Fax: (504) 838-5349
Web site: http://www.lsbn.state.la.us/

Maine
Maine State Board of Nursing
158 State House Station
Augusta, ME 04333
Phone: (207) 287-1133
Fax: (207) 287-1149
Web site: http://www.maine.gov/boardofnursing/

Maryland
Maryland Board of Nursing
4140 Patterson Avenue
Baltimore, MD 21215
Phone: (410) 585-1900
Fax: (410) 358-3530
Web site: http://www.mbon.org/

Massachusetts
Massachusetts Board of Registration in Nursing
Commonwealth of Massachusetts
239 Causeway Street, Second Floor
Boston, MA 02114
Phone: (617) 973-0800 or (800) 414-0168
Fax: (617) 973-0984

Michigan
Michigan DCH/Bureau of Health Professions
Ottawa Towers North
611 W. Ottawa, 1st Floor
Lansing, MI 48933
Phone: (517) 335-0918
Fax: (517) 373-2179
Web site: http://www.michigan.gov/healthlicense

Minnesota
Minnesota Board of Nursing
2829 University Avenue SE
Minneapolis, MN 55414
Phone: (612) 617-2270
Fax: (612) 617-2190
Web site: http://www.nursingboard.state.mn.us/

Mississippi
Mississippi Board of Nursing
1935 Lakeland Drive, Suite B
Jackson, MS 39216-5014
Phone: (601) 987-4188
Fax: (601) 364-2352
Web site: http://www.msbn.state.ms.us/

Missouri
Missouri State Board of Nursing
3605 Missouri Blvd.
P.O. Box 656
Jefferson City, MO 65102-0656
Phone: (573) 751-0681
Fax: (573) 751-0075
Web site: http://www.pr.mo.gov/nursing.asp

Montana
Montana State Board of Nursing
301 South Park
P.O. Box 200513
Helena, MT 59620-0513
Phone: (406) 841-2340
Fax: (406) 841-2305
Web site: http://www.discoveringmontana.com/dli/bsd/license/bsd_boards/nur_board/board_page.htm

Nebraska
Nebraska Department of Health and Human Services
Regulation and Licensure, Nursing and Nursing Support
301 Centennial Mall South
Lincoln, NE 68509-4986
Phone: (402) 471-4376
Fax: (402) 471-1066
Web site: http://www.hhs.state.ne.us/crl/nursing/nursingindex.htm

Nevada
Nevada State Board of Nursing
License Certification & Education
5011 Meadowood Mall #201
Reno, NV 89502-6547
Phone: (775) 688-2620
Fax: (775) 688-2628
Web site: http://www.nursingboard.state.nv.us/

New Hampshire
New Hampshire Board of Nursing
21 South Fruit Street
Suite 16
Concord, NH 03302-2341
Phone: (603) 271-2323
Fax: (603) 271-6605
Web site: http://www.state.nh.us/nursing/

New Jersey
New Jersey Board of Nursing
P.O. Box 45010
124 Halsey Street, 6th Floor
Newark, NJ 07101
Phone: (973) 504-6586
Fax: (973) 648-3481
Web site: http://www.state.nj.us/lps/ca/medical.htm

New Mexico
New Mexico Board of Nursing
6301 Indian School Road, NE
Suite 710
Albuquerque, NM 87109
Phone: (505) 841-8340
Fax: (505) 841-8347
Web site: http://www.state.nm.us/clients/nursing

New York
New York State Board of Nursing
Education Bldg.
89 Washington Avenue
2nd Floor, West Wing
Albany, NY 12234
Phone: (518) 474-3817, ext. 280
Fax: (518) 474-3706
Web site: http://www.nysed.gov/prof/nurse.htm

North Carolina
North Carolina Board of Nursing
3724 National Drive, Suite 201
Raleigh, NC 27602
Phone: (919) 782-3211
Fax: (919) 781-9461
Web site: http://www.ncbon.com/

North Dakota
North Dakota Board of Nursing
919 South 7th Street, Suite 504
Bismarck, ND 58504
Phone: (701) 328-9777
Fax: (701) 328-9785
Web site: http://www.ndbon.org/

Ohio
Ohio Board of Nursing
17 South High Street, Suite 400
Columbus, OH 43215-3413
Phone: (614) 466-3947
Fax: (614) 466-0388
Web site: http://www.nursing.ohio.gov/

Oklahoma
Oklahoma Board of Nursing
2915 N. Classen Blvd., Suite 524
Oklahoma City, OK 73106
Phone: (405) 962-1800
Fax: (405) 962-1821
Web Site: http://www.youroklahoma.com/nursing

Oregon
Oregon State Board of Nursing
800 NE Oregon Street, Box 25
Suite 465
Portland, OR 97232
Phone: (503) 731-4745
Fax: (503) 731-4755
Web site: http://www.osbn.state.or.us/

Pennsylvania
Pennsylvania State Board of Nursing
P.O. 2649
Harrisburg, PA 17105-2649
Phone: (717) 783-7142
Fax: (717) 783-0822
Web site: http://www.dos.state.pa.us/bpoa/cwp/view.asp?a = 1104&q = 432869

Puerto Rico
Commonwealth of Puerto Rico
Board of Nurse Examiners
800 Roberto H. Todd Ave.
Room 202, Stop 18
Santurce, PR 00908
Phone: (787) 725-7506
Fax: (787) 725-7903

Rhode Island
Rhode Island Board of Nurse Registration and Nursing Education
105 Cannon Building
Three Capitol Hill
Providence, RI 02908
Phone: (401) 222-5700
Fax: (401) 222-3352
Web site: http://www.healthri.gov/

South Carolina
South Carolina State Board of Nursing
110 Centerview Drive
Suite 202
Columbia, SC 29210
Phone: (803) 896-4550
Fax: (803) 896-4525
Web site: http://www.llr.state.sc.us/pol/nursing

South Dakota
South Dakota Board of Nursing
4305 South Louise Ave., Suite 201
Sioux Falls, SD 57106-3115
Phone: (605) 362-2760
Fax: (605) 362-2768
Web site: http://www.state.sd.us/dcr/nursing/

Tennessee
Tennessee State Board of Nursing
425 Fifth Avenue North
1st Floor—Cordell Hull Building
Nashville, TN 37247
Phone: (615) 532-5166
Fax: (615) 741-7899
Web site: http://www.tennessee.gov/health

Texas
Texas Board of Nurse Examiners
333 Guadalupe, Suite 3-460
Austin, TX 78701
Phone: (512) 305-7400
Fax: (512) 305-7401
Web site: http://www.bne.state.tx.us/

Utah
Utah State Board of Nursing
Heber M. Wells Bldg., 4th Floor
160 East 300 South
Salt Lake City, UT 84111
Phone: (801) 530-6628
Fax: (801) 530-6511
Web site: http://www.commerce.state.ut.us/

Vermont
Vermont State Board of Nursing
81 River Street
Heritage Building
Montpelier, VT 05609-1106
Phone: (802) 828-2396
Fax: (802) 828-2484
Web site: http://www.vtprofessionals.org/opr1/nurses/

Virgin Islands
Virgin Islands Board of Nurse Licensure
Veterans Drive Station
St. Thomas, VI 00803
Phone: (340) 776-7397
Fax: (340) 777-4003

Virginia
Virginia Board of Nursing
6603 West Broad Street
5th Floor
Richmond, VA 23230-1712
Phone: (804) 662-9909
Fax: (804) 662-9512
Web Site: http://www.dhp.virginia.gov/

Washington
Washington State Nursing Care Quality Assurance Commission
Department of Health
HPQA #6
310 Israel Rd. SE
Tumwater, WA 98501-7864
Phone: (360) 236-4700
Fax: (360) 236-4738
Web site: http://wws2.wa.gov/doh/hpqa-licensing/HP56/Nursing/default.htm

West Virginia
West Virginia Board of Examiners for Registered Professional Nurses
101 Dee Drive
Charleston, WV 25311
Phone: (304) 558-3596
Fax: (304) 558-3666
Web site: http://www.state.wv.us/nurses/rn/

Wisconsin
Wisconsin Department of Regulation and Licensing
1400 E. Washington Avenue RM 173
Madison, WI 53708
Phone: (608) 266-0145
Fax: (608) 261-7083
Web site: http://www.drl.state.wi.us/

Wyoming
Wyoming State Board of Nursing
2020 Carey Avenue, Suite 110
Cheyenne, WY 82002
Phone: (307) 777-7601
Fax: (307) 777-3519
Web site: http://nursing.state.wy.us/

NANDA nursing diagnoses

This list contains the 2005-2006 nursing diagnoses developed by the North American Nursing Diagnosis Association (NANDA). The diagnoses are classified alphabetically according to their domains.

Domain: Activity/Rest

- Activity intolerance
- Bathing or hygiene self-care deficit
- Decreased cardiac output
- Deficient diversional activity
- Delayed surgical recovery
- Disturbed energy field
- Disturbed sleep pattern
- Dressing or grooming self-care deficit
- Dysfunctional ventilatory weaning response
- Fatigue
- Feeding self-care deficit
- Impaired bed mobility
- Impaired physical mobility
- Impaired spontaneous ventilation
- Impaired transfer ability
- Impaired walking
- Impaired wheelchair mobility
- Ineffective breathing pattern
- Ineffective tissue perfusion (specify type: renal, cerebral, cardiopulmonary, gastrointestinal, peripheral)
- Readiness for enhanced sleep
- Risk for activity intolerance
- Risk for disuse syndrome
- Sedentary lifestyle
- Sleep deprivation
- Toileting self-care deficit

Domain: Comfort

- Acute pain
- Chronic pain
- Nausea
- Social isolation

Domain: Coping/Stress tolerance

- Anticipatory grieving
- Anxiety
- Autonomic dysreflexia
- Chronic sorrow
- Compromised family coping
- Death anxiety
- Decreased intracranial adaptive capacity
- Defensive coping
- Disabled family coping
- Disorganized infant behavior
- Dysfunctional grieving
- Fear
- Impaired adjustment
- Ineffective community coping
- Ineffective coping
- Ineffective denial
- Posttrauma syndrome
- Rape-trauma syndrome
- Rape-trauma syndrome: Compound reaction
- Rape-trauma syndrome: Silent reaction
- Readiness for enhanced community coping
- Readiness for enhanced coping
- Readiness for enhanced family coping
- Readiness for enhanced organized infant behavior
- Relocation stress syndrome
- Risk for autonomic dysreflexia
- Risk for disorganized infant behavior
- Risk for dysfunctional grieving
- Risk for posttrauma syndrome
- Risk for relocation stress syndrome

Domain: Elimination/Exchange

- Bowel incontinence
- Constipation
- Diarrhea
- Functional urinary incontinence
- Impaired gas exchange
- Impaired urinary elimination
- Perceived constipation
- Readiness for enhanced urinary elimination
- Reflex urinary incontinence
- Risk for constipation
- Risk for urge urinary incontinence
- Stress urinary incontinence
- Total urinary incontinence
- Urge urinary incontinence
- Urinary retention

Domain: Growth/Development

- Adult failure to thrive
- Delayed growth and development
- Risk for delayed development
- Risk for disproportionate growth

Domain: Health promotion

- Effective therapeutic regimen management
- Health-seeking behaviors (specify)
- Impaired home maintenance
- Ineffective community therapeutic regimen management
- Ineffective family therapeutic regimen management
- Ineffective health maintenance
- Ineffective therapeutic regimen management
- Readiness for enhanced management of therapeutic regimen
- Readiness for enhanced nutrition

Domain: Life principles

- Decisional conflict (specify)
- Impaired religiosity
- Noncompliance (specify)
- Readiness for enhanced religiosity
- Readiness for enhanced spiritual well-being
- Risk for impaired religiosity
- Risk for spiritual distress
- Spiritual distress

Domain: Nutrition

- Deficient fluid volume
- Excess fluid volume
- Imbalanced nutrition: Less than body requirements
- Imbalanced nutrition: More than body requirements
- Impaired swallowing
- Ineffective infant feeding pattern
- Readiness for enhanced fluid balance
- Risk for deficient fluid volume
- Risk for imbalanced fluid volume
- Risk for imbalanced nutrition: More than body requirements

Domain: Perception/Cognition

- Disturbed sensory perception (specify: visual, auditory, kinesthetic, gustatory, tactile, olfactory)
- Impaired environmental interpretation syndrome
- Impaired verbal communication
- Readiness for enhanced communication
- Unilateral neglect
- Wandering

Domain: Role relationships

- Caregiver role strain
- Dysfunctional family processes: Alcoholism
- Effective breast-feeding
- Impaired parenting
- Impaired social interaction
- Ineffective breast-feeding
- Ineffective role performance
- Interrupted breast-feeding
- Interrupted family processes
- Parental role conflict
- Readiness for enhanced family processes
- Readiness for enhanced parenting
- Risk for caregiver role strain
- Risk for impaired parent/infant/child attachment
- Risk for impaired parenting

Domain: Safety/Protection

- Hyperthermia
- Hypothermia
- Impaired dentition
- Impaired oral mucous membrane
- Impaired skin integrity
- Impaired tissue integrity
- Ineffective airway clearance

- Ineffective protection
- Ineffective thermoregulation
- Latex allergy response
- Risk for aspiration
- Risk for falls
- Risk for imbalanced body temperature
- Risk for impaired skin integrity
- Risk for infection
- Risk for injury
- Risk for latex allergy response
- Risk for other-directed violence
- Risk for perioperative-positioning injury
- Risk for peripheral neurovascular dysfunction
- Risk for poisoning
- Risk for self-directed violence
- Risk for self-mutilation
- Risk for sudden infant death syndrome
- Risk for suffocation
- Risk for suicide
- Risk for trauma
- Self-mutilation

Domain: Self-perception

- Chronic low self-esteem
- Disturbed body image
- Disturbed personal identity
- Hopelessness
- Powerlessness
- Readiness for enhanced self-concept
- Risk for loneliness
- Risk for powerlessness
- Risk for situational low self-esteem
- Situational low self-esteem

Domain: Sexuality

- Ineffective sexuality patterns
- Sexual dysfunction

Recommended childhood and adolescent immunization schedule United States, 2005

Vaccines are listed under routinely recommended ages. The bars below indicate range of recommended ages for immunization. Any doses not given at the recommended age should be given as a "catch-up" immunization at any subsequent visit when indicated and feasible. Ovals indicate vaccines to be given if previously recommended doses were missed or given earlier than the recommended minimum age.

	AGE											
VACCINE	BIRTH	1 MONTH	2 MONTHS	4 MONTHS	6 MONTHS	12 MONTHS	15 MONTHS	18 MONTHS	24 MONTHS	4 to 6 YEARS	11 to 12 YEARS	13 to 18 YEARS
Hepatitis B	Hep B #1											
			Hep B #2			Hep B #3					HepB Series	
Diptheria, tetanus, pertussis			DTaP	DTaP	DTaP			DTaP		DTaP	Td	Td
Haemophilus influenzae type b			Hib	Hib	Hib	Hib						
Inactivated poliovirus			IPV	IPV		IPV				IPV		
Measles, mumps, rubella						MMR #1				MMR#2	MMR#2	
Varicella							Varicella				Varicella	
Pneumococcal			PCV	PCV	PCV	PCV			PCV		PPV	
Influenza						Influenza (Yearly)					Influenza (Yearly)	
Vaccines below this line are for selected populations												
Hepatitis A											Hep A Series	

This schedule indicates the recommended ages for routine administration of currently licensed childhood vaccines, as of December 1, 2004, for children through age 18 years. Any dose not administered at the recommended age should be administered at any subsequent visit when indicated and feasible.

(Oval) Indicates age groups that warrant special effort to administer those vaccines not previously administered. Additional vaccines may be licensed and recommended during the year. Licensed combination vaccines may be used whenever any components of the combination are indicated and other components of the vaccine are not contraindicated.

Providers should consult the manufacturers' package inserts for detailed recommendations. Clinically significant adverse events that follow immunization should be reported to the Vaccine Adverse Event Reporting System (VAERS). Guidance about how to obtain and complete a VAERS form is available at *www.vaers.org* or by telephone, 800-822-7967.

- Range of recommended ages for immunization
- Preadolescent assessment
- Only if mother has HBsAg(−)
- Catch-up immunization

Centers for Disease Control and Prevention. Approved by the Advisory Committee on Immunization Practices, the American Academy of Pediatrics, and the American Academy of Family Physicians.

1. Hepatitis B (HepB) vaccine. All infants should receive the first dose of HepB vaccine soon after birth and before hospital discharge; the first dose may also be administered by age 2 months if the mother is hepatitis B surface antigen (HBsAg) negative. Only monovalent HepB may be used for the birth dose. Monovalent or combination vaccine containing HepB may be used to complete the series. Four doses of vaccine may be administered when a birth dose is given. The second dose should be administered at least 4 weeks after the first dose, except for combination vaccines which cannot be administered before age 6 weeks. The third dose should be given at least 16 weeks after the first dose and at least 8 weeks after the second dose. The last dose in the vaccination series (third or fourth dose) should not be administered before age 24 weeks.

Infants born to HBsAg-positive mothers should receive HepB and 0.5 ml of hepatitis B immune globulin (HBIG) at separate sites within 12 hours of birth. The second dose is recommended at age 1 to 2 months. The final dose in the immunization series should not be administered before age 24 weeks. These infants should be tested for HBsAg and antibody to HBsAg (anti-HBs) at age 9 to 15 months.

Infants born to mothers whose HBsAg status is unknown should receive the first dose of the HepB series within 12 hours of birth. Maternal blood should be drawn as soon as possible to determine the mother's HBsAg status; if the HbsAg test is positive, the infant should receive HBIG as soon as possible (no later than age 1 week). The second dose is recommended at age 1 to 2 months. The last dose in the immunization series should not be administered before age 24 weeks.

2. Diphtheria and tetanus toxoids and acellular pertussis (DTaP) vaccine. The fourth dose of DTaP may be administered as early as age 12 months, provided 6 months have elapsed since the third dose and the child is unlikely to return at age 15 to 18 months. The final dose in the series should be given at age ≥ 4 years. **Tetanus and diphtheria toxoids (Td)** is recommended at age 11 to 12 years if at least 5 years have elapsed since the last dose of tetanus and diphtheria toxoid-containing vaccine. Subsequent routine Td boosters are recommended every 10 years.

3. *Haemophilus influenzae* type b (Hib) conjugate vaccine. Three Hib conjugate vaccines are licensed for infant use. If PRP-OMP (PedvaxHIB® or ComVax® [Merck]) is administered at ages 2 and 4 months, a dose at age 6 months is not required. DTaP/Hib combination products should not be used for primary immunization in infants at ages 2, 4 or 6 months but can be used as boosters after any Hib vaccine. The final dose in the series should be administered at age ≥ 12 months.

4. Measles, mumps, and rubella vaccine (MMR). The second dose of MMR is recommended routinely at age 4 to 6 years but may be administered during any visit, provided at least 4 weeks have elapsed since the first dose and both doses are administered beginning at or after age 12 months. Those who have not previously received the second dose should complete the schedule by age 11 to 12 years.

5. Varicella vaccine. Varicella vaccine is recommended at any visit at or after age 12 months for susceptible children (i.e., those who lack a reliable history of chickenpox). Susceptible persons age ≥ 13 years should receive 2 doses administered at least 4 weeks apart.

6. Pneumococcal vaccine. The heptavalent pneumococcal conjugate vaccine (PCV) is recommended for all children aged 2 to 23 months and for certain children age 24 to 59 months. The final dose in the series should be given at age ≥ 12 months. **Pneumococcal polysaccharide vaccine (PPV)** is recommended in addition to PCV for certain high-risk groups. See *MMWR* 2000;49(RR-9):1-35.

7. Influenza vaccine. Influenza vaccine is recommended annually for children age ≥ 6 months with certain risk factors (including, but not limited to, asthma, cardiac disease, sickle cell disease, human immunodeficiency virus [HIV], and diabetes), healthcare workers, and other persons (including household members) in close contact with persons in groups at high risk (see *MMWR* 2004;53[RR-6]:1-40). In addition, healthy children age 6 to 23 months and close contacts of healthy children age 0 to 23 months are recommended to receive influenza vaccine because children in this age group are at substantially increased risk for influenza-related hospitalizations. For healthy persons age 5 to 49 years, the intranasally administered, live, attenuated influenza vaccine (LAIV) is an acceptable alternative to the intramuscular trivalent inactivated influenza vaccine (TIV). See *MMWR* 2004;53(RR-6):1-40. Children receiving TIV should be administered a dosage appropriate for their age (0.25 ml if age 6 to 35 months or 0.5 ml if age ≥ 3 years). Children age ≤ 8 years who are receiving influenza vaccine for the first time should receive 2 doses (separated by at least 4 weeks for TIV and at least 6 weeks for LAIV).

8. Hepatitis A vaccine. Hepatitis A vaccine is recommended for children and adolescents in selected states and regions and for certain high-risk groups; consult your local public health authority. Children and adolescents in these states, regions, and high-risk groups who have not been immunized against hepatitis A can begin the hepatitis A immunization series during any visit. The 2 doses in the series should be administered at least 6 months apart. See *MMWR* 1999;48(RR-12):1-37.

Common bacterial, fungal, and parasitic infections

This chart provides information about the characteristic signs and symptoms and nursing interventions for common bacterial, fungal, and parasitic infections.

CONDITION	SIGNS AND SYMPTOMS	NURSING CARE
Bacterial infection		
Impetigo contagiosa (from *Staphylococcus* or *Streptococcus*)	Red macule initially; vesicles that coalesce and rupture easily, leaving superficial moist lesion; spreads easily in sharply marginated but irregular lesions; exudate dries to form heavy, honey-colored crusts; pruritus	• Wash lesions 2 or 3 times daily with soap and water; stubborn crusts may require a compress of saline or diluted soap solutions. • Apply topical antibiotic ointment (mupirocin). • Administer systemic antibiotics (usually a penicillinase-resistant penicillin, cephalosporin, or erthyromycin)for 10 days.
Fungal infections		
Ringworm Tinea capitis (head)	Scalp pruritus, scaly patches, erythematous scaling patches that clear centrally and spread peripherally, scalp lesions (may spread to hairline and neck), temporary hair loss; usually contracted from household pets (puppies and kittens) or person to person	• Administer oral griseofulvin. • Administer ketoconazole for resistant cases. • Recommend frequent shampoos and haircuts.
Tinea corporis (body)	Lesions (same as those in tinea capitis); contracted from household pets	• Administer oral griseofulvin. • Apply tolnaftate ointment.
Tinea cruris (jock itch)	Skin response similar to that in tinea corporis; usually limited to crural fold and medial proximal thigh, but may involve scrotum	• Apply tolnaftate liquid locally. • Recommend wet compresses or sitz baths.
Tinea pedis (athlete's foot)	Pruritus, maceration, and fissures between toes; patches with pinhead-size vesicles on soles	• Administer oral griseofulvin. • Apply tolnaftate liquid or antifungal powder. • Apply compresses or soaks for 15 minutes, followed by steroid creams. • Tell the client to wear light-weight socks and well-ventilated shoes. • Advise the client not to wear the same shoes every day.

CONDITION	SIGNS AND SYMPTOMS	NURSING CARE
Parasitic infections		
Hookworm (GI, pulmonary)	Anemia, weight loss, pruritus, malnutrition, coughing, dyspnea	• Tell the client to avoid going barefoot and to wear gloves when gardening; tell a pediatric client not to play in the dirt. • Administer mebendazole, or albendozole. • Teach hygienic measures, as with pinworm and roundworm.
Pinworm (gastrointestinal)	Intense perianal and (in women and girls) perivaginal pruritus; occasionally causes appendicitis	• Perform a cellophane tape test: Press the tape's sticky side tightly over the perianal area; then seal the tape on a slide and view with a microscope to identify the presence of and type of worm. • Prevent the infection from spreading by: – decontaminating the client's bed linens and clothing by washing in hot water, using strong soap and chlorine bleach. – cutting the client's fingernails short. – teaching the client to wash hands on arising and after toileting. – administering piperazine, pyrantel, mebendazole, or albendozole as ordered. • Treat other family members.
Pediculosis (lice) Capitis	Severe scalp pruritus, white eggs (nits) firmly attached to hair (visible upon close examination of scalp); excoriation on scalp may develop into secondary infection; children with long hair are more frequently affected	• Wear gloves and protective cap during examination and treatment. • Apply pyrethrins solution or permethrin cream. • Rinse hair and comb it with a fine-tooth comb dipped in vinegar to remove nits. • Decontaminate clothing and bed linen, as with pinworm and roundworm. • Have the client bathe with soap and water to remove lice from the body.
Corporis	Pruritus; erythematous macules, wheals, and excoriated patches (usually found on the upper back and pressure areas from tight clothing)	• Thoroughly launder clothing and bed linen in hot water; ironing and dry cleaning are also effective. • Administer lindane cream in severe cases.
Roundworm (GI, pulmonary)	Anorexia, enlarged belly, weight loss, fever, intestinal colic; may progress to intestinal obstruction, appendicitis, perforation, obstructive jaundice, pneumonitis	• Teach the client hygienic measures, as with pinworm. Reinfection is common. • Administer pyrantel or piperazine. • Collect stool specimens and keep them warm to test for ova and parasites.

Drug administration rights, calculations, and equivalents

Drug administration rights

When administering any drug, remember to use the five rights:

1. right client
2. right drug
3. right dose
4. right route
5. right time.

Basic calculations

To calculate the number of doses in a specified amount of medicine:

$$\text{Number of doses} = \frac{\text{Total amount}}{\text{Size of dose}}$$

To calculate the size of each dose, using a specified amount of medication and the number of doses it contains:

$$\text{Size of dose} = \frac{\text{Total amount}}{\text{Number of doses}}$$

To calculate the amount of a medicine, using the number of doses it contains and the size of each dose:

$$\text{Total amount} = \text{Number of doses} \times \text{Size of dose}$$

Short formula for determining rate of I.V. solution infusion:

$$\frac{\text{Volume of solution}}{\text{Time interval in minutes} \times \text{Drop factor}} = \text{Drops/minute}$$

Dimensional analysis

Dimensional analysis (also known as *factor analysis* or *factor labeling*) is an alternative method of solving mathematical problems. It eliminates the need to memorize formulas and requires only one equation to determine an answer. To compare the ratio-and-proportion method and dimensional analysis at a glance, read the following problem and solutions.

The doctor prescribes 0.25 g streptomycin sulfate I.M. The vial reads 2 ml = 1 g. How many milliliters should you administer?

Dimensional analysis

$$\frac{0.25\text{ g}}{1} \times \frac{2\text{ ml}}{1\text{ g}} = 0.5\text{ ml}$$

Ratio and proportion

$$1\text{ g} : 2\text{ ml} :: 0.25\text{ g} : X$$

$$2\text{ ml} \times 0.25\text{ g} = 1\text{ g} \times X$$

$$\frac{2\text{ ml} \times 0.25\cancel{\text{g}}}{1\cancel{\text{g}}} = X$$

$$0.5\text{ ml} = X$$

When using dimensional analysis, the problem solver arranges a series of ratios, called *factors,* in a single fractional equation. Each factor, written as a fraction, consists of two quantities and their units of measurement that are related to each other in a given problem. For instance, if 1,000 ml of a drug should be administered over 8 hours, the relationship between 1,000 ml and 8 hours is expressed by the fraction:

$$\frac{1{,}000 \text{ ml}}{8 \text{ hours}}$$

When a problem includes a quantity and its unit of measurement that are unrelated to any other factor in the problem, they serve as the numerator of the fraction, and 1 (implied) becomes the denominator.

Some mathematical problems contain all of the information needed to identify the factors, set up the equation, and find the solution. Other problems require the use of a conversion factor. Conversion factors are equivalents (for example, 1 g = 1,000 mg) that the nurse can memorize or obtain from a conversion chart. Because the two quantities and units of measurement are equivalent, they can serve as the numerator or the denominator; thus, the conversion factor 1 g = 1,000 mg can be written in fraction form as:

$$\frac{1{,}000 \text{ mg}}{1 \text{ g}} \text{ or } \frac{1 \text{ g}}{1{,}000 \text{ mg}}$$

The factors given in the problem plus any conversion factors necessary to solve the problem are called *knowns.* The quantity of the answer, of course, is *unknown.* When setting up an equation in dimensional analysis, work backward, beginning with the unit of measurement of the answer. After plotting all the knowns, find the solution by following this sequence:

1. Cancel similar quantities and units of measurement.
2. Multiply the numerators.
3. Multiply the denominators.
4. Divide the numerator by the denominator.

Mastering dimensional analysis can take practice, but you may find your efforts well rewarded. To understand more fully how dimensional analysis works, review the following problem and the steps taken to solve it.

The doctor prescribes X grains (gr) of a drug. The pharmacy supplies the drug in 300-mg tablets (tab). How many tablets should you administer?

1. Write down the unit of measurement of the answer, followed by an "equal to" symbol (=).

$$\text{tab} =$$

2. Search the problem for the quantity with the same unit of measurement (if one doesn't exist, use a conversion factor); place this in the numerator and its related quantity and unit of measurement in the denominator.

$$\text{tab} = \frac{1 \text{ tab}}{300 \text{ mg}}$$

3. Separate the first factor from the next with a multiplication symbol (×).

$$\text{tab} = \frac{1 \text{ tab}}{300 \text{ mg}} \times$$

4. Place the unit of measurement of the denominator of the first factor in the numerator of the second factor. Search the problem for the quantity with the same unit of measurement. (If one doesn't exist, as in this example, use a conversion factor.) Place this number in the numerator and its related quantity and unit of measurement in the denominator; and follow with a multiplication symbol. Repeat this step until all known factors are included in the equation.

$$\text{tab} = \frac{1 \text{ tab}}{300 \text{ mg}} \times \frac{60 \text{ mg}}{1 \text{ gr}} \times \frac{10 \text{ gr}}{1}$$

Alternatively, you can treat the equation as a large fraction, using these steps:

1. First, cancel similar units of measurement in the numerator and the denominator (what remains should be what you began with — the unit of measurement of the answer; if not, recheck your equation to find and correct the error).
2. Multiply the numerators and then the denominators.
3. Divide the numerator by the denominator.

$$\text{tab} = \frac{1 \text{ tab}}{300 \cancel{\text{mg}}} \times \frac{60 \cancel{\text{mg}}}{1 \cancel{\text{gr}}} \times \frac{10 \cancel{\text{gr}}}{1}$$

$$= \frac{60 \times 10 \text{ tab}}{300}$$

$$= \frac{600 \text{ tab}}{300}$$

$$= 2 \text{ tablets}$$

Equivalents

Metric weight equivalents	Conversions	Metric volume equivalents
1 kg = 1,000 g	1 oz = 30 g	1 L = 1,000 ml
1 g = 1,000 mg	1 lb = 453.6 g	1 dl = 100 ml
1 mg = 0.001 g	2.2 lb = 1 kg	
1 mcg or µg = 0.001 mg		

Liquid measures

Household		Apothecaries'		Metric
1 tsp	=	1 fluid dram	=	4 or 5 ml
1 tbs	=	4 fluid drams	=	15 or 16 ml
2 tbs	=	1 fl oz	=	30 ml
1 cup	=	8 fl oz	=	240 ml
1 pt	=	16 fl oz	=	500 ml
1 qt	=	32 fl oz	=	1,000 ml

Although the fluid dram is about 4 ml, in prescriptions it's considered equivalent to the teaspoon (which is 5 ml).

Temperature conversion

Celsius to Fahrenheit	Fahrenheit to Celsius
(° C × 9/5) + 32 = ° F	(° F – 32) × 5/9 = ° C

Common drug prototypes

This chart is a general review of some of the more common drug classes. Each drug class is presented with a prototype drug, actions, indications, and nursing considerations. This chart should be used only for a review; a drug handbook should be used for more in-depth information about the medications.

CLASSIFICATION	PROTOTYPE	ACTIONS	INDICATIONS	NURSING CONSIDERATIONS
Alkylating agent	cisplatin	Probably cross-links strands of cellular deoxyribonucleic acid (DNA) and interferes with ribonucleic acid (RNA) transcription, causing growth imbalance that leads to cell death; kills selected cancer cells	◆ Adjunct therapy in metastatic testicular and ovarian cancer ◆ Advanced bladder and esophageal cancer ◆ Head, neck, and cervical cancers ◆ Non–small cell lung cancer ◆ Brain tumor ◆ Osteogenic sarcoma or neuroblastoma	◆ Monitor for adverse reactions, such as peripheral neuritis, seizures, tinnitus, hearing loss, nausea and vomiting, severe renal toxicity, myelosuppression, leukopenia, thrombocytopenia, anemia, and anaphylactoid reaction. ◆ Assess the underlying neoplastic disease before therapy, and reassess regularly throughout therapy.
Alpha-adrenergic blocker	prazosin	Inhibits alpha-adrenergic receptors, causing arterial and venous dilation, which reduces peripheral vascular resistance	◆ Mild to moderate hypertension	◆ Monitor for adverse reactions, such as dizziness, first-dose syncope, palpitations, or nausea. ◆ Monitor pulse rate and blood pressure frequently. ◆ Advise the client to arise slowly and to avoid abrupt position changes.

CLASSIFICATION	PROTOTYPE	ACTIONS	INDICATIONS	NURSING CONSIDERATIONS
Aminoglycoside	gentamicin	Inhibits protein synthesis by binding directly to the 30S ribosomal subunit; usually bactericidal	◆ Serious infections caused by susceptible organisms ◆ Endocarditis prophylaxis for GI and genitourinary procedures or surgery	◆ Monitor for adverse reactions, such as seizures, ototoxicity, nephrotoxicity, apnea, anaphylaxis, leukopenia, thrombocytopenia, and agranulocytosis. ◆ Obtain peak gentamicin level 1 hour after I.M. injection or 30 minutes after I.V. infusion; check trough levels prior to next dose.
Angiotensin-converting enzyme inhibitor	captopril	Prevents the conversion of angiotensin I to angiotensin II; decreases vasoconstriction, reducing peripheral arterial resistance; causes inhibition of angiotensin II and decreases adrenocortical secretion of aldosterone; results in decreased sodium and water retention and extracellular fluid volume	◆ Hypertension ◆ Management of symptomatic heart failure	◆ Monitor for adverse reactions, such as hypotension, dry cough, and angioedema. ◆ Monitor serum potassium levels and complete blood count with differential.
Angiotensin II receptor blocker	losartan	Inhibits vasoconstricting and aldosterone-secreting effects of angiotensin II by selectively blocking binding of angiotensin II to receptor sites in many tissues, including vascular smooth muscle and adrenal glands	◆ Reduction of blood pressure	◆ Monitor blood pressure before therapy and regularly thereafter. ◆ Regularly assess the client's kidney function (creatinine and blood urea nitrogen [BUN] levels).

CLASSIFICATION	PROTOTYPE	ACTIONS	INDICATIONS	NURSING CONSIDERATIONS
Antacids	aluminum hydroxide	Reduces total acid load in the GI tract; elevates gastric pH to reduce pepsin activity; strengthens the gastric mucosal barrier; increases esophageal sphincter tone	◆ Relief of GI discomfort	◆ When administering through a nasogastric (NG) tube, make sure that the tube is patent and placed correctly; after instilling, flush the tube with water to ensure passage to the stomach and to clear the tube. ◆ Don't give other oral drugs within 2 hours of antacid administration because antacids may cause premature release of enteric-coated drugs in the stomach.
Antiarrhythmic (class 1A)	quinidine gluconate	Causes direct and indirect effects on cardiac tissue; decreases automaticity, conduction velocity, and membrane responsiveness; prolongs effective refractory period; reduces vagal tone	◆ Atrial fibrillation and flutter ◆ Atrial tachycardia; premature atrial and ventricular contractions ◆ Paroxysmal supra ventricular tachycardia	◆ Monitor for adverse reactions, such as vertigo, headache, arrhythmias, hypotension, heart failure, tinnitus, diarrhea, nausea, vomiting, hematologic disorders, hepatotoxicity, respiratory arrest, angioedema, fever, and cinchonism. ◆ Monitor pulse and blood pressure frequently. ◆ Administer anticoagulants before treatment, if ordered.
Antiarrhythmic (class 1B)	lidocaine	Decreases depolarization, automaticity, and excitability in the ventricles during the diastole phase by direct action on the tissues (especially the Purkinje network)	◆ Ventricular arrhythmias	◆ Monitor for adverse reactions, such as confusion, tremor, restlessness, seizures, hypotension, new arrhythmias, cardiac arrest, tinnitus, blurred vision, respiratory depression, and anaphylaxis. ◆ Monitor serum lidocaine levels for toxicity. ◆ Monitor electrolytes, BUN, and creatinine levels.

CLASSIFICATION	PROTOTYPE	ACTIONS	INDICATIONS	NURSING CONSIDERATIONS
Antiarrhythmic (class 1C)	propafenone	Reduces inward sodium current in Purkinje and myocardial cells; decreases excitability, conduction, velocity, and automaticity in atrioventricular (AV) nodal, His-Purkinje, and intraventricular tissues; prolongs refractory period in AV nodal tissue	◆ Ventricular arrhythmias	◆ Notify prescriber if QRS complex widens by more than 20%. ◆ During use with digoxin, monitor ECG and digoxin levels frequently.
Antiarrhythmic (class III)	amiodarone	Thought to prolong refractory period and duration of action and decrease depolarization	◆ Life-threatening ventricular arrhythmias ◆ Suppression of supraventricular tachycardia	◆ Monitor liver function studies and pulmonary function studies. ◆ Monitor for impaired vision. ◆ Administer oral loading dose in three equal doses, and give with meals. ◆ If giving I.V., monitor cardiac function closely and keep resuscitation equipment available.
Antibiotic antineoplastic	doxorubicin hydrochloride	Thought to interfere with DNA-dependent RNA synthesis by intercalation (chemical effect unknown); hinders or kills certain cancer cells	◆ Bladder, breast, lung, ovarian, stomach, testicular, and thyroid cancers ◆ Hodgkin's disease ◆ Acute lymphoblastic and myeloblastic leukemia ◆ Wilms' tumor ◆ Neuroblastoma, lymphoma, and sarcoma	◆ Monitor for adverse reactions, such as arrhythmias, leukopenia, thrombocytopenia, myelosuppression, alopecia, and anaphylaxis. ◆ Assess the underlying neoplastic disease before therapy, and reassess regularly throughout therapy. ◆ Follow facility policy for reconstitution and administration.

CLASSIFICATION	PROTOTYPE	ACTIONS	INDICATIONS	NURSING CONSIDERATIONS
Anticholinergic	atropine	Antagonizes actions of acetylcholine and other cholinergic agonists at muscarinic and nicotinic receptors within the parasympathetic nervous system and smooth muscles that lack cholinergic innervation	◆ Symptomatic bradycardia ◆ Given preoperatively to diminish secretions and block cardiac vagal reflexes ◆ Adjunct treatment for peptic ulcer disease; treatment for functional GI disorders	◆ Monitor for adverse reactions, such as headache, restlessness, insomnia, urine retention, urinary hesitancy, dizziness, blurred vision, dry mouth, constipation, anaphylaxis, and urticara. ◆ Recommend monitoring the client's vital signs, urine output, and vision, and for signs of impending toxicity. ◆ Constipation may be relieved by stool softeners or bulk laxatives.
Anticoagulant	heparin and heparin derivatives	Accelerates formation of antithrombin III–thrombin complex and deactivates thrombin; prevents conversion of fibrinogen to fibrin	◆ Treatment for deep vein thrombosis (DVT), myocardial infarction (MI), pulmonary embolism, and consumption coagulopathy ◆ Prevention of DVT and pulmonary embolism	◆ Monitor for adverse reactions, such as hemorrhage, prolonged clotting time, thrombocytopenia, and hypersensitivity reactions. ◆ Regularly inspect the client for bleeding gums, bruises, petechiae, epistaxis, tarry stools, hematuria, and hematemesis. ◆ Effects can be neutralized by protamine sulfate. ◆ Monitor partial thromboplastin time regularly.
	warfarin	Inhibits vitamin K–dependent activation of clotting factors II, VII, IX, and X formed in the liver	◆ Prevention of pulmonary embolism caused by DVT, MI, rheumatic fever, prosthetic heart valves, or chronic atrial fibrillation	◆ Monitor for adverse reactions, such as hemorrhage, prolonged clotting time, rash, fever, diarrhea, and hepatitis. ◆ Regularly inspect the client for bleeding gums, bruises, petechiae, epistaxis, tarry stools, hematuria, and hematemesis. ◆ Monitor prothrombin time regularly. ◆ Adminster vitamin K to neutralize effects of drug, if ordered.

CLASSIFICATION	PROTOTYPE	ACTIONS	INDICATIONS	NURSING CONSIDERATIONS
Anticonvulsant	phenytoin	Stabilizes neuronal membranes and limits seizure activity by either increasing efflux or decreasing influx of sodium ions across cell membranes in the motor cortex during generation of nerve impulses	◆ Control of tonic-clonic and complex partial seizures ◆ Status epilepticus ◆ Prevention of and treatment for seizures during neurosurgery	◆ Monitor for adverse reactions, such as ataxia, slurred speech, mental confusion, nystagmus, blurred vision, gingival hyperplasia, nausea, vomiting, hematologic disorders, hepatitis, Stevens-Johnson syndrome, and hirsutism. ◆ Don't withdraw suddenly; seizures may occur. ◆ Monitor drug levels as ordered; therapeutic levels range from 10 to 20 μg/ml.
Antidiarrheal	loperamide	Inhibits peristaltic activity, prolonging transit of intestinal contents	◆ Diarrhea	◆ Monitor the drug's effect on bowel movements. ◆ If giving by NG tube, flush the tube to clear it and to ensure the drug's passage to the stomach. ◆ Check dosage carefully because oral liquids are available in different concentrations. ◆ For children, consider an oral liquid that doesn't contain alcohol.
Antihistamine	diphenhydramine	Competes with histamine for H_1-receptor sites on the smooth muscle of the bronchi, GI tract, uterus, and large blood vessels, binding to the cellular receptors and preventing access and subsequent activity of histamine; doesn't directly alter histamine or prevent its release; antagonizes the action of histamine that causes increased capillary permeability and resultant edema and suppresses flare and pruritus associated with the endogenous release of histamine	◆ Rhinitis ◆ Allergy symptoms ◆ Motion sickness ◆ Parkinson's disease	◆ Monitor for adverse reactions, such as drowsiness, sedation, seizures, nausea, dry mouth, thrombocytopenia, agranulocytosis, thickening of secretions, and anaphylactic shock. ◆ Use with extreme caution in clients with prostatic hyperplasia, asthma, chronic obstructive pulmonary disease, hyperthyroidism, cardiovascular disease, and hypertension.

CLASSIFICATION	PROTOTYPE	ACTIONS	INDICATIONS	NURSING CONSIDERATIONS
Antilipemic	atorvastatin	Inhibits 3-hydroxy-3-methylglutaryl-coenzyme A reductase, an early (and rate-limiting) step in cholesterol biosynthesis	◆ Treatment for various dyslipidemias	◆ Monitor for adverse reactions, such as headache and muscle aches. ◆ Monitor lipid profile and liver enzymes periodically.
Antimetabolite	methotrexate	Prevents the reduction of folic acid to tetrahydrofolate by binding to dihydrofolate reductase; kills certain cancer cells and reduces inflammation	◆ Trophobalstic tumors (choriocarcinoma, hydatiform mole) ◆ Acute lymphoblastic and lymphatic leukemia; meningeal leukemia ◆ Burkitt's lymphoma (stage I or stage II) ◆ Lymphosarcoma (stage III) ◆ Osteosarcoma	◆ Monitor for adverse reactions, such as stomatitis, diarrhea, intestinal perforation, nausea, vomiting, renal failure, anemia, leukopenia, thrombocytopenia, acute hepatic toxicity, pulmonary fibrosis, urticaria, and sudden death. ◆ Assess the underlying neoplastic disease before therapy, and reassess regularly throughout therapy. ◆ Follow facility policy for reconstitution and administration.
Antiparkinsonian	carbidopa-levodopa	Converts to dopamine in the CNS; increases dopamine levels in the brain (levodopa); inhibits peripheral decarboxylation of levodopa without affecting its metabolism within CNS, leaving more to be decarboxylated to dopamine in the brain (carbidopa)	◆ Parkinson's disease ◆ Symptomatic parkinsonism resulting from carbon monoxide or manganese toxicity	◆ Monitor for adverse reactions, such as choreiform, dystonic, dyskinetic movements; involuntary grimacing; head movements; myoclonic jerks; ataxia; suicidal tendencies; hypotension; dry mouth; nausea; vomiting; hematologic disorders; and hepatotoxicity. ◆ Withhold the dose and notify the prescriber if the client's vital signs or mental status change significantly. A reduced dosage or discontinuation may be necessary. ◆ Advise clients on long-term therapy of the need for testing for acromegaly and diabetes.

CLASSIFICATION	PROTOTYPE	ACTIONS	INDICATIONS	NURSING CONSIDERATIONS
Antitubercular	isoniazid	Appears to inhibit cell-wall biosynthesis by interfering with lipid and deoxyribonucleic acid (DNA) synthesis	◆ Tuberculosis	◆ Monitor for adverse reactions, such as peripheral neuropathy, seizures, hematologic disorders, hepatitis, and hypersensitivity reactions. ◆ Always give with other antituberculotics to prevent development of resistant organisms.
Antiviral	acyclovir	Interferes with DNA synthesis and inhibits viral multiplication	◆ Treatment for herpes simplex viruses types 1 and 2; varicella	◆ Monitor for adverse reactions, such as malaise, headache, encephalopathy, renal failure, thrombocytopenia, and pain at injection site.
Barbiturate	phenobarbital	Induces imbalance in central inhibitory and facilitatory mechanisms, which influence cerebral cortex and reticular formation; decreases presynaptic and postsynaptic membrane excitability; exact mechanism of action unknown, and which cellular and synaptic actions result in sedative-hypnotic effects not clear; produces all levels of CNS depression (mild sedation to coma to death); exerts its effect by facilitating the actions of gamma-aminobutyric acid (GABA); exerts a central effect, which depresses respiration and GI motility; has no analgesic action but may increase the reaction to painful stimuli at subanesthetic doses; reduces nerve transmission and decreases excitability of the nerve cell as its principal anticonvulsant mechanism of action; raises the seizure threshold	◆ Epilepsy ◆ Febrile seizures ◆ Sedation	◆ Monitor for adverse reactions, such as drowsiness, lethargy, hangover, respiratory depression, apnea, Stevens-Johnson syndrome, and angioedema. ◆ Don't withdraw abruptly because seizures may worsen. ◆ Watch for signs of toxicity: coma, asthmatic breathing, cyanosis and clammy skin.

CLASSIFICATION	PROTOTYPE	ACTIONS	INDICATIONS	NURSING CONSIDERATIONS
Benzodiazepine	alprazolam	Sites and mechanisms of action unknown; enhances or facilitates the action of GABA, an inhibitory neurotransmitter in the CNS; acts at the limbic, thalamic, and hypothalamic levels of the CNS; produces anxiolytic, sedative, hypnotic, skeletal muscle relaxant, and anticonvulsant effects; CNS-depressant activities; individual derivatives act more selectively at specific sites, allowing them to be subclassified into five categories based on their predominant clinical use	◆ Anxiety ◆ Panic disorders	◆ Monitor for adverse reactions, such as drowsiness, lightheadedness, depression, dry mouth, diarrhea, and constipation. ◆ Drug isn't recommended for long-term use. ◆ Don't withdraw abruptly because seizures may occur.
Beta-adrenergic blocker	metoprolol	Competes with beta agonists for available beta-receptor sites	◆ Hypertension ◆ Angina pectoris	◆ Monitor for adverse reactions, such as fatigue, dizziness, bradycardia, hypotension, heart failure, and AV block. ◆ Withhold the drug if apical pulse is less than 60 beats/minute, as ordered. ◆ Monitor blood pressure frequently.
Bulk-forming laxative	psyllium	Absorbs water and expands to increase bulk and moisture content of stool, thus encouraging peristalsis and bowel movements	◆ Constipation	◆ Mix the drug with at least 8 oz (240 ml) of cold liquid, such as orange juice, to mask grittiness. Stir only a few seconds. Have the client drink the mixture immediately, before it congeals. Follow administration with another glass of liquid. ◆ Note that psyllium may reduce the client's appetite if taken before meals. ◆ Advise the client with diabetes to check the drug's label and to use a brand that doesn't contain sugar.

CLASSIFICATION	PROTOTYPE	ACTIONS	INDICATIONS	NURSING CONSIDERATIONS
Calcium channel blocker	verapamil	Inhibits calcium influx across the slow channels of myocardial and vascular smooth muscle cells; reduces intracellular calcium concentrations; dilates coronary arteries, peripheral arteries, and arterioles, and slows cardiac conduction	◆ Vasospasm angina ◆ Hypertension ◆ Supraventricular arrhythmias	◆ Monitor for adverse reactions, such as hypotension, heart failure, constipation, and ventricular asystole or fibrillation. ◆ Monitor cardiac rhythm and blood pressure during the start of therapy and with dose adjustments.
Cardiac glycoside	digoxin	Inhibits sodium potassium-activated adenosine triphosphate; promotes movement of calcium from extracellular to intracellular cytoplasm and strengthens myocardial contraction; acts on CNS to enhance vagal tone, slowing contraction through the sinoatrial and AV nodes and providing an anti-arrhythmic effect	◆ Heart failure ◆ Atrial fibrillation and flutter ◆ Supraventricular tachycardia	◆ Monitor for adverse reactions, such as fatigue, agitation, hallucinations, arrhythmias, anorexia, and nausea. ◆ Withhold drug if apical pulse is less than 60 beats/minute, as ordered. ◆ Monitor serum potassium and digoxin levels periodically.
Centrally acting sympatholytic	clonidine	Inhibits central vasomotor centers, decreasing sympathetic outflow to the heart, kidneys, and peripheral vasculature; decreases peripheral vascular resistance; decreases systolic and diastolic blood pressure; decreases heart rate	◆ Reduction of blood pressure	◆ Advise the client that the drug will need to be adjusted according to blood pressure and tolerance. ◆ When stopping therapy in a client receiving clonidine and a beta-adrenergic blocker, gradually withdraw the beta-adrenergic blocker first to minimize adverse reactions. ◆ Note that clonidine isn't generally discontinued for surgery.

CLASSIFICATION	PROTOTYPE	ACTIONS	INDICATIONS	NURSING CONSIDERATIONS
Cephalosporin (first-generation)	cefazolin	Inhibits cell wall synthesis, promoting osmotic instability; usually bactericidal	◆ Infection caused by susceptible organisms	◆ Monitor for adverse reactions, such as diarrhea, hematologic disorders, rash, and hypersensitivity reactions. ◆ With large doses or prolonged treatment, monitor for superinfections. ◆ Obtain specimen for culture and sensitivity before first dose; therapy may begin before results.
Corticosteroid	prednisone	Decreases inflammation; stabilizes leukocyte lysosomal membranes; suppresses immune response; stimulates bone marrow; and influences protein, fat, and carbohydrate metabolism	◆ Severe inflammation, immunosuppression	◆ Monitor for adverse reactions, such as euphoria, insomnia, seizures, heart failure, arrhythmias, thromboembolism, peptic ulcers, pancreatitis, and acute adrenal insufficiency. ◆ Monitor the client's weight, blood pressure, and serum electrolyte levels. ◆ Note that prednisone may mask signs of infection. ◆ Keep in mind that the dose must be gradually reduced after long-term therapy.
Diuretic, loop	furosemide	Inhibits sodium and chloride reabsorption in the ascending loop of Henle, thus increasing renal excretion of sodium, chloride, and water; like thiazide diuretics, increases excretion of potassium; produces greater maximum diuresis and electrolyte loss than a thiazide diuretic	◆ Acute pulmonary edema ◆ Edema ◆ Hypertension	◆ Monitor for adverse reactions, such as pancreatitis, hematologic disorders, and electrolyte imbalances (especially hypokalemia). ◆ Monitor weight and blood pressure frequently. ◆ Monitor for signs of hypokalemia, including leg cramps and muscle aches.

CLASSIFICATION	PROTOTYPE	ACTIONS	INDICATIONS	NURSING CONSIDERATIONS
Diuretic, thiazide	hydrochlorothiazide	Interferes with sodium transport across tubules of the cortical diluting segment of the nephron; increases renal excretion of sodium, chloride, water, potassium, and calcium; increases bicarbonate, magnesium, phosphate, bromide, and iodide excretion; decreases excretion of ammonia, causing increased serum ammonia levels	◆ Edema ◆ Hypertension	◆ Monitor for adverse reactions, such as pancreatitis, hematologic disorders, and electrolyte imbalances (especially hypokalemia). ◆ Monitor weight and blood pressure frequently. ◆ Monitor for signs of hypokalemia, including leg cramps and muscle aches.
Emollient laxative	docusate	Reduces surface tension of interfacing liquid contents of the bowel, promoting incorporation of additional liquid into stool, thus forming a softer mass	◆ Stool softener for clients who should avoid straining during a bowel movement	◆ Monitor the drug's effect on bowel movements. ◆ Discontinue the drug and notify the prescriber if abdominal cramping occurs.
Estrogen	conjugated estrogenic substances	Increases synthesis of DNA, RNA, and protein in responsive tissues; reduces release of follicle-stimulating hormone and luteinizing hormone from the pituitary gland	◆ Abnormal uterine bleeding ◆ Palliative treatment of breast cancer at least 5 years after menopause ◆ Female castration ◆ Primary ovarian failure ◆ Osteoporosis ◆ Hypogonadism ◆ Vasomotor menopausal symptoms ◆ Atrophic vaginitis, kraurosis vulvae, vulvar and vaginal atrophy ◆ Palliative treatment of inoperable prostate cancer	◆ Monitor lipid levels, liver function tests, blood pressure, and body weight. ◆ Withhold the drug if a thromboembolic event is suspected.

CLASSIFICATION	PROTOTYPE	ACTIONS	INDICATIONS	NURSING CONSIDERATIONS
Histamine-2 receptor antagonist	famotidine	Inhibits histamine's action at H_2 receptors in gastric parietal cells; reduces gastric acid output and concentration regardless of the stimulatory agent (histamine, food, insulin, caffeine, betazole, pentagastrin) or basal conditions	◆ Gastroesophageal reflux disease ◆ Zollinger-Ellison syndrome ◆ Duodenal ulcer ◆ Gastric ulcer ◆ Heartburn	◆ Monitor for adverse reactions such as headache. ◆ Monitor for signs of GI bleeding such as blood in the stool.
Hypoglycemic agent	glyburide	Stimulates insulin release from the pancreatic beta cells and reduces glucose output by the liver; extrapancreatic effect increases peripheral sensitivity to insulin and causes a mild diuretic effect	◆ Type 2 diabetes mellitus	◆ Monitor for adverse reactions, such as hypoglycemia, angioedema, and hematologic disorders. ◆ During times of stress, clients may need insulin. Monitor for signs of hypoglycemia.
	insulin	Increases glucose transport across muscle and fat cell membranes to reduce blood glucose levels; promotes conversion of glucose to its storage form, glycogen; triggers amino acid uptake and conversion to protein in muscle cells and inhibits protein degradation; stimulates triglyceride formation and inhibits release of free fatty acids from adipose tissue; stimulates lipoprotein lipase activity, which converts circulating lipoproteins to fatty acids	◆ Type 1 diabetes mellitus ◆ Adjunct treatment in type 2 diabetes mellitus ◆ Diabetic ketoacidosis	◆ Monitor for adverse reactions, such as hypoglycemia and hypersensitivity reactions.

CLASSIFICATION	PROTOTYPE	ACTIONS	INDICATIONS	NURSING CONSIDERATIONS
Leukotriene modifier	zafirlukast	Selectively competes for leukotriene receptor sites, blocking inflammatory action	◆ Prophylaxis and long-term management of asthma	◆ Note that this drug isn't indicated for reversing bronchospasm in acute asthma attacks. ◆ Give cautiously to elderly clients and those with hepatic impairment. ◆ Drug absorption is decreased by food; give drug 1 hour before or 2 hours after meals. ◆ Monitor liver function studies in clients with suspected hepatic dysfunction. This drug may need to be discontinued if hepatic dysfunction is confirmed.
Lubricant laxative	mineral oil	Increases water retention in stool by creating a barrier between the colon wall and feces that prevents colonic reabsorption of fecal water	◆ Constipation	◆ Monitor the drug's effect on bowel movements. ◆ Give the drug on an empty stomach. ◆ Give the drug with fruit juice or a carbonated drink to disguise its taste.
Natural penicillin	penicillin G sodium	Inhibits cell wall synthesis during microorganism multiplication; resists penicillinase enzymes produced by bacteria that convert penicillin to inactive penicillic acid	◆ Bacterial infection caused by non-penicillinase-producing strains of gram-positive and gram-negative aerobic cocci, spirochetes, or certain gram-positive aerobic and anaerobic bacilli	◆ Monitor the client for adverse reactions, such as seizures, anaphylaxis, leukopenia, and thrombocytopenia. ◆ Obtain a specimen for culture and sensitivity tests before giving the first dose. Therapy may begin pending results.
Nitrate	nitroglycerin	Relaxes vascular smooth muscle; causes generalized vasodilation	◆ Acute or chronic anginal attacks	◆ Monitor for adverse reactions, such as headache, dizziness, orthostatic hypotension, tachycardia, flushing, palpitations, and hypersensitivity reactions. ◆ Monitor vital signs closely. ◆ Treat headaches with acetaminophen or aspirin.

CLASSIFICATION	PROTOTYPE	ACTIONS	INDICATIONS	NURSING CONSIDERATIONS
Nonsteroidal anti-inflammatory drug (NSAID)	ibuprofen	Interferes with the prostaglandins involved in pain; appears to sensitize pain receptors to mechanical stimulation or other chemical mediators (such as bradykinin and histamine); inhibits synthesis of prostaglandins peripherally and, possibly, centrally; inhibits prostaglandin synthesis and release during inflammation; antipyretic effect due to suppression of prostaglandin synthesis in the CNS	◆ Rheumatoid arthritis ◆ Osteoarthritis ◆ Juvenile arthritis ◆ Mild to moderate pain ◆ Fever	◆ Monitor for adverse reactions, such as bronchospasm, Stevens-Johnson syndrome, hematologic disorders, and aseptic meningitis. ◆ Be advised that full anti-inflammatory effects may take 1 to 2 weeks to occur. ◆ Note that NSAIDs may mask the signs and symptoms of infection.
Opioid agonist	morphine	Acts on opiate receptors in the CNS	◆ Pain	◆ Monitor for adverse reactions, such as sedation, euphoria, seizures, dizziness, nightmares, bradycardia, shock, cardiac arrest, nausea, constipation, vomiting, thrombocytopenia, and respiratory depression. ◆ Keep opioid antagonist (naloxone) and resuscitation equipment available.
Proton pump inhibitor	omeprazole	Inhibits activity of acid (proton) pump and binds to hydrogen-potassium adenosinetriphosphatase, located at the secretory surface of the gastric parietal cells, to block formation of gastric acid	◆ Gastroesophageal reflux disease ◆ Zollinger-Ellison syndrome ◆ Duodenal ulcer ◆ Gastric ulcer ◆ *Helicobacter pylori* infection	◆ Monitor for adverse reactions, such as headache, dizziness, and nausea. ◆ Administer 30 minutes before meals.

CLASSIFICATION	PROTOTYPE	ACTIONS	INDICATIONS	NURSING CONSIDERATIONS
Selective serotonin reuptake inhibitor	fluoxetine	Presumed to be linked to the inhibition of CNS neuronal uptake of serotonin	◆ Depression ◆ Treatment of binge eating and vomiting behaviors in clients with moderate to severe bulimia nervosa ◆ Premenstrual dysphoric disorder ◆ Anorexia nervosa ◆ Panic disorder ◆ Alcohol dependence	◆ Monitor for adverse reactions, such as anxiety, nervousness, insomnia, drowsiness, nausea, diarrhea, dry mouth, and respiratory distress. ◆ Give the drug in the morning to prevent insomnia. ◆ Warn the client to avoid hazardous activities that require alertness and psychomotor coordination until the CNS effects of the drug are known.
Skeletal muscle relaxant	baclofen	Unknown action; appears to reduce transmission of impulses from the spinal cord to skeletal muscle; relieves muscle spasms	◆ Spasticity in multiple sclerosis and spinal cord injury	◆ Give with meals to prevent GI distress ◆ Avoid abrupt discontinuation of intrathecal baclofen because high fever, altered mental status, exaggerated rebound spasticity, and muscle rigidity can result. In rare instances, these effects may progress to rhabdomyolysis, multisystem organ failure, and death.
Stimulant laxative	bisacodyl	Increases peristalsis, probably by acting directly on the smooth muscle of the intestine; thought to irritate musculature or stimulate colonic intramural plexus; promotes fluid accumulation in the colon and small intestine	◆ Constipation ◆ Emptying of the bowel before general surgery, sigmoidoscopic or proctoscopic procedures, and radiologic procedures	◆ Don't give tablets within 1 hour of milk or antacids. ◆ Insert a suppository as high as possible into the rectum, and try to position it against the rectal wall. Avoid embedding it in the fecal material (onset may be delayed). ◆ Soft-formed stool is usually produced 15 to 60 minutes after rectal administration.

CLASSIFICATION	PROTOTYPE	ACTIONS	INDICATIONS	NURSING CONSIDERATIONS
Sulfonamide	co-trimoxazole	Bacteriostatic; mechanism of action correlates directly to the structural similarities it shares with para-aminobenzoic acid; inhibits biosynthesis of folic acid; susceptible bacteria are those that synthesize folic acid	◆ Infections of the urinary tract, respiratory tract, and ear caused by susceptible organisms ◆ Chronic bacterial prostatitis ◆ Prevention of "traveler's diarrhea" and recurrent urinary tract infection in women	◆ Monitor for adverse reactions, such as seizures, nausea, vomiting, diarrhea, hematologic disorders, Stevens-Johnson syndrome, toxic nephrosis, and hypersensitivity reactions. ◆ Reduce dosages, as needed, in clients with renal and hepatic impairment. ◆ With large doses or prolonged treatment, monitor for superinfections. ◆ Obtain specimen for culture and sensitivity before first dose; therapy may begin before results.
Tetracycline	tetracycline	Bacteriostatic but may be bactericidal against certain organisms; binds reversibly to 30S and 50S ribosomal subunits; inhibits bacterial protein synthesis; bacterial resistance to tetracyclines usually mediated by plasmids (R-factor resistance), which decrease bacterial cell wall permeability	◆ Infections caused by susceptible organisms ◆ Gonorrhea	◆ Monitor for adverse reactions, such as nausea, vomiting, diarrhea, hematologic disorders, Stevens-Johnson syndrome, intracranial hypertension, rash, photosensitivity, and hypersensitivity reactions. ◆ With large doses or prolonged treatment, monitor for superinfections. ◆ Obtain specimen for culture and sensitivity before first dose; therapy may begin before results.
Thrombolytic	streptokinase	Lyses clots by converting plasminogen to plasmin; in contrast, anticoagulants act by preventing thrombi from developing	◆ Venous thrombosis, pulmonary embolism, arterial thrombosis, and embolism ◆ Lysis of a clot during MI	◆ Monitor for adverse reactions, such as arrhythmias, bleeding, pulmonary edema, and hypersensitivity reaction. ◆ Monitor vital signs and for bleeding frequently.

CLASSIFICATION	PROTOTYPE	ACTIONS	INDICATIONS	NURSING CONSIDERATIONS
Thyroid hormone	levothyroxine	Stimulates metabolism of all body tissues by accelerating rate of cellular oxidation	◆ Cretinism ◆ Myxedema coma ◆ Thyroid hormone replacement	◆ Monitor for adverse reactions, such as nervousness, insomnia, tremor, tachycardia, palpitations, angina, arrhythmias, and cardiac arrest. ◆ Use with extreme caution in elderly clients and those with cardiovascular disorders.
Tricyclic antidepressant	imipramine	May inhibit the reuptake of norepinephrine and serotonin in CNS nerve terminals (presynaptic neurons), thus enhancing the concentration and activity of neurotransmitters in the synaptic cleft; exerts antihistaminic, sedative, anticholinergic, vasodilatory, and quinidine-like effects	◆ Depression ◆ Enuresis in children older than age 6	◆ Monitor the client for adverse reactions, such as sedation, anticholinergic effects, and orthostatic hypotension. ◆ Don't withdraw the drug abruptly; gradually reduce the dosage over several weeks. ◆ Warn the client to avoid hazardous activities that require alertness and psychomotor coordination until the CNS effects of the drug are known.
Vasodilator	nitroprusside	Relaxes arteriolar and venous smooth muscle	◆ Reduction of blood pressure; reduction of preload and afterload	◆ Monitor thiocyanate levels every 72 hours; excessive doses or rapid infusion (more than 15 mcg/kg/minute) can cause cyanide toxicity. ◆ Monitor for adverse reactions and signs of cyanide toxicity, including profound hypotension, metabolic acidosis, dyspnea, headache, loss of consciousness, ataxia, and vomiting. ◆ Monitor blood pressure every 5 minutes at start of infusion and every 15 minutes thereafter. ◆ Wrap I.V. infusion in aluminum foil because it's sensitive to light.

Posttest 1

INSTRUCTIONS

Four posttests have been included to help you evaluate your nursing skills and knowledge as you prepare to take the NCLEX-RN. These posttests can also be used for review by nurses returning to active practice after an absence and by those moving to a different clinical area of practice.

The posttests are based on the same question-and-response format used on the NCLEX–RN. The questions on the posttests focus primarily on a practical application of nursing principles rather than on a simple recall of facts.

Each posttest contains 75 questions, written in the format used in the computerized examination. Like the NCLEX–RN, the Springhouse Review posttests don't contain deliberately misleading questions. Be sure to read each question and all possible answers carefully; then select the best answer. Remember that on the computerized examination, you will *not* be able to go back to a question or go on to the next question without selecting an answer choice. Take no more than 75 minutes to complete each posttest.

Before beginning the first posttest, select a quiet room where you'll be undisturbed and set a timer for 75 minutes. After you've completed the first posttest or the 75-minute time limit expires, check your responses against the answers and rationales that follow. Carefully study the rationales for any questions you answered incorrectly. Doing so will give you an additional opportunity to recall important nursing information. Repeat the steps described above for the three remaining posttests.

QUESTIONS

1. A client had an abdominal hysterectomy 10 hours ago. Which position should a nurse teach the client to avoid?

- ☐ **1.** High Fowler's
- ☐ **2.** Lateral recumbent
- ☐ **3.** Supine
- ☐ **4.** Side-lying

2. A physician orders an upper GI series for a client with GI complaints. The nurse teaches the client about the upper GI series. Which statement indicates that the client understands the instructions?

- ☐ **1.** "I'll have a special instrument passed through my mouth into my stomach."
- ☐ **2.** "I'll take several tablets the night before the test."
- ☐ **3.** "I'll drink a contrast medium while X-rays are taken."
- ☐ **4.** "I'll have a CT scan taken after I'm injected with a radioactive substance."

3. A client returns from surgery. Which nursing diagnosis takes priority at this time?

- ☐ **1.** Ineffective breathing pattern
- ☐ **2.** Deficient fluid volume
- ☐ **3.** Imbalanced nutrition: Less than body requirements
- ☐ **4.** Diarrhea

4. A client had abdominal surgery 2 days ago. Which nursing assessment finding suggests that the client has developed a postoperative complication?

- ☐ **1.** Serous wound drainage
- ☐ **2.** Weakness when ambulating
- ☐ **3.** Abdominal distention
- ☐ **4.** Muscle soreness

5. Shortly after a multigravida client is admitted to the hospital in labor, her amniotic membranes rupture. Which action should the nurse take first?

☐ **1.** Check fetal heart tones.
☐ **2.** Turn the client onto her left side.
☐ **3.** Take the client's blood pressure.
☐ **4.** Change the pad under the client's buttocks.

6. A client is scheduled to receive a blood transfusion. During the transfusion, the nurse should observe for which sign or symptom of a transfusion reaction?

☐ **1.** Dizziness
☐ **2.** Chills
☐ **3.** Hypothermia
☐ **4.** Hyperreflexia

7. A 2-year-old child with cystic fibrosis is admitted to the hospital with pneumonia. The child receives aerosol treatments followed by percussion and postural drainage four times per day. Which nursing diagnosis takes priority for this client?

☐ **1.** Imbalanced nutrition: Less than body requirements related to appetite loss
☐ **2.** Anxiety (parental and child) related to acute illness
☐ **3.** Anticipatory grieving related to life-threatening illness
☐ **4.** Ineffective airway clearance related to tenacious tracheobronchial secretions

8. Which reflex should the nurse discuss and demonstrate to educate the parents about providing a safe environment for their neonate?

☐ **1.** Babinski's
☐ **2.** Stepping
☐ **3.** Tonic neck
☐ **4.** Prone crawl

9. A client with status asthmaticus is in severe respiratory distress. The nurse should maintain the client in which position?

☐ **1.** Sitting upright
☐ **2.** Side-lying
☐ **3.** Supine
☐ **4.** Prone

10. A client is admitted to the hospital with symptoms of left-sided heart failure. The physician prescribes digoxin (Lanoxin), 0.125 mg daily, and a low-sodium diet. When assessing this client, the nurse should expect to find which sign or symptom?

☐ **1.** Tingling sensation in the fingers
☐ **2.** Dyspnea
☐ **3.** Abdominal distention
☐ **4.** Engorged neck veins

11. A physician informs a client that he'll need heart surgery. Later, the client tells the nurse angrily, "When you deal with surgeons, you can only expect they'll want to cut you up." Which response by the nurse would be most appropriate?

☐ **1.** "I'm sure the surgeons know what they're doing."
☐ **2.** "I think you're too upset to think clearly."
☐ **3** "You're wondering if the surgery is necessary."
☐ **4.** "You're concerned about the skill of the surgeon."

12. A client has been placed on a low-sodium diet. The client would show an understanding of the dietary instructions by selecting which food as having the lowest sodium content?

☐ **1.** Canned tomato soup
☐ **2.** Broiled lobster
☐ **3.** Tapioca pudding
☐ **4.** Fresh string beans

13. A child undergoes a tonsillectomy and adenoidectomy. During the early postoperative period, the nurse should observe the child closely for which finding?

☐ **1.** Frequent swallowing
☐ **2.** Intermittent moaning
☐ **3.** Incontinence
☐ **4.** Lethargy

14. A primgravida client's husband asks the nurse what his role should be during labor because his wife seems so uncomfortable. The nurse explains that the coach has what primary role?

☐ **1.** An active support person throughout the labor
☐ **2.** An observer who primarily participates during delivery
☐ **3.** A witness to the labor and delivery experience
☐ **4.** An information giver to all other family members not present at the birth

15. A client is admitted to the hospital with signs and symptoms of a stroke. The client is unconscious on admission. The health team inserts a central venous catheter and starts an I.V. infusion. When the client is admitted to the nursing unit, the nurse should assign highest priority to which goal?

☐ **1.** Preventing skin breakdown
☐ **2.** Promoting urinary elimination
☐ **3.** Maintaining a patent airway
☐ **4.** Preserving muscle function

16. A child is scheduled for a tonsillectomy and adenoidectomy. Preoperatively, which nursing assessment is essential?

☐ **1.** Examining for loose teeth
☐ **2.** Comparing the apical and radial pulse rates
☐ **3.** Checking the function of the facial nerve
☐ **4.** Determining the range of motion of the head and neck

17. A client begins to sob uncontrollably after learning that a tumor removed from the lung is cancerous. How should the nurse deal with this situation?

☐ **1.** Remain with the client and allow him to cry.
☐ **2.** Leave the room and find out if the client can have a sedative.
☐ **3.** Ask the client exactly what the physician said.
☐ **4.** Explain that it's important for the client not to cry now.

18. A physician prescribes an I.V. infusion of 1,000 ml of dextrose 5% in water every 12 hours for a client. The I.V. setup delivers 15 gtt/ml. Approximately how many drops should be administered each minute?

☐ **1.** 18
☐ **2.** 21
☐ **3.** 24
☐ **4.** 27

19. Two hours after a client delivers a neonate, a nurse assesses the mother to determine if she's ready for transfer to the postpartum unit. Which assessment finding warrants immediate nursing intervention?

☐ **1.** Temperature of 99.8° F (37.7° C); heart rate of 70 beats/minute
☐ **2.** Breasts soft and not tender; colostrum present
☐ **3.** Uterine fundus soft and located left of midline
☐ **4.** Moderate lochia rubra containing small clots

20. A client is receiving clonidine (Catapres). Which nursing action is appropriate for this client?

☐ **1.** Teach the client to change position slowly.
☐ **2.** Give the medication before meals.
☐ **3.** Instruct the client to take the medication with orange juice.
☐ **4.** Offer the client a cup of tea with meals.

21. While visiting a client who is recovering from a stroke, the client's husband asks the nurse, "Why does my wife have a splint on her hand?" The nurse explains that the splint is necessary to prevent which condition?

☐ **1.** Injury to the hand
☐ **2.** Deformity of the hand
☐ **3.** Muscle wasting in the hand
☐ **4.** Edema of the hand

22. A client requires tracheal suctioning through the nose. Which nursing action would be correct?

☐ **1.** Lubricating the catheter with sterile water before beginning
☐ **2.** Applying suction when inserting the catheter in the nose
☐ **3.** Suctioning for 30 seconds
☐ **4.** Rotating the catheter when inserting it

23. A client with emphysema is to receive oxygen by nasal cannula. Which measure should the nurse take when caring for this client?

☐ **1.** Maintain the oxygen flow rate at no more than 3 L/minute.
☐ **2.** Increase the oxygen flow rate up to 6 L/minute, if required.
☐ **3.** Teach the client to adjust the oxygen flow rate as needed.
☐ **4.** Change the oxygen tubing at each shift.

24. As a nurse assists a client with breathing exercises, the client says, "I don't feel any better. Why should I bother learning how to do these exercises?" How should the nurse respond?

☐ **1.** Tell the client that the physician ordered the exercises.
☐ **2.** Encourage the client to express feelings.
☐ **3.** Ask if the client would like to do the exercises at another time.
☐ **4.** Inform the physician of the client's statements.

25. A client is admitted to the hospital with a tentative diagnosis of acute pyelonephritis. To assess for risk factors for pyelonephritis, the nurse should ask the client which question?

☐ **1.** "Do you have pain in your back?"
☐ **2.** "Have you had a sore throat lately?"
☐ **3.** "Do you hold your urine for a long time before voiding?"
☐ **4.** "Have you taken any analgesics recently?"

26. A child is in skin traction. To help prevent one of the most common complications of immobility, the nurse should include which measure in the child's care plan?

☐ **1.** Provide a high-fiber diet.
☐ **2.** Keep a soft light glowing in the corner of the room.
☐ **3.** Measure abdominal girth routinely.
☐ **4.** Perform range-of-motion (ROM) exercises to the legs at every shift.

27. A law student who has been preparing for final exams comes to the student health center. Sobbing hysterically and hyperventilating, she says, "I haven't slept all night. I just can't go on." Which response by the nurse would be appropriate?

☐ **1.** "Relax, we all feel this way sometimes. You'll get through it."
☐ **2.** "Perhaps you need more time to study. Have you discussed this with your advisor?"
☐ **3.** "Studying for finals can be very stressful. Let's work on a plan that might be helpful."
☐ **4.** "You need to calm down. Students have to learn to take a lot of stress."

28. A client has been in the manic phase of bipolar disorder for the past 8 days. During this time, he has been hyperactive, hasn't sat down to eat meals, and has slept only 2 hours each night. Which strategy should the nurse use to help the client get adequate rest?

☐ **1.** Establish a bedtime routine.
☐ **2.** Place the client in seclusion during the night.
☐ **3.** Prevent the client from sleeping during the day.
☐ **4.** Encourage the client to catnap throughout the day.

29. A client's son is 1 day old. She's upset because he sleeps most of the day and doesn't look at her often. Her interpretation is that her baby doesn't like her. Which response by the nurse would be best in this situation?

☐ **1.** "Babies have no likes or dislikes; he'll like you later as his mother."
☐ **2.** "Babies sleep up to 20 hours per day. You'll notice him staying awake longer each week."
☐ **3.** "Babies sleep when they're getting sick; I'll take him to the nursery for the pediatrician to examine."
☐ **4.** "Don't worry; he's just a baby."

30. A 2-year-old child is in Bryant's traction. Which measure should the nurse take to feed this child?

☐ **1.** Adjust the traction so the child can be turned to one side to eat.
☐ **2.** Temporarily stop the traction so the child can sit upright to eat.
☐ **3.** Ask the child's mother about the child's favorite eating position.
☐ **4.** Maintain the child in proper traction alignment during meals.

31. A nurse is caring for a postpartum client. To assess for thrombophlebitis, which periodic assessment should the nurse perform?

☐ **1.** Checking for blood pressure discrepancy between the right and left legs
☐ **2.** Assessing for pain when the feet are dorsiflexed
☐ **3.** Assessing for limited range-of-motion in the legs
☐ **4.** Checking for pitting edema in the lower extremities

32. A client is admitted to the hospital after falling at home. X-rays confirm a fracture of the right hip; the client is placed in Buck's traction and scheduled for an open reduction and internal fixation. During Buck's traction, which nursing action is appropriate?

☐ **1.** Elevate the head of the bed 45 degrees.
☐ **2.** Make sure the client's right heel touches the bed.
☐ **3.** Remove the weights when bathing the client's legs.
☐ **4.** Allow the weights to hang freely at the foot of the bed.

33. A client undergoes an open reduction and internal fixation to treat a fractured right hip. Five hours after surgery, the nurse should maintain the client's affected leg in which position?

☐ **1.** External rotation
☐ **2.** Abduction
☐ **3.** Flexion
☐ **4.** Hyperextension

34. A nurse on a psychiatric unit is assigned to stay with a severely depressed client. The nurse needs to go to the lavatory. How should the nurse manage this situation?

☐ **1.** Have another staff member inform the nurse manager of the need for a replacement.
☐ **2.** Tell the client that the nurse will return in a few minutes.
☐ **3.** Ask another client to sit in for awhile.
☐ **4.** Discontinue observation only when the client states that the depression has lifted.

35. A pregnant client is in the first stage of labor. The nurse should include which instructions in the client's care plan during this stage?

☐ **1.** Encourage the client to lie on her left side.
☐ **2.** Instruct the client to ambulate.
☐ **3.** Urge the client to accept pain medication.
☐ **4.** Advise the client to use learned breathing techniques.

36. A child is receiving prednisone. The nurse knows that the mother understands the teaching about her child's prednisone therapy if she makes which statement?

☐ **1.** "I'll be sure to count my child's pulse every day."
☐ **2.** "I can't feed my child her favorite oatmeal for breakfast any more."
☐ **3.** "I'll keep my child away from people with colds."
☐ **4.** "I'll make sure my child rests in bed every afternoon."

37. A 5-year-old child with leukemia has a platelet count of 20,000/µl. Based on this information, the nurse should include which measure in the care plan?

☐ **1.** Provide a diet high in iron.
☐ **2.** Use hypoallergenic soap when bathing the child.
☐ **3.** Change the child's position every 2 hours.
☐ **4.** Inspect the child's skin for ecchymosis.

38. When measuring a client's blood pressure, the nurse sees that the client is having carpal spasms. Which action should the nurse take next?

☐ **1.** Assess for Babinski's reflex.
☐ **2.** Check for Chvostek's sign.
☐ **3.** Evaluate the client's apical pulse.
☐ **4.** Determine the client's level of consciousness.

39. A client who is scheduled for a frozen section biopsy and a possible mastectomy has difficulty understanding the surgeon's instructions. What's the most likely cause of her difficulty?

☐ **1.** She lacks knowledge of anatomy and physiology.
☐ **2.** She isn't interested in details.
☐ **3.** She has a high anxiety level.
☐ **4.** She has a limited mental ability.

40. At 38 weeks' gestation, a pregnant client comes to the clinic because her amniotic membranes have ruptured and she isn't having contractions. To confirm membrane rupture, the nurse should assess which characteristic of the amniotic fluid?

☐ **1.** Glucose
☐ **2.** pH
☐ **3.** Color
☐ **4.** Albumin

41. After a mastectomy, a client returns to her room with a wound drain attached to a Hemovac closed drainage system. The nurse caring for the client should take which measure?

☐ **1.** Clamp the wound catheter when emptying the Hemovac chamber.
☐ **2.** Flush the Hemovac chamber with sterile saline solution if it becomes clogged.
☐ **3.** Apply pressure around the wound catheter to promote drainage.
☐ **4.** Assess the client if the Hemovac chamber fills rapidly.

42. A client undergoes a mastectomy. Several days later, which finding by the nurse suggests that the client has accepted the alteration to her body?

☐ **1.** She's eager to be discharged.
☐ **2.** She asks when her sutures will be removed.
☐ **3.** She sits at the edge of the bed when the physician removes her dressing.
☐ **4.** She looks at the incision when the dressing is being changed.

43. After a cataract extraction, a client receives instructions on self-care. Which statement by the client indicates an understanding of the instructions?

☐ **1.** "I'll cover my mouth when I cough."
☐ **2.** "I'll get someone to pick up heavy objects from the floor."
☐ **3.** "I'll practice Valsalva's maneuver daily."
☐ **4.** "I'll sleep with two pillows under my head."

44. A client with Alzheimer's disease is at a group reality-orientation session. Several members of the group discuss the party they all just attended. Which outcome suggests that the client is benefiting from this session?

☐ **1.** The client is quiet when others talk about the party.
☐ **2.** The client tells the group she wasn't at the party.
☐ **3.** The client says she wants to have a party now.
☐ **4.** The client talks about something that happened at the party.

45. A child is admitted to the hospital with a tentative diagnosis of acute lymphocytic leukemia. What is a common sign of leukemia in children?

☐ **1.** Maculopapular rash
☐ **2.** Low-grade fever
☐ **3.** Photosensitivity
☐ **4.** Polydipsia

46. When obtaining a history from a client with cholelithiasis, the nurse should ask which question relating to this disorder?

☐ **1.** "Are you more comfortable when you sleep in a sitting position?"
☐ **2.** "Do you get heartburn after a spicy meal?"
☐ **3.** "Do you have an intolerance to fatty foods?"
☐ **4.** "Do you have less flatus after taking an antacid?"

47. A client underwent abdominal surgery 6 hours ago. At 6 p.m., the client receives an order of meperidine (Demerol), 50 mg, as needed. Two hours later, the client complains of incisional pain. Which action should the nurse take?

☐ **1.** Place a heating pad against the client's abdomen.
☐ **2.** Repeat the meperidine dose.
☐ **3.** Turn the client onto his side and place a pillow behind his back.
☐ **4.** Give the client half the ordered dosage of meperidine.

48. After a cholecystectomy with a choledochostomy, a client returns to the medical-surgical unit with a T tube in place. The nurse should take which action related to the T tube?

☐ **1.** Irrigate it periodically.
☐ **2.** Connect it to a straight drainage system.
☐ **3.** Attach it to a low-suction apparatus.
☐ **4.** Aspirate it at least four times per day.

49. A client with a normal pregnancy visits the clinic. When teaching the client about nutrition, the nurse should provide which instruction?

☐ **1.** "Avoid salt whenever possible, and don't use salt when cooking."
☐ **2.** "Limit your intake of carbohydrates, such as bread, to improve your protein metabolism."
☐ **3.** "Peanut butter is a good source of protein to include in your diet."
☐ **4.** "Avoid eating fatty foods until after your baby is born."

50. A client with tuberculosis is to take isoniazid (INH) and rifampin (Rifadin). Which comment by the client indicates correct understanding of the medication regimen?

☐ **1.** "I'll take the medications until I regain my strength."
☐ **2.** "I'll take the medications as prescribed for over a year."
☐ **3.** "I'll take the medications with citrus juice."
☐ **4.** "I'll take the medications until my white blood cell count is normal."

51. A client, age 76, is admitted to the hospital with a diagnosis of osteoarthritis. At a conference to discuss the client's progress, the nursing staff reports that the client looks at them intently when being questioned and answers inappropriately at times. Based on this information, the client should be evaluated for which possible condition?

☐ **1.** Hearing loss
☐ **2.** Perceptual defect
☐ **3.** Shortened attention span
☐ **4.** Cerebral oxygen deficit

52. A client with heart failure is to be maintained on bed rest. What's the main purpose of bed rest for this client?

☐ **1.** To improve the heart's pumping action
☐ **2.** To enhance oxygenation of body tissues
☐ **3.** To decrease blood volume throughout the body
☐ **4.** To reduce the work load of the heart

53. A schizophrenic client experiences auditory hallucinations. He tells the nurse that voices from another planet are commanding him to collect all metal cups. When responding, the nurse should tell the client that:

- ☐ **1.** It's all right for him to do what the voices tell him to do.
- ☐ **2.** The nurse doesn't hear the voices.
- ☐ **3.** Listening to music will obliterate the voices.
- ☐ **4.** The client doesn't hear the voices.

54. The nurse encourages a postoperative client to move his legs. Contracting the leg muscles helps to prevent which postoperative complication?

- ☐ **1.** Pleurisy
- ☐ **2.** Portal hypertension
- ☐ **3.** Hypostatic pneumonia
- ☐ **4.** Pulmonary embolism

55. When assessing a dehydrated infant, the nurse is most likely to detect which sign?

- ☐ **1.** A heart rate of 100 beats/minute
- ☐ **2.** Absence of tears when crying
- ☐ **3.** Distended neck veins
- ☐ **4.** A bulging anterior fontanel

56. A client who suspects she's pregnant has a pregnancy test. The presence of which hormone would confirm the pregnancy?

- ☐ **1.** Human chorionic gonadotropin
- ☐ **2.** Progesterone
- ☐ **3.** Follicle-stimulating hormone
- ☐ **4.** Luteinizing hormone

57. The nurse should instruct the client with Parkinson's disease to avoid which activity?

- ☐ **1.** Walking in an indoor shopping mall
- ☐ **2.** Sitting on the deck on a cool summer evening
- ☐ **3.** Walking to the car on a cold winter day
- ☐ **4.** Sitting on the beach in the sun on a summer day

58. Shortly after a neonate is delivered, erythromycin is instilled into the neonate's eyes. This drug is given to prevent which condition?

- ☐ **1.** Ophthalmia neonatorum
- ☐ **2.** Retrolental fibroplasia
- ☐ **3.** Corneal keratitis
- ☐ **4.** Acute uveitis

59. A client with type 1 diabetes mellitus is taking NPH insulin. The client sometimes engages in strenuous exercise. Which preexercise instructions should the nurse consider including in client teaching?

- ☐ **1.** Take extra insulin.
- ☐ **2.** Have a simple carbohydrate source available.
- ☐ **3.** Rest for an hour.
- ☐ **4.** Stretch and bend for 10 minutes.

60. A client with newly diagnosed type 2 diabetes mellitus seems anxious when receiving instructions in self-care. The client tells the nurse, "What's the use? I can't be cured, so what's the sense in you telling me all this nonsense?" Which response by the nurse would be appropriate?

- ☐ **1.** "Getting tense and discouraged will only aggravate your condition."
- ☐ **2.** "Take one step at a time. None of us knows what will happen from day to day."
- ☐ **3.** "It's true, you'll have to modify your lifestyle. But the quality of it doesn't have to decline."
- ☐ **4.** "Don't feel so negative about the future. We're trying to help you better care for yourself."

61. A client receives instructions about high-calcium foods. The client shows an understanding of these instructions by selecting which food as highest in calcium?

- ☐ **1.** Liver
- ☐ **2.** Yogurt
- ☐ **3.** Bran muffin
- ☐ **4.** Carrots

62. A female client is diagnosed with gonorrhea. The nurse should assess her for which symptom?

- ☐ **1.** Lower abdominal pain
- ☐ **2.** Muscle rigidity
- ☐ **3.** An unsteady gait
- ☐ **4.** Reddish rash on the inner thighs

63. During labor, a client's amniotic membranes rupture. The nurse sees the umbilical cord protruding from the vagina. Which action should the nurse take?

- ☐ **1.** Encourage the client to breathe deeply.
- ☐ **2.** Turn the client onto her left side.
- ☐ **3.** Place the client in Trendelenburg's position.
- ☐ **4.** Place sterile pads under the client's buttocks.

64. A client is to receive 8 mg of morphine sulfate. The ampule contains 15 mg/ml. Approximately how much morphine should the nurse administer?

☐ **1.** 0.5 ml
☐ **2.** 0.7 ml
☐ **3.** 1.0 ml
☐ **4.** 1.5 ml

65. Which of the following conditions can cause tachycardia?

☐ **1.** Vagal stimulation
☐ **2.** Fear, anger, or pain
☐ **3.** Stress, pain, or vomiting
☐ **4.** Vomiting or suctioning

66. A 63-year-old male is admitted to the medical-surgical floor preoperatively and is scheduled for a left carotid endarterectomy. The nurse is completing an admission assessment. What preexisting condition might the nurse expect to find with the client?

☐ **1.** Renal disease
☐ **2.** Atherosclerosis
☐ **3.** Crohn's disease
☐ **4.** Cervical dysplasia

67. A child, age 5, is admitted to the hospital for an elective tonsillectomy and adenoidectomy. During the admission assessment, the nurse makes all of the following observations. Which observation calls for further evaluation?

☐ **1.** The child is chewing on his fingernails.
☐ **2.** The child is clutching a ragged teddy bear.
☐ **3.** The child is avoiding eye contact with the nurse.
☐ **4.** The child is sneezing frequently.

68. A client who has suffered a myocardial infarction (MI) is in the coronary care unit. The nurse suspects that the client is denying the seriousness of the medical condition. Which behavior supports this suspicion?

☐ **1.** The client refuses to eat solid food.
☐ **2.** The client says that tea made from heart-shaped leaves helps the heart.
☐ **3.** The client expects to return to work within 2 weeks.
☐ **4.** The client plans to do an oil painting for his daughter.

69. A client who was hospitalized for a myocardial infarction is being prepared for discharge. Which statement by the client indicates an understanding of the nurse's discharge instructions?

☐ **1.** "I'll stop walking when my pulse rate exceeds 80 beats/minute."
☐ **2.** "I'll wait about 1 hour after a meal before walking."
☐ **3.** "I'll use a ramp to walk the four steps into my house."
☐ **4.** "I'll walk for 10 minutes every 2 hours while awake."

70. A client is admitted to the hospital with a diagnosis of acute upper GI bleeding. Which nursing diagnosis takes highest priority for this client?

☐ **1.** Deficient fluid volume related to bleeding
☐ **2.** Impaired tissue integrity related to mucosal damage
☐ **3.** Impaired physical mobility related to weakness secondary to blood loss
☐ **4.** Anxiety related to critical illness

71. A client in an alcohol treatment center admits to drinking two to three cases of beer every weekend and reports experiencing several blackouts in the past few months. Which recommendation by a nurse would be appropriate?

☐ **1.** Monitor alcohol intake for the next 3 months.
☐ **2.** Reduce alcohol intake and attend Alcoholics Anonymous meetings.
☐ **3.** Limit drinking to special occasions only.
☐ **4.** Abstain from alcohol altogether.

72. The cervix of a client in labor is dilated 8 cm. The nurse notes that the client bears down during contractions and teaches her to avoid doing this. Which observation during the client's next contraction indicates that the teaching was effective?

☐ **1.** The client pants when breathing.
☐ **2.** The client holds her breath.
☐ **3.** The client holds on to the side rails firmly.
☐ **4.** The client maintains a supine position.

73. To help prevent an infant from contracting infectious diarrhea, the nurse should instruct the mother in which topic?

☐ **1.** When to introduce solid foods into the infant's diet
☐ **2.** How to prepare, handle, and store infant formula
☐ **3.** When to have the child immunized
☐ **4.** When to bring the infant to the clinic for routine checkups

74. A nurse is evaluating the following telemetry strip frm one of her clients. What arrhythmia should the nurse document?

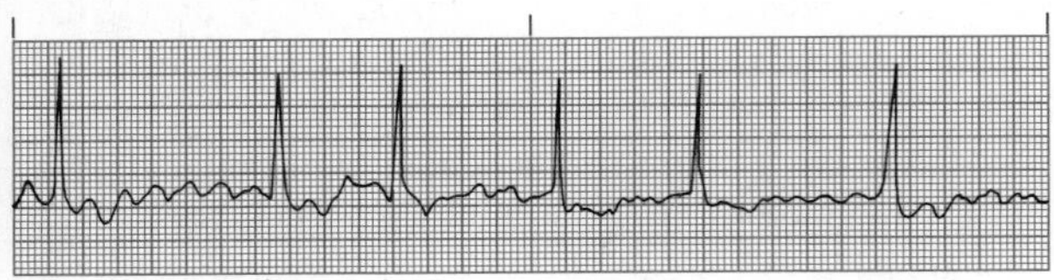

☐ **1.** Atrial fibrillation
☐ **2.** Atrial tachycardia
☐ **3.** Normal sinus rhythm with PACs
☐ **4.** Atrial flutter

75. A client has a history of aortic stenosis. Identify the area where the nurse should place the stethoscope to best hear the murmur.

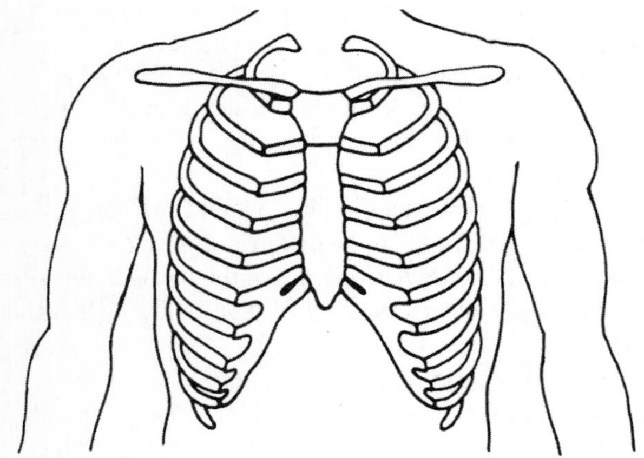

ANSWERS AND RATIONALES

In the posttest answers, the question number appears in boldface type, followed by the number of the correct answer. Rationales for correct answers and, where appropriate, for incorrect options follow. To help you evaluate your knowledge base and application of nursing behaviors, each rationale is classified according to:

- nursing process step
- client needs category
- client needs subcategory
- cognitive level.

1. CORRECT ANSWER: 1
High Fowler position may cause pelvic congestion. The other options don't contribute to pelvic congestion and are desirable positions for this client.
Nursing process step: Planning
Client needs category: Physiological integrity
Client needs subcategory: Reduction of risk potential
Cognitive level: Analysis

2. CORRECT ANSWER: 3
In an upper GI series, the client swallows barium and has X-rays of the stomach taken. Options 1, 2, and 4 don't apply to an upper GI series. A gastroscope is passed through the mouth into the stomach to observe the gastric mucosa to perform gastroscopy. The night before a gallbladder series, a client takes radiopaque tablets. A computed tomography (CT) scan isn't a component of an upper GI series.
Nursing process step: Evaluation
Client needs category: Safe, effective care environment
Client needs subcategory: Management of care
Cognitive level: Application

3. CORRECT ANSWER: 1
An ineffective breathing pattern is a dangerous complication that can occur in a client recovering from general anesthesia. Option 2 may cause a problem but doesn't take priority over an ineffective breathing pattern. Options 3 and 4 aren't immediate postoperative problems.
Nursing process step: Nursing diagnosis
Client needs category: Safe, effective care environment
Client needs subcategory: Safety and infection control
Cognitive level: Application

4. CORRECT ANSWER: 3
Postoperatively, persistent abdominal distention may indicate paralytic ileus. The other options are expected during the postoperative period.
Nursing process step: Assessment
Client needs category: Physiological integrity
Client needs subcategory: Reduction of risk potential
Cognitive level: Application

5. Correct answer: 1
When the amniotic membranes rupture, fluid is expelled through the vaginal canal and the cord may prolapse, possibly impeding the fetal blood supply. The nurse should check fetal heart tones to assess fetal status. A position change (option 2) isn't required unless the fetal heart rate is abnormal. Recording the client's blood pressure (option 3) would be necessary only with signs of maternal distress. Changing the pad under the client (option 4) would be done after checking the fetal heart tones.
Nursing process step: Implementation
Client needs category: Health promotion and maintenance
Client needs subcategory: None
Cognitive level: Comprehension

6. Correct answer: 2
Chills are a classic symptom of a transfusion reaction. The other options aren't associated with transfusion reactions.
Nursing process step: Assessment
Client needs category: Physiological integrity
Client needs subcategory: Pharmacological and parenteral therapies
Cognitive level: Comprehension

7. Correct answer: 4
In cystic fibrosis, thick, tenacious tracheobronchial secretions may obstruct the airway. Ensuring a patent airway is the highest priority. Cystic fibrosis and pneumonia may cause fatigue and loss of energy, which may decrease the appetite and reduce food intake; however, option 1 isn't the highest priority. Options 2 and 3 are also appropriate nursing concerns and should be addressed in the care plan; however, they're secondary to ineffective airway clearance.
Nursing process step: Nursing diagnosis
Client needs category: Physiological integrity
Client needs subcategory: Physiological adaptation
Cognitive level: Analysis

8. Correct answer: 4
The neonate is capable of making crawling-forward movements. Discussion and demonstration of this neonate capability is important so that parents realize the danger of placing the neonate on a bed or changing table without sides. Babinski's, stepping, and tonic neck reflexes aren't specifically related to a safety concern that should be taught to the parents.
Nursing process step: Implementation
Client needs category: Safe, effective care environment
Client needs subcategory: Safety and infection control
Cognitive level: Application

9. Correct answer: 1
A client in status asthmaticus should be placed in the position that best promotes air exchange. Sitting upright eases the motion of the diaphragm and promotes a patent airway. The other options don't promote air exchange.
Nursing process step: Implementation
Client needs category: Physiological integrity
Client needs subcategory: Basic care and comfort
Cognitive level: Analysis

10. Correct answer: 2
When the left side of the heart fails, fluid accumulates in the lungs, causing dyspnea. The other options are signs and symptoms of right-sided, not left-sided, heart failure.
Nursing process step: Assessment
Client needs category: Physiological integrity
Client needs subcategory: Pharmacological and parenteral therapies
Cognitive level: Comprehension

11. Correct answer: 3
This response encourages the client to express feelings. Option 1 denies the client's feelings. Option 2 is judgmental. Option 4 is inappropriate because the client hasn't expressed concern about the skill of the surgeon.
Nursing process step: Implementation
Client needs category: Psychosocial integrity
Client needs subcategory: None
Cognitive level: Application

12. Correct answer: 4
Fresh vegetables have the lowest sodium content of the foods listed. The other options have more than 150 mg of sodium in an average portion and should be avoided by a client on a low-sodium diet.
Nursing process step: Evaluation
Client needs category: Physiological integrity
Client needs subcategory: Basic care and comfort
Cognitive level: Comprehension

13. Correct answer: 1
Frequent swallowing may indicate that the child is swallowing blood, a sign of excessive bleeding (hemorrhage). The other options may be expected during the early postoperative period.

Nursing process step: Assessment
Client needs category: Physiological integrity
Client needs subcategory: Reduction of risk potential
Cognitive level: Comprehension

14. CORRECT ANSWER: 1
The primary role of the labor coach is to be actively involved in the birth process by providing emotional and physical support during labor and delivery. The coach does witness the events of the labor and birth and commonly is the one who shares this information with other family members but these actions aren't the primary role.
Nursing process step: Implementation
Client needs category: Psychosocial integrity
Client needs subcategory: None
Cognitive level: Application

15. CORRECT ANSWER: 3
Maintaining a patent airway is a priority for any client who's unconscious. Although the other options are appropriate goals for an unconscious client, they aren't priorities.
Nursing process step: Planning
Client needs category: Physiological integrity
Client needs subcategory: Reduction of risk potential
Cognitive level: Application

16. CORRECT ANSWER: 1
Examining for loose teeth is essential because, during the anesthetic phase of surgery, a loose tooth is likely to become completely dislodged and may be aspirated. The other options aren't essential preoperative assessments for this client.
Nursing process step: Assessment
Client needs category: Safe, effective care environment
Client needs subcategory: Safety and infection control
Cognitive level: Analysis

17. CORRECT ANSWER: 1
Crying is an appropriate reaction to hearing distressing news; the nurse should remain with the client to provide comfort, as needed. The nurse shouldn't leave the room; giving a sedative at this time would be premature. When a client is obviously distressed, it's the wrong time to try to obtain information. The client is venting feelings by crying and should be allowed to do so.
Nursing process step: Implementation
Client needs category: Psychosocial integrity
Client needs subcategory: None
Cognitive level: Application

18. CORRECT ANSWER: 2
About 21 drops/minute should be administered, based on the following calculation:

$$\frac{\text{Volume of infusion in ml} \times \text{Drop factor (gtt/ml)}}{\text{Time of infusion in minutes}} = \text{Drops/minute}$$

Therefore:

$$\frac{\dfrac{1{,}000 \cancel{\text{ml}}}{1} \times \dfrac{15 \text{ gtt}}{1 \cancel{\text{ml}}}}{720 \text{ min}} = \frac{15{,}000 \text{ gtt}}{720 \text{ min}} = \begin{matrix}20.8 \text{ or} \\ 21 \text{ drops/minute}\end{matrix}$$

Nursing process step: Implementation
Client needs category: Physiological integrity
Client needs subcategory: Pharmacological and parenteral therapies
Cognitive level: Application

19. CORRECT ANSWER: 3
A soft (relaxed) uterine fundus may lead to excessive bleeding; uterine displacement may result from a distended bladder. The other options are within normal limits for a client 2 hours postpartum.
Nursing process step: Assessment
Client needs category: Health promotion and maintenance
Client needs subcategory: None
Cognitive level: Comprehension

20. CORRECT ANSWER: 1
A client receiving clonidine or another antihypertensive medication should change position slowly to prevent orthostatic hypotension. Clonidine can be taken before or after meals. No therapeutic justification exists for taking it with orange juice. Overconsumption of tea and other stimulants should be discouraged in hypertensive clients.
Nursing process step: Implementation
Client needs category: Physiological integrity
Client needs subcategory: Pharmacological and parenteral therapies
Cognitive level: Application

21. CORRECT ANSWER: 2
After a stroke affecting the arm, fingers of the affected hand should be extended and the hand and wrist placed in a functional position to prevent deformity. (Be aware that in some instances handsplints may increase spasticity.)
Nursing process step: Implementation
Client needs category: Physiological integrity
Client needs subcategory: Basic care and comfort
Cognitive level: Application

22. CORRECT ANSWER: 1
The catheter should be lubricated to prevent injury and ease its passage through the nose. Suctioning shouldn't continue for more than 12 seconds; suctioning for 30 seconds causes hypoxia. Suction should only be applied when withdrawing the catheter — not inserting it. The catheter should also be rotated when it's withdrawn, not inserted, to ensure that secretions are removed.
Nursing process step: Implementation
Client needs category: Safe, effective care environment
Client needs subcategory: Safety and infection control
Cognitive level: Application

23. CORRECT ANSWER: 1
A client with emphysema who requires oxygen should receive a maximum of 3 L/minute. A flow rate of 6 L/minute (option 2) would be excessive. The client shouldn't adjust the oxygen flow rate (option 3). Changing the tubing at each shift (option 4) is unnecessary.
Nursing process step: Implementation
Client needs category: Safe, effective care environment
Client needs subcategory: Safety and infection control
Cognitive level: Application

24. CORRECT ANSWER: 2
A client who's upset with the treatment regimen should be given the opportunity to express feelings. The other options don't provide this opportunity.
Nursing process step: Implementation
Client needs category: Psychosocial integrity
Client needs subcategory: None
Cognitive level: Application

25. CORRECT ANSWER: 1
Pyelonephritis is a complication of a lower urinary tract infection, such as cystitis or urethritis. Back pain is a common symptom. The other options might elicit information about other renal problems but not about pyelonephritis.
Nursing process step: Assessment
Client needs category: Physiological integrity
Client needs subcategory: Reduction of risk potential
Cognitive level: Application

26. CORRECT ANSWER: 1
A high-fiber diet helps prevent constipation, a common complication of immobility. Options 2 and 3 wouldn't prevent complications of immobility. Performing ROM exercises (option 4) is impossible without interrupting traction, which is undesirable.
Nursing process step: Planning
Client needs category: Physiological integrity
Client needs subcategory: Reduction of risk potential
Cognitive level: Application

27. CORRECT ANSWER: 3
This response provides support, reassurance, and a concrete plan for dealing with the issues. Option 1 invalidates the client's feelings and gives false reassurance. Option 2 is unrealistic; a client in severe anxiety can't think coherently enough to respond to such a suggestion. Option 4 negates the client's feelings and may cause further anxiety.
Nursing process step: Implementation
Client needs category: Psychosocial integrity
Client needs subcategory: None
Cognitive level: Application

28. CORRECT ANSWER: 4
The client's energy level is so high that a complete night's sleep is probably impossible. The nurse should encourage the client to sleep or rest at any time to prevent physical exhaustion. The client's sleep pattern, including a bedtime routine, can be repatterned when the client comes "down" from the manic phase of the disorder (option 1). During the manic phase, the client's energy level is so high that enforcing seclusion during the night isn't likely to promote sleep (option 2).
Nursing process step: Planning
Client needs category: Safe, effective care environment
Client needs subcategory: Management of care
Cognitive level: Analysis

29. CORRECT ANSWER: 2
The nurse should tell the mother that neonates sleep up to 20 hours per day. This neonate is exhibiting normal behavior. The mother needs to be reassured that her baby is acting appropriately. Likes and dislikes are learned as children have experiences with people. These occur later as children develop. Because the neonate's behavior is normal, discussion of illness is inappropriate in response to this mother's comments. Mothers need reassurance. Telling a mother not to worry leads to more concern.
Nursing process step: Implementation
Client needs category: Psychosocial integrity
Client needs subcategory: None
Cognitive level: Application

30. CORRECT ANSWER: 4
For Bryant's traction to be effective, it must be continuous, with the child in proper traction alignment at all times. Options 1 and 2 interfere with proper traction. Option 3 is inappropriate because the child must remain in proper traction alignment when eating, regardless of the favorite eating position.
Nursing process step: Implementation
Client needs category: Safe, effective care environment
Client needs subcategory: Management of care
Cognitive level: Application

31. CORRECT ANSWER: 2
Pain elicited by dorsiflexing the foot (positive Homans' sign) indicates thrombophlebitis. A blood pressure discrepancy between the right and left legs (option 1), limited range of motion in the legs (option 3), and dependent edema (option 4) aren't signs of thrombophlebitis.
Nursing process step: Assessment
Client needs category: Health promotion and maintenance
Client needs subcategory: None
Cognitive level: Comprehension

32. CORRECT ANSWER: 4
Weights on a traction apparatus should hang freely and unobstructed. The head of the bed should be elevated no more than 30 degrees (option 1). The affected heel should be raised off the bed (option 2). The weights shouldn't be removed from the traction apparatus (option 3).
Nursing process step: Planning
Client needs category: Physiological integrity
Client needs subcategory: Basic care and comfort
Cognitive level: Application

33. CORRECT ANSWER: 2
After surgery for a fractured hip, the affected leg should be placed in abduction, using an abduction splint or pillows placed between the legs to separate them. The other options may cause dislocation.
Nursing process step: Implementation
Client needs category: Physiological integrity
Client needs subcategory: Basic care and comfort
Cognitive level: Application

34. CORRECT ANSWER: 1
A depressed client is at great risk for committing suicide and needs continuous observation. This client must not be left alone (options 2 and 4). The nurse must not relinquish responsibilities to another client (option 3).
Nursing process step: Implementation
Client needs category: Safe, effective care environment
Client needs subcategory: Management of care
Cognitive level: Application

35. CORRECT ANSWER: 2
During the first stage of labor, ambulation helps to stimulate labor. Lying down (option 1) and taking pain medication (option 3) may slow early labor. The client should use learned breathing techniques only when she can no longer talk during contractions (option 4).
Nursing process step: Planning
Client needs category: Health promotion and maintenance
Client needs subcategory: None
Cognitive level: Application

36. CORRECT ANSWER: 3
Because prednisone increases susceptibility to infections, the child should be kept away from persons with infections. The other options describe limitations or activities that aren't necessary during prednisone therapy.
Nursing process step: Evaluation
Client needs category: Physiological integrity
Client needs subcategory: Pharmacological and parenteral therapies
Cognitive level: Analysis

37. CORRECT ANSWER: 4
A normal platelet count for a 5-year-old child ranges from 150,000 to 400,000/µl. Leukemia typically causes an extremely low platelet count, predisposing the child to hemorrhage. The nurse should check the child frequently for ecchymosis and other signs and symptoms of hemorrhage. The other options aren't relevant for a client with a below-normal platelet count.
Nursing process step: Assessment
Client needs category: Physiological integrity
Client needs subcategory: Reduction of risk potential
Cognitive level: Analysis

38. CORRECT ANSWER: 2
Hypocalcemia is a possible cause of carpal spasm. To determine if the client has hypocalcemia, the nurse should check for Chvostek's sign by tapping the facial nerve; in a positive response, indicating hypocalcemia, the facial muscles twitch. Babinski's reflex indicates damage to the central nervous system, not hypocalcemia (option 1). Options 3 and 4 don't elicit information relevant to carpal spasms.

Nursing process step: Planning
Client needs category: Physiological integrity
Client needs subcategory: Reduction of risk potential
Cognitive level: Comprehension

39. CORRECT ANSWER: 3
The client who faces a possible mastectomy is obviously apprehensive and anxious about the possibility of having cancer and losing a breast. A high anxiety level limits concentration and learning ability. No data suggest that the client lacks knowledge of anatomy and physiology (option 1), isn't interested in details (option 2), or has a limited mental ability (option 4).
Nursing process step: Assessment
Client needs category: Psychosocial integrity
Client needs subcategory: None
Cognitive level: Application

40. CORRECT ANSWER: 2
To confirm rupture of the amniotic membranes the nurse assesses the pH of the vaginal fluid using Nitrazine Paper. With amniotic fluid, which is alkaline, the paper turns blue. Testing amniotic fluid for glucose (option 1), color (option 3), or albumin (option 4) doesn't confirm membrane rupture.
Nursing process step: Assessment
Client needs category: Health promotion and maintenance
Client needs subcategory: None
Cognitive level: Application

41. CORRECT ANSWER: 4
If the Hemovac chamber fills rapidly, it's typically filling with blood, indicating hemorrhage. To empty the chamber, the nurse simply opens it; clamping the catheter isn't necessary (option 1). Because patency of the Hemovac is maintained by suction, a saline solution flush isn't needed (option 2). Suction from the Hemovac, rather than pressure applied around the catheter, is used to promote drainage (option 3).
Nursing process step: Implementation
Client needs category: Physiological integrity
Client needs subcategory: Physiological adaptation
Cognitive level: Application

42. CORRECT ANSWER: 1
A client who's eager to be discharged typically has accepted the alteration to her body and is willing to deal with the reaction of family and friends to the removal of her breast. Options 2 and 3 don't necessarily indicate such willingness. Option 4 isn't conclusive because it doesn't indicate the client's reaction when looking at the incision.
Nursing process step: Evaluation
Client needs category: Psychosocial integrity
Client needs subcategory: None
Cognitive level: Comprehension

43. CORRECT ANSWER: 2
After cataract surgery, the client must not stoop, bend, cough, or strain because these activities increase intraocular pressure and may damage the surgical site. The other options describe activities that increase intraocular pressure.
Nursing process step: Evaluation
Client needs category: Physiological integrity
Client needs subcategory: Reduction of risk potential
Cognitive level: Application

44. CORRECT ANSWER: 4
The purpose of the reality-orientation session is to focus on the topic at hand. Talking about a specific event suggests that the client is following the discussion. Option 1 doesn't indicate whether the client is following the discussion. Option 2 doesn't reveal whether she's oriented to the present. Option 3 doesn't indicate if she's aware of the discussion or is merely responding to the word "party."
Nursing process step: Evaluation
Client needs category: Psychosocial integrity
Client needs subcategory: None
Cognitive level: Analysis

45. CORRECT ANSWER: 2
Most children with acute lymphocytic leukemia have a low-grade fever. The other options aren't common signs of leukemia.
Nursing process step: Assessment
Client needs category: Physiological integrity
Client needs subcategory: Physiological adaptation
Cognitive level: Knowledge

46. CORRECT ANSWER: 3
Bile is necessary for fat digestion. Gallstones may block the common bile duct, leaving no bile available for digesting fat; this leads to an intolerance to fatty foods. Options 1 and 2 don't relate to fat digestion. Stools are accompanied by flatus (from lack of bile product), which is unrelated to antacids (option 4).

Nursing process step: Assessment
Client needs category: Physiological integrity
Client needs subcategory: Physiological adaptation
Cognitive level: Application

47. CORRECT ANSWER: 3
Changing the client's position is the most appropriate action because the pain may result from pressure on the incision. A position change may also promote drainage. Placing a heating pad on the abdomen is unlikely to ease incisional pain (option 1). Options 2 and 4 might be appropriate if a change in position isn't effective, but they require a physician's order.
Nursing process step: Implementation
Client needs category: Physiological integrity
Client needs subcategory: Basic care and comfort
Cognitive level: Application

48. CORRECT ANSWER: 2
The nurse should connect the T tube to a collection bag, which collects drainage by gravity (straight drainage system). There's no need to irrigate the tube (option 1), attach it to suction (option 3), or aspirate it (option 4) after surgery. The physician may perform sterile saline irrigation if the client has thick bile or inadequate drainage.
Nursing process step: Implementation
Client needs category: Safe, effective care environment
Client needs subcategory: Safety and infection control
Taxonomic level: Application

49. CORRECT ANSWER: 3
Peanuts and other nuts are a good source of protein. Options 1, 2, and 4 are incorrect because salt, carbohydrates, and fats are important to the diet of a pregnant woman.
Nursing process step: Implementation
Client needs category: Physiological integrity
Client needs subcategory: Basic care and comfort
Cognitive level: Application

50. CORRECT ANSWER: 2
Most clients must take antituberculosis medications for 18 to 24 months. Typically, they must continue to take these medications even if they no longer have symptoms (options 1 and 4). Isoniazid is best taken on an empty stomach; vitamin C, such as from citrus juice, doesn't affect absorption of rifampin or isoniazid (option 3).
Nursing process step: Evaluation
Client needs category: Physiological integrity
Client needs subcategory: Pharmacological and parenteral therapies
Cognitive level: Application

51. CORRECT ANSWER: 1
Many older persons have a degenerative hearing loss. They may try to read lips and then misinterpret what has been said. No data suggest that the client has a perceptual defect (option 2), shortened attention span (option 3), or cerebral oxygen deficit (option 4).
Nursing process step: Assessment
Client needs category: Physiological integrity
Client needs subcategory: Reduction of risk potential
Cognitive level: Application

52. CORRECT ANSWER: 4
Bed rest reduces the work load of the heart by decreasing tissue demands for oxygen. Cardiac glycosides, not bed rest, are used to improve the heart's pumping action (option 1). Oxygen therapy is used to enhance oxygenation of body tissues (option 2). Diuretics are prescribed to decrease the blood volume (option 3).
Nursing process step: Planning
Client needs category: Physiological integrity
Client needs subcategory: Reduction of risk potential
Cognitive level: Application

53. CORRECT ANSWER: 2
The nurse must not reinforce the client's hallucinations. Telling the client to listen to the voices would reinforce the hallucinations (option 1). The nurse shouldn't say things that may not be true (option 3). The voices are real to the client; telling him that he doesn't hear them isn't therapeutic (option 4).
Nursing process step: Implementation
Client needs category: Psychosocial integrity
Client needs subcategory: None
Cognitive level: Application

54. CORRECT ANSWER: 4
Contracting the leg muscles helps to prevent pulmonary embolism, which occurs when a piece of a thrombus breaks off and enters the lung. Bed rest and inactivity promote such thrombus formation. Pleurisy, an inflammation of the lung pleura, typically results from spread of an infection from the lung (option 1). Portal hypertension usually is caused by liver damage (option 2). Hypostatic

pneumonia results from inhibition of normal lung clearing mechanisms, such as coughing (option 3).
Nursing process step: Planning
Client needs category: Physiological integrity
Client needs subcategory: Reduction of risk potential
Cognitive level: Application

55. CORRECT ANSWER: 2
Absence of tears in a crying infant indicates dehydration, which causes a rapid heart rate (above 160 beats/minute in an infant). A heart rate of 100 beats/minute is within normal limits (option 1). Distended neck veins (option 3) and bulging fontanels (option 4) are signs of overhydration.
Nursing process step: Assessment
Client needs category: Physiological integrity
Client needs subcategory: Physiological adaptation
Cognitive level: Analysis

56. CORRECT ANSWER: 1
Human chorionic gonadotropin is produced by the placenta and appears in maternal blood or urine 10 to 12 days after conception. Progesterone (option 2), follicle-stimulating hormone (option 3), and luteinizing hormone (option 4) are hormones of the menstrual cycle. (Progesterone is an important hormone of pregnancy as well.)
Nursing process step: Assessment
Client needs category: Health promotion and maintenance
Client needs subcategory: None
Cognitive level: Knowledge

57. CORRECT ANSWER: 4
The client with Parkinson's disease may be hypersensitive to heat, which increases the risk of hyperthermia, and he should be instructed to avoid sun exposure during hot weather.
Nursing process step: Planning
Client needs category: Health promotion and maintenance
Client needs subcategory: None
Cognitive level: Application

58. CORRECT ANSWER: 1
Erythromycin is an antibiotic used to prevent ophthalmia neonatorum (ocular gonorrheal infection). It doesn't prevent other eye disorders, such as retrolental fibroplasia (option 2), corneal keratitis (option 3), or acute uveitis (option 4).
Nursing process step: Implementation
Client needs category: Physiological integrity
Client needs subcategory: Pharmacological and parenteral therapies
Cogntive level: Application

59. CORRECT ANSWER: 2
During exercise, the body uses more circulating glucose and calories, increasing the risk for a hypoglycemic reaction. Therefore, the client should make sure to have a simple carbohydrate source available to consume during exercise. Taking extra insulin before exercising would lower the blood glucose level further (option 1). Resting (option 3) and stretching and bending (option 4) before exercising wouldn't alter the client's need for glucose during exercise.
Nursing process step: Planning
Client needs category: Health promotion and maintenance
Client needs subcategory: None
Cognitive level: Application

60. CORRECT ANSWER: 3
Type 1 diabetes mellitus is compatible with a good quality of life as long as the client modifies his diet and uses insulin properly. A client who follows the prescribed regimen has few limitations. The other options don't convey this information and therefore are inappropriate responses.
Nursing process step: Implementation
Client needs category: Psychosocial integrity
Client needs subcategory: None
Cognitive level: Application

61. CORRECT ANSWER: 2
Milk, milk products, and some green vegetables are good sources of calcium. The other options are lower in calcium.
Nursing process step: Evaluation
Client needs category: Health promotion and maintenance
Client needs subcategory: None
Cognitive level: Application

62. CORRECT ANSWER: 1
Signs and symptoms of gonorrhea in females include lower abdominal pain, pain on urination, and vaginal discharge.

Nursing process step: Assessment
Client needs category: Physiological integrity
Client needs subcategory: Physiological adaptation
Cognitive level: Application

63. CORRECT ANSWER: 3
When the umbilical cord prolapses, pressure placed on the cord by the fetus may impede the fetal oxygen supply. The nurse should take measures to help prevent pressure on the cord, such as placing the client's head lower than her legs (Trendelenburg's position). The other options wouldn't relieve pressure on the cord.
Nursing process step: Implementation
Client needs category: Physiological integrity
Client needs subcategory: Physiological adaptation
Cognitive level: Application

64. CORRECT ANSWER: 1
The nurse should administer about 0.5 ml of morphine, as indicated by the following formula:

Amount desired/Amount on hand × Quantity = Amount to administer

Therefore:

$$\frac{8\text{ mg}}{1} \div \frac{15\text{ mg}}{1\text{ ml}} = \frac{8\cancel{\text{mg}}}{1} \times \frac{1\text{ ml}}{15\cancel{\text{mg}}} = \frac{8\text{ ml}}{15} = 0.53\text{ or }0.5\text{ ml}$$

Nursing process step: Implementation
Client needs category: Physiological integrity
Client needs subcategory: Pharmacological and parenteral therapies
Cognitive level: Comprehension

65. CORRECT ANSWER: 2
Tachycardia (overly rapid heart rate) may occur as a result of fear, anger, or pain. Bradycardia (slowed heart rate) can result from vomiting, suctioning (causing vagal nerve stimulation), and certain medications.
Nursing process step: Assessment
Client needs category: Health promotion and maintenance
Client needs subcategory: None
Cognitive level: Comprehension

66. CORRECT ANSWER: 2
Arterial occlusive disease, which narrows the carotid artery, is a common complication of atherosclerosis and is treated with left carotid endarterectomy. Predisposing factors include smoking, hypertension, hyperlipidemia, and diabetes. The other conditions aren't directly related to arterial occlusive disease.
Nursing process step: Assessment
Client needs category: Physiological integrity
Client needs subcategory: Reduction of risk potential
Cognitive level: Knowledge

67. CORRECT ANSWER: 4
Frequent sneezing may indicate an allergy or infection, such as a cold. If an infection is present, surgery is usually postponed. The other options suggest mild anxiety — not uncommon in a 5-year-old who is in a new situation.
Nursing process step: Assessment
Client needs category: Physiological integrity
Client needs subcategory: Reduction of risk potential
Cognitive level: Analysis

68. CORRECT ANSWER: 3
A client who has had a MI must return to a modified routine slowly, with the physician determining how well the heart is tolerating increasing demands. Expecting to return to work within 2 weeks is unrealistic.
Nursing process step: Evaluation
Client needs category: Psychosocial integrity
Client needs subcategory: None
Cognitive level: Application

69. CORRECT ANSWER: 2
After a meal, the circulatory system (including the heart) must carry more blood to the stomach for digestion. Exercise, such as walking, also increases demands on the heart. To prevent both demands from occurring at once, the client should wait about 1 hour after a meal before exercising. The client need not measure the pulse rate when walking (option 1). The client should be able to walk the four steps to the house without a ramp, although the pace may be slow (option 3). Although the client should be encouraged to exercise, a rigid exercise schedule isn't desirable (option 4).
Nursing process step: Evaluation
Client needs category: Health promotion and maintenance
Client needs subcategory: None
Cognitive level: Application

70. CORRECT ANSWER: 1
Deficient fluid volume reflects a physiological need that's critical for life; using Maslow's hierarchy of needs, this

need takes highest priority. The other options are less essential and therefore take lower priority.
Nursing process step: Nursing diagnosis
Client needs category: Physiological integrity
Client needs subcategory: Physiological adaptation
Cognitive level: Comprehension

71. CORRECT ANSWER: 4
This client is addicted to alcohol and can't control what happens once consumption begins. Therefore, the client must abstain altogether.
Nursing process step: Planning
Client needs category: Safe, effective care environment
Client needs subcategory: Management of care
Cognitive level: Analysis

72. CORRECT ANSWER: 1
It isn't possible to bear down and pant at the same time. Holding her breath may help the client to bear down rather than preventing this (option 2). The client can hold on to the side rails (option 3) or maintain a supine position (option 4) while bearing down.
Nursing process step: Evaluation
Client needs category: Health promotion and maintenance
Client needs subcategory: None
Cognitive level: Application

73. CORRECT ANSWER: 2
Infants most commonly contract infectious diarrhea through improper preparation, handling, or storage of formula. The other options are important topics to discuss with mothers of infants but don't relate directly to preventing infectious diarrhea.
Nursing process step: Implementation
Client needs category: Health promotion and maintenance
Client needs subcategory: None
Cognitive level: Application

74. CORRECT ANSWER: 4
This is atrial fibrillation with aberrant ventricular conduction. The rhythm is irregular; the atrial rate can't be determined; the ventricular rate is 60 beats/minute; the P wave is absent; coarse fibrillatory waves are present; the PR interval is indiscernible; the duration of the QRS complex is 0.12 second; the T wave is indiscernible; and the QT interval is unmeasureable.
Nursing process step: Assessment
Client needs category: Physiological integrity
Client needs subcategory: Physiological adaptation
Cognitive level: Analysis

75. CORRECT ANSWER:

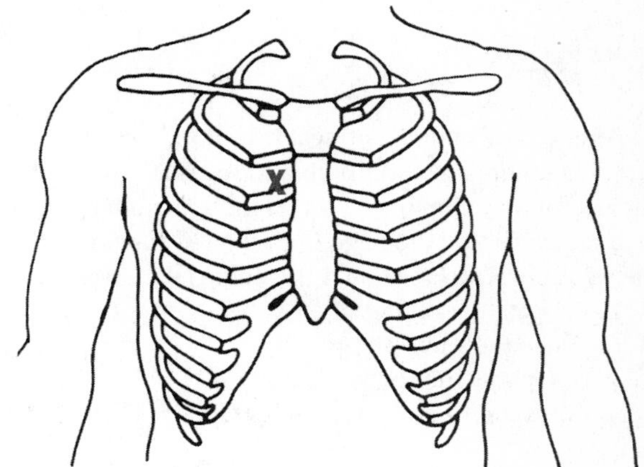

The murmur of aortic stenosis is low-pitched, rough, and rasping. It's heard loudest in the second intercostal space to the right of the sternum.
Nursing process step: Assessment
Client needs category: Physiological integrity
Client needs subcategory: Physiological adaptation
Cognitive level: Application

Posttest 2

QUESTIONS

1. After an abdominal perineal resection, a client returns to the nursing unit with a nasogastric (NG) tube attached to intermittent suction. Eight hours after surgery, the nurse notes that drainage from the NG tube has stopped. Which action should the nurse take first?

☐ **1.** Irrigate the tubing.
☐ **2.** Have the client sit upright.
☐ **3.** Check the tubing for kinks.
☐ **4.** Turn the suction to CONSTANT.

2. A client with type 1 diabetes mellitus is admitted to the hospital with a diagnosis of ketoacidosis. Which client behavior is most likely to contribute to the development of ketoacidosis?

☐ **1.** Increasing the length of daily walks
☐ **2.** Neglecting to take insulin regularly
☐ **3.** Failing to adhere to the prescribed diet
☐ **4.** Working 8 hours per day

3. A client has been in a psychiatric facility for 6 months. During this time, she's been unable to meet her own hygiene and grooming needs. She spends most of her time alone and usually is nonverbal. When a staff member approaches her, she turns away. She's standing in the hall when the nurse notices a large, damp, red area on the seat of her pants. The nurse assumes the client has begun to menstruate. Which response is most appropriate for the nurse to make at this time?

☐ **1.** "You have begun your period. I want you to come into the bathroom with me."
☐ **2.** "Your pants are bloody, and you'll need to go and change your clothes now."
☐ **3.** "You have started your period. Do you want me to get you some supplies?"
☐ **4.** "Did you know that you have started your period?"

4. A nurse instructs a client to eat foods high in protein. The client shows an understanding of these instructions by selecting which food from a sample menu?

☐ **1.** Eggs
☐ **2.** Gelatin dessert
☐ **3.** Rice
☐ **4.** Banana

5. Which intervention should a nurse include in the care plan for a young child in Bryant's traction?

☐ **1.** Bathe the child with a mild soap daily.
☐ **2.** Test the urine for acetone once each shift.
☐ **3.** Check the toes for warmth and color every 2 hours.
☐ **4.** Pad the side rails of the child's crib.

6. A client tells a nurse, "My husband and I have been married for 60 years. I don't understand why I always get cystitis and he doesn't." The nurse's explanation should include which information?

☐ **1.** The female urethra is shorter and closer to the rectum than the male urethra.
☐ **2.** Males have a greater resistance to bacterial organisms than females.
☐ **3.** The sphincter of the female meatus doesn't contract as tightly as that of the male.
☐ **4.** Toilet tissue is more likely to irritate the female meatus than the male meatus.

7. When preparing to administer NPH insulin to a client, a nurse should take which action?

☐ **1.** Rotate the vial between the hands.
☐ **2.** Warm the vial to body temperature by running hot water over it.
☐ **3.** Invert the vial for a few minutes.
☐ **4.** Aspirate the insulin without injecting air into the vial.

8. Which medication should the nurse have on hand to counteract adverse effects of heparin sodium?

- ☐ **1.** Calcium gluconate
- ☐ **2.** Protamine sulfate
- ☐ **3.** Chlorambucil
- ☐ **4.** Lithium carbonate

9. After a transurethral prostatic resection, a client returns to the unit with an indwelling urethral catheter attached to a continuous bladder irrigating system. Within several hours, the client complains of bladder spasms. Which action should the nurse take initially?

- ☐ **1.** Determine if clots are obstructing the catheter.
- ☐ **2.** Support the client in a side-lying position.
- ☐ **3.** Assess the client's vital signs.
- ☐ **4.** Administer prescribed pain medication.

10. On the 3rd day after a partial thyroidectomy, a client exhibits muscle twitching and hyperirritability of the nervous system. When questioned, the client reports numbness and tingling of the mouth and fingertips. Suspecting a life-threatening electrolyte disturbance, the nurse notifies the surgeon immediately. Which electrolyte disturbance most commonly follows thyroid surgery?

- ☐ **1.** Hypocalcemia
- ☐ **2.** Hyponatremia
- ☐ **3.** Hyperkalemia
- ☐ **4.** Hypermagnesemia

11. A nurse teaches a client about warfarin sodium (Coumadin). Which statement by the client indicates the need for further instruction?

- ☐ **1.** "I'll use an electric razor when shaving."
- ☐ **2.** "I'll need to have periodic blood coagulation tests."
- ☐ **3.** "I'll expect my urine to be dark brown."
- ☐ **4.** "I'll check my skin to see if I'm bruising more easily."

12. A client with a displaced fracture of the left femur is placed in balanced-suspension skeletal traction. The client complains of a sharp pain when the nurse dorsiflexes the affected foot. How should the nurse interpret this complaint?

- ☐ **1.** The client has thrombophlebitis.
- ☐ **2.** Osteomyelitis has set in.
- ☐ **3.** The client has developed compartment syndrome.
- ☐ **4.** Fragments of the fracture are displaced.

13. Which nursing measure is most likely to prevent further excoriation of an infant's bright red buttocks?

- ☐ **1.** Exposing the affected area to air.
- ☐ **2.** Applying baby lotion to the affected area.
- ☐ **3.** Using only disposable diapers.
- ☐ **4.** Washing the affected area with warm water only.

14. Which finding should the nurse expect when assessing the neonate of a diabetic mother?

- ☐ **1.** Hypertonia
- ☐ **2.** Hyperactivity
- ☐ **3.** Macrosomia
- ☐ **4.** Scaly skin

15. A nurse is obtaining a history from a client with suspected peptic ulcer disease. Which history finding is most likely to contribute to ulcer development?

- ☐ **1.** The client takes ibuprofen daily for arthritis pain.
- ☐ **2.** The client operates a photocopy machine 8 hours per day, 5 days per week.
- ☐ **3.** The client has been on a strict vegetarian diet.
- ☐ **4.** The client has a family history of severe psoriasis.

16. A client with cervical cancer is receiving internal radiation treatment. The intensity of radiation is estimated by using the principle of the inverse square rule. If the nurse is 4′ from the radiation source, the exposure would be:

- ☐ **1.** ½ of the exposure at 1′.
- ☐ **2.** ¼ of the exposure at 1′.
- ☐ **3.** ⅛ of the exposure at 1′.
- ☐ **4.** 1/16 of the exposure at 1′.

17. A client in a nursing home has Alzheimer's disease. She's very forgetful and frequently asks what time it is. How should the nurse respond the next time the client asks the time?

- ☐ **1.** Ask the client what time it was the last time she asked.
- ☐ **2.** Ask the client why she can't remember the time.
- ☐ **3.** Tell the client the correct time.
- ☐ **4.** Tell the client this is the last time she'll be told.

18. A nurse is administering the prescribed morning dose of NPH insulin to a diabetic client. Within 30 minutes after administering NPH insulin, the nurse should assign highest priority to which action?

☐ **1.** Testing the client's urine for glucose
☐ **2.** Observing the client for a skin reaction
☐ **3.** Checking the injection site for drug absorption
☐ **4.** Instructing the client to eat breakfast

19. While on the examining table, a client who is 19 weeks pregnant tells the nurse that she's experiencing quickening. Which action should the nurse take?

☐ **1.** Inform the charge nurse of the client's symptom.
☐ **2.** Turn the client onto her left side.
☐ **3.** Tell the client that quickening is normal.
☐ **4.** Remind the client that she soon may have bloody show.

20. A client is recovering from abdominal surgery. Which finding indicates that the client is ready for removal of the nasogastric (NG) tube?

☐ **1.** The client no longer complains of feeling nauseated.
☐ **2.** The client burps after taking a sip of clear fluids.
☐ **3.** Drainage from the client's stomach has diminished in volume.
☐ **4.** The client has been passing flatus.

21. A 2-month-old infant who has been vomiting formula and passing watery green stools is admitted to the pediatric unit. The physician diagnoses infectious diarrhea and dehydration. An I.V. infusion is started in a scalp vein and all oral intake is withheld. The nurse assigned to care for the child should take which action first?

☐ **1.** Obtain a stool specimen.
☐ **2.** Measure the infant's axillary temperature.
☐ **3.** Place the infant on isolation precautions.
☐ **4.** Test urine specific gravity.

22. A client is receiving digoxin. Which adverse reaction should the nurse watch for during digoxin therapy?

☐ **1.** Blurred vision
☐ **2.** Hand tremors
☐ **3.** Urine retention
☐ **4.** Hearing loss

23. For a client with osteoporosis, the nurse should provide which dietary instruction?

☐ **1.** "Decrease your intake of red meat."
☐ **2.** "Decrease your intake of popcorn, nuts, and seeds."
☐ **3.** "Eat more fruits to increase your potassium intake."
☐ **4.** Eat more dairy products to increase your calcium intake."

24. A client undergoes an abdominal-perineal resection and a permanent colostomy in the descending colon. Postoperatively, a nasogastric tube is attached to low intermittent suction and a urethral catheter is attached to straight drainage. Two hours after surgery, the nurse notes that the perineal dressing is saturated with serosanguineous drainage. The nurse's next action should be based on the conclusion that the drainage resulted from which ocurrence?

☐ **1.** An abrupt movement by the client
☐ **2.** Slippage of the suture holding the stoma in place
☐ **3.** A properly functioning Penrose drain
☐ **4.** A displaced urinary catheter

25. A client with benign prostatic hyperplasia undergoes transurethral prostatic resection. Postoperatively, an indwelling catheter is in place. During the immediate postoperative period, the nurse should expect which assessment finding?

☐ **1.** Discomfort when urinating
☐ **2.** A distended bladder
☐ **3.** A neurogenic bladder
☐ **4.** Bloody urinary drainage

26. A physician prescribes ferrous gluconate (Fergon) in liquid form for a client with iron-deficiency anemia. How should the nurse administer this preparation?

☐ **1.** Undiluted, with a dropper onto the tongue
☐ **2.** Undiluted, from a teaspoon
☐ **3.** Diluted with milk, in a glass
☐ **4.** Diluted with water, through a straw

27. A physician orders 1,000 ml of dextrose 5% in water every 8 hours for a client. The I.V. setup delivers 20 gtt/ml. About how many drops should be administered per minute?

☐ **1.** 27
☐ **2.** 35
☐ **3.** 42
☐ **4.** 50

28. A client is admitted to an alcohol treatment clinic. During the first meeting with the nurse, the client says, "Why am I meeting with you? You can't make me stop drinking." Which response by the nurse would be most therapeutic?

- ☐ **1.** "What makes you think I want to make you stop drinking?"
- ☐ **2.** "That's true. Quitting is truly your decision."
- ☐ **3.** "It's your life. I hope you'll give the program a fair try."
- ☐ **4.** "Your family really cares about you, and I think you care, too."

29. Which action by a nurse may help prevent a urinary tract infection in a client who is in labor?

- ☐ **1.** Providing the client with ice chips
- ☐ **2.** Encouraging the client to void frequently
- ☐ **3.** Testing the client's urine for glycosuria
- ☐ **4.** Providing frequent perineal care

30. A 4-year-old girl is scheduled for a bone marrow aspiration. Which nursing action would help prepare her for this procedure?

- ☐ **1.** Using a doll to show her what will happen during the procedure
- ☐ **2.** Telling her a story about a little girl who had the procedure
- ☐ **3.** Discussing the procedure with her parents and letting them explain it to her
- ☐ **4.** Asking her parents if she knows anyone who has had this procedure

31. A client with rectal cancer is scheduled for an abdominal-perineal resection. Before surgery, the nurse tells the client that this procedure will cause a change in which area?

- ☐ **1.** Urine output
- ☐ **2.** Eating habits
- ☐ **3.** Physical activity
- ☐ **4.** Body image

32. A physician prescribes an intramuscular injection of iron dextran (DexFerrum) for a client with anemia. Which nursing action applies to administering this medication?

- ☐ **1.** Asking if the client drinks alcoholic beverages
- ☐ **2.** Finding out if the client is allergic to fish oil
- ☐ **3.** Giving the medication by the Z-track method
- ☐ **4.** Using a 1″ 25G needle to inject the medication

33. A client with rectal cancer is scheduled for an abdominal-perineal resection. The client is placed on a low-residue diet initially, then he's switched to a liquid diet for 24 hours before surgery. The nurse teaches the client that the low-residue and liquid diets are needed for what reason?

- ☐ **1.** To eliminate stress in the diseased bowel
- ☐ **2.** To empty the bowel of fecal material
- ☐ **3.** To reduce bowel motility
- ☐ **4.** To decrease pain in the diseased bowel

34. A client is to take ferrous sulfate (Feosol). Which adverse reaction can this preparation cause?

- ☐ **1.** Tinnitus
- ☐ **2.** Ataxia
- ☐ **3.** Blurred vision
- ☐ **4.** Black stools

35. A depressed client talks, walks, and moves at a slow pace. Which measure should a nurse include in the care plan?

- ☐ **1.** Try to slow the pace of care activities.
- ☐ **2.** Encourage the client to move at a faster pace.
- ☐ **3.** Remind the client that this behavior isn't appropriate.
- ☐ **4.** Provide the client with a more stimulating environment.

36. A nurse teaches a client with anemia to eat iron-rich foods. The client shows an understanding of the dietary instructions by selecting which snack?

- ☐ **1.** 1 cup of popcorn
- ☐ **2.** ½ cup of raisins
- ☐ **3.** ½ cup of blueberries
- ☐ **4.** 1 cup of hot chocolate

37. A multigravida client has her urine tested for protein. The purpose of this test is to help determine if the client has which problem?

- ☐ **1.** Gestational hypertension
- ☐ **2.** Ketoacidosis
- ☐ **3.** Placenta previa
- ☐ **4.** Gestational diabetes

38. After learning that their child has acute lymphocytic leukemia, the child's parents become angry and hostile toward the staff. How should the nurse respond to the parents?

- ☐ **1.** Tell them that their behavior isn't helping their child.
- ☐ **2.** Give them a chance to talk and help them cope with their feelings.
- ☐ **3.** Limit their visiting time with their child.
- ☐ **4.** Tell them that everything is being done to restore their child's health.

39. A client with iron-deficiency anemia reports episodes of feeling dizzy and faint. To manage these episodes, the nurse should include which intervention in the care plan?

- ☐ **1.** Have the client lie down until the episode is over.
- ☐ **2.** Instruct the client to do breathing exercises when an episode occurs.
- ☐ **3.** Advise the client to drink highly sweetened beverages when an episode occurs.
- ☐ **4.** Teach the client to rise slowly from a lying or sitting position to a standing position.

40. After a client has a sigmoidoscopy, the nurse should observe for which potential complication of this procedure?

- ☐ **1.** Muscle atony of the colon
- ☐ **2.** Fissure of the anal sphincter
- ☐ **3.** Perforation of the intestinal wall
- ☐ **4.** Intestinal hyperactivity

41. A client with iron-deficiency anemia is most likely to express which complaint?

- ☐ **1.** "My skin feels warm."
- ☐ **2.** "I get short of breath."
- ☐ **3.** "My tongue is swollen."
- ☐ **4.** "I've lost my sense of smell."

42. A nurse teaches a client how to prepare for a barium enema. Which statement by the client indicates a correct understanding of the teaching?

- ☐ **1.** "I'll cleanse my bowel with laxatives and enemas before the test."
- ☐ **2.** "I'll receive a muscle relaxant during the test."
- ☐ **3.** "I'll drink a contrast medium during the test."
- ☐ **4.** "I'll stop eating red meat 3 days before the test."

43. A client receives instructions on breast-feeding. Which statement indicates that she understands the instructions?

- ☐ **1.** "I should pull my baby's mouth from my nipple gently to detach him from my breast."
- ☐ **2.** "I should use cold compresses to relieve breast discomfort between feedings."
- ☐ **3.** "I should clean my nipples with soap and water gently after each feeding."
- ☐ **4.** "I should alternate breasts with each feeding."

44. Which behavior modification technique is useful in the treatment of phobias?

- ☐ **1.** Aversion therapy
- ☐ **2.** Imitation or modeling
- ☐ **3.** Positive reinforcement
- ☐ **4.** Systematic desensitization

45. A client is found sitting in a car with the motor running in an enclosed garage. When brought to the emergency department by the rescue squad, the client is unresponsive and hypotensive, with a respiratory rate of 6 breaths/minute, with bright red skin. Which nursing diagnosis takes highest priority for this client?

- ☐ **1.** Ineffective coping related to depression
- ☐ **2.** Ineffective tissue perfusion (peripheral) related to decreased cardiac output
- ☐ **3.** Ineffective tissue perfusion (cerebral) related to depressed neurological functioning
- ☐ **4.** Ineffective breathing pattern related to depressed respirations

46. An 18-month-old infant falls down a flight of stairs and is admitted to the hospital with a fractured right femur. The infant is placed in Bryant's traction. The nurse makes the following observations of the infant and the traction system. Which one necessitates intervention?

- ☐ **1.** The weights are hanging freely over the foot of the crib.
- ☐ **2.** The infant's buttocks are resting on the crib mattress.
- ☐ **3.** The ropes are resting in the pulley grooves.
- ☐ **4.** The infant's legs are flexed at a 90-degree angle to the body.

47. Which goal of nursing care takes priority for a female client with cystitis?

☐ **1.** Increasing urine alkalinity
☐ **2.** Maintaining a balanced fluid intake and output
☐ **3.** Providing instructions on perineal hygiene
☐ **4.** Screening urine for sedimentation

48. A nurse teaches a client about a high-fiber diet. The client shows an understanding of the instructions by selecting which food from a sample menu?

☐ **1.** Cheese
☐ **2.** White bread
☐ **3.** Grapefruit
☐ **4.** Broccoli

49. A client had abdominal surgery 2 days ago. Which observation indicates that peristaltic activity has returned?

☐ **1.** The client is belching.
☐ **2.** The client is hungry.
☐ **3.** The client is passing flatus.
☐ **4.** The client is thirsty.

50. A client complains of irritability and poor concentration. These symptoms indicate which level of anxiety?

☐ **1.** Mild
☐ **2.** Moderate
☐ **3.** Severe
☐ **4.** Panic

51. A client with emphysema is scheduled for discharge. During discharge preparation, the nurse reminds the client to stop smoking. The client replies angrily, "Who are you to tell me what to do? I'm older than you." Which response by the nurse would be most appropriate?

☐ **1.** "I'm giving you this information in your best interest."
☐ **2.** "You have the right to make your own decisions."
☐ **3.** "I don't mean to be disrespectful."
☐ **4.** "If you don't want to take my advice, do whatever you wish."

52. A nurse is assessing a child, age 2, for signs of increased intracranial pressure (ICP). These signs include which finding?

☐ **1.** Increasing irritability
☐ **2.** Tachycardia
☐ **3.** Narrowing pulse pressure
☐ **4.** Pinpoint pupils

53. A client in the first phase of labor is connected to an external electronic fetal monitor. Her cervix is dilated 9 cm. Which electronic fetal monitor finding warrants immediate intervention?

☐ **1.** Consistent variability of the baseline fetal heart rate (FHR)
☐ **2.** A change in the FHR that mirrors the uterine contraction
☐ **3.** FHR deceleration with delayed recovery after a uterine contraction
☐ **4.** FHR acceleration of 15 beats/minute that lasts 15 seconds

54. A physician prescribes promethazine hydrochloride (Phenergan) for a client who's being prepared for surgery. What's the purpose of administering this drug to this client?

☐ **1.** To provide sedation
☐ **2.** To inhibit oral secretions
☐ **3.** To prevent bleeding problems
☐ **4.** To enhance wound healing

55. After being admitted for diagnostic tests to rule out a cardiac problem, a client complains of nervousness, irritability, and an upset stomach. To best assist the client, the nurse should have which understanding?

☐ **1.** The client's symptoms are an inappropriate reaction to the diagnostic tests.
☐ **2.** A client may invent symptoms to gain the nurse's attention.
☐ **3.** The client's symptoms may indicate increased anxiety.
☐ **4.** An exaggerated reaction to unpleasant situations is common.

56. A client is receiving a transfusion of whole blood. Which assessment finding indicates that a hemolytic reaction is occurring?

☐ **1.** Lower back pain
☐ **2.** Positive Homans' sign
☐ **3.** Hyperreflexia
☐ **4.** Hematemesis

57. A child is scheduled for surgery. Which statement by the child indicates the need for more preoperative teaching?

☐ **1.** "I'll wake up in another room and then come back to my room."
☐ **2.** "I'll see Mom and Dad after the operation."
☐ **3.** "I'll have my favorite ice cream after I wake up."
☐ **4.** "I'll feel sleepy for a while after the operation."

58. Immediately after a neonate's birth, which goal of nursing care takes priority?

☐ **1.** Clearing the neonate's airway
☐ **2.** Determining the neonate's Apgar score
☐ **3.** Initiating the neonate's identification
☐ **4.** Maintaining the neonate's body temperature

59. A 74-year-old client has vascular disease. Which nursing intervention would be most appropriate for this client?

☐ **1.** Encourage him to avoid caffeine and nicotine.
☐ **2.** Advise him to wear knee-length stockings.
☐ **3.** Instruct him to soak both feet in cool water.
☐ **4.** Caution him not to exercise daily.

60. A client undergoes a left-sided mastectomy with removal of the axillary lymph nodes. During discharge preparation, the nurse should provide which instruction?

☐ **1.** "Wear an elastic bandage on your left arm at all times."
☐ **2.** "Don't let anyone draw blood from your left arm or take blood pressure on that arm."
☐ **3.** "Avoid sleeping on your left side or putting pressure on your left arm."
☐ **4.** "Keep your left arm elevated or in a sling most of the day."

61. After a tonsillectomy and adenoidectomy, a child returns to the pediatric unit. Until fully awake, the child should be maintained in which position?

☐ **1.** Side-lying
☐ **2.** Supine
☐ **3.** Knee-to-chest
☐ **4.** Lithotomy

62. Which intervention would the nurse recommend to a client having severe heartburn during her pregnancy?

☐ **1.** Eat several small meals daily.
☐ **2.** Eat crackers on waking every morning.
☐ **3.** Drink small amounts of milk frequently.
☐ **4.** Drink orange juice frequently during the day.

63. A client who's 40-weeks' pregnant is scheduled for a cesarean delivery because of cephalopelvic disproportion. Which intervention should be included in her preoperative care plan?

☐ **1.** Activity: may be up and about or side-lying in bed
☐ **2.** Nutrition: may have clear fluids as desired because of planned spinal anesthesia
☐ **3.** Vital signs: taken every half hour until surgery
☐ **4.** Pain medication: given as directed

64. A client's daughter tells the nurse, "Since I found out that my mother needs heart surgery, I've had trouble eating and sleeping." Which response by the nurse is best?

☐ **1.** "You must keep up your strength."
☐ **2.** "Your mother's condition is upsetting you."
☐ **3.** "Don't be concerned. These operations are common now."
☐ **4.** "I have the opposite reaction when I'm troubled."

65. Which response pattern best describes Babinski's reflex?

☐ **1.** Flexion of the foot when the Achilles tendon is tapped
☐ **2.** Extension of the leg when the patellar tendon is struck
☐ **3.** Tremor of the foot following brisk, forcible dorsiflexion
☐ **4.** Dorsiflexion of the great toe when the sole is scratched

66. Which assessment finding would indicate that a client's abdominal ascites is decreasing?

☐ **1.** The amount of ankle edema remains the same.
☐ **2.** Abdominal skin becomes shinier.
☐ **3.** Urine output per void increases.
☐ **4.** The pulse rate increases over time.

67. At the change of shift, an 18-month-old infant is being placed in Bryant's traction after a fall down a flight of stairs. What position would the infant be in for this type of traction?

- ☐ **1.** Flat in bed with the affected leg extended wrapped in an elastic bandage with traction applied
- ☐ **2.** Flat in bed with a padded sling under the knee on the affected leg with traction applied
- ☐ **3.** Both legs at a 90-degree angle with buttocks off the bed with traction applied
- ☐ **4.** Affected leg at a 90-degree angle with a skeletal pin inserted in the distal end of the femur with traction applied

68. A client is recovering from abdominal surgery. During the immediate postoperative period, which action should the nurse take to help prevent hypostatic pneumonia?

- ☐ **1.** Splint the incisional area while the client breathes deeply.
- ☐ **2.** Have the client use an incentive spirometer four times daily.
- ☐ **3.** Encourage the client to exhale through pursed lips.
- ☐ **4.** Support the client in an orthopneic position.

69. Which action by the nurse helps prevent thrombophlebitis in the calves of a postoperative client?

- ☐ **1.** Obtaining an order for the use of elastic stockings
- ☐ **2.** Keeping the knee gatch of the bed in a slightly elevated position
- ☐ **3.** Elevating the client's legs higher than the heart
- ☐ **4.** Encouraging the client to dorsiflex his feet three times daily

70. Which nursing action is especially important in the secondary prevention of violence and abuse?

- ☐ **A.** Helping participants discuss the problem and develop alternatives for dealing with the tension that could lead to violence
- ☐ **B.** Identifying "red flag" behaviors, including isolation and depression
- ☐ **C.** Emphasizing safety as a top priority
- ☐ **D.** Teaching clients the importance of respect and caring for family members

71. The mother of a child who has been hospitalized for status asthmaticus stands outside the child's room crying. Which comment by the nurse would be most therapeutic?

- ☐ **1.** "This must be upsetting for you."
- ☐ **2.** "Talking to the doctor will help."
- ☐ **3.** "Most mothers of asthmatic children feel this way."
- ☐ **4.** "Come talk with other parents in the waiting room who are experiencing similar situations."

72. A client with type 1 diabetes mellitus is taking NPH insulin. Which dietary instruction should the nurse provide?

- ☐ **1.** "When you skip a meal, reduce your insulin dosage."
- ☐ **2.** "Substitute 1 oz of fat for 2 oz of protein."
- ☐ **3.** "Eat your meals and snacks on schedule."
- ☐ **4.** "Use artificial sweeteners instead of complex sugars."

73. Based on multiple referrals, the nurse determines that childhood injuries are increasing in the community in which she practices. What's the first step the nurse should take in developing an educational program?

- ☐ **1.** Assessing for a decrease in referrals following a pediatric safety class
- ☐ **2.** Assessing the strengths and needs of the community while identifying barriers to learning
- ☐ **3.** Choosing a health promotion or health belief model as a framework
- ☐ **4.** Developing and implementing a specific plan to decrease childhood injuries

74. A neonate is 8 hours old. Which assessment finding indicates that the neonate is in satisfactory condition? Select all that apply.

- ☐ **1.** Axillary temperature of 96° F (35.5° C)
- ☐ **2.** Apical pulse rate of 124 beats/minute
- ☐ **3.** Slight yellowish tinge to the sclera
- ☐ **4.** Respiratory grunting on expiration
- ☐ **5.** Respiratory rate of 44 breaths/minute

75. A physician prescribes ibuprofen (Motrin) for a client with osteoarthritis. The nurse should instruct the client to take this drug with which of the following? Select all that apply.

- ☐ **1.** Food
- ☐ **2.** An antacid
- ☐ **3.** Milk
- ☐ **4.** Aspirin
- ☐ **5.** Apple juice

ANSWERS AND RATIONALES

In the posttest answers, the question number appears in boldface type, followed by the number of the correct answer. Rationales for correct answers and, where appropriate, for incorrect options follow. To help you evaluate your knowledge base and application of nursing behaviors, each rationale is classified according to:

- nursing process step
- client needs category
- client needs subcategory
- cognitive level.

1. CORRECT ANSWER: 3
Drainage should be present when an NG tube is attached to suction. If drainage stops, the nurse first should check for external causes of tube malfunction, such as kinked tubing. Options 1 and 2 may be appropriate later but aren't priorities. Option 4 requires a physician's order.
Nursing process step: Implementation
Client needs category: Physiological integrity
Client needs subcategory: Physiological adaptation
Cognitive level: Analysis

2. CORRECT ANSWER: 2
Ketoacidosis (accumulation of ketones in the body) results from insufficient endogenous insulin and an elevated blood glucose level, such as from neglecting to take insulin regularly. Option 1 is more likely to cause hypoglycemia. Option 3 may cause hypoglycemia or hyperglycemia. Option 4 isn't a potential cause of ketoacidosis.
Nursing process step: Evaluation
Client needs category: Physiological integrity
Client needs subcategory: Reduction of risk potential
Cogntive level: Analysis

3. CORRECT ANSWER: 1
This response orients the client to reality and provides the structure the client needs to solve the immediate problem. The client is too anxious and regressed to engage in the problem solving required by options 2 and 3. Option 4 is inane because the client is unable to provide self-care as a result of severe anxiety that interferes with problem solving and prevents awareness of reality.
Nursing process step: Implementation
Client needs category: Psychosocial integrity
Client needs subcategory: None
Cognitive level: Analysis

4. CORRECT ANSWER: 1
Eggs, meat, fish, and poultry are good sources of protein. Eggs have 6.1 g of protein. A gelatin dessert has 1.6 g of protein, rice has 4 g, and bananas have 1.2 g.
Nursing process step: Evaluation
Client needs category: Health promotion and maintenance
Client needs subcategory: None
Cognitive level: Comprehension

5. CORRECT ANSWER: 3
Bryant's traction is applied with elastic bandages; if wrapped too tightly, these bandages may impair circulation. Checking the toes for warmth and color verifies adequate circulation.
Nursing process step: Implementation
Client needs category: Physiological integrity
Client needs subcategory: Reduction of risk potential
Cognitive level: Application

6. CORRECT ANSWER: 1
Women are more susceptible than men to lower urinary tract infections, such as cystitis, because the female urethra is shorter and closer to the rectum, making it more vulnerable to bacteria.
Nursing process step: Implementation
Client needs category: Health promotion and maintenance
Client needs subcategory: None
Cognitive level: Application

7. CORRECT ANSWER: 1
The active principle in NPH insulin is in the milky white precipitate. To ensure complete dispersion of the precipitate, the nurse must rotate the vial gently between the hands. Insulin should be administered at room temperature, not warmed (option 2). The nurse shouldn't invert the vial for a few minutes (option 3) because this would allow the precipitate to settle. Inserting air into the vial is the correct procedure for insulin administration (option 4).
Nursing process step: Implementation
Client needs category: Physiological integrity
Client needs subcategory: Pharmacological and parenteral therapies
Cognitive level: Application

8. CORRECT ANSWER: 2
Protamine sulfate is the antidote for heparin sodium. When given I.V., it binds with heparin, rendering it inef-

fective within 5 minutes. The other options aren't heparin antidotes or antagonists.
Nursing process step: Planning
Client needs category: Physiological integrity
Client needs subcategory: Pharmacological and parenteral therapies
Cognitive level: Comprehension

9. CORRECT ANSWER: 1
The presence of clots in the urethral catheter may obstruct urine flow and cause bladder distention, resulting in bladder spasms.
Nursing process step: Implementation
Client needs category: Physiological integrity
Client needs subcategory: Reduction of risk potential
Cognitive level: Analysis

10. CORRECT ANSWER: 1
Hypocalcemia may follow thyroid surgery if the parathyroid glands were removed accidentally. Signs and symptoms of hypocalcemia may be delayed for up to 7 days after surgery. Thyroid surgery doesn't directly cause serum sodium, potassium, or magnesium abnormalities. Hyponatremia may occur if the patient inadvertently received too much fluid; however, this can happen to any surgical patient receiving I.V. fluid therapy, not just one recovering from thyroid surgery. Hyperkalemia and hypermagnesemia usually are associated with reduced renal excretion of potassium and magnesium.
Nursing process step: Evaluation
Client needs category: Safe, effective care environment
Client needs subcategory: Management of care
Cognitive level: Comprehension

11. CORRECT ANSWER: 3
Dark brown urine (hematuria) is an unexpected finding indicating bleeding of the urinary tract, which may signal an overdose of warfarin, an anticoagulant. During warfarin therapy, the client should use an electric razor to reduce the risk of injury (option 1). The client must have periodic coagulation tests to determine if clotting time is satisfactory (option 2). Bruising may be a sign of bleeding into the skin, another potential sign of warfarin overdose (option 4).
Nursing process step: Evaluation
Client needs category: Physiological integrity
Client needs subcategory: Reduction of risk potential
Cognitive level: Analysis

12. CORRECT ANSWER: 3
Increasing pain on passive movement signals compartment syndrome, which results from increased venous pressure and decreased arterial perfusion in a confined space, leading to anoxia. Dorsiflexing the affected foot increases muscle stretching, worsening anoxia and pain. Unlike compartment syndrome, which causes sharp pain, thrombophlebitis causes dull, constant pain (option 1). Osteomyelitis usually causes continuous pain (option 2). No assessment data suggest that the traction apparatus is functioning improperly; therefore, the nurse has no reason to suspect that fragments of the fracture are displaced (option 4).
Nursing process step: Assessment
Client needs category: Physiological integrity
Client needs subcategory: Reduction of risk potential
Cognitive evel: Comprehension

13. CORRECT ANSWER: 1
Exposure to air allows the skin to dry and heal. Bacteria grow best in a warm, moist environment, which is encouraged by applying baby lotion (option 2) and using only occlusive disposable diapers (option 3). Option 4 doesn't remove the offending bacteria.
Nursing process step: Implementation
Client needs category: Physiological integrity
Client needs subcategory: Basic care and comfort
Cognitive level: Application

14. CORRECT ANSWER: 3
The neonate of a diabetic mother typically is large (macrosomia) but physically immature. This neonate also may have hypocalcemia, hypoglycemia, hyperbilirubinemia, polycythemia, congestive anomalies, and renal thrombosis.
Nursing process step: Assessment
Client needs category: Health promotion and maintenance
Client needs subcategory: None
Cognitive level: Analysis

15. CORRECT ANSWER: 1
Ibuprofen is a nonsteroidal anti-inflammatory drug that can erode through the gastric mucosal barrier, predisposing the client to ulcer formation.
Nursing process step: Assessment
Client needs category: Physiological integrity
Client needs subcategory: Reduction of risk potential
Cognitive level: Analysis

16. CORRECT ANSWER: 4
The exposure to radiation at 4′ from the source is determined by squaring $^1/_4$. To receive $^1/_2$ the exposure at 1′ (option 1), the nurse would have to be 1.415′ from the client; to receive $^1/_4$ the exposure (option 2), the nurse would have to be 2′ from the client; to receive $^1/_8$ the exposure (option 3), the nurse would have to be 2.83′ from the client.
Nursing process step: Assessment
Client needs category: Safe, effective care environment
Client needs subcategory: Safety and infection control
Cognitive level: Comprehension

17. CORRECT ANSWER: 3
Alzheimer's disease typically affects the memory, so the nurse should tell the client the time whenever she asks. Option 1 is demeaning. Option 2 would upset the client. Option 4 is threatening and nontherapeutic.
Nursing process step: Implementation
Client needs category: Psychosocial integrity
Client needs subcategory: None
Cognitive level: Application

18. CORRECT ANSWER: 4
NPH insulin starts to act within 2 hours after administration. Eating breakfast 30 minutes after administration ensures that the blood glucose level will be elevated. Hypoglycemia could result if the client didn't eat after NPH administration. The urine glucose level doesn't reliably reflect the blood glucose level (option 1). Insulin injection doesn't cause a skin reaction (option 2). Drug absorption is rarely a problem with insulin (option 3).
Nursing process step: Planning
Client needs category: Safe, effective care environment
Client needs subcategory: Safety and infection control
Cognitive level: Analysis

19. CORRECT ANSWER: 3
Quickening, the pregnant woman's first awareness of fetal movement, normally is felt between 16 and 20 weeks. Options 1, 2, and 4 are inappropriate nursing actions for a patient who's experiencing quickening.
Nursing process step: Implementation
Client needs category: Health promotion and maintenance
Client needs subcategory: None
Cognitive level: Comprehension

20. CORRECT ANSWER: 4
Anesthesia and surgery impede intestinal peristalsis, leading to gas accumulation in the intestine and distention. An NG tube is inserted to prevent distention. The tube can be removed when the bowel resumes normal function, as indicated by passing flatus.
Nursing process step: Assessment
Client needs category: Physiological integrity
Client needs subcategory: Physiological adaptation
Cognitive level: Comprehension

21. CORRECT ANSWER: 3
Infectious diarrhea is highly contagious, and all persons on the pediatric unit should be protected from exposure. Options 1 and 2 are appropriate measures to take after isolating the infant. Option 4 may also be required but isn't done first.
Nursing process step: Planning
Client needs category: Safe, effective care environment
Client needs subcategory: Safety and infection control
Cognitive level: Application

22. CORRECT ANSWER: 1
Adverse reactions of digoxin include nausea, vomiting, anorexia, and vision disturbances, such as blurred or yellow vision.
Nursing process step: Evaluation
Client needs category: Physiological integrity
Client needs subcategory: Pharmacological and parenteral therapies
Cognitive level: Comprehension

23. CORRECT ANSWER: 4
Osteoporosis causes a severe, general reduction in skeletal bone mass. To offset this reduction, the nurse should advise the patient to increase calcium intake by consuming more dairy products, which provide about 75% of the calcium in the average diet. None of the other options would prevent osteoporosis from worsening.
Nursing process step: Implementation
Client needs category: Physiological integrity
Client needs subcategory: Basic care and comfort
Cognitive level: Comprehension

24. CORRECT ANSWER: 3
The wound site is the probable source of serosanguineous drainage. After an abdominal-perineal resection, a Penrose drain is generally used to drain the wound site, and serosanguineous drainage on the perineal dressing is normal.

Nursing process step: Implementation
Client needs category: Physiological integrity
Client needs subcategory: Physiological adaptation
Cognitive level: Application

25. CORRECT ANSWER: 4
During a transurethral prostatic resection, the surgeon removes prostate tissue through the urethra with a resectoscope, cutting away slices of the prostate bit by bit. Bloody urinary drainage is expected during the immediate postoperative period. During this time, the client has a catheter attached to an irrigation system that continuously drains urine, so discomfort on urination (option 1) and a distended bladder (option 2) shouldn't occur. A neurogenic bladder (option 3) develops secondary to central or peripheral nervous system lesions.
Nursing process step: Planning
Client needs category: Physiological integrity
Client needs subcategory: Physiological adaptation
Cognitive level: Comprehension

26. CORRECT ANSWER: 4
Ferrous gluconate should be well diluted and administered through a straw or placed on the back of the client's tongue with a dropper to prevent staining and to mask the taste. This preparation shouldn't be administered undiluted (options 1 and 2). Although it may be mixed with water, it isn't compatible with milk (option 3).
Nursing process step: Implementation
Client needs category: Physiological integrity
Client needs subcategory: Pharmacological and parenteral therapies
Cognitive level: Application

27. CORRECT ANSWER: 3
The I.V. should deliver about 42 drops/minute, as indicated by the following formula:

$$\frac{\text{Volume of infusion in ml} \times \text{Drop factor (gtt/ml)}}{\text{Time of infusion in minutes}} = \text{Drops/minute}$$

Therefore:

$$\frac{\frac{1{,}000\ \cancel{\text{ml}}}{1} \times \frac{20\ \text{gtt}}{1\ \cancel{\text{ml}}}}{480\ \text{min}} = \frac{20{,}000\ \text{gtt}}{480\ \text{min}} = \begin{matrix}41.6\ \text{or}\\ 42\ \text{drops/minute}\end{matrix}$$

Nursing process step: Implementation
Client needs category: Physiological integrity
Client needs subcategory: Pharmacological and parenteral therapies
Cognitive level: Comprehension

28. CORRECT ANSWER: 2
This response places the responsibility for recovery squarely on the client. Option 1 sounds like a dare. Options 3 and 4 suggest that others are also responsible for the client's recovery.
Nursing process step: Implementation
Client needs category: Psychosocial integrity
Client needs subcategory: None
Cognitive level: Application

29. CORRECT ANSWER: 4
Keeping the perineal area clean reduces the risk of an infection that ascends the urinary tract. The nurse encourages the client to void frequently to provide more space for the descending fetus (option 2). Options 1 and 3 don't prevent an infection.
Nursing process step: Planning
Client needs category: Physiological integrity
Client needs subcategory: Basic care and comfort
Cognitive level: Comprehension

30. CORRECT ANSWER: 1
Typically, a 4-year-old child is at the preoperational level of cognitive development and has trouble understanding anything beyond her own experience. Using a doll provides a near-life experience, giving the child an understanding of the procedure and a sense of control. Options 2, 3, and 4 require abstract thinking, which is beyond the cognitive developmental level of a 4-year-old.
Nursing process step: Implementation
Client needs category: Safe, effective care environment
Client needs subcategory: Management of care
Cognitive level: Application

31. CORRECT ANSWER: 4
Because an abdominal-perineal resection commonly necessitates a colostomy and prevents defecation through the rectum, it causes a permanent change in body image to which the client must adapt. Although the client may have a catheter postoperatively and may need to restrict the diet and activity level, these changes are only temporary.

Nursing process step: Planning
Client needs category: Psychosocial integrity
Client needs subcategory: None
Cognitive level: Application

32. CORRECT ANSWER: 3
The nurse should use the Z-track method to give iron dextran to prevent drug leakage along the needle track and brown staining of subcutaneous tissue. Options 1 and 2 are unrelated to iron dextran administration. Option 4 is incorrect because iron dextran must be injected deep into the muscle mass, so the nurse should use a 2″ or 3″ 19G or 20G needle.
Nursing process step: Implementation
Client needs category: Physiological integrity
Client needs subcategory: Pharmacological and parenteral therapies
Cognitive level: Application

33. CORRECT ANSWER: 2
These diets rid the bowel of bacteria and reduce feces formation. They don't eliminate stress in the bowel (option 1), reduce bowel motility (option 3), or decrease pain (option 4).
Nursing process step: Implementation
Client needs category: Physiological integrity
Client needs subcategory: Reduction of risk potential
Cognitive level: Comprehension

34. CORRECT ANSWER: 4
Ferrous sulfate may cause black or dark green stools.
Nursing process step: Assessment
Client needs category: Physiological integrity
Client needs subcategory: Pharmacological and parenteral therapies
Cognitive level: Comprehension

35. CORRECT ANSWER: 1
Slowing the pace of care activities will help the client feel more in touch. A depressed client can't move at a faster pace (option 2) and lacks the energy to change behavior (option 3). A highly stimulating environment isn't helpful to a depressed client and may make the client even more conscious of the depression (option 4).
Nursing process step: Planning
Client needs category: Psychosocial integrity
Client needs subcategory: None
Cognitive level: Analysis

36. CORRECT ANSWER: 2
Iron-rich foods include raisins and other dried fruits, liver, meat, dark green vegetables, and egg yolks.
Nursing process step: Evaluation
Client needs category: Health promotion and maintenance
Client needs subcategory: None
Cognitive level: Comprehension

37. CORRECT ANSWER: 1
Proteinuria (protein in the urine) is a cardinal sign of gestational hypertension. It doesn't occur in ketoacidosis (option 2), placenta previa (option 3), or gestational diabetes (option 4).
Nursing process step: Assessment
Client needs category: Health promotion and maintenance
Client needs subcategory: None
Cognitive level: Analysis

38. CORRECT ANSWER: 2
Parents of a child with a catastrophic illness typically feel guilty about the child's illness and wonder whether something they did (or failed to do) might have caused it. To cope with their guilt feelings, they may become angry at those around them — particularly health care providers. The nurse should let them talk and help them cope with their feelings. Options 1 and 3 serve only to chastise the parents, not help them. Option 4 doesn't respond to their needs.
Nursing process step: Planning
Client needs category: Psychosocial integrity
Client needs subcategory: None
Cognitive level: Application

39. CORRECT ANSWER: 1
A client with iron-deficiency anemia may become dizzy and faint from lack of hemoglobin, which in turn reduces oxygen to the brain. Lying down improves circulation, reduces oxygen demands, and promotes safety. Options 2 and 3 wouldn't alleviate the symptoms. Option 4 would be appropriate to alleviate dizziness from hypotension but wouldn't aid in preventing symptoms of iron-deficiency anemia.
Nursing process step: Planning
Client needs category: Physiological integrity
Client needs subcategory: Reduction of risk potential
Cognitive level: Application

40. CORRECT ANSWER: 3
In sigmoidoscopy, an endoscope is inserted into the rectum. Improper insertion may cause perforation of the intestinal wall. The other options aren't potential complications of sigmoidoscopy.
Nursing process step: Assessment
Client needs category: Physiological integrity
Client needs subcategory: Physiological adaptation
Cognitive level: Application

41. CORRECT ANSWER: 2
Iron-deficiency anemia is characterized by decreased hemoglobin in the blood, which reduces the amount of oxygen transported to body tissues. Therefore, the client may complain of shortness of breath. Other signs and symptoms of iron-deficiency anemia include chills, pallor, faintness, and appetite loss.
Nursing process step: Assessment
Client needs category: Physiological integrity
Client needs subcategory: Physiological adaptation
Cognitive level: Comprehension

42. CORRECT ANSWER: 1
Barium sulfate is administered rectally. To ensure that it adheres to the lower portion of the intestine, the area must be properly cleaned, using laxatives and enemas. A muscle relaxant (option 2) isn't administered during the test. Barium sulfate isn't administered orally (option 3). The client is put on a liquid diet the night before the procedure and receives nothing by mouth the morning of the procedure (option 4).
Nursing process step: Evaluation
Client needs category: Safe, effective care environment
Client needs subcategory: Safety and infection control
Cognitive level: Application

43. CORRECT ANSWER: 4
Alternating breasts with each breast-feeding session promotes emptying of milk from the breasts. Pulling the infant from the breast before suction is broken may cause nipple trauma (option 1). Warm compresses are more effective in relieving breast discomfort than cold compresses (option 2). Soap and water may dry the nipples (option 3).
Nursing process step: Evaluation
Client needs category: Health promotion and maintenance
Client needs subcategory: None
Cognitive level: Application

44. CORRECT ANSWER: 4
Systematic desensitization is a common behavior modification technique successfully used to help treat phobias. Aversion therapy and positive reinforcement aren't behavior modification techniques used in the treatment of phobias (options 1 and 3). The techniques of imitation or modeling are social learning techniques, not behavior modification techniques (option 2).
Nursing process step: Implementation
Client needs category: Psychosocial integrity
Client needs subcategory: None
Cognitive level: Application

45. CORRECT ANSWER: 4
Respiratory problems always take highest priority. Options 1, 2, and 3 have lower priority.
Nursing process step: Planning
Client needs category: Physiological integrity
Client needs subcategory: Physiological adaptation
Cognitive level: Analysis

46. CORRECT ANSWER: 2
Proper countertraction occurs when the child's buttocks are raised approximately 2″ (5 cm) above the mattress. Options 1 and 3 describe proper traction. Option 4 describes correct alignment for a child in Bryant's traction.
Nursing process step: Evaluation
Client needs category: Safe, effective care environment
Client needs subcategory: Safety and infection control
Cognitive level: Analysis

47. CORRECT ANSWER: 3
The nurse should teach a client with cystitis to wipe from front to back after using the toilet to avoid bacterial contamination caused by close proximity of the urethra and rectum. An acidic, not alkaline, urine helps to discourage bacterial growth.
Nursing process step: Planning
Client needs category: Physiological integrity
Client needs subcategory: Physiological adaptation
Cognitive level: Analysis

48. CORRECT ANSWER: 4
One cup of cooked broccoli contains a moderate amount of total dietary fiber. Cheese (option A), white bread (option B), and grapefruit (option C) contain smaller amounts of fiber.

Nursing process step: Evaluation
Client needs category: Health promotion and maintenance
Client needs subcategory: None
Cognitive level: Application

49. CORRECT ANSWER: 3
The return of peristaltic activity is signaled by movement in the bowel, which causes expulsion of bowel contents (usually gas). Belching (option 1), hunger (option 3), and thirst (option 4) don't indicate movement in the entire bowel.
Nursing process step: Assessment
Client needs category: Physiological integrity
Client needs subcategory: Physiological adaptation
Cognitive level: Comprehension

50. CORRECT ANSWER: 2
Irritability and poor concentration are associated with a moderate anxiety level. Mild anxiety doesn't cause irritability and poor concentration (option 1). Severe anxiety and panic cause more marked symptoms. For instance, a client with panic-level anxiety typically is out of touch with reality.
Nursing process step: Assessment
Client needs category: Psychosocial integrity
Client needs subcategory: None
Cognitive level: Comprehension

51. CORRECT ANSWER: 3
When a client becomes angry and resents advice from a younger health care provider to give up a lifelong habit, the nurse should apologize and assure the client that no disrespect was intended. The other options would antagonize the client rather than reduce anger.
Nursing process step: Implementation
Client needs category: Psychosocial integrity
Client needs subcategory: None
Cognitive level: Analysis

52. CORRECT ANSWER: 1
In a 2-year-old child, increasing irritability suggests increased ICP. The other options describe findings opposite those expected in a child with increased ICP.
Nursing process step: Assessment
Client needs category: Physiological integrity
Client needs subcategory: Reduction of risk potential
Cogntive level: Comprehension

53. CORRECT ANSWER: 3
A deceleration of the FHR with delayed recovery after a uterine contraction indicates fetal hypoxia, a finding that warrants immediate intervention. An irregular baseline FHR and occasional short accelerations are normal (option 1). Option 2 is a sign of fetal head compression, which is normal during the first phase of labor. An FHR acceleration of 15 beats/minute that lasts 15 seconds is normal (option 4).
Nursing process step: Evaluation
Client needs category: Health promotion and maintenance
Client needs subcategory: None
Cognitive level: Analysis

54. CORRECT ANSWER: 1
Promethazine hydrochloride, an antihistamine, has prominent sedative effects. It doesn't inhibit oral secretions (option 2), prevent bleeding problems (option 3), or enhance wound healing (option 4).
Nursing process step: Planning
Client needs category: Safe, effective care environment
Client needs subcategory: Safety and infection control
Cognitive level: Comprehension

55. CORRECT ANSWER: 3
Fear of the unknown may cause anxiety, which may manifest in such symptoms as irritability, nervousness, and upset stomach (as well as pain). The client's anxiety isn't inappropriate (option 1). Anxiety causes real symptoms, not imaginary ones (option 2). No evidence suggests that the client's anxiety is an exaggerated reaction (option 4).
Nursing process step: Planning
Client needs category: Psychosocial integrity
Client needs subcategory: None
Cognitive level: Analysis

56. CORRECT ANSWER: 1
A hemolytic reaction to a blood transfusion usually results from blood group incompatibility. Signs and symptoms include back pain, reduced blood pressure, decreased urine output, tightness in the chest, dyspnea, and shock.
Nursing process step: Assessment
Client needs category: Physiological integrity
Client needs subcategory: Physiological adaptation
Cognitive level: Comprehension

57. Correct answer: 3

After awakening, the child will receive sips of water and a clear liquid diet, including ice popsicles. Milk products are rarely given immediately. The child will probably go to the postanesthesia care unit immediately after surgery (option 1) and will be allowed to see the parents (option 2). The child will feel drowsy from the effects of general anesthesia (option 4).

Nursing process step: Evaluation
Client needs category: Physiological integrity
Client needs subcategory: Physiological adaptation
Cognitive level: Analysis

58. Correct answer: 1

Clearing the neonate's airway takes priority. Although important, the other options have lower priorities.

Nursing process step: Planning
Client needs category: Health promotion and maintenance
Client needs subcategory: None
Cognitive level: Application

59. Correct answer: 1

The client should be taught to avoid caffeine and nicotine because they constrict blood vessels and would further impair the circulation. Wearing knee-length stockings would impair circulation (option 2). Clients with peripheral vascular disease should keep the extremities warm and dry, therefore option 3 is incorrect. The client should exercise daily, not avoid exercise (option 4).

Nursing process step: Implementation
Client needs category: Physiological integrity
Client needs subcategory: Reduction of risk potential
Cognitive level: Analysis

60. Correct answer: 2

Because the client's axillary lymph nodes were removed, the risk of lymphedema is high. Therefore, the client must avoid any actions that carry a risk of constriction, such as using a tourniquet or a blood pressure cuff. Wearing an elastic bandage may decrease circulation and cause edema, leading to skin breakdown (option 1). The client's position and movement need not be restricted (options 3 and 4).

Nursing process step: Implementation
Client needs category: Physiological integrity
Client needs subcategory: Reduction of risk potential
Cognitive level: Application

61. Correct answer: 1

A side-lying position helps prevent aspiration. The other options don't provide this advantage.

Nursing process step: Implementation
Client needs category: Physiological integrity
Client needs subcategory: Reduction of risk potential
Cognitive level: Comprehension

62. Correct answer: 1

Eating small, frequent meals places less pressure on the esophageal sphincter, reducing the likelihood of regurgitation of stomach contents into the lower esophagus. None of the other suggestions would reduce heartburn.

Nursing process step: Planning
Client needs category: Physiological integrity
Client needs subcategory: Basic care and comfort
Cognitive level: Application

63. Correct answer: 1

The weight of the pregnant uterus compresses the abdominal aorta and may cause a decrease in blood pressure, so the recommended positions include walking, side-lying, and sitting for short periods of time. Even though epidural anesthesia is anticipated, fluids are restricted in case general anesthesia is required. Vital signs and pain medication would be more important after the procedure.

Nursing process step: Implementation
Client needs category: Physiological integrity
Client needs subcategory: Basic care and comfort
Cognitive level: Analysis

64. Correct answer: 2

This response shows respect for the daughter's feelings and encourages her to express these feelings further. Giving advice is inappropriate and doesn't acknowledge the daughter's feelings (option 1). Telling the daughter not to worry denies her the right to her feelings (option 3). The nurse's response should focus on the daughter's feelings, not the nurse's (option 4).

Nursing process step: Implementation
Client needs category: Psychosocial integrity
Client needs subcategory: None
Cognitive level: Analysis

65. Correct Answer: 4

Babinski's reflex is characterized by dorsiflexion of the great toe, and fanning of the other toes when the sole is stimulated. This reflex is usually absent in adults and in

children older than age 24 months; its presence may indicate damage to pyramidal tracts. Option 1 describes the Achilles reflex. Option 2 describes the patellar reflex. Option 3 occurs with ankle clonus.
Nursing process step: Assessment
Client needs category: Physiological integrity
Client needs subcategory: Physiological adaptation
Cognitive level: Comprehension

66. CORRECT ANSWER: 3
Increased urine output means ascitic fluid is being absorbed into the circulation and then excreted. As this fluid is absorbed, ankle edema should decrease, not remain the same (option 1), and abdominal skin should become less shiny, not shinier (option 2). With decreasing ascites, lower fluid volume would cause the pulse rate to slow, not to increase (option 4).
Nursing process step: Assessment
Client needs category: Physiological integrity
Client needs subcategory: Physiological adaptation
Cognitive level: Comprehension

67. CORRECT ANSWER: 3
Bryant's traction may be used in infants and children weighing 25 to 30 lb (11 to 13.5 kg) to reduce a fractured femur. It's also used to reduce congenital hip dislocation. Flat in bed with an elastic wrap is Buck's extension; flat in bed with a pad under the knee is a Russell traction; traction with a pin or wire is skeletal traction.
Nursing process step: Assessment
Client needs category: Safe, effective care environment
Client needs subcategory: Management of care
Cognitive level: Knowledge

68. CORRECT ANSWER: 1
During the immediate postoperative period, breathing deeply is essential to preventing hypostatic pneumonia and other complications. However, many clients are afraid to breathe deeply because this may cause incisional pain; therefore, the nurse must support the incisional area. The other options don't enhance expansion and air exchange in the lungs and, therefore, don't help prevent hypostatic pneumonia.
Nursing process step: Implementation
Client needs category: Physiological integrity
Client needs subcategory: Reduction of risk potential
Cognitive level: Application

69. CORRECT ANSWER: 1
Thrombophlebitis refers to clot formation in a vein, caused by such conditions as venous stasis. It may result from lying in bed, which causes pooling of blood. Elastic stockings compress superficial blood vessels, promoting circulation. The other options are less effective than elastic stockings in preventing thrombophlebitis.
Nursing process step: Implementation
Client needs category: Physiological integrity
Client needs subcategory: Reduction of risk potential
Cognitive level: Application

70. CORRECT ANSWER: 1
Nursing measures in the secondary prevention of violence and abuse are intended to reduce the further incidence of violence and abuse once those behaviors have occurred. Nursing interventions in these situations are aimed at helping the participants, notably the victim, discuss the problem, seek alternative actions, and move to a safe haven, if needed.
Nursing process step: Assessment
Client needs category: Safe, effective care environment
Client needs subcategory: Management of care
Cognitive level: Analysis

71. CORRECT ANSWER: 1
Because this comment reflects the mother's feelings, it encourages her to express her feelings further, thereby reducing her anxiety. The nurse should avoid giving false reassurance (option 2). Option 3 belittles the mother's feelings by implying that they aren't unique. Although sharing feelings in a group session may be helpful, this client's mother is too upset to talk with other parents, who aren't necessarily experiencing similar emotions (option 4).
Nursing process step: Implementation
Client needs category: Psychosocial integrity
Client needs subcategory: None
Cognitive level: Application

72. CORRECT ANSWER: 3
An intermediate-acting insulin, NPH insulin starts to act within 2 hours and peaks in 8 to 10 hours. To ensure adequate blood glucose control, the client must eat meals or snacks at scheduled times. The client should not skip a meal (option 1). One ounce of fat isn't an equal exchange for 2 oz of protein (option 2). The client should use artificial sweeteners instead of simple sugars, not complex sugars.

Nursing process step: Implementation
Client needs category: Health promotion and maintenance
Client needs subcategory: None
Cognitive level: Application

73. CORRECT ANSWER: 2
Following the identification of a learning need, the first step is to assess the strengths and needs of the community while identifying barriers to learning.
Nursing process step: Planning
Client needs category: Safe, effective care management
Client needs subcategory: Management of care
Cognitive level: Analysis

74. CORRECT ANSWER: 2, 5
For a neonate, a normal apical pulse rate ranges from 120 to 160 beats/minute. The normal respiratory rate ranges between 30 and 50 breaths/minute. The axillary temperature (option 1) should measure 97.7° F (36.5° C) to 98.6° F (37° C). The sclera (option 3) should be white, not yellowish. Respiratory grunting (option 4) may be a sign of respiratory obstruction or distress.
Nursing process step: Assessment
Client needs category: Health promotion and maintenance
Client needs subcategory: None
Cognitive level: Analysis

75. CORRECT ANSWER: 1, 2, 3, 5
Concomitant use of aspirin and ibuprofen isn't recommended. To reduce the risk of adverse GI effects, the client can take ibuprofen with food, an antacid, milk, or apple juice.
Nursing process step: Implementation
Client needs subcategory: Physiological integrity
Client needs subcategory: Pharmacological and parenteral therapies
Cognitive level: Application

Posttest 3

QUESTIONS

1. Which treatment is the definitive one for a ruptured aneurysm?

☐ **1.** Antihypertensive medication administration
☐ **2.** Aortogram
☐ **3.** Beta-adrenergic blocker administration
☐ **4.** Surgical intervention

2. Which recurring condition most commonly occurs in clients with cardiomyopathy?

☐ **1.** Heart failure
☐ **2.** Diabetes mellitus
☐ **3.** Myocardial infarction
☐ **4.** Pericardial effusion

3. Which percentage represents the amount of damage the myocardium must sustain before signs and symptoms of cardiogenic shock develop?

☐ **1.** 10%
☐ **2.** 25%
☐ **3.** 40%
☐ **4.** 90%

4. Myocardial oxygen consumption increases as which of the following parameters increase?

☐ **1.** Preload, afterload, and cerebral blood flow
☐ **2.** Preload, afterload, and contractility
☐ **3.** Preload, afterload, contractility, and heart rate
☐ **4.** Preload, afterload, cerebral blood flow, and heart rate

5. Which symptom of hypertension is most common?

☐ **1.** Blurred vision
☐ **2.** Epistaxis
☐ **3.** Headache
☐ **4.** Peripheral edema

6. A 36-year-old client complains of fatigue, weight loss, and a low-grade fever. He also has pain in his fingers, elbows, and ankles. Which condition is suspected?

☐ **1.** Anemia
☐ **2.** Leukemia
☐ **3.** Rheumatic arthritis
☐ **4.** Systemic lupus erythematosus (SLE)

7. When examining a preschool-age child, the nurse finds multiple contusions over the body. Child abuse is suspected. Which statement indicates which findings should be documented?

☐ **1.** Contusions confined to one body area are typically suspicious.
☐ **2.** All lesions, including location, shape, and color, should be documented.
☐ **3.** Natural injuries usually have straight linear lines, while injuries from abuse have multiple curved lines.
☐ **4.** The depth, location, and amount of bleeding that initially occurs is constant, but the sequence of color change is variable.

8. Although a client's physiologic response to a health crisis is important to the health outcome, which nursing intervention also must be addressed?

☐ **1.** Teach the family how to care for the client.
☐ **2.** Help the client effectively cope with the crisis.
☐ **3.** Maintain I.V. access, medications, and diet.
☐ **4.** Teach the client basic information about the illness.

9. A client was infected with tuberculosis (TB) bacillus 10 years ago but never developed the disease. He's now being treated for cancer. The client begins to develop signs of TB. This is known as which type of infection?

- ☐ **1.** Active infection
- ☐ **2.** Primary infection
- ☐ **3.** Superinfection
- ☐ **4.** Tertiary infection

10. A client has active tuberculosis (TB). Which symptom will he most likely exhibit?

- ☐ **1.** Chest and lower back pain
- ☐ **2.** Chills, fever, night sweats, and hemoptysis
- ☐ **3.** Fever of more than 104° F (40° C) and nausea
- ☐ **4.** Headache and photophobia

11. Which measure best determines that a chest tube is no longer needed for a client who had a pneumothorax?

- ☐ **1.** The drainage from the chest tube is minimal.
- ☐ **2.** Arterial blood gas (ABG) levels are obtained to ensure proper oxygenation.
- ☐ **3.** It's removed and the client is assessed to see if he's breathing adequately.
- ☐ **4.** No fluctuation in the water seal chamber occurs when no suction is applied.

12. Nursing management of a client with a pulmonary embolism focuses on which action?

- ☐ **1.** Assessing oxygenation status
- ☐ **2.** Monitoring the oxygen delivery device
- ☐ **3.** Monitoring for other sources of clots
- ☐ **4.** Determining whether the client requires another ventilation-perfusion scan

13. A client with a subdural hematoma was given mannitol to decrease intracranial pressure (ICP). Which result would best show the mannitol was effective?

- ☐ **1.** Urine output increases.
- ☐ **2.** Pupils are 8 mm and nonreactive.
- ☐ **3.** Systolic blood pressure remains at 150 mm Hg.
- ☐ **4.** Blood urea nitrogen (BUN) and creatinine levels return to normal.

14. Which nursing intervention should be used to prevent foot drop and contractures in a client recovering from a subdural hematoma?

- ☐ **1.** High-topped sneakers
- ☐ **2.** Low-dose heparin therapy
- ☐ **3.** Physical therapy consultation
- ☐ **4.** Sequential compression device

15. A client who had a transsphenoidal hypophysectomy should be watched carefully for hemorrhage, which may be shown by which of the following signs?

- ☐ **1.** Bloody drainage from the ears
- ☐ **2.** Frequent swallowing
- ☐ **3.** Guaiac-positive stools
- ☐ **4.** Hematuria

16. Why is vasopressin given I.M. after a hypophysectomy?

- ☐ **1.** To prevent GI bleeding
- ☐ **2.** To prevent the syndrome of inappropriate antidiuretic hormone (SIADH)
- ☐ **3.** To reduce cerebral edema and lower intracranial pressure
- ☐ **4.** To replace antidiuretic hormone (ADH) normally secreted from the pituitary

17. The treatment for osteoarthritis commonly includes salicylates. Salicylates can be dangerous in older people because they can cause which adverse reaction?

- ☐ **1.** Hearing loss
- ☐ **2.** Increased pain in joints
- ☐ **3.** Decreased calcium absorption
- ☐ **4.** Increased bone demineralization

18. Clients with osteoarthritis may be on bed rest for prolonged periods. Which nursing intervention would be appropriate for these clients?

- ☐ **1.** Encourage coughing and deep breathing, and limit fluid intake.
- ☐ **2.** Provide only passive range of motion, and decrease stimulation.
- ☐ **3.** Have the client lie as still as possible, and give adequate pain medicine.
- ☐ **4.** Turn the client every 2 hours, and encourage coughing and deep breathing.

19. A client describes a foul odor from his cast. Which response or interventions would be most appropriate?

☐ **1.** Assess further because this may be a sign of infection.

☐ **2.** Teach him proper cast care, including hygiene measures.

☐ **3.** This is normal, especially when a cast is in place for a few weeks.

☐ **4.** Assess further because this may be a sign of neurovascular compromise.

20. Which substance is most likely to cause gastritis?

☐ **1.** Milk

☐ **2.** Bicarbonate of soda, or baking soda

☐ **3.** Enteric-coated aspirin

☐ **4.** Nonsteroidal anti-inflammatory drugs (NSAIDs)

21. Which task should be included in the immediate postoperative management of a client who has undergone gastric resection?

☐ **1.** Monitoring gastric pH to detect complications

☐ **2.** Assessing for bowel sounds

☐ **3.** Providing nutritional support

☐ **4.** Monitoring for symptoms of hemorrhage

22. Which treatment should be included in the immediate management of acute gastritis?

☐ **1.** Reducing work stress

☐ **2.** Performing gastric resection

☐ **3.** Treating the underlying cause

☐ **4.** Administering enteral tube feedings

23. Which nursing intervention should be performed for a client who complains of nausea and vomits 1 hour after taking his morning glyburide (DiaBeta)?

☐ **1.** Give glyburide again.

☐ **2.** Give subcutaneous insulin, and monitor blood glucose.

☐ **3.** Monitor blood glucose closely, and look for signs of hypoglycemia.

☐ **4.** Monitor blood glucose, and assess for symptoms of hyperglycemia.

24. Which chronic complication is associated with diabetes mellitus?

☐ **1.** Dizziness, dyspnea on exertion, and angina

☐ **2.** Retinopathy, neuropathy, and coronary artery disease (CAD)

☐ **3.** Leg ulcers, cerebral ischemic events, and pulmonary infarcts

☐ **4.** Fatigue, nausea, vomiting, muscle weakness, and cardiac arrhythmias

25. Rotating injection sites when administering insulin prevents which complication?

☐ **1.** Insulin edema

☐ **2.** Insulin lipodystrophy

☐ **3.** Insulin resistance

☐ **4.** Systemic allergic reactions

26. What tests should be ordered if hypothyroidism is suspected?

☐ **1.** Liver function tests

☐ **2.** Hemoglobin A_{1C}

☐ **3.** T_4 and thyroid-stimulating hormone (TSH)

☐ **4.** 24-hour urine free-cortisol measurement

27. A client with hypothyroidism may exhibit which signs or symptoms?

☐ **1.** Polyuria, polydipsia, and weight loss

☐ **2.** Heat intolerance, nervousness, weight loss, and hair loss

☐ **3.** Coarsening of facial features and extremity enlargement

☐ **4.** Tiredness, cold intolerance, weight gain, and constipation

28. Which statement best explains why it's important to empty the bowel before treatment with intracavitary radiation for cancer of the cervix?

☐ **1.** Feces in the bowel increase the risk of ileus.

☐ **2.** An empty bowel allows the applicator to be positioned with little or no discomfort.

☐ **3.** Bowel movements increase the risk for inadvertent contamination of the vagina and urethra.

☐ **4.** Pressure changes in the pelvis associated with bowel movements can alter the position of the applicator and the radiation source.

29. A nurse enters the room of a client who had a left modified mastectomy 8 hours earlier. Which observation indicates that the nursing assistant assigned to the client needs further instruction and guidance?

☐ **1.** The client is squeezing a ball in her left hand.
☐ **2.** The client is wearing a robe with elastic cuffs.
☐ **3.** The client's affected arm is elevated on a pillow.
☐ **4.** A blood pressure cuff is on the client's right arm.

30. For which symptoms should a client at risk for evisceration be monitored after an abdominal hysterectomy?

☐ **1.** Tachycardia accompanied by a weak, thready pulse
☐ **2.** Hypotension with a decreased level of consciousness (LOC)
☐ **3.** Shallow, rapid respirations and increasing vaginal drainage
☐ **4.** Low-grade fever with increasing serosanguineous incisional drainage

31. Which finding indicates that oxycodone (Percodan) given to a client with breast cancer metastasized to the bone is exerting the desired effect?

☐ **1.** Respiratory rate is decreased.
☐ **2.** Pain is 0 to 2 on a 10-point scale.
☐ **3.** Anxiety is decreased.
☐ **4.** Serum drug level is within normal range.

32. Which adverse reaction may be caused by the use of isotretinoin (Accutane)?

☐ **1.** Birth defects
☐ **2.** Nausea and vomiting
☐ **3.** Vaginal yeast infection
☐ **4.** Gram-negative folliculitis

33. A client complains of small, red, pruritic dots between his fingers and toes. Which condition is the most likely diagnosis?

☐ **1.** Contusion
☐ **2.** Herpes zoster
☐ **3.** Scabies
☐ **4.** Varicella

34. A client is examined and found to have pinpoint, pink-to-purple, nonblanching macular lesions 1 to 3 mm in diameter. Which term best describes these lesions?

☐ **1.** Ecchymosis
☐ **2.** Hematoma
☐ **3.** Petechiae
☐ **4.** Purpura

35. A 50-year-old client is scheduled for electroconvulsive therapy (ECT). The nurse knows that ECT is most commonly prescribed for which condition?

☐ **1.** Major depression
☐ **2.** Antisocial personality disorder
☐ **3.** Chronic schizophrenia
☐ **4.** Somatoform disorder

36. A patient with bipolar disorder becomes verbally aggressive in a group therapy session. Which response by the nurse would be best?

☐ **1.** "You're behaving in an unacceptable manner and you need to control yourself."
☐ **2.** "If you continue to talk like that, no one will want to be around you."
☐ **3.** "You're frightening everyone in the group. Leave the room immediately."
☐ **4.** "Other people are disturbed by your profanity. I'll walk with you down the hall to help release some of that energy."

37. Which measure should be included when teaching a client strategies to help him sleep?

☐ **1.** Keep the room warm.
☐ **2.** Eat a large meal before bedtime.
☐ **3.** Schedule bedtime for when you feel tired.
☐ **4.** Avoid caffeine, excessive fluid intake, alcohol, and stimulating drugs before bedtime.

38. A client with sleep terror disorder might have autonomic signs of intense anxiety. Which autonomic sign or symptom should the nurse monitor?

☐ **1.** Tachycardia
☐ **2.** Pupil constriction
☐ **3.** Cool, clammy skin
☐ **4.** Decreased muscle tone

39. Which question should a nurse ask to determine how agoraphobia affects the life of a client who has panic attacks with agoraphobia?

☐ **1.** "How realistic are your goals?"
☐ **2.** "Are you able to go shopping?"
☐ **3.** "Do you struggle with impulse control?"
☐ **4.** "Who else in your family has panic disorder?"

40. Which fact about the relationship between substance abuse and panic attacks would be helpful to a client considering lifestyle changes as part of a behavior modification program to treat his panic attacks?

☐ **1.** Cigarettes can trigger panic episodes.
☐ **2.** Fermented foods can cause panic attacks.
☐ **3.** Hormonal therapy can induce panic attacks.
☐ **4.** Tryptophan can predispose a person to panic attacks.

41. Which short-term client outcome is appropriate for a client with panic disorder?

☐ **1.** Identify childhood trauma.
☐ **2.** Monitor nutritional intake.
☐ **3.** Institute suicide precautions.
☐ **4.** Decrease episodes of disorientation.

42. Which pathophysiological change in the brain causes the symptoms of Alzheimer's disease?

☐ **1.** Glucose inadequacy
☐ **2.** Atrophy of the frontal lobe
☐ **3.** Degeneration of the cholinergic system
☐ **4.** Intracranial bleeding in the limbic system

43. Which assessment finding shows impairment in abstract thinking and reasoning?

☐ **1.** The client can't repeat a sentence.
☐ **2.** The client has difficulty calculating simple problems.
☐ **3.** The client doesn't know the name of the President of the United States.
☐ **4.** The client can't find similarities and differences between related words or objects.

44. Which intervention would help a client diagnosed with Alzheimer's disease perform activities of daily living (ADLs)?

☐ **1.** Have the client perform all basic care without help.
☐ **2.** Tell the client morning care must be done by 9 a.m.
☐ **3.** Give the client a written list of activities he's expected to do.
☐ **4.** Encourage the client, and give ample time to complete basic tasks.

45. Which factor or condition is the most common cause of amnestic disorders?

☐ **1.** Delirium
☐ **2.** Metabolic factors
☐ **3.** Organic factors
☐ **4.** Thiamine deficiency related to alcohol abuse

46. Which nursing diagnosis is appropriate for a client diagnosed with an amnestic disorder?

☐ **1.** Anticipatory grieving related to loss of functional ability
☐ **2.** Denial
☐ **3.** Ineffective individual coping
☐ **4.** Risk for injury related to impaired cognition

47. Which condition indicates impairment in a client's ability to learn new information?

☐ **1.** Anterograde amnesia
☐ **2.** Korsakoff's syndrome
☐ **3.** Retrograde amnesia
☐ **4.** Wernicke's encephalopathy

48. A nurse is assessing a client who has been actively abusing alcohol for 20 years. Which of the following conditions might be seen during the assessment?

☐ **1.** Agitated behavior
☐ **2.** Paranoid thoughts
☐ **3.** Ritualistic behaviors
☐ **4.** Cognitive impairment

49. A nurse has a meeting with the family of a recovering client. The client tells a family member, "You made it easy for me to use alcohol. You always made excuses for my behavior." Which important issue should the family be encouraged to address?

☐ **1.** Giving up enabling behaviors
☐ **2.** Managing the client's self-care
☐ **3.** Dealing with negative behaviors
☐ **4.** Evaluating the home environment

50. Which short-term goal should be a priority for a client with a deficient knowledge about the effects of alcohol on the body?

- ☐ **1.** Test blood chemistries daily.
- ☐ **2.** Verbalize health consequences of substance use.
- ☐ **3.** Talk to a pharmacist about the substance.
- ☐ **4.** Attend a weekly aerobic exercise program.

51. The nurse observes that the alter personality of the client with a dissociative identity disorder is in control. The client is sitting in the dayroom, interacting with others. Which action would be most appropriate?

- ☐ **1.** Allow the client to continue interacting with others in the dayroom.
- ☐ **2.** Ask to speak to one of the adult alter personalities of the host personality.
- ☐ **3.** Remove the client from the dayroom, and allow the client to play with toys.
- ☐ **4.** Remove the client from the dayroom, and reorient her that she's in a safe place.

52. Which feeling or background history is most commonly reported by clients with dissociative identity disorder (DID) who seek help?

- ☐ **1.** Feelings of loneliness
- ☐ **2.** Supportive family system
- ☐ **3.** Feelings of profound sadness
- ☐ **4.** An almost uncontrollable urge to kill the abuser

53. A client tells the nurse she's having her menstrual period every 2 weeks and it lasts for 1 week. Which condition is best defined by this menstrual pattern?

- ☐ **1.** Amenorrhea
- ☐ **2.** Dyspareunia
- ☐ **3.** Menorrhagia
- ☐ **4.** Metrorrhagia

54. Which aspect might be a major stressor for a couple being treated for infertility?

- ☐ **1.** Examinations
- ☐ **2.** Giving specimens
- ☐ **3.** Scheduling intercourse
- ☐ **4.** Finding out which partner is infertile

55. A 38-year-old woman must undergo a hysterectomy for uterine cancer. The nurse planning her care should include which action to meet the woman's body image changes?

- ☐ **1.** Ask her if she's having pain.
- ☐ **2.** Refer her to a psychotherapist.
- ☐ **3.** Don't discuss the subject with her.
- ☐ **4.** Encourage her to verbalize her feelings.

56. Which communication strategy is best to use with a client with anorexia nervosa who's having problems with peer relationships?

- ☐ **1.** Use concrete language and maintain a focus on reality.
- ☐ **2.** Direct the client to talk about what's causing the anxiety.
- ☐ **3.** Teach the client to communicate feelings and express self appropriately.
- ☐ **4.** Confront the client about being depressed and self-absorbed.

57. A nurse is working with a family who has a member with anorexia nervosa. Which information is essential to teach this family?

- ☐ **1.** How to be supportive
- ☐ **2.** How to encourage grieving
- ☐ **3.** How to set limits on behavior
- ☐ **4.** How to monitor social interactions

58. A client with anorexia nervosa tells a nurse she always feels fat. Which intervention is the best for this client?

- ☐ **1.** Talk about how important the client is.
- ☐ **2.** Encourage her to look at herself in a mirror.
- ☐ **3.** Address the dynamics of the disorder.
- ☐ **4.** Talk about how she's different from her peers.

59. Which condition is common in pregnant clients in the second trimester?

- ☐ **1.** Mastitis
- ☐ **2.** Metabolic alkalosis
- ☐ **3.** Physiologic anemia
- ☐ **4.** Respiratory acidosis

60. A 21-year-old client who is 6 weeks pregnant is diagnosed with hyperemesis gravidarum. This excessive vomiting during pregnancy commonly results in which condition?

- ☐ **1.** Bowel perforation
- ☐ **2.** Electrolyte imbalance
- ☐ **3.** Spontaneous abortion
- ☐ **4.** Gestational hypertension

61. Clients with gestational diabetes are usually managed by which therapy?

- ☐ **1.** Diet
- ☐ **2.** Long-acting insulin
- ☐ **3.** Oral antidiabetic drugs
- ☐ **4.** Oral antidiabetic drugs and insulin

62. Magnesium sulfate is given to clients with gestational hypertension to prevent seizure activity. Which magnesium level is therapeutic for clients with gestational hypertension?

- ☐ **1.** 4 to 7 mEq/L
- ☐ **2.** 8 to 10 mEq/L
- ☐ **3.** 10 to 12 mEq/L
- ☐ **4.** Greater than 15 mEq/L

63. A client is receiving I.V. magnesium sulfate for severe preeclampsia. Which adverse reaction is associated with magnesium sulfate?

- ☐ **1.** Anemia
- ☐ **2.** Decreased urine output
- ☐ **3.** Hyperreflexia
- ☐ **4.** Increased respiratory rate

64. The antagonist for magnesium sulfate should be readily available to any client receiving I.V. magnesium. Which drug is the antagonist for magnesium toxicity?

- ☐ **1.** Calcium gluconate (Kalcinate)
- ☐ **2.** Hydralazine hydrochloride (Apresoline)
- ☐ **3.** Naloxone hydrochloride (Narcan)
- ☐ **4.** Rh_o(D) immune globulin (RhoGAM)

65. What laboratory result would be critical for a client admitted to the labor-and-delivery unit?

- ☐ **1.** Blood type
- ☐ **2.** Calcium
- ☐ **3.** Iron
- ☐ **4.** Oxygen saturation

66. Which fetal heart rate would be expected in the fetus of a woman in labor who is full-term?

- ☐ **1.** 80 to 100 beats/minute
- ☐ **2.** 100 to 120 beats/minute
- ☐ **3.** 120 to 160 beats/minute
- ☐ **4.** 160 to 180 beats/minute

67. A laboring client has external electronic fetal monitoring in place. Which assessment data can be determined by examining the fetal heart rate strip produced by the external electronic fetal monitor?

- ☐ **1.** Gender of the fetus
- ☐ **2.** Fetal position
- ☐ **3.** Labor progress
- ☐ **4.** Oxygenation

68. Which description is correct for an endocardial cushion defect?

- ☐ **1.** Absent tricuspid valve
- ☐ **2.** Opening or hole in the atrial septum
- ☐ **3.** Opening or hole in the ventricular septum
- ☐ **4.** Involvement of the mitral valve, tricuspid valve, atria, and ventricles

69. Which cardiac anomaly is most common in children with Down syndrome (trisomy 21)?

- ☐ **1.** Atrial septal defect
- ☐ **2.** Pulmonic stenosis
- ☐ **3.** Ventricular septal defect
- ☐ **4.** Endocardial cushion defect

70. The skin in the diaper area of a 6-month-old infant is excoriated and red. Which instruction would the nurse give to the mother?

- ☐ **1.** Change the diaper more often.
- ☐ **2.** Apply talcum powder with diaper changes.
- ☐ **3.** Wash the area vigorously with each diaper change.
- ☐ **4.** Decrease the infant's fluid intake to decrease saturating diapers.

71. A 9-year-old child is being discharged from the hospital after severe urticaria caused by an allergy to nuts. Which instruction would be included in discharge teaching for the child's parents?

☐ **1.** Use emollient lotions and baths.
☐ **2.** Apply topical steroids to the lesions as needed.
☐ **3.** Apply over-the-counter products such as diphenhydramine hydrochloride (Benadryl).
☐ **4.** Use an epinephrine administration kit and follow up with an allergist.

72. A nurse would expect an elderly client with pneumonia to manifest which symptom first?

☐ **1.** Altered mental status and dehydration
☐ **2.** Fever and chills
☐ **3.** Hemoptysis and dyspnea
☐ **4.** Pleuritic chest pain and cough

73. If a client with a fat embolism continues to be hypoxic after therapy with positive end-expiratory pressure, what can be done to reduce oxygen demand?

☐ **1.** Give diuretics.
☐ **2.** Give neuromuscular blockers.
☐ **3.** Lower the head of the bed to a flat position.
☐ **4.** Use bronchodilators.

74. A client has a cervical spine injury at the level of C5. Which condition would the nurse anticipate during the acute phase? Select all that apply.

☐ **1.** Absent corneal reflex
☐ **2.** Decerebrate posturing
☐ **3.** Movement of only the right or left half of the body
☐ **4.** The need for mechanical ventilation
☐ **5.** The need for an indwelling urinary catheter

75. A physician prescribes 100 mg Dilantin oral suspension t.i.d. for a client with seizures. The label reads *Dilantin 125 mg/ml.* How many milliliters should the nurse give?

____

ANSWERS AND RATIONALES

In the posttest answers, the question number appears in boldface type, followed by the number of the correct answer. Rationales for correct answers and, where appropriate, for incorrect options follow. To help you evaluate your knowledge base and application of nursing behaviors, each rationale is classified according to:

- nursing process step
- client needs category
- client needs subcategory
- cognitive level.

1. CORRECT ANSWER: 4

When the vessel ruptures, surgery is the only intervention that can repair it. Administration of antihypertensive medications and beta-adrenergic blockers can help control hypertension, reducing the risk of rupture. An aortogram is a diagnostic tool used to detect an aneurysm.
Nursing process step: Implementation
Client needs category: Physiological integrity
Client needs subcategory: Basic care and comfort
Cognitive level: Application

2. CORRECT ANSWER: 1

Because the structure and function of the heart muscle is affected, heart failure most commonly occurs in clients with cardiomyopathy. Myocardial infarction results from atherosclerosis. Pericardial effusion is most predominant in clients with pericarditis. Diabetes mellitus is unrelated to cardiomyopathy.
Nursing process step: Assessment
Client needs category: Physiological integrity
Client needs subcategory: Physiological adaptation
Cognitive level: Comprehension

3. CORRECT ANSWER: 3

At least 40% of the heart muscle must be involved for cardiogenic shock to develop. In most circumstances, the heart can compensate for up to 25% damage. An infarction involving 90% of the heart would result in death.
Nursing process step: Assessment
Client needs category: Physiological integrity
Client needs subcategory: Physiological adaptation
Cognitive level: Comprehension

4. CORRECT ANSWER: 3
Myocardial oxygen consumption increases as preload, afterload, contractility, and heart rate increase. Cerebral blood flow doesn't directly affect myocardial oxygen consumption.
Nursing process step: Assessment
Client needs category: Physiological integrity
Client needs subcategory: Physiological adaptation
Cognitive level: Comprehension

5. CORRECT ANSWER: 3
An occipital headache is typical of hypertension secondary to continued increased pressure on the cerebral vasculature. Epistaxis (nosebleed) occurs far less frequently than a headache but can also be a diagnostic sign of hypertension. Blurred vision can result from hypertension due to the arteriolar changes in the eye. Peripheral edema can also occur from an increase in sodium and water retention but is usually a latent sign.
Nursing process step: Evaluation
Client needs category: Health promotion and maintenance
Client needs subcategory: None
Cognitive level: Comprehension

6. CORRECT ANSWER: 3
Fatigue, weight loss, and a low-grade fever are all early signs of many immune system diseases, including anemia, leukemia, and SLE. However, only rheumatic arthritis is associated with pain in the fingers, elbows, wrists, ankles, and knees.
Nursing process step: Assessment
Client needs category: Health promotion and maintenance
Client needs subcategory: None
Cognitive level: Application

7. CORRECT ANSWER: 2
An accurate precise examination must be properly documented as a legal document. Injuries from normal falls aren't usually linear in nature. The bleeding can cause variations, but the color change is consistent. Contusions that result from falls are typically confined to a single body area and are considered a reasonable finding of a child still learning to walk.
Nursing process step: Assessment
Client needs category: Health promotion and maintenance
Client needs subcategory: None
Cognitive level: Application

8. CORRECT ANSWER: 2
Although all of the answers are important in the care of the client, if the individual can't cope with the emotional, spiritual, and psychological aspects of his crisis, the other components of care may be ineffective as well.
Nursing process step: Implementation
Client needs category: Psychosocial integrity
Client needs subcategory: None
Cognitive level: Application

9. CORRECT ANSWER: 1
Some people carry dormant TB infections that may develop into active disease. In addition, primary sites of infection containing TB bacilli may remain latent for years and then activate when the client's resistance is lowered, as when a client is being treated for cancer. There's no such thing as tertiary infection, and superinfection doesn't apply in this case.
Nursing process step: Application
Client needs category: Physiological integrity
Client needs subcategory: Physiological adaptation
Cognitive level: Application

10. CORRECT ANSWER: 2
Typical signs and symptoms are chills, fever, night sweats, and hemoptysis. Clients with TB typically have low-grade fevers, not higher than 102° F (38.9° C). Chest pain may be present from coughing, but isn't usual. Nausea, headache, and photophobia aren't usual TB symptoms.
Nursing process step: Assessment
Client needs category: Physiological integrity
Client needs subcategory: Physiological adaptation
Cognitive level: Application

11. CORRECT ANSWER: 4
The chest tube isn't removed until it's determined that the client's lung has adequately reexpanded and will stay that way. One indication of reexpansion is the cessation of fluctuation in the water seal chamber when suction isn't applied. After the lung stays expanded, the chest tube is removed. Drainage should be minimal before the chest tube is removed. An ABG test may be done to ensure proper oxygenation but isn't necessary if clinical assessment criteria are met.
Nursing process step: Implementation
Client needs category: Physiological integrity
Client needs subcategory: Physiological adaptation
Cognitive level: Application

12. CORRECT ANSWER: 1
Nursing management of a client with a pulmonary embolism focuses on assessing oxygenation status and ensuring treatment is adequate. If the client's status begins to deteriorate, it's the nurse's responsibility to contact the physician and attempt to improve oxygenation. Monitoring for other clot sources and ensuring the oxygen delivery device is working properly are other nursing responsibilities, but they aren't the focus of care.
Nursing process step: Implementation
Client needs category: Physiological integrity
Client needs subcategory: Physiological adaptation
Cognitive level: Application

13. CORRECT ANSWER: 1
Mannitol promotes osmotic diuresis by increasing the pressure gradient in the renal tubules. No information is given about abnormal BUN and creatinine levels or that mannitol is being given for renal dysfunction or blood pressure maintenance. Fixed and dilated pupils are symptoms of increased ICP or cranial nerve damage.
Nursing process step: Evaluation
Client needs category: Physiological integrity
Client needs subcategory: Physiological adaptation
Cognitive level: Application

14. CORRECT ANSWER: 1
High-topped sneakers are used to prevent foot drop and contractures in neurologic clients. Low-dose heparin therapy and sequential compression boots will prevent deep vein thrombosis. Although a consultation with physical therapy is important to prevent foot drop, a nurse may use high-topped sneakers independently.
Nursing process step: Implementation
Client needs category: Physiological integrity
Client needs subcategory: Reduction of risk potential
Cognitive level: Application

15. CORRECT ANSWER: 2
Frequent swallowing after brain surgery may indicate fluid or blood leaking from the sinuses into the oropharynx. Guaiac-positive stools indicate GI bleeding, blood or fluid draining from the ear may indicate a basilar skull fracture, and hematuria may result from cystitis or other urologic complications.
Nursing process step: Assessment
Client needs category: Physiological integrity
Client needs subcategory: Physiological adaptation
Cognitive level: Analysis

16. CORRECT ANSWER: 4
After hypophysectomy, or removal of the pituitary gland, the body can't synthesize ADH. Although vasopressin tannate may be used I.V. to decrease portal pressure, it isn't correct in this instance. SIADH results from excessive ADH secretion. Mannitol or corticosteroids are used to decrease cerebral edema.
Nursing process step: Implementation
Client needs category: Physiological integrity
Client needs subcategory: Pharmacological and parenteral therapies
Cognitive level: Application

17. CORRECT ANSWER: 1
Many elderly people already have diminished hearing, and salicylate use can lead to further or total hearing loss. Salicylates can cause fluid retention and edema, which is worrisome in older clients, especially those with heart failure. Salicylates don't increase bone demineralization, decrease calcium absorption, or increase pain in joints.
Nursing process step: Assessment
Client needs category: Physiological integrity
Client needs subcategory: Pharmacological and parenteral therapies
Cognitive level: Comprehension

18. CORRECT ANSWER: 4
A bedridden client needs to be turned every 2 hours, have adequate nutrition, and cough and deep-breathe. Adequate pain medication, active and passive ROM, and hydration are also appropriate nursing measures. The client shouldn't lie as still as possible or limit his fluid intake.
Nursing process step: Implementation
Client needs category: Safe, effective care environment
Client needs subcategory: Management of care
Cognitive level: Application

19. CORRECT ANSWER: 1
A foul odor from a cast may be a sign of infection. The nurse must assess for fever, malaise and, possibly, an elevation in white blood cells. Odor from a cast is never normal, and it isn't a sign of neurovascular compromise, which would include decreased pulses, coolness, and paresthesia.
Nursing process step: Assessment
Client needs category: Health promotion and maintenance
Client needs subcategory: None
Cognitive level: Analysis

20. CORRECT ANSWER: 4
NSAIDs are a common cause of gastritis because they inhibit prostaglandin synthesis. Milk, once thought to help reduce gastritis, has little effect on the stomach mucosa. Bicarbonate of soda, or baking soda, may be used to neutralize stomach acid but it should be used cautiously because it may lead to metabolic acidosis. Aspirin with enteric coating shouldn't contribute significantly to gastritis because the coating limits the aspirin's effect on the gastric mucosa.
Nursing process step: Assessment
Client needs category: Physiological integrity
Client needs subcategory: Reduction of risk potential
Cognitive level: Knowledge

21. CORRECT ANSWER: 4
The client should be monitored closely for signs and symptoms of hemorrhage, such as bright red blood in the nasogastric tube suction, tachycardia, or a drop in blood pressure. Gastric pH may be monitored to evaluate the need for histamine-2 receptor antagonists. Bowel sounds may not return for up to 72 hours postoperatively. Nutritional needs should be addressed soon after surgery.
Nursing process step: Assessment
Client needs category: Physiological integrity
Client needs subcategory: Reduction of risk potential
Cognitive level: Comprehension

22. CORRECT ANSWER: 3
Discovering and treating the cause of gastritis is the most beneficial approach. Reducing or eliminating oral intake until the symptoms are gone and reducing the amount of stress are important in the recovery phase. A gastric resection is only an option when serious erosion has occurred.
Nursing process step: Assessment
Client needs category: Safe, effective care environment
Client needs subcategory: Safety and infection control
Cognitive level: Comprehension

23. CORRECT ANSWER: 3
When a client who has taken an oral antidiabetic agent vomits, the nurse would monitor glucose and assess him frequently for signs of hypoglycemia. Most of the medication has probably been absorbed. Therefore, repeating the dose would further lower glucose levels later in the day. Giving insulin also will lower glucose levels, causing hypoglycemia. The client wouldn't have hyperglycemia if the glyburide was absorbed.
Nursing process step: Assessment
Client needs category: Physiological integrity
Client needs subcategory: Pharmacological and parenteral therapies
Cognitive level: Analysis

24. CORRECT ANSWER: 2
Retinopathy, neuropathy, and CAD are all chronic complications of diabetes mellitus. Dizziness, dyspnea on exertion, and angina are symptoms of aortic valve stenosis. Hyperparathyroidism causes fatigue, nausea, vomiting, muscle weakness, and cardiac arrhythmias. Leg ulcers, cerebral ischemic events, and pulmonary infarcts are complications of sickle cell anemia.
Nursing process step: Assessment
Client needs category: Physiological integrity
Client needs subcategory: Reduction of risk potential
Cogntive level: Knowledge

25. CORRECT ANSWER: 2
Insulin lipodystrophy produces fatty masses at the injection sites, causing unpredictable absorption of insulin injected into these sites. Insulin edema is generalized retention of fluid, sometimes seen after normal blood glucose levels are established in a client with prolonged hyperglycemia. Insulin resistance occurs mostly in overweight clients and is due to insulin binding with antibodies, decreasing the amount of absorption. Systemic allergic reactions range from hives to anaphylaxis; rotating injection sites won't prevent these reactions.
Nursing process step: Planning
Client needs category: Health promotion and maintenance
Client needs subcategory: None
Cognitive level: Comprehension

26. CORRECT ANSWER: 3
Levels of TSH and T_4 should be measured if hypothyroidism is suspected. Hemoglobin A_{1C} measurement is used to assess hyperglycemia. Liver function tests are used to determine liver disease. As part of the screening process for Cushing's syndrome, a 24-hour urine-free cortisol measurement is completed.
Nursing process step: Planning
Client needs category: Physiological integrity
Client needs subcategory: Physiological adaptation
Cognitive level: Knowledge

27. CORRECT ANSWER: 4
Tiredness, cold intolerance, weight gain, and constipation are signs and symptoms of hypothyroidism, secondary to a decrease in cellular metabolism. Polyuria, polydipsia, and weight loss are signs and symptoms of type 1 diabetes mellitus. Hyperthyroidism has signs and symptoms of heat intolerance, nervousness, weight loss, and hair loss. Coarsening of facial features and extremity enlargement are signs of acromegaly.
Nursing process step: Assessment
Client needs category: Physiological integrity
Client needs subcategory: Physiological adaptation
Cognitive level: Application

28. CORRECT ANSWER: 4
A position change of the radioactive implant could deliver more radiation to healthy tissue and less to the malignant lesion. Such radiation increases the risk of injury to healthy tissue and decreases the effectiveness of treatment on the cancer. Feces in the bowel increase the likelihood of a bowel movement, which can change the position of the applicator and radiation source. Feces in the bowel don't increase the risk for ileus or inadvertant contamination of the vagina and urethra from a bowel movement. All applicators are inserted under anesthesia in the operating room.
Nursing process step: Planning
Client needs category: Physiological integrity
Client needs subcategory: Reduction of risk potential
Cognitive level: Comprehension

29. CORRECT ANSWER: 2
Elastic cuffs can contribute to the development of lymphedema and should be avoided. Blood pressure measurements in the affected arm also should be avoided. Simple exercises such as squeezing a ball help promote circulation and should be started as soon as possible after surgery. Elevation of the affected arm promotes venous and lymphatic return from the extremity.
Nursing process step: Evaluation
Client needs category: Safe, effective care environment
Client needs subcategory: Management of care
Cognitive level: Analysis

30. CORRECT ANSWER: 4
Signs of impending evisceration are low-grade fever and increasing serosanguineous drainage. Tachycardia; weak, thready pulse; shallow, rapid respirations; vaginal drainage; hypotension; and decreased LOC after abdominal hysterectomy are all unrelated to impeding evisceration, although they may be associated with other serious problems such as shock.
Nursing process step: Planning
Client needs category: Physiological integrity
Client needs subcategory: Reduction of risk potential
Cognitive level: Comprehension

31. CORRECT ANSWER: 2
Oxycodone is an opioid analgesic used for alleviating severe pain, especially in terminal illness. If a client's pain has decreased to 0 to 2 on a 10-point scale (where 0 is no pain and 10 is the worst pain), the medication is working as desired. The drug isn't used to relieve anxiety and its effect isn't measured by drug levels or respiratory rates.
Nursing process step: Evaluation
Client needs category: Physiological integrity
Client needs subcategory: Pharmacological and parenteral therapies
Cognitive level: Analysis

32. CORRECT ANSWER: 1
Even small amounts of Accutane are associated with severe birth defects. Most female clients are also prescribed oral contraceptives. Clindamycin phosphate (Cleocin T Gel), another medicine used in the treatment of acne, can cause diarrhea and gram-negative folliculitis. Tetracycline is associated with yeast infections.
Nursing process step: Assessment
Client needs category: Health promotion and maintenance
Client needs subcategory: None
Cognitive level: Knowledge

33. CORRECT ANSWER: 3
Scabies are seen as linear burrows between the fingers and toes caused by a mite. Contusions don't have small, pruritic dots. The varicella zoster virus causes herpes zoster, characterized by papulovesicular lesions that erupt along a dermatome, usually with hyperesthesia, pain, and tenderness. The papulovesicular lesions of varicella are distributed over the trunk, face, and scalp and don't follow a dermatome.
Nursing process step: Assessment
Client needs category: Physiological integrity
Client needs subcategory: Physiological adaptation
Cognitive level: Knowledge

34. CORRECT ANSWER: 3
Petechiae are small macular lesions 1 to 3 mm in diameter. Ecchymosis is a purple-to-brown bruise, macular or papular, and varied in size. A hematoma is a collection of blood from ruptured blood vessels more than 1 cm in diameter. Purpura are purple macular lesions larger than 1 cm.
Nursing process step: Assessment
Client needs category: Physiological integrity
Client needs subcategory: Physiological adaptation
Cognitive level: Knowledge

35. CORRECT ANSWER: 1
ECT is most commonly used for the treatment of major depression in clients who haven't responded to antidepressants or who have medical problems that contraindicate the use of antidepressants. ECT isn't commonly used for treatment of personality disorders. ECT doesn't appear to be of value to individuals with chronic schizophrenia and isn't the treatment of choice for clients with dissociative disorders.
Nursing process step: Planning
Client needs category: Safe, effective care environment
Client needs subcategory: Management of care
Cognitive level: Knowledge

36. CORRECT ANSWER: 4
This response informs the client that, although the behavior is unacceptable, the client is still worthy of help. The other responses indicate that the client is in control of the behavior.
Nursing process step: Implementation
Client needs category: Safe, effective care environment
Client needs subcategory: Management of care
Cognitive level: Application

37. CORRECT ANSWER: 4
Caffeine, excessive fluid intake, alcohol, and stimulating drugs act as stimulants; avoiding them should promote sleep. Excessive fullness or hunger may interfere with sleep. Setting a regular bedtime and wake-up time facilitates physiological patterns. Maintaining a cool temperature in the room will better facilitate sleeping.
Nursing process step: Implementation
Client needs category: Health promotion and maintenance
Client needs subcategory: None
Cognitive level: Application

38. CORRECT ANSWER: 1
Autonomic arousal includes tachycardia, which should be closely monitored by the nurse to prevent the occurrence of further complications such as arrhythmia. Sweating, increased muscle tone, and pupillary dilation are responses that may also occur but aren't considered life-threatening.
Nursing process step: Assessment
Client needs category: Physiological integrity
Client needs subcategory: Physiological adaptation
Cognitive level: Application

39. CORRECT ANSWER: 2
The client with agoraphobia commonly restricts himself to home and can't carry out normal socializing and life-sustaining activities. Clients with panic disorder are able to set realistic goals and tend to be cautious and reclusive rather than impulsive. Although there's a familial tendency toward panic disorder, information about client needs must be obtained to determine how agoraphobia affects the client's life.
Nursing process step: Planning
Client needs category: Psychosocial integrity
Client needs subcategory: None
Cognitive level: Comprehension

40. CORRECT ANSWER: 1
Cigarettes are considered stimulants and can trigger panic attacks. None of the other options cause panic attacks.
Nursing process step: Implementation
Client needs category: Psychosocial integrity
*Client needs subcategory:*None
Cognitive level: Comprehension

41. CORRECT ANSWER: 3
Clients with panic disorder are at risk for suicide. Childhood trauma is associated with posttraumatic stress disorder, not panic disorder. Nutritional problems don't typically accompany panic disorder. Clients aren't typically disoriented; they may have a temporarily altered sense of reality, but that lasts only for the duration of the attack.
Nursing process step: Analysis
Client needs category: Psychosocial integrity
Client needs subcategory: None
Cognitive level: Comprehension

42. CORRECT ANSWER: 3
Research related to Alzheimer's disease indicates the enzyme needed to produce acetylcholine is dramatically

reduced. The other pathophysiological changes don't cause the symptoms of Alzheimer's.
Nursing process step: Assessment
Client needs category: Physiological integrity
Client needs subcategory: Physiological adaptation
Cognitive level: Analysis

43. CORRECT ANSWER: 4
Abstract thinking is assessed by noting similarities and differences between related words or objects. Not knowing the name of the President of the United States is a deficiency in general knowledge. Not being able to do a simple calculation shows a client's inability to concentrate and focus on thoughts.
Nursing process step: Assessment
Client needs category: Physiological integrity
Client needs subcategory: Physiological adaptation
Cognitive level: Analysis

44. CORRECT ANSWER: 4
Clients with Alzheimer's disease respond to the affect of those around them. A gentle, calm approach is comforting and nonthreatening, and a tense, hurried approach may agitate the client. The client has problems performing independently. These expectations may lead to frustration.
Nursing process step: Implementation
Client needs category: Safe, effective care environment
Client needs subcategory: Management of care
Cognitive level: Application

45. CORRECT ANSWER: 4
The most common cause is thiamine deficiency related to alcohol abuse. The diagnosis can't be made if amnesia occurs only during delirium. Metabolic and organic factors can cause amnestic disorders, but they aren't the most common causes.
Nursing process step: Assessment
Client needs category: Health promotion and maintenance
Client needs subcategory: None
Cognitive level: Knowledge

46. CORRECT ANSWER: 4
Changes in cognitive ability place a client at high risk for injury. The client isn't aware of a loss and therefore doesn't grieve for it. The client isn't aware of a need to cope.
Nursing process step: Nursing diagnosis
Client needs category: Safe, effective care environment
Client needs subcategory: Safety and infection control
Cognitive level: Analysis

47. CORRECT ANSWER: 1
Anterograde amnesia refers to impairment in the ability to learn new information. Retrograde amnesia refers to the inability to recall previously remembered knowledge. Korsakoff's syndrome is an amnestic syndrome caused by thiamine deficiency. Wernicke's encephalopathy is associated with Korsakoff's syndrome, in which the client experiences confusion, ataxia, and ophthalmoplegia.
Nursing process step: Assessment
Client needs category: Physiological integrity
Client needs subcategory: Physiological adaptation
Cognitive level: Knowledge

48. CORRECT ANSWER: 4
A long-term effect of alcohol is cognitive impairment. Agitated behavior occurs when the client is withdrawing from alcohol, not during active use. Paranoid thoughts and ritualistic behaviors aren't typically seen in a client actively abusing alcohol.
Nursing process step: Assessment
Client needs category: Psychosocial integrity
Client needs subcategory: None
Cognitive level: Comprehension

49. CORRECT ANSWER: 1
Enabling behaviors of family members allows the client to continue the addiction by rationalizing, denying, or otherwise excusing the problem. Managing the client's self-care isn't an issue that needs to be addressed based on the client's statement. Dealing with negative behaviors and evaluating the home environment don't address the client's statement about the family's enabling behavior.
Nursing process step: Implementation
Client needs category: Psychosocial integrity
Client needs subcategory: None
Cognitive level: Comprehension

50. CORRECT ANSWER: 2
It's important for the client to talk about the health consequences of continued alcohol use. Testing blood chemistries daily gives the client minimal knowledge about the effects of alcohol on the body and isn't the

most useful information in a teaching plan. A pharmacist isn't the appropriate health care professional to educate the client about the effects of alcohol. Although exercise is an important goal of self-care, it doesn't address the client's knowledge deficit.
Nursing process step: Nursing diagnosis
Client needs category: Psychosocial integrity
Client needs subcategory: None
Cognitive level: Application

51. CORRECT ANSWER: 4
Removing the client at this time may protect her from future embarrassment. Reorienting the client discourages dissociation and encourages integration. Asking to speak to another alter personality encourages dissociation. Allowing the client to play with toys also reinforces this behavior and encourages dissociation.
Nursing process step: Implementation
Client needs category: Safe, effective care environment
Client needs subcategory: Safety and infection control
Cognitive level: Analysis

52. CORRECT ANSWER: 3
Many clients with DID initially experience problems with depression. Commonly the memories of abuse are repressed; the client may not have conscious awareness of being angry with the abuser. Although clients with DID may feel lonely, this is secondary to sadness. Typically, the family is dysfunctional and unlikely to be supportive.
Nursing process step: Assessment
Client needs category: Psychosocial integrity
Client needs subcategory: None
Cognitive level: Knowledge

53. CORRECT ANSWER: 3
Menorrhagia is an excessive menstrual period. Dyspareunia is painful intercourse. Metrorrhagia is uterine bleeding from another cause other than menstruation. Amenorrhea is a lack of menstruation.
Nursing process step: Assessment
Client needs category: Physiological integrity
Client needs subcategory: Reduction of risk potential
Cognitive level: Knowledge

54. CORRECT ANSWER: 3
The major cause of stress in infertile couples is planning sexual intercourse to correlate to fertility cycles. The inconvenience and discomfort of producing specimens and receiving examinations isn't a major stressor. Most couples undergoing fertility treatment understand that one partner is usually infertile.
Nursing process step: Implementation
Client needs category: Health promotion and maintenance
Client needs subcategory: None
Cognitive level: Application

55. CORRECT ANSWER: 4
Encourage the client to verbalize her feelings because loss of one's reproductive organs may bring on feelings of loss of sexuality. Referring her to a psychotherapist may be premature; the client should be given time to work through her feelings. Avoidance of the subject isn't a therapeutic nursing intervention. Pain is a concern after surgery, but it has no bearing on body image.
Nursing process step: Implementation
Client needs category: Psychosocial integrity
Client needs subcategory: None
Cognitive level: Application

56. CORRECT ANSWER: 3
Clients with anorexia nervosa commonly communicate on a superficial level and avoid expressing feelings. Identifying feelings and learning to express them are initial steps in decreasing isolation. Clients with anorexia nervosa are usually able to discuss abstract and concrete issues. Confrontation usually isn't an effective communication strategy because the client may withdraw and become more depressed.
Nursing process step: Implementation
Client needs category: Psychosocial integrity
Client needs subcategory: None
Cognitive level: Application

57. CORRECT ANSWER: 1
The most important intervention to teach the family is how to be there for the client and express their support. These clients need to be encouraged to handle all feelings, not just grief. The client commonly needs encouragement to express negative feelings appropriately, especially anger. Setting limits may prevent important dialogue from occurring. Social interactions are usually limited because the client is withdrawn and self-absorbed. The client needs to develop peer relationships.
Nursing process step: Implementation
Client needs category: Psychosocial integrity
Client needs subcategory: None
Cognitive level: Comprehension

58. CORRECT ANSWER: 3
The client can benefit from understanding the underlying dynamics of the eating disorder. The client with anorexia nervosa has low self-esteem and won't believe the positive statements. Although the client may look at herself in the mirror, in her mind she'll still see herself as fat. Pointing out differences will only diminish her already low self-esteem.
Nursing process step: Implementation
Client needs category: Psychosocial integrity
Client needs subcategory: None
Cognitive level: Application

59. CORRECT ANSWER: 3
Hemoglobin values and hematocrit decrease during pregnancy as the increase in plasma volume exceeds the increase in red blood cell production. Alterations in acid-base balance during pregnancy result in a state of respiratory alkalosis, compensated by mild metabolic acidosis. Mastitis is an infection in the breast characterized by a swollen tender breast and flulike symptoms. This condition is most frequently seen in breast-feeding clients.
Nursing process step: Assessment
Client needs category: Health promotion and maintenance
Client needs subcategory: None
Cognitive level: Knowledge

60. CORRECT ANSWER: 2
Excessive vomiting in clients with hyperemesis gravidarum commonly causes weight loss and fluid, electrolyte, and acid-base imbalances. Gestational hypertension and bowel perforation aren't related to hyperemesis. The effects of hyperemesis on the fetus depend on the severity of the disorder. Clients with severe hyperemesis may have a low-birth-weight infant, but the disorder is generally not life-threatening.
Nursing process step: Assessment
Client needs category: Physiological integrity
Client needs subcategory: Reduction of risk potential
Cognitive level: Analysis

61. CORRECT ANSWER: 1
Clients with gestational diabetes are usually managed by diet alone to control their glucose intolerance. Oral antidiabetic drugs are contraindicated in pregnancy. Long-acting insulin usually isn't needed for blood glucose control in the client with gestational diabetes.
Nursing process step: Implementation
Client needs category: Health promotion and maintenance
Client needs subcategory: None
Cognitive level: Knowledge

62. CORRECT ANSWER: 1
The therapeutic level of magnesium for clients with gestational hypertension is 4 to 7 mEq/L. A serum level of 8 to 10 mEq/L may cause the absence of reflexes in the client. Serum levels of 10 to 12 mEq/L may cause respiratory depression, and a serum level of magnesium greater than 15 mEq/L may result in respiratory paralysis.
Nursing process step: Assessment
Client needs category: Physiological integrity
Client needs subcategory: Pharmacological and parenteral therapies
Cognitive level: Knowledge

63. CORRECT ANSWER: 2
Decreased urine output may occur in clients receiving I.V. magnesium and should be monitored closely to keep urine output at greater than 30 ml/hour because magnesium is excreted through the kidneys and can easily accumulate to toxic levels. Anemia isn't associated with magnesium therapy. The client should be monitored for respiratory depression and paralysis when serum magnesium levels reach approximately 15 mEq/L. Magnesium infusions may cause depression of deep tendon reflexes.
Nursing process step: Assessment
Client needs category: Physiological integrity
Client needs subcategory: Pharmacological and parenteral therapies
Cognitive level: Analysis

64. CORRECT ANSWER: 1
Calcium gluconate is the antidote for magnesium toxicity. Ten milliliters of 10% calcium gluconate is given I.V. push over 3 to 5 minutes. Hydralazine is given for sustained elevated blood pressures in preeclamptic clients. Rh_o(D) immune globulin is given to women with Rh-negative blood to prevent antibody formation from Rh-positive conceptions. Naloxone is used to correct narcotic toxicity.
Nursing process step: Planning
Client needs category: Physiological integrity
Client needs subcategory: Reduction of risk potential
Cognitive level: Analysis

65. CORRECT ANSWER: 1
Blood type would be a critical value to have because the risk of blood loss is always a potential complication during the labor and delivery process. Approximately 40% of a woman's cardiac output is delivered to the uterus; therefore, blood loss can occur quite rapidly in the event of uncontrolled bleeding. Calcium and iron aren't critical values, and oxygen saturation isn't a laboratory value.
Nursing process step: Planning
Client needs category: Physiological integrity
Client needs subcategory: Reduction of risk potential
Cognitive level: Analysis

66. CORRECT ANSWER: 3
A rate of 120 to 160 beats/minute in the fetal heart is appropriate for filling the heart with blood and pumping it out to the system. Faster or slower rates don't accomplish perfusion adequately.
Nursing process step: Assessment
Client needs category: Health promotion and maintenance
Client needs subcategory: None
Cognitive level: Knowledge

67. CORRECT ANSWER: 4
Oxygenation of the fetus may be indirectly assessed through fetal monitoring by closely examining the fetal heart rate strip. Accelerations in the fetal heart rate strip indicate good oxygenation, while decelerations in the fetal heart rate sometimes indicate poor fetal oxygenation. The fetal heart rate strip can't determine the gender of the fetus or assess fetal position. Labor progress can be directly assessed only through cervical examination although, commonly, the woman's body language can give some indication of the progression of labor.
Nursing process step: Assessment
Client needs category: Physiological integrity
Client needs subcategory: Reduction of risk potential
Cognitive level: Comprehension

68. CORRECT ANSWER: 4
An endocardial cushion defect develops early in fetal life due to inappropriate fusion of the endocardial cushions. It usually involves the mitral valve, tricuspid valve, atria, and ventricles. An opening in the atria is considered an atrial septal defect. An opening in the ventricles is considered a ventricular septal defect. An absent tricuspid valve is considered tricuspid atresia.
Nursing process step: Evaluation
Client needs category: Health promotion and maintenance
Client needs subcategory: None
Cognitive level: Knowledge

69. CORRECT ANSWER: 4
Endocardial cushion defects are seen most in children with Down syndrome, asplenia, or polysplenia. Ventricular septal defects are the most common of the cardiac anomalies. Atrial septal defects account for about 10% of all cardiac anomalies. Pulmonic stenosis is responsible for about 8% of all cardiac anomalies.
Nursing process step: Evaluation
Client needs category: Health promotion and maintenance
Client needs subcategory: None
Cognitive level: Knowledge

70. CORRECT ANSWER: 1
Simply decreasing the amount of time the skin comes in contact with wet, soiled diapers will help heal the irritation. Gentle cleaning of the irritated skin should be encouraged. Infants shouldn't have fluid intake restrictions. Talc is contraindicated in children because of the risks of inhaling the fine powder.
Nursing process step: Assessment
Client needs category: Safe, effective care environment
Client needs subcategory: Safety and infection control
Cognitive level: Application

71. CORRECT ANSWER: 4
Children who have urticaria in response to nuts, seafood, or bee stings should be warned about the possibility of anaphylactic reactions to future exposure. The use of epinephrine pens should be taught to the parents and older children. Other treatment choices, such as Benadryl, topical steroids, and emollients, are for the treatment of mild urticaria.
Nursing process step: Planning
Client needs category: Health promotion and maintenance
Client needs subcategory: None
Cognitive level: Application

72. CORRECT ANSWER: 1
Fever, chills, hemoptysis, dyspnea, cough, and pleuritic chest pain are the common symptoms of pneumonia, but elderly clients may first appear with only an altered mental status and dehydration due to a blunted immune response.

Nursing process step: Assessment
Client needs category: Physiological integrity
Client needs subcategory: Physiological adaptation
Cognitive level: Application

73. CORRECT ANSWER: 2
Neuromuscular blockers cause skeletal muscle paralysis, reducing the amount of oxygen used by the restless skeletal muscles, which should improve oxygenation. Bronchodilators may be used, but they typically don't have enough of an effect to reduce the amount of hypoxia present. The head of the bed should be partially elevated to facilitate diaphragm movement, and diuretics can be administered to reduce pulmonary congestion. However, bronchodilators, diuretics, and head elevation would improve oxygen delivery, not reduce oxygen demand.
Nursing process step: Implementation
Client needs category: Physiological integrity
Client needs subcategory: Physiological adaptation
Cognitive level: Application

74. CORRECT ANSWER: 4, 5
The diaphragm is stimulated by nerves at the level of C4. Initially, this client may need mechanical ventilation due to cord edema. This may resolve in time. The client will also require an indwelling urinary catheter to closely monitor fluid status. Decerebrate posturing, hemiplegia, and absent corneal reflexes occur with brain injuries, not spinal cord injuries.
Nursing process step: Planning
Client needs category: Physiological integrity
Client needs subcategory: Physiological adaptation
Cognitive level: Application

75. CORRECT ANSWER: 4
Set up the following ratio for X:

X:100 mg::5ml:125 mg
X = 4 ml

Nursing process step: Planning
Client needs category: Physiological integrity
Client needs subcategory: Pharmacological and parenteral therapies
Cognitive level: Application

Posttest 4

QUESTIONS

1. A nurse is caring for a client who underwent open reduction and internal fixation of a fractured left hip 1 day ago. Which intervention takes priority for this client during the first postoperative day?

☐ **1.** Assessing and controlling pain
☐ **2.** Assisting the client with full weight bearing and walking
☐ **3.** Allowing the client to perform activities of daily living (ADLs) independently
☐ **4.** Removing the client's surgical staples

2. A nurse removes a client's nasogastric (NG) tube according to a physician's order. The nurse should watch for which complication after removing an NG tube?

☐ **1.** Abdominal distention
☐ **2.** Flatulence
☐ **3.** Constipation
☐ **4.** Presence of bowel sounds

3. A nurse instructs the nursing assistant to feed a client who has developed dysphagia after being admitted with a stroke. How should the nursing assistant position the client based on the nurse's instruction?

☐ **1.** On his left side
☐ **2.** On his right side
☐ **3.** In bed with the head of the bed elevated to 30 degrees
☐ **4.** In bed with the head of the bed elevated to at least 45 degrees

4. Which task can a nurse appropriately delegate to a nursing assistant?

☐ **1.** Obtaining vital signs on a client who has just returned from undergoing a colonoscopy
☐ **2.** Feeding a client for the first time after he has experienced a stroke
☐ **3.** Administering feedings through a nasogastric (NG) tube
☐ **4.** Encouraging a client to drink fluids

5. A 70-year-old client who's alert and oriented refuses to take his regularly scheduled medications. Which action should the nurse take?

☐ **1.** Explain to the client that he must take the medications because his physician prescribed them.
☐ **2.** Tell the client that his health will deteriorate if he doesn't take his medications.
☐ **3.** Inform the physician; chart the medications as not given in the medication administration record, and document the reasons the client refused to take them.
☐ **4.** Explain to the client's family that he refused to take his medications.

6. A nurse notes that a client coughs frequently while eating. Which health team member should be notified of this finding?

☐ **1.** Respiratory therapist
☐ **2.** Speech therapist
☐ **3.** Enterostomal therapist
☐ **4.** Smoking-cessation counselor

7. Which scenario requires the licensed practical nurse (LPN) to notify the registered nurse (RN) immediately?

☐ **1.** A decrease in a client's blood pressure from 160/90 mm Hg to 140/84 mm Hg
☐ **2.** A complaint of pain that rates 7 on a 1-to-10 pain-rating scale
☐ **3.** Apical pulse rate of 90 beats/minute with a radial pulse rate of 70 beats/minute
☐ **4.** Family inquiry about the client's discharge time

8. A nurse is caring for a group of clients on a medical-surgical floor. Which client should she attend to first?

☐ **1.** The client whose lower leg is red and swollen
☐ **2.** The client whose apical pulse is 80 beats/minute
☐ **3.** The client who's concerned about going home
☐ **4.** The client who's concerned about receiving his breakfast tray

9. Which client requires further assessment by a nurse?

☐ **1.** The client whose respiratory rate is 21 breaths/minute
☐ **2.** The client whose blood pressure is 140/78 mm Hg
☐ **3.** The client whose apical pulse rate is 84 beats/minute
☐ **4.** The client who is restless

10. A nurse is admitting a client to the medical-surgical floor. She asks the client if he has an advance directive. The client responds by saying, "I don't know what you mean." How should the nurse respond?

☐ **1.** "An advance directive is a document that states your wishes about health care."
☐ **2.** "An advance directive tells us your wishes should you die during hospitalization."
☐ **3.** "An advance directive is much like a last will and testament; it states your financial wishes should you become disabled."
☐ **4.** "An advance directive states your wishes concerning your personal items."

11. A nurse hears the facility code that indicates an infant has been abducted from the nursery. Which action should the nurse take?

☐ **1.** Go immediately to the nursery and inquire about what happened.
☐ **2.** Inform the police department about the incident.
☐ **3.** Report to an exit and be alert for anyone carrying packages.
☐ **4.** Document the names of all visitors on the medical-surgical floor.

12. Several clients are brought to the emergency department after sustaining injuries in a building explosion. According to disaster management principles, which client should be triaged first?

☐ **1.** A 57-year-old with a clavicle fracture
☐ **2.** A 62-year-old with tachypnea
☐ **3.** A 37-year-old with a scalp laceration
☐ **4.** A 10-month-old infant who's crying uncontrollably

13. A client who's scheduled for surgery asks the nurse to keep $50 for him until he returns from surgery. How should the nurse respond?

☐ **1.** "I'll put your money in an envelope and keep it in my locker until you return from surgery."
☐ **2.** "I'll notify your physician about the money."
☐ **3.** "I'll notify the business office to make arrangements for your money to be placed in the hospital safe."
☐ **4.** "You can place the money in your bedside drawer; it will be safe there."

14. A nurse is teaching a client with right-sided weakness proper cane use. Which instruction should the nurse include in her teaching?

☐ **1.** "Hold the cane on the same side as the injury."
☐ **2.** "Hold the cane on the opposite side from the injury."
☐ **3.** "Don't use the cane when climbing stairs."
☐ **4.** "Use the cane when walking further than 50 feet."

15. Several residents in a long-term care facility ask a nurse if they can share their aromatherapy with other clients in the dining area. Why shouldn't the nurse permit them to practice aromatherapy in a group environment?

☐ **1.** Some residents may have an adverse sensitivity to the oils and fragrances.
☐ **2.** The nurse should have no reason for concern because the oils and fragrances are mild.
☐ **3.** There's no scientific evidence to support the use of aromatherapy.
☐ **4.** Aromatherapy can suppress appetite.

16. A nurse is caring for a client who practices reflexology. When collecting client data, the nurse notes that the client's ankles are edematous. Which intervention by the nurse supports the client's beliefs in reflexology and helps reduce edema?

☐ **1.** Lowering the client's legs
☐ **2.** Elevating the client's legs
☐ **3.** Abducting the client's legs
☐ **4.** Adducting the client's legs

17. A physician asks a nurse to join him to discuss palliative care options with a terminally ill client and his family. Which statement by the nurse indicates an understanding of palliative care?

- ☐ **1.** "I'll assist the client with his spiritual needs."
- ☐ **2.** "I'll assist the client with his pain management needs."
- ☐ **3.** "I'll assist the client with his physical needs."
- ☐ **4.** "I'll assist the client with his total needs."

18. A nurse is caring for a dying client who is receiving comfort measures. Which intervention by the nurse is most effective in promoting comfort?

- ☐ **1.** Offering the client fluids every 30 minutes
- ☐ **2.** Changing the client's linens every shift
- ☐ **3.** Combing the client's hair
- ☐ **4.** Maintaining silence when caring for the client

19. A nurse is caring for a recently married, 29-year-old woman who was diagnosed with acute lymphoblastic leukemia (ALL). The client is preparing for an allogeneic bone marrow transplant. Which statement by the client demonstrates an understanding of the physician's explanation about the diagnosis and treatment?

- ☐ **1.** "I should be able to finally start a family after I'm finished with the chemo."
- ☐ **2.** "I've always had a good appetite; even with chemo, I shouldn't have to make any changes to my diet."
- ☐ **3.** "I'll have to remain in the hospital for about 3 months after my transplant."
- ☐ **4.** "I'll only need chemotherapy before receiving my bone marrow transplant."

20. A client is admitted to the emergency department with complaints of right lower quadrant pain. Blood specimens are drawn and sent to the laboratory. Which laboratory finding should be reported to the physician immediately?

- ☐ **1.** Hematocrit 42%
- ☐ **2.** White blood cell count 22.8/mm^3
- ☐ **3.** Serum potassium 4.2 mEq/L
- ☐ **4.** Serum sodium 135 mEq/L

21. A newly hired graduate nurse and her preceptor are establishing priorities for their morning assessments. Which client should they assess first?

- ☐ **1.** The newly admitted client with acute abdominal pain
- ☐ **2.** The client who underwent surgery 3 days ago who requires a dressing change
- ☐ **3.** The client receiving continuous tube feedings who needs the tube-feeding residual checked
- ☐ **4.** The sleeping client who received pain medication 1 hour ago

22. A nurse asks a client who had abdominal surgery 3 days ago if he moved his bowels since surgery. The client states, "I haven't moved my bowels, but I am passing gas." How should the nurse intervene?

- ☐ **1.** Apply moist heat to the client's abdomen.
- ☐ **2.** Encourage the client to ambulate at least three times a day.
- ☐ **3.** Administer a tap water enema.
- ☐ **4.** Notify the physician.

23. A client who underwent abdominal surgery begins to complain of abdominal pain that he describes as "feeling full and uncomfortable." Which assessment should the nurse perform first?

- ☐ **1.** Measuring abdominal girth
- ☐ **2.** Auscultating bowel sounds
- ☐ **3.** Assessing patency of the nasogastric (NG) tube
- ☐ **4.** Assessing vital signs

24. A client requested a do-not-resuscitate order (DNR) upon admission to the hospital. He now tells the nurse that he wants to have everything possible done to help him get better and is concerned about the DNR order. Which response by the nurse is best?

- ☐ **1.** "It's too late to change your mind now."
- ☐ **2.** "We'll have to ask your physician if this is possible."
- ☐ **3.** "Why do you want to do this?"
- ☐ **4.** "It isn't a problem to rescind your DNR order; I'll let your physician know your wishes right away."

25. A 26-year-old client is diagnosed with a brain tumor. As the nurse assists her from the bed to the chair, the client begins having a generalized seizure. Which action should the nurse take first?

☐ **1.** Initiate the code team response.
☐ **2.** Put a padded tongue blade into the client's mouth, and restrain her extremities.
☐ **3.** Record the type of seizure and the time that it occurred.
☐ **4.** Assist the client to the floor, in a side-lying position, and protect her with linens.

26. A child who had bacterial meningitis is scheduled to have his hearing tested before discharge. The mother asks a nurse why this test is necessary. Which response by the nurse is appropriate?

☐ **1.** "It's necessary to make sure your child is developing appropriately."
☐ **2.** "The test will identify attention deficit problems that may occur as a result of his illness."
☐ **3.** "It's necessary to make sure the steroid therapy your child received hasn't affected his hearing."
☐ **4.** "Some children with bacterial meningitis suffer damage to the nerve responsible for hearing."

27. An 18-month-old is admitted to the emergency department with a diagnosis of seizure. Upon assessment, his vital signs are temperature of 104° F (40° C), respiratory rate of 26 breaths/minute, pulse rate of 120 beats/minute, and blood pressure of 90/69 mm Hg. Which action should the nurse take first?

☐ **1.** Give a tepid sponge bath.
☐ **2.** Administer phenytoin (Dilantin).
☐ **3.** Obtain a fingerstick glucose level.
☐ **4.** Obtain a blood specimen to check electrolyte levels.

28. A 9-year-old is admitted with weakness in his legs and a history of the flu. He's diagnosed with Guillain-Barré syndrome. The nurse must notify the physician immediately of which finding?

☐ **1.** Tingling in the hands
☐ **2.** Increasing hoarseness
☐ **3.** Weak muscle tone in the arms
☐ **4.** Weak muscle tone in the legs

29. An infant is diagnosed with patent ductus arteriosus. Which drug may be administered to achieve pharmacologic closure of the defect?

☐ **1.** Digoxin (Lanoxin)
☐ **2.** Prednisone (Deltasone)
☐ **3.** Furosemide (Lasix)
☐ **4.** Indomethacin (Indocin)

30. A mother brings her 12-month-old to the pediatrician's office for a check-up. Which finding suggests that the infant has cystic fibrosis?

☐ **1.** Presence of fat in the stool
☐ **2.** Decreased appetite
☐ **3.** Decreased respiratory rate
☐ **4.** Weight gain

31. Two days after cesarean delivery, a client is diagnosed with deep vein thrombosis. A nurse should monitor this client closely for which complication?

☐ **1.** Endometritis
☐ **2.** Pulmonary embolism
☐ **3.** Hematoma
☐ **4.** Mastitis

32. After an Rh-negative woman experiences a spontaneous abortion, a nurse should expect to administer which medication?

☐ **1.** Magnesium sulfate
☐ **2.** Rh_o (D) immune globulin human (RhoGAM)
☐ **3.** Terbutaline (Brethine)
☐ **4.** Betamethasone (Celestone)

33. A pregnant client develops a chlamydia infection. Which drug is considered the treatment of choice for pregnant clients infected with chlamydia?

☐ **1.** Doxycycline (Vibramycin)
☐ **2.** Azithromycin (Zithromax)
☐ **3.** Acyclovir (Zovirax)
☐ **4.** Miconazole (Monistat)

34. A client reports to a nurse that she feels like she's losing her mind. This fear is most commonly associated with which disorder?

☐ **1.** Social phobia
☐ **2.** Panic disorder
☐ **3.** Generalized anxiety disorder
☐ **4.** Myctophobia

35. A client with schizophrenia who began taking haloperidol (Haldol) 1 week ago now exhibits jerking movements of the neck and mouth. These findings are associated with which adverse reaction to the drug?

- ☐ **1.** Dystonia
- ☐ **2.** Psychosis
- ☐ **3.** Akathisia
- ☐ **4.** Parkinsonism

36. What should a nurse teach the parents of a child who's receiving methylphenidate (Ritalin)?

- ☐ **1.** Monitor the child's blood glucose level because the drug increases the risk of diabetes.
- ☐ **2.** Monitor the child's growth closely because the drug may interfere with growth and development.
- ☐ **3.** Have the child undergo IQ testing because the drug may decrease intelligence.
- ☐ **4.** Have the child's hearing tested because the drug can cause hearing loss.

37. A nurse caring for an 8-month-old infant diagnosed with respiratory syncytial virus can't read a medication dosage written in the infant's medical record. What's the only ethical solution for the nurse?

- ☐ **1.** Erase the original order, and rewrite it more clearly.
- ☐ **2.** Call the physician, and ask for a verbal order to clarify the dosage.
- ☐ **3.** Ask another nurse what she thinks the dosage should be.
- ☐ **4.** Ask the mother what dosage the infant takes at home.

38. The registered nurse (RN) on the adolescent unit delegates a task to the licensed practical nurse (LPN). After delegating the task, what should the RN do?

- ☐ **1.** Allow adequate time for the task to be completed, then follow-up with the LPN.
- ☐ **2.** Document in the chart that the task has been completed.
- ☐ **3.** Keep asking the LPN if the task has been completed.
- ☐ **4.** Assume the task has been completed to her satisfaction.

39. A teenage girl arrives in the emergency department after a physical assault. How could the nurse best protect her rights during the physical examination?

- ☐ **1.** Leave the door open.
- ☐ **2.** Have another female health care worker present.
- ☐ **3.** Keep the suspected attacker from the examination room.
- ☐ **4.** Keep her friends, waiting in the lounge area, informed of her medical condition.

40. An elderly client becomes extremely agitated and attempts to remove his endotracheal tube. The physician orders physical restraints. Which of the following indicates that the nurse has applied the restraints correctly?

- ☐ **1.** A quick-release knot is used to tie the restraint.
- ☐ **2.** The restraint is attached to the bed side rails.
- ☐ **3.** Leather restraints are applied.
- ☐ **4.** The hands are restrained tightly and can't be moved.

41. A client is prescribed digoxin (Lanoxin) 0.125 mg P.O to be administered immediately. The pharmacy dispenses digoxin 0.25 mg. A nurse promptly administers the medication, then realizes she administered the wrong dose. How should the nurse proceed?

- ☐ **1.** Obtain the client's vital signs, then notify the physician and nursing supervisor immediately of the error.
- ☐ **2.** Obtain a copy of the physician's order, and inform the pharmacy of their dispensing error.
- ☐ **3.** Immediately inform the pharmacist of his dispensing error, and document the incident.
- ☐ **4.** Inform the pharmacist and the nursing supervisor of the error, and document the incident.

42. A nurse is teaching a client about three medications he'll receive after discharge. While performing the discharge teaching, the nurse notices that the client suddenly becomes withdrawn and appears anxious. The nurse reviews the client's medical record and notes that he doesn't have a prescription plan and his finances are limited. What action should the nurse take?

- ☐ **1.** Notify the physician, and request that he change the prescription.
- ☐ **2.** Inform the physician, and request a social services consult.
- ☐ **3.** Request that the physician prescribe generic alternatives.
- ☐ **4.** Explore with the client whether he can purchase the medications over time.

43. A 15-year-old client comes to the clinic requesting a test for human immunodeficiency virus (HIV) exposure. The adolescent is concerned that her parents might be notified of her test results. Which response by the nurse is best?

☐ **1.** "HIV testing is very serious; we must notify your parents of the results."
☐ **2.** "Discussing testing with your parents can be frightening, but I can stay with you while you tell them."
☐ **3.** "HIV testing is confidential; after we get the test results we'll discuss your options."
☐ **4.** "Your parents must sign the consent form before we can test you."

44. A 14 year-old client with type 1 diabetes is admitted with ketoacidosis for the second time in 3 months. The mother explains, "I don't know why this keeps happening." Which response by the nurse is best?

☐ **1.** "Adolescents need strict rules to make sure they adhere to their treatment plan."
☐ **2.** "Adolescents sometimes become overwhelmed by adhering to dietary restrictions and taking medication."
☐ **3.** "You'll need to keep a closer eye on your child to make sure she adheres to the treatment plan."
☐ **4.** "You should notify the school nurse so she can monitor your daughter closely while she's at school."

45. A nurse observes a gun under the jacket of a young man visiting a 17-year-old client. Which action should the nurse take first?

☐ **1.** Confront the visitor, and ask him to give her the gun.
☐ **2.** Immediately evacuate the unit to ensure the safety of the other clients and staff.
☐ **3.** Notify security immediately.
☐ **4.** Do nothing because the visitor isn't threatening anyone with the weapon.

46. The nursing staff is developing a care plan for a client who's receiving palliative care for end-stage leukemia. The client is experiencing break-through pain, which she rates as a 5 on a pain scale of 1 to 10. Which action by the nurse should be included in the client's care plan?

☐ **1.** Meeting with the pain management team to devise a more effective pain control plan
☐ **2.** Explaining that pain relief may not be possible because she's receiving maximum doses of pain medications
☐ **3.** Assessing whether the client is abusing the pain medications
☐ **4.** Providing nonpharmacologic pain measures only, because maximum doses of pain medications are ineffective

47. Which statement by a client would lead a nurse to suspect depression?

☐ **1.** "My daughter said she isn't coming to visit today because she needs to work late."
☐ **2.** "I just know my daughter doesn't love me any more."
☐ **3.** "I'm very sad about losing my job, but I know things will turn around for me."
☐ **4.** "At least not everything in my life is bad."

48. A nurse is assessing a client with a history of multiple substance abuse. The client reports that he has been experiencing nausea, vomiting, and diarrhea. The nurse observes flushing, piloerection, increased lacrimation, and rhinorrhea. These signs and symptoms most likely indicate withdrawal from what substance?

☐ **1.** Alcohol
☐ **2.** Amphetamines
☐ **3.** Opioids
☐ **4.** Cocaine

49. A nurse is caring for a client who's taking alprazolam (Xanax) 1 mg twice per day for panic attacks. The nurse knows that the client understands teaching about the drug when the client makes which statement?

☐ **1.** "I'll stop taking the drug immediately if I experience any side effects."
☐ **2.** "I'll go to my physician's office to have blood work done weekly to monitor drug levels."
☐ **3.** "I'll skip a dose if I'm not having any panic attacks."
☐ **4.** "I'll discuss my plans for pregnancy with my physician."

50. How should a nurse measure the length of the feeding tube that should be inserted?
- ☐ **1.** Measure from the mouth to the upper curvature of the stomach.
- ☐ **2.** Measure from the mouth to the xiphoid process.
- ☐ **3.** Measure from the tip of the nose to the upper curvature of the stomach.
- ☐ **4.** Measure from the tip of the nose to the xiphoid process.

51. Which finding would lead a nurse to suspect that a client has developed hypovolemic shock caused by postpartum hemorrhage?
- ☐ **1.** Respiratory rate of 22 breaths/minute
- ☐ **2.** Pale, pink, moist skin
- ☐ **3.** Urine output less than 25 ml/hour
- ☐ **4.** Bounding peripheral pulses

52. A nurse is collecting data on a neonate. Which finding indicates that the neonate's fontanels are normal?
- ☐ **1.** They're soft to the touch.
- ☐ **2.** They're depressed.
- ☐ **3.** They're bulging.
- ☐ **4.** They're large and flat.

53. A client is diagnosed with prehypertension. Which therapy option would most likely be included in the client's treatment plan?
- ☐ **1.** Diuretics
- ☐ **2.** Lifestyle modification instructions
- ☐ **3.** Beta-adrenergic blockers
- ☐ **4.** Angiotensin-converting enzyme inhibitors

54. A nurse should suspect an abdominal aortic aneurysm in an average-weight client who complains of generalized steady abdominal pain when it's accompanied by which finding?
- ☐ **1.** Pulsating mass in the periumbilical area
- ☐ **2.** Elevated cardiac enzymes
- ☐ **3.** Positive Babinski's sign
- ☐ **4.** Pink, frothy sputum

55. A nurse notes that the report from her client's echocardiograph shows vegetation on the client's heart valves. Heart valve vegetation can result from which condition?
- ☐ **1.** Bacterial invasion
- ☐ **2.** Inadequate nutrition
- ☐ **3.** Hypertension
- ☐ **4.** Diabetes mellitus

56. Which characteristic suggests that the client's chest pain is pleuritic in nature?
- ☐ **1.** Resolves with sublingual nitroglycerin
- ☐ **2.** Occurs only during sleep
- ☐ **3.** Increases with deep inspiration, and decreases when the client leans forward
- ☐ **4.** Resolves with a deep breath

57. The night shift nurse reports that a client admitted with a myocardial infarction has normal capillary refill. What capillary refill time would the nurse expect to find if the client's refill time remains normal?
- ☐ **1.** 11 to 15 seconds
- ☐ **2.** 7 to 10 seconds
- ☐ **3.** 4 to 6 seconds
- ☐ **4.** 1 to 3 seconds

58. A client is prescribed tamoxifen 20 mg P.O. b.i.d. for treatment of breast cancer. The client complains to the nurse that she has worsening bone pain. Which response by the nurse is best?
- ☐ **1.** "Acute worsening of bone pain commonly indicates that the drug will produce a good response."
- ☐ **2.** "I'll get you something for pain immediately."
- ☐ **3.** "I'll notify your physician immediately to see if he wants to change your treatment plan."
- ☐ **4.** "I'll withhold the next dose, and we'll see if your bone pain lessens."

59. A nurse in a long-term care facility notes a change in the color, shape, and texture of a nevus located on a client's shoulder. The nurse knows that this finding might suggest:
- ☐ **1.** multiple myeloma.
- ☐ **2.** malignant melanoma.
- ☐ **3.** a sign that the nevus is healing.
- ☐ **4.** acute leukemia.

60. A client diagnosed with leukemia asks the nurse why he must undergo bone marrow aspiration. Which response by the nurse is best?
- ☐ **1.** "It's needed to determine the type of leukemia; your physician will explain it to you in more detail."
- ☐ **2.** "It's needed to examine your platelets."
- ☐ **3.** "It helps to measure the amount of marrow in the bone."
- ☐ **4.** "It helps to measure the white blood cell count."

61. A client with metastatic cancer is experiencing neuropathic pain. Which alternative therapy is most beneficial in treating this type of pain?

☐ **1.** Cryotherapy
☐ **2.** Biofeedback
☐ **3.** Herbal therapy
☐ **4.** Transcutaneous electrical nerve stimulation (TENS)

62. Which drug should be prescribed with nonsteroidal anti-inflammatory drugs (NSAIDs) in elderly cancer clients to reduce the risk of GI adverse reactions?

☐ **1.** Misoprostol (Cytotec)
☐ **2.** Methadone (Dolphine)
☐ **3.** Aspirin
☐ **4.** Naloxone (Narcan)

63. A client who underwent surgery 2 days ago can't tolerate anything by mouth and is experiencing mild to moderate cancer pain. Which nonsteroidal anti-inflammatory drug (NSAID) can the nurse safely administer by the I.M. route?

☐ **1.** Ibuprofen (Motrin)
☐ **2.** Indomethacin (Indocin)
☐ **3.** Ketorolac (Toradol)
☐ **4.** Diclofenac sodium (Voltaren)

64. Which position would best aid breathing in a client with acute pulmonary edema?

☐ **1.** Lying flat in bed
☐ **2.** Left side-lying position
☐ **3.** High Fowler's position
☐ **4.** Semi-Fowler's position

65. A client with blood type B needs a blood transfusion. Which type of blood can this client receive?

☐ **1.** Type A or type O blood
☐ **2.** Type B or type O blood
☐ **3.** Type AB or type O blood
☐ **4.** Type A or type B

66. A client's blood studies reveal a deficiency in all of the blood's formed elements. The physician suspects that the client's bone marrow is failing to generate enough new cells. Which disorder is most likely affecting this client?

☐ **1.** Sickle cell anemia
☐ **2.** Folic acid deficiency anemia
☐ **3.** Aplastic anemia
☐ **4.** Iron deficiency anemia

67. Which nursing instruction can help the parents of a child with hemophilia provide a safe home environment?

☐ **1.** "Pad the corners of coffee tables when your child is a toddler, and provide kneepads for sports when the child is older."
☐ **2.** "Establish a written emergency plan, including what to do in specific situations and the names and phone numbers of emergency contacts."
☐ **3.** "Be a role model to your child by wearing a helmet when riding a bike so your child will, too."
☐ **4.** "Talk to your child about home safety, and have him problem-solve hypothetical situations about his health."

68. A 56-year-old woman diagnosed with acquired immunodeficiency syndrome (AIDS) is admitted with a closed head injury after being found unconscious on the kitchen floor by her neighbor. Based on information from the client's neighbor, the staff suspects domestic abuse. The client has a restraining order against her husband, yet her husband repeatedly attempts to visit her. Which nursing action ensures client safety?

☐ **1.** Place the client in a reverse isolation room, and post an isolation sign on the door restricting visitors.
☐ **2.** Instruct the client that she should put on her call light if her husband enters her room.
☐ **3.** Admit the client to the pediatric unit under an assumed name so that the husband can't find her.
☐ **4.** Inform hospital security personnel of the restraining order, and formulate an action plan with security that protects the client.

69. The charge nurse on the pediatric unit informs the staff nurse that four of her clients require attention. Which client should the nurse see first?

☐ **1.** An 8-year-old client admitted from the postanesthesia care unit who's complaining of pain
☐ **2.** A 10-year-old client with asthma whose oxygen saturation levels are dropping
☐ **3.** A 7-year-old client whose mother is waiting for discharge instructions
☐ **4.** A 9-year-old client with a broken leg who wants help moving from the bed to the chair

70. The coordinator from the organ procurement agency is leading a meeting with a physician, nurse, and mother of a client with confirmed brain death. The client's driver's license indicates that he's an organ donor. After the meeting, the client's mother states, "I just can't make the decision to let him die." Which response by the nurse is best?

- ☐ **1.** "I understand it's a hard choice."
- ☐ **2.** "You can't let him live like this."
- ☐ **3.** "The decision is whether or not you want to honor his wishes concerning organ donation."
- ☐ **4.** "Organ donation brings a positive to death."

71. A 46-year-old client with status asthmaticus requires endotracheal intubation and mechanical ventilation. Twenty-four hours after intubation, the client is started on the insulin infusion protocol. The nurse must monitor the client's blood glucose levels hourly and watch for which early signs and symptoms associated with hypoglycemia?

- ☐ **1.** Sweating, tremors, and tachycardia
- ☐ **2.** Dry skin, bradycardia, and somnolence
- ☐ **3.** Bradycardia, thirst, and anxiety
- ☐ **4.** Polyuria, polydipsia, and polyphagia

72. A nurse is caring for a client who was visiting from out-of-state when he developed severe acute respiratory syndrome (SARS). The nurse receives a phone call from a person who identifies herself as the client's wife. The caller is tearful and requests information about the client. Which response by the nurse is best?

- ☐ **1.** "How soon can you come? He has SARS."
- ☐ **2.** "Only the physician can give you that information."
- ☐ **3.** "I really don't know. I haven't had a chance to look at his chart."
- ☐ **4.** "I'm sorry, but for confidentiality reasons I can't give you information over the phone."

73. The client with SARS privately informs the nurse that he doesn't want to be placed on a ventilator if his condition worsens. The client's wife and children have repeatedly expressed their desire that everything be done for the client. The most appropriate action by the nurse would be to:

- ☐ **1.** inform the family of the client's wishes.
- ☐ **2.** assure the family that everything possible will be done.
- ☐ **3.** support the client's decision.
- ☐ **4.** assure the client that everything possible will be done.

74. When a nurse enters a client's room, she finds him slumped over in his chair. What actions should the nurse take? Rank the options in ascending, chronological order. Use all the options.

1. Activate the resuscitation team.
2. Establish unresponsiveness.
3. Check breathing; if absent, give two breaths.
4. Place the client on a firm surface.
5. Check pulse; if absent, begin compressions.
6. Open the client's airway.

75. A 64-year-old client has just had total hip replacement surgery. The physician orders heparin 8,000 units to be administered subcutaneously. The label on the heparin vial reads: heparin 10,000 units/ml. How many milliliters of heparin should the nurse draw up in the syringe to administer the correct dose?

____

ANSWERS AND RATIONALES

In the posttest answers, the question number appears in boldface type, followed by the number of the correct answer. Rationales for correct answers and, where appropriate, for incorrect options follow. To help you evaluate your knowledge base and application of nursing behaviors, each rationale is classified according to:

- nursing process step
- client needs category
- client needs subcategory
- cognitive level.

1. CORRECT ANSWER: 1
During the first postoperative day, assessing and controlling pain takes priority. Recovery may be delayed by uncontrolled pain. The client must progress to full weight bearing but, during the immediate postoperative period, he requires an assistive device to avoid full weight bearing. The nurse should assist the client with ADLs during the immediate postoperative period. Staples are typically removed by the surgeon and shouldn't be removed for several days after surgery.
Nursing process step: Implementation
Client needs category: Physiological integrity
Client needs subcategory: Reduction of risk potential
Cognitive level: Application

2. CORRECT ANSWER: 1
After removing an NG tube, the nurse should assess the client for such complications as abdominal distention, nausea, and vomiting. Flatulence indicates that gas from the small intestine is passing through the colon. Constipation isn't a complication associated with removing an NG tube. Bowel sounds occur when peristalsis is present, which indicates that the GI tract is functioning.
Nursing process step: Planning
Client needs category: Physiological integrity
Client needs subcategory: Reduction of risk potential
Cognitive level: Application

3. CORRECT ANSWER: 4
The client with dysphagia should be positioned upright (with the head of the bed elevated to at least 45 degrees) to prevent aspiration. Placing the client on his left or right side or lowering the head of the bed to 30 degrees or less will increase the risk of aspiration.
Nursing process step: Planning
Client needs category: Physiological integrity
Client needs subcategory: Reduction of risk potential
Cognitive level: Application

4. CORRECT ANSWER: 4
The nurse can safely delegate the task of encouraging a client to drink fluids. The nurse shouldn't delegate obtaining the vital signs of a client who just underwent a colonoscopy because the client might be unstable and require nursing intervention. Vital signs can be delegated when the client's condition stabilizes. The client newly diagnosed with a stroke must undergo swallowing studies before feeding. After swallowing studies verify that the client is able to eat, licensed personnel should assist the client with eating for the first time. Nursing assistants aren't qualified to administer feedings through an NG tube.
Nursing process step: Implementation
Client needs category: Safe, effective care environment
Client needs subcategory: Management of care
Cognitive level: Application

5. CORRECT ANSWER: 3
The client has the right to refuse his medication. Therefore, the nurse should inform the physician that the client refused his medications. She should also chart them as not given in the medication administration record, and document in the medical record why the client refused them. The nurse should educate the client about his medications, but she can't force him to take them. Forcing a client to take medications is considered assault. Telling a client that his health will deteriorate if the medications aren't taken is making a medical judgment and is outside the scope of practice for a nurse. Informing the client's family is a breach of client confidentiality.
Nursing process step: Implementation
Client needs category: Safe, effective care environment
Client needs subcategory: Management of care
Cognitive level: Application

6. CORRECT ANSWER: 2
Frequent coughing while eating may indicate a problem with swallowing. Therefore, the nurse should notify the speech therapist, who can then perform a swallowing evaluation. The respiratory therapist should be consulted for problems concerning this client's breathing pattern. The enterostomal therapist should be consulted for ostomy and wound care issues. The nurse can't assume that the client smokes simply because he coughs while eating.
Nursing process step: Planning
Client needs category: Safe, effective care environment
Client needs subcategory: Management of care
Cognitive level: Analysis

7. CORRECT ANSWER: 3
The LPN should immediately report an apical pulse rate of 90 beats/minute associated with a radial pulse rate of 70 beats/minute, which indicates a pulse deficit of 20 beats/minute. This finding signifies an irregular heartbeat that might lead to a decrease in cardiac output. Option 1 is a positive finding and doesn't need to be reported immediately. The LPN can assess pain and administer pain medications as prescribed. The LPN can provide the family with an estimated discharge time without consulting the RN.
Nursing process step: Implementation
Client needs category: Safe, effective care environment
Client needs subcategory: Management of care
Cognitive level: Application

8. CORRECT ANSWER: 1
The nurse should first attend to the client whose lower leg is red and swollen. This client may have deep vein thrombosis caused by immobility, which should be investigated further. An apical pulse rate of 80 beats/minute is within normal limits. The nurse should address the clients' concerns about going home and receiving the breakfast tray; however, those concerns don't take priority.
Nursing process step: Planning
Client needs category: Safe, effective care environment
Client needs subcategory: Management of care
Cognitive level: Analysis

9. CORRECT ANSWER: 4
The nurse should further assess the client who's restless because restlessness is an early sign of hypoxia. A respiratory rate of 21 breaths/minute, blood pressure of 140/78 mm Hg, and an apical pulse rate of 84 beats/minute are within normal limits and don't require further assessment at this time.
Nursing process step: Assessment
Client needs category: Safe, effective care environment
Client needs subcategory: Management of care
Cognitive level: Analysis

10. CORRECT ANSWER: 1
An advance directive is a written document that states a client's health care wishes should certain conditions occur. The document includes wishes regarding withdrawing treatment, resuscitation measures, life support, and end-of-life care. Options 2, 3, and 4 might be included in a last will and testament; however, these wishes aren't included in an advance directive.
Nursing process step: Implementation
Client needs category: Safe, effective care environment
Client needs subcategory: Management of care
Cognitive level: Application

11. CORRECT ANSWER: 3
The nurse should report to an exit and be alert for anyone carrying packages. The abductor could conceal an infant in a package to remove it from the facility. Going to the nursery to ask what happened interferes with the nursery investigation and prevents the nurse from securing an exit. The facility should have a policy in which a hospital security officer is responsible for notifying the police when necessary; it isn't appropriate for the nurse to do so. It isn't necessary for the nurse to document the names of visitors visiting the medical-surgical floor.
Nursing process step: Implementation
Client needs category: Safe, effective care environment
Client needs subcategory: Management of care
Cognitive level: Comprehension

12. CORRECT ANSWER: 2
The nurse should immediately attend to the client with tachypnea. Abnormally rapid breathing takes priority over a clavicle fracture or scalp laceration. An infant who's crying uncontrollably needs comforting but not immediate medical attention.
Nursing process step: Assessment
Client needs category: Safe, effective care environment
Client needs subcategory: Management of care
Cognitive level: Application

13. CORRECT ANSWER: 3
It's the nurse's obligation to keep the client's belongings safe, but she shouldn't personally keep the money for the client. Instead, the nurse should notify the business office and make arrangements for the client's money to be placed in the hospital safe. The physician doesn't require notification that the client has money in his possession. Placing the client's money in the bedside drawer doesn't keep the money secure.
Nursing process step: Implementation
Client needs category: Safe, effective care environment
Client needs subcategory: Management of care
Cognitive level: Application

14. CORRECT ANSWER: 2
The nurse should instruct the client to hold the cane in the hand opposite the affected extremity; the only exception is when the client is physically unable to hold the cane in that hand. A cane helps maintain balance; so the client should be encouraged to use the cane when navigating stairs. The cane should be used when walking any distance to prevent injury from falls.
Nursing process step: Implementation
Client needs category: Safe, effective care environment
Client needs subcategory: Safety and infection control
Cognitive level: Application

15. CORRECT ANSWER: 1
The nurse shouldn't permit the clients to perform aromatherapy in a group environment because some clients may experience adverse reactions to the oils and fragrances. Studies have shown that aromatherapy can, in fact, improve mood and promote relaxation. Aromatherapy hasn't been shown to suppress appetite.
Nursing process step: Planning
Client needs category: Safe, effective care environment
Client needs subcategory: Safety and infection control
Cognitive level: Application

16. CORRECT ANSWER: 2
Reflexology is based on the theory that fluid in interstitial spaces blocks oxygen supply to tissues. Therefore, elevating the client's legs helps decrease fluid in the ankles, thereby increasing oxygen supply to the tissues. Lowering, abducting, or adducting the client's legs won't lessen edema or promote reflexology.
Nursing process step: Implementation
Client needs category: Physiological integrity
Client needs subcategory: Basic care and comfort
Cognitive level: Application

17. CORRECT ANSWER: 4
Providing palliative care involves taking care of the client's total needs, which include spiritual, emotional, and pain management and other physical needs. Options 1, 2, and 3 each describe only one aspect of palliative care.
Nursing process step: Planning
Client needs category: Physiological integrity
Client needs subcategory: Basic care and comfort
Cognitive level: Application

18. CORRECT ANSWER: 3
Gently combing the client's hair is soothing and helps maintain the client's dignity. Offering the client fluids every 30 minutes and changing linens every shift unnecessarily disturbs the client. Fluids should be offered at appropriate intervals and linens should be changed when damp or soiled to prevent skin breakdown. The nurse should speak to the client while providing care to allay anxiety.
Nursing process step: Planning
Client needs category: Physiological integrity
Client needs subcategory: Basic care and comfort
Cognitive level: Application

19. CORRECT ANSWER: 4
Most clients receive chemotherapy before undergoing bone marrow transplantation. Most women older than age 26 can't bear children after undergoing treatment because they experience the early onset of menopause. Clients who undergo chemotherapy or radiation must avoid all fresh fruits and vegetables and all foods should be cooked to avoid bacterial contamination. Clients who undergo bone marrow transplantation typically remain hospitalized for 20 to 25 days.
Nursing process step: Evaluation
Client needs category: Physiological integrity
Client needs subcategory: Reduction of risk potential
Cognitive level: Application

20. CORRECT ANSWER: 2
The nurse should report the elevated white blood cell count, which is evident in option 2. This finding, which is a sign of infection, indicates that the client's appendix might have ruptured. Hematocrit of 42%, serum potassium of 4.2 mEq/L and serum sodium of 135 mEq/L are within normal limits. Alterations in these levels aren't indicative of appendicitis.
Nursing process step: Implementation
Client needs category: Safe, effective care environment
Client needs subcategory: Management of care
Cognitive level: Analysis

21. CORRECT ANSWER: 1
The graduate nurse and her preceptor should assess the new admission with an acute abdominal pain first because he just arrived on the floor and might be unstable. Next, they should change the abdominal dressing for the postoperative client or measure feeding tube residual in the client with continuous tube feedings. These tasks are

of equal importance. They should assess the sleeping client who received pain medication 1 hour ago last because he just received relief from his pain and is able to sleep.
Nursing process step: Planning
Client needs category: Safe, effective care environment
Client needs subcategory: Management of care
Cognitive level: Analysis

22. CORRECT ANSWER: 2
The nurse should encourage the client to ambulate at least 3 times a day. Ambulating stimulates peristalsis, which helps the bowels to move. It isn't appropriate to apply heat to a surgical wound. Moreover, heat application can't be initiated without a physician's order. A tap water enema is typically administered as a last resort after other methods fail. A physician's order is also needed with a tap water enema. Notifying the physician isn't necessary at this point because the client is exhibiting bowel function by passing flatus.
Nursing process step: Implementation
Client needs category: Safe, effective care environment
Client needs subcategory: Management of care
Cognitive level: Application

23. CORRECT ANSWER: 3
When an NG tube is no longer patent, stomach contents collect in the stomach, giving the client a sensation of fullness. Therefore, the nurse should begin by assessing patency of the NG tube. The nurse can measure abdominal girth, auscultate bowels, and assess vital signs, but she should check NG tube patency first to help relieve the client's discomfort.
Nursing process step: Assessment
Client needs category: Safe, effective care environment
Client needs subcategory: Management of care
Cognitive level: Application

24. CORRECT ANSWER: 4
The client is allowed to rescind a DNR order at any time. The client makes the decision about a DNR order, with input from the physician. Questioning a client's motives can make the client feel defensive and shut down his communication with the nurse.
Nursing process step: Planning
Client needs category: Safe, effective care environment
Client needs subcategory: Management of care
Cognitive level: Analysis

25. CORRECT ANSWER: 4
The nurse should protect the client from injury by assisting her to the floor in a side-lying position while protecting her from harm by padding the floor with bed linens. There's no need to initiate a response from the code team because seizures are self-limiting. As long as the client's airway is protected, cardiopulmonary status isn't affected. The nurse shouldn't force anything into the mouth of a client during a seizure; doing so may cause injury. Documenting seizure activity is important, but it doesn't take priority over client safety.
Nursing process step: Implementation
Client needs category: Physiological integrity
Client needs subcategory: Reduction of risk potential
Cognitive level: Application

26. CORRECT ANSWER: 4
The most common neurologic complications associated with bacterial meningitis include hearing loss, mental retardation, seizures, visual impairment, and behavioral problems. Therefore, the appropriate response by the nurse is to explain that the hearing test is necessary because some children with bacterial meningitis suffer damage to the nerve responsible for hearing. The hearing test isn't used to monitor childhood development or to identify attention deficit problems. Steroid therapy doesn't cause hearing loss.
Nursing process step: Implementation
Client needs category: Physiological integrity
Client needs subcategory: Physiological adaptation
Cognitive level: Application

27. CORRECT ANSWER: 1
The child's seizure was most likely caused by his fever. Therefore, the nurse should try to lower the child's core body temperature by giving him a tepid sponge bath. Phenytoin isn't prescribed for fever-related seizures. It isn't necessary to obtain a fingerstick glucose level or a blood specimen for electrolytes at this time.
Nursing process step: Implementation
Client needs category: Physiological integrity
Client needs subcategory: Physiological adaptation
Cognitive level: Analysis

28. CORRECT ANSWER: 2
The most serious complication of Guillain-Barré syndrome is respiratory failure, which occurs as paralysis progresses to the nerves that innervate the thoracic area. Increasing hoarseness may be a sign of impending respiratory dis-

tress. Tingling in the hands and weak muscle tone in the arms and legs are findings that commonly occur with Guillain-Barré syndrome as part of the disease's progression. It isn't necessary to notify the physician immediately of these findings.
Nursing process step: Planning
Client needs category: Physiological integrity
Client needs subcategory: Physiological adaptation
Cognitive level: Analysis

29. CORRECT ANSWER: 4
Indomethacin is administered to an infant with patent ductus arteriosus in an effort to close the defect. Digoxin, prednisone, and furosemide aren't effective in closing the defect.
Nursing process step: Implementation
Client needs category: Physiological integrity
Client needs subcategory: Pharmacological and parenteral therapies
Cognitive level: Knowledge

30. CORRECT ANSWER: 1
Cystic fibrosis causes thick secretions that block the pancreatic ducts and prevent essential pancreatic enzymes from reaching the duodenum. This condition causes stools that are greasy, foul-smelling, and frothy from undigested fats. The infant will have weight loss (not weight gain), despite an increased appetite, and dyspnea (not a decreased respiratory rate).
Nursing process step: Assessment
Client needs category: Physiological integrity
Client needs subcategory: Physiological adaptation
Cognitive level: Analysis

31. CORRECT ANSWER: 2
The nurse should monitor the client closely for pulmonary embolism. Pulmonary embolism occurs when the clot breaks off and travels to the pulmonary vascular bed, interfering with gas exchange. Endometritis, hematoma, and mastitis aren't associated with deep vein thrombosis.
Nursing process step: Assessment
Client needs category: Physiological integrity
Client needs subcategory: Reduction of risk potential
Cognitive level: Application

32. CORRECT ANSWER: 2
A woman who is Rh-negative should receive Rh_o (D) immune globulin human (RhoGAM) after a spontaneous abortion to reduce the risk of possible isoimmunization of the fetus in a future pregnancy. Magnesium sulfate, terbutaline, and betamethasone aren't indicated for this use.
Nursing process step: Planning
Client needs category: Physiological integrity
Client needs subcategory: Pharmacological and parenteral therapies
Cognitive level: Knowledge

33. CORRECT ANSWER: 2
Chlamydia infection in the pregnant client is treated with azithromycin or amoxicillin. Doxycycline isn't indicated for chlamydia infection in a pregnant client. Acyclovir and miconazole aren't indicated for chlamydia.
Nursing process step: Planning
Client needs category: Physiological integrity
Client needs subcategory: Pharmacological and parenteral therapies
Cognitive level: Application

34. CORRECT ANSWER: 2
Anxiety severe enough to cause the client to fear she's losing her mind occurs with panic disorder. Social phobia, generalized anxiety disorder, and myctophobia may have a panic component to them, but the anxiety is less severe.
Nursing process step: Assessment
Client needs category: Psychosocial integrity
Client needs subcategory: None
Cognitive level: Application

35. CORRECT ANSWER: 1
Haloperidol and other high-potency conventional antipsychotic drugs cause a high incidence of dystonia and other extrapyramidal adverse reactions. Dystonia is marked by prolonged, repetitive muscle contractions that cause twisting or jerking movements—especially of the neck, mouth, and tongue. Schizophrenia is a type of psychosis.
Akathisia is also an adverse reaction of haloperidol; however, it's characterized by restlessness, pacing, and the inability to rest or sit still. Drug-induced parkinsonism results from abnormally slow movements, muscle rigidity, shuffling gait, stooped posture, flat facial affect, tremors, and drooling. It's also associated with haloperidol therapy.
Nursing process step: Assessment
Client needs category: Physiological integrity
Client needs subcategory: Pharmacological and parenteral therapies
Cognitive level: Application

36. CORRECT ANSWER: 2
The nurse should teach the parents to monitor their child's growth regularly because the drug can cause a temporary delay in growth. The drug doesn't increase the risk of diabetes, decrease intelligence, or impair hearing.
Nursing process step: Planning
Client needs category: Physiological integrity
Client needs subcategory: Pharmacological and parenteral therapies
Cognitive level: Application

37. CORRECT ANSWER: 2
Clarification of written orders must come from the physician or health care provider who wrote the order. A verbal order should be obtained and then entered into the medical record on a separate line. Assuming what the prescriber intended could lead to a medication error. Medical records are legal documents; information should never be altered or erased. The nurse shouldn't ask the mother; the mother may not be reliable and the physician may have prescribed a different dose during hospitalization.
Nursing process step: Implementation
Client needs category: Safe, effective care environment
Client needs subcategory: Management of care
Cognitive level: Application

38. CORRECT ANSWER: 1
The RN remains accountable for all of the client's care including that which has been delegated to the LPN. The RN should allow the LPN ample time to complete the task, then check with the LPN to ensure the task has been completed. The LPN can document the task after it has been satisfactorily completed. After the task has been delegated, it's important to allow the team members the authority to complete the assigned task. The RN is responsible for following-up to make sure the task has been completed satisfactorily and can't assume that this has occurred.
Nursing process step: Evaluation
Client needs category: Safe, effective care environment
Client needs subcategory: Management of care
Cognitive level: Analysis

39. CORRECT ANSWER: 2
Another female health care provider should be present to observe the examination, particularly when it's performed by a male health care provider. Leaving the door open and informing her friends violates her right to privacy and confidentiality. The suspected attacker should be kept from the examination room; however, having another female health care worker present during the examination best protects the client's rights.
Nursing process step: Planning
Client needs category: Safe, effective care environment
Client needs subcategory: Management of care
Cognitive level: Application

40. CORRECT ANSWER: 1
A quick-release knot is always used when fastening a restraint to allow the restraint to be removed quickly in an emergency. Restraints should only be fastened to the bed frame, not the side rails. Soft (not leather) restraints should be used to prevent client injury. Restraints should be applied as loosely as possible to allow movement, but tight enough to ensure client safety.
Nursing process step: Implementation
Client needs category: Safe, effective care environment
Client needs subcategory: Safety and infection control
Cognitive level: Application

41. CORRECT ANSWER: 1
The nurse should obtain vital signs, then notify the physician and nursing supervisor of the error. An incident report should then be completed to document the occurrence. The nurse administering the drug is legally responsible to ensure that she calculates and administers the correct dose. She shouldn't immediately inform the pharmacist. The incident will be shared with the pharmacy supervisor after completion of the incident report.
Nursing process step: Implementation
Client needs category: Safe, effective care environment
Client needs subcategory: Management of care
Cognitive level: Application

42. CORRECT ANSWER: 2
The nurse should inform the physician of the client's financial concerns and request a social services consult to help the client with his financial concerns. The nurse shouldn't request that prescriptions be changed. Treatment shouldn't be delayed by purchasing medications over time.
Nursing process step: Implementation
Client needs category: Safe, effective care environment
Client needs subcategory: Management of care
Cognitive level: Analysis

43. CORRECT ANSWER: 3
State laws may vary, but in most states an adolescent that understands informed consent can consent to HIV testing. The adolescent may not wish to discuss testing with her parents. If the adolescent does, however, the nurse should support the adolescent. If the test results are positive, it's important for the adolescent to have parental support for the treatment regimen.
Nursing process step: Implementation
Client needs category: Psychosocial integrity
Client needs subcategory: None
Cognitive level: Application

44. CORRECT ANSWER: 2
The nurse should explain that some adolescents simply become overwhelmed or tired of taking medication and adhering to dietary restrictions. These feeling should be recognized as normal. Referral to a support group may help the child and her parents cope with the diagnosis and its implications. Adolescents shouldn't be given strict rules. Strict rules cause rebellion and don't allow the adolescent to develop her own decision-making process. Having the mother and school nurse keep a closer eye on the adolescent may cause rebellion. The adolescent needs support from these individuals, not close monitoring, which might be overwhelming and lead to rebellion. Close monitoring might also diminish communication between the adolescent and her parents.
Nursing process step: Implementation
Client needs category: Physiological integrity
Client needs subcategory: Reduction of risk potential
Cognitive level: Analysis

45. CORRECT ANSWER: 3
The nurse should notify security immediately because they're trained to handle the situation. Direct confrontation by the nurse may startle him and provoke threatening behavior. It isn't necessary to evacuate the unit because the visitor isn't threatening anyone with the weapon. Staff should take measures to prevent people from entering the client's room until the situation is controlled. It's neglectful for the nurse to do nothing about the situation.
Nursing process step: Implementation
Client needs category: Safe, effective care environment
Client needs subcategory: Safety and infection control
Cognitive level: Comprehension

46. CORRECT ANSWER: 1
Patient comfort is the top priority in palliative care. The nurse should meet with the pain management team to devise a plan to control the client's pain. Typically, doses are increased above the normal maximum doses to meet the client's needs. Clients who require opioids long-term develop drug tolerance, so it's necessary to increase dosages. There's no need to assess the client for drug abuse. The nursing staff should also incorporate nonpharmacologic measures to relieve pain into the client's care plan, but they shouldn't be the only measures used to control pain.
Nursing process step: Implementation
Client needs category: Physiological integrity
Client needs subcategory: Basic care and comfort
Cognitive level: Application

47. CORRECT ANSWER: 2
People who are depressed typically have cognitive distortions. They commonly jump to negative conclusions (as in option 2) without facts to validate the conclusions. They also tend to have all-or-nothing thinking, in which they label all of life's events as "bad," predict negative events, and commonly assume that another person thinks or feels a certain way.
Nursing process step: Assessment
Client needs category: Psychosocial integrity
Client needs subcategory: None
Cognitive level: Analysis

48. CORRECT ANSWER: 3
Typical symptoms of opioid withdrawal include flushing, piloerection, nausea, vomiting, abdominal cramps, increased lacrimation, and rhinorrhea. The nurse must be aware of symptoms of opioid withdrawal because of the risk of abusing opioids, such as heroin and hydrocodone. Alcohol withdrawal symptoms include tachycardia, disorientation, confusion, agitation, and inability to sleep. Cocaine withdrawal symptoms include depression with possible suicidal ideation, sleep disturbances, poor concentration, and cocaine craving. Amphetamine withdrawal symptoms are similar to those of cocaine but not as pronounced.
Nursing process step: Assessment
Client needs category: Psychosocial integrity
Client needs subcategory: None
Cognitive level: Analysis

49. CORRECT ANSWER: 4
Alprazolam is contraindicated in pregnancy; therefore, the client should be instructed to discuss plans for pregnancy with the physician. A client should be advised that adverse reactions may subside with time and not to stop taking the drug. Weekly blood tests aren't indicated with alprazolam. A client should be advised not to skip doses.
Nursing process step: Evaluation
Client needs category: Physiological integrity
Client needs subcategory: Pharmacological and parenteral therapies
Cognitive level: Application

50. CORRECT ANSWER: 4
To determine the correct tube length needed to reach the stomach, first extend the distal end of the tube from the tip of the patient's nose to his earlobe. Coil this portion of the tube around your fingers so the end will remain curved until you insert it. Then, extend the uncoiled portion from the earlobe to the xiphoid process.
Nursing process step: Planning
Client needs category: Physiological integrity
Client needs subcategory: Basic care and comfort
Cognitive level: Application

51. CORRECT ANSWER: 3
A urine output less than 25 ml/hour suggests hypovolemic shock secondary to decreased renal perfusion associated with blood loss. Other findings include rapid, shallow respirations; pale, cold, clammy skin; rapid, thready peripheral pulses; mean arterial pressure below 60 mm Hg; and narrowed pulse pressure.
Nursing process step: Assessment
Client needs category: Physiological integrity
Client needs subcategory: Reduction of risk potential
Cognitive level: Application

52. CORRECT ANSWER: 1
The fontanels of a neonate should be soft to touch. Soon after birth, the anterior fontanel should be diamond shaped and measure approximately 5 cm. The posterior fontanel should be triangular and smaller than the anterior fontanel. A depressed fontanel indicates dehydration. A full, bulging fontanel indicates tumor, infection, or hemorrhage. A large, flat, soft fontanel is characteristic of hydrocephalus.
Nursing process step: Assessment
Client needs category: Health promotion and maintenance
Client needs subcategory: None
Cognitive level: Comprehension

53. CORRECT ANSWER: 2
Prehypertension signals the need for teaching about lifestyle modifications and the prevention of developing hypertension. Lifestyle modifications may include changes in diet, adoption of relaxation techniques, regular exercise, smoking cessation, limited intake of alcohol, and restricted sodium and saturated fat intake. Diuretics, beta-adrenergic blockers, and angiotensin-converting enzyme inhibitors are used to treat hypertension.
Nursing process step: Planning
Client needs category: Health promotion and maintenance
Client needs subcategory: None
Cognitive level: Application

54. CORRECT ANSWER: 1
Signs of abdominal aortic aneurysm include gnawing, generalized, steady abdominal pain; lower back pain that's unaffected by movement; gastric or abdominal fullness; pulsating mass in the periumbilical area (if the client isn't obese), systolic bruit over the aorta on auscultation of the abdomen; bruit over the femoral arteries; and hypotension (with aneurysm rupture). Elevated cardiac enzymes indicate heart muscle damage. A positive Babinski's sign indicates damage to the pyramidal tract of the central nervous system. Pink, frothy sputum is a sign of pulmonary edema.
Nursing process step: Assessment
Client needs category: Physiological integrity
Client needs subcategory: Physiological adaptation
Cognitive level: Analysis

55. CORRECT ANSWER: 1
Bacterial invasion produces vegetative growths on the heart valves, the endocardial lining of heart chamber, or the endothelium of a blood vessel. These growths may embolize to the spleen, kidneys, central nervous system, extremities, and lungs. Vegetation doesn't result from inadequate nutrition, hypertension, or diabetes mellitus.
Nursing process step: Assessment
Client needs category: Physiological integrity
Client needs subcategory: Physiological adaptation
Cognitive level: Comprehension

56. CORRECT ANSWER: 3
Pleuritic pain increases with deep inspiration and decreases when the client sits up and leans forward. This decrease occurs because leaning forward pulls the heart away from the diaphragmatic pleurae of the lungs. Pain associated with stable angina resolves with sublingual ni-

troglycerin. Pleuritic pain doesn't occur only during sleep, and it doesn't resolve with a deep breath.
Nursing process step: Assessment
Client needs category: Physiological integrity
Client needs subcategory: Physiological adaptation
Cognitive level: Application

57. CORRECT ANSWER: 4
A capillary refill time lasting longer than 3 seconds is considered delayed and indicates decreased perfusion.
Nursing process step: Assessment
Client needs category: Physiological integrity
Client needs subcategory: Reduction of risk potential
Cognitive level: Knowledge

58. CORRECT ANSWER: 1
The nurse should reassure the client that acute worsening of bone pain commonly indicates that the drug will produce a good response. After reassuring the client, the nurse should offer pain medication to the client, as prescribed. It isn't necessary to notify the physician unless the client has nothing prescribed for treatment of pain. The nurse shouldn't withhold a dose of the medication without a physician's order.
Nursing process step: Implementation
Client needs category: Physiological integrity
Client needs subcategory: Pharmacological and parenteral therapies
Cognitive level: Application

59. CORRECT ANSWER: 2
A change in a nevus is a sign of malignant melanoma, not a sign that the nevus is healing. Multiple myeloma produces vision disturbances, headaches, somnolence, irritability, confusion, cold intolerance, renal failure, and skeletal pain. Findings associated with acute leukemia include infection, fever, bleeding, anemia, malaise, fever, lethargy, paleness, weight loss, and night sweats.
Nursing process step: Assessment
Client needs category: Physiological integrity
Client needs subcategory: Physiological adaptation
Cognitive level: Analysis

60. CORRECT ANSWER: 1
Bone marrow aspiration determines what type of immature white blood cell count is involved to determine the type of leukemia and direct the type of treatment. The nurse should offer a simple explanation and tell the client that the physician will explain fully before informed consent is obtained. It isn't performed to examine platelets, measure white blood cell count, or measure the amount of marrow in the bone.
Nursing process step: Implementation
Client needs category: Physiological integrity
Client needs subcategory: Reduction of risk potential
Cognitive level: Application

61. CORRECT ANSWER: 4
TENS alters the client's perception of pain by blocking painful stimuli traveling over nerve fibers. It may be effective in treatment of cancer pain by reducing muscle spasm, decreasing edema, and raising the pain threshold. The therapy appears to be most effective in treating neuropathic pain. Cryotherapy is effective for treating acute injuries, such as an ankle sprain, by reducing inflammation. Biofeedback has been found to reduce cancer pain through the client's learned conscious control of the body's responses to pain. However, this method of pain control isn't the most beneficial in treating neuropathic pain. Herbal therapy isn't most effective in treating neuropathic pain.
Nursing process step: Implementation
Client needs category: Physiological integrity
Client needs subcategory: Basic care and comfort
Cognitive level: Application

62. CORRECT ANSWER: 1
NSAIDs should be administered with omeprazole (Prilosec), ranitidine (Zantac), or misoprostol in the elderly or those with a history of GI bleeding to reduce the risk of GI adverse reactions. Methadone is sometimes administered with NSAIDs to further control pain. Aspirin also causes GI adverse reactions and isn't commonly administered with NSAIDs. Naloxone is an opioid antagonist, which is administered to reverse opioid-induced respiratory depression.
Nursing process step: Planning
Client needs category: Physiological integrity
Client needs subcategory: Pharmacological and parenteral therapies
Cognitive level: Application

63. CORRECT ANSWER: 3
Currently, ketorolac is the only NSAID that can be administered parenterally in the United States. Ketorolac may be used for up to 5 days to control mild to moderate cancer pain. Ibuprofen, indomethacin, and diclofenac sodium are all NSAIDs, but they can't be administered parenterally.

Nursing process step: Planning
Client needs category: Physiological integrity
Client needs subcategory: Pharmacological and parenteral therapies
Cognitive level: Knowledge

64. CORRECT ANSWER: 3
High Fowler's position promotes ventilation and facilitates breathing by reducing venous return. A flat or side-lying position would worsen the client's breathing and increase the workload of the heart. Semi-Fowler's position won't reduce the workload of the heart as effectively as high Fowler's position.
Nursing process step: Implementation
Client needs category: Physiological integrity
Client needs subcategory: Basic care and comfort
Cognitive level: Comprehension

65. CORRECT ANSWER: 2
Type B blood contains B antigens and anti-A antibodies, but no anti-B antibodies. Therefore, a client with type B blood can receive type B or type O blood (which contains neither anti-A nor anti-B antibodies).
Nursing process step: Planning
Client needs category: Physiological integrity
Client needs subcategory: Pharmacological and parenteral therapies
Cognitive level: Comprehension

66. CORRECT ANSWER: 3
Aplastic anemia usually results from injury or destruction of stem cells in bone marrow or the bone marrow matrix, causing pancytopenia (anemia, granulocytopenia, thrombocytopenia) and bone marrow hypoplasia (bone marrow becomes fatty). In sickle cell anemia, a defective hemoglobin molecule (HbS) causes red blood cells (RBCs) to roughen and become sickle-shaped and more fragile. Folic acid deficiency anemia results from a decreased level or lack of folate, a vitamin that's essential for RBC production and maturation. With iron deficiency anemia, an inadequate supply of iron for optimal formation of RBCs results in smaller cells.
Nursing process step: Assessment
Client needs category: Physiological integrity
Client needs subcategory: Physiological adaptation
Cognitive level: Application

67. CORRECT ANSWER: 2
Establishing a written emergency plan that includes what to do in specific situations helps the family provide safety measures for their child with hemophilia. Option 1 doesn't help provide a safe home environment for children of all ages. Option 3 is only applicable to children who are old enough to emulate their parents' behaviors. Option 4 doesn't help provide a safe environment; it just addresses problem solving.
Nursing process step: Planning
Client needs category: Safe, effective care environment
Client needs subcategory: Safety and infection control
Cognitive level: Application

68. CORRECT ANSWER: 4
The nurse should inform hospital security personnel about the restraining order and formulate an action plan with security that protects the client. Option 1 isolates the client and doesn't incorporate protective measures. Option 2 may alert hospital staff but doesn't allow for implementation of safety measures. Measures should be in place to stop the husband before he enters the client's room. Option 3 doesn't protect the client from harm.
Nursing process step: Planning
Client needs category: Safe, effective care environment
Client needs subcategory: Safety and infection control
Cognitive level: Application

69. CORRECT ANSWER: 2
Decreasing oxygen saturation levels indicate difficulty breathing and increased work of breathing. Airway, breathing, and circulation always take priority. Administration of pain medication and reviewing discharge instructions can be delegated to another registered nurse. Moving a client from the bed to the chair can be delegated to a nursing assistant.
Nursing process step: Planning
Client needs category: Safe, effective care environment
Client needs subcategory: Management of care
Cognitive level: Analysis

70. CORRECT ANSWER: 3
Because the client meets the criteria for brain death, the client can be pronounced dead. The mother should be redirected to the decision at hand, which is whether or not she wants to honor her son's decision to be an organ donor. Even though the client indicated that he wishes to

be a donor on his driver's license, the family is still asked to sign a consent form. Options 1 and 2 don't address the fact that the client has already been declared brain dead. Option 4 offers false reassurance without addressing the mother's concerns.
Nursing process step: Planning
Client needs category: Safe, effective care environment
Client needs subcategory: Management of care
Cognitive level: Application

71. CORRECT ANSWER: 1
Sweating, tremors, and tachycardia are early signs of hypoglycemia. Dry skin, bradycardia, and somnolence are signs and symptoms associated with hypothyroidism. In option 3, thirst and anxiety are signs of hypoglycemia, but bradycardia isn't. Polyuria, polydipsia, and polyphagia are signs and symptoms of diabetes mellitus.
Nursing process step: Evaluation
Client needs category: Safe, effective care environment
Client needs subcategory: Safety and infection control
Cognitive level: Application

72. CORRECT ANSWER: 4
Health Insurance Portability and Accountability Act (HIPAA) regulations and confidentiality prohibit the nurse from providing information over the phone to an unknown caller. Option 1 is incorrect because it breeches confidentiality. Options 2 and 3 are incorrect because they ignore the caller's concerns.
Nursing process step: Implementation
Client needs category: Safe, effective care environment
Client needs subcategory: Management of care
Cognitive level: Analysis

73. CORRECT ANSWER: 3
The nurse is obligated to act as a client advocate. The nurse shouldn't discuss the issue with the client's family unless the client gives permission. Options 2 and 4 oppose the client's wishes and don't demonstrate client advocacy.
Nursing process step: Implementation
Client needs category: Safe, effective care environment
Client needs subcategory: Management of care
Cognitive level: Application

74. CORRECT ANSWER:

2. Establish unresponsiveness.
1. Activate the resuscitation team.
4. Place the client on a firm surface.
6. Open the client's airway.
3. Check breathing; if absent, give two breaths.
5. Check pulse; if absent, begin compressions.

The nurse should first establish unresponsiveness. After confirming unresponsiveness, the nurse should activate the resuscitation team. Next, she should place the client on a firm surface, open his airway, and check for breathing. If the client isn't breathing, the nurse should give two slow breaths using a pocket mask or bag mask. Next, the nurse should check for signs of circulation (breathing, coughing, movement, or presence of carotid pulse). If there are no signs of circulation, the nurse should initiate chest compressions.
Nursing process step: Implementation
Client needs category: Physiological integrity
Client needs subcategory: Reduction of risk potential
Cognitive level: Analysis

75. CORRECT ANSWER: 0.8
The following formula is used to calculate drug dosages:

$$\frac{\text{dose on hand}}{\text{quantity on hand}} = \frac{\text{dose desired}}{X}$$

In this example, the equation is as follows:

$$\frac{10{,}000 \text{ units}}{\text{ml}} = \frac{8{,}000 \text{ units}}{X}$$

$$X = 0.8 \text{ ml}$$

Nursing process step: Implementation
Client needs category: Physiological integrity
Client needs subcategory: Pharmacological and parenteral therapies
Cognitive level: Application

Glosssary of key terms

ABDOMINAL AORTIC ANEURYSM An aneurysm that affects part of the abdominal aorta

ABRUPTIO PLACENTAE The premature separation of a normally positioned placenta in a pregnancy of at least 20 weeks' gestation, before or during labor but before delivery; it can result in hemorrhage and death of the mother, the fetus, or both

ABUSE A wrong or improper action taken toward another that mistreats and injures

ACNE VULGARIS A form of acne common during puberty and adolescence, characterized by comedones, cysts, papules, and pustules on the face, back, and chest

ACQUIRED IMMUNE DEFICIENCY SYNDROME (AIDS) A disorder of the immune system caused by infection with human immunodeficiency virus and characterized by an inability to mount a successful defense against infection, such as by organisms that usually aren't pathogenic (opportunistic infections)

ACROCYANOSIS The bluish discoloration of a neonate's extremities

ACROMEGALY A metabolic disorder occurring in a middle-aged person that results from excess secretion of somatotropin and is characterized by progressive enlargement of the head, hands, and feet

ACTIVITY THEORY The social theory that a client is satisfied with becoming older and living a middle-age lifestyle

ACUTE HEAD INJURY A head injury caused by an incident that leads to brain injury or bleeding within the brain

ACUTE LYMPHOCYTIC LEUKEMIA (ALL) A common type of leukemia in children that's marked by extreme proliferation of immature lymphocytes (blast cells)

ACUTE POSTSTREPTOCOCCAL GLOMERULONEPHRITIS An inflammatory kidney disease involving the glomeruli and characterized by the sudden onset of facial edema, hematuria, proteinuria, and decreased urine output; it occurs as a late complication of pharyngitis caused by streptococcal infection (beta-hemolytic streptococci)

ACUTE RENAL FAILURE The inability of a kidney to excrete metabolites at normal plasma levels under conditions of normal loading or the inability to retain electrolytes under conditions of normal intake; marked by uremia and usually by oliguria or anuria, with hyperkalemia and pulmonary edema

ACUTE RESPIRATORY DISTRESS SYNDROME (ARDS) A fulminant, pulmonary interstitial and alveolar edema, hemorrhage, and acute hypoxemia, which usually develops a few days after the initiating trauma

ACUTE RESPIRATORY FAILURE Failure of the cardiac and pulmonary systems to adequately exchange oxygen and carbon dioxide in the lungs

ADDISON'S DISEASE Disease when the adrenal gland fails to secrete sufficient mineralocorticoids, glucocorticoids, and androgens

ADDISONIAN CRISIS Critical deficiency of mineralocorticoids and glucocorticoids

ADHESION Band of granulation tissue that binds tissues and organs, causing loss of function or other complications

ADMINISTRATIVE LAW The enforcement of government agencies' rules and regulations

ADRENERGIC FIBERS The nerve fibers in the sympathetic nervous system that release norepinephrine

ADVANCE DIRECTIVE A legally binding document that gives instructions for which treatments should and shouldn't be performed if the person is incapacitated

ADVOCACY POWER The particular ability nurses have to speak for patients and to work to remove obstacles because they're acknowledged as patient advocates

AFFECT A feeling, emotion, or mood

AFFECTIVE INAPPROPRIATENESS An inappropriate emotional response to a situation; for example, laughing when sad or crying when happy

AGORAPHOBIA Fear of being alone or in public places

AGRANULOCYTOSIS An abnormal condition of the blood characterized by a severe reduction in the number of granulocytes, resulting in fever, sore throat, and bleeding ulcers of the rectum, mouth, and vagina; it may arise as an adverse reaction to neuroleptic drugs or other medications

ALPHA PARTICLES One of the primary types of radiation associated with radioactivity; heavy, slow moving, charged particles that travel only one or two inches in air and can be stopped by a piece of paper or the dead, outside layers of skin

ALOPECIA The absence or loss of hair

ALZHEIMER'S TYPE DEMENTIA Disease that causes an irreversible, global impairment of cognitive functioning, memory, and personality

AMBIVALENCE The simultaneous existence of two opposing feelings, needs, or wishes

AMENORRHEA The absence or cessation of menstruation

AMNIOCENTESIS Procedure that involves transabdominal insertion of a spinal needle into the uterus to aspirate amniotic fluid

AMNION Thin, tough, inner fetal membrane that lines the amniotic sac

AMYOTROPHIC LATERAL SCLEROSIS (ALS) An incurable disease affecting the spinal cord and the medulla and cortex of the brain, characterized by progressive degeneration of motor neurons, and leading to weakness and wasting of muscles, increased reflexes, and severe muscle spasms

ANAPHYLAXIS A type of distributive shock that's dramatic and widespread, resulting in a systemic reaction to a previously encountered antigen

ANEMIA A reduction either in the volume of red blood cells or in hemoglobin concentration that diminishes the blood's capacity to carry oxygen, therefore reducing the amount of oxygen available to tissue

ANESTHESIA The loss of the ability to feel pain sensation caused by the administration of a drug, which may be general, regional, or local

ANGINA Chest pain that results from myocardia ischemia; an imbalance between myocardial oxygen supply and demand; the most common symptom of coronary artery disease

ANHEDONIA The inability to experience pleasure from acts that normally give it

ANKYLOSING SPONDYLITIS Spinal arthritis that resembles rheumatoid arthritis, sometimes progressing to fusion of the involved vertebrae

ANKYLOSIS The fixation or immobility of a joint, usually from cartilage destruction

ANOREXIA NERVOSA Disorder characterized by starvation or binge eating and purging in hopes of losing or maintaining weight

ANTICIPATORY GUIDANCE The initiation of interventions before an event occurs to prevent potential problems

ANTICIPATORY PLANNING The act of preparing for potential situations and outcomes

AORTIC INSUFFICIENCY A defective functioning of the aortic valve with incomplete closure resulting in aortic regurgitation

AORTIC STENOSIS A narrowing or fusion of the aortic valve that interferes with left ventricular outflow

APGAR SCORE The physical assessment of heart rate, respiratory effort, muscle tone, reflexes, and color of a neonate at 1 and 5 minutes to test his adjustment to extrauterine life; a score of 0 to 3 reveals severe distress, a score of 4 to 7 reveals moderate distress, and a score of 7 to 10 reveals no distress

APLASTIC ANEMIA Immune-medicated illness that results from suppression, damage, or infiltration of the bone marrow

APPENDICITIS A disorder that causes inflammation of the vermiform appendix

ARRHYTHMIAS A variation from the normal rhythm of the heartbeat encompassing abnormal regular and irregular rhythms as well as loss of rhythm

ARTERIAL OCCLUSIVE DISEASE An obstruction or narrowing of the lumen of the aorta and its major branches, which interrupts blood flow, usually to the legs and feet; the disease may affect the carotid, vertebral, innominate, subclavian, mesenteric, and celiac arteries

ASBESTOSIS A chronic disease of the lungs characterized by inflammation, leading to fibrotic changes in lung tissue; it results from inhalation of asbestos fibers and is most common among asbestos miners and workers

ASPHYXIA A condition characterized by impairment or cessation of oxygen and carbon dioxide exchange in the body, resulting in a critically insufficient blood oxygen level and a significantly increased carbon dioxide level

ASSAULT The threat of imminent harmful or offensive bodily contact

ASSOCIATIVE LOOSENESS The illogical connection of thoughts, so that verbalization is nonsensical or confusing to the listener

ASTHMA A respiratory disorder characterized by recurrent attacks of paroxysmal dyspnea, bronchospasm, wheezing on expiration, and coughing; triggers may include pollutants, vigorous exercise, emotional stress, and infection

ATAXIA Poorly coordinated muscle movement

ATELECTASIS The collapse of lung tissue or incomplete expansion of a lung, caused by the absence of air in a portion of the lung or in the entire lung

ATONY A lack of normal muscle tone or strength

ATOPIC DERMATITIS A skin inflammation occurring in individuals with a genetic predisposition to allergies, characterized by intense itching, maculopapular lesions, and excoriation

ATRESIA The complete closure of a tube or body opening

ATRIAL SEPTAL DEFECT A defect stemming from a patent foramen ovale or the failure of a septum to develop completely between the atria

ATTENTION DEFICIT HYPERACTIVITY DISORDER (ADHD) Previously called *attention deficit disorder*, this disorder includes hyperactivity, impulsiveness, and inattention, which can result in intrusive and disruptive behavior

ATTITUDINAL ISOLATION A type of isolation that results from societal rejection

AUSCULTATION The method of listening for sounds from within the body by applying the ear directly to a bare surface or by using an instrument such as a stethoscope

AUTHORITARIAN A style of leadership and management that's characterized by structure, order, and a greater emphasis on task accomplishment than on the people who perform the tasks (a useful style in a crisis such as a "code blue")

AUTISTIC WITHDRAWAL Retreat from the external environment through hallucinations, delusions, verbal abuse, refusal to speak, catatonia, or excitation

AUTOLOGOUS BLOOD TRANSFUSION The process of reinfusing the client with his own blood

BARLOW'S SIGN Test in which a click is felt when the infant is placed supine with hips flexed 90 degrees, knees fully flexed, and the hip brought into midabduction

BASAL CELL EPITHELIOMA Tumor commonly caused by prolonged exposure to the sun

BATTERY Bodily contact with another person without the person's permission or consent

B CELLS Also known as *lymphocytes*, B cells are any of the mononuclear, nonphagocytic leukocytes found in the blood, lymph, and lymphoid tissues that are responsible for the body's humoral immunity

BEHAVIORAL ISOLATION Isolation that results from social withdrawal because of unacceptable social behavior, such as confusion, incontinence, or erratic behavior

BELL'S PALSY Unilateral facial paralysis of sudden onset, resulting from trauma to the facial nerve, from compression of the nerve by a tumor, or from an unknown cause

BENIGN PROSTATIC HYPERPLASIA (BPH) An age-related disorder characterized by the enlargement of the prostate resulting from proliferation of glandular and stromal elements; it may cause urethral compression and obstruction

BETA PARTICLES High-energy electrons emitted by the nucleus in nuclei that contain too many or too few neutrons

BINGE-PURGE CYCLE Uncontrolled ingestion of large amounts of food followed by vomiting

BIPOLAR DISORDER Also known as *manic-depression*, a severe disturbance in affect, manifested by episodes of extreme sadness alternating with episodes of euphoria

BLOOD TYPE The specific ABO blood group; consists of four major blood types: O, A, B, and AB; this classification depends on the presence or absence of two major antigens, A and B; type O occurs when neither is present and type AB occurs when both are present

BORDERLINE PERSONALITY DISORDER A condition that results in a pattern of instability in a person's mood, interpersonal relationships, self-esteem, self-identity, behavior, and cognition; impulsiveness is its most prominent characteristic

BRACHYTHERAPY Radiation therapy whereby sealed radionuclide sources are placed within or near malignant tumors

BRAIN ABSCESS A free or capsulated collection of pus that can occur in the brain and is usually due to a secondary infection, such as otitis media, sinusitis, dental abscess, or mastoiditis

BRAIN TUMOR A neoplasm of the brain characterized by uncontrolled and progressive cell multiplication Brain tumors are usually invasive but don't cross the cerebrospinal axis

BRAXTON HICKS CONTRACTIONS Painless uterine contractions that occur throughout pregnancy

BREACH OF DUTY A failure to provide the expected reasonable standard of care under the circumstances

BRONCHIECTASIS A chronic condition of the bronchial tree marked by irreversible dilation and destruction of the bronchial walls, resulting in a paroxysmal, mucus-producing cough

BRONCHIOLITIS An infection of the lower respiratory tract that produces inflammation and obstruction of the lungs by thick mucus and edema

BRUDZINSKI'S SIGN In meningitis, flexion of the neck usually results in flexion of the hip and knee

BULIMIA NERVOSA Disorder characterized by episodic bingeing on food, followed by purging in the form of vomiting, in the hopes of losing or maintaining weight

CANCER A large group of diseases characterized by a malfunction of the cell growth process, which causes the uncontrolled growth of abnormal cells

CARDIAC TAMPONADE Compression of the heart resulting from increased intrapericardial pressure secondary to accumulating fluid or blood in the pericardial sac (resulting from cardiac rupture or a penetrating wound)

CARDIOGENIC SHOCK Occurs when the heart fails to pump adequately, thereby reducing cardiac output and compromising tissue perfusion, as in acute myocardial infarction, heart failure, or severe cardiomyopathy

CARDIOMYOPATHY Primarily, a noninflammatory disease of the myocardium

CARPAL TUNNEL SYNDROME A painful disorder of the wrist and hand resulting from rapid, repetitive use of the fingers or from steady wrist-shaking vibrations, resulting in compression of the median nerve inside the carpal tunnel

CATARACT Disorder of the eye where the normally clear, transparent crystalline lens becomes opaque

CATATONIC SCHIZOPHRENIA A state of pronounced psychomotor disturbance in which the individual remains immobile with extreme muscle rigidity or, less commonly, exhibits uncontrolled excessive movement

CELLULITIS A diffuse, commonly infectious inflammation of the skin and underlying tissue, characterized by pain, redness, edema, and heat

CEPHALOCAUDAL Pertaining to the long axis of the body, in a direction from head to tail, as in the development of an organism (for example, an infant gains control of his head before his trunk and extremities)

CEPHALOPELVIC DISPROPORTION (CPD) The incompatibility of the fetal head with the diameter of the maternal pelvis

CEREBRAL ANEURYSM A saclike dilation of the wall of a cerebral artery, typically resulting from weakness of the wall

CEREBRAL PALSY A permanent disorder of motor function resulting from nonprogressive brain damage

CERTIFIED NURSE-MIDWIFE An advanced practice nurse who provides care to low-risk perinatal and gynecologic clients

CHADWICK'S SIGN Change in color of the vaginal walls from normal light pink to deep violet

CHEILOPLASTY Plastic surgery performed to correct a deformity of the lips

CHEMICAL CARCINOGENESIS The development of cancer caused by chemical substances, such as hydrocarbons, asbestos, and vinylchoride

CHEMOTHERAPY Treatment that uses cytoxic drugs to destroy cancer cells

CHLAMYDIA A genus of bacteria of the *Chlamydiaceae* family, occurring as gram-negative organisms, which are common animal pathogens and cause various diseases in humans

CHLOASMA Irregular facial pigmentation—usually on the cheeks, forehead, and nose—that occurs during pregnancy

CHORION Fetal membrane closest to the uterine wall; gives rise to the placenta

CHRONIC BRONCHITIS A persistent respiratory disease marked by increased production of mucus by the glands of the trachea and bronchi; it's characterized by a cough with expectoration for at least 3 months of the year for more than 2 consecutive years

CHRONIC GLOMERULONEPHRITIS An inflammation of the glomerulus of the kidney, characterized by decreased urine production, blood and protein in the urine, and edema; it may follow acute glomerulonephritis or occur secondary to a systemic disease and may lead to renal failure

CHRONIC OBSTRUCTIVE PULMONARY DISEASE (COPD) A disorder that's marked by reduced inspiratory and expiratory capacity of the lungs; COPD is progressive and irreversible and causes such symptoms as dyspnea on exertion, difficulty inhaling or exhaling deeply and, sometimes, a chronic cough

CHRONIC RENAL FAILURE The inability of a kidney to perform its essential functions of excreting wastes, concentrating urine, and conserving electrolytes

CHRONIC VENOUS INSUFFICIENCY A condition resulting from inadequate circulation, resulting in decreased blood flow

CIRRHOSIS A liver disease characterized by diffuse interlacing bands of fibrous tissue dividing the hepatic parenchyma into micronodular or macronodular areas

CIVIL LAW A wide range of legal issues that are unrelated to criminal acts

CLEFT LIP A facial malformation that results from failure of the premaxillary process to merge during gestational weeks 7 and 8; the malformation may be unilateral or bilateral and range from a notch in the vermilion border of the lip to a separation extending to the floor of the nose

CLEFT PALATE A congenital fissure of the roof of the mouth that results from failure of the palatal process to fuse from the 7th to the 12th week of gestation

CLUB FOOT A congenital deformity in which the foot is twisted out of shape or position

COARCTATION OF THE AORTA A narrowing of the aortic arch that's usually distal to the ductus arteriosus beyond the left subclavian artery

COCAINE USE DISORDER Disorder in which a person is addicted to the potent euphoric effects of cocaine

COGNITIVE DEVELOPMENT The acquisition of increasingly complex knowledge, thought processes, reasoning, judgment, memory, and problem-solving skills

COGNITIVE DISORDERS The result of any condition that alters or destroys brain tissue and, in turn, impairs cerebral functioning

COLICYSTITIS Inflammation of the bladder resulting from *Escherichia coli* infection

COLOSTRUM The first breast milk, which is high in antibodies that provide passive immunization to the neonate; production begins early in pregnancy and continues for 1 to 2 days after delivery of the neonate

COMPARTMENT SYNDROME Compromised circulation, in many cases to an extremity, due to swelling and inflammation as a result of trauma or burns

COMPENSATORY DAMAGES Reimbursement awarded to the plaintiff for expenses, rehabilitation, and pain and suffering related to the injury

COMPULSION A repetitive behavior that's performed to decrease escalating anxiety

CONFABULATION The fabrication of "stories" to fill in memory gaps or to answer questions; the individual considers the "stories" to be factual

CONGENITAL Existing at birth

CONJUNCTIVITIS Inflammation and redness of the conjunctiva of the eye as a result of infection, allergy, or a chemical reaction

CONSCIOUS SEDATION The state when medication is administered I.V. to reduce the intensity or awareness of pain while maintaining defensive reflexes

CONTINUITY THEORY The social theory whereby the client adjusts successfully to the aging process by continuing the patterns of living that he has established over his lifetime

CONTRACT A written or oral agreement between two or more individuals that has several elements to its formation, interpretation, and enforcement

CONTRACTURE Shortening or tightening of tissues, causing deformity

CONVERSION DISORDER A condition that's characterized by symptoms that suggest a physical disorder, but evaluation and observation can't determine a physiologic cause

CORNEA Transparent, dome-shaped structure covering the front of the eye that consists of five layers of cells and proteins and refracts light

CORNEAL ABRASION The wearing away of the outer layers of the cornea

CORONARY ARTERY DISEASE (CAD) A disease characterized by atherosclerosis of the coronary arteries, which may cause angina pectoris, myocardial infarction, and sudden death; genetically determined and avoidable risk factors contribute to CAD, including hypercholesterolemia, hypertension, smoking, diabetes mellitus, and low levels of high-density lipoproteins

COR PULMONALE A heart condition in which hypertension of the pulmonary circulation leads to enlargement of the right ventricle

CORPORATE LIABILITY An employer's responsibility for injury caused by an employee who acted according to the employer's decisions

CRIMINAL LAW A set of laws that define wrongs against society

CROHN'S DISEASE A chronic granulomatous inflammatory disease of unknown etiology involving any part of the GI tract from the mouth to the anus, but commonly involving the terminal ileum with scarring and thickening of the bowel wall

CROUP A condition resulting from inflammation of the larynx that commonly occurs in young children and is characterized by a barking, resonant cough

CUSHING'S SYNDROME Hyperactivity of the adrenal cortex, resulting in excessive secretion of glucocorticoids, particularly cortisol

CUSHING'S TRIAD The triad of hypertension, bradycardia, and Cheyne-Stokes respiration (irregular breathing) in patients with head injuries

CYSTIC FIBROSIS (CF) A disease that affects the pancreas and causes a generalized dysfunction of the exocrine glands; thickened and tenacious secretions occlude glandular ducts and cause dysfunction in many organ systems

CYSTITIS An inflammation of the urinary bladder

DAMAGES Physical or psychological injury; also monetary compensation awarded to the plaintiff for incurring the injury

DEFAMATION The act of injuring the plaintiff's reputation in the community as the result of a false statement, either spoken (slander) or written (libel)

DEHISCENCE The partial or complete separation of wound edges

DELIRIUM Disturbance of consciousness accompanied by a change in cognition that can't be attributed to preexisting dementia

DELUSION A false belief to which an individual adheres despite contradictory evidence

DELUSIONAL DISORDER A condition where a client holds firmly to false beliefs, despite contradictory information

DEMOCRATIC STYLE A style of leadership and management characterized by high productivity and group participation and collaboration in decision making

DENIAL The unconscious ego defense mechanism whereby an individual refrains from acknowledging stressful aspects about himself or his environment to ease anxiety

DEPENDENT PERSONALITY DISORDER A disorder in which the client experiences an extreme need to be taken care of, which leads to submissive, clinging behavior and fear of separation

DEVELOPMENT The increasingly complex functioning that progresses sequentially (for instance, the attainment of cognitive, psychosocial, motor, and communication skills)

DEVELOPMENTAL DYSPLASIA OF THE HIP The abnormal development of the hip socket that occurs when the head of the femur is cartilaginous and the acetabulum (socket) is shallow; as a result, the head of the femur comes out of the hip socket

DIABETES INSIPIDUS A metabolic disorder marked by extreme polyuria and polydipsia, resulting from deficient secretion or production of antidiuretic hormone (ADH) or the inability of the renal tubules to respond to ADH

DIABETES MELLITUS A disorder of carbohydrate metabolism characterized by insufficient insulin to allow glucose to cross the cell membrane

DISORGANIZED SCHIZOPHRENIA A type of schizophrenia in which clients have a flat or inappropriate affect and incoherent thoughts

DISPLACEMENT Placing one's emotions toward something on another less-threatening person, object, or situation

DISSEMINATED INTRAVASCULAR COAGULATION Syndrome that occurs as a complication of disease and conditions that accelerate clotting, causing small blood vessel occlusion, organ necrosis, depletion of circulating clotting factors and platelets, and activation of the fibrinolytic system

DIVERTICULITIS A disease that causes inflammation of a diverticulum, especially inflammation related to colonic diverticula, which may cause perforation with abscess formation

DIVERTICULOSIS The presence of diverticula, particularly of colonic diverticula, in the absence of inflammation

DOWN SYNDROME A chromosomal disorder marked by varying degrees of mental retardation and physical characteristics that include a sloping forehead, low-set ears, and short, broad hands with a single palmar crease

DRUG DEPENDENCE A physical or psychological need to use a drug to experience its effects or avoid the discomfort of its absence

DUAL DIAGNOSIS A diagnosis that reveals an addictive disorder and a psychiatric disorder in a client

DUCHENNE'S MUSCULAR DYSTROPHY A degenerative disease characterized by weakness and progressive atrophy of skeletal muscles with no evidence of involvement of the nervous system

DURABLE POWER OF ATTORNEY A legal document in which a client identifies a proxy, or surrogate, decision maker in case the client becomes incapacitated; this document should also be included in the client's medical record

DUTY The nurse's legal obligation to provide nursing care to a client

DYSTOCIA Abnormally difficult labor

ECLAMPSIA The most serious form of toxemia of pregnancy, marked by hypertension, proteinuria, edema, generalized tonic-clonic seizures, and coma

ECTODERM Embryonic germ layer that generate the epidermis, nervous system, pituitary glad, salivary glands, optic lens, lining of the lower portion of the anal canal, hair, and tooth enamel

ECTOPIC PREGNANCY Implantation of a fertilized ovum outside the uterine cavity

EFFACEMENT The thinning and shortening (obliteration) of the cervix during labor, which is reported in percentages from 0% to 100%

ELECTRONIC FETAL MONITORING (EFM) The use of a direct or indirect device to assess fetal status and uterine activity

EMPHYSEMA A chronic, irreversible lung disorder marked by the enlargement of air spaces distal to terminal bronchioles due to destruction of the alveolar walls; it results in decreased elastic recoil of the lungs

EMPYEMA The accumulation of pus in a cavity of the body

ENABLING Helping a chemically dependent client so that the consequences of drug use can be avoided

ENCEPHALITIS An inflammatory condition of the brain, usually caused by an arbovirus infection transmitted by the bite of an infected mosquito

ENDODERM Embryonic germ layer that generates the epithelial lining of the larynx, trachea, bladder, urethra, prostate gland, auditory canal, liver, pancreas, and alimentary canal

ENDOGENOUS Growing from within the body

EGO The part of the personality that keeps an individual oriented to reality, enables the individual to solve problems, and mediates between the id and superego

EPILEPSY A disorder characterized by excessive neuronal discharge, recurrent seizures, and some alteration of consciousness

EPISTAXIS A nosebleed

ERYTHROCYTES Also called *red blood cells,* erythrocytes are one of the elements found in peripheral blood

ESOPHAGEAL ATRESIA The proximal end of the esophagus ends in a blind pouch, blocking food from the esophagus to enter the stomach

EVISCERATION The protrusion of abdominal contents through a surgical incision

EXPECTED DATE OF DELIVERY (EDD) The due date established by calculations, ultrasound, or amniocentesis

EXTRACORPOREAL Occurring outside of the body

EXUDATIVE PLEURAL EFFUSION Condition that results when capillaries exhibit increased permeability with or without changes in hydrostatic and colloid osmotic pressures, allowing protein-rich fluid to leak into the pleural space

FAILURE TO THRIVE A condition in which an infant or young child not only fails to gain weight, but may also lose it as a result of physical and psychosocial causation

FALSE IMPRISONMENT Unlawful restraint of a person against his will

FAMILIAL CARCINOGENESIS The development of cancer as a result of autosomal dominant traits, such as breast cancer, retinoblastoma, familial polyposis, xeroderma pigmentosum, and Wilms' tumor

FELONY A type of crime that entails more serious offenses and warrants lengthy prison sentences

FETAL STATION The relationship of the fetal presenting part to the maternal ischial spines, which is measured in centimeters

FISTULA An abnormal opening between two organs

FLIGHT OF IDEAS A nearly continuous flow of rapid speech that jumps from topic to topic

FREE-FLOATING ANXIETY Anxiety that occurs without cause and produces acute psychic discomfort

GAMETOGENESIS Production of specialized sex cells called *gametes*

GAMMA RAYS Electromagnetic radiation of short wavelengths emitted by the nucleus of an atom during a nuclear reaction; consist of high energy photons, have no mass and no electric charge, and travel with the speed of light and are usually associated with beta rays

GASTRITIS An inflammation of the stomach and stomach lining

GASTROENTERITIS An inflammation of the stomach lining and intestines that accompanies numerous GI disorders and is characterized by anorexia, weakness, abdominal pain, nausea, and diarrhea

GASTROESOPHAGEAL REFLUX DISEASE (GERD) A backflow of stomach and duodenum contents into the esophagus that may result from an incompetent lower esophageal sphincter

GATE CONTROL THEORY Theory on pain in which the idea is that only one major stimulus can be transmitted at a time

GENERALIZED ANXIETY DISORDER A disorder in which the client worries excessively and experiences tremendous anxiety almost daily

GESTATIONAL DIABETES MELLITUS Elevated blood glucose levels in an individual as a result of the stress of pregnancy

GESTATIONAL HYPERTENSION Condition during pregnancy where the client has hypertension, proteinuria, and edema

GIGANTISM Abnormal stature or overgrowth of the body or any of its parts, caused most commonly by oversecretion of pituitary growth hormone

GLAUCOMA Disorder of visual field loss due to damage to the optic nerve resulting from increased intraocular pressure caused by impaired flow of aqueous humor

GOITER An enlarged thyroid gland, usually evident as a pronounced swelling in the front of the neck

GONORRHEA A sexually transmitted disease that commonly infects the genitourinary tract and, occasionally, the pharynx, conjunctiva, or rectum; caused by *Neisseria gonorrhoeae*

GOODELL'S SIGN Softening of the cervix

GOUT A group of disorders associated with inborn errors of metabolism that affect purine and pyrimidine use; it causes increased uric acid production or interferes with its excretion and results in hyperuricemia, recurrent acute inflammatory arthritis, deposition of urate crystals in the joints of the extremities, and uric acid urolithiasis

GOWERS' SIGN In a child, characteristic use of hands to rise from the floor or a low-sitting position to compensate for proximal muscle weakness

GRANULOMA Nodular inflammatory lesions containing compactly grouped modified phagocytes, giant cells, and other macrophages

GRAVIDA A pregnant woman; also, the number of pregnancies, including the current one

GROWTH A quantitative increase in size resulting from an increase in the number or size of cells, or both

GUILLAIN-BARRÉ SYNDROME An acute febrile polyneuritis that occurs after a viral infection and is marked by rapidly ascending paralysis that begins as paresthesia of the feet

HALLUCINATION A sensory experience where no external stimuli exist

HEAD LICE *Pediculosis capitis* infestation resulting in lice feeding on human blood and laying their eggs (nits) in body hair on the head; it's commonly due to overcrowded conditions, is common in children, and spreads by sharing hats, combs, hairbrushes, or clothing

HEART FAILURE The inability of the heart to pump blood at an adequate rate to fill tissue's metabolic requirements or the ability to do so only at an elevated filling pressure

HEGAR'S SIGN Softening of the lower uterine segment that may be present at 6 to 8 weeks' gestation

HEMIPARESIS Muscle weakness in half of the body

HEMOPHILIA A bleeding disorder characterized by failure of the blood clotting mechanism; it's an inherited condition that occurs almost exclusively in males

HEMOTHORAX An accumulation of blood in the pleural cavity, resulting from a traumatic injury or from the rupture of small blood vessels in individuals with inflammatory or malignant lung diseases

HEPATITIS A disease that causes inflammation of the liver, usually due to a viral infection but may also result from exposure to toxic agents

HERNIA Outward bulging of part or structure through the tissues normally containing it

HERNIATED DISK Intervertebral disk rupture, causing a protrusion of the nucleus pulposus into the spinal canal

HERPES SIMPLEX VIRUS (HSV) An infection caused by herpes virus type 1 or 2 and characterized by painful, itching lesions consisting of tiny blisters, which commonly appear around the mouth or on the skin and mucous membranes of the genitals

HERPES ZOSTER An acute infection characterized by pain resulting from inflammation of the ganglia and dorsal nerve roots as well as the eruption of painful lesions that occur on one side of the body, following the course of a nerve

HIATAL HERNIA The herniation of an abdominal organ, usually the stomach, through the esophageal hiatus of the diaphragm

HIRSCHSPRUNG'S DISEASE A disease in which a portion of the colon lacks ganglionic cells and the peristatic waves that are needed to pass feces through that segment of the colon

HODGKIN'S DISEASE Disease in which Reed-Sternberg cells proliferate in a single lymph node and travel contiguously through the lymphatic system to other lymphatic nodes and organs

HOMANS' SIGN Pain on passive dorsiflexion of the foot; a sign of thrombosis of deep calf veins

HOMEOSTASIS A state of constancy or equilibrium within the body

HOSPICE A multidisciplinary approach to provide comfort and care to a client with a terminal illness

HUMAN IMMUNODEFICIENCY VIRUS (HIV) A virus of the genus *Lentivirus,* separated into two serotypes (HIV-1 and HIV-2), that is the etiologic agent of acquired immunodeficiency syndrome

HUNTINGTON'S DISEASE A hereditary disease in which degeneration in the cerebral cortex and basal ganglia causes chronic progressive chorea (involuntary and irregular movements) and cognitive deterioration, ending in dementia

HYDATIDIFORM MOLE A commonly benign neoplasm that occurs at the end of a degenerating pregnancy and arises from enlarged chorionic villi and the proliferation of trophoblastic tissue

HYDROCEPHALUS An increase in the amount of cerebrospinal fluid in the ventricles and subarachnoid spaces of the brain

HYPERCAPNIA Elevated partial pressure of carbon dioxide in the blood

HYPEREMESIS GRAVIDARUM Severe and prolonged vomiting during pregnancy to such a degree that weight loss and fluid and electrolyte imbalance occur

HYPERPYREXIA Also known as *malignant hyperthermia,* a body temperature elevation that may be produced as a reaction to an infection or as a complication of surgery

HYPERTENSION A persistent, abnormal elevation in blood pressure, usually defined as systolic pressure exceeding 140 mm Hg or diastolic pressure exceeding 90 mm Hg

HYPERTHYROIDISM An abnormality of the thyroid gland in which secretion of thyroid hormone is increased, resulting in a hypermetabolic state

HYPERVOLEMIA An abnormal fluid volume increase, usually in the circulatory (blood) system

HYPOCHONDRIASIS A mental disorder characterized by a preoccupation with the state of one's physical health

HYPOSPADIAS Opening of the urethra on the ventral surface of the penis

HYPOTHYROIDISM A state of low serum thyroid hormone resulting from hypothalamic, pituitary, or thyroid insufficiency that can progress to myxedema coma

HYPOVOLEMIA An abnormal fluid volume decrease, usually in the circulatory (blood) system

HYPOVOLEMIC SHOCK A shock state that results from decreased intravascular volume due to fluid loss, causing circulatory dysfunction and inadequate tissue perfusion

HYPOXEMIA A deficient blood oxygen level, usually resulting from a ventilation-perfusion imbalance

ID The part of the personality that houses an individual's needs, drives, and wishes and that has no regard for reality

IDEAS OF REFERENCE The assumption by a client that the words and actions of another person refer directly to himself

IDENTIFICATION An unconscious ego defense mechanism whereby an individual takes on characteristics of one or more people

IMMOBILITY To be fixed in one position or to be rendered incapable of movement; casts, splints, or surgical fixation are examples of induced immobility

IMMUNITY A state of protection against a disease, especially one of infectious origin

IMMUNOGLOBULIN (Ig) One of a class of structurally related glycoproteins that function as antibodies (IgA, IgD, IgE, IgG, and IgM)

INCENTIVE SPIROMETRY The promotion of deep breathing and full expansion of the alveoli by means of a mechanical device that measures the amount of air the client inhales and exhales

INFECTIVE ENDOCARDITIS Endocarditis caused by infection with microorganisms, especially bacteria and fungi

INFORMED CONSENT The client's involvement in and agreement with treatment decisions based on careful consideration of all information pertinent to the client's condition

INSPECTION Observing a client during an examination

INTEGRATIVE POWER The ability to help a client return to his normal life with the recognition that adaptations may be necessary because of illness or injury

INTENTIONAL INFLICTION OF EMOTIONAL DISTRESS Extreme, outrageous, or intolerable conduct toward another, causing emotional harm

INTENTIONAL TORT A willful act that injures another person or his property

INTERFERON A class of glycoproteins that are produced after cells are exposed to a virus; interferon therapy is a potentially valuable treatment for various viral infections because interferons prevent viral replication in noninfected cells

INTERMITTENT CLAUDICATION The periodic pain and lameness in a limb brought on by activity and relieved by rest; commonly found in arterial peripheral vascular disease

INTESTINAL OBSTRUCTION A blockage, clogging, or stricture of the lumen in any area of the bowel that prevents the normal passage of intestinal contents

INTRACRANIAL PRESSURE (ICP) The pressure of the cerebrospinal fluid in the subarachnoid space between the skull and the brain

INTROJECTION An unconscious ego defense mechanism by which a client incorporates positive or negative aspects of another person or object into his own ego (this is the mechanism by which anger is turned inward)

INVASION OF PRIVACY Also known as a *breach of confidentiality,* the act of revealing personal information about a client to an unauthorized person

IRIS Thin, circular pigmented muscular structure in the eye that gives color to the eye, divides the space between the cornea and lens into anterior and posterior chambers, and controls the amount of light admitted to the retina

IRON DEFICIENCY ANEMIA Anemia resulting from an iron insufficiency in the serum, decreased iron stores in the bone marrow, and elevated serum iron binding

IRRITABLE BOWEL SYNDROME A condition characterized by diarrhea and resulting from increased bowel motility

ISCHEMIA Decreased blood supply to a body part caused by an obstruction or constriction in a blood vessel

ISOLATION The unconscious ego defense mechanism that enables an individual to remain unaware of the emotions associated with a thought

KAPOSI'S SARCOMA A malignant tumor that begins as a soft, brownish or purple nodule, usually on the feet and spreading slowly in the skin, metastasizing to lymph nodes and internal organs

KELOID Excessive growth of scar tissue

KERNICTERUS The abnormal toxic accumulation of bilirubin in the brain tissues resulting from hyperbilirubinemia, which may cause brain damage and neonatal death

KERNIG'S SIGN A sign of meningitis; the client can easily and completely extend the leg when in dorsal decubitus position but not when in the sitting posture or when lying with the thigh flexed upon the abdomen

LACRIMATION The secretion and discharge of tears

LAISSEZ-FAIRE A style of leadership and management — also known as *permissive* — that's characterized by minimal, if any, direction or control (a useful style when leading highly motivated professional groups such as a research project team)

LANUGO The fine downy hair that appears on the fetal body at about 20 weeks' gestation

LECITHIN-SPHINGOMYELIN RATIO (L/S RATIO) The ratio of lecithin to sphingomyelin in amniotic fluid; it's useful in predicting fetal lung maturity

LEGIONNAIRES' DISEASE An acute flulike disease caused by *Legionella pneumophila;* signs and symptoms include high fever, GI distress, headache, and pneumonia and may involve the liver, kidney, and nervous system

LENS Biconvex, avascular, colorless, transparent structure that's suspended behind the iris by the ciliary zonulae and focuses light

LEUKEMIA A progressive malignant disease of the blood-forming organs characterized by abnormal numbers or forms of immature circulating white blood cells, with infiltration of the lymph nodes, liver, spleen, and other sites

LEUKOCYTES Also called *white blood cells,* leukocytes are a colorless ameboid cell mass

LEUKOCYTOSIS Increased production of white blood cells

LEUKOPENIA Abnormally low white blood cell count (below 5,000 µl)

LIABILITY The legal responsibility for failure to act or an action that fails to meet standards of care and causes another person harm

LIVING WILL A document in which a client instructs family members and health care professionals about medical care that should or shouldn't be provided if the client becomes incapacitated

LOCHIA The postpartum vaginal discharge containing debris from the uterus, such as blood, decidual tissue, mucus, and epithelial cells

LOOSE EGO BOUNDARY The failure to adequately distinguish between one's thoughts, wishes, and needs and those of others

LUND AND BROWDER CHART Method of estimating body surface area that has been burned; accounts for changes in body proportion that occur with age

LYMPHOMA Any neoplastic disorder of the lymphoid tissue

MAJOR DEPRESSIVE DISORDER Syndrome of depressed mood that's present for most of the day, nearly every day for at least 2 weeks

MALPRACTICE Negligence by a member of a profession, differing from negligence only in that the standard or duty owed is a professional one, based on special knowledge and skills

MANIPULATION Behaviors directed at getting one's needs met at the expense of another person

MELANOMA Neoplasm that arises from melanocytes; spreads through the lymph and vascular systems and metastasizes to the lymph nodes, skin, liver, lungs, and central nervous system

MÉNIÈRE'S DISEASE A chronic inner ear disease characterized by recurrent episodes of vertigo, progressive unilateral nerve deafness, and tinnitus

MENINGITIS An inflammation of the brain and spinal cord, usually as the result of a bacterial infection

MENINGOCELE The protrusion of the meninges outside the body through a defect in the vertebral column; the protruding sac is filled with spinal fluid

MESODERM Embryonic germ layer that generates the connective and sclerous tissues; the blood and vascular system; the musculature; teeth (except enamel); mesothelia lining of the pericardial, pleural, and peritoneal cavities; kidneys; and ureters

METABOLIC ACIDOSIS A state of excess acid accumulation and deficient base bicarbonate

METABOLIC ALKALOSIS A clinical state marked by decreased amounts of acid or increased amounts of base bicarbonate

METASTASIS Spread of cancer from the primary site through the blood or lymphatic circulation to distant sites of the body

MISDEMEANOR An offense that's considered less serious than a felony and carries with it a lesser penalty, usually a fine or imprisonment for less than 1 year

MITRAL INSUFFICIENCY A defective functioning of the mitral valve with incomplete closure, causing mitral regurgitation

MITRAL STENOSIS A narrowing of the left atrioventricular orifice

MITRAL VALVE PROLAPSE (MVP) A prolapse of the mitral valve, commonly with regurgitation, associated with myxomatous proliferation of the leaflets of the mitral valve

MULTIPLE MYELOMA Abnormal proliferation of plasma cells that are immature and malignant

MULTIPLE SCLEROSIS (MS) A disease in which there are foci of demyelination of various sizes throughout the white matter of the central nervous system, sometimes extending into the gray matter; typically, the symptoms include weakness, incoordination, paresthesia, speech disturbances, and visual complaints

MYASTHENIA GRAVIS (MG) A disorder of neuromuscular function due to the presence of antibodies to acetylcholine receptors at the neuromuscular junction and characterized by fatigue and exhaustion of the muscular system; the disorder has a tendency to fluctuate in severity and can affect any muscle of the body

MYDRIATIC A drug that dilates the pupil

MYELOMENINGOCELE A meningocele that contains a portion of the spinal cord and spinal nerves in the sac

MYOCARDIAL INFARCTION (MI) A condition in which gross necrosis of the myocardium occurs as a result of interruption of the blood supply to the area; usually caused by atherosclerosis or an embolism of the coronary arteries

MYOCARDITIS Inflammation of the myocardium, which may arise from a number of conditions, including viral, bacterial, or fungal infection; serum sickness; rheumatic fever; a chemical agent; or a complication of a collagen disease

NEGLIGENCE An unintentional tort involving four elements: duty, breach of duty, proximate cause, and damages

NEPHRITIS Inflammation and abnormal function of the kidneys

NEPHROTIC SYNDROME Condition that develops when large amounts of plasma protein are lost in urine because of increased glomerular permeability

NEUROGENIC BLADDER The loss of bladder control from lesions or damage to the nervous system

NEUROGENIC SHOCK Also known as *spinal shock*, a form of distributive shock that causes loss of sympathetic (vasomotor) tone

NEUROLEPTIC MALIGNANT SYNDROME A potentially fatal reaction to neuroleptic (antipsychotic) drugs characterized by fluctuating vital signs, altered consciousness, fever, muscle rigidity, diaphoresis, drooling, and an increased white blood cell count

NOMINAL DAMAGES Reimbursement awarded to the plaintiff that indicates a defendant's wrongdoing when little, if any, injury occurred

NO-SUICIDE CONTRACT Agreement stating that the client will seek out a person with whom to talk out suicidal feelings, rather than acting on them

NYSTAGMUS Rapid, involuntary rolling or vertical movement of the eyeballs

OBSESSION Ideas or thoughts that a person can't put out of his consciousness

OBSESSIVE-COMPULSIVE DISORDER (OCD) A disorder characterized by recurrent obsessions (intrusive thoughts, images, and impulses) and compulsions (repetitive behaviors in response to an obsession)

OLIGURIA An abnormally low urine output (less than 500 ml/day) such that metabolic wastes can't be excreted

OPHTHALMOSCOPE An instrument used to examine the internal structures of the eye

OPTIC NERVE Nerve located at the posterior portion of the eye that transmits visual impulses from the retina to the brain

ORTOLANI'S SIGN Test in which a click can be felt at the hip area as the femur head snaps out of and back into the acetabulum

OSTEOARTHRITIS Degeneration of cartilage in weight-bearing joints, such as the spine, knees, and hips

OSTEOMYELITIS An infection of the bone and bone marrow

OSTEOPOROSIS Metabolic bone disorder in which the rate of bone resorption accelerates while the rate of bone formation slows down, causing a progressive loss of bone mass

OTITIS MEDIA Inflammation of the middle ear that may be accompanied by infection; fluid pressing on the tympanic membrane results in pain and leads to possible rupture or perforation

OTOSCLEROSIS Abnormal overgrowth of the ear's spongy bone around the oval window and stapes footplate

OTOSCOPE An instrument used to examine the ear canal and tympanic membrane

OXYTOCIN A posterior pituitary hormone that stimulates uterine contractions and also initiates the let-down reflex of lactation

PALLIATIVE Relieving symptoms rather than curing a condition

PALPATION Examining a client by use of the hands to feel the shape, texture, consistency, and location of parts of the body

PANCREATITIS An inflammation, either acute or chronic, of the pancreas

PANIC DISORDER A disorder in which the client experiences a nonspecific feeling of terror and dread, accompanied by symptoms of physiologic stress

PARALYTIC ILEUS A temporary paralysis of the intestines, causing abdominal distention and signs of bowel obstruction

PARANOIA An intense, irrational suspicion that can't be changed by giving facts or explaining reality

PARANOID PERSONALITY DISORDER A disorder characterized by extreme distrust of others

PARANOID SCHIZOPHRENIA A disorder characterized by delusions unrelated to reality; in many cases, the client displays bizarre behavior, is easily angered, and is at high risk for violence

PARESTHESIA An abnormal sensation (such as numbness, tingling, or burning) that lacks an objective cause

PARKINSON'S DISEASE A slowly progressive disease that's characterized by tremor of resting muscles, a slowing of voluntary movements, a festinating gait, peculiar posture, and muscle weakness

PASSIVE IMMUNITY A form of acquired resistance to an infection resulting from transfer of antibodies either naturally through the placenta to a fetus or through the colostrum to an infant, or artificially by inoculation of antiserum

PATENT DUCTUS ARTERIOSUS (PDA) A defect resulting from the failure of the ductus to close causing shunting of blood to the pulmonary artery

PATHOLOGIC JAUNDICE A yellowness of the skin caused by hyperbilirubinemia that occurs within the first 24 hours after birth

PATIENT'S BILL OF RIGHTS A document that defines a person's rights while receiving health care; it's designed to protect such basic rights as human dignity, privacy, confidentiality, informed consent, and refusal of treatment; the American Hospital Association, the National League for Nursing, the American Civil Liberties Union, and other organizations and health care facilities have prepared patient's bills of rights, and concepts expressed in these documents may be incorporated into law; although bills of rights issued by health care facilities and professional organizations don't have the force of law, nurses should regard them as professionally binding

PEPTIC ULCER An ulceration of the mucous membrane of the esophagus, stomach, or duodenum caused by the action of gastric acid

PERCUSSION The act of striking the body with the fist or finger (for example, directly striking the kidney area) or the act of using both hands, by placing either the palm or middle finger on the client and striking with the other fist or finger indirectly (for example, percussing the thorax)

PERCUTANEOUS ANEMIA Chronic, progressive, macrocytic anemia caused by a deficiency of intrinsic factor, a substance normally secreted by the stomach

PERICARDIOCENTESIS Needle aspiration of the pericardial sac

PERICARDITIS An inflammation of the pericardium, which may be caused by trauma, neoplasm, infection, uremia, myocardial infarction, or collagen disease

PERINATAL PERIOD The time from conception through postpartum; also, the time extending from completion of the 20th to 28th week of gestation and ending 28 days after birth

PERITONITIS An inflammation of the peritoneum that can be produced by bacteria or irritating substances introduced into the abdominal cavity by a penetrating wound or an organ perforation

PERSONAL LIABILITY Responsibility for one's acts

PHALEN'S WRIST-FLEXION TEST Test to see if holding the forearms vertically and allowing both hands to drop into complete flexion at the wrists for 1 minute reproduces symptoms of carpal tunnel syndrome

PHOBIA Irrational fear of something that, in reality, can cause little, if any, harm

PHYSICAL CARCINOGENESIS The development of cancer as a result of environmental and other elements, such as ultraviolet radiation, precancerous lesions, acquired disorders (cirrhosis and hepatitis), dietary factors, and obesity

PLACENTA PREVIA Implantation of the placenta so that it adjoins or covers the internal os of the uterine cervix

PLAINTIFF A person who files a civil lawsuit initiating a legal action; in criminal actions, the prosecution is the plaintiff acting on behalf of the people in the jurisdiction

PLEURAL EFFUSION An accumulation of fluid in the interstitial and air spaces of the lung

PLEURISY An inflammation of the pleura characterized by dyspnea and stabbing pain, leading to restriction of breathing

PNEUMOCYSTIS CARINII PNEUMONIA Infection with the parasite *P. carinii,* which produces an interstitial plasma cell pneumonia commonly seen in debilitated or immunosuppressed clients

PNEUMONIA An acute infection of the lung parenchyma causing impaired gas exchange

PNEUMOTHORAX A collection of air in the pleural space that may result from an open chest wound that permits the entrance of air or from the rupture of a vesicle on the surface of the lung

POINT OF MAXIMAL IMPULSE (PMI) The location at the 4th or 5th left intercostal space, or the midclavicular line, where the heart is usually heard the loudest through a stethoscope

POLYCYTHEMIA VERA Chronic myeloproliferative disorder characterized by increased red blood cell mass, leukocytosis, thrombocytosis and increased hemoglobulin concentration with normal or increased plasma volume

POSTTRAUMATIC STRESS DISORDER (PTSD) A group of symptoms that develop after a traumatic event

PRESENTATIONAL ISOLATION Social withdrawal that results from changes in body image, mental or physical functional loss, or self-consciousness

PRESSURED SPEECH Frantic speech that's due to a person's attempt to keep up with racing thoughts

PRIMARY GAIN The control of anxiety through manifestation of symptoms

PROJECTION The unconscious defense mechanism of the ego whereby an individual attributes unacceptable ideas, feelings, and impulses to the external environment or to someone else

PROXIMATE CAUSE The causal connection between the breach of duty and the resulting injury

PROXIMODISTAL The point from the nearest to the farthest, as in the development of an organism (for instance, infants gain control of the arm before the hand)

PSORIASIS A common, chronic dermatologic condition with polygenic inheritance; marked by rounded red lesions covered by grayish or silvery white dry scales, psoriasis is caused by an overabundance of epithelial cells; affected areas include nails, the scalp, genitalia, and the lumbosacral region

PSYCHOMOTOR AGITATION The continuous movement or performance of an activity designed to relieve distress

PSYCHOMOTOR RETARDATION The slowing of movements to such an extent that the individual appears to perform all physical activity in slow motion; also, slow and difficult movement that approaches inactivity

PSYCHOSIS A condition characterized by major disturbances in ego functioning

PULMONARY ARTERY STENOSIS A narrowing or fusing of valve leaflets at the entrance of the pulmonary artery that interferes with right ventricular outflow

PULMONARY EDEMA The abnormal accumulation of fluid in the pulmonary tissues and air spaces due to changes in hydrostatic forces in the capillaries or to increased capillary permeability

PULMONARY EMBOLISM Foreign matter that forms a blockage in a pulmonary artery and can be caused by fat, air, tumor tissue, or a thrombus that usually arises from a peripheral vein

PULSE OXIMETRY A noninvasive monitoring of the oxygen saturation of arterial blood; a sensor is placed on a finger, toe, or earlobe to determine hemoglobin saturation

PUNITIVE DAMAGES Compensation awarded to the plaintiff in special circumstances, usually to punish the defendant for an especially egregious or outrageous act

PUPIL Circular aperture in the iris that changes size as the iris adapts to the amount of light entering the eye

PYLORIC STENOSIS A disorder in which hyperplasia of the circular muscle at the pylorus causes a narrowing of the pyloric canal, preventing the stomach from emptying normally

QUICKENING Fetal movement as perceived by the pregnant woman; first noticed between 16 and 20 weeks' gestation

RADIATION THERAPY Localized treatment that uses high-energy, ionizing radiation to destroy cancer cells

RADIOLABELED ANTIBODIES Tumor-specific antibodies coupled with radioactive isotopes that can be used to maximize tumor cell kill while sparing healthy tissue

RATIONALIZATION The unconscious defense mechanism whereby an individual justifies thoughts, wishes, needs, drives, or actions that would otherwise be unacceptable to himself or others

RAYNAUD'S DISEASE Intermittent bilateral ischemic attacks of the fingers or toes and, sometimes, the ears or nose, characterized by severe pallor and usually accompanied by paresthesia and pain

REACTION FORMATION An unconscious defense mechanism whereby an individual develops behaviors and attitudes that directly oppose the individual's underlying feelings and attitudes

REFRAMING Altering one's view of a situation

REGRESSION An unconscious defense mechanism whereby an individual returns to an earlier, less mature level of functioning

REGURGITATION Backward flow of fluid or solids from a cavity or tube (for instance, the backward flow of blood through a defective heart valve, or stomach contents flowing into the throat and mouth)

RELAPSE A return to using a drug after a period of sobriety has occurred

RENAL CALCULI Stones formed in the kidneys

REPRESSION An unconscious defense mechanism whereby an individual keeps unacceptable ideas, impulses, or feelings from conscious awareness

RESPIRATORY ACIDOSIS An acid-base disturbance caused by reduced alveolar ventilation; this condition is characterized by an excess of carbon dioxide in the blood (hypercapnia) and increased plasma hydrogen-ion concentrated

RESPIRATORY ALKALOSIS An acid-base disturbance characterized by decreased carbon dioxide in the blood (hypocapnia), a decreased hydrogen-ion concentration, and increased pH

RESPIRATORY SYNCYTIAL VIRUS (RSV) A species of viruses belonging to the genus *Pneumovirus* that causes respiratory disease and that can be severe in infants; RSV can lead to pneumonia and bronchiolitis

RESPONDEAT SUPERIOR The principle that addresses an employer's responsibility for injuries caused by an employee's negligent acts if those acts were performed within the scope of employment and when an employment relationship existed

RETICULAR ACTIVATING SYSTEM (RAS) A functional system in the brain that controls the overall degree of the central nervous system, including wakefulness, attention, concentration, and introspection

RETINA Thin, semitransparent layer of nerve tissue that lines the back of the eye

RETINAL CONES Visual cell segments responsible for visual acuity and color discrimination

RETINAL RODS Visual cell segments responsible for peripheral vision under decreased light conditions

REYE'S SYNDROME Acute encephalopathy and fatty infiltration of the internal organs following acute viral infections, such as influenza B, chickenpox (varicella), the enteroviruses, and Epstein-Barr virus; it has been associated with administration of aspirin and other salicylates in children

RHEUMATIC FEVER An inflammatory disease that occurs if a group A beta-hemolytic streptococcal infection is inadequately treated

RHEUMATIC HEART DISEASE A disease that causes damage to the heart muscle and valves as a result of rheumatic fever

RHEUMATOID ARTHRITIS A chronic, systemic collagen disease marked by inflammation, stiffness, and pain in the joints and related structures that result in crippling deformities

RISK MANAGEMENT A system for anticipating, acquiring, and maintaining the skills and resources needed to prevent mishaps and to respond effectively when a mishap occurs

ROLE THEORY A theoretical framework for describing, analyzing, and understanding social interaction

RULE OF NINES Method used to estimate the size of a burned area; person's skin is divided into several sections, each representing 9% or multiples of 9%

SARCOIDOSIS A disease in which granulomatous lesions affect organs and tissues of the body

SCHIZOPHRENIA A brain disorder characterized by neurotransmitter imbalances and structural changes within the brain

SCLERODERMA A relatively rare autoimmune disease characterized by a chronic hardening and thickening of the skin and degeneration of the connective tissue of the skin, lungs, and internal organs

SCOLIOSIS A lateral curvature of the spine

SECLUSION An extreme last course of action taken to maintain client safety by placing the person in a room where the nurse can provide protection and intensive monitoring

SECONDARY GAIN Any benefit that an individual experiences as a result of having a symptom or illness

SEIZURE DISORDER Also called *epilepsy,* seizure disorder is characterized by paroxysmal transient disturbances of brain function that may be manifested as episodic impairment or loss of consciousness, abnormal motor phenomena, psychic or sensory disturbances, or perturbation of the autonomic nervous system

SELF-MUTILATION An action that causes pain or injury without actually attempting to kill oneself

SEPTIC SHOCK The result of bacterial infection that causes inadequate blood perfusion and circulatory collapse

SICKLE CELL ANEMIA A chronic and incurable hereditary disorder occurring in people homozygous for hemoglobin S, resulting in erythrocyte fragility

SITUATION REPETITION The repetition of bothersome or problematic behavior during the course of therapy

SOMATOFORM DISORDER A disorder characterized by the literal transference of inner conflict onto a body part, commonly resulting in paralysis; clients with somatoform disorders channel anxiety through a body system

SOUFFLE The soft, blowing sound auscultated as fetal blood flows through the umbilical arteries (fundic souffle) or as maternal blood enters the uterine arteries (uterine souffle)

SPECIFICITY THEORY Traditional theory of pain perceptions and interpretation

SPINA BIFIDA A congenital cleft of the vertebral column with hernial protrusion of the meninges and, sometimes, the spinal cord

SPINAL CORD INJURY A traumatic disruption of the spinal cord, usually accompanied by extensive musculoskeletal involvement

SPONTANEOUS ABORTION Expulsion of the fetus from the uterus before the 20th week of gestation as a result of fetal abnormalities or maternal environment

SQUAMOUS CELL CARCINOMA Malignant neoplasm derived from stratified squamous epithelium

STATE ANXIETY Anxiety experienced under specific conditions

STENOSIS The narrowing of the lumen of a tube or body opening

STEREOTACTIC EXTERNAL-BEAM IRRADIATION A type of radiation that uses a three-dimensional distribution of the radiation beam in the treatment of relatively small intracranial benign lesions, such as arteriovenous malformations, or malignant astrocytomas and brain metastases

STOMATITIS An inflammation of the oral mucous membrane

STRICTURE Scar tissue that encircles a tubular structure, such as the esophagus, producing a narrowing

STROKE Sudden disruption in normal cerebral circulation from occlusion of an intracranial or extracranial blood vessel or hemorrhage in the brain from rupture of an intracranial blood vessel

SUBLIMATION The process of substituting acceptable activities for impulses that aren't socially acceptable

SUBSTANCE ABUSE DISORDER A disorder characterized by a maladaptive pattern of substance use manifested by recurrent and significant adverse consequences related to the repeated use of substances

SUBSTITUTED CONSENT Decisions made by surrogate decision-makers if a person lacks the capacity to make informed decisions

SUDDEN INFANT DEATH SYNDROME (SIDS) The sudden, unexpected, and inexplicable death of an infant that appears healthy; it occurs during sleep, typically in infants between ages 3 weeks and 5 months

SUPEREGO A part of the personality that's commonly called the *conscience* or the *moral component* of the personality

SYNDROME OF INAPPROPRIATE ANTIDIURETIC HORMONE Osmolality, associated with the release of vasopressin in amounts excessive for the state of hydration

SYPHILIS An infectious disease, usually transmitted by sexual contact or acquired in utero, that's caused by the spirochete *Treponema pallidum*

SYSTEMIC LUPUS ERYTHEMATOSUS (SLE) A chronic inflammatory multisystemic disorder of connective tissue characterized principally by involvement of the skin, joints, kidneys, and serosal membranes

TARDIVE DYSKINESIA A serious, irreversible adverse effect of long-term phenothiazine therapy; symptoms include gait disturbances and involuntary, bizarre movements of the face, tongue, neck, trunk, or pelvis

T CELLS Also known as *lymphocytes,* T cells are any of the mononuclear, nonphagocytic leukocytes found in the blood, lymph, and lymphoid tissues, that are responsible for the body's cellular immunity

TERATOGEN A substance that causes severely deformed fetal parts

TETANY Twitching, cramps, and muscle spasms that are caused by hypocalcemia

TETRALOGY OF FALLOT A congenital anomaly of the heart characterized by pulmonic stenosis, ventricular septal defect, overriding position or dextroposition of the aorta, and compensatory right ventricular hypertrophy

THORACIC AORTIC ANEURYSM An aneurysm that affects part of the thoracic aorta

THROMBOCYTES Blood platelets

THROMBOPHLEBITIS Inflammation of a vein that's commonly associated with clot formation

THYROIDITIS An inflammation of the thyroid gland; acute thyroiditis is caused by infections, such as staphylococcal or streptococcal infections; it's painful and symptoms include abscesses

TINEL'S SIGN Tingling over the median nerve on light percussion

TINNITUS Ringing or crackling in one or both ears

TONIC-CLONIC SEIZURE A spasm or seizure consisting of a convulsive twitching of the muscles

TORT A private wrong or a breach of a legal duty to the rights and interests of another

TRACHEOESOPHAGEAL FISTULA An abnormal passage between the esophagus and the trachea

TRAIT ANXIETY Anxiety experienced most of the time regardless of the circumstances

TRANSFORMATIONAL POWER The ability to assist a client to change his self-image or his self-care strategies

TRANSILLUMINATION The act of observing a body part by shining a light through the part and viewing the quality and quantity of light on the other side

TRANSPOSITION OF THE GREAT VESSELS A developmental cardiac anomaly characterized by the aorta arising from the right ventricle and the pulmonary artery arising from the left ventricle

TRANSUDATIVE PLEURAL EFFUSION An ultrafiltrate of plasma containing low concentrations of protein; results when excessive hydrostatic pressure or decreased osmotic pressure causes excessive amounts of fluid to pass across intact capillaries

TRENDELENBURG'S TEST Test in which the opposite pelvis dips to maintain erect posture when the infant or child stands on the affected leg

TRICUSPID INSUFFICIENCY The incomplete closure of the tricuspid valve resulting in tricuspid regurgitation

TRICUSPID VALVULAR ATRESIA A defect characterized by absence of the tricuspid valve and no blood flow between the right atrium and right ventricle, a small right ventricle and large left ventricle, and diminished pulmonary circulation

TRIGEMINAL NEURALGIA Also called *tic douloureux,* a painful disorder of one or more branches of the fifth cranial (trigeminal) nerve that produces paroxysmal attacks of excruciating facial pain precipitated by stimulation of a trigger zone

TUBERCULOSIS (TB) An infectious disease caused by a species of *Myobacterium* and characterized by the formation of tubercles and caseous necrosis in the tissues; the lung is the major organ affected in TB

ULCERATIVE COLITIS A chronic, recurrent ulceration in the colon, commonly of the mucosa and submucosa, characterized by cramping abdominal pain, rectal bleeding, and loose discharges of blood, pus, and mucus with scanty fecal particles

UNDOING An unconscious ego defense mechanism whereby an individual acts to reverse the effects of a previous act

UNINTENTIONAL TORT An act that fails to meet a duty owed to another person (the plaintiff) and leads to the person's injury

URINARY TRACT INFECTION (UTI) A bacterial infection most commonly caused by *Escherichia coli* or a species of *Klebsiella, Proteus, Pseudomonas,* or *Enterobacter* and affecting one or more parts of the urinary tract

VALVULAR HEART DISEASE A disorder characterized by stenosis of a cardiac valve, resulting in obstruction of the flow of blood, or degeneration of the valve, which leads to reflux of blood

VASCULAR DEMENTIA Also called *multi-infarct dementia;* disorder that impairs the client's cognitive functioning, memory, and personality, but doesn't affect the level of consciousness

VASCULITIS A disorder in which the blood vessels are inflamed, either from an allergic reaction or as a result of disease

VENTRICULAR SEPTAL DEFECT A defect that occurs when the ventricular septum fails to complete its formation between the ventricles, resulting in a left-to-right shunt

VENTRICULOPERITONEAL SHUNT A diversion of cerebrospinal fluid from the cerebral ventricles to the peritoneal cavity using a one-way flow valve and a tubing system

VERNIX A cheesy substance that covers and protects the fetal body

VICARIOUS LIABILITY A type of liability by which one is found to have responsibility for the actions of another because a relationship exists between those individuals, such as an employer-employee relationship

VIRAL CARCINOGENESIS The development of cancer as a result of viral illnesses, such as hepatitis B and hepatocellular carcinoma, herpes virus, herpes simplex type 2, human papillomavirus, and T-cell leukemia or lymphoma

VITREOUS BODY Clear, transparent, avascular, gelatinous fluid that fills the space in the posterior portion of the eye and maintains the transparency and form of the eye

WAIVER Situation in which a client tells a physician that he doesn't want to know the appropriate information

WITHDRAWAL An adverse physical or psychological reaction to abstinence from a substance to which the individual has become addicted

Selected references

Fundamentals of Nursing

Alfaro-LeFevre, R. *Applying Nursing Process: A Tool for Critical Thinking,* 6th ed. Philadelphia: Lippincott Williams & Wilkins, 2005.

Bickley, L.S. *Bates' Guide to Physical Examination and History Taking,* 9th ed. Philadelphia: Lippincott Williams & Wilkins, 2005.

Carpenito-Moyet, L.J. *Nursing Diagnosis: Application to Clinical Practice,* 11th ed. Philadelphia: Lippincott Williams & Wilkins, 2006.

Craven, R.F., and Hirnle, M.N. *Fundamentals of Nursing: Human Health and Function,* 4th ed. Philadelphia: Lippincott Williams & Wilkins, 2004.

Evans-Smith, P. *Taylor's Clinical Nursing Skills: A Nursing Process Approach.* Philadelphia: Lippincott Williams & Wilkins, 2004.

Kozier, B., et al. *Fundamentals of Nursing: Concepts, Process, and Practice,* 7th ed. Upper Saddle River, N.J.: Prentice Hall, 2004.

Malloch, K., and Porter-O'Grady, T. *Introduction to Evidence-Based Practice in Nursing and Health Care.* Sudbury, Mass.: Jones & Bartlett Publishers, Inc., 2006.

Medical Terms and Abbreviations, 2nd ed. Lippincott Professional Guides Series. Philadelphia: Lippincott Williams & Wilkins, 2002.

Nettina, S.M. *Lippincott Manual of Nursing Practice,* 8th ed. Philadelphia: Lippincott Williams & Wilkins, 2005.

Nursing Procedures, 4th ed. Philadelphia: Lippincott Williams & Wilkins, 2004.

Pathophysiology Made Incredibly Easy, 3rd ed. Philadelphia: Lippincott Williams & Wilkins, 2006.

Smith-Temple, A.J., and Johnson, J.Y. *Nurse's Guide to Clinical Procedures,* 5th ed. Philadelphia: Lippincott Williams & Wilkins, 2005.

Taylor, C., et al. *Fundamentals of Nursing: The Art and Science of Nursing Care,* 5th ed. Philadelphia: Lippincott Williams & Wilkins, 2004.

Taylor, C., et al. *Skills Checklist to Accompany Fundamentals of Nursing: The Art and Science of Nursing Care,* 5th ed. Philadelphia: Lippincott Williams & Wilkins, 2004.

Medical-Surgical Nursing

Abrams, A.C. *Clinical Drug Therapy: Rationales for Nursing Practice,* 7th ed. Philadelphia: Lippincott Williams & Wilkins, 2003.

Alexander, M, and Corrigan A. *Core Curriculum for Infusion Nursing.* Philadelphia: Lippincott Williams & Wilkins, 2004.

American Diabetes Association. *American Diabetes Association Complete Guide to Diabetes,* 3rd ed. Alexandria, Va.: American Diabetes Association, 2002.

Arcangelo, V.P., and Peterson, A.M. *Pharmacotherapeutics for Advanced Practice: A Practical Approach,* 2nd ed. Philadelphia: Lippincott Williams & Wilkins, 2005.

Assessment Made Incredibly Easy, 3rd ed. Philadelphia: Lippincott Williams & Wilkins, 2005.

Behan, E. *Therapeutic Nutrition: A Guide to Patient Education.* Philadelphia: Lippincott Williams & Wilkins, 2006.

Childs, B.P. *Complete Nurses Guide to Diabetes Care.* Alexandria, Va.: American Diabetes Association, 2005.

Complete Guide to Documentation. Philadelphia: Lippincott Williams & Wilkins, 2003.

Fischbach, F.T. *A Manual of Laboratory and Diagnostic Tests,* 7th ed. Philadelphia: Lippincott Williams & Wilkins, 2003.

Handbook of Diagnostic Tests, 3rd ed. Philadelphia: Lippincott Williams & Wilkins, 2003.

Handbook of Diseases, 3rd ed. Philadelphia: Lippincott Williams & Wilkins, 2004.

Handbook of Geriatric Nursing Care, 2nd ed. Philadelphia: Lippincott Williams & Wilkins, 2003.

Handbook of Medical-Surgical Nursing, 4th ed. Philadelphia: Lippincott Williams & Wilkins, 2006.

Hess, C.T. *Clinical Guide: Wound Care,* 5th ed. Philadelphia: Lippincott Williams & Wilkins, 2005.

Holloway, N.M. *Medical-Surgical Care Planning,* 4th ed. Philadelphia: Lippincott Williams & Wilkins, 2003.

I.V. Therapy Made Incredibly Easy, 3rd ed. Philadelphia: Lippincott Williams & Wilkins, 2006.

Ignatavicius, D., and Workman, M.L. *Medical-Surgical Nursing: Critical Thinking for Collaborative Care,* 5th ed. Philadelphia: W.B. Saunders Co., 2006.

Lundy, K.S., and Janes, S. *Community Health Nursing: Caring for the Public's Health.* Sudbury, Mass.: Jones and Bartlett Publishers, Inc., 2001.

Nurse's Quick Check: Diagnostic Tests, Philadelphia: Lippincott Williams & Wilkins, 2005.

Nursing I.V. Drug Handbook, 8th ed. Philadelphia: Lippincott Williams & Wilkins, 2003.

Nursing Procedures, 4th ed. Philadelphia: Lippincott Williams & Wilkins, 2004.

Nursing2006 Drug Handbook, 26th ed. Philadelphia: Lippincott Williams & Wilkins, 2006.

Pagana, K.D., and Pagana, T.J. *Mosby's Diagnostic and Laboratory Test Reference.* 7th ed. St. Louis: C.V. Mosby–Year Book, Inc., 2005.

Professional Guide to Diseases, 8th ed. Philadelphia: Lippincott Williams & Wilkins, 2005.

Rice, R. *Home Care Nursing Practice: Concepts and Application.* C.V. Mosby-Year Book, Inc., 2006.

Smeltzer, S.C., and Bare, B.G. *Brunner and Suddarth's Textbook of Medical-Surgical Nursing,* 10th ed. Philadelphia: Lippincott Williams & Wilkins, 2005.

Tierney, L.M., et al., eds. *2005 Current Medical Diagnosis & Treatment.* New York: McGraw-Hill, 2005.

Maternal-Neonatal Nursing

Core Curriculum for Maternal-Newborn Nursing, 3rd ed. Philadelphia: W.B. Saunders Co., 2004.

Core Curriculum for Neonatal Intensive Care Nursing, 3rd ed. Philadelphia: W.B. Saunders Co., 2004.

Klossner, N.J., and Hatfield, N. *Introductory Maternity & Pediatric Nursing.* Philadelphia: Lippincott Williams & Wilkins, 2005.

Ladewig, P.W., et al. *Contemporary Maternal-Newborn Nursing Care,* 6th ed. Upper Saddle River, N.J.: Prentice Hall, 2006.

Lippincott's Maternity Nursing Video Series. Philadelphia: Lippincott Williams & Wilkins, 2006.

Littleton, L.Y., and Engebreston, J. *Maternity Nursing Care.* Clifton Park, N.Y.: Delmar Learning, 2005.

Luxner, K.L. *Delmar's Maternal Nursing Care Plans,* 2nd ed. Clifton Park, N.Y.: Delmar Learning, 2005.

Martin's Quick-E OB: Obstetric Clinical Nursing Reference, 2nd ed. Orlando, Fla.: Bandido Books, 2005.

Maternal-Neonatal Facts Made Incredibly Quick. Philadelphia: Lippincott Williams & Wilkins, 2005.

McKinney, E.S., et al. *Maternal-Child Nursing,* 2nd ed. Philadelphia: W.B. Saunders Co., 2005.

Nursing Procedures, 4th ed. Philadelphia: Lippincott Williams & Wilkins, 2004.

Pathophysiology Made Incredibly Easy, 3rd ed. Philadelphia: Lippincott Williams & Wilkins, 2006.

Pillitteri, A. *Maternal & Child Nursing: Care of the Childbearing and Childrearing Family,* 4th ed. Philadelphia: Lippincott Williams & Wilkins, 2003.

Straight A's in Maternal-Neonatal Nursing. Philadelphia: Lippincott Williams & Wilkins, 2004.

White, L. *Foundations of Maternal and Pediatric Nursing,* 2nd ed. Clifton Park, N.Y.: Delmar Learning, 2004.

Wong, D.L., et al. *Maternal Child Nursing Care,* 2nd ed. St. Louis: Mosby–Year Book, Inc., 2002.

Pediatric Nursing

Broyles, B. *Clinical Decision Making: Case Studies in Pediatrics.* Clifton Park, N.Y.: Delmar Learning, 2005.

Hockenberry, M.J. *Wong's Clinical Manual of Pediatric Nursing,* 6th ed. St. Louis: C.V. Mosby-Year Book, Inc., 2004.

Hockenberry, M.J. *Wong's Essentials of Pediatric Nursing,* 7th ed. St. Louis: C.V. Mosby-Year Book, Inc., 2005.

Lippincott's Pediatric Nursing Video Series. Philadelphia: Lippincott Williams & Wilkins, 2006.

Nursing Procedures, 4th ed. Philadelphia: Lippincott Williams & Wilkins, 2004.

Pediatric Nursing Made Incredibly Easy. Philadelphia: Lippincott Williams & Wilkins, 2004.

Samour, P.Q., et al. *Handbook of Pediatric Nutrition,* 3rd ed. Sudbury, Mass.: Jones & Bartlett Publishers, Inc., 2005.

Straight A's in Pediatric Nursing. Philadelphia: Lippincott Williams & Wilkins, 2003.

Psychiatric and Mental Health Nursing

Boyd, M.A. *Psychiatric Nursing: Contemporary Practice,* 3rd ed. Philadelphia: Lippincott Williams & Wilkins, 2004.

Eby, L.A., and Brown, N.J. *Mental Health Nursing Care.* Upper Saddle River, N.J.: Prentice Hall, 2005.

Frisch, N.C., and Frisch, L.E. *Psychiatric Mental Health Nursing,* 3rd ed. Clifton Park, N.Y.: Delmar Learning, 2002.

Harrison, M., et al. *Acute Mental Health Nursing: From Acute Concerns to the Capable Practitioner.* Thousand Oaks, Calif.: SAGE Publications, 2004.

Isaacs, A. *Mental Health and Psychiatric Nursing, 4th ed.* Philadelphia: Lippincott Williams & Wilkins, 2005.

Mohr, W.K. *Johnson's Psychiatric-Mental Health Nursing,* 6th ed. Philadelphia: Lippincott Williams & Wilkins, 2005.

Pilgrim, D. *Key Concepts in Mental Health.* Thousand Oaks, Calif.: SAGE Publications, 2005.

Psychiatric Nursing Made Incredibly Easy. Philadelphia: Lippincott Williams & Wilkins, 2003.

Schultz, J.M., and Videbeck, S.L. *Lippincott's Manual of Psychiatric Nursing Care Plans,* 7th ed. Philadelphia: Lippincott Williams & Wilkins, 2004.

Shives, L.R. *Basic Concepts of Psychiatric-Mental Health Nursing,* 6th ed. Philadelphia: Lippincott Williams & Wilkins, 2004.

Townsend, M.C. *Essentials of Psychiatric Mental Health Nursing,* 3rd ed. Philadelphia: F.A. Davis Co., 2005.

Townsend, M.C. *Psychiatric Mental Health Nursing: Concepts of Care,* 4th ed. Philadelphia: F.A. Davis Co., 2003.

Varcarolis, E.M. *Manual of Psychiatric Nursing Care Plans: Diagnoses, Clinical Tools, and Psychopharmacology,* 2nd ed. Philadelphia: W.B. Saunders Co., 2004.

Videbeck, S.L. *Psychiatric Mental Health Nursing,* 2nd ed. Philadelphia: Lippincott Williams & Wilkins, 2004.

Womble, D.M. *Introductory Mental Health Nursing.* Philadelphia: Lippincott Williams & Wilkins, 2005.

Client Needs

Broyles, B. *Clinical Decision Making: Case Studies Pediatrics.* Clifton Park, N.Y.: Thomson Delmar Learning, 2005.

Carpenito-Moyet, L.J. *Handbook of Nursing Diagnosis,* 11th ed. Philadelphia: Lippincott Williams & Wilkins, 2006.

Carpenito-Moyet, L.J. *Nursing Diagnosis: Application to Clinical Practice,* 11th ed. Philadelphia: Lippincott Williams & Wilkins, 2006.

Ladwig, G.B., and Ackley, B.J. *Mosby's Guide to Nursing Diagnosis.* St, Louis: C.V. Mosby, 2006.

Luxner, K.L., and Phinney, D.J. *Delmar's Maternal Nursing Care Plans,* 2nd ed. Clifton Park, N.Y.: Delmar Learning, 2005.

NCLEX-RN Review Made Incredibly Easy. 3rd ed. Philadelphia: Lippincott Williams & Wilkins, 2005.

Varcarolis, E.M. *Manual of Psychiatric Nursing Care Plans: Diagnoses, Clinical Tools, and Psychopharmacology,* 2nd ed. Philadelphia: W.B. Saunders Co., 2004.

The Nursing Process

Ackley, B.J., and Ladwig, G.B. *Nursing Diagnosis Handbook: A Guide to Planning Care,* 6th ed. St. Louis: Mosby–Year Book, Inc., 2004.

Alfaro-LeFevre, R. *Applying Nursing Process: A Tool for Critical Thinking,* 6th ed. Philadelphia: Lippincott Williams & Wilkins, 2005.

Broyles, B. *Clinical Decision Making: Case Studies in Pediatrics.* Clifton Park, N.Y.: Delmar Learning, 2005.

Carpenito, L.J. *Handbook of Nursing Diagnosis,* 10th ed. Philadelphia: Lippincott Williams & Wilkins, 2003.

Carpenito-Movet, L.J. *Handbook of Nursing Diagnosis,* 11th ed. Philadelphia: Lippincott Williams & Wilkins, 2006.

Carpenito-Movet, L.J. *Nursing Diagnosis: Application to Clinical Practice,* 11th ed. Philadelphia: Lippincott Williams & Wilkins, 2005.

Doenges, M.E., et al. *Nursing Care Plans: Guidelines for Individualizing Patient Care,* 6th ed. Philadelphia: F.A. Davis Co., 2002.

Gordon, M. *Manual of Nursing Diagnosis,* 10th ed. St. Louis: Mosby–Year Book, Inc., 2002.

Luxner, K.L., and Phinney, D.J. *Delmar's Maternal Nursing Care Plans,* 2nd ed. Clifton Park, N.Y.: Delmar Learning, 2004.

McCloskey, J.C., and Bulechek, G.M. *Nursing Interventions Classifications,* 4th ed. St. Louis: Mosby–Year Book, Inc., 2004.

Morehead, S., et al. *Nursing Outcomes Classification (NOC),* 3rd ed. St. Louis: Mosby–Year Book, Inc., 2004.

Sparks, S.M., and Taylor, C.M. *Nursing Diagnosis Reference Manual,* 6th ed. Philadelphia: Lippincott Williams & Wilkins, 2005.

Varcarolis, E.M. *Manual of Psychiatric Nursing Care Plans: Diagnoses, Clinical Tools, and Psychopharmacology,* 2nd ed. Philadelphia: W.B. Saunders Co., 2004.

Index

i refers to an illustration; t refers to a table.

D

i refers to an illustration; t refers to a table.

i refers to an illustration; t refers to a table.

i refers to an illustration; t refers to a table.

M

N

O

i refers to an illustration; t refers to a table.

i refers to an illustration; t refers to a table.

i refers to an illustration; t refers to a table.

i refers to an illustration; t refers to a table.

ABOUT THE CD-ROM

The *Springhouse Review for NCLEX-RN®* CD-ROM is a review-and-test program that gives you unprecedented flexibility in preparing for the NCLEX-RN. This program contains more than 1,500 NCLEX-style questions. It's designed to pose questions randomly, so you can test yourself repeatedly. You can tailor your test or review to cover any combination of 29 nursing topics, 5 nursing process steps, or 4 client needs categories. The program provides the correct answer and rationales for the correct and incorrect answers after each question and a performance appraisal at the end of the test. This feature allows you to review any weak areas identified in the performance appraisal.

MINIMUM SYSTEM REQUIREMENTS

To operate the *Springhouse Review for NCLEX-RN®* CD-ROM, we recommend that you have the following minimum computer equipment:

- Windows 98
- Pentium 166
- 128 MB RAM
- 8 MB of free hard-disk space
- SVGA monitor with High Color (16-bit)
- CD-ROM drive
- mouse.

INSTALLATION

Before installing the CD-ROM, make sure that your monitor is set to High Color (16-bit) and your display area is set to 800 × 600. If it isn't, consult your monitor's user's manual for instructions about changing the display settings. (The display settings are typically found in Start/Settings/Control Panel/Display/Settings tab.)

To run this program, you must install it onto the hard drive of your computer, following these three steps:

1. Start Windows 98 (minimum).
2. Place the CD-ROM in your CD-ROM drive. After a few moments, the install process will automatically begin. *Note:* If the install process doesn't automatically begin, click the Start menu and select Run. Type D:\setup.exe (where D: is the letter of your CD-ROM drive) and then click OK.
3. Follow the on-screen instructions for installation.

TECHNICAL SUPPORT

For technical support, call toll-free 1-800-638-3030, Monday through Friday, 8:30 a.m. to 5 p.m. Eastern Time. You may also write to Lippincott Williams & Wilkins Technical Support, 351 W. Camden Street, Baltimore, MD 21201-2436, or e-mail us at techsupp@lww.com.